SALEM HEALTH

MAGILL'S
MEDICAL
GUIDE

SALEM HEALTH

MAGILL'S MEDICAL GUIDE

Ninth Edition

Volume 4

N95 masks – Systems and organs

Medical Editors

Anubhav Agarwal, MD
Mount Sinai South Nassau

Michael A. Buratovich, PhD
Spring Arbor University

Paul Moglia, PhD
Mount Sinai South Nassau

John N. Morley, MD
NYS Department of Health

SALEM PRESS
A Division of EBSCO Information Services, Inc.
Ipswich, Massachusetts

GREY HOUSE PUBLISHING

Magill's Medical Guide: Health and Illness, 1995
Supplement, 1996
Magill's Medical Guide, revised edition, 1998
Second revised edition, 2002
Third revised edition, 2005
Fourth revised edition, 2008
Sixth edition, 2011
Seventh edition, 2014
Eighth edition, 2018
Ninth edition, 2022

∞ The paper used in these volumes conforms to the American National Standard for Permanence of Paper for Printed Library Materials, Z39.48 1992 (R2009).

Note to Readers

The material presented in *Magill's Medical Guide* is intended for broad informational and educational purposes. Readers who suspect that they suffer from any of the physical or psychological disorders, diseases, or conditions described in this set should contact a physician without delay; this work should not be used as a substitute for professional medical diagnosis or treatment. This set is not to be considered definitive on the covered topics, and readers should remember that the field of health care is characterized by a diversity of medical opinions and constant expansion in knowledge and understanding.

Publisher's Cataloging-in-Publication Data
(Prepared by The Donohue Group, Inc.)

Names: Anubhav Agarwal, MD, editor.
Title: Magill's medical guide / medical editors: Anubhav Agarwal, MD, Mount Sinai South Nassau [and three others].
Other Titles: Salem health (Pasadena, Calif.)
Description: Ninth Edition. | Ipswich, Massachusetts : Salem Press, a division of EBSCO Information Services, Inc. ; Amenia, NY : Grey House Publishing, 2022. | Includes bibliographical references and index. | Contents: Volume 1. Abdomen–Cytopathology — Volume 2. Deafness–Gynecomastia — Volume 3. Hair–Myringotomy — Volume 4. N95 masks–Systems and organs — Volume 5. Tapeworms–Zoonoses, Appendixes, Indexes.
Identifiers: ISBN 9781637001073 (set) | ISBN 9781637001097 (v.1) | ISBN 9781637001103 (v.2) | ISBN 9781637001110 (v.3) | ISBN 9781637001127 (v.4) | ISBN 9781637001134 (v.5)
Subjects: LCSH: Medicine—Encyclopedias.
Classification: LCC RC41 .M345 2018 | DDC 610.3—dc23

First Printing

Printed in the United States of America

Complete Table of Contents

Volume 1

Volume 2

Volume 3

Volume 4

Shading indicates current volume.

Shading indicates current volume.

Shading indicates current volume.

Volume 5

SALEM HEALTH

MAGILL'S
MEDICAL
GUIDE

N

N95 MASKS

Category: Personal Protective Equipment
Definition: N95 masks are respirators designed to filter small particles in the air, thus protecting the wearer from airborne chemicals, particulate matter (i.e., smoke), bacteria, and viruses.

INDICATIONS

Historically, N95 masks have been used in health care settings to protect workers from aerosolized biologic material such as tuberculosis and industrial and agriculture settings. With the onset of the COVID-19 pandemic, the use of N95 masks has rapidly increased due to their protection from this aerosolized ribonucleic acid (RNA) virus.

CRITERIA

N95 masks filter airborne particles approximately 0.3 micrometers in size, offering more protection to the wearer than traditional surgical masks, which typically filter particles of 0.5 micrometers or larger. The precursor "N" denotes that these masks are not oil resistant, and "95" delineates that it filters 95 percent of particles in the surrounding air. To determine whether a mask meets the filtration characteristics to be considered an N95 mask, it must undergo a rigorous testing process overseen by a regulatory body (i.e., National Institute of Occupational Health and Safety (NIOSH) in the United States). If a mask has met the testing criteria to be considered an N95 mask, the mask and/or its packaging will contain a NIOSH-approved label or be listed as approved by NIOSH resources. For example, masks designated as "KN95" do not undergo NIOSH testing and do not contain the NIOSH label.

CONSIDERATIONS FOR USAGE

The N95 mask requires an appropriate seal with the wearer's face to ensure that the mask has filtered the inhaled air. If a significant amount of air can pass unfiltered between the sides of the mask and the face of the wearer, it negates the mask's efficacy. Facial hair or anything obstructing the seal between the N95 and skin (i.e., a mask placed under the N95) prevents the mask from protecting the wearer. N95 masks are not currently approved for use in children. They are generally not recommended in populations with

Personal Protective Equipment (PPE) N95 face mask. Image via iStock/Gregi69. [Used under license.]

conditions that affect their breathing ability. Fit testing is also required to determine the appropriate N95 make and size for the wearer's facial structure. Health care workers typically undergo fit testing annually to ensure that they use the mask to maximum benefit since their facial structure can change with weight changes, age, or cosmetic procedures.

FIT TESTING

Fit testing consists of ensuring appropriate mask seal and ensuring wearer comfort and safety. Mask should fit securely, and the wearer is encouraged to move their head in all directions to test whether the fit is secure and mask placement remains appropriate. The mask should not obstruct vision, particularly while the wearer looks down to reduce their visual field while performing procedures or surgeries. While wearing the mask, there should be adequate space for glasses or eye protection.

Safety: Fit testing should also ensure that the mask is safe for the wearer. Individuals with cardiac or respiratory issues must consult their health care provider before wearing an N95 mask, as they may not breathe adequately. Some mechanisms to ensure wearer safety during fit testing require the subject to breathe deeply and speak by requiring them to recite standardized text or count backward. Subjects are instructed to remove the mask if they feel lightheaded or breathless. They are referred to their health care provider for further evaluation.

Maximizing protection: Fit testing also involves ensuring an appropriate mask seal to the participant's face with minimal leakage. The Occupational Safety and Health Administration (OSHA) in the United States has certain protocols to ensure that the mask fits the wearer appropriately with minimal leakage. Qualitative tests are most often used in health care settings, which rely on whether the participant can taste or smell a particular solution while wearing the mask. For example, in the saccharine solution protocol for fit testing, participants wearing the N95 mask are placed in an apparatus that encloses their head/neck region. The solution is sprayed within that apparatus. If the participant can taste the solution, the mask does not fit appropriately, and an alternative model should be used. Quantitative mask fit tests may also be used, which rely on a fit factor to determine the appropriate seal, calculated by the quantity of the test agent measured inside and outside the mask. Each aspect of fit testing ensures that the N95 mask is worn comfortably and safely and provides adequate protection from aerosolized pathogens.

UTILIZATION

Masks are intended for single-use, and they are meant to be changed at least daily or if visibly soiled or saturated with fluid. The wearer should initially put on the mask with clean hands, following the directions on mask packaging if applicable. The wearer should adjust the superior portion of the mask to form a seal with the skin in the nasal and peri-nasal region. Once the mask has been used, it should be taken off with care so as not to disperse any particles clinging to the mask surface and immediately discarded. After handling the mask, the wearer should disinfect their hands to eliminate any pathogenic material transferred from the mask.

CURRENT PERSPECTIVES: COVID-19 PANDEMIC

Within the context of the COVID-19 pandemic, the demand for N95 masks increased dramatically. The mask protects the wearer from the aerosolized virus. If the wearer becomes infected, it also significantly minimizes the likelihood of spreading to those they encounter. In addition to protecting health care personnel, N95 masks are also used by laypeople to minimize the risk of infection.

COVID-19 pandemic mask shortages: N95 masks are intended for single-use, but in times of critical N95 mask shortages where masks are unavailable for essential personnel, NIOSH recommends a maximum of five donnings of the same mask to preserve fit and filtration. In critical mask shortages where no replacement masks are available, disinfection is recommended between uses, and proposed disinfection mechanisms include ultraviolet light and moist heat. Alcohol or sanitizing wipes are not recommended for resanitizing masks, as they compromise the filtration capacity of the mask. NIOSH, Centers for Disease Control and Prevention (CDC), and US Food and Drug Administration (FDA) may be consulted for the most up-to-date guidelines in addition to the resources listed below.

—*Caroline Campbell, MD*

For Further Information:
Center for Devices and Radiological Health. "N95 Respirators, Surgical Masks, Face Masks, & Barrier Face Coverings." *US Food and Drug Administration*, FDA, 15 Sept. 2021, www.fda.gov/medical-devices/personal-protective-equipment-infection-control/n95-respirators-surgical-masks-face-masks-and-barrier-face-coverings#cdc.
"Covid-19 Decontamination and Reuse of Filtering Facepiece Respirators." *Centers for Disease Control and Prevention*, CDC, 19 Oct. 2020, www.cdc.gov/coronavirus/2019-ncov/hcp/ppe-strategy/decontamination-reuse-respirators.html.
"Fit Testing Procedures." *Occupational Safety and Health Administration*, US Department of Labor, www.osha.gov/laws-regs/regulations/standardnumber/1910/1910.134AppA.
"Masks and Respirators." *Centers for Disease Control and Prevention*, 28 Jan. 2022, www.cdc.gov/coronavirus/2019-ncov/prevent-getting-sick/types-of-masks.html.
"NIOSH-Approved N95 Particulate Filtering Facepiece Respirators." *The National Personal Protective Technology Laboratory (NPPTL)*, CDC, 7 Jan. 2022, www.cdc.gov/niosh/npptl/topics/respirators/disp_part/N95list1.html.

NAIL REMOVAL

Category: Procedure
Anatomy or system affected: Feet, hands, nails
Specialties and related fields: Emergency medicine, family medicine, internal medicine, pediatrics, podiatry, sports medicine
Definition: The partial or total removal of either fingernails or toenails.

INDICATIONS AND PROCEDURES

Nail removal is one of the most common office procedures seen in primary care. Nail disorders leading to removal occur most often in toenails, but they can also occur in fingernails. Common reasons for removal are infection, ingrown nails, or trauma. Patients usually experience pain and inability to function in their normal activities. Rarely are there any systemic signs or symptoms, such as fever, chills, or nausea, unless the cause is a serious infection.

The patient's foot or hand is first cleansed and draped. Sterile techniques are used throughout the procedure. Patients undergoing partial or total nail removal require adequate anesthesia, which is usually done through a digital block. This procedure is performed at the base of the digit with lidocaine or a similar anesthetic to numb the entire finger or toe. The provider should wait five minutes for the anesthesia to become effective. A tourniquet may be applied to minimize bleeding and enhance anesthesia. An instrument is then used to separate the nail from the nail bed with the least trauma possible. In a complete removal, the nail is gently pulled away from the nail bed. In a partial removal, scissors are used to cut the desired amount of nail away from the intact nail. Some providers will also chemically destroy the nail matrix in the area of the partial removal to prevent recurrent ingrown nails, if clinically indicated.

Compression for a few minutes may be needed to slow any bleeding from the nail removal. Topical antibiotic ointment may be applied with gauze and a compression dressing. When a toenail is removed, patients may walk immediately after the procedure and resume any activity as tolerated. Local wound care instructions are given, and if the procedure is performed secondary to an infected digit, oral antibiotics may be ordered. The procedure usually takes approximately fifteen minutes to complete.

USES AND COMPLICATIONS
Partial nail removal or trimming may also be performed in diabetic patients or those unable to perform routine nail care. Fungal infections cannot be cured with nail removal alone, though in severe or painful cases, the procedure may be performed in conjunction with the administration of antifungal agents.

Nail removal has few complications if performed properly. Pain is one of the most common complications of the procedure, especially if the digit was already infected. Bacterial infection may also occur after the procedure without proper wound care management. Bleeding may occur, as epinephrine is not used in digital blocks. Adequate compression or cautery usually stops any continued bleeding after the procedure. Patients must also be warned that the nail may not grow back with the same shape prior to removal. Nails should be cut straight across without curvature to prevent any ingrown nail recurrence.

—*Jeffrey R. Bytomski, DO*

See also Bacterial infections; Diabetes mellitus; Feet; Lower extremities; Nails; Podiatry; Upper extremities; Wounds.

For Further Information:
Clark, Robert E., and Whitney D. Tope. "Nail Surgery." In *Cutaneous Surgery*, edited by Roland G. Wheeland. Philadelphia: W. B. Saunders, 1994.
"Nail Diseases." *MedlinePlus*, April 11, 2013.
Woods, Michael, et al. "Ingrown Toenail Removal." *Health Library*, May 2, 2013.
Zuber, Thomas J. "Ingrown Toenail Removal." *American Family Physician* 65, no. 12 (June 15, 2002): 2547-2554.

NAILS

Category: Anatomy
Anatomy or system affected: Hands, feet, skin
Specialties and related fields: Dermatology, histology
Definition: The thin, horny plates covering the dorsal ends of the fingers or toes.
Key terms:
cuticle: cutaneous or skin tissue that surrounds the nail plate on its proximal sides and provides a protective barrier to the nail bed; it is attached to the proximal nail fold and to the nail plate
hyponychium: cutaneous tissue underlying the free nail at its point of separation from the nail bed; structurally similar to the cuticle
keratinocytes: matrix basal epithelial cells that differentiate, fill with keratin, and form the dead horny substance making up the nail plate
lunula: a whitish, crescent-shaped area at the end of the proximal nail fold that marks the end of the nail matrix and is the site of mitosis and nail growth
onychomycosis: common nail disorder in which fungal organisms invade the nail bed causing progressive changes in the color, texture, and structure of the nail

STRUCTURE AND FUNCTIONS
Nails function to protect fingers and toes against bumps and trauma. Fine touch is amplified and skillful manipulation of small objects with the fingers is enabled by the presence of nails. Nails also provide the ability to scratch, both as a temporary relief of an itch and in personal defense. Nails are important social communicators of beauty and sexuality and hence are the focus of a major cosmetic industry.

Biologically, nails are characterized as plates of tightly packed, hard epidermis cells filled with a protein called keratin. Nails are normally seen on the dorsal side (the side opposite the palm or sole) of all fingers and toes. The anatomy of the normal nail consists of a nail plate, proximal nail fold, nail bed, matrix, and hyponychium. These components are epithelial-derived structures, like skin and hair, which emerge from the live germinative zone of the epidermis. In nails, these cells differentiate and form the horny layer, which is considered to be dead.

The nail plate is a relatively hard and flat, transparent, horny structure that is rectangular in shape. It rests on the underlying nail bed but typically extends beyond the bed as an unattached, free-growing edge reaching toward or beyond the tip of the finger or toe. On the fingers, the thickness of the plate in adults increases from about 0.7 millimeters at the proximal edge to about 1.6 millimeters at the distal edge. The terminal tip thickness varies considerably between persons.

Normally, a pinkish nail bed is seen through the transparent nail plate. Frequently in the thumbnail and sometimes in the other fingernails, a whitish, semi-moon-shaped structure called the lunula is seen that extends under the proximal nail fold. The borders of the nail plate are covered by skin structures: two lateral folds and a single proximal fold.

The proximal nail fold is the cutaneous or skin structure that is in continuity with the visible proximal border of the nail but overlies part of the nail root. The ventral side (underside) of the proximal nail fold provides physical protection to the germinative zone of the nail and aids in the physical attachment of the nail plate. About a fourth of the total surface area of the nail plate is located under the proximal fold. The cuticle is a layer of epidermis extending from the proximal nail fold and attached to the dorsal side of the nail. The cuticle functions to provide a physical seal against microbes and chemical irritants, which may otherwise enter the matrix and affect nail production.

The nail bed is the portion of the digit upon which the nail rests. The nail bed is highly vascular, with numerous capillaries. It consists of epithelial tissue and extends from the lunula to the point where the bed separates from the nail. A series of fine longitudinal folds in the nail bed corresponds to the undersurface structure of the nail. This arrangement enhances the adherence of the nail plate to the nail bed.

The nail matrix is generally considered the most proximal part of the nail bed and is bordered by the proximal nail fold. On the distal end it is bordered by the distal margin of the lunula. The nail matrix epithelium cells consist predominantly of keratinocytes in both a basal and a spinous layer. Melanocytes and Langerhans cells are intermingled with keratinocytes. It is within the matrix that the germinating center of nail growth is found. Basal epithelial cells increase in number through mitosis, or division, and then differentiate into keratinocytes, which are epithelial cells filled with keratin protein. These keratinocytes condense their cytoplasm, lose their nucleus, and form flat, horny-looking dead cells. As further cell division occurs in the nail matrix, more distal keratinocytes are pushed out to form the nail plate.

The hyponychium consists of epidermis tissue that underlies the edge of the nail plate and extends from the nail bed to the distal groove. It functions to pro-

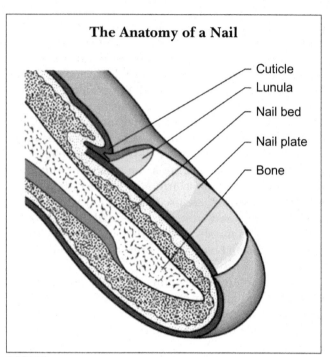

The Anatomy of a Nail

- Cuticle
- Lunula
- Nail bed
- Nail plate
- Bone

©EBSCO

vide a defense against entry of bacteria under the free edge of the nail plate. Excessively vigorous cleaning may damage the hyponychium and allow for bacteria to enter more readily under the nail plate.

The turnover rate of matrix cells determines the growth rate of the nail. This rate varies with age, environmental conditions, nutritional status, and the specific digit. The growth rate proportionately increases with the length of the digit; thus the middle finger nail grows the fastest while the growth rate in the little finger is the slowest. Fingernails grow three times as rapidly as toenails. The growth rate is more rapid in the winter than in the summer. Furthermore, nails grow faster in young children than in older adults. It takes about six months for a fingernail to completely grow in. Male nails grow faster than female nails. Nails on the dominant hand grow faster than those on the other hand.

If nails are protected and untrimmed, they can grow to considerable lengths. Such long nails were prized by the wealthy classes in imperial Chinese culture as an indication of status. The practice of painting toenails red may have originated in the Ottoman seraglio, where it was a signal of menstrual status.

Nails continue to grow throughout life without a resting phase. Contrary to folk belief, nails cease growing when an individual dies. The matrix cells stop producing deoxyribonucleic acid (DNA) and dividing soon after death, and thus the nail bed cannot grow longer. The appearance of nail growth after death is due to a retraction or shrinkage of nail matrix tissue, resulting in the apparent lengthening of the nail plate.

Professional grooming of the nails for both men and women is termed a manicure. Manicure procedures include cutting the nails according to fashion standards to improve their cosmetic appearance. A pedicure is the term applied to grooming the toenails. Typically, the nails are first soaked in a soapy solution to soften the nail plate and to remove dirt and debris. It is often fashionable to trim the nails to a delicate arc at the middle of the fingertip. The corners of the nail are typically filed. While this shape is attractive in creating the illusion of longer, slender fingers, it heightens the probability of nail plate fractures, hangnails, or ingrown nails. The cuticle, considered to be unattractive by manicurists, is typically minimized, partially removed, or traumatized. This may increase the incidence of fungal invasion and disease. Most of the problems associated with a manicure arise from excessive manipulation of the cuticle.

Nail polish typically consists of pigments suspended in a volatile solvent that also contains a film-forming agent. When the polish is applied to the finger, a covering film develops over the nail. The film is permeable to oxygen, which allows gas exchange to occur between the atmosphere and the nail plate. Resins and plasticizers are added to the polish to increase the flexibility of the film and to minimize chipping. The variety in nail polish color is due to the addition of coloring agents. Deep red nail polishes can cause a temporary yellowish staining of the nail plate.

Nail adornments are sometimes used. Frequently, small nail jewels or ribbons are applied to the fingernails immediately before the nail polish dries, allowing the decoration to adhere to the nail plate. Since some people frequently develop contact dermatitis in reaction to nickel, gold or nickel-free jewels should be selected. Artificial nail tips made of plastic also are glued to the nail tip to create the illusion of an elongated natural nail tip. The gluing may cause nail problems, since a portion of the natural nail is occluded by the glue. This occlusion inhibits oxygen transfer and stresses the nail plate. Frequently, the nail may thin and be unable to support its own weight after the plastic tip is removed. Removal of the plastic tip may result in nail pitting.

DISORDERS AND DISEASES
Nails are useful indicators of skin disease and internal disorders. An abnormally pigmented band in the nail may indicate a malignant melanoma. A yellow nail may indicate psoriasis or a fungal infection. Pulmonary disease or smoking may also cause yellow or brownish nails. Antimalarial drugs may cause the nail to darken in appearance. Frequently, psoriasis causes pitting of nails and an acceleration in their growth rate. Chronic chest disease or a cyanotic congenital

heart disorder is frequently associated with club-shaped deformity of the nail plate. Beau's lines, which are transverse depressions in the nail plates, are associated with illnesses such as coronary thrombosis, pneumonia, and severe injuries. Drug treatment may cause nail breakdown or destruction or complete shedding of the nail plate.

An unexplained aspect of nail physiology is its relationship to lung physiology. Hippocrates first described a connection between lung parenchymal disorders and an edema in the connective tissue beneath the lunula that results in clubbing. The relationship has long been recognized, but the causal link is still unknown.

An ingrown nail results when a deformed nail grows improperly into the skin or when the skin around the nails engulfs part of the nail. Wearing narrow, tight shoes can cause or worsen this pathology. Initially, symptoms may be slight or mild, but with time may come increasing pain. The affected area becomes reddish and, if not treated, may become infected. If infected, the area becomes swollen, inflamed, and painful. Blisters may develop. Treatment involves trimming away the nail from the infected area, allowing the inflammation to decline and the area to heal.

Clubbing is a disorder characterized by a bulblike enlargement of the nail with increased horizontal and longitudinal curvatures. Clubbing involves both fingers and toes and commonly begins at puberty. The disorder may be genetically inherited or acquired. Clubbed nails often have a spongy feel when pressure is placed on the proximal nail fold. This is due to the expanded soft tissue that underlies the nail. Acquired clubbing is often associated with another clinical pathology, most commonly pulmonary or cardiovascular disease. However, at times it is also associated with gastrointestinal inflammatory disease or cystic fibrosis.

A fungal infection is the cause of onychomycosis, which is the most common nail disorder. About half of all nail problems can be linked to this disease, which affects as many as 15 to 20 percent of people in North America. It is uncommon in children and more frequently seen in aged adults.

Several fungi may cause onychomycosis, although most belong to the group called dermatophytes. The fungi are present in soil, and indirect transmission to humans frequently occurs through public swimming pools and shower floors. Some yeasts and molds are also thought to cause this clinical condition. Alternatively, this infection is associated with athlete's foot infection. Typically this condition is found in toenails more frequently than fingernails. The presence of the fungus is further evidenced by scaling on the plantar surface of the foot, where it is often harbored.

In onychomycosis, the fungal organism invades the nail bed, causing a progressive change in the color, texture, and structure of the nail. The nail may turn white, thicken, and even detach from the nail bed. Debris from the infected nail often collects under its free edge. If untreated, the pathology may involve the entire nail plate, and rarely will the nail unit spontaneously heal itself.

Since several organisms may induce the pathology, effective treatment depends on matching the curative with the causal agent. Topically applied antifungals are seldom effective because most cannot penetrate the nail-plate barrier to reach the causal organism. Systemically (orally) administered antifungal therapy frequently uses one of several drugs such as griseofulvin, thiabendazole, or ketoconazole. These drugs are generally effective in halting further invasion of the fungus. While treatment continues, the new nail growth is usually normal, so treatment typically continues until the old nail is replaced by new nail and is then discontinued.

More than seventy tumors have been associated with parts of the nail. They may originate from the epidermis, dermis, subcutaneous tissues, or bone and may be found in the nail bed, nail matrix, hyponychium, or nail fold. The tumors may take various forms, including warts, erosion or ulceration of the nail bed, malignant neoplasms from underlying melanocytes, benign fibromas of the connective tissue, or squamous cell carcinomas. Diagnosis usually is made by taking a biopsy of the affected area. Treatment typically involves surgical removal of the tumor.

PERSPECTIVE AND PROSPECTS

The earliest cellular growth leading to nail formation can be seen histologically at eight weeks of human development, the end of the embryonic period. Microscopically, the cells forming the proximal edge of the nail field and the future matrix can be distinguished at this time. The earliest gross anatomical appearance of nails is seen on the finger digit surface at about nine weeks of development, the very early fetal stage. By eleven weeks of age, the nail field is seen clearly on the hand digits of the fetus. By twenty weeks of age, the fetus shows a nail plate and bed and a proximal cuticle. By thirty-two weeks, the third trimester of pregnancy, adult-type nail structures are visible in the fetus, including a nail plate, matrix, and bed and a forming hyponychium.

Aging results in changes and disorders in nails. When people get older, the color, contour, growth rate, surface texture, and thickness of the nail plate change. Some disorders are more prevalent with aging, such as brittle nails, splitting or fissuring of the nail plate, and increased infections. Aged nails appear dull and opaque, with their color varying from yellow to gray. Frequently in older persons, the lunula is decreased in size or is absent. The growth rate of nails decreases with aging. The most rapid period of growth is during the first thirty years, after which the rate steadily declines. Nail plate thickness frequently increases with advanced age, in combination with discoloration and loss of translucency of the nail plate.

For many years, blood and urine specimens have been used to detect and measure body concentrations of therapeutic drugs or drugs of abuse. During the past decade, alternative biological specimens such as nails and hair have been frequently used as the basis for drug detection. The basis for drug detection in nail clippings is that the dividing epidermal cells that form the nail plate also incorporate drugs from the systemic circulation. The subsequent cornification of these cells traps the drug within the forming nail plate. Drug-detection methods involve taking a sample of nail clippings and extracting and identifying drug molecules via immunochemical or chromatographic techniques. These techniques are extremely sensitive and capable of detecting minute quantities of drug in the samples; as little as ten milligrams of nail clippings is required to detect the presence of drugs. Twenty-first-century drug-screening methods have detected amphetamines and cocaine in nail clippings. Using nail clippings for drug analysis and screening provides a long-term measure of drug exposure that may potentially represent months of drug use. Furthermore, nail clippings are relatively easy to collect and involve a noninvasive procedure; samples are easily stored, and once incorporated in the nail tissue, most of the drugs are presumably stable.

Modern medicine in the early twenty-first century still lacks adequate descriptive science as well as understanding of the molecular mechanisms that control nail development and growth. To date, the specific genes or gene products that initiate nail growth have not been identified. The molecular basis for brittle nails, clubbing, and other nail pathologies is not known. Is onychomycosis affected by a systemic immune deficit? What causes yellow nail syndrome? Answers to these questions as well as additional information about the molecular control of nail physiology will greatly increase understanding and lead to better treatments for nail disorders.

—*Roman J. Miller, PhD*

See also Feet; Fungal infections; Lower extremities; Nail removal; Pulmonary diseases; Skin; Skin disorders; Upper extremities.

For Further Information:

Baran, R., et al., eds. *Baran and Dawber's Diseases of the Nails and Their Management.* 3d ed. Malden, Mass.: Blackwell Science, 2001.

Du Vivier, Anthony. *Atlas of Clinical Dermatology.* 4th ed. Edinburgh: Churchill Livingstone, 2012.

"Fingernails: Dos and Don'ts for Healthy Nails." *Mayo Clinic*, December 8, 2011.

Hordinsky, Maria K., Marty E. Sawaya, and Richard K. Scher, eds. *Atlas of Hair and Nails*. Philadelphia: Churchill Livingstone, 2000.

Mix, Godfrey F. *The Salon Professional's Guide to Foot Care*. Albany: Milday SalonOvations, 1999.

"Nail Diseases." *MedlinePlus*, July 9, 2013.

Porter, Robert S., et al., eds. *The Merck Manual Home Health Handbook*. Whitehouse Station, N.J.: Merck Research Laboratories, 2009.

Standring, Susan, et al., eds. *Gray's Anatomy*. 40th ed. New York: Churchill Livingstone/Elsevier, 2008.

Zaias, Nardo. *The Nail in Health and Disease*. 2d ed. Norwalk, Conn.: Appleton & Lange, 1992.

NARCOLEPSY

Category: Disease/Disorder
Anatomy or system affected: Brain, nervous system, psychic-emotional system
Specialties and related fields: Neurology
Definition: An apparently inherited disorder of the nervous system characterized by brief, numerous, and overwhelming attacks of sleepiness throughout the day.

Key terms:

cataplexy: brief periods of partial or total loss of skeletal muscle tone, usually triggered by emotional stimuli, which can cause the person to collapse

electroencephalogram (EEG): a recording of brain wave activity using electrodes attached to the scalp

excessive daytime sleepiness: a strong tendency to fall asleep, accompanied by reduced energy and lack of alertness during the entire day

hypnogogic hallucination: a bizarre, sometimes frightening, dreamlike occurrence just as one is falling asleep or just after waking

maintenance of wakefulness test: a polysomnographic technique to measure a person's ability to remain awake during repeated trials throughout the day

multiple sleep latency test: a polysomnographic technique to measure how quickly one falls asleep during repeated trials throughout the day

polysomnography: the continuous recording of brain waves, eye movements, skeletal muscle movements, and other body functions to determine bodily changes during the stages of sleep

REM sleep: a period of intense brain activity, often associated with dreams; named for the rapid eye movements that typically occur during this time

sleep paralysis: an inability to move voluntarily, occurring just at the beginning of sleep or upon awakening

CAUSES AND SYMPTOMS

Narcolepsy (*narco* meaning "numbness" and *lepsy* meaning "seizure") consists primarily of attacks of irresistible sleepiness in the daytime. The sleepiness is extreme; it has been described as the feeling that most people would experience if they tried to add columns of numbers in the middle of the night after forty-eight hours without sleep.

The narcoleptic's day is broken up by a series of brief and repetitive sleep attacks, perhaps even two hundred attacks in a single day. These transient, overpowering attacks of sleepiness may last from a few seconds to thirty minutes, with an average spell lasting two minutes. It is excruciatingly difficult, and frequently impossible, to ignore the urge to sleep, no matter how inconvenient or inappropriate. Narcoleptics typically fall asleep suddenly, on the job, in conversation, standing up, and even while eating, driving, or making love.

These sleep attacks result from an abrupt failure in resisting sleep, as opposed to a sudden surge in sleepiness, because narcoleptics are actually sleepy all day. The misconception that their daytime sleepiness is caused by insufficient nighttime sleep prompts undiagnosed patients to spend inordinately long hours in bed. Narcoleptics will be sleepy during the day regardless of how much sleep they get at night.

One of the most prominent and troubling features of narcolepsy is cataplexy, a sudden loss of muscle tone that causes the person to collapse. Cataplexy, the second most common symptom of narcolepsy, is experienced by approximately 70 percent of those diagnosed with the disorder. It occurs during the daytime while the person is awake. It may involve all the muscles at once or only a select few, so the severity may range from total collapse to the ground to partial collapse of a limb or the jaw. The cataplectic sometimes remains conscious, able to think, hear, and see, although vision may be blurred. At other times, there is a brief loss of consciousness, associated with an experience of dreaming. Although most attacks of cataplexy last less than a minute, occasionally they go on for several minutes or more. Cataplexy is often triggered by enjoyable feelings, laughter, or excitement during which the person suddenly crumples into a heap. For other patients, a strong negative emotion, such as fear or anger, precipitates an attack.

Many narcoleptics notice the symptom of excessive daytime sleepiness (EDS) for as much as a year before the onset of cataplexy. After many years of experiencing cataplexy, some patients find that less emotional stimulus is required to induce the muscle collapse and that increasingly more muscles are involved. Others find that this symptom diminishes, possibly because they have become adept at anticipating and avoiding the situations that trigger attacks. It has been noted that other hypersomnias-that is, other diseases of excessive sleepiness-do not include cataplexy; only narcoleptics suffer from this embarrassing and troubling symptom of muscle collapse.

Many narcoleptics also experience hypnogogic hallucinations, dreams that intrude into the waking state. In normal sleep, dreaming generally occurs approximately ninety minutes after falling asleep; narcoleptics begin their sleeping episodes with vivid dreams. These hallucinations are extremely realistic and often violent. The patient sees someone else in the room or hears someone calling his or her name, for the hallucinations are nearly always visual and are usually auditory. The vivid sights, sounds, and feelings characteristic of hypnogogic hallucinations are thought to occur while the person is awake, both during the day and just at the edges of nighttime sleep. Since narcoleptics typically fall asleep dozens if not hundreds of times a day, they can experience these disturbing hallucinations with great frequency.

Narcoleptics may suffer from another frightening symptom: sleep paralysis. This condition occurs at the beginning or end of sleep and renders immobile virtually every voluntary muscle, except those around the eyes. During sleep paralysis, the mind is awake and one is aware of the external surroundings, but the muscles refuse to move. The paralysis usually lasts only a few seconds, but it may continue for as long as twenty minutes. Sleep researchers find that almost everyone has an episode of sleep paralysis that lasts a few seconds some time during his or her lifetime. When the paralysis continues for more than a few seconds, however, it is usually a sign of narcolepsy. Although either sleep paralysis or hypnogogic hallucinations alone are distressing enough, they may happen simultaneously. However, it is estimated that only 10 to 25 percent of narcoleptics experience all four major symptoms of this sleep disorder.

Because of their frequent, irresistible sleep attacks, narcoleptics often wobble back and forth between sleep and wakefulness in a state that has been likened to sleepwalking and is termed automatic behavior.

When in this state, the person seems to behave normally but later does not remember extended periods of time. For example, narcoleptics might find themselves in a different building or several exits farther down a highway than they last remembered. Obviously, automatic behavior is very anxiety-producing; it is very troubling to narcoleptics to be unable to remember what they have done in the minutes or hours that have just passed.

In addition to these memory difficulties, some narcoleptics experience constant eye fatigue, difficulty focusing, and double vision. They also have a higher incidence of the heart abnormality called mitral valve prolapse, which affects blood flow to the left ventricle.

Although narcolepsy is an illness of excessive daytime sleepiness, the nighttime sleep of those afflicted is far from normal as well. It is often troubled by restlessness and frequent awakenings, which are brief or may last for hours. Patients also experience many nightmares. Many narcoleptics talk, cry out, or thrash about periodically during the night.

One narcoleptic in ten has the added complication of suffering from sleep apnea. This sleep disorder consists of recurrent interruptions in breathing during sleep. This further disturbance of nighttime sleep aggravates the narcoleptic's tendency to excessive daytime sleepiness.

Narcolepsy was once thought to be extremely rare. By the late twentieth century, however, it became one of the most diagnosed sleep disorders, behind insomnia, obstructive sleep apnea, and restless legs syndrome. Nevertheless, many medical officials consider narcolepsy to be an underdiagnosed condition.

Males and females are equally affected by narcolepsy. Although the disorder has been diagnosed in a five-year-old, its symptoms most frequently appear for the first time during adolescence. In about 75 percent of cases, the attacks begin between the ages of fifteen and twenty-five; only 5 percent of cases begin before the age of ten. Onset is rare after the age of forty; if narcolepsy seems to appear in an older person, it has probably existed undiagnosed for years. Sleep researchers believe that the extra need for sleep characteristic of adolescence may make this stage of development particularly vulnerable for the onset of narcolepsy. Thus, this disorder may typically begin in adolescence because it is somehow triggered by the brain changes associated with sexual maturation.

While many members of the general population have scattered episodes of excessive daytime sleepiness, they are not considered narcoleptics. It is not until a person has one to several attacks each day that narcolepsy is suspected.

TREATMENT AND THERAPY

Narcolepsy is a disease of the nervous system. Although incurable, it can be successfully treated with various medications once it has been diagnosed. The diagnosis of narcolepsy, however, is often slow to occur. The average interval between the first appearance of symptoms and diagnosis is often as long as thirteen years. Because early symptoms are usually mild, narcoleptics typically spend years wondering whether they are sick or whether they merely lack initiative. They are often called lazy because they repeatedly nap during the day and are lethargic even when awake. Diagnosis is made more difficult by the wide range of severity of symptoms. For example, excessive daytime sleepiness may trouble a person for ten or twenty years before cataplexy appears. Patients may even occasionally experience a temporary or partial remission in their condition. Narcoleptics often fight off their sleep attacks by ingesting large amounts of caffeine and never realize that they have an actual disease until years later.

If narcolepsy is suspected, a polysomnographic study is done at a sleep disorders center to confirm the diagnosis. The most reliable confirmation of narcolepsy can be obtained by what is called the multiple sleep latency test (MSLT). The MSLT is easy, convenient, inexpensive, and very informative. The person is given four or five opportunities to lie down and fall asleep during the daytime. Normal individuals take fifteen to thirty minutes to fall asleep. In the MSLT, falling asleep in less than five minutes is considered abnormal. Those afflicted with narcolepsy always fall asleep in less than five minutes and often within a minute. The maintenance of wakefulness test (MOWT) is also used in the confirmation of narcolepsy. In the MOWT, the person is kept all day in a comfortable reclining position. Polysomnography is used to measure the patient's ability to stay awake and how many times he or she falls asleep.

Along with the MSLT and the MOWT, a thorough physical examination is needed to discover if the person has some other disorder that can mimic narcolepsy; an underactive thyroid gland, diabetes, chronic low blood sugar, anemia, and a malfunctioning liver can each cause excessive daytime sleepiness. Similarly, drug use, poor nutrition, emotional frustration, dissatisfaction, or poor motivation can also result in the type of sleepiness that a narcoleptic experiences.

When the diagnosis of narcolepsy is confirmed, treatment usually consists of stimulant medications such as dextroamphetamine, pemoline, or methylphenidate (Ritalin) during the daytime. These stimulant drugs can increase alertness and cut down the number of sleep attacks from perhaps several per day to several per month. Unfortunately, patients can quickly develop tolerance to these medications.

Even on low doses, some patients become irritable, aggressive, or nervous, or they may develop obesity and sexual problems. It is very important, therefore, to monitor a narcoleptic carefully, determining the lowest effective dose and the best times of day to take it. It may be months before the positive effects of drug therapy are fully experienced. The MSLT will often be given on a day that one takes the medication and on another when it is not taken, in order to evaluate the success of a given treatment.

Because specific drug and dosage schedules may have to be altered frequently, patients may repeatedly have to face drug withdrawal symptoms such as intensified sleepiness and disturbing dreams. To prevent adverse reactions, narcoleptics must often avoid certain foods and common medications. Their use of stimulant drugs may even be viewed as morally wrong, in these days of widespread drug abuse, by neighbors or coworkers who do not comprehend that narcolepsy is a disabling disease.

If cataplexy is present, medications other than amphetamines or Ritalin are required and useful. The class of drugs called tricyclic antidepressants, including protriptyline and imipramine, or the class of drugs called monoamine oxidase inhibitors may alleviate cataplexy. These medicines can often reduce attacks-for example, from three a day to three a month. In addition, effective treatment for cataplexy usually also relieves sleep paralysis and hypnogogic hallucinations.

Since the development of tolerance is common and these drugs can aggravate the symptom of sleepiness, determining the best timing and dose is critical. Another side effect of cataplexy drugs is impaired sexual function in males. Some men even discontinue these medications periodically for a day or two in order to sustain sexual relations. In addition, none of the drugs used for any symptoms of narcolepsy are safe to take during pregnancy.

In some cases, narcoleptics can be treated without medication if they carefully space naps during the day to relieve excessive sleepiness. Patients keep nap diaries to rate their alertness at regular intervals during the day. They then schedule short, strategically timed naps during those daytime periods when their sleep attacks are most likely to occur.

Naps are particularly valuable in treating children with narcolepsy because the consequences of a lifetime of medication on their development or on the course of their illness is unknown. Some children who show hyperactive behavior actually have narcolepsy; they are working frantically to overcome their persistent sleepiness and to keep themselves awake. Children with narcolepsy may also justifiably fear falling asleep, day or night, because of hallucinations and sleep paralysis.

It is evident that supportive counseling must be a strong component of treatment, whatever the patient's age. Sensitive medical monitoring can offer narcoleptics a measure of satisfactory daily living, but the use of stimulants to improve alertness may also make them more aware of their limitations and, therefore, more frustrated. Depression is not the cause of narcolepsy but may result primarily from the disruption in their lives and the feeling that they are denied the right to a "normal" life. Their constant sleepiness engenders feelings of inferiority and inadequacy. Narcoleptics usually refrain from mentioning their hallucinations and try to hide their automatic behavior for fear of being labeled insane. Loss of work, broken marriages, and social isolation are often witnesses to the crippling effects of narcolepsy.

Of all the people with narcolepsy seen at major sleep disorders centers, more than one-half have been completely disabled with respect to regular employment by the age of forty. With part-time, homebound, or self-employment, however, most narcoleptics can gain self-respect and help support themselves through work that is safe and tailored to their needs. They must be given tasks that can be divided into parts performed in relatively short time periods.

Drug and nap therapy can do little for narcoleptics without education of their families, friends, acquaintances, employers, and coworkers about the reality of this neurological disease. Most people find it hard to accept the notion that sleepiness cannot be controlled and insist that narcoleptics could be more alert if they tried harder. Narcoleptics are often stigmatized as slackers or incompetents, or assumed to be drug abusers or closet drinkers. It is most important that patients and all the people in their lives comprehend that excessive daytime sleepiness is not the patients' "fault."

Further help for narcoleptics seems to lie in animal studies, which may fill in many important pieces of the narcolepsy puzzle. The effects of the disease on behavior, the way in which it is inherited, and the benefits and risks of specific drugs continue to be evaluated in narcoleptic dogs.

PERSPECTIVE AND PROSPECTS

Once viewed as "all in the mind," narcolepsy is now recognized as a neurological disorder. Its origin is unknown, but research has already discovered evidence of possible causes. An understanding of narcolepsy both depended on and advanced the understanding of normal sleep and of other sleep disorders. Scientists define sleep as a reduction in awareness of and interaction with the environment, lowered movement and muscle activity, and partial or complete suspension of voluntary behavior and consciousness.

Although narcolepsy was named and described in 1880, it could not be genuinely studied until the 1930s, when the electroencephalograph (EEG) was developed to record brain activity during the various stages of sleep. By the 1940s, this advancement led to a description of the narcoleptic tetrad, the four usual symptoms of narcolepsy: excessive daytime sleepiness, cataplexy, sleep paralysis, and hypnogogic hallucinations.

In the 1950s, narcolepsy still only rated a paragraph in one neurology textbook, which mistakenly called it a rare variety of epilepsy. A major discovery occurred in 1960: Narcoleptics bypass the normal stages of light and deep sleep and fall directly into rapid eye movement (REM) sleep. Thus, sudden-onset REM period (or SOREMP) became the major distinguishing feature of this brain disorder.

It was soon noted that relatives of narcoleptics are sixty times more likely to have the disease than members of the general population. Clearly, there is a hereditary factor involved, and geneticists have joined the hunt for narcolepsy's cause. The hereditary aspects of the disease are particularly important to counselors because parents with narcolepsy may feel guilty if their child develops it. (Indeed, some patients abandon plans to have children.) Geneticists have found a gene that may be responsible for narcolepsy. Since the gene produces an antigen called DR2 on patients' white blood cells, which is not found in nonnarcoleptics, immunologists have also begun to search for the origins of narcolepsy.

Rapid advances have been made in the last few years in determining the cause of narcolepsy. The disease is thought to arise from a biochemical imbalance in the brain that disturbs the mechanism that activates the on/off cycle of sleep. Biochemists are studying the possible relationship of various brain chemicals called neurotransmitters to narcolepsy. A defect in the way in which the body produces or uses dopamine, acetylcholine, or some other neurotransmitter is suspected to precipitate narcolepsy, which never spontaneously disappears once it is developed. The newest discovery has been the finding of abnormalities in the structure and function of a particular group of nerve cells, called hypocretin neurons, in the brains of patients with narcolepsy. The molecules implicated in narcolepsy are neuropeptides known as orexins (originally described as hypocretins). Researchers discovered that changes in the hypocretin receptor 2 and preprohypocretin genes are able to produce narcolepsy in animals. In one study involving nine human subjects, hypocretin could not be detected in seven of the subjects. Other studies have produced hypocretin knockout mice, which have symptoms that are quite similar to those found in human narcoleptics.

Hypocretins have been found to occur normally in the regions of the central nervous system that appear to be involved in the regulation of sleep. An autosomal recessive mutation has been discovered in narcoleptic dogs that alters the hypocretin receptor 2 gene. In humans, a similar disruption or deficiency in hypocretin is associated with most cases of narcolepsy, although it is still unclear as to what underlies the exact genetic predisposition to the disease. Scientists speculate that they one day may cure narcolepsy or reduce its effects with drugs mimicking secretions of the missing nerve cells or even with brain-cell transplants.

Two interesting discoveries may help in the diagnosis of narcolepsy even before the classical clinical symptoms develop. There is some evidence that REM sleep is entered with abnormal rapidity years before the disorder develops. The drug physostigmine salicylate has no effect on normal dogs but elicits cataplexy in puppies with narcolepsy. Both these discoveries may be useful in screening the children of narcoleptics.

Because narcolepsy involves the fundamental processes of sleep, the combined efforts of neuroscientists, geneticists, biochemists, immunologists, and other scientists to unravel its mysteries will continue to yield important information about the basic mechanism of sleep-that state in which humans spend almost one-third of their lives.

—*Grace D. Matzen*

See also Apnea; Brain; Electroencephalography (EEG); Hallucinations; Memory loss; Nervous system; Neurology; Neurology, pediatric; Paralysis; Sleep; Sleep disorders; Sleeping sickness; Unconsciousness.

For Further Information:
Bassetti, Claudio L., Michel Billiard, and Emmanuel Mignot, eds. *Narcolepsy and Hypersomnia.* New York: Informa Healthcare, 2007.
Caldwell, J. Paul. *Sleep: The Complete Guide to Sleep Disorders and a Better Night's Sleep.* Rev. ed. Toronto, Ont.: Firefly Books, 2003.
Dement, William C. *The Sleepwatchers.* 2d ed. Menlo Park, Calif.: Stanford Alumni Association, 1996.
Hartmann, Ernest. *The Sleep Book: Understanding and Preventing Sleep Problems in People over Fifty.* Glenview, Ill.: Scott, Foresman, 1987.
Hollenstein, Jenna, and Rimas Lukas. "Narcolepsy." *Health Library,* Sept. 30, 2012.
Jasmin, Luc, David C. Dugdale III, and David Zieve. "Narcolepsy." *MedlinePlus,* Sept. 26, 2011.
Kryger, Meir H., Thomas Roth, and William C. Dement, eds. *Principles and Practices of Sleep Medicine.* 5th ed. Philadelphia: Saunders/Elsevier, 2011.
"Sleep Disorders." *MedlinePlus,* May 14, 2013.
"Narcolepsy Fact Sheet." *National Institute of Neurological Disorders and Stroke,* Dec. 28, 2011.
"About Narcolepsy." *Narcolepsy Network,* 2013.
Poceta, J. Steven, and Merrill Mitler, eds. *Sleep Disorders: Diagnosis and Treatment.* Totowa, N.J.: Humana Press, 1998.
Reite, Martin, John Ruddy, and Kim E. Nagel. *Concise Guide to Evaluation and Management of Sleep Disorders.* 3d ed. Washington, DC: American Psychiatric Press, 2002.
Walsleben, Joyce A., and Rita Baron-Faust. *A Woman's Guide to Sleep: Guaranteed Solutions for a Good Night's Rest.* New York: Crown, 2001.
"What Is Narcolepsy?" *National Heart, Lung, and Blood Institute,* Nov. 1, 2010.

NARCOTICS

Category: Treatment
Anatomy or system affected: Brain, spinal cord and peripheral nerves
Specialties and related fields: Pharmacology
Definition: Narcotics are drugs, which mimic the action of the body's own painkilling substances, to treat pain, anxiety, coughing, diarrhea, and insomnia.
Key terms:
agonist: a drug that mimics the effects of a hormone or neurotransmitter normally found in the body
analgesia: relief of pain; analgesics are compounds that stop the neurotransmission of pain messages
antagonist: a drug that acts to block the effects of a hormone or neurotransmitter normally found in the body
brainstem: the region between the brain and spinal cord that controls vital functions such as breathing and heart rate
central nervous system: the brain and spinal cord
dependence: a craving for a drug
endogenous: something naturally found in the body, such as neurotransmitters
exogenous: something originating outside the body and administered orally or by injection
neurotransmitter: a chemical substance released by one nerve cell to stimulate or inhibit the function of an adjacent nerve cell; a chemical message released from a neuron
opioids: endogenous or exogenous substances (opiates) that relieve pain and cause euphoria
opiates: drugs made from the opium flower, such as opium, morphine, and codeine
synthetically made neuron: a nerve cell that can conduct electrical impulses from one region of the body to another; it is capable of releasing neurotransmitters
tolerance: diminished effect of a drug over time due to its chronic use
withdrawal: the body's response, both physical and mental, when an addictive substance is reduced or not given to the body

THE EFFECTS OF NARCOTICS

Narcotics are drugs commonly used to treat pain (analgesics), suppress coughing, control diarrhea, and aid in anesthesia. These drugs are some of the oldest and most commonly used agents in medicine. They have psychoactive effects on the body which either block (an antagonist) or mimic (an agonist) the effects of naturally occurring chemicals. Researchers have studied the many effects of opiates, such as morphine, codeine, and heroin in comparison to the body's own endogenous opioids. Naturally occurring opioids, such as endorphins, dynorphins, and enkephalins, act as neurotransmitters, which send chemical signals throughout the human nervous system to relieve pain and increase euphoria.

To understand how opioids affect the body's response to pain, one must first understand the physiology of pain. When tissues are damaged, they release chemical substances into the space outside of the damaged cell, known as the extracellular space. Sensory neurons that have the ability to detect these chemicals are known as pain neurons. Once the chemicals bind to receptors on a pain neuron, the neuron is stimulated to send an ascending electrical message from the peripheral nerve, to the spinal cord and eventually to the brain. One type of neurotransmitter that transfers this message is called substance P. Once released and transmitted, two actions occur when the message arrives to the brain. The first is an immediate initiation of a reflex, which attempts to remove the tissue from the source of injury. For example, when one accidentally places an arm on a hot stove, a neural reflex causes the muscles of the limb to retract the arm from the burner. This is accomplished when the pain neuron releases a descending chemical message (neurotransmitter) from the brain to the spinal cord which then stimulates peripheral neurons that control the muscles of the affected limb. The second action of sensory pain occurs in terms of memory where appropriate behavioral modification can take place. For example, one may become more cautious around the kitchen after burning one's arm on the stove.

Regulation of pain occurs via neurotransmitters such as 5-hydroxytryptamine (5-HT) receptors, glycine, gamma-aminobutyric acid (GABA), and opioids. Morphine acts as an exogenous opioid, dampening the transmission of pain messages at various sites in the nervous system. One of the most clinically important places is within the spinal cord at the region where the pain neurons release substance P. Opioids are known to reduce the amount of substance P that is released and thereby decreasing the stimulatory message in the neural pathway to the brain. If the pain impulses traveling to the brain are reduced, so is one's perception of pain. The second area of the nervous system known to be involved in regulating the perception of pain is a dense area of neurons located between the brain and spinal cord referred to as the brainstem. When researchers stimulated a particular region of the brainstem, pain impulses traveling to the brain were reduced by the modulation of endogenous opioids.

Considering exogenous opioids mimic endogenous opioids, one may wonder why there is a need for narcotic drugs if the body already produces opioids such as endorphins and enkephalins. The answer is that every individual has a different degree of pain tolerance. How much pain one can endure also changes with certain circumstances. For example, one hardly notices the pain of a cut when participating in an exciting outdoor game. If the same wound occurs while one's attention is focused on it, however, the cut becomes noticeably painful. Perhaps the best explanation for the differing interpretation of pain during these activities and among different people is the endogenous opioid system. It is postulated that the analgesic effects of acupuncture are a result of stimulating neurons to release endorphins, enkephalins, and dynorphins. In the same way, with the administration of narcotics, one artificially increases the amount of opioids in the body in order to block pain impulses.

Opioids also act on the brainstem to modulate other pathways not associated with pain. They suppress coughing in a way that is similar to their effect on neural signals to decrease pain messages to the brain. Narcotics appear to inhibit the release of neurotransmitters responsible for the cough reflex. Unfortunately, opiates can simultaneously activate other areas of the brainstem responsible for nausea and vomiting. This unwanted side effect is related to the dose and type of drug used. Therefore, physicians can usually diminish the vomiting response with appropriate treatment selections. Perhaps the most dangerous problem with opioid usage is the effect on the brainstem's regulation of respiration. When the brainstem senses that the level of carbon dioxide is too high, breathing is increased to rid the body of this excess gas. Narcotics decrease the responsiveness of the brainstem to carbon dioxide. Therefore, breathing rates tend to be inappropriately low, causing a buildup of carbon dioxide.

Constriction of the pupils of the eyes is a very common side effect of opiates on the visual system. In fact, this constriction serves as an important diagnostic clue in examining a patient who has taken an overdose of a narcotic.

Opiates have a constipating effect, indirectly through the central nervous system and directly through their influence on the intestines. Opiates cause a decrease in peristalsis, concerted muscular contractions of the intestinal wall that would normally move food toward the anus.

Most opiate analgesics have no direct effect on the heart and blood vessels. Thus, they do not alter heart rate or blood pressure to any significant degree. The only noticeable effect on the cardiovascular system is a flushing and warming of the skin because of a slight increase in blood flow. Occasionally, this is accompanied by sweating. Kidney function tends to be depressed by opiates, which may be attributable to a decrease in the amount of blood that is filtered through the kidneys. There is also a decrease in the ability to urinate, as these drugs increase contraction of the muscle that prevents urine from leaving the bladder.

USES AND COMPLICATIONS

Medical personnel utilize narcotics to alter the body for the patient's advantage. Narcotics such as opiates are used for the relief of pain and anxiety, adjuncts for anesthesia, reduction of coughing, and control of diarrhea.

Opiate analgesics are among the most effective and valuable medications for the treatment of acute and chronic pain. They are often used to treat pain in the postoperative period, in which they effectively reduce or eliminate the short-term pain from tissue trauma that is caused by surgery. When pain is reduced, patients tend to eat, sleep, and recover much more rapidly. Physicians often prescribe narcotics such as morphine or codeine for an as-needed basis ("PRN"). By doing so, the patient, who knows firsthand the effectiveness of the drug, can control the frequency of analgesic administration. In fact, patients are usually advised to administer a small dose before the pain becomes too intense, thus decreasing the pain message before it reaches a higher level, requiring a higher dosage for relief.

A painful sensation consists of the neural response to the tissue damage and the patient's reaction to the stimulus. The analgesic properties of narcotics are related to their ability to diminish both pain perception and the reaction of the patient to pain. These drugs effectively raise the threshold for pain, perhaps because of the euphoria experienced by patients given opioids. For example, a patient in pain who is given morphine experiences a pleasant floating sensation with a great reduction in distress and anxiety. It is interesting to note, however, that some subjects do not experience euphoria when given morphine. In fact, they tend to have an unpleasant response known as dysphoria, which often includes restlessness and a feeling of general discomfort.

Physicians and other health care workers must achieve a delicate balance between alleviating pain from known causes and masking pain as a warning signal from unexpected sources. For example, a patient having abdominal surgery would likely require relatively high doses of analgesics to reduce the postoperative pain. Yet the administration of an analgesic could mask the pain from an unexpected abdominal infection. Therefore, if used excessively, narcotics may prevent the early recognition of complications.

In addition to their analgesic effects, opiates tend to have a sedative effect and are often used as an adjunct to anesthesia. Potent opiates are used in relatively large doses to achieve general anesthesia, particularly in patients undergoing heart surgery. These narcotics are also commonly used during other surgeries in which it is important that heart function be affected only minimally. Examples of narcotic agents used in anesthesia include fentanyl (Sublimaze), sufentanil, alfentanil, and propofol.

Suppression of the cough reflex is a clinically useful effect of opiates. Therapeutic doses needed to reduce coughing are much lower than doses to achieve analgesia. The opioid derivatives most commonly used to suppress the cough reflex are codeine, dextromethorphan, and noscapine. The exact mechanism of action is unknown; however, it is thought to act on the brainstem.

Diarrhea from almost any cause can be controlled with opiates. Diphenoxylate (Lomotil) and loperamide (Imodium) are commonly used to treat diarrhea and do not possess analgesic properties. These drugs appear to act on the nerves within the intestinal tract to decrease muscular activity.

Like all drugs, narcotics have both beneficial and undesired effects. The toxic effects of an opioid depend on the dosage, the agent used, the clinical condition in which it is used, and an individual patient's response to the drug. Some of the more common unwanted side effects include restlessness and hyperactivity instead of sedation, respiratory depression, nausea and vomiting, increased pressure within the brain, low blood pressure, constipation, urinary retention, and itching around the nose. Most of these conditions are of short duration and resolve after the drug has been discontinued.

Patients on chronic opiate therapy may develop tolerance and become physically and mentally dependent upon these agents. Many people abuse narcotics in high dosages in order to experience euphoric effects. With chronic use, the euphoric effects diminish and the user eventually requires higher doses to achieve the same euphoria. Physiological adaptation to the long-term use of opioids (two to three weeks) causes the development of tolerance towards these drugs.

Exogenous opioids take the place of endogenous ones. Therefore, the nervous system and other physiological systems attempt to bring the levels of these neurotransmitters back to normal. First, the liver speeds up its metabolism of the drugs to eliminate them from the system more rapidly. Second, the regions of the nervous system that respond to opioids become desensitized by reducing the number of neural receptors that are available. Finally, after a few weeks of high levels of opiates, changes in other areas of the brain attempt to compensate for the rising opioid levels. Individuals who abruptly stop taking the drugs enter a period of withdrawal in which they experience symptoms similar to a bad case of influenza. Morphine and heroine withdrawal symptoms usually start within twelve hours of the last dose. Peak symptoms of narcotic withdrawal occur after one to two days. Most symptoms gradually subside and resolve after one week. It should be emphasized that, under a physician's direction, the abuse potential of narcotics is very low.

There are certain clinical conditions in which opiates should not be used or should be used with extreme caution. Because of the potential for respiratory depression with opiate treatment, these drugs should not be administered to patients with head injuries or impaired lung function. Most opioid drugs can cross the placenta and therefore should be avoided during pregnancy; with long-term use, the infant can be born addicted to narcotics.

Fortunately, some drugs can reverse the effects of narcotics when required. Three commonly used opioid antagonists are nalmefene, naloxone (Narcan), and naltrexone (Trexan). When these agents are given in the absence of an opioid agonist, they have no noticeable effect. When administered to a morphine-treated patient, however, they completely reverse the opioid effects almost immediately. These narcotic antagonists are particularly useful in treating patients who have taken an overdose of opiates. Such patients often arrive in the hospital emergency room with severe respiratory depression or in a coma. These antagonists will normalize respiration, restore consciousness, and counteract other opioid effects. Interestingly, individuals who have become tolerant to and dependent upon opioids will immediately experience withdrawal symptoms when given naloxone or naltrexone.

PERSPECTIVE AND PROSPECTS
Narcotic drugs were originally found in the opium poppy five thousand years ago. Opium is obtained from the milky fluid of the unripe seed capsules of the poppy plant. The juice is dried in the air and forms a brown, sticky substance. With continued drying, the mass can be pulverized into powder. It is this powder that opiates are derived from. Morphine,

codeine, and papaverine are the natural opiates that are used clinically. Most other narcotics are chemically derived.

The opium poppy, Papaver somniferum, was named after the Roman god of sleep, Somnis. Ancient Egyptian medical texts listed opium as a cure for illness and as a poison. Although opium was used extensively, the abuse potential was low because the poppy has a very bitter taste. Smoking opium became popular in eighteenth century China as a treatment for severe diarrhea and was also a socially acceptable drug used mainly for its euphoric effects.

The opium poppy contains more than twenty distinct agents with a variety of potencies and unwanted side effects. In 1806, a pharmacist refined opium into one active substance, morphine, which was found to be ten times as potent. Morphine was named after Morpheus, the Greek god of dreams, because of its powerful sedative effects. The discovery of other medically active agents quickly followed. Codeine and papaverine were identified next and found to be slightly less potent than morphine. At this time, clinicians used these purified products rather than the crude opium juice.

Shortly after purified narcotics became available, so did the widespread use of hypodermic needles. This allowed physicians to administer narcotics directly into the bloodstream. The injected opioids would rapidly travel via the blood to the brain and exert its effects. In the United States, morphine found widespread use as an analgesic for wounded soldiers during the Civil War. It was one of the most powerful painkillers available to physicians, but its unrestricted availability created great potential for addiction with long-term use.

Opioid derivations became so popular that hundreds of medications became available to the public in many different forms. Tonics promised to cure everything from "tired blood" to common aches and pains. Their widespread unregulated usage allowed for potential addiction. At the beginning of the twentieth century, the U.S. government attempted to address this issue by making it illegal to buy any opiate-containing compound without a prescription. Chemists then tried to synthesize compounds with morphine-like characteristics but without the addictive effects.

Physicians now have a vast selection of narcotics with different pharmacological properties to choose from. For example, there are drugs without addictive, euphoric, or sedative properties that can treat coughing or diarrhea. Narcotic analgesics can only be prescribed and administered under the direction of a physician. With proper medical supervision, the benefit of narcotics can be maximized and the side effects, including addiction, can be minimized. Morphine is still used as a potent pain reliever, and when used appropriately, there is less potential for addiction. With further research into opioids and pain pathways, the potential for further medical usage remains an endless possibility.

—Matthew Berria, PhD;
updated by Cristina Cesaro, DO,
and Jimmy Bajaj, DO

See also Addiction; Anesthesia; Anesthesiology; Coughing; Diarrhea and dysentery; Marijuana; Over-the-counter medications; Pain; Pain management; Pharmacology; Prescription drug abuse; Self-medication; Substance abuse

For Further Information:

Acker, Caroline Jean. *Creating the American Junkie: Addiction Research in the Classic Era of Narcotic Control.* Baltimore: Johns Hopkins University Press, 2002. A fascinating examination of how the construction of addiction in the early twentieth century was influenced by a nexus of actors and events: psychiatrists, pharmacologists, and the American Medical Association's campaign to reduce prescriptions of opiates.

Davenport-Hines, Richard. *The Pursuit of Oblivion: A Global History of Narcotics.* New York: W.W. Norton, 2002. Blends social, political, and cultural history to trace the evolution of drugs, their role in society, and addiction.

Griffith, H. Winter. *Complete Guide to Prescription and Nonprescription Drugs.* Revised and updated by Stephen Moore. New York: Penguin Group, 2010. A complete guide to both prescription and nonprescription drugs, including major uses, unwanted effects, precautions, and interactions with other drugs. A highly organized, useful tool for the nonscientist.

Inaba, Darryl S., William E. Cohen, and Michael E. Holstein. *Uppers, Downers, All Arounders: Physical and Mental Effects of Psychoactive Drugs.* 6th ed. Ashland, OR: CNS, 2007. Mainly covers drug abuse, but also contains brief descriptions of the history and medical uses for drugs with abuse potential. A reader-friendly book that offers numerous statements from drug addicts regarding their addiction and, in some cases, their recovery.

Ling, W., and D.R. Wesson. "Drugs of Abuse: Opiates." *Western Journal of Medicine* 152 (May, 1990): 565-572. This article reviews the ways that addiction can be treated. Also addresses the use of narcotic antagonists in the treatment of drug overdose.

Liska, Ken. *Drugs and the Human Body, with Implications for Society.* 8th ed. Upper Saddle River, NJ: Pearson/Prentice Hall, 2009. Examines the use of drugs in the North American culture by discussing such topics as what constitutes a drug and where drugs come from, federal laws, drug metabolism, and the different classifications of drugs.

Voth, Eric A., Robert L. Dupont, and Harold M. Voth. "Responsible Prescribing of Controlled Substances." *American Family Physician* 44 (November, 1991): 1673-1680. This article details some of the important problems in prescribing narcotics. Gives a description of characteristics that both health care workers and nonprofessionals can watch for in their attempts to identify drug abusers.

NASAL POLYP REMOVAL

Category: Procedure
Anatomy or system affected: Head, nose
Specialties and related fields: Family medicine, general surgery, otorhinolaryngology
Definition: The excision of benign growths that project from the mucous membrane lining the nasal cavity.

INDICATIONS AND PROCEDURES

Nasal polyps are swollen masses that project from the nasal wall. These benign structures are commonly found in patients with allergies. They may cause chronic nasal obstruction, which results in diminished air flow through the nasal cavity.

Once a polyp is detected, the physician may prescribe a nasal spray to reduce its size, such as the corticosteroids beclometasone or flunisolide. This treatment is usually effective for small nasal polyps that cause only minor symptoms. When pharmacological management is not successful, the polyps should be removed surgically.

Surgical removal of nasal polyps (nasal polypectomy) is typically done as an outpatient procedure. It requires either general anesthesia or local anesthesia with sedation. After the patient is asleep or sedated, the lining of the nasal cavity is injected with a combination of local anesthesia and epinephrine to control pain and bleeding. The surgeon (usually an otorhinolaryngologist) visualizes the polyps with a headlight, and the polyps are removed with specialized long surgical instruments inserted into the nasal

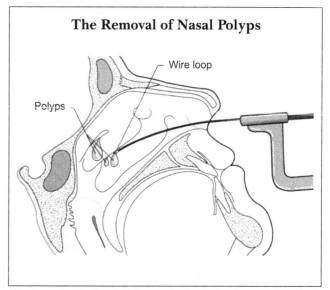

The Removal of Nasal Polyps

Allergies or chronic sinus infections can lead to the development of nasal polyps, distended areas of the nasal lining. If they interfere with breathing or the sense of smell or if they cause frequent nosebleeds, the polyps may be removed with a wire loop. ©EBSCO

cavity. After the polyps are removed, the nasal passages are packed with ointment-coated gauze to help control bleeding and aid in the healing of the nasal mucosa. The gauze is removed in the physician's office a few days after the surgery. Once the packing is removed, the patient enjoys improved breathing through the nasal passages.

USES AND COMPLICATIONS

There are relatively few complications associated with nasal polyp removal. Some of the more common complications include bleeding from the surgical site, nasal and ear discomfort or anxiety as a result of the packing, and nausea from the anesthesia. The recurrence of nasal polyps after polypectomy is not unusual. Patients with cystic fibrosis have a high rate of occurrence of nasal polyps and often have recurrent problems.

—*Matthew Berria, PhD and Douglas Reinhart, MD*

See also Allergies; Nasopharyngeal disorders; Oral and maxillofacial surgency; Otorhinolaryngology; Polyps; Sense organs; Sinusitis; Smell.

For Further Information:
Adelman, Daniel C., Thomas B. Casale, and Jonathan Corren, eds. *Manual of Allergy and Immunology.* 5th ed. Philadelphia: Wolters Kluwer Health/Lippincott Williams & Wilkins, 2012.
Benjamin, Bruce, et al. *A Colour Atlas of Otorhinolaryngology.* Edited by Michael Hawke. Philadelphia: J. B. Lippincott, 1995.
Bull, P. D. *Lecture Notes: Diseases of the Ear, Nose and Throat.* 10th ed. Malden, Mass.: Blackwell Science, 2007.
PDxMD. *PDxMD Ear, Nose, and Throat Disorders.* Philadelphia: Author, 2003.
Icon Health. *Nasal Polyps: A Medical Dictionary, Bibliography, and Annotated Research Guide to Internet References.* San Diego, Calif.: Author, 2004.
Kimball, Chad T. *Colds, Flu, and Other Common Ailments Sourcebook.* Detroit, Mich.: Omnigraphics, 2001.
Lewy, Jennifer, and Marcin Chwistek. "Nasal Polyp." *Health Library,* March 15, 2013.
Morelock, Michael, and J. B. Vap. *Your Guide to Problems of the Ear, Nose, and Throat.* Philadelphia: Lippincott Williams & Wilkins, 1985.
"Nasal Polyps." *Mayo Clinic,* February 19, 2011.
Settipane, Guy A., et al., eds. *Nasal Polyps: Epidemiology, Pathogenesis and Treatment.* Providence, R.I.: OceanSide, 1997.
Vorvick, Linda J., Seth Schwartz, and David Zieve. "Nasal Polyps." *MedlinePlus,* August 31, 2011.

NASOPHARYNGEAL DISORDERS

Category: Disease/Disorder
Anatomy or system affected: Nose, respiratory system, throat
Specialties and related fields: Family medicine, occupational health, otorhinolaryngology
Definition: Disorders of the nose, nasal passages (sinuses), and pharynx (mouth, throat, and esophagus).
Key terms:
acute disease: a short and sharp disease process
chronic disease: a lingering illness
esophagus: the tube that leads from the pharynx to the stomach
larynx: the organ that produces the voice, which lies between the pharynx and the trachea; commonly called the voice box
nasopharyngeal: referring to the nose and pharynx (the upper part of the throat that leads from the mouth to the esophagus)
trachea: a tube that leads from the throat to the lungs; commonly called the windpipe

CAUSES AND SYMPTOMS

Nasopharyngeal disorders are all the diseases that can be present in the nasal cavity and the pharynx. These include the common cold, pharyngitis (sore throat), laryngitis (inflammation of the larynx), epiglottitis (inflammation of the lid over the larynx), tonsillitis (inflammation of the lymph nodes at the rear of the mouth), sinusitis (inflammation of the sinus cavities that surround the nose), otitis media (earache that is often associated with nasopharyngeal infection), nosebleed, nasal obstruction, halitosis (bad breath), and various other disorders.

The common cold is one of the most prevalent diseases that afflict humankind. Pharyngitis, or sore throat, often accompanies the common cold, or it may appear by itself. Acute infections can be caused by viruses or bacteria, often by certain streptococcus strains-hence the common term for the disorder, strep throat. Acute pharyngitis can also be caused by chemicals or radiation. As a chronic disorder, pharyngitis can be caused by lingering infection in other organs such as the lungs and sinuses, or it can be attributable to constant irritation from smoking, drinking alcohol, or breathing polluted air. The usual symptoms of pharyngitis include sore throat, difficulty swallowing, and fever. The infected area appears red and swollen.

Ordinarily, pharyngitis is not serious. If certain strains of streptococcus are the cause, however, then the infection may progress to rheumatic fever. This disease appears to be the result of an immune system reaction to some streptococcus bacteria. It can have painful effects in many parts of the body, including the joints, and can do permanent damage to parts of the heart. In rare cases, rheumatic fever can be fatal.

Acute laryngitis is usually caused by a viral infection, but bacteria, outside irritants, or misuse of the voice are other causes. Ordinarily, the vocal cords produce sounds by vibrating in response to the air passing over them. When inflamed or irritated, they swell, causing distortion in the sounds produced. The affected person's voice becomes hoarse and raspy and may even diminish to a soft whisper. This distortion of sound is the main symptom of laryngitis; other possible symptoms include a sore throat and congestion that causes constant coughing. The condition generally resolves itself and requires no treatment. Chronic laryngitis has the same symptoms but does not go away spontaneously. It may be caused by an infectious agent but more likely is attributable to some irritant activity, such as constantly misusing one's voice, smoking, drinking alcohol, or breathing contaminated air.

The epiglottis is a waferlike tissue covered by a mucous membrane that sits on top of the larynx. It can become infected by such microorganisms as the bacteria *Haemophilus influenzae* type b, causing a condition called epiglottitis. Although the symptoms of epiglottitis can resemble those of pharyngitis, the infection can quickly progress to a very serious, life-threatening disorder. Epiglottitis usually afflicts children from two to four years of age, but adults can also be affected. The infection can begin rapidly, causing the epiglottis to swell and obstruct the airway to the lungs, creating a major medical emergency. Within twelve hours of the onset of symptoms, 50 percent of patients require hospitalization and intubation (insertion of a breathing tube into the trachea). The symptoms are high fever, severe sore throat, difficulty breathing, difficulty swallowing, and general malaise. As the airway becomes more and more occluded, the patient begins to gasp for air. The lack of oxygen may cause cyanosis (blue color in the lips, fingers, and skin), exhaustion, and shock.

Another disease associated with the larynx is croup, or laryngotracheobronchitis. As the medical name indicates, croup involves the larynx, the trachea, and the bronchi (the large branches of the lung). It is usually caused by a virus, but some cases are attributable to bacterial infection. Children from three to five years of age are the usual victims. This disease causes the airways to narrow due to inflammation of the inner mucosal surfaces. Inflammation causes coughing, but the narrowed airway causes the cough to be sharp and brassy, like the barking of a seal. Croup is usually relatively benign, but sometimes it progresses to a severe disease requiring hospitalization.

Various other disorders can afflict the larynx, such as damage to the vocal cords because of infection by bacteria, fungi, or other microorganisms. The vocal cords can also be damaged by misusing one's voice, smoking, or breathing contaminated air. Polyps (masses of tissue growing on the surface), nodes (little knots of

---

INFORMATION ON NASOPHARYNGEAL DISORDERS

Causes: May include bacterial or viral infection, nasal obstruction (polyps), environmental allergens or toxins

Symptoms: Sore throat; inflamed lymph nodes, larynx, and sinus cavities; earache or ear infection; nosebleeds; nasal obstruction; fever; difficulty breathing or swallowing; general malaise; bad breath

Duration: Acute to chronic

Treatments: Antibiotics, over-the-counter medications, surgery; if severe, emergency intubation

---

tissue), or so-called singer's nodules may develop. Sores called contact ulcers may form on the vocal cords.

Tonsillitis is an inflammation of the tonsils, two large lymph nodes located at the back of the throat. It may also involve the adenoids, lymph nodes located at the top of the throat. The function of these lymph nodes is to remove harmful pathogens (disease-causing organisms) from the nasopharyngeal cavity. At times, the load of microorganisms that they absorb becomes more than they can handle, and they become infected. The tonsils and adenoids may then become enlarged. A sore throat develops, along with a headache, fever, and chills. Glands of the neck and throat feel sore and may become enlarged. Young adults can also suffer from quinsy, or peritonsillar abscess. In this condition, one of the tonsils becomes infected and pus forms between the tonsil and the soft tissue surrounding it. Quinsy is characterized by pain in the throat or the soft palate, pain on swallowing, fever, and a tendency to lean one's head toward the affected side.

The nasal sinuses are four pairs of cavities in the bone around the nose. There are two maxillary sinuses, so called because they are found in the maxilla, or upper jaw. Slightly above and behind them are the ethmoid sinuses, and behind them are the sphenoid sinuses. Sitting over the nose in the lower part of the forehead are the two frontal sinuses. All these sinuses are lined with a mucous membrane and have small openings that lead into the nasal passages. Air moves in and out of the sinuses and allows mucus to drain into the nose. In acute sinusitis, infection builds up in the mucous membrane of any or all of the sinuses. The membrane lining the sinus swells and shuts the opening into the nasal passages. At the same time, membranes of the nose swell and become congested. Mucus and pus build up inside the sinuses, causing pain and pressure. Most often, sinusitis accompanies the common cold: the mucous membrane that lines the nose extends into the sinuses, so the infection of a cold can readily spread into the sinuses. The various viruses responsible for the common cold may be involved, as well as a wide group of bacteria. Chronic sinusitis can be caused by repeated infections that have allowed scar tissue to build up, closing the sinus openings and impeding mucus drainage, or it may be the result of allergies.

According to the Centers for Disease Control and Prevention, chronic sinusitis is the most common long-term illness in the United States, surpassing the rates for asthma, arthritis, and congestive heart disease and causing nearly fourteen million doctor's office visits per year. For reasons that are not yet understood, sinusitis sufferers are often beset with inflammation of the ducts, trapping mucus, bacteria, and viruses inside and allowing nasal polyps to develop. Researchers have been very interested in finding causes and effective treatments for sinusitis. In the late twentieth century, most chronic cases of sinusitis were treated with fiber-optic surgery that allowed access to the cramped sinus passageways. However, patients often returned within weeks or months with ongoing problems. This fact has recently prompted a reconsideration of the problem and its underlying causes as well as a struggle to redefine sinusitis. Some medical experts suspect that inflammation or the responses of the immune system are the culprit but note that additional research must be completed before any definitive answers are found.

Tissues in the nasopharyngeal cavity may be affected by conditions occurring in other parts of the body. For example, vocal cord paralysis may be caused by vascular accidents, certain cancers, tissue trauma, and other events.

Some infections in the nasopharyngeal cavity can spread to the ear through the eustachian tubes that connect the two areas. Chief among the diseases of the ear that can be associated with nasopharyngeal disorders are the various forms of acute otitis media, an earache occurring in the central part of the ear. There are four basic types of otitis media. In the first type, serous otitis media, there is usually no infection, but fluid accumulates inside the middle ear because of the blockage of the eustachian tube or the overproduction of fluid; the condition is usually mild, with some pain and temporary loss of hearing. The second type is otitis media with effusion; with this condition comes both infection and accumulation of fluid. The third form is acute purulent otitis media, the most serious type. Pus builds up inside the middle ear, and its pressure may rupture the eardrum, allowing discharge of blood and pus. The fourth type is secretory otitis media, which usually occurs after several bouts of otitis media. Cells within the middle ear start producing a fluid that is thicker than normal and produced in greater amounts.

Chronic otitis media is bacterial in origin. It is characterized by a perforation of the eardrum and chronic pus discharge. The eardrum is a flat, pliable disk of tissue that vibrates to conduct sounds from the outside to the inner-ear structures. The perforation that occurs in chronic otitis media can be one of two types: a relatively benign perforation occurring in the central part of the eardrum or a potentially dangerous perforation occurring near the edges of the eardrum. The latter perforation can be associated with loss of hearing, increased discharge of pus and other fluids, facial paralysis, and the spread of infection to other tissues. When the perforation of chronic otitis media is near the edges of the eardrum, something called a cholesteatoma develops. This accumulation of matter grows in the inner ear and can be destructive to bone and other tissue.

The same organisms that cause otitis media can be responsible for a condition called mastoiditis. The mastoid process is a bone structure lined with a mucous membrane. Infection from otitis media can spread to this area and in severe cases can destroy the

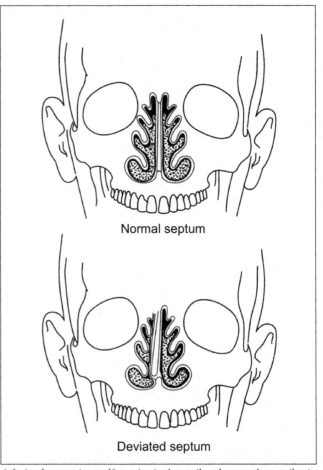

Normal septum

Deviated septum

A deviated septum is a malformation in the cartilage between the nostrils, either present at birth or caused by a blow to the nose. ©EBSCO

bone. Mastoiditis used to be a leading cause of death in children.

Nosebleeds are common and most often result from a blow to the nose, but they can also be caused by colds, sinusitis, and breathing dry air. The septum (the cartilaginous tissue that separates the nostrils) and the surrounding intranasal mucous membrane contain many tiny blood vessels that are easily ruptured. If an individual receives a blow to the nose, these vessels can break and bleed. They can also rupture due to irritation from a cold or other condition. Breathing very dry air sometimes causes the nasal mucous membrane to crust over, and bleeding can follow. Nosebleeds are not usually serious, but sometimes they are indicative of an underlying condition, such as hypertension (high blood pressure), a tumor, or another disease.

Nasal obstruction is common during colds and allergy attacks, but it can also be caused by a deviated septum, a malformation in the cartilage between the nostrils that can be congenital or caused by a blow to the nose. Nasal obstruction can also be attributable to nasal polyps, nasal tumors, or swollen adenoids. A common source of nasal obstruction is overuse of nasal decongestants. These agents relieve nasal congestion by reducing intranasal inflammation and swelling. If used too often or for too long, however, they can cause the very problem that they were intended to cure: intranasal blood vessels dilate, the area swells, secretions increase, and the nose becomes blocked. This is known as rebound congestion or, in medical terminology, rhinitis medicamentosa (nasal inflammation that is caused by a medication).

Halitosis, or bad breath, can be considered a nasopharyngeal disorder in the sense that it can originate in the mouth. It can be caused by diseases of the teeth or gums, but the most common causes are smoking or eating aromatic foods such as onions and garlic. Bad breath may also be a sign of disease conditions in other parts of the body, such as certain lung disorders or cancer of the esophagus. Hepatic failure, a liver dysfunction, may be accompanied by a fishy odor on the breath. Azotemia, the retention of nitrogen in the blood, may give rise to an ammonia-like odor. A sweet, fruity odor on the breath of diabetic patients may accompany ketoacidosis, a condition that occurs when there are high levels of glucose in the blood. Sometimes, young children stick foreign objects or other materials into their noses; it has been reported that these materials can fester, causing severe halitosis. Bad breath is rarely apparent to the individual who has it, however offensive it may be to others. A good way to check one's breath is to lick the back of one's hand and smell the spot; malodor, if it exists, will usually be apparent.

TREATMENT AND THERAPY

Nasopharyngeal disorders are most often mild illnesses that can be treated at home. For example, acute pharyngitis, or sore throat, is easily managed most of the time. The patient is advised to rest, gargle with warm salt water several times a day, and soothe the pain with lozenges or anesthetic gargles. If the infection is caused by a virus, it usually will clear without further treatment. If the physician suspects that the infection is bacterial in origin, throat smears may be taken so that the organism can be identified. If bacteria are discovered, antibiotic therapy will be undertaken to eradicate the pathogens. This is particularly important if the infection is caused by certain strains of streptococcus bacteria. In this case, it is vital to destroy the organism in order to avoid the development of rheumatic fever.

In cases of acute laryngitis caused by viral infection, the patient is advised to rest his or her voice, inhale steam, and drink warm liquids. If bacteria are the cause of the laryngitis, antibiotic therapy is undertaken. In treating chronic laryngitis, the physician must discover the cause and remove it. If allergy is the cause, antihistamine therapy could help. If the cause is bacterial, antibiotic therapy is used. If smoking or drinking alcohol is the problem, the patient should be counseled to stop. The simple palliative measures used for acute laryngitis-resting the voice, drinking warm liquids, and breathing steam-are also useful for chronic laryngitis.

Symptoms of epiglottitis are often similar to those of sore throat. If there is any evidence of difficulty in breathing, however, the patient should be seen by a physician quickly, as an emergency situation may be developing. If epiglottitis is obstructing the airway, the patient should be treated in an intensive care setting. Antibiotics must be given to the patient to treat the infection. It is important to make an airway for the patient, and it may be necessary to insert a tube into the trachea to allow the patient to breathe.

Before the age of antibiotics, tonsillitis was often treated surgically, with both tonsils and adenoids removed. This procedure is now rare, as the infection usually responds to antibiotic therapy. Similarly, in the case of peritonsillar abscess or quinsy, antibiotics usually clear the condition satisfactorily. In some cases, accumulations of pus may be removed surgically. If the abscesses return, it may be advisable to remove the tonsils.

As a rule, a child with croup is treated at home. Because the disease is usually caused by viruses, antibiotics are not used unless bacteria are known to be involved. Steam is often used to help liquefy mucus deposits on the interior walls of the trachea, the larynx, and the bronchi. The patient is given warm liquids to drink and is closely watched so that any signs that the condition is getting worse will be detected. The following symptoms should alert the caregiver to the possibility that an emergency situation is developing and that medical help is needed quickly: drooling, difficulty breathing or swallowing, inability to bend the neck forward, blue or dark color in the lips, high-pitched sounds when inhaling, rapid heartbeat, and loss of consciousness.

The main goals of therapy for sinusitis are to control infection, relieve the blockage of the sinus openings to permit drainage, and relieve pain. When sinusitis is known to be of bacterial origin, an appropriate antibiotic will be used to eradicate the organism. Often, however, sinusitis is attributable to viral infection, and other procedures are used to treat it. Inhaling steam is useful for thinning secretions and promoting drainage, as are mucolytic agents such as guaifenesin. Decongestant sprays and oral decongestants reduce swelling and open passages. Analgesics can be given for pain. In certain circumstances, the sinuses are drained surgically.

Acute otitis media is most often diagnosed with the aid of an otoscope, an instrument that the doctor uses to look at the eardrum and surrounding tissues. The eardrum will be a dull red color, bulging, and perhaps perforated. While a viral infection may precede otitis media, the causative microorganisms for this and related ear infections, such as mastoiditis, are usually bacteria. Antibiotics are used both to treat the infections and to prevent the spread of disease to other areas. The drugs are usually taken orally. Penicillin and its derivatives are used, as are erythromycin and sulfisoxazole. Antibiotic therapy for acute otitis media is usually continued for ten days to two weeks. Sometimes pus and other fluids and solid matter build up in the inner ear, and it may be necessary to pierce the eardrum in order to remove these deposits. To help relieve blockage of the eustachian tubes, a topical vasoconstrictor may be used in the nose to reduce the swelling of blood vessels. Antihistamines could be helpful to patients with allergies but are otherwise not indicated.

For chronic otitis media, it is necessary to clean both the outer ear canal and the middle ear thoroughly. A mild acetic acid solution with a corticosteroid is used for a week to ten days. Meanwhile, aggressive oral antibiotic therapy is undertaken to eradicate the pathogen. The perforated eardrum associated with chronic otitis media can usually be repaired surgically with little or no loss of function, and the cholesteatoma must be surgically removed.

Simple nosebleeds can be treated by pinching the nose with the fingers and breathing through the mouth for five or ten minutes to allow the blood to clot. Also, a plug of absorbent paper or cloth can be inserted into the bleeding nostril. A nosebleed that does not stop easily should be seen by a physician.

Nasal obstruction resulting from colds or allergies is treated by appropriate medications, decongestants for colds and antihistamines for allergies. A deviated septum may require surgery. The only therapy for rhinitis medicamentosa, or rebound congestion caused by overuse of nasal decongestants, is to stop the medication and endure the congestion for as long as it takes the condition to clear. Sometimes it is necessary to consult a physician.

For simple halitosis caused by smoking or food, breath fresheners (with or without "odor-fighting" chemicals) are often used, even though they usually simply replace a "bad" odor with a "good" one. Some people believe that chewing parsley or other leaves rich in chlorophyll will counteract the smell of garlic. When halitosis is attributable to tooth or gum disease, it will persist until the condition is cured. Halitosis may be of diagnostic value in certain situations where a characteristic odor could alert the physician to the possibility of a disease condition.

PERSPECTIVE AND PROSPECTS

Diseases and infections of the nasal cavity and throat have always been common among human populations, as have therapies to deal with them. Until the advent of antibiotics, some of these disorders were quite serious, especially in young children, but modern medications and surgeries, where appropriate, have greatly lessened the danger. The widespread use of a vaccine against *Haemophilus influenzae* type b, the most common causative organism of epiglottitis, has made this life-threatening disease a rarity. Many over-the-counter drugs are used to combat sore throats, sinus congestion, and other nasopharyngeal symptoms of the common cold, although colds themselves remain incurable because of the hundreds or thousands of different microorganisms that may be responsible.

Despite the numerous medications that can be taken, however, more serious infections or diseases, such as chronic tonsillitis or laryngitis, require a doctor's care, with more potent prescription drugs and surgery if needed. The treatments available to physicians and patients for the symptoms of nasopharyngeal disorders are many, but the search continues for better drugs and perhaps preventive measures such as vaccinations to address the causes of these conditions.

—*C. Richard Falcon*

See also Allergies; Antihistamines; Choking; Common cold; Decongestants; Ear infections and disorders; Ears; Earwax; Esophagus; Halitosis; Hearing; Hearing loss; Laryngectomy; Laryngitis; Mouth and throat cancer; Multiple chemical sensitivity syndrome; Nasal polyp removal; Nosebleeds; Oral and maxillofacial surgery; Otorhinolaryngology; Pharyngitis; Pharynx; Plastic surgery; Respiration; Rhinitis; Rhinoplasty and submucous resection; Sinusitis; Smell; Sore throat; Strep throat; Taste; Tonsillectomy and adenoid removal; Tonsillitis; Tonsils; Voice and vocal cord disorders.

For Further Information:
Friedman, Ellen M., and James P. Barassi. *My Ear Hurts! A Complete Guide to Understanding and Treating Your Child's Ear Infections*. Darby, Pa.: Diane, 2004.
Greene, Alan R. *The Parent's Complete Guide to Ear Infections*. Allentown, Pa.: People's Medical Society, 1999.
Kimball, Chad T. *Colds, Flu, and Other Common Ailments Sourcebook*. Detroit: Omnigraphics, 2001.
Litin, Scott C., ed. *Mayo Clinic Family Health Book*. 4th ed. New York: HarperResource, 2009.
PDxMD. *PDxMD Ear, Nose, and Throat Disorders*. Philadelphia: Author, 2003.
Wagman, Richard J., ed. *The New Complete Medical and Health Encyclopedia*. 4 vols. Chicago: J. G. Ferguson, 2002.

NATIONAL CANCER INSTITUTE (NCI)

Category: Organization
Definition: A federal agency devoted to the study of cancer, as well as communication and education about this condition.

Key terms:
carcinogenesis: the biological process of the initiation, promotion, and progression of cancer
epidemiology: the study of the relationships between a host, an agent, and an environment that lead to a condition or disease

OVERVIEW

The US Department of Health and Human Services (HHS) is the federal agency responsible for public health. The HHS includes eleven divisions, one of which is the National Institutes of Health (NIH). The National Cancer Institute (NCI) is one of twenty-seven institutes and centers within the NIH. The institute was established in 1937 under the National Cancer Institute Act and in 1944 was made part of the National Institutes of Health under the Public Health Service Act. NCI is the principal federal agency for cancer research and training. Following special legislation in 1971 that amended the Public Health Service Act and created the National Cancer Act, the scope of the NCI has continued to broaden through new initiatives and legislation.

The purpose of the NCI is to eliminate cancer as far as possible and to discover treatment for those cancers which cannot be eradicated. The NCI approaches these goals by supporting research, coordinating efforts in prevention and treatment, facilitating the movement of research findings into medicine, and providing education and resources for patients and their families, health educators, and scientists. The NCI conducts research in its own laboratories and clinics in Bethesda, Maryland, but also supports and coordinates research projects conducted by universities, hospitals, research foundations, and businesses throughout the United States and many other countries.

THE ORGANIZATION AND FOCUS OF THE NCI

The NCI is organized by the Office of the Director into nearly thirty centers, offices, and divisions. Each of the intiatives specializes in a different aspect of cancer research, although there is overlap among them. The Office of Cancer Centers, for example, supports cancer research at academic and research institutions across the United States, while the Office of Cancer Genomics specifically supports research programs that focus on the molecular components of cancer.

Another group, the Office of Cancer Nanotechnology Research, is in charge of the NCI Alliance for Nanotechnology in Cancer Program, which works to develop nanotechnology-based tools for research, detection, treatment, monitoring, and prevention. The Center to Reduce Cancer Health Disparities works through research, training, and partnerships to reduce cancer disparities among diverse populations. The Center for Global Health fosters international collaboration and sharing of research resources among government agencies, nongovernment organizations, biotechnology companies, and pharmaceutical companies. In 1998, the Office of Cancer Complementary and Alternative Medicine was established to coordinate research and communication activities in the arena of complementary and alternative medicine, both within the NCI and with other agencies.

The main purpose of the NCI's basic, clinical intramural research program, the Center for Cancer Research, is to improve the lives of those affected by cancer as well as by HIV/AIDS. The NCI's other intramural initiative is the Division of Cancer Epidemiology and Genetics, whose goal is prevention. This division focuses on the factors that could lead to cancer growth, namely genetic predisposition, lifestyle factors, environmental contaminants, occupational exposures, medications, radiation, and infectious agents; the group also works on epidemiological methods development.

Research in cancer cell biology, such as carcinogenesis and cancer immunology, falls within the realm of the extramural Division of Cancer Biology. This division also examines the biological and health effects of exposures to ionizing and nonionizing radiation. The efforts of the Division of Cancer Prevention center on early detection methods and the efficacy of nutritional or life-

2006 • National Cancer Institute (NCI)

style changes on cancer prevention. The results of research in this area led to the 5 a Day for Better Health program. Initiated in 1991, this program is a collaborative effort between the food industry and the NCI, which encourages Americans to eat five or more servings of vegetables and fruits each day as part of a low-fat, high-fiber diet. The goal of this type of diet is to prevent the risk of cancer, heart disease, diabetes, and stroke. The Division of Cancer Treatment and Diagnosis includes programs in biomedical imaging, cancer diagnosis, cancer therapy evaluation, developmental therapeutics, and radiation research. The Division of Cancer Control and Population Sciences supports a wide array of research in the areas of surveillance, genetics, epidemiology, and behavior.

The mission of the Coordinating Center for Clinical Trials (CCCT), established in 2006, is to facilitate the bringing of new scientific discoveries and tools to the medical clinic. Research areas supported by the CCCT include cancer genetics, cancer vaccines and immunotherapy, molecular therapeutics, experimental transplantation, and advanced technology. The clinical cancer genetics program integrates all aspects of clinical and laboratory medicine, particularly in studies of breast, colon, renal, and prostate cancer. Processes include molecular diagnostics, novel imaging techniques, and the molecular assessment of normal tissues in at-risk populations. The cancer vaccines and immunotherapy program investigates the clinical feasibility of using vaccines against known conditions associated with cancer, such as the human papillomavirus (HPV vaccines Cervarix and Gardasil) and human immunodeficiency virus (HIV), as well as with cancer-specific products, such as in melanoma and in lymphomas. The molecular therapeutics program is concerned with most clinical trial experiments. Important discoveries include the development of paclitaxel (Taxol) as an effective anticancer agent, the development of zidovudine (AZT, Retrovir) as an important anti-HIV drug, and the use of adoptive immunotherapy in the treatment of malignant melanoma. The scientific thrust of the molecular therapeutics program is the belief that the analysis of the molecular profile of individual cancers will help determine the most effective chemotherapeutic approaches. The experimental transplantation program examines bone marrow biology in order to advance transplantation techniques and the effectiveness of this approach.

Integrating many programs and divisions is the advanced technology initiative. New technology is an essential key to identifying genetic elements involved in cancer initiation and progression, as well as in drug efficacy and drug resistance. Although many drugs have been discovered that inhibit the growth of cancer cells

successfully, they also affect healthy cells. This causes side effects that have a negative impact on patients' health and quality of life. New therapeutics and technology have been investigated to minimize or eliminate these side effects and enhance the effectiveness of therapy.

Another division of the NCI is the Division of Extramural Activities, which is responsible for handling all applications for funding and for monitoring research that has received funding from the NCI. Extramural activities also include the oversight of scientific communications. To enhance communication, the NCI has a number of advisory boards and groups that provide the institute with input from the public, medical, and research communities.

The NCI has helped strengthen the information base for cancer care decision making. Researchers, medical providers, and patients seek to better understand what constitutes quality cancer care. The Cancer Information Service, established in 1975, is the section of the NCI that is the link to the public, attempting to explain research findings in a clear, timely, and understandable manner. To this end, the Cancer Information Service helps develop education efforts that target minority audiences and people with limited access to health care information or services.

PERSPECTIVE AND PROSPECTS

To be successful in managing this range of responsibilities and breadth of mission, the NCI has a budget in the billions of dollars. Although cancer is the second leading cause of death in the United States and is a leading cause of death worldwide, through the years, the work of the NCI has led to a decline in the number of deaths due to this disease. Creative and dedicated scientists at the NCI are committed to lowering its numbers even further.

—*Karen Chapman-Novakofski, RD, LDN, PhD*

See also Cancer; Chemotherapy; Clinical trials; Department of Health and Human Services; Environmental diseases; Environmental health; Epidemiology; Genetics and inheritance; National Institutes of Health (NIH); Nutrition; Oncology; Preventive medicine; Radiation therapy.

For Further Information:
"About NCI." *National Cancer Institute*, 2013.
"Cancer." *World Health Organization*, Jan. 2013.
"Cancer: Addressing the Cancer Burden at a Glance." *Centers for Disease Control and Prevention*, 30 Aug. 2012.
Hewitt, Maria Elizabeth, et al., eds. *Ensuring Quality Cancer Care*. Washington, DC: National Academy Press, 1999.
Lerner, Barron H. *The Breast Cancer Wars: Fear, Hope, and the Pursuit of a Cure in Twentieth-Century America*. New York: Oxford University Press, 2003.
National Cancer Institute. *The Cancer Information Service: A Fifteen-Year History of Service and Research*. Bethesda, Md.: Author, 1993.

National Cancer Institute. *National Cancer Institute's Research Programs: Pursuing the Central Questions of Cancer Research*. Bethesda, Md.: Author, 1999.

National Cancer Institute. *NCI Fact Book*. Bethesda, Md.: Author, 1979.

"NCI Mission Statement." National Cancer Institute, 2013.

"NCI Organization." *National Cancer Institute*, 2013.

Reuben, Suzanne H. *Assessing Progress, Advancing Change: 2005-2006 Annual Report*. Bethesda, Md.: National Institutes of Health, National Cancer Institute, 2006.

Varmus, Harold. "Professional Judgment Budget 2013." *National Cancer Institute*, 2013.

NATIONAL INSTITUTES OF HEALTH (NIH)

Category: Organization

Definition: The National Institutes of Health (NIH), composed of more than twenty-five separate institutes, centers, and offices, is one of eight agencies constituting the U.S. Department of Health and Human Services.

Key terms:

AIDSLINE: a database that is part of the National Library of Medicine (NLM) and is devoted to the topic of research on acquired immunodeficiency syndrome (AIDS)

CATLINE: the online catalog of books and manuscripts in the NLM

grant proposals: research plans that outline scientific methods to pursue new knowledge, the required budget, and the resulting products and significance of that work

institute: a specific subagency of the NIH that has the charge of advancing scientific discovery and clinical practice in a specific area of medical science

MEDLINE: a database that is available via the Internet featuring current and historical medical literature, research articles, monographs, presentations, and abstracts

HISTORY AND MISSION

The National Institutes of Health (NIH) is a US federal agency that occupies a multibuilding campus in Bethesda, Maryland. It consists of a variety of offices, institutes focused on specific medical problems, research laboratories and centers, a center for scientific review, and a national medical library. Its main goal is to discover knowledge that will improve the state of public health for all persons, especially those in the United States. This goal extends to all medical conditions afflicting men, women, and children of all ethnic backgrounds. It also extends to seeking knowledge in areas of basic biological research, clinical research, and research on policy and practice in health care.

The National Institute of Health (precursor to the NIH) was formally established by the Ransdell Act of 1930, which bestowed the name on what was formerly called the Hygienic Laboratory (HL) of the Marine Hospital Service (MHS) in New York. The Ransdell Act also allowed for the establishment of fellowships for basic medical and biological research. The very beginnings of the NIH extend back to 1887, however, when basic laboratory work into medical problems was pursued by the MHS, the founding body of the United States Public Health Service (PHS). The MHS was formed in 1798 to provide hospital care for seamen, but by the 1880s it had shifted its focus to screening ship passengers for infectious diseases capable of starting epidemics.

New European research in the 1880s suggesting that microorganisms caused such diseases spurred American interest in medical research and helped form the original HL. Work by the HL continued, with the laboratory eventually moving from the MHS to its own Washington, DC, campus. The study of microorganisms continued, extending from study of individual persons to studying the effects of bacteria on water and air pollution. Progress for such work was rewarded in 1901 with governmental money for the construction of a building (completed in 1904) to house the HL and further foster work focused on advancing the public health. Because the value of such work was not well established, however, no permanent funding was provided, leaving the organization subject to ongoing evaluation and supplemental funding.

In 1902 the MHS was reorganized and renamed the Public Health and Marine Hospital Service (PH-MHS); in 1912 it adopted the shortened name of the Public Health Service (PHS). During the intervening time, the HL continued its work and expanded to work in chemistry, pharmacology, zoology, immunology, and the regulation and production of vaccines and antitoxins. Additionally, new scientific staff were added to the staff of medical doctors already on board. Changes in the mission of the organization in 1912 also opened the door for the pursuit of research on noncontagious diseases and water pollution. This work continued during World War I in the form of examining sanitation, anthrax outbreaks, smallpox, tetanus, influenza, and other combat-related conditions. The success of the PHS's work in these areas caught the attention of legislators and resulted in the Ransdell Act of 1930, which established both the National Institute of Health and the practice of setting aside public monies for funding medical research. In 1937, the National Cancer Institute (NCI) was created. In 1944, the PHS formally designated the NCI as a component of the NIH, setting the pattern of a problem-focused structure within the NIH that continues to the present.

World War II led the NIH to focus almost exclusively on war-related problems. This involved examinations of fitness for military service and issues such as dental problems and syphilis. The effects of hazardous substances and conditions on workers in war industries; risks armed service professionals faced from lack of oxygen, cold temperatures, and blood clots while flying; burns, shock, bacterial infections, and fever; and the development of vaccines and therapies for tropical diseases such as malaria also composed much of its work during this time.

Successes established during the wars by such medical research led the PHS to take the 1944 Public Health Service Act to Congress. This act led to grant-funding mechanisms being extended from the NCI alone to the entire National Institute of Health. Additionally, an increasing public interest in health organizations caused Congress to create additional institutes for research on mental health, dental diseases, and heart disease between 1946 and 1949. In 1948, the National Heart Act allowed for the formal pluralization of the National Institutes of Health, rather than a singular institute with the NCI as a subinstitute. The Public Health Service Act of 1944 also provided funding for the Warren Grant Magnuson Clinical Center, which opened in 1953 to focus exclusively on clinical research on health.

From this point forward, each of the individual institutes now composing the NIH came into being. By 1960 there were ten institutes, and by 2013 there were twenty-seven institutes and centers. As different health interests develop and advances in medical knowledge are needed, the NIH has responded by allocating its resources to pursue goals in those areas. This has been done both by developing institutes and also by creating specialized offices to pursue contemporary medical problems.

Illness and medicine know no boundaries, however, so the NIH has also maintained an interest in global public health issues. Such interest was formally shown in 1947, when grants were first awarded to investigators abroad. Similarly, in 1968, the John E. Fogarty International Center (FIC) was created to coordinate international research efforts, involving liaisons with the World Health Organization and a variety of international research organizations. The FIC also supports language translation, documentation, and reviews of new health findings. It facilitates biomedical communications through its maintenance of the National Library of Medicine (NLM), MEDLINE, CATLINE, AIDSLINE, and numerous other databases for researchers, physicians, and the public at large. Similarly, focused consensus development conferences, where investigators and clinicians from around the world can meet to evaluate new and existing therapies, are another way in which international interests are pursued.

In keeping with its practical focus, the NIH has strived to seek out knowledge that yields new drugs, devices, and procedures that are useful not just for the government but for the public at large as well. In 1986, the Technology Transfer Act allowed for a partnership between NIH-funded research and the private sector. Encouraging researchers to examine possible commercial and practical applications of basic medical research to wide-reaching clinical or research use benefits overall scientific and health progress. Partnering with business allows private industries to take over the process of marketing and developing products in a manner more affordable to them than to the government, allowing the government to focus on development while benefiting through the use of the eventual marketed products.

ORGANIZATIONAL STRUCTURE AND METHOD
The NIH is organized to accomplish its goals by using its offices, institutes, and research centers. Research is conducted on the NIH campus in its own funded laboratories as well as in the labs of scientists supported by NIH funding, who are stationed in institutes of higher education, teaching hospitals, and research institutions in the United States and other countries. In addition to supporting ongoing research, the NIH also supports research infrastructure by maintaining a library and a variety of printed and electronic resources to facilitate communication among its researchers, the larger scientific community, policymakers, and the public. Scientific research also is supported through development of one of the most valuable resources known to medicine: new researchers. The NIH sponsors a variety of training programs focusing on medical training and research in order to keep a large body of high-quality scholars and investigators in development. Such programs extend from career development for postdoctoral researchers and predoctoral training, to high school level learning in the sponsoring of internships and other learning experiences for teenagers interested in medical science careers.

Funding for research and training programs outside the NIH campus and research centers is facilitated through grant proposal programs that distribute federal tax monies devoted to such endeavors. Applicants to such programs are able to submit independent proposals for work related to the goals of the NIH that they believe is demanded by the state of science and knowledge. They are also able to submit proposals in response to program announcements and calls for proposals on specific topics as outlined by the institutes and offices of the NIH. Many different grant mechanisms exist for such proposals, including grants supporting the work of individual trainees, training programs for cohorts of researchers at different stages of career development, the ongoing work of career scientists, small grants for new or experimental work, focused projects, and even centers of research excellence where many researchers focus on the same topic of study. In addition, grant support is offered to sponsor conferences and academic meetings on special topics in health research and training.

To receive this funding, those wishing to be considered must submit proposals for confidential peer review through the Center for Scientific Review (CSR), which is part of the NIH structure. Proposals are reviewed by panels of experts who evaluate the research plans, goals, staff, environment, and overall innovation and merit of the work proposed. In addition, ethical considerations about the proposed research are reviewed and considered for both animal welfare and the welfare of human research participants. Emphasis on ethical issues has been a long-standing issue for medical research. It was, however, highlighted in the 1960s, when grantees receiving NIH grant monies were required to state the ethical principles guiding their research on humans, and in 1979, when written guidelines for research on human subjects were established. Once through peer review, proposals are reviewed again by a national advisory council to determine the priority of the work in addressing the goals of the NIH and its institutes and offices. After the proposals are approved by this council for advancement, the individual institutes (sometimes cooperating with specific NIH offices) work to fund them with the monies allotted. Unfortunately, not all proposals can be funded. It should be noted that even after funding, the work of the NIH continues so as to ensure that proper research ethics are followed through the life of the research.

Research funded by the NIH is facilitated by the various institutions and research offices that fall under its organizational umbrella, each focusing on a discrete area of health interest. Some of the institutions involved include the NCI; the National Eye Institute; the National Heart, Lung, and Blood Institute; and the National Human Genome Research Institute. Also included are the National Institutes on Aging, Alcohol Abuse and Alcoholism, Allergy and Infectious Diseases, Arthritis and Musculoskeletal and Skin Diseases, Child Health and Human Development, Deafness and Other Communication Disorders, Dental and Craniofacial Research, Diabetes and Digestive and Kidney Diseases, Drug Abuse, Environmental Health Sciences, Mental Health, Minority Health and Health Disparities, and Neurological Disorders and Stroke.

In addition to these institutes, the NIH has numerous offices focusing on specific issues or populations that need to be addressed in health research. These offices focus on contemporary issues of importance for research and include the Offices of Technology Transfer, AIDS Research, Research on Women's Health, Behavioral and Social Sciences Research, Dietary Supplements, Rare Diseases, Science Policy, Biotechnology Activities, Science Education, and Information Technology. There are also offices that focus on the management of research, specific organizational issues at the NIH, or the communication of information from the NIH to members of the public. These include the Offices of Intramural Research, Extramural Research, Evaluation, Human Resources, Financial Management, Acquisition and Logistics Management, Management Assessment, and Communications and Public Liaison as well as the NIH Legal Advisor and the Freedom of Information Act Office.

PERSPECTIVE AND PROSPECTS

The NIH has been responsible for supporting some very influential research for more than one hundred years, garnering more than eighty Nobel Prizes for NIH-supported work. More vaccines against infectious diseases are available than ever before. The successful mapping of the human genome has set the stage for enhanced genetic testing and the development of gene therapies. Substantial decreases in mortality rates have been achieved for heart disease and strokes. Survival rates for individuals afflicted by cancer have increased, as have survival rates for infants with respiratory distress syndrome. Recovery from spinal cord injuries has been enhanced so as to lessen the probability of long-term disability. Advances in the pharmacological and behavioral treatment of mental health problems such as depression, anxiety, bipolar disorders, and schizophrenia have been achieved. Preventive approaches in dentistry have been highly successful in stopping and slowing dental problems.

Given such successes, billions of dollars of federal tax monies continue to be devoted to the NIH budget to foster continued scientific advances. New work focused on improving prevention, screening, assessment, diagnosis, and treatment for conditions such as AIDS, alcoholism and drug dependence, Alzheimer's disease, arthritis, blindness, communication disorders, diabetes, heart disease, kidney disease, lung cancer, lupus, mental illnesses, Parkinson's disease, stroke, and other persisting conditions continues on a daily basis. While great successes have been achieved to date, new research is needed that will focus on specialized approaches that may enhance health for women, minorities, youth, and the elderly. The combination of these needs, past successes, and governmental commitment to improving the state of the public health ensures that the NIH will continue onward with its mission for the foreseeable future.

—*Nancy A. Piotrowski, PhD*

See also Childhood infectious diseases; Department of Health and Human Services; Disease; Environmental diseases; Environmental health; Epidemics and pandemics; Epidemiology; Health Canada; Immunization and vaccination; National Cancer Institute (NCI); Occupational health; World Health Organization.

For Further Information:
Desalle, Rob. *Epidemic! The World of Infectious Disease*. New York: New Press, 1999.
Eberhart-Philips, Jason. *Outbreak Alert: Responding to the Increasing Threat of Infectious Diseases*. Oakland, Calif.: New Harbinger, 2000.
Garrett, Laurie. *Betrayal of Trust: The Collapse of Global Public Health*. New York: Hyperion, 2001.
Guest, Charles, et al. Oxford Handbook of Public Health Practice. 3d ed. Oxford: Oxford University Press, 2013.
Institute of Medicine. *Scientific Opportunities and Public Needs: Improving Priority Setting and Public Input at the National Institutes of Health*. Washington, DC: National Academy Press, 1998.
Lee, Philip R., and Carroll L. Estes, eds. *The Nation's Health*. 7th ed. Sudbury, Mass.: Jones and Bartlett, 2003.
National Institutes of Health. "About NIH." US Department of Health and Human Services, June 6, 2013.
National Institutes of Health. "Institutes, Centers, and Offices." US Department of Health and Human Services, August 1, 2013.
Shnayerson, Michael, and Mark J. Plotkin. *The Killers Within: The Deadly Rise of Drug Resistant Bacteria*. Boston: Little, Brown, 2003.
Tulchinsky, Theodore H., and Elena A. Varavikova. *The New Public Health: An Introduction for the Twenty-first Century*. San Diego, Calif.: Academic Press, 2000.

NAUSEA AND VOMITING

Category: Disease/Disorder
Anatomy or system affected: Brain, gastrointestinal system, nervous system, stomach
Specialties and related fields: Gastroenterology, otorhinolaryngology
Definition: Nausea is an unpleasant subjective sensation, accompanied by epigastric and duodenal discomfort, which often culminates in vomiting, the regurgitation of the contents of the stomach.
Key terms:
affect: the emotional reactions associated with experience
antiemetics: drugs that prevent or relieve the symptoms of nausea and/or vomiting
chemoreceptor trigger zone: a sensory nerve ending in the brain that is stimulated by and reacts to certain chemical stimulation localized outside the central nervous system
emesis: the act of vomiting
psychogenic: of mental origin
psychotropics: drugs that affect psychic function, behavior, or experience

CAUSES AND SYMPTOMS

Nausea is defined as a subjectively unpleasant sensation associated with awareness of the urge to vomit. It is usually felt in the back of the throat and epigastrium and is accompanied by the loss of gastric tone, duodenal contractions, and reflux of the intestinal contents into the stomach. Retching is defined as labored, spasmodic, rhythmic contractions of the respiratory muscles (including the diaphragm, chest wall, and abdominal wall muscles) without the expulsion of gastric contents. Vomiting, or emesis, is the forceful expulsion of gastric contents from the mouth and is brought about by the powerful sustained contraction of the abdominal muscles, the descent of the diaphragm, and the opening of the gastric cardia (the cardiac orifice of the stomach).

Nausea and vomiting are important defense mechanisms against the ingestion of toxins. The act of emesis involves a sequence of events that can be divided into three phases: preejection, ejection, and postejection. The preejection phase includes the symptoms of nausea, along with salivation, swallowing, pallor, and tachycardia (an abnormally fast heartbeat). The ejection phase comprises retching and vomiting. Retching is characterized by rhythmic, synchronous, inspiratory movements of the diaphragm, abdominal, and external intercostal muscles, while the mouth and the glottis are kept closed. As the antral (cavity) portion of the stomach contracts, the proximal (nearest the center) portion relaxes and the gastric contents oscillate between the stomach and the esophagus. During retching, the hiatal portion of the diaphragm does not relax, and intra-abdominal pressure increases are associated with a decrease in intrathoracic pressure.

In contrast, relaxation of the hiatal portion of the diaphragm (near the esophagus) permits a transfer of intra-abdominal pressure to the thorax during the act of vomiting. Contraction of the muscles of the anterior abdominal wall, relaxation of the esophageal sphincter, an increase in intrathoracic and intragastric pressure, reverse peristalsis (movement of the contents of the alimentary canal), and an open glottis and mouth result in the expulsion of gastric contents. The postejection phase consists of autonomic and visceral responses that return the body to a quiescent phase, with or without residual nausea.

The complex act of vomiting, involving coordination of the respiratory, gastrointestinal, and abdominal musculature, is controlled by what researchers label the emetic center. This center in the brain stem has access to the motor pathways responsible for the visceral and somatic output involved in vomiting, and stimuli from several areas within the central nervous system can affect this center. These include afferent (inward-directed) nerves from the pharynx and gastrointestinal tract, as well as afferents from the higher cortical centers (including the visual center) and the chemoreceptor trigger zone (CTZ) in the area postrema (a highly vascularized area of the brain stem). The CTZ can be activated by chemical stimuli received through the blood or the cerebrospinal fluid. Direct electrical stimulation of the CTZ, however, does not result in emesis.

Clinical assessment of nausea and vomiting usually focuses on the occurrence of vomiting, that is, the frequency and number of episodes. Nausea, however, is a subjective phenomenon unobservable by another. Few data collection instruments that measure separately the patient's experience of nausea and vomiting and his or her symptom distress have been reported in the literature. In fact, the Rhodes Index of Nausea and Vomiting (INV) Form 2 is the only available tool that measures the individual components of nausea, vomiting, and retching. This index measures the patient's perception of the duration, frequency, and distress from nausea. The frequency, amount, and distress from vomiting; and the frequency, amount, and distress from retching (dry heaves). The INV score provides a measurement of the total symptom experience of the patient.

While the causes of nausea and vomiting are numerous-they include gastrointestinal diseases, infections, intracranial disease, toxins, radiation sickness, psychological trauma, migraines, and circulatory syncope-three of the most common causes are motion sickness (air, sea, land, or space), pregnancy, and anesthesia administered during operative procedures.

The sequence of symptoms and signs that constitute motion sickness is fairly characteristic. Premonitory symptoms often include yawning or sighing, lethargy, somnolence, and a loss of enthusiasm and concern for the task at hand. Increasing malaise is directed toward the epigastrium, a sensation best described as "stomach awareness," which progresses to nausea. Diversion of the blood flow from the skin toward the muscles results in pallor. A feeling of warmth and a desire for cool air is often accompanied by sweating. Frontal headache and a sensation of disorientation, dizziness, or light-headedness may also occur. As symptoms progress, vomiting occurs early in the sequence of symptoms for some; in others, malaise is severe and prolonged and vomiting is delayed. After vomiting, there is often a temporary improvement in well-being;

INFORMATION ON NAUSEA AND VOMITING

Causes: May include gastrointestinal diseases, infections, intracranial disease, toxins, radiation sickness, migraines, motion sickness, pregnancy, anesthesia, psychological trauma

Symptoms: Increased salivation and swallowing, pallor, rapid heartbeat, sweating

Duration: Typically acute; can be recurrent with acute episodes

Treatments: Depends on cause; may include drug therapy, diet regulation, lifestyle change, emotional support

however, with continued provocative motion, symptoms build again and vomiting recurs. The symptoms may last for minutes, hours, or even days.

The most coherent explanation for the development of motion sickness is provided by sensory conflict theory. Motion sickness is generally thought to occur as the result of a "sensory conflict" between information arising from the semicircular canals and organs of the vestibular system, visual and other sensory input, and the input that is expected on the basis of past experience or exposure history. It is argued that conflicts between current sensory inputs are by themselves insufficient to produce motion sickness since adaptation occurs even though the conflicting inputs continue to be present. Visual input alone, however, can produce symptoms of motion sickness, such as watching motion pictures shot from a moving vehicle or looking out of the side window (as opposed to the front window) of a moving vehicle.

Nausea and/or vomiting in the early morning during pregnancy, so-called morning sickness, is so common that it is accepted as a symptom of normal pregnancy. Occurring soon after waking, it is often retching rather than actual vomiting and usually does not disturb the woman's health or her pregnancy. The symptoms nearly always cease before the fourteenth week of pregnancy. In a much smaller proportion of cases, approximately one in one thousand births, the vomiting becomes more serious and persistent, occurring throughout the day and even during the night. The term "hyperemesis gravidarum" is given to this serious form of vomiting. Theories on the etiology of morning sickness have tended to be grouped under four main areas: endocrine (caused by estrogen and progesterone levels), psychosomatic (a conscious or unconscious wish not to be pregnant), allergic (a histamine reaction), and metabolic (a lack of potassium).

Nausea and vomiting occur frequently as unpleasant side effects of the administration of anesthesia in many clinical procedures. Most postoperative vomiting is mild, and only in a few cases will the problem persist so as to cause electrolyte disturbances and dehydration. The factors affecting postoperative nausea and vomiting may be divided into two categories: by the type of patient and surgery, and by the anesthetic and preoperative and postoperative medication uses. Patients with a history of motion sickness have a predisposition to postoperative vomiting. Nearly 43 percent of patients who vomited following previous surgery vomited again, whereas slightly more than 14 percent of those who did not vomit previously had an emetic episode at their next operation. Patients undergoing their first anesthetic procedure had an incidence of vomiting of approximately 30 percent.

No direct association between vomiting and age has been found. That vomiting may be hormonally related, however, is suggested by the higher incidence of nausea and vomiting in the latter half of the menstrual cycle. Other factors that may affect nausea and vomiting associated with anesthesia include patient weight (female obese patients being particularly more vulnerable), amount of hydration, metabolic status, and psychological state.

With regard to the type of surgery performed, the highest incidence of nausea and vomiting appears to be associated with abdominal surgery, as well as ear, nose, and throat surgery, with middle-ear surgery being the major category. The length of surgery, and therefore the duration of anesthesia, also has a direct effect on nausea and vomiting. Short (thirty-minute to sixty-minute) operations using cyclopropane had an emetic incidence of 17.5 percent, while operations lasting one and a half to three and a half hours had an incidence of 46.4 percent.

Most of the causes of vomiting associated with general anesthesia are expected to be eliminated with regional or spinal anesthesia. The type of anesthesia used also has an effect on nausea and vomiting. Research indicates that cyclopropane, ether, and nitrous oxide are potent emetics.

TREATMENT AND THERAPY

Since the generation of sensory conflict underlies all motion environments that give rise to motion sickness, practical measures that reduce conflict are likely to reduce motion sickness incidence. Motion sickness can be minimized if the subject has the widest possible view of a visual reference in which the earth is stable. Passengers aboard ships are less likely to be seasick if they remain on deck at midship, where vertical motion is minimized, and view the horizon. In a car or bus, individuals should be in a position to see the road directly ahead, since the movement of this visual scene will correlate with the changes in the direction of the vehicle. While head movements in a rotating

environment are known to precipitate motion sickness, there is no clear experimental evidence that they elicit nausea in mild linear oscillation. Thus, some nonpharmacologic remedies for motion sickness are restricting head movements, lying in a supine position, or closing the eyes. In addition, the use of acupressure wrist bands has proven effective in combating motion sickness.

Pharmacologically, the drug hyoscine hydrobromide (also called hyoscine or scopolamine) emerged as a valuable prophylactic drug following extensive research during World War II into the problems of motion sickness in troops transported in aircraft, ships, and landing craft. It remains one of the most effective drugs for short-duration exposures to provocative motion. Doses in excess of 0.6 milligram, however, are very likely to lead to drowsiness, and there is much experimental evidence that hyoscine impairs short-term memory. Hyoscine can be absorbed transdermally, and in order to extend the duration of action, a controlled-release patch was developed to deliver 1.2 milligrams on application and 0.01 milligram hourly thereafter. There is substantial evidence of its sustained effectiveness, but, perhaps as a result of variable absorption rates, there is an increased risk of blurred vision after more than twenty-four hours of use.

Amphetamines, ephedrine, and a number of antihistamines (such as dimenhydrinate) have been found to be clinically useful in motion sickness. Following oral administration, these drugs are generally slower than hyoscine in reaching their peak efficacy, but they have a longer duration of action.

For most susceptible subjects whose exposure to motion sickness-inducing stimuli is infrequent, prophylactic drugs offer the only useful treatment. When exposure to provocative stimuli is more frequent, as for example in professional aircraft pilots, spontaneous adaption occurs during training and an initially high incidence of motion sickness decreases with time.

In medical conditions in which the cause is relatively unknown, it is usual to find a wide variety of suggested therapies; nausea and vomiting during pregnancy and hyperemesis gravidarum (the serious, persistent form of vomiting in pregnancy) are no exception. Prior to 1968, treatments numbered approximately thirty. In subsequent years, however, suggested therapy has been mainly drugs of the antiemetic variety. Yet since the thalidomide tragedy (in which severe deformities occurred in the children of women who took this drug), there has been a reluctance to use drugs of any kind during early pregnancy. Probably the only value of drug therapy is at the stage of morning sickness, when antiemetics or mild sedatives may counter the feeling of nausea and prevent women from experiencing excessive vomiting and entering the vicious cycle of dehydration, starvation, and electrolyte imbalance. Once the patient has reached the stage of hyperemesis gravidarum, much more basic therapy is required, and the regimen calls for correction of dehydration, carbohydrate deficiency, and ionic deficiencies. This program is best managed by intravenous therapy, with or without the addition of vitamin supplements and sedative agents.

Nonpharmacologic self-care actions for morning sickness fall into the three broad categories of manipulating diet, adjusting behavior, and seeking emotional support. Some of the most effective self-care actions are getting rest, eating several small meals rather than three large ones, avoiding bad smells, avoiding greasy or fried foods, avoiding cooking, and receiving extra attention and support.

In terms of postoperative nausea and vomiting caused by anesthesia, it has been found that routine antiemetic prophylaxis of patients undergoing elective surgical procedures is not indicated, since fewer than 30 percent of patients experience postoperative nausea and vomiting. Of those who develop these symptoms, many have transient nausea or only one or two bouts of emesis and do not require antiemetic therapy. In addition, commonly used antiemetic drugs can produce significant side effects, such as sedation. Nevertheless, antiemetic prophylaxis may be justified in those patients who are at greater risk for developing postoperative nausea and/or vomiting. Such therapy is often given to patients with a history of motion sickness or to those undergoing gynecologic procedures, inner-ear procedures, oral surgery (in which the jaws are occluded by wires, causing a high risk of breathing in vomitus), and operations on the ear or eye and plastic surgery operations (in order to avoid disruption of delicate surgical work).

Many different antiemetic drugs are available for the treatment of postoperative nausea and vomiting. Researchers have found it difficult to interpret the results of antiemetic drug studies because the severity of postoperative vomiting and the response to therapeutic agents can be influenced by many variables in addition to the antiemetic drug being studied. Even with the use of the same drugs in a homogeneous population undergoing the same procedure, the severity of emesis varies from individual to individual.

Because antiemetic drugs have differing sites of action, better results can be obtained by using a multidrug approach. If a combination of drugs with a similar site of action is used, however, the incidence of side effects may be increased. There are few data regarding combination antiemetic prophylaxis or therapy for postoperative nausea and emesis. Drug combinations have been avoided in postsurgical patients because of concerns about additive central nervous sys-

tem toxicity. An exception is the combination of low-dose droperidol and metoclopramide, which appears to be more effective than droperidol alone for outpatient gynecologic procedures.

Although a full stomach is best avoided before any operative procedure, with situations such as emergencies, in which danger from vomiting is acute, a rapid sequence of administering anesthesia (induction) and clearing the air passage (intubation) remains the method of choice to avoid nausea and vomiting in patients with a full stomach. After the procedure, it is recommended that the patient minimize movement in order to avoid nausea and vomiting. Also, it has been found that avoiding eating solid food for at least eight hours after a surgical procedure is helpful in preventing postoperative nausea and vomiting.

PERSPECTIVE AND PROSPECTS

Though it has existed for as long as there have been human beings, the symptom of nausea has never received much attention in health care practice or research. In fact, until the early 1970s the sensation of nausea was frequently dismissed as merely a passing phenomenon. The rationale for this dismissal was most likely the understanding that nausea is self-limiting (it always passes with time), is never life-threatening in itself, is probably psychogenic in nature (at least to some degree), and, being subjective, is very difficult to measure. In addition, in the past the most predictable nausea was related to pregnancy, which may also explain the lack of attention given to nausea.

Until the late 1980s, there was still little research being conducted on the nausea associated with pregnancy, although it is a common symptom. The historical lack of interest in nausea and vomiting during pregnancy may be traced to the fact that, since the symptoms generally persist only through the first trimester, health care professionals have viewed the problem as relatively insignificant. As more pregnant women work outside the home in demanding positions, however, these women have exhibited less tolerance for illness. Demands upon the health care industry and upon personal physicians for more research and effective treatment have become more widespread.

While it is surprising that nausea has received scant attention in the history of clinical research, it is even more astonishing that vomiting, an observable behavior, has received so little attention as well. Although vomiting is a primitive neurologic process that has remained almost unchanged in the evolution of animals, the mechanisms that regulate the behavior remain virtually unknown.

One reason for the paucity of information on the subject of nausea in particular stems from the lack of a reliable animal model. This fact has hampered research aimed at establishing the etiological basis for nausea and its relationship to vomiting. While some species of lower animals, for example rats, cannot vomit, it is not known whether rats experience the phenomenon of nausea. Thus no effective means of measuring nausea in lower animals has been devised.

Since the early 1970s, there has been a noticeable increase in research on nausea as a drug side effect because it was so frequently seen in cancer chemotherapy clinical trials sponsored by the National Cancer Institute and the American Cancer Society. As more powerful chemotherapy agents and aggressive combinations were clinically investigated, patients began to experience severe, potentially life-threatening nausea and vomiting. Older drugs such as antihistamines, phenothiazines, and benzodiazepines are still used for their antiemetic characteristics, but they are augmented by newer agents such as benzamides, neurokinin-1-receptor antagonists, and serotonin antagonists.

Aside from the pharmacological investigations of new drugs and drug combinations in the treatment of nausea and vomiting, an interesting branch of scientific investigation has begun the process of exploring alternative ways of managing these symptoms. Behavioral interventions, such as progressive muscle relaxation, biofeedback, imagery, or music therapy, have been used to alleviate postchemotherapy anxiety. These methods may also be used to treat other patients suffering from the symptoms of nausea and vomiting, such as pregnant women.

Another noninvasive, nonpharmacologic measure that has been considered in the relief of nausea and vomiting is transcutaneous electrical nerve stimulation (TENS). Several research studies indicate that TENS may be useful in alleviating chemotherapy-related nausea and vomiting, including delayed nausea and vomiting. Side effects from using TENS units are negligible, and with further study they may prove to be an acceptable, helpful relief measure.

—*Genevieve Slomski, PhD*

See also Acid reflux disease; Anesthesia; Appetite loss; Botulism; Bulimia; Chemotherapy; Colitis; Crohn's disease; Diaphragm; Digestion; Eating disorders; Esophagus; Food biochemistry; Food poisoning; Gastroenteritis; Gastroenterology; Gastroenterology, pediatric; Gastrointestinal disorders; Gastrointestinal system; Heartburn; Indigestion; Influenza; Lactose intolerance; Motion sickness; Multiple chemical sensitivity syndrome; Noroviruses; Poisoning; Poisonous plants; Pregnancy and gestation; Radiation sickness; Rotavirus; Salmonella infection; Stomach, intestinal, and pancreatic cancers; Ulcer surgery; Ulcers; Vagotomy.

For Further Information:

Blum, Richard H., and W. LeRoy Heinrichs. *Nausea and Vomiting: Overview, Challenges, Practical Treatments, and New Perspectives*. Philadelphia: Whurr, 2000.
Casey, Georgina. "Treating Nausea and Vomiting." *Kai Tiaki Nursing New Zealand* 18, no. 11 (December, 2012): 20-24.
Edmundowicz, Steven A., ed. *Twenty Common Problems in Gastroenterology*. New York: McGraw-Hill, 2002.
Funk, Sandra G., et al., eds. *Key Aspects of Comfort: Management of Pain, Fatigue, and Nausea*. New York: Springer, 1989.
Hesketh, Paul J., ed. *Management of Nausea and Vomiting in Cancer and Cancer Treatment*. Sudbury, Mass.: Jones and Bartlett, 2005.
Kucharczyk, John, David J. Stewart, and Alan D. Miller, eds. *Nausea and Vomiting: Recent Research and Clinical Advances*. Boca Raton, Fla.: CRC Press, 1991.
Litin, Scott C., ed. *Mayo Clinic Family Health Book*. 4th ed. New York: HarperResource, 2009.
Palatty, Princy Lous, et al. "Ginger in the Prevention of Nausea and Vomiting." *Critical Reviews in Food Science and Nutrition* 53, no. 7 (2013): 659.
Rao, Kamakshi V., and Aimee Faso. "Chemotherapy-Induced Nausea and Vomiting: Optimizing Prevention and Management." *American Health and Drug Benefits* 5, no. 4 (July, 2012): 232-240.
Sleisenger, Marvin H., ed. *The Handbook of Nausea and Vomiting*. New York: Caduceus Medical/Parthenon, 1993.

NECK INJURIES AND DISORDERS. SEE HEAD AND NECK DISORDERS.

NECROSIS

Category: Disease/Disorder
Also known as: Gangrene, mortification
Anatomy or system affected: Bones, cells
Specialties and related fields: Oncology, orthopedics
Definition: Tissue damage occurring as a result of cell death.

CAUSES AND SYMPTOMS

Necrosis refers to the degeneration of cells or tissues after cell death occurs for any reason, generally in localized regions of the body. Thus, necrosis is tissue degeneration, which occurs secondary to cell death from any cause. Necrosis is most commonly the result of ischemia, traumatic injury, bacterial infection, or toxins (including excessive steroids or alcohol).

In its earliest stage, there are often no symptoms of necrosis. Tissue damage begins to occur within twelve hours of cell death. When symptoms do begin to occur, they range from atrophy to decreased range of motion and pain to the development of gangrenous tissue.

TREATMENT AND THERAPY

The damage done to the tissue resulting from cell death is permanent. Any treatment of necrosis is aimed at minimizing further cell death and tissue injury. In the case of heart disease, treatment of the

INFORMATION ON NECROSIS

Causes: Cell death leading to degeneration of tissue over time
Symptoms: Pain, tissue decay
Duration: Permanent, irreversible
Treatments: Pain relievers (NSAIDs), surgery

underlying condition to alleviate hypoxia prevents further cell death from ischemia. In the case of bacterial infection, antibiotics are used to treat the infection and prevent cell death and tissue damage. In the case of necrosis of bone tissue from decreased blood supply, the aim of treatment is to minimize further bone loss. This type of necrosis, known as "avascular necrosis" or "osteonecrosis," is treated with nonsteroidal anti-inflammatory drugs (NSAIDs) to relieve pain, exercise to improve range of motion, electrical treatment to stimulate bone growth, or surgery to reshape or graft bone or to replace joints.

PERSPECTIVE AND PROSPECTS

The term "necrosis" was used nearly two thousand years ago in ancient Greek textbooks to refer to changes within tissue, long after cell death had occurred, that were visible to the naked eye. With the advent of light microscopy, the tissue damage following cell death became visible within twelve to twenty-four hours.

In 1859, Rudolf Virchow, in his renowned text *Cellular Pathology as Based upon Physiological and Pathological Histology*, discussed degeneration, necrosis, mortification, and gangrene, using these terms more or less synonymously. It should be noted that he used the term "necrosis" to refer to an advanced stage of tissue breakdown. At this point, the breakdown had to be visible to the naked eye, since light microscopy had not yet been developed. Today, using the microscope, tissue damage resulting from cell death is obvious and often identical whether caused by ischemia, traumatic injury, bacteria, or toxins.

—*Robin Kamienny Montvilo, RN, PhD*

See also Cells; Circulation; Gangrene; Ischemia; Necrotizing fasciitis; Osteonecrosis; Pathology; Vascular medicine; Vascular system.

For Further Information:
A.D.A.M. Medical Encyclopedia. "Necrosis." *MedlinePlus*, March 23, 2013.
"Cell Death." In *Pathology: Clinicopathologic Foundations of Medicine*, edited by Raphael Rubin, David Sheldon Strayer, and Emanuel Rubin. 6th ed. Baltimore: Lippincott, 2012.
Majno, G., and I. Joris. "Apoptosis, Oncosis, and Necrosis: An Overview of Cell Death." *American Journal of Pathology* 146, no. 1 (1995): 3-15.
"Necrosis." In *Taber's Cyclopedic Medical Dictionary*, edited by Donald Venes. 21st ed. Philadelphia: F. A. Davis, 2010.
Parker, J. N., and P. M. Parker. *The Official Patient's Sourcebook on Avascular Necrosis*. San Diego, Calif.: Icon Health, 2002.

NECROTIZING FASCIITIS

Category: Disease/Disorder
Anatomy or system affected: Blood vessels, muscles, skin
Specialties and related fields: Bacteriology, critical care, dermatology, emergency medicine, epidemiology, histology, plastic surgery, vascular medicine
Definition: An invasive bacterial infection that occurs in the connective tissue between the skin and muscle known as the "fascia," cutting off blood flow and causing death of tissues (necrotizing); it must be urgently treated surgically and, even in the best circumstances, has a high mortality rate.

CAUSES AND SYMPTOMS

Although it had been identified in the past, in 1994 there were numerous headline newspaper reports describing a new "flesh-eating bacteria." These articles detailed the devastating effect of seemingly minor wounds, such as cuts and scrapes, infected with streptococcal bacteria. Patients quickly become very sick, with a rapidly progressive downward course, as multiplication and movement of these streptococcal bacteria and their toxins into the bloodstream produces a shock-like state.

In nonpenetrating injuries, such as a deep muscle bruise or strain, it is likely that the bacteria were already present in the blood and then entered the site of damage. Most of these patients, however, did not recall any prior recent infection that may have made them susceptible. Penetrating injuries, where the normally protective barrier of the skin has been broken, were often minor and not originally treated as contaminated or infected. Other cases of necrotizing fasciitis are caused by surgical infections and bowel contamination. These cases are rarer and often found to have a mixture of bacteria, such as staphylococci or *Escherichia coli* (*E. coli*).

Patients with necrotizing fasciitis can have fever, low blood pressure, inflammation, severe pain, redness, and blistering at the site of infection. How does one tell the difference between a skin infection and deeper tissue involvement of necrotizing fasciitis? One of the hallmark features is intense pain and tenderness over the involved skin and muscle. Because of the presence of gas producing bacteria, there can sometimes be crepitus (crackling sound from the tissue).

Lack of skin sensation may also occur as bacteria multiply, due to the formation of blood clots, which deprives the skin of nutrients and oxygen, subsequently leading to skin necrosis (death). Once this occurs, the nerves are destroyed and the patient no longer feels pain or sensation. The skin at this point appears to be "eaten away." A major concern for necrotizing fasciitis is that underlying muscle and the adjacent fascia will become infected, subsequently leading to muscle death. The extremities and the area around the genitals and anus (perineum) are most commonly and extensively involved. The most frequent comorbidities of necrotizing fasciitis include diabetes and cardiovascular disease.

Diagnosis is made through surgical exploration, with physical analysis of each layer of tissues: skin, fascia, and muscle. This helps establish the presence of infection and extent of tissue involvement, allowing the ability to intervene to stop infection.

TREATMENT AND THERAPY
The only lifesaving treatment available is extensive surgery to remove all necrotic (dead) tissue and slow the spread of the bacteria. The patient with necrotizing fasciitis must be stabilized quickly in an intensive care unit, where fluids can be administered and heart and lung condition can be closely monitored. Antibiotics including penicillin, clindamycin, and gentamicin are given to help eradicate the pathogen. Due to increasing drug resistance, however, stronger broader based antibiotics such as carbapenems can be used. Because the infection spreads so rapidly, death often results even with heroic surgical and drug therapy unless the condition is diagnosed and treated early. Fortunately, these infections remain relatively rare.

—*Oghuz Anwar, OMS-III*

See also: Antibiotics; Bacterial infections; Bacteriology; Connective tissue; Dermatology; Epidemiology; Fascia; Necrosis; Shock; Skin; Skin disorders; Streptococcal infections; Toxic shock syndrome; Wounds.

For Further Information:
Berman, Kevin. "Necrotizing Soft Tissue Infection." *MedlinePlus*, 22 Nov. 2011.

Biddle, Wayne. *A Field Guide to Germs*. 3rd ed., New York: Anchor Books, 2010.
Forbes, Betty A., Daniel F. Sahm, and Alice S. Weissfeld. *Bailey and Scott's Diagnostic Microbiology*. 12th ed., Mosby/Elsevier, 2007.
Lille, S. T., T. T. Sato, L. H. Engrav, et al. "Necrotizing Soft Tissue Infections: Obstacles in Diagnosis." *Journal of the American College of Surgeons*, vol. 182, no. 1, 1995, pp. 7-11.
MedlinePlus. "Streptococcal Infections." *MedlinePlus*, 7 May 2013.
Olafsson, E. J., T. Zeni, and D. S. Wilkes. "A 46-Year-Old Man with Excruciating Shoulder Pain." *Chest*, vol. 127, no. 3, 2005, pp. 1039-44.
Roemmele, Jacqueline A., and Donna Batdorff. *Surviving the Flesh-Eating Bacteria: Understanding, Preventing, Treating, and Living with the Effects of Necrotizing Fasciitis*. Avery, 2000.
Snyder, Larry, et al. *Molecular Genetics of Bacteria*. 4th ed., ASM Press, 2013.
Stevens, D. L., A. L. Bisno, H. F. Chambers, et al. "Practice Guidelines for the Diagnosis and Management of Skin and Soft Tissue Infections: 2014 Update the Infectious Diseases Society of America." *Clinical Infectious Diseases*, vol. 59, no. 2, 2014, pp. 147-59.
van Stigt S. F., J. de Vries J. B. Bijker, et al. "Review of 58 Patients with Necrotizing Fasciitis in the Netherlands." *World Journal of Emergency Surgery*, vol. 11, 2016, p. 21.
Wilson, Brenda A., Abigail A. Salyers, et al. *Bacterial Pathogenesis: A Molecular Approach*. 3rd ed., ASM Press, 2011.
Wilson, Michael, Brian Henderson, and Rod McNab. *Bacterial Disease Mechanisms: An Introduction to Cellular Microbiology*. Cambridge UP, 2002.

NEONATAL BRACHIAL PLEXUS PALSY

Category: Disease/Disorder
Also known as: Erb's palsy, obstetric brachial plexus palsy, birth brachial plexus palsy
Anatomy or system affected: Arms, nerves
Specialties and related fields: Neonatology, neurology, obstetrics, organizations and programs, orthopedics, pediatrics, perinatology, physical therapy, plastic surgery, psychology, radiology
Definition: A motor disability evident early in life that manifests as weakness of the affected arm due to stretching or compression of the nerves of the brachial plexus during the perinatal period, with passive range of motion greater than active.
Key terms:
brachial plexus: complex of nerves that carry motor and sensory function to the arm
contractures: permanent shorting of muscles or joints
Erb's palsy: stereotyped clinical presentation of neonatal brachial plexus palsy resulting from injury to the C5, C6, and sometimes C7 spinal nerve roots

Horner's syndrome: ptosis (eyelid drooping), miosis (abnormal constriction of the pupil of the eye), and anhydrosis (decreased sweating on the face)

incidence: the rate at which a certain event occurs or the number of new cases of a specific disorder occurring during a certain period in a population at risk

pan-plexopathy: a form of neonatal brachial plexus palsy comprising of injury to all of the spinal nerve roots manifesting as a flaccid arm

perinatal period: the period immediately before and after birth, commencing at 20 weeks of gestation and ending at 28 weeks after birth (140 days total)

range of motion: movement of a joint from full flexion to full extension

shoulder dystocia: diagnosed when the delivery of the fetal head is not followed by the emergence of the shoulder due to impaction of the fetus' shoulder in the birth canal

CAUSES AND SYMPTOMS

Children with neonatal brachial plexus palsy (NBPP) have a weak or paralyzed arm, and their passive range of motion is greater than their active range of motion. NBPP becomes evident early in life and usually results from stretching or compression of the nerves of the brachial plexus during the perinatal period. NBPP occurs with an incidence of 1.5 cases per 1000 live births, with or without shoulder dystocia at the time of both vaginal and cesarean delivery. Risk factors for NBPP include abnormal positioning of the fetus, labor abnormalities, artificial labor induction, large fetus, and shoulder dystocia. However, except for shoulder dystocia, none of these risk factors are statistically significant clinical predictors for the occurrence of NBPP.

Compression or stretching of the nerves of the brachial plexus can occur during development in the uterus or during the descent and emergence of the fetus from the uterus and pelvis with maternal pushing and naturally expulsive forces. Biomechanically, nerve injury can result from forces applied by clinicians, or natural physical events that move the fetus from the uterus through the birth canal and out of the mother's pelvis. No one force or factor seems to be responsible for the cause of NBPP, but the available data do suggest that the occurrence of NBPP may be a multifactorial event.

The brachial plexus is a very complex structure that connects the spinal nerves in the neck to their terminal branches in the arm and is divided into 5 zones: (1) C5 through T1 spinal nerve roots; (2) upper, middle, and lower trunks; (3) anterior and posterior divisions of each trunk; (4) lateral, posterior, and medial cords; and (5) terminal branches. These nerves carry the signals necessary for the normal movement and sensation in the entire arm. The brachial plexus is

analogous to a set of intersecting highways with overpasses, underpasses, and multiple merging traffic intersections, with several roads leading into (analogous to the spinal nerve roots) and out of (analogous to the terminal branches) the intersections. However, for simplicity, the nerve roots can be indexed to the muscles in the following fashion: C5-shoulder movement, C6-elbow flexion, C7-elbow extension, C8/T1-hand and finger movement.

Not all cases of NBPP are the same, and the symptoms may be radically different depending on which parts of the brachial plexus are injured. The intricate intersecting nature of the brachial plexus implies that thousands of potentially different palsies can ensue, but in reality, only a few variations actually occur. The most useful classification scheme for clinical presentation of NBPP is the Narakas Grade system that represents the extent of the spinal nerve root injury: only C5 and C6 nerve roots are injured in Grade 1, C5, C6, C7 nerve roots in Grade 2, and C5 through T1 injured in Grade 3 (without Horner's syndrome) and Grade 4 (with Horner's syndrome). When this classification system is used in 2-4 week old affected babies, it may guide the prognosis for spontaneous recovery, since up to 90 percent of the patients with Grade 1 NBPP regain functional use of the affected arm, but less than 5 percent of the patients with Grade 4 NBPP regain functional use without medical and/or surgical intervention.

Other classification systems are based on the clinical manifestations of NBPP. Erb's palsy, the most common type of NBPP, is synonymous with an "upper" plexus palsy that specifically results from damage to C5, C6, and sometimes C7 spinal nerve roots. Patients with Erb's palsy present a "waiter's tip" posture when their affected arm is pulled toward the midline of the body, an internally rotated shoulder, flexed wrist, extended fingers that result from loss of both shoulder control and elbow bending. Contrastingly, the extremely rare Klumpke's palsy is synonymous with a "lower" plexus palsy characterized by a flaccid hand attached to an otherwise active arm. Total plexus palsy or pan-plexopathy is equivalent to Narakas Grade 3 and 4 and is recognized by loss of total function of the arm.

TREATMENT AND THERAPY

Lack of normal arm movement observed during the perinatal period warrants confirmation of the diagnosis of NBPP by a specialist. Possible skeletal injuries or fractures should be confirmed by clinical and radiographic evaluation since these injuries may preclude early occupational/physical therapy. Immobilization of the arm is not recommended except in the case of skeletal injuries.

With regard to the specific motor function of the affected arm, the treating physician assesses the passive and active range of motion of the affected arm. Available assessment scales of motor function in NBPP are used to determine the extent and severity of nerve injury, to prognosticate potential functional recovery, and to guide and assess the outcomes from further treatment. Traditional scales focus only upon the affected arm, but more recently, assessment methods are focusing upon the overall function of the child. Supplementing the physical examination with electrodiagnostic / electromyographic (EMG) and radiographic (magnetic resonance imaging, MRI) findings are helpful to decide whether surgical nerve reconstruction will be beneficial.

Early referral of those babies with severe or extensive NBPP to interdisciplinary specialty clinics can improve overall functional outcomes as the baby grows. Regardless of the need for surgical intervention, rehabilitation management is critical. Occupational/physical therapy to maintain the normal passive range of motion in all upper extremity joints (especially shoulder external rotation and forearm rotation) facilitates successful functional recovery. Parents and caregivers should consider themselves to be the patient's primary therapist by performing range of motion exercises regularly, with multimedia assistance if available (e.g., during every diaper change). Reinforced use of the affected arm while constraining the normal arm (similar to patching a lazy eye) can aid the child's recognition of the arm and strengthen the arm through increased

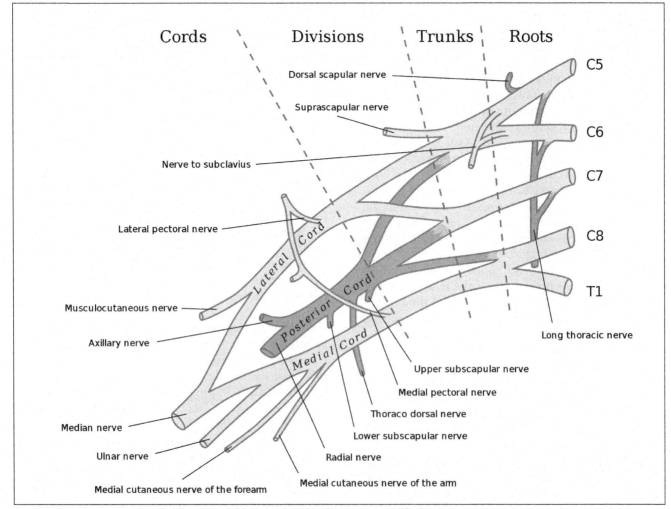

Brachial plexus. Erb's palsy primarily affects C5 and C6. Image via Wikimedia Commons. [Public domain.]

arm use during age-appropriate activities. Normal childhood developmental milestones must be encouraged, including crawling. Splinting may be used during sleep to avoid contractures or to protect floppy joints. As the child grows, recreational activities like swimming, dance, sports, and potentially therapist-designed video game platforms can help to sustain the goals of formal occupational/physical therapy.

For NBPP patients who do not recover with conservative management, surgical nerve reconstruction may be an option, usually occurring between 3-9 months of age. Although the indications and timing for nerve reconstruction have not been absolutely established, most practitioners agree that babies with the extensive total brachial plexus palsy and those with the severe Erb's palsy will benefit from nerve surgery. The goal of nerve reconstruction is not to regain a normal arm, but surgical intervention is a step towards a functional arm with adequate movement, if not power. Nerve repair using autologous nerve graft and/or nerve transfer (using a good nerve to re-innervate an injured one) constitute the primary options for reconstructing the function of the brachial plexus. As nerve repair and transfer rely upon regrowth of the normal portions of the nerve through the residual pathways after injured nerve is cleared away (Wallerian degeneration), and as this nerve regeneration is very slow, the ultimate functional outcome from nerve reconstruction surgery may not be apparent for 1-3 years.

Toddlers and older children with incomplete recovery following neurosurgical or conservative treatment may have functional limitations because of residual muscle weakness and soft tissue contractures, especially around the shoulder and elbow. MRI imaging can guide the decision to pursue orthopedic intervention. Internal rotation contracture of the shoulder is most common and can be associated with progressive shoulder joint deformity and instability. Indications for surgical intervention include persistent internal rotation contracture despite aggressive nonsurgical therapy, progressive joint deformity, and obvious joint dislocation. Surgical options include muscle lengthening combined with tendon transfers, corrective bone surgery (osteotomies), and open or arthroscopic reduction of the shoulder joint.

For children with residual elbow, forearm, and hand problems, secondary procedures by a hand surgeon may be appropriate. These procedures include soft tissue releases, joint fusions, muscle transfers, and corrective osteotomies. The usual age for secondary reconstruction of the elbow/forearm function is 4-6 years of age, and for wrist/hand function is 6-13 years of age.

For all surgical interventions, the most important factor in producing the optimal result is a cooperative child with intense investment from assertive parents/caretakers. The parents must understand the objectives of the surgical procedure and work hard with their children in postoperative rehabilitation-and maintenance of function by being their children's primary therapists. Surgery alone without subsequent rehabilitation management and therapy is unlikely to yield the desired outcome.

PERSPECTIVE AND PROSPECTS

Overall, the majority of infants with NBPP have a good prognosis for recovering adequate functional use of the affected arm-with rehabilitation management and therapy, supplemented with surgical intervention when and where appropriate and desired by the patient and parents/caretakers. Early occupational/physical therapy can support the spontaneous recovery of function and minimize consequent musculoskeletal comorbidities along with more efficient recovery of function after surgery. Despite the similar incidence of NBPP to cerebral palsy, public awareness of this perinatal disorder and its lifelong implications (medical and psychosocial) for the more extensively/severely affected children are significantly lacking. Similarly, published research studies regarding NBPP number only a fraction of that regarding cerebral palsy. Therefore, current efforts exist not only to find new medical treatment techniques but also to increase awareness, to address and improve the quality of life for patients with NBPP via traditional and recent technology-assisted modalities. Early referral to an interdisciplinary specialty brachial plexus clinic can avail the patient of the most current treatment paradigms to achieve the optimal outcome.

—*Lynda J.-S. Yang, MD, PD, FAANS*

See also Neonatology; Neurology; Neurology, pediatric; Obstetrics; Occupational health; Orthopedics; Physical rehabilitation

For Further Information:

Bowerson, M., V.S. Nelson, and L.J. Yang. "Diaphragmatic Paralysis Associated with Neonatal Brachial Plexus Palsy." *Pediatric Neurology* 42, no. 3 (March 2010) 234-236. Case study of a NBPP baby whose diaphragm was also paralyzed.

Chung, Kevin C., Lynda J.-S.Yang, and John E. McGillicuddy, eds. *Practical Management of Pediatric and Adult Brachial Plexus Palsies.* London: Elsevier, 2011. Extensive overview of the medical and surgical techniques for managing disorders of the brachial plexus. Presents a multidisciplinary approach to pediatric brachial plexus palsy treatment and rehabilitation, obstetric considerations, and other timely topics in the field (includes DVD).

Mehta, S.H., and B. Gonik. "Neonatal Brachial Plexus Injury: Obstetrical Factors and Neonatal Management." *Journal of Pediatric Rehabilitation Medicine* 4, no. 2 (2011) 113-118. A review of the potential causes of and risk factors for NBPP.

Murphy, K.M., L. Rasmussen, S.L. Hervey-Jumper, D. Justice, V.S. Nelson, and L.J. Yang. "An Assessment of the Compliance and Utility of a Home Exercise DVD for Caregivers of Children and Adolescents with Brachial Plexus Palsy: A Pilot Study." *PM & R* 4, no. 3 (March 2012) 190-197. Small, initial study of the efficacy of home exercises for NBPP children.

Piatt, J.H., Jr. "Birth Injuries of the Brachial Plexus." *Clinical Perinatology* 32, no. 1 (March 2005) 39-59. Excellent summary of the classification of various types of NBPP.

Squitieri, L.. B.P. Larson, K.W. Chang, L.J. Yang, and K.C. Chung. "Medical Decision-Making among Adolescents with Neonatal Brachial Plexus Palsy and Their Families: A Qualitative Study." *Plastic and Reconstructive Surgery* 131, no. 6 (June, 2013): 880e-887e. A study that examines why patients make particular treatment choices and stresses the need for proper patient education.

NEONATOLOGY

Category: Specialty
Anatomy or system affected: All
Specialties and related fields: Cardiology, critical care, embryology, genetics, obstetrics, pediatrics, perinatology
Definition: A subspecialty of pediatrics that involves the care of newborn infants from birth through the first month of life, especially those infants with life-threatening conditions such as prematurity, genetic defects, and serious illnesses.

Key terms:

congenital disorders: abnormalities present at birth that occurred during fetal development as a result of genetic errors, exposure to toxins and microorganisms, or maternal illness

incubator: in the nursery, a plexiglass unit that encloses the premature or sick infant to allow strict temperature regulation

intrauterine growth retardation: the condition of infants who are born significantly smaller than the standard for the number of weeks that they have spent in the uterus

neonatal intensive care unit: a hospital nursery with advanced equipment and specially trained staff to maintain the vital functions of sick newborns and to monitor their progress closely

neonatal period: the first month of life; derived from the Greek *neo* (meaning "new") and the Latin *natum* (meaning "birth")

prematurity: strictly defined, birth before a full-term pregnancy (thirty-eight weeks); more commonly associated with birth before thirty-five weeks

respirator: a machine that inflates and deflates the lungs, imitating normal breathing; connected to the patient through a tube placed into the windpipe (endotracheal tube)

respiratory distress syndrome: a life-threatening illness primarily of premature infants; immature lungs lack surfactant, a vital substance that keeps the tiny air sacs (alveoli) from collapsing upon exhalation

SCIENCE AND PROFESSION

Neonatology has grown dramatically since its beginnings in the late 1960s, and neonatologists have become an integral part of the obstetric-pediatric team at major medical centers throughout the world. In addition to being cared for by physicians who specialize in neonatology, some neonatal infants, in particular those who are critically ill or premature, are cared for by nurse practitioners with the specialty certification of neonatal nurse practitioner (NNP). In large part because of an ever-expanding technological base and marked advances in scientific research, these health care professionals have changed the outlook for premature and sick newborns.

As a subspecialty of pediatrics, neonatology is concerned with the most critical time of transition and adjustment-the first four weeks of life, or the neonatal period-whether the infant is healthy (a normal birth) or sick (as a result of genetic problems, obstetric complications, or medical illness). By the early 1970s, it became increasingly clear to health administrators that hospitals throughout the United States had varying abilities to care for medical and pediatric cases requiring the most sophisticated staff and equipment. Consequently, they developed a system that designated hospitals as either level I (small, community hospitals), level II (larger hospitals), or level III (major regional medical centers, also called tertiary care centers). It was in the last group that the most advanced neonatal care could be delivered. In these major centers, there are two types of nurseries, separating the normal healthy infant from the sick or high-risk infant: the routine nursery and the neonatal intensive care unit (NICU).

Routine nurseries are the temporary home of the vast majority of newborns. The services of the neonatologist are rarely needed here, and the general pediatrician or family practitioner observes and examines the infant for twenty-four to forty-eight hours to be sure that it has made a smooth transition from intrauterine to extrauterine life. These babies soon leave the hospital for their homes. Those neonates with minor problems arising from multiple births, difficult deliveries, mild prematurity, and minor illness are easily managed by a primary care physician in consultation with a neonatologist, perhaps at another hospital. It is in the neonatal intensive care unit, however, that the most difficult situations present themselves. Here several teams of pediatric subspecialists-surgeons, cardiologists, anesthesiologists, and highly trained nurses, along with many other health professionals-are led by a neonatologist, who coordinates the team's efforts. These newborns have life-threatening conditions, often as a result of extreme prematurity (more than six weeks earlier than the expected date of delivery), major birth defects (genetic or developmental), severe illness (such as overwhelming infections), or being born to drug- or alcohol-addicted mothers. They require the most advanced technological and medical interventions, often to sustain life artificially until the underlying problem is corrected. It is in this setting that the most dramatic successes of neonatology are found.

After hours of being inside a forcefully contracting uterus and sustaining the stress of passing through a narrow birth canal, the newborn emerges into a dry, cold, and hostile environment. The umbilical cord, which has provided oxygen and nutrients, is clamped and cut; the fluid-filled lungs must now exchange air instead, and the respiratory center of the infant's brain begins a lifetime of spontaneous breathing, usually heralded by crying. The vast majority of neonates make this extraordinary adjustment to extrauterine life without difficulty. At one minute and again at five minutes, the newborn is evaluated and scored on five physical signs: heart rate, breathing, muscle tone, reflexes, and skin tone. The healthy infant is vigorously moving, crying, and pink regardless of race. These Apgar scores, named for neonatology pioneer Virginia Apgar, evaluate the need for immediate resuscitation. A brief physical examination follows, which can identify other life-threatening abnormalities.

It is essential to remember that the medical history of a neonate is in fact the medical and obstetric history of its mother, and seemingly normal infants may develop problems shortly after birth. Risk factors include very young or middle-aged mothers; difficult deliveries; babies with Rh-negative blood types; mothers with diabetes mellitus, kidney disease, or heart disease; and concurrent infections in either the mother or the baby. Anticipating these problems of the healthy newborn by using the Apgar scores and the results of the physical examination allows the proper assignment of the infant to the nursery or NICU.

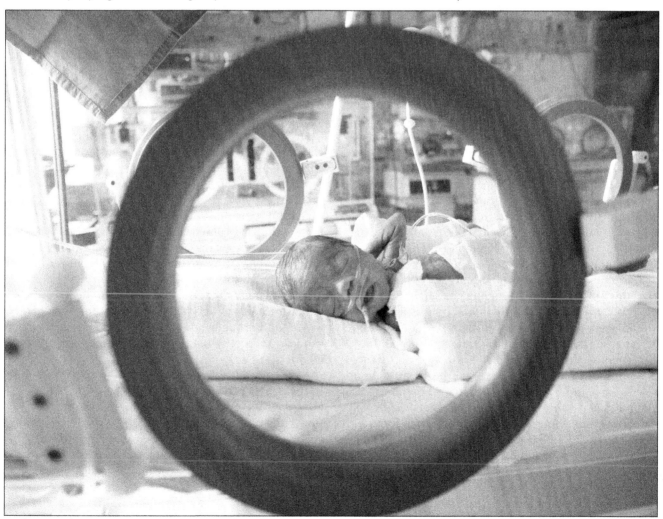

Newborns at risk may require a special environment such as an incubator. Photo via iStock/IvanJekic. [Used under license.]

The NICU is a daunting place containing high-tech equipment, a tangle of wires and tubes, the sounds of beeps and alarms, and tiny, fragile infants. All this technology serves two simple purposes: to monitor vital functions and to sustain malfunctioning or nonfunctioning organ systems. Looked at individually, however, the machines and attachments become much more understandable. The incubator, perhaps the most common device, maintains a warm, moist environment of constant temperature at 37 degrees Celsius (98.6 degrees Fahrenheit). Small portholes with rubber gloves allow people to touch the child safely. Generally, the infants will have small electrodes taped on their chests, connected to video monitors that record the heart and breathing rates and that will sound alarms if significant deviations occur. These monitors will also record blood pressure through an arm or thigh cuff. To ensure immediate access to the blood, for delivering medications and taking blood for testing, catheters (plastic tubes) are placed into larger arteries or veins near the umbilicus, neck, or thigh (in adults, intravenous access is found in the arms).

The remaining equipment is used for the very serious business of life support, in particular the support of the respiratory system. Maintaining adequate oxygenation is critical and can be accomplished in several ways, depending on the baby's needs. The least stressful are tubes placed in the nostrils or a face mask, but these methods require that breathing be spontaneous although inadequate. More often, unfortunately, neonates with the types of problems that bring them to an intensive care unit cannot breathe on their own. In these cases, a tube must be connected from the artificial respirator into the windpipe (the endotracheal tube). Warm, moistened, oxygen-rich air is delivered under pressure and removed from the lungs rhythmically to simulate breathing. Tranquilizers and paralytic agents are used to calm and immobilize the infant. Sick or premature infants are also generally unable to feed or nurse naturally, by mouth. Again, several methods of feeding can be employed, depending on the problems and the length of time that such feedings will be needed. For the first few days, simple solutions of water, sugar, and protein can be given through the intravenous catheters. These lines, because of the very small, fragile blood vessels of the newborn, are seldom able to carry more complex solutions. A second method, known as gavage feeding, employs tubing that is inserted through the nose directly into the stomach. Through that tube, infant formula (water, sugar, protein, fat, vitamins, and minerals) and, if available, breast milk can be given.

As the underlying problems are resolved, the infant is slowly weaned, first feeding orally and then breathing naturally. Next, the infant will be placed in an open crib, and gradually the tangled web of tubes and wires will clear. With approval from the neonatologist, the baby is transferred to the routine nursery, a transitional home until discharge from the hospital is advisable.

DIAGNOSTIC AND TREATMENT TECHNIQUES

Neonatology has amassed an enormous body of knowledge about normal neonatal anatomy and physiology, disease processes, and, most important, how to manage the wide variety of complications that can occur. Specific treatment protocols have been developed that are practiced uniformly in all neonatal intensive care units. Short-term stays (twenty-four to forty-eight hours) are meant to observe and monitor the infant with respiratory distress at birth that required immediate intervention. Long-term stays, lasting from several weeks to months, are the case for the sickest newborns, most commonly those with severe prematurity and low birth weight (less than 1,500 grams), respiratory distress syndrome (also known as hyaline membrane disease), congenital defects, and drug or alcohol addictions.

Infants born prematurely make up the major proportion of all infants at high risk for disability and death, and each passing decade has seen younger and younger babies being kept alive. While many maternal factors can lead to preterm delivery, often no explanation can be found. The main problem of prematurity lies in the functional and structural immaturity of vital organs. Weak sucking, swallowing, and coughing reflexes lead to an inability to feed and to the danger of choking. Lungs that lack surfactant, a substance that coats the millions of tiny air sacs (alveoli) in each lung to keep them from collapsing and sticking together after air is exhaled, cause severe breathing difficulty as the infant struggles to reinflate the lungs. When premature delivery is inevitable but not immediate, lung maturity can be increased by administration of steroids to the mother. An immature immune system cannot protect the newborn from the many viruses, bacteria, and other microorganisms that exist. Inadequate metabolism causes low body temperature and inadequate use of food or medications. Neurological immaturity can lead to intellectual disability, blindness, and deafness.

Aggressive management of the preterm baby begins in the delivery room, with close cooperation between the obstetrician and the neonatologist. Severely preterm infants, some born after only twenty weeks of pregnancy, require immediate respiratory and cardiac support. Placement of the endotracheal tube, assisted ventilation with a handheld bag, and delicate chest compressions similar to the cardiopulmonary resuscitation (CPR) performed on adults to stimulate the heartbeat are each accomplished quickly. Once the respiratory and circulatory systems have been stabilized, excess fluid will be suctioned, while a brief physical examination is performed to note any abnormalities that require immediate attention. As soon as transport is considered safe, the newborn is sent to the NICU. If the infant has been delivered at a small community hospital, this may involve ambulance or even helicopter transport to the nearest tertiary care center.

Once in the unit, the neonate will be placed in an incubator and attached to video monitors that record heart rate, breathing, and blood pressure. The endotracheal tube can now be attached to the respirator machine, and intravenous or intra-arterial catheters will be placed to allow the fluid and medication infusions and the blood drawing for the battery of tests that the neonatologist requires. Feeding methods can be set up as soon as the infant has stabilized. Within a short time after delivery, the premature newborn has had a flurry of activity about it and is surrounded by the most sophisticated equipment and staff available. Supporting the immature organs becomes the first priority, although the ethical issues of saving very sick infants must soon be addressed as complications begin to occur. Nearly 15 percent of surviving preterm infants whose birth weights were less than 2,000 grams have serious physical and mental disabilities after discharge. The majority, however, grow to lead normal, healthy lives.

Congenital defects are common, and it is estimated that the majority of miscarriages are a direct result of congenital defects that are incompatible with life. Many infants that do survive development and delivery die shortly after birth despite the most sophisticated and heroic attempts to intervene. The causes of such defects are arbitrarily assigned to two broad categories, although a combination of these factors is the most likely explanation: genetic errors (such as breaks, doubling, and mutations) and environmental insults (such as chemicals, drugs, viruses, radiation, and malnutrition). In the United States, among the most common birth defects that require immediate intervention are heart problems, spina bifida (an open spine), and tracheoesophageal fistulas and esophageal atresias (wrongly connected or incomplete wind and food pipes).

The birth of a malformed infant is rarely expected, and the neonatologist's team plays a key role in its survival. Congenital heart disease is the most prevalent life-threatening defect. During development in utero, the umbilical cord supplies the necessary oxygen; it is not until birth, when that lifeline is cut, that the neonate's circulatory and respiratory systems acquire full responsibility. At delivery, all may appear normal, and the one-minute Apgar score may be high. Several minutes later, however, the pink skin color may begin to

darken to a purplish blue (cyanosis), indicating that insufficient oxygen is being extracted from the air. Immediately, the infant receives rescue breathing from the bag mask. Upon admission to the neonatal unit, the source of the cyanosis must be determined. A chest x-ray may provide significant information about the anatomy of the heart and lungs, but special tests are usually needed to pinpoint the problem. Catheters that are threaded from neck or leg vessels into the heart can reveal the pressure and oxygen content of each chamber in the heart and across its four valves. Echocardiograms, video pictures similar to sonograms generated by sound waves passing through the chest, enhance the data provided by the x-rays and catheterizations, and a diagnosis is made. Based on the physical signs and symptoms of the newborn, a treatment plan is devised.

Because of the nature of congenital defects and structural abnormalities, their correction generally requires surgery. Openings between the heart's chambers (septal defects), valves that are too narrow or do not close properly, and blood vessels that leave or enter the heart incorrectly are all common defects treated by the pediatric heart surgeon. Because of the delicacy of the operation and the vulnerability of the newborn, surgery may be postponed until the baby is larger and stronger while it is provided with supplemental oxygen and nutrients. The risk of such operations is high, and depending on the degree of abnormality, several operations may be required.

Another group of infants who have benefited from advances in neonatology are those born to drug-addicted women. The lives of these infants are often complicated by congenital defects and life-threatening withdrawal symptoms. For example, heroin-addicted babies are quite small, are extremely irritable and hyperactive, and develop tremors, vomiting, diarrhea, and seizures. The newborn must be carefully monitored in the unit, and sedatives and antiseizure medications are given, sometimes for as long as six weeks. Cocaine and its derivatives frequently cause premature labor, fetal death, and maternal hemorrhaging during delivery. Infants that do survive often have serious congenital defects and suffer withdrawal symptoms. The risk of acquired immunodeficiency syndrome (AIDS) adds another dimension to an already complicated picture.

PERSPECTIVE AND PROSPECTS
Throughout human history, maternal and neonatal deaths have been staggering in number. Ignorance and unsanitary conditions frequently resulted in uterine hemorrhaging and overwhelming infection, killing both mother and baby. Highly inaccurate records at the beginning of the twentieth century in New York

City show maternal death averaging 2 percent; in fact, the rate was probably greater, since most births occurred at home. Neonatal deaths from respiratory failure, congenital defects, prematurity, and infection loom large in these medical records. The expansion of medical, obstetric, and pediatric knowledge and technology that began after World War II has dramatically lowered maternal and infant mortality. It should not be forgotten, however, that nonindustrialized nations, the majority in the world, remain devastated by the neonatal problems that have plagued civilization for thousands of years.

Ironically, the problems associated with neonatology in Western nations are now at the other end of the spectrum: saving and prolonging life beyond what is natural or "reasonable." As neonatology advanced scientifically and technically, saving life took precedence over ethical issues. The famous and poignant story of Baby Doe in the early 1980s illustrates the dilemmas that occur daily in neonatal intensive care units. Baby Doe was a six-pound, full-term male born with Down syndrome and severe congenital defects of the heart, trachea, and esophagus. These malformations were deemed surgically correctable, although the underlying problem of Down syndrome, a disease characterized by intellectual disabilities and particular facial and body features, would remain. The parents did not agree to any operations and requested that all treatment be withheld. Baby Doe was given only medication for sedation and died within a few days. The case was later related by the attending physician in a letter to *The New England Journal of Medicine*, sparking enormous controversy. On July 5, 1983, a law was passed in effect stating that all newborns with disabilities, no matter how seriously afflicted, should receive all possible life-sustaining treatment, unless it is unequivocally clear that imminent death is inevitable or that the risks of treatment cannot be justified by its benefit. The legislators believed that Baby Doe had been allowed to die because of his underlying condition of Down syndrome.

Since then, attorneys, ethicists, juries, and courts have used the example of Baby Doe, and the law that grew from it, to interpret many cases that have come to light. Life-and-death decisions are made on a daily basis in the neonatal care unit. They are always difficult, but they usually remain a private matter between the parents and the neonatologist. These cases become public matters, however, when the family disagrees with the medical staff. Then the question of what is in the best interest of the child is compounded by who will pay for the treatments and who will care for the baby after it is discharged.

Such ethical dilemmas will continue as expertise and technology grow. A multitude of questions, previously relegated to philosophy and religion, will arise, and the benefits of saving a life will have to be weighed against its quality and the resources necessary to maintain it.

—*Connie Rizzo, MD, PhD;*
updated by Alexander Sandra, MD

See also Apgar score; Birth defects; Blue baby syndrome; Bonding; Cardiology, pediatric; Cesarean section; Childbirth; Childbirth complications; Chlamydia; Circumcision, male; Cleft lip and palate; Cleft lip and palate repair; Cognitive development; Colic; Congenital disorders; Congenital heart disease; Craniosynostosis; Critical care, pediatric; Cystic fibrosis; Developmental disorders; Developmental stages; Down syndrome; Embryology; Endocrinology, pediatric; Failure to thrive; Fetal alcohol syndrome; Fetal surgery; Gastroenterology, pediatric; Genetic diseases; Genetics and inheritance; Hematology, pediatric; Hemolytic disease of the newborn; Hydrocephalus; Intraventricular hemorrhage; Jaundice, neonatal; Metabolic disorders; Motor skill development; Multiple births; Nephrology, pediatric; Neurology, pediatric; Obstetrics; Orthopedics, pediatric; Pediatrics; Perinatology; Phenylketonuria (PKU); Polydactyly and syndactyly; Premature birth; Pulmonary medicine, pediatric; Rh factor; Shunts; Sudden infant death syndrome (SIDS); Surgery, pediatric; Tay-Sachs disease; Teratogens; Toxoplasmosis; Urology, pediatric; Well-baby examinations.

For Further Information:
Behrman, Richard E., Robert M. Kliegman, and Hal B. Jenson, eds. *Nelson Textbook of Pediatrics.* 18th ed. Philadelphia: Saunders/Elsevier, 2007.
Bradford, Nikki. *Your Premature Baby: The First Five Years.* Toronto, Ont.: Firefly Books, 2003.
Crisp, Stuart, and Jo Rainbow, eds. *Emergencies in Paediatrics and Neonatology.* 2d ed. Oxford: Oxford University Press, 2013.
Cunningham, Nicholas, ed. *Columbia University College of Physicians and Surgeons: Complete Guide to Early Child Care.* New York: Crown, 1990.
Levin, Daniel L., and Frances C. Morriss, eds. *Essentials of Pediatric Intensive Care.* 2d ed. New York: Churchill Livingstone, 1997.
MacDonald, Mhairi G., Mary M. K. Seshia, and Martha D. Mullett, eds. *Avery's Neonatology: Pathophysiology and Management of the Newborn.* 6th ed. Philadelphia: Lippincott Williams & Wilkins, 2005.
Martin, Richard J., Avroy A. Fanaroff, and Michele C. Walsh, eds. *Fanaroff and Martin's Neonatal-Perinatal Medicine: Diseases of the Fetus and Infant.* 2 vols. 8th ed. Philadelphia: Mosby/Elsevier, 2006.
Meeks, Maggie, Maggie Hallsworth, and Helen Yeo, eds. *Nursing the Neonate.* 2d ed. Malden: Wiley-Blackwell, 2013.
Moore, Keith L., and T. V. N. Persaud. *The Developing Human.* 8th ed. Philadelphia: Saunders/Elsevier, 2008.
Ruhlman, Michael. *Walk on Water: Inside an Elite Pediatric Surgery Unit.* New York: Viking-Penguin, 2003.
Sadler, T. W. *Langman's Medical Embryology.* 11th ed. Philadelphia: Lippincott Williams & Wilkins, 2009.
Sinha, Sunil, Lawrence Miall, and Luke Jardine. *Essential Neonatal Medicine.* 5th ed. Malden: Wiley-Blackwell, 2012.
Woolf, Alan D., et al., eds. *The Children's Hospital Guide to Your Child's Health and Development.* Cambridge, Mass.: Perseus, 2002.

NEPHRECTOMY

Category: Procedure
Anatomy or system affected: Abdomen, kidneys, urinary system
Specialties and related fields: General surgery, nephrology, oncology, urology
Definition: The removal of the kidney, which may be performed to treat disorders and disease or for the purpose of transplantation.
Key terms:
adrenal gland: a small hormone-producing gland which is adjacent to the upper pole of the kidney
donor nephrectomy: a procedure in which a kidney is removed for transplantation into another patient; the kidney can be removed from a person who is brain-dead but whose heart is still beating (cadaveric donor nephrectomy) or from a relative of the recipient (a living related donor)
nephroureterectomy: a procedure similar to a radical nephrectomy, with the additional removal of the ureter and a cuff of the bladder; performed to treat transitional cell carcinomas of the ureters and the pelvis of the kidneys
radical nephrectomy: a procedure in which a kidney is removed along with the covering layers of tissue and the adjacent adrenal gland; performed with cancerous conditions
renal cell carcinoma (RCC): cancer of the small tubules of the kidney; generally known as kidney cancer
simple nephrectomy: a procedure in which a kidney is removed but the covering layers of tissue and the adjacent adrenal gland are left intact; usually performed to treat benign (noncancerous) conditions
transitional cell carcinoma (TCC): cancer arising from the lining of the urine-collecting system of the kidneys, ureters, and bladder
ureters: the tubes that drain urine from the kidneys to the bladder

INDICATIONS AND PROCEDURES

A kidney may be removed for several reasons, including congenital defects, trauma, cancer, inflammation, and transplantation. Congenital problems, or birth defects, associated with thekidneys include abnormal development, nonfunctional cysts, blockage, tumors, and cysts that leave the kidneys functional but which cause difficulty in breathing because of their large size. A kidney may be removed if the organ or its main blood vessels have been damaged beyond repair by trauma, such as a gunshot wound. Cancer is one of the most common reasons for nephrectomy; kidney cancers include renal cell carcinomas, transitional cell carcinomas, and tumors in the capsules of the kidneys or in

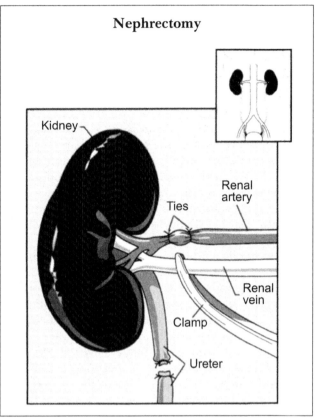

Nephrectomy

Kidney

Renal artery

Ties

Renal vein

Clamp

Ureter

The removal of a kidney may be necessary because of disease or because the kidney is intended for transplantation into another patient; the inset shows the location of the kidneys. ©EBSCO

surrounding layers of tissue. Infections or abscesses in the kidney that are beyond medical treatment and that become life-threatening may also necessitate a nephrectomy. Finally, a kidney may be removed from a donor for transplantation.

Simple nephrectomies involve removal of the kidney only, whereas radical nephrectomies include removal of the kidney and surrounding glands. Depending on the underlying disease and the surgeon's preference and experience, the kidney can be approached from the front, side, or back. The incisions used to reach the kidney are similar for simple, radical, and donor nephrectomies, but the steps that follow differ once the abdomen has been entered. For a nephroureterectomy, in which the kidney, the connecting ureter, and a part of the bladder are removed, the surgeon makes either one long, S-shaped incision starting in the flank and ending near the bladder, or two separate incisions.

In the frontal approach to nephrectomy, the patient lies on his or her back and the abdomen and peritoneal cavity are opened. The intestines near the kidney are pushed to the side, and the kidney is approached from the front. The advantage of this approach includes better evaluation of the liver and the structures surrounding the kidney, better control of the blood vessels, and easy removal of clots from veins if necessary. The disadvantages of this approach are the possibility of adhesions developing in the intestines and lung complications after the surgery. The frontal approach may also be laparoscopic, in which a number of small incisions are made in the abdomen; a camera is fed through one incision, and surgical tools through another; one of the incisions is then made larger for the removal of the kidney. A laparoscopic nephrectomy takes longer to perform but has a shorter recovery period with less postoperative discomfort.

In the side approach, the patient is placed on his or her side and the incision is made through the eleventh or twelfth ribs. The kidney is approached from behind. This type of incision involves cutting into muscle and results in significant postoperative pain. The main advantage is that the peritoneal cavity is not entered.

In the back approach, known as a dorsal lumbotomy, the patient is placed face-down and a muscle-splitting incision is used. The kidney is approached from behind. This method is usually used for a simple nephrectomy. Its primary advantages are less postoperative pain and avoidance of the peritoneal cavity. Its main disadvantage is a limited view of the surgery site.

In a simple nephrectomy, after the kidney has been exposed, Gerota's fascia (the covering envelope of the kidney) is opened, and the fat around the kidney is dissected. The adjacent blood vessels and the connecting ureter are tied and cut, and the kidney is removed. In a radical nephrectomy, the adjacent adrenal gland and surrounding lymph glands are also removed in the one block. For a nephroureterectomy, the ureter is not cut close to the kidney but is removed all the way down to the bladder. A 2-centimeter cuff of bladder is cut off, the entire specimen is removed, and the hole in the bladder is closed.

The techniques used with kidney transplantation differ for cadaveric (deceased) donor nephrectomy and living related donor (LRD) nephrectomy. For cadaveric donor nephrectomy, the abdominal aorta (the main artery bringing blood to the kidney) and the inferior vena cava (the main vein taking blood away from the kidney) are isolated above and below the kidneys and cannulated with pipes to irrigate both kidneys with cold preservation fluid. Both kidneys and ureters, along with their related blood vessels, are removed. For LRD nephrectomy, the kidney is dissected along with its blood vessels and ureter. Great care is taken to obtain the maximum length of ureter and blood vessels without causing damage to the donor.

USES AND COMPLICATIONS

The major complications of nephrectomy during surgery are bleeding, damage to surrounding structures, and problems related to anesthesia. Therefore, there is significant evaluation of the patient before surgery. A battery of tests may be performed, including blood testing, urinalysis, electrocardiography, and x-rays. A thorough medical examination is done to determine whether the patient can be placed under anesthesia safely. The patient's blood is also typed and cross-matched in the event that a transfusion is required. Good surgical skills, the availability of blood for transfusion, and proper anesthesia techniques usually ensure that any complications that occur are not life-threatening. Nevertheless, the patient may also experience complications during the procedure that are not directly related to the surgery, such as a heart attack.

After a nephrectomy, the patient is at some risk for other problems. These complications may include bleeding, infection, intestinal obstruction, blood clots in the legs or lungs, or a heart attack.

PERSPECTIVE AND PROSPECTS

Significant advances have been made in nephrectomy since the first such procedure was performed by Gustav Simmons in 1869. Thorough preoperative evaluation; improved anesthesia techniques; a greater understanding of anatomy, physiology, and pathology (including the nature of infections and microorganisms); and the discovery of antibiotics have all led to better surgical techniques. As a result, the death rate for nephrectomy operations is only 1 percent.

—*Saeed Akhter, MD*

See also Adrenalectomy; Dialysis; Hemolytic uremic syndrome; Kidney cancer; Kidney disorders; Kidney transplantation; Kidneys; Nephritis; Nephrology; Nephrology, pediatric; Transplantation.

For Further Information:
Brenner, Barry M., et al., ed. *Brenner and Rector's The Kidney.* 9th ed. Philadelphia: Saunders/Elsevier, 2012.
Danovitch, Gabriel M., ed. *Handbook of Kidney Transplantation.* 5th ed. Philadelphia: Lippincott Williams & Wilkins, 2010.
Hinman, Frank, Jr. *Atlas of Urologic Surgery.* 2d ed. Philadelphia: W. B. Saunders, 1998.
"Kidney Removal." *MedlinePlus,* October 9, 2012.
Kohnle, Diana. "Nephrectomy." *Health Library,* May 23, 2013.
Marshall, Fray F., ed. *Textbook of Operative Urology.* Philadelphia: W. B. Saunders, 1996.
"Nephrectomy (Kidney Removal)." *Mayo Clinic,* May 23, 2012.
Novick, Andrew C., and Stevan B. Streem. "Surgery of the Kidney." In *Campbell-Walsh Urology,* edited by Patrick Walsh et al. 9th ed. 4 vols. Philadelphia: Saunders/Elsevier, 2007.
Schrier, Robert W., ed. *Diseases of the Kidney and Urinary Tract.* 8th ed. Philadelphia: Wolters Kluwer Health/Lippincott Williams & Wilkins, 2007.

Nephritis

Category: Disease/Disorder
Anatomy or system affected: Blood vessels, immune system, kidneys
Specialties and related fields: Immunology, internal medicine, nephrology
Definition: An inflammatory response of the kidneys, particularly of the glomeruli, to infectious agents or immunological challenges.
Key terms:
albuminuria: excretion in the urine of the protein albumin, usually as a result of changes occurring in the glomeruli
amyloidosis: the deposition of immunoglobulin fibrils in various tissues, including the kidneys
dialysis: the use of artificial membranes to remove metabolites from the blood when the kidneys fail; the peritoneum can also be used (peritoneal dialysis)
filtration rate: the amount of fluid passing per minute from blood across the glomerular capillaries to form glomerular fluid
glomeruli: structures consisting mainly of capillary blood vessels contained in a capsule, across whose walls water and solutes pass (filter) to form glomerular fluid
glomerulonephritis: inflammation of glomeruli
hematuria: the presence of red blood cells or red blood cell casts in the urine
immunoglobulins: proteins associated with immune responses
nephrotic syndrome: a condition involving edema, the retention of water and of sodium and chloride ions, urinary protein losses greater than 3 grams per day, and hypoalbuminemia
proteinuria: the presence of proteins, including globulins, in the urine; usually considered a sign of changes in the glomerular structures
renal blood flow: the amount of whole blood entering the renal arteries per minute; a fraction of water and solutes is removed to form urine
renal failure: severe kidney insufficiency requiring the use of dialysis or transplantation to return and maintain composition of body fluids at or near normal values
renal insufficiency: the inability of the kidneys to maintain a normal internal environment of the body and its fluids
streptococci: bacteria responsible for the development of some cases of acute glomerulonephritis, but without infection of the kidneys
tubules: hollow structures conducting glomerular fluid to the collecting ducts and the renal pelvis; they produce composition and volume changes of glomerular fluid passing through them and may reabsorb some of the protein that crosses the glomerular capillaries

CAUSES AND SYMPTOMS

Nephritis means any inflammatory responses of the kidney, whether the cause is infectious or immunological. Generally, it involves mainly the glomeruli, where the initial formation of urine takes place. The term is therefore equivalent in meaning to glomerulonephritis. Pathological changes may also occur in the interstitium (the extravascular, extracellular domain in which the tubules are embedded) and affect tubular functions. This condition, referred to as tubulointerstitial nephritis, is associated with localized cellular infiltrates and the accumulation of fluid.

The classic cause of acute glomerulonephritis is an infection in the throat or of the skin by a nephritogenic strain of Group A streptococci. The clinical presentation can be dramatic and can be associated not only with a sore throat but also with headaches, shortness of breath, and swelling of the ankles. Physical examination may find hypertension, rales in the lungs, peripheral pitting edema, and changes in the retinal vessels. In the chronic form, the onset is usually insidious; an infection may have been forgotten or ignored, without specific complaints except for some ankle edema, tiredness, and perhaps pallor. The physical findings for chronic glomerulonephritis are similar to but less striking than in the acute form.

The diagnosis in each type of nephritis is presumed on the basis of urinalysis, with a finding of blood (hematuria) in the acute form; proteinuria (actually mainly albuminuria, although globulins may also be present); and a decreased glomerular filtration rate. Diagnosis is established on the basis of renal biopsy with examination by both light and electron microscopy. Throat cultures and streptococcal group determination are appropriate if an infection is suspected.

Both conditions may be followed by the development of nephrotic syndrome, which is characterized by major losses of albumin in the urine, decreased serum albumin concentrations (hypoalbuminemia), the retention of water and of sodium and chloride ions, and massive edema and ascites (fluid leakage from blood vessels into the abdomen). Nephrotic syndrome may also appear without any history or evidence of a preceding episode of acute glomerulonephritis. On renal biopsy, essentially no changes or only minimal changes may be noted on inspection by light microscopy (minimal change disease), although characteristic changes are found with electron microscopy affecting particularly the foot processes (podocytes) of the glomeruli.

INFORMATION ON NEPHRITIS

Causes: Inflammation of kidney from bacterial infection (often streptococcal) or immune disorder

Symptoms: In acute form, sore throat, headache, shortness of breath, ankle swelling, hypertension, edema; in chronic form, ankle swelling, fatigue, pallor; either may lead to nephrotic syndrome (loss of albumin in urine, decreased serum albumin, water retention, sodium and chloride ion retention, massive edema and ascites)

Duration: Acute or chronic

Treatments: Usually none needed for acute form; for nonresolving or chronic form, dietary control (decreased protein and potassium), steroids, hemodialysis or peritoneal dialysis, kidney transplantation

Acute glomerulonephritis resolves spontaneously and rapidly in about 95 percent of cases, without detectable residual damage to kidney functions. Apart from control of hypertension, no specific treatment is available. The edema is rarely sufficient to warrant the use of diuretics. Antibiotics are not indicated unless there is evidence of an infection. Patients can be considered to be cured but should nonetheless be followed in the event of a reappearance of symptoms or manifestations.

In nonresolving acute glomerulonephritis and in chronic glomerulonephritis, there can be progression of damage to the glomeruli so that the number of functioning glomeruli (normally, about one million in each kidney) diminishes. This process may be gradual or may occur as a part of acute exacerbations that subside but leave the patient with diminished renal functions. As a result, glomerular filtration is decreased and the accumulation of metabolic end-products, particularly urea, occurs in the blood and tissue fluids. Abnormalities of acid-base regulation appear with decreased blood pH (acidemia), decreased serum bicarbonate concentration, and increased potassium concentration. Generally, a significant anemia exists, and renal blood flow is decreased so that the metabolic activities of the renal tubule cells are affected. Renal insufficiency is established, and dietary control is instituted, with decreased intakes of protein and potassium. Paradoxically, with decreased glomerular function, proteinuria decreases, serum albumin increases, and edema decreases or disappears.

Unfortunately, the progression of glomerular dysfunction continues, and dietary measures provide insufficient control of metabolic abnormalities. Resort is then made to hemodialysis or peritoneal dialysis to control the metabolic abnormalities and lift dietary restrictions to some degree while the patient awaits kidney transplantation. During this waiting period, stimulants of the bone marrow, such as erythropoietin, are administered in the expectation of maintaining the red cell count and the hematocrit at a satisfactory level. Transplants will require the use of immunosuppressive agents to prevent rejection unless an identical twin is the donor.

Other diseases in which glomerular damage can occur include diabetes mellitus, amyloidosis, systemic lupus erythematosus (SLE), Wegener's granulomatosis, Goodpasture's syndrome, syphilis, and human immunodeficiency virus (HIV) infection. Common problems associated with glomerular damage of any etiology are hypertension, strokes, heart failure, pulmonary edema, arteriolar vasoconstriction and sclerosis, impaired vision from exudates, pericarditis, and pericardial effusions.

TREATMENT AND THERAPY

Acute glomerulonephritis is characterized by the disappearance of signs and symptoms, or at least their marked reduction, in most patients. In 90 to 95 percent of cases, there is no progression and no recurrence. In some patients, the problems may reappear after apparent complete remission, while in others the disease progresses, often to nephrotic syndrome. This phase, too, disappears as the disease worsens, reaching the stage where hemodialysis or peritoneal dialysis becomes necessary. A renal biopsy can aid in determining the appropriate treatment. For example, if the biopsy confirms that poststreptococcal nephritis is present, then no specific treatment is available. If progressive glomerulonephritis is the diagnosis, then steroids may be indicated.

Hemodialysis depends on an arteriovenous shunt being created, usually in the forearm, so that the patient's blood can pass through a dialysis machine, which functions in a manner similar to glomeruli. Usually, several sessions, two or three times per week for several hours at a time, are required. Peritoneal dialysis involves the introduction of large amounts of fluid into the peritoneal cavity and its withdrawal after adequate exchanges with body fluids across the peritoneal surfaces have occurred. Hemodialysis requires going to a hospital or specialized facility, while pertoneal dialysis can be performed at home. Both procedures require careful and frequent monitoring of the patient's acid-base, electrolyte, and metabolic statuses.

While arrangements can usually be made for local dialysis, patients on dialysis lose a significant degree of mobility and independence. This independence can be regained to a considerable degree through kidney transplantation. Kidneys may be obtained from cadavers, unrelated living donors, and related living donors, such as identical twins. Except with the latter group, rejection phenomena may occur. Infections can occur with the use of immunosuppressive agents. Rarely, malignancies can be introduced with transplanted kidneys.

A low protein intake is recommended in the later stages of glomerulonephritis because too high a protein intake may accelerate the progression of the disease. Lack of control of water intake may lead to edema. Anemia is common in the later stages and may require the administration of erythropoietin.

In the nephrotic phase and in minimal change disease, control of edema is sought through one or more of the following measures: salt restriction, diuretics, intravenous (IV) administration of concentrated human serum albumin, corticosteroids (such as prednisone, which is more likely to be effective in minimal change disease), and other immunosuppressive agents. Nephrotic syndrome may occur in the presence of other underlying diseases, such as lupus, diabetes mellitus, HIV infection, syphilis, amyloidosis, and microvascular angiopathies. Specific treatments should be used when applicable.

PERSPECTIVE AND PROSPECTS

The monograph *Reports of Medical Cases* by Richard Bright, published in 1827, marks the first clear description of nephritis through clinical findings (edema), laboratory assessment (proteinuria), and gross structural changes in the kidneys at postmortem. For many years, nephritis was referred to as Bright's disease. Apart from the measurement of blood constituents such as urea and creatinine, functional assessment was limited until the development, by Donald D. Van Slyke, of the clearance concept, defined as the amount of a given substance excreted in the urine per unit time relative to its concentration in plasma or blood. Van Slyke focused on the clearance of urea, while P. B. Rehberg in Denmark proposed that the clearance of creatinine could be used as a measure of the glomerular filtration rate. Glomerular fluid had been shown by Newton Richards to have the same composition as an ultrafiltrate of plasma. Accordingly, if creatinine was neither secreted nor reabsorbed by the tubules, then its clearance would be equivalent to the glomerular filtration rate.

The assumptions with respect to creatinine were shown to be incorrect, and inulin, a polyfructoside studied by Homer Smith, was found to be a reliable and correct indicator for measuring the glomerular filtration rate. Smith and his collaborators systematized and advanced knowledge of the kidney as a whole organ in a quantitative manner. Detailed understanding of the components of the whole organ progressed rapidly with the discovery of the significance of countercirculation in establishing the solute concentration gradient from cortex to medulla reported by H. Wirz and B. Hargitay. Functions of limited segments of the tubules (and later of individual cells) have provided additional important information on transport and metabolic processes in the kidneys.

On the clinical side, the introduction of renal biopsies and of hemodialysis (and later peritoneal dialysis) by way of an arteriovenous shunt made for more accurate diagnoses and longer life expectancies for patients with chronic renal disease. Further encouragement was provided by the development of techniques for successful renal transplants, first from identical twins, then from living donors and cadavers. Problems of rejection remain. Another major challenge is to find the means of delaying or arresting the progression of chronic renal disease before dialysis and transplants become necessary.

A study published in the *Journal of Epidemiology and Community Health* in May 2013 reported that half of over 1,100 adults treated for stroke in Boston, Massachusetts between 1999 and 2004 lived in close proximity to a major roadway. According to researchers, there is evidence that air pollution caused by traffic can cause harm to the arteries that supply blood to the kidneys.

—*Francis P. Chinard, MD*

See also Bacterial infection; End-stage renal disease; Hemolytic uremic syndrome; Kidney cancer; Kidney disorders; Kidneys; Nephrectomy; Nephrology; Nephrology, pediatric; Proteinuria; Pyelonephritis; Renal failure; Stone removal; Stones; Streptococcal infection; Systemic lupus erythematosus (SLE); Transplantation.

For Further Information:
Brenner, Barry M. "Retarding the Progression of Renal Disease." *Kidney International* 64 (2003): 370-378.
———, ed. *Brenner and Rector's The Kidney.* 8th ed. Philadelphia: Saunders/Elsevier, 2008.
Cameron, J. Stewart, and Richard J. Glassock, eds. *The Nephrotic Syndrome.* New York: Marcel Dekker, 1988.
D'Amico, G., and C. Bazzi. "Pathophysiology of Proteinuria." *Kidney International* 63 (2003): 809-825.
Eddy, A. A., and J. M. Symons. "Nephrotic Syndrome in Children." *The Lancet* 362 (2003): 629-639.
Hricik, D. E., M. Chung-Park, and J. R. Sedor. "Glomerulonephritis." *New England Journal of Medicine* 339 (1998): 888-899.
Lue, Shih-Ho. "Residential Proximity to Major Roadways and Renal function."Â *Journal of Epidemiology and Community Health*. 10.1136 (2012). Print.

NEPHROLOGY

Category: Specialty
Anatomy or system affected: Abdomen, blood, kidneys, urinary system
Specialties and related fields: Biochemistry, biotechnology, endocrinology, genetics, hematology, internal medicine, urology
Definition: The field of medicine that deals with the anatomy and physiology of the kidneys.
Key terms:

analyte: any chemical substance undergoing measurement; includes charged electrolytes found in the blood, such as sodium or potassium

creatinine: a nitrogen-containing by-product of metabolism; levels of creatinine may be indicative of kidney function

endocrine: referring to a process in which cells from an organ or gland secrete substances into the blood; these substances in turn act on cells elsewhere in the body

glomerulonephritis: inflammation of the glomeruli, the clusters of blood vessels and nerves found throughout the kidney

nephritis: any disease or pathology of the kidney that results in inflammation

nephron: the structural and functional unit of the kidney; composed of the renal corpuscle, the loop of Henle, and renal tubules

nephrotic syndrome: an abnormal condition of the kidneys characterized by a variety of conditions, including edema and proteinuria; often accompanies glomerular dysfunction and diabetes

renal: pertaining to the kidney

urea: a waste product of protein metabolism that represents the form in which nitrogen is eliminated from the body

SCIENCE AND PROFESSION

Nephrology is the branch of medicine that deals with the function of the kidneys. As a consequence, a nephrologist frequently deals with problems related to homeostasis, that is, the maintenance of the internal environment of the body. The most obvious function of the kidneys is their ability to regulate the excretion of water and minerals from the body, at the same time serving to eliminate nitrogenous wastes in the form of urea. While such waste material, produced as by-products of cell metabolism, is removed from the circulation, essential nutrients from body fluids are retained within the renal apparatus. These nutrients include proteins, carbohydrates, and electrolytes, some of which help maintain the proper acid-base balance within the blood. In addition, cells in the kidneys regulate red blood cell production through the release of the hormone erythropoietin.

The human excretory system includes two kidneys, which lie in the rear of the abdominal cavity on opposite sides of the spinal column. Urine is produced by the kidneys through a filtration network composed of 2 million nephrons, the actual functional units within each kidney. Two ureters, one for each kidney, serve to remove the collected urine and transport this liquid to the urinary bladder. The urethra drains urine from the bladder, voiding the liquid from the body.

Each adult human kidney is approximately 11 centimeters in length, with a shape resembling a bean. When the kidney is sectioned, three anatomical regions are visible: a light-colored outer cortex; a darker inner region, called the medulla; and the renal pelvis, the lowest portion of the kidney. The cortex consists primarily of a network of nephrons and associated blood capillaries. Tubules extending from each nephron pass into the medulla. The medulla, in turn, is visibly divided into about a dozen conical masses, or pyramids, with the base of the pyramid at the junction between the cortex and medulla and the apex of the pyramid extending into the renal pelvis. The loops (such as the loop of Henle) and tubules within the medulla carry out the reabsorption of nutrients and fluids that have passed through the capsular network of the nephron. The tubules extend through the medulla and return to the cortical region.

There are approximately 1 million nephrons in each kidney. Within each nephron, the actual filtration of blood is carried out within a bulb-shaped region, Bowman's capsule, which surrounds a capillary network, the glomerulus. In most individuals, a single renal artery brings the blood supply to the kidney. Since the renal artery originates from a branch of the aorta, the body's largest artery, the blood pressure within this region of the kidney is high. Consequently, hypotension, a significant lowering of blood pressure, may also result in kidney failure.

The renal artery enters the kidney through the renal pelvis, branching into progressively smaller arterioles and capillaries. The capillary network serves both to supply nutrition to the cells that make up the kidney and to collect nutrients or fluids reabsorbed from the loops and tubules of the nephrons. Renal capillaries also enter the Bowman's capsules in the form of balls or coils, the glomeruli. Since blood pressure remains high, the force filtration in a nephron pushes about 20 percent of the fluid volume of the glomerulus into the cavity portion of the capsule. Most small materials dissolved in the blood, including proteins, sugars, electrolytes, and the nitrogenous waste product urea, pass along within the fluid into the capsule. As the filtrate passes through the series of convoluted tubules extending from the Bowman's capsule, most nutrients and salts are reabsorbed and reenter the capillary network. Approximately 99 percent of the water that has passed through the capsule is also reabsorbed. The material which remains, much of it waste such as urea, is excreted from the body.

Nephrology is the branch of medicine that deals with these functions of the kidney. Loss of kidney function can quickly result in a buildup of waste material in the blood; hence kidney failure, if untreated, can result in serious illness or death. Within the purview of nephrology, however, is more than the function of the kidneys as filters for the excretion of wastes. The kidneys are also endocrine organs, structures that secrete hormones into the bloodstream to act on other, distal organs. The major endocrine functions of the kidneys involve the secretion of the hormones renin and erythropoietin.

Renin functions within the renin-angiotensin system in the regulation of blood pressure. It is produced within the juxtaglomerular complex, the region around Bowman's capsule in which the arteriole enters the structure. Cells within the tubules of the nephron closely monitor the blood pressure within the incoming arterioles. When blood pressure drops, these cells stimulate the release of renin directly into the blood circulation.

Renin does not act directly on the nephrons. Rather, it serves as a proteolytic enzyme that activates another protein, angiotensin, the precursor of which is found in the blood. The activated angiotensin, called angiotensin II, has several effects on kidney function that involve the regulation of blood pressure. First, by decreasing the glomerular filtration rate, it allows more water to be retained. Second, angiotensin II stimulates the release of the steroid hormone aldosterone from the adrenal glands, located in close association with the kidneys. Aldosterone acts to increase sodium retention and transport by cells within the tubules of the nephron, resulting in increased water reabsorption. The result of this complex series of hormone interactions within the kidney is a close monitoring of both salt retention and blood pressure and volume. In this manner, nephrology also relates to the pathophysiology of hypertension-high blood pressure.

The kidneys also regulate the production of erythrocytes, red blood cells, through the production of the hormone erythropoietin. Erythropoietin is secreted by the peritubular cells associated with regions outside the nephrons in response to lowered oxygen levels in the blood, also monitored by cells within the kidney. The hormone serves to stimulate red cell production within the bone marrow. Approximately 85 percent of the erythropoietin in blood fluids is synthesized within the kidneys, the remainder by the liver.

Since proper kidney function is related to a wide variety of body processes, from the regulation of nitrogenous waste disposal to the monitoring and control of blood pressure, nephrology may deal with a number of disparate syndromes. The kidney may represent the primary site of a disease or pathology, an example being the autoimmune phenomenon of glomerulonephritis. Renal failure may also result from the indirect action of a more general systemic syndrome, as is the case with diabetes mellitus. In many cases, the decrease in kidney function may result from any number of disorders, which poses many problems for the nephrologist.

Proper function of the kidney is central to numerous homeostatic processes within the body. Thus nephrology by necessity deals with a variety of pathophysiological disorders. Renal dysfunction may involve disorders of the organ itself or pathology associated with individual structures within the kidneys, the glomeruli or tubules. Likewise, the disorder within the body may be of a more general type, with the kidney being a secondary site of damage. This is particularly true of immune disorders such as lupus (systemic lupus erythematosus) or diabetes. Conditions that affect proper kidney function may result from infection or inflammation, the obstruction of tubules or the vascular system, or neoplastic disorders (cancers).

Immune disorders are among the more common processes that result in kidney disease. They may be of two types: glomerulonephritis or the more general nephrotic syndrome. Glomerulonephritis can result either from a direct attack on basement membrane tissue by host antibodies, such as with Goodpasture's syndrome, or indirectly through deposits of immune (antigen-antibody) complexes, such as with lupus. Nephritis may also be secondary to high blood pressure. In any of these situations, inflammation resulting from the infiltration of immune complexes and/or from the activation of the complement system may result in a decreased ability of the glomeruli to function. Treatment of such disorders often involves the use of corticosteroids or other immunosuppressive drugs to dampen the immune response. Continued recurrence of the disease may result in renal failure, requiring dialysis treatment or even kidney transplantation.

Activation of the complement system as a result of immune complex deposition along the glomeruli is a frequent source of inflammation. Complement consists of a series of some dozen serum proteins, many of which are pharmacologically active. Intermediates in the complement pathway include enzymes that activate subsequent components in a cascade fashion. The terminal proteins in the pathway form a "membrane attack complex," capable of significantly damaging a target (such as the basement membrane of a Bowman's capsule). Activation of the initial steps in the pathway begins with either the deposition of immune complexes along basement membranes or the direct binding of antibodies on glomerular surfaces. The end result can be extensive nephrotic destruction.

Nephrotic syndrome, which can also result in extensive damage to the glomeruli, is often secondary to other disease. Diabetes is a frequent primary disorder in its development; approximately one-third of insulin-dependent diabetics are at risk for significant renal failure. Other causes of nephrotic syndrome may include cancer or infectious agents and toxins.

DIAGNOSTIC AND TREATMENT TECHNIQUES

Nephrologists can measure glomerular function using a variety of tests. These tests are based on the ability of the basement membranes associated with the glomeruli to act as filters. Blood cells and large materials such as proteins dissolved in the blood are unable to pass through these filters. Plasma, the liquid portion of the blood containing dissolved factors involved in blood-clotting mechanisms, is able to pass through the basement membrane, the driving force for filtration being the hydrostatic pressure of the blood (blood pressure).

The glomerular filtration rate (GFR) is defined as the rate by which the glomeruli filter the plasma during a fixed period of time. Generally, the rate is determined by measuring either the time of clearance of the carbohydrate inulin from the blood or the rate of clearance of creatinine, a nitrogenous by-product of metabolism. Though the rate may vary with age, it generally is about 125 to 130 milliliters of plasma filtered per minute.

Any significant decrease in the GFR is indicative of renal failure and can result in significant disruptions of acid-base or electrolyte balance in the blood. A decrease in the GFR can sometimes be observed through measurements of urine output. Healthy individuals usually excrete from 1 to 2 liters of urine per day. If the urine output drops to less than 500 milliliters (0.5 liter) per day, a condition known as oliguria, the body suffers a diminished capacity to remove metabolic waste products (urea, creatinine, or acids). Taken to an extreme, in which the filtering capacity is completely shut down and urine formation drops below 100 milliliters per day (anuria), the resulting uremia may cause death in a matter of days.

Anuria may have a variety of causes: kidney failure; hypotension, in which blood pressure is insufficient to maintain glomerular filtration; or a blockage in the urinary tract. As waste products, fluids, and electrolytes (especially sodium and potassium) build up, the person may appear puffy, be feverish, and exhibit muscle weakness. Heart arrhythmia or failure may also

occur. Mediation of the problem, in addition to attempts to alleviate the reasons for kidney dysfunction, include regulation of fluid, protein, and electrolyte uptake. Medications are also used to increase the excretion of potassium and tissue fluids, assuming that the cause is not a urinary blockage.

The nephrologist or other physician may also monitor kidney function through measurements of serum analytes or through observation of certain chemicals within the urine. The levels of blood, urea, and nitrogen (BUN), nitrogenous substances in the blood, present a rough measure of kidney function. Generally, BUN levels change significantly only after glomerular filtration has been significantly disrupted. The levels are also dependent on the amount of protein intake in the diet. When changes occur as a result of renal dysfunction, BUN levels can be a useful marker for the progression of the disease. A more specific indicator of renal function can be the creatinine concentration within the blood. Serum creatinine, unlike BUN levels, is not related to the diet. In the event of renal failure, however, changes in BUN levels usually can be detected earlier than those of creatinine.

As the glomeruli lose their ability to distinguish large from small molecules during filtration, protein can begin to appear in the urine, the condition known as proteinuria. Usually, the level of protein in the urine is negligible (less than 250 milligrams per day). A transient proteinuria can result from heavy exercise or minor illness, but persistent levels of more than 1 gram per day may be indicative of renal dysfunction or even complications of hypertension. Generally, if the problem resides in the loss of tubular reabsorption, levels of protein generally are below 1 to 2 grams per day, with that amount usually consisting of small proteins. If the problem is a result of increased glomerular permeability caused by inflammation, levels may reach greater than 2 grams per day. In cases of nephrotic syndrome, excretion of protein in the urine may exceed 5 grams per day.

Measurement of urine protein is a relatively easy process. A urine sample is placed on a plastic stick with an indicator pad capable of turning colors, depending on the protein concentration. Analogous strips may be used for detection of other materials in urine, including acid, blood, or sugars. The presence of either red or white blood cells in urine can be indicative of infection or glomerulonephritis.

In addition to the filtration of blood fluids through the nephrons, the reabsorption of materials within the tubules results in increased urine concentration. A normal GFR within a healthy kidney produces a urine concentration three or four times as great as that found within serum. As kidney failure progresses, the concentration of urine begins to decrease, with the urine becoming more dilute. The kidneys compensate for the decreased concentration by increasing the amount of urine output: The frequency of urination may increase, as well as the volume excreted (polyuria). In time, if renal failure continues, the GFR will decrease, resulting in the retention of both analytes and water.

Determination of urine concentration is carried out following a brief period of dehydration: deprivation of fluids for about fifteen hours prior to the test. This dehydration will result in increased production by the hypothalamus of antidiuretic hormone (ADH), or vasopressin, a chemical that decreases the production of urine through increased renal tubule reabsorption of water. The result is a more concentrated urine. Following the dehydration period, the patient's urine is collected over a period of three hours and assessed for concentration. Significantly low values may be indicative of kidney disease.

A battery of tests in addition to those already described may be utilized in the diagnosis of kidney disease. These may include intravenous pyelography (in which a contrast medium is injected into the blood and followed as it passes through the kidneys), kidney biopsy, and ultrasound examinations. Diagnosis and course of treatment depend on an evaluation of these tests.

PERSPECTIVE AND PROSPECTS

The roots of modern nephrology date from the seventeenth century. In the early decades of that century, the English physician William Harvey demonstrated the principles of blood circulation and the role of the heart in that process. Harvey's theories opened the door for more extensive analysis of organ systems, both in humans and in other animals. As a result, in 1666, Italian anatomist Marcello Malpighi, while exploring organ structure with the newly developed microscope, discovered the presence of glomeruli (what he called Malpighian corpuscles) within the kidneys. Malpighi thought that these structures were in some way connected with collecting ducts in the kidneys that had recently been found by Lorenzo Bellini. Malpighi also suspected that these structures played a role in urine formation.

Sir William Bowman, in 1832, was the first to describe the true relationship of the corpuscles discovered by Malpighi to urine secretion through the tubules. Bowman's capsule, as it is now called, is a filter that allows only the liquid of the blood, as well as dissolved salts and urea within the blood, into the tubules, from which the urine is secreted. It remained for Carl Ludwig, in 1842, to complete the story. Ludwig suggested that the corpuscles function in a passive manner, in that the filtrate is filtered by means of hydrostatic pressure through the capsule into the tubules and from there concentrated as water and solutes that are reabsorbed.

The first definitive work on urine formation, *The Secretion of the Urine*, was published by Arthur Robertson Cushny in 1917. In the monograph, Cushny offered a thorough analysis of the data published on kidney function. Though Cushny was incorrect in some of his conclusions, the work catalyzed intensive research activity on the functions of the kidney. A colleague of Cushny, E. Brice Mayrs, made the first attempt to determine the glomerular filtration rate, measuring the clearance of sulfate in rabbits. In 1926, the Danish physiologist Poul Brandt Rehberg demonstrated the superiority of creatinine as a marker for glomerular filtration; the "guinea pig" for the experiment was Rehberg himself.

A pioneer in renal physiology, Homer William Smith, began his research while serving in the United States Army during World War I. Until he retired in 1961, Smith was involved in much of the research related to renal excretion. It was Smith who developed inulin clearance as a measure of the GFR; his later years dealt with studies on mechanisms of solute excretion.

With the newer technology of the late twentieth century, more accurate methods for analysis became available. These have included ultrasound scanning, intravenous pyelography, and angiography. In addition, better understanding of immediate causes of many kidney problems has served to control or prevent some forms of renal failure.

—Richard Adler, PhD

See also Abdomen; Abdominal disorders; Adrenalectomy; Blood and blood disorders; Cysts; Diabetes mellitus; Dialysis; Edema; End-stage renal disease; Hemolytic uremic syndrome; Internal medicine; Kidney cancer; Kidney disorders; Kidney transplantation; Kidneys; Lithotripsy; Nephrectomy; Nephritis; Nephrology, pediatric; Polycystic kidney disease; Pyelonephritis; Renal failure; Stone removal; Stones; Systemic lupus erythematosus (SLE); Terminally ill: Extended care; Transplantation; Urinalysis; Urinary system; Urology; Urology, pediatric.

For Further Information:
Brenner, Barry M., ed. *Brenner and Rector's The Kidney*. 8th ed. Philadelphia: Saunders/Elsevier, 2008.
Cameron, Stewart. *Kidney Disease: The Facts*. 2d ed. New York: Oxford University Press, 1990.
Floege, Jurgen, Richard J. Johnson, and John Feehally. *Comprehensive Clinical Nephrology: Expert Consult*. St. Louis: Mosby/Elsevier, 2010.
Hricik, Donald E., R. Tyler Miller, and John R. Sedor, eds. *Nephrology Secrets*. 2d ed. Philadelphia: Hanley & Belfus, 2003.
Legrain, Marcel, et al. *Nephrology*. Trans. M. Cavaillé-Coll. New York: Masson, 1987.

Lerma, Edgar, and Allen R. Nissenson. *Nephrology Secrets*. 3d ed. Philadelphia: Elsevier Mosby, 2011.

Marieb, Elaine N. *Essentials of Human Anatomy and Physiology*. 9th ed. San Francisco: Pearson/Benjamin Cummings, 2009.

Mitchell, Rosner H, and Edgar V. Lerma. *Clinical Decisions in Nephrology, Hypertension and Kidney Transplantation*. New York: Springer, 2013.

O'Callaghan, Chris A., and Barry M. Brenner. *The Kidney at a Glance*. Boston: Blackwell Scientific, 2000.

Tanagho, Emil A., and Jack W. McAninich, eds. *Smith's General Urology*. 17th ed. New York: McGraw-Hill, 2008.

Wallace, Robert A., Gerald P. Sanders, and Robert J. Ferl. *Biology: The Science of Life*. 4th ed. New York: HarperCollins, 1996.

Whitworth, Judith A., and J. R. Lawrence, eds. *Textbook of Renal Disease*. 2d ed. New York: Churchill Livingstone, 1994.

NERVOUS SYSTEM

Category: Anatomy
Anatomy or system affected: Ears, nerves, spine
Specialties and related fields: Neurology
Definition: The major control system of the body, which synchronizes physiologic activity by interpreting incoming stimuli and which is responsible for memory and reasoning; it is composed of the central nervous system (the brain and spinal cord) and the peripheral nervous system (nerve processes, sensory receptors, and ganglia).

Key terms:

cerebrospinal fluid (CSF): the extracellular fluid of the central nervous system; it flows through the ventricles of the brain and the central canal of the spinal cord, circulating nutrients and providing a cushion for the brain

effector: a general term referring to skeletal, smooth, and cardiac muscles or glands that respond to impulses produced by the nervous system

glial cells: nonexcitable cells of the nervous system; they include astrocytes, microglial cells, oligodendrocytes, and Schwann cells

receptors: membrane-bound proteins with specific binding sites for neurotransmitters

synapse: a juncture between neurons or between neurons and muscle

STRUCTURE AND FUNCTIONS

The nervous system serves as the major control system of the human body. It is responsible for the synchronization of body parts, the integration of physiologic activity, the interpretation of incoming stimuli, and all intellectual activity, including memory and abstract reasoning. The nervous system regulates these activities by communication between various nerve cells; by controlling the actions of skeletal, smooth, and cardiac muscle; and by stimulating the secretion of products from various glands of the body.

Anatomically, the nervous system is divided into the central nervous system, which is composed of the brain and the spinal cord, and the peripheral nervous system, which includes all nervous structures outside the central nervous system-primarily nerve processes, sensory receptors, and a limited number of cells of the nervous system that are located in special structures known as ganglia. Ganglia are found at various locations throughout the body. They are the only locations of neurons outside the central nervous system. Information from incoming cells can be transmitted to the ganglion cells, which in turn can transmit that information to other locations.

Although the brain and the spinal cord contain several different types of cells that are morphologically unique, there is only one type of functional cell present, which by convention is always referred to as the neuron. The neuron is one of the few cells in the body that cannot reproduce; a fixed number of these cells develop in infancy, and the number never increases, though it can decrease in the event of injury or disease.

The neuron consists of a cell body that is similar to that of the typical animal cell familiar to most people. In addition, the neuron has extensions called processes. In the typical neuron, there are two types of processes: dendrites and axons.

Usually a neuron has many dendrites. Dendrites are very short; they receive information from nearby cells and relay that information to the cell body. Each cell has only a single axon, which may be very long, extending up and down the spinal cord or from the spinal cord to the ends of the fingers or toes. The axons conduct information from the cell bodies to the effectors-that is, the muscles and glands-or to other neurons.

Functionally, the nervous system is divided into two areas: the somatic nervous system and the autonomic nervous system. The somatic system controls posture and locomotion by stimulating the skeletal muscles. It is responsible for knowing where the body is in space and for ensuring that there is sufficient muscle contraction (tone) to maintain posture. Responses of the somatic system occur through the motor neurons.

The autonomic nervous system regulates internal activities through the innervation, or nerve stimulation, of the smooth muscles or the glands. It is anatomically different from the somatic nervous system in that the stimulation of body parts always involves two neurons. The cell body of the second neuron in the sequence is located in a ganglion outside the central nervous system.

The autonomic nervous system is broken down further into two divisions: the sympathetic and the parasympathetic. The sympathetic system is also known as the "fight or flight" reaction, since it evolved from the mechanism in lower animals by which an animal would prepare to fight a predator or run from it. More commonly, it is referred to in humans as the adrenaline response, which is active during stressful situations, strenuous physical activity, public performance, or competition.

The parasympathetic system, which is responsible for the digestive functions of the body, controls stimulation of salivary gland secretions, increased blood flow to digestive organs, and movement of material through the digestive system. The sympathetic and parasympathetic systems usually function in balance; the parasympathetic system predominates after meals, and the sympathetic system predominates during periods of stress or physical activity.

Neurons communicate with other neurons or effectors through the release of chemical messengers known as neurotransmitters. At the termination of the axon, there is a widened area known as the synaptic knob, which produces and stores neurotransmitters. The effects of neurotransmitters are always localized and of short duration. There are many types of neurotransmitters, some of which are well known, such as acetylcholine and norepinephrine.

Neurotransmitters are released in response to an electrical impulse that is conducted along the axon. Once released, a neurotransmitter binds to cells that have appropriate receptors on their dendrites. Neurotransmitters may either stimulate or inhibit the activity of the second cell. If there is significant stimulation of the second cell, it will conduct the information along its axon and release a neurotransmitter from the axon terminal, which will in turn stimulate or inhibit the next neuron or effector. There must be a mechanism for the immediate removal of neurotransmitters from the synaptic cleft if the stimulation of the second neuron is to cease and if other impulses are to be conducted.

Neurotransmitters can influence only those cells that have the appropriate receptors on their surfaces. It is through the neurotransmitter-receptor complex that neurotransmitters are able to influence cells, and any alteration of the number or type of receptors on a cell membrane will lead to an alteration of cellular functioning.

The axons of some neurons are covered with multiple layers of a cell membrane known as myelin. The myelin is produced by specialized cells in the brain known as oligodendrocytes and by cells in the peripheral axons known as Schwann cells. Myelin serves as an insulator for axons and is effective in speeding up the

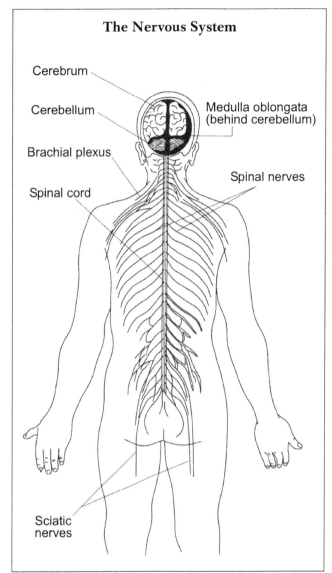

The Nervous System

Cerebrum

Cerebellum

Brachial plexus

Spinal cord

Medulla oblongata (behind cerebellum)

Spinal nerves

Sciatic nerves

©EBSCO

conduction of nerve impulses. It is essential for the normal functioning of the nervous system.

The brain and spinal cord are enclosed by three membranes of dense connective tissue called the meninges, which separate the nervous system from other tissue and from the skull and spinal cord. From the outside inward, they are the dura mater, the arachnoid mater, and the pia mater. Many of the blood vessels of the brain travel through the meninges; therefore, the surface of the brain is very vascular and is subject to bleeding or clotting after trauma.

DISORDERS AND DISEASES
Diseases of the nervous system can be arranged into several general categories: infections, congenital diseases, seizure disorders, circulatory diseases, traumatic injury, demyelinating diseases, degenerative diseases, mental diseases, and neoplasms.

Infections of the nervous system are described according to the tissues infected. If the meninges are infected, the disease is known as meningitis; if the brain tissue is infected, the disease is referred to as encephalitis. The development of abscesses in the nervous tissue can also occur. The conditions described can be caused by viruses, bacteria, protozoa, or other parasites.

In most cases, the organism that causes meningitis is spread via the bloodstream. It is also possible for infections to be spread via an infected middle ear or paranasal sinus, a skull fracture, brain surgery, or a lumbar puncture. The infectious agent can usually be determined by analyzing the spinal fluid. Bacterial infections are treated with antibiotics, while viral infections receive only supportive treatment.

An abscess of nervous tissue is usually a complication resulting from an infection at some other anatomical site, particularly from middle-ear infections or sinus infections. Abscesses may also occur following penetrating injuries. The abscess can create pressure inside the skull and, if left untreated, may rupture and lead to death.

Viral encephalitis is an acute disease that is often spread to humans by arthropods from animal hosts. After a carrier insect bites a human, the virus is spread to the brain of the human via the bloodstream. The specific causative agent often goes undiagnosed. Some well-known forms of encephalitis are herpes simplex encephalitis, poliomyelitis, rabies, and cytomegalovirus encephalitis. In addition, some forms of encephalitis fall into the category of slow virus infections, which have latent periods as long as several years between the time of infection and the development of encephalitis.

Other serious infections include neurosyphilis, which occurs in the late stages of untreated syphilis infections; toxoplasmosis, a protozoan infection that is extremely dangerous to fetuses but rarely causes serious problems in adults; cerebral malaria; and African trypanosomiasis, which is also known as sleeping sickness.

Congenital diseases of the brain vary in the degree of malfunction they produce. Spina bifida is a general term for a group of disorders in which the vertebrae do not develop as they should. As a result, the spinal cord may protrude from the lower back. In some cases, the effects may be so minimal as to produce no symptoms; in other cases, however, these malformations may lead to major neurologic impairment.

Hydrocephalus is another congenital malformation, one that may lead to an increase in the size of the ventricles of the brain. It may be caused by blockage of the flow of spinal fluid in the fetus. In some cases, the spinal fluid produced by the nervous system fills the ventricles and limits the space available for the growing brain and nervous tissue. The result under these conditions is the presence of larger-than-normal ventricles and a smaller-than-normal amount of nervous tissue.

A seizure disorder is any sudden burst of excess electrical activity in the neurons of the brain. Epilepsy is a general term for seizure disorders. The condition may be mild and have only minimal effects, or it may be severe, leading to convulsions. The cause is often unknown, but epilepsy may result from infection, trauma, or neoplasms.

Cerebrovascular accident (CVA) is the term used to describe a variety of malfunctions of blood circulation in the nervous system that are not a result of trauma. More commonly, the term *stroke* is used to describe the condition. Strokes have many causes that generally fall into two categories: ischemic and hemorrhagic.

Ischemic strokes are those in which the nervous tissue is deprived of oxygen as a result of an impairment of blood flow to the area. An ischemic stroke is most commonly the result of a blood clot that blocks the blood vessels leading to the brain or the blood vessels in the brain itself. Since the cells can live for only a few minutes without oxygen, an ischemic stroke can result in neurological impairment or even death.

In hemorrhagic strokes, there is bleeding in the brain itself. It may be caused by hypertension or by the rupture of a weakened blood vessel, which is known as an aneurysm. Both ischemic and hemorrhagic strokes lead to the death of neurons in the affected area. The degree of damage to the brain is determined by the number of cells destroyed by the oxygen deprivation.

Traumatic injury to the brain can generally be classified as penetrating or nonpenetrating. Penetrating injuries produce a risk of infection as well as bleeding at the site of the wound. Since many large blood vessels are located in the meninges, even injuries that penetrate only into the meninges may be sufficient to cause serious injury. Nonpenetrating injuries may also cause bleeding of the meninges, which can limit blood flow to the nervous tissue or put excessive pressure on the tissue.

Injury to the spinal cord may result in severing the spinal cord from the brain. If this should occur, communications between the brain and any structures below the area of the injury are lost, as is all sensory and motor function in those areas. Since neurons are unable to regenerate and axon repair is limited, there is little hope for reversal of this condition, although extensive research is being conducted in this area.

Demyelinating diseases are those that result in changes in the myelin sheaths of neurons. The most common example is multiple sclerosis, which affects myelin in the central nervous system but not in the peripheral nervous system. Although there are varying degrees of severity, the condition causes limb weakness, impaired perception, and optic neuritis, among other things. Some cases present only mild symptoms, while others are degenerative and can lead to death, sometimes within months. Many patients, however, survive for more than twenty years. The cause of these diseases is not yet clear, although viral infections have been associated with some demyelinating diseases.

Degenerative diseases are those in which there is a gradual decline in nervous function. The disease may be hereditary, as in the case of Huntington's disease, or may occur without any apparent genetic basis, as in the case of Parkinson's disease. Parkinson's disease involves the death of certain neurons in the brain and a decreased concentration of neurotransmitters. As the disease progresses, there is a gradual loss of motor ability and, ultimately, a complete loss of motor function. Not much is known about neurotransmitter replacement or mechanisms to stop degenerative diseases.

Little is known about mental diseases such as schizophrenia and manic depression. They appear to involve abnormal levels of neurotransmitters or errors in the membrane receptors associated with those neurotransmitters. Success in localizing the causes of these diseases has been slow in coming; there has been much more success in the development of medications to treat them.

Cancer of the brain can be primary or metastatic. Metastatic tumors, the more common variety, can arise from any source. Of the primary neoplasms, the most common are those derived from glial cells, which are responsible for more than 65 percent of all primary neoplasms. The second most common are neoplasms resulting from transformation of cells of the meninges. Since neurons cannot divide, neuron tumors are almost nonexistent except in children.

PERSPECTIVE AND PROSPECTS

When the control system of the body experiences a malfunction, the effects are wide ranging. Since the nervous system is responsible for regulating so many diverse activities, nervous-system injury or disease must be treated immediately if the patient is to survive. This problem is further complicated by the fact that the brain is a difficult organ to study, because of its location within the skull and because its cells are vital and can be studied only after they have died.

Disease or injury of the cells of the nervous system, especially the brain, creates problems that are unique to that organ for several reasons, including the fact that those cells cannot repair themselves and cannot divide. In addition, the cells of the brain are restricted

to a limited area. The cells of the nervous system are unique in that they are so highly specialized that they are not capable of cell division. As a result, humans have the greatest number of neurons during early childhood. Any neural injury or disease that kills cells results in a decreased number of neurons. Furthermore, the space in the skull is tightly packed with cells and cerebrospinal fluid, leaving no room for blood that might result from an injury or fluid accumulation due to tissue infection or tumors. Any of these conditions will increase the pressure within the skull and will also increase the extent of the injury to the nervous tissue.

Although there is no mechanism for replacing cells that have died, the prognosis is not totally bleak. There are cells in the brain that can, in the event of disease or injury, assume the responsibilities of the dead cells. For example, a person who has lost the capacity to speak following a stroke may be retaught to speak using cells that previously did not perform that function.

Among the problems with which the nervous system must cope, there are many things that can go wrong at the synapse of a neuron. The cell may produce too little or too much neurotransmitter. It is possible that the neurotransmitter may not be released on cue or that, if it is released, the postsynaptic cells will not have the appropriate receptors. There also may be no mechanism for removal of the neurotransmitter from the synaptic cleft. These are only a few of the problems that can interfere with communication between different neurons or between neurons and other effectors. As science learns more about the communication system of neurons, efforts to correct these problems will intensify. Already there are many drugs available that can alter activity at the synapse. Correcting these errors can lead to methods for the treatment of mental diseases.

Someday it may be possible to transplant healthy neurons from one person to another. This procedure may permit physicians to prevent total paralysis in a person who has suffered a broken neck or total loss of motor function in an individual who suffers from Parkinson's disease. In 1990, normal neurons were grown in tissue culture for the first time. Such scientific breakthroughs will lead to more and better treatments for individuals who suffer from diseases of the nervous system.

—Annette O'Connor, PhD

See also Acupressure; Acupuncture; Alzheimer's disease; Amnesia; Amputation; Anesthesia; Anesthesiology; Aneurysmectomy; Aneurysms; Anxiety; Aphasia and dysphasia; Apnea; Aromatherapy; Ataxia; Autism; Balance disorders; Behçet's disease; Bell's palsy; Biofeedback; Botox; Brain; Brain damage; Brain disorders; Brain tumors; Caffeine; Carpal tunnel syndrome; Cells; Cerebral palsy; Cluster headaches; Coma; Computed tomography (CT) scanning; Concussion; Craniotomy; Cysts; Deafness; Dementias; Disk removal; Dizziness and fainting; Dyslexia; Ear infections and disorders; Ear surgery; Ears; Electrical shock; Electroencephalography (EEG); Electromyography; Encephalitis; Epilepsy; Fetal alcohol syndrome; Fetal tissue transplantation; Ganglion removal; Guillain-Barré syndrome; Hallucinations; Head and neck disorders; Headaches; Hearing loss; Hemiplegia; Huntington's disease; Hydrocephalus; Hypothalamus; Intellectual disability; Intraventricular hemorrhage; Laminectomy and spinal fusion; Lead poisoning; Learning disabilities; Leprosy; Leukodystrophy; Lower extremities; Lumbar puncture; Memory loss; Meningitis; Migraine headaches; Motor neuron diseases; Motor skill development; Multiple sclerosis; Narcolepsy; Neuralgia, neuritis, and neuropathy; Neurofibromatosis; Neuroimaging; Neurology; Neurology, pediatric; Neurosurgery; Numbness and tingling; Paget's disease; Palsy; Paralysis; Paraplegia; Parkinson's disease; Physical rehabilitation; Poisoning; Poliomyelitis; Porphyria; Premenstrual syndrome (PMS); Quadriplegia; Rabies; Reflexes, primitive; Restless legs syndrome; Sciatica; Seizures; Sense organs; Shingles; Shock therapy; Skin; Sleep disorders; Snakebites; Spina bifida; Spinal cord disorders; Spine, vertebrae, and disks; Strokes; Sympathectomy; Systems and organs; Tetanus; Tics; Touch; Toxicology; Transient ischemic attacks (TIAs); Tremors; Unconsciousness; Upper extremities; Vagotomy; Vagus nerve.

For Further Information:
Afifi, Adel K., and Ronald A. Bergman. *Functional Neuroanatomy: Text and Atlas.* 2d ed. New York: Lange Medical Books/McGraw-Hill, 2005.

"Autonomic Nervous System Disorders." *MedlinePlus*, April 17, 2013.

Barondes, Samuel H. *Molecules and Mental Illness.* 2d ed. New York: Scientific American, 1999.

Bear, Mark F., Barry W. Connors, and Michael A. Paradiso. *Neuroscience: Exploring the Brain.* 3d ed. Philadelphia: Lippincott Williams & Wilkins, 2007.

Bloom, Floyd E., M. Flint Beal, and David J. Kupfer, eds. *The Dana Guide to Brain Health: A Practical Family Reference from Medical Experts.* New York: Dana Press, 2006.

Goldman, Steven A. "Biology of the Nervous System." *Merck Manual Home Health Handbook*, November 2007.

McCance, Kathryn L., and Sue M. Huether. *Pathophysiology: The Biologic Basis for Disease in Adults and Children.* 6th ed. St. Louis, Mo.: Mosby/Elsevier, 2010.

McLendon, Roger E., Marc K. Rosenblum, and Darell D. Bigner, eds. *Russell and Rubinstein's Pathology of Tumors of the Nervous System.* 7th ed. 2 vols. London: Hodder Arnold, 2006.

"Neurologic Diseases." *MedlinePlus*, July 4, 2013.

Nicholls, John G., et al. *From Neuron to Brain.* 5th ed. Sunderland, Mass.: Sinauer, 2012.

Underwood, J. C. E., and S. S. Cross, eds. *General and Systematic Pathology.* 5th ed. New York: Churchill Livingstone/Elsevier, 2009.

Woolsey, Thomas A., Joseph Hanaway, and Mokhtar H. Gado. *The Brain Atlas: A Visual Guide to the Human Central Nervous System.* 3d ed. Hoboken, N.J.: Wiley, 2007.

NEURALGIA, NEURITIS, AND NEUROPATHY

Category: Disease/Disorder
Anatomy or system affected: Nerves, nervous system, spine
Specialties and related fields: Neurology
Definition: Pathological conditions affecting the peripheral nerves of the body and interfering with the proper functioning of those nerves.
Key terms:

autonomic neuropathy: a disorder involving the nerves that work independently of conscious control, and including those nerves that go to small blood vessels, sweat glands, the urinary bladder, the gastrointestinal tract, and the genital organs

axon: the portion of a neuron that carries electrical impulses away from the nerve cell body

mononeuropathy: a neuropathy involving only one peripheral nerve

nerve: a bundle of sensory and motor neurons held together by layers of connective tissue

neuralgia: pain associated with a nerve, often caused by inflammation or injury

neuritis: inflammation of a nerve

neuron: a nerve cell that is capable of conducting electrical impulses; several different types of neurons exist, including motor neurons, sensory neurons, and interneurons

neuropathy: a disorder that causes a functional disturbance of a peripheral nerve, brought about by any cause

peripheral nervous system: the portion of the nervous system found outside the brain and spinal cord

polyneuropathy: a disease that involves a disturbance in the function of several peripheral nerves

CAUSES AND SYMPTOMS

Peripheral nerves, those nerves found outside the brain and spinal cord, function to carry information between the central nervous system and the other portions of the body. These peripheral nerves consist of a bundle of nerve cells, also called neurons, which are wrapped in a protective sheath of connective tissue. A nerve consisting only of neurons that carry impulses toward the central nervous system is termed a sensory nerve. Nerves that contain only neurons that carry information from the central nervous system to the periphery of the body are called motor nerves, because they usually carry information telling a particular body part to move. Most nerves, however, consist of both sensory and motor neurons and are thus called mixed nerves.

The nerves of the peripheral nervous system can be divided into two different categories, cranial nerves and spinal nerves. Cranial nerves come directly out of the brain and supply information to and about the head and neck. There are twelve pairs of cranial nerves. Spinal nerves come directly out of the spinal cord and provide information to and from the arms, legs, chest, gut, and all other parts of the body not supplied by cranial nerves. In humans, there are usually thirty-one pairs of spinal nerves. Both cranial and spinal nerves can be affected by neuropathies.

Neurons (nerve cells) are highly specialized structures designed to convey information from one part of the body to another. This information is passed along in the form of electrical impulses. Neurons consist of three main parts: a cell body, which contains the nucleus and is the control center of the entire neuron; dendrites, which are slender, fingerlike extensions that convey electrical impulses toward the cell body; and an axon, which is a slender extension that carries electrical impulses away from the cell body.

Most of the dendrites and axons of peripheral nerves are covered with a white, fatty substance called myelin. Myelin acts to protect and insulate axons and dendrites. By insulating the axons and dendrites, myelin actually speeds up the rate at which an electrical impulse can be carried along these two structures. Damage to the myelin sheath surrounding axons and dendrites can greatly impair the function of a nerve.

Often, when a nerve becomes pinched, damaged, or inflamed, the result is excessive electrical stimulation of the nerve, which will be registered as pain. The pain associated with the damaged nerve is referred to as neuralgia. One of the most common forms of neuralgia occurs upon the striking of the "funny bone." This area around the elbow is the spot where the ulnar nerve is easily accessible. The ulnar nerve runs from just under the shoulder to the little finger, and when the ulnar nerve is struck near the elbow it is compressed or pinched, leading to pain or a tingling sensation from the elbow down to the little finger.

Compression of nerves for prolonged periods can also lead to neuralgia. The most common example of compression neuralgia is carpal tunnel syndrome. In this syndrome, the median nerve becomes compressed at the wrist, usually as a result of an inflammation of the sheaths of the tendons located on either side of the median nerve. The swelling of these tendon sheaths causes the compression of the median nerve, which may initially lead to neuralgia. As this condition progresses, it can lead to a loss of feeling along the palm side of the thumb and the index and middle fingers. This condition is most common in people who use their fingers for rigorous work over prolonged periods of time, such as typing.

INFORMATION ON NEURALGIA, NEURITIS, AND NEUROPATHY

Causes: Wide ranging; may include toxic exposure to solvents, pesticides, or heavy metals; viral infection; certain medications; excessive alcohol use; vitamin deficiency; loss of blood to nerve; carpal tunnel syndrome; injury; disease (e.g., leprosy, shingles, diabetes)

Symptoms: Pain; inflammation; tingling, prickling, and burning sensations; inability to perceive touch, heat, cold, or pressure; localized muscle weakness

Duration: Acute to chronic

Treatments: Depends on cause; may include antibiotics, anti-inflammatory drugs, surgery

---

Sciatica is another common form of neuralgia, in which pain is associated with the sciatic nerve. The sciatic nerve is the longest nerve in the human body, running from the pelvis down the back of the thigh to the lower leg and then down to the soles of the feet. The symptoms of sciatica include sharp pains along the sciatic nerve. The pain may involve the buttocks, hip, back, posterior thigh, leg, ankle, and foot. Sciatica can result from many different causes, but the most common cause is from a ruptured intervertebral disk that puts pressure on, or causes a pinching of, the sciatic nerve.

Neuritis is defined as the inflammation of a nerve or of the connective tissue that surrounds the nerve. Many diseases can lead to the inflammation of peripheral nerves. Perhaps the most common disease leading to neuritis is shingles. Shingles are caused by the occurrence of herpes zoster, a virus that attacks the dorsal root ganglion, a place near the spinal cord that houses the cell bodies of neurons. A rash, swelling, and pain progress from the dorsal root ganglion along one or more spinal nerves. The rash along the course of the spinal nerves usually disappears within a few days to a couple of weeks, but the pain along this path can persist for months.

Leprosy is another disease that leads to the inflammation of nerves. Leprosy is a bacterial disease caused by *Mycobacterium leprae*. These bacteria invade the cells that make up the myelin sheath that surrounds the nerve. The result is a noticeable swelling of the nerves affected, primarily those that are close to the skin. Many times, this swelling will lead to neuralgia and, if left untreated, to muscle wasting.

"Neuropathy" is a general term used to describe a decrease in the function of peripheral nerves, which may be caused by many factors. The first signs of a neuropathy are usually a tingling, prickling, or burning sensation in some part of the body. This is followed by a sensory loss; the inability to perceive touch, heat, cold, or pressure; and a weakness in the muscles in the area affected. This weakness may eventually lead to a loss of muscle termed muscular atrophy. Neuropathies may affect sensory neurons, motor neurons, or both and can occur in both spinal and cranial nerves. A neuropathy may develop over a few days or many years. Neuropathies can be caused by a number of factors, including toxic exposure to solvents, pesticides, or heavy metals; viral illness; certain medications; metabolic disturbances such as diabetes mellitus; excessive use of alcohol; vitamin deficiency; loss of blood to the nerve; or cold exposure.

Neuropathies can be categorized based on the number of nerves that they affect, whether it is the myelin sheath surrounding the axon that is affected or the axon itself is destroyed, and the amount of time before symptoms of the neuropathy occur and progress. Thus, neuropathies are usually broken down into four different types: polyneuropathy, in which more than one nerve is affected; mononeuropathy, in which only one nerve is affected; axonal neuropathy, in which the axon is affected and degenerates; and demyelinating neuropathy, in which the myelin sheath surrounding the nerve is destroyed. Each of the four categories can be further subdivided based on the time frame in which the symptoms occur. Those neuropathies that appear over days are termed acute, those that appear over weeks are termed subacute, and those neuropathies whose symptoms slowly appear over months or years are termed chronic.

Another type of neuropathy is autonomic neuropathy, a condition that affects the nerves of the autonomic nervous system. These are the peripheral nerves that go to the sweat glands, small blood vessels, gastrointestinal tract, urinary bladder, and genital organs. These nerves are referred to as autonomic since they automatically provide information between these organs and the central nervous system without the individual's conscious effort. The symptoms associated with this form of neuropathy include loss of control over urination, difficulty swallowing food, occasional stomach upset, diarrhea, impotence, and excessive sweating.

The most common cause of neuropathies in the Western world is diabetes mellitus, while leprosy is the more common cause of neuropathies elsewhere. It is estimated that at least 70 percent of all diabetics have some degree of peripheral neuropathy. In most of these cases, the neuropathy is very slight and causes the patient no noticeable symptoms. In about 10 percent of those diabetics with a neuropathy, however, the symptoms will be serious.

TREATMENT AND THERAPY

Often, the first notable feature of a neuropathy that prompts a patient to seek medical attention is a tingling, prickling, or burning sensation in a particular area of the body. The occurrence of these sensations without any external stimuli is termed paresthesias. Since diabetes is the most common cause of neuropathy in the Western world, the sensations experienced by a diabetic patient can serve as an example of the symptoms that are associated with common neuropathies. These patients may first notice the above-mentioned symptoms in the balls of the feet or tips of the toes. As the neuropathy progresses, patients may lose feeling in their feet and experience a weakness in the muscles of the feet, leading to a difficulty in flexing the toes upward. This makes walking difficult, and many patients remark that they feel as if they are walking on stumps. This condition may lead to difficulties in maintaining balance. The neuropathy will begin to affect the legs above the ankles and then travel up the legs, eventually leading to atrophy of the leg muscles.

As the neuropathy worsens, it is critical that patients seek help because they can no longer feel pain. This situation is dangerous, as the patient may no longer sense the pain that can be caused by injuries from sharp objects or even a pebble in the shoe. If unnoticed, these injuries lead to ulcers that can easily become infected.

The first step in treating a neuropathy is to diagnose the type of neuropathy affecting the patient. A patient's medical history is taken to identify any recent viral or bacterial illness, any exposure to toxic substances such as pesticides or heavy metals, the patient's habits concerning alcohol use, or any other illness or injury that might have brought about a possible neuropathy. Next, a physical exam will be performed to determine if the patient's sensations regarding touch, pain, pressure, or temperature have been affected, as well as the ability of the patient to react to these stimuli. The physician may also feel the affected area to determine if the nerve or nerves are inflamed and enlarged.

If the patient's history and the physical examination point toward a neuropathy, further testing using electrodiagnostic tests will be performed. These tests measure the speed at which an electrical impulse travels down a nerve, which is called the nerve conduction velocity. Motor nerve conduction velocity is measured by stimulating the nerve with electrodes placed on the skin above the nerve. Stimulation of the nerve is typically done at two different sites. Using the arm as an example, one electrode would be placed on the inside of the arm at the elbow. The time that it takes for the impulse to reach a recording electrode on the thumb would be measured. A second site at the wrist would be tested to determine the time that it takes for the electrical impulse to reach the recording electrode on the thumb. The time that it took for the impulse to travel from the wrist to thumb would be subtracted from the amount of time that it took for the impulse to go from the inside of the arm at the elbow to the thumb. The resulting value would then be divided by the distance between the site at the wrist and the site at the elbow, giving a nerve conduction velocity value measured in meters per second.

The typical nerve conduction velocity for the motor and sensory peripheral nerves of adults is approximately 40 to 80 meters per second. If a neuropathy is the result of demyelination, the affected nerve will have a much slower nerve conduction velocity. If the neuropathy is a result of axonal damage, then the nerve conduction velocity is usually not altered from normal. Thus, electrodiagnostic testing helps to determine if the neuropathy is a demyelination neuropathy or an axonal neuropathy. Such a determination is important because the different neuropathies are caused by different diseases and are thus treated differently. Electrodiagnostic tests can also provide useful information regarding the site of the neuropathy and whether the neuropathy is affecting sensory neurons, motor neurons, or both.

The last diagnostic test to be performed, if other methods are inconclusive, is a biopsy of the affected nerve. This procedure involves the surgical removal of a portion of the afflicted nerve. The small sample of nerve will be placed under a microscope and examined for specific changes in the nerve. The nerve sample may also be subjected to various biochemical studies to determine if metabolic disturbances have occurred. Nerve biopsies are rarely performed, however, and are usually not recommended.

Once the type of neuropathy afflicting the patient has been determined, treatment can begin. Unlike axons in the central nervous system, axons in the peripheral nervous system are capable of regenerating under certain conditions. If the neuropathy is the result of exposure to toxic substances such as pesticides or heavy metals, removal of the patient from the exposure to such substances is the simple cure. If the neuropathy is the result of viral or bacterial infections, the treatment and recovery from these infections will also usually correct the neuropathy. The same principle applies to neuropathies caused by metabolic diseases and vitamin deficiencies: corrections of these problems will lead to the correction of the neuropathy.

Should the neuropathy be of the mononeuropathy type and caused by trauma, anti-inflammatory drugs such as corticosteroids may be used or surgery may be performed to repair the nerve. If the mononeuropathy

is caused by compression, as in carpal tunnel syndrome, surgery may also be needed to increase the space around the nerve and thus relieve the compression. Surgery is also used to remove tumors on the nerve that might be causing a neuropathy.

The time required to recover from a neuropathy is dependent on the severity and type of neuropathy. Recovery from demyelination is typically quicker than recovery from axonal neuropathies. If only the myelin surrounding the axon is damaged, and not the axon itself, the axon can quickly replace the damaged myelin. Demyelinating neuropathies usually require three to four weeks for recovery. In contrast, recovery from axonal neuropathies may take from two months to more than a year, depending on the severity of the neuropathy.

PERSPECTIVE AND PROSPECTS

Perhaps the earliest documentation of peripheral neuropathies occurred during biblical times, when the term "leprosy" was coined. It is likely, however, that this term was employed rather loosely, as it was used to describe not only the disease leprosy but also a number of skin diseases not involving neuropathies, such as psoriasis.

The actual diagnosis of neuropathies and their subsequent categorization did not occur until the advent of electrical diagnostic testing. The earliest use of electricity to study nerve function occurred in 1876 when German neurologist Wilhelm Erb noted that the electrical stimulation of a damaged peripheral nerve below the site of injury resulted in muscular contraction. In contrast, electrical stimulation at a site above the injured nerve brought about no activity in the muscle. Erb concluded that the injury blocked the flow of electrical impulses down the nerve.

The actual use of electrical diagnostic testing did not take place until the late 1940s, when electrodes and an oscilloscope, an instrument that measures electrical activity, were used to measure the rate at which an electrical impulse could travel down a nerve. This discovery allowed the testing of nerve function and would become useful in the discrimination between axonal and demyelinating neuropathies. During this period, the invention of the electron microscope and the discovery of better nerve-staining techniques enhanced the ability of scientists to study the physiological and anatomical changes that occur in nerves with the onset of neuropathies.

Neuropathies received considerable attention in 1976 when approximately five hundred cases of the neuropathy called Guillain-Barré syndrome occurred in the United States following a national vaccination program for swine flu. The reason that the swine flu vaccine caused this neuropathy has never been discovered, but this syndrome often occurs after an upper respiratory tract or gastrointestinal infection.

Those suffering from neuropathies that result from exposure to toxic substances, viral or bacterial infections, or metabolic diseases have a good prognosis of recovery if the underlying cause of the neuropathy is treated. The prognosis of recovery is not as good for those who suffer neuropathies as a result of hereditary diseases. Advances made in genetic research and continued research in gene therapy may someday greatly increase the prognosis of recovery for those suffering from hereditary neuropathies.

—*David K. Saunders, PhD*

See also Batten's disease; Botox; Carpal tunnel syndrome; Cerebral palsy; Chiari malformations; Cluster headaches; Diabetes mellitus; Electromyography; Encephalitis; Epilepsy; Guillain-Barré syndrome; Hallucinations; Headaches; Hemiplegia; Huntington's disease; Lead poisoning; Leprosy; Leukodystrophy; Meningitis; Migraine headaches; Motor neuron diseases; Multiple sclerosis; Nervous system; Neuroimaging; Neurology; Neurology, pediatric; Neurosurgery; Numbness and tingling; Pain; Palsy; Paralysis; Paraplegia; Parkinson's disease; Quadriplegia; Radiculopathy; Restless legs syndrome; Sciatica; Seizures; Shingles; Sympathectomy; Tics; Vagotomy; Vagus nerve.

For Further Information:

"Conditions." *Facial Neuralgia Resources*, Jan. 31, 2007.

Kandel, Eric R., James H. Schwartz, and Thomas M. Jessell, eds. *Principles of Neural Science*. 5th ed. Norwalk, Conn.: Appleton and Lange, 2006.

"Knowledge Base." *TNA Facial Pain Association*, Apr. 18, 2013.

Margolis, Simeon, and Hamilton Moses III, eds. *The Johns Hopkins Medical Handbook: The One Hundred Major Medical Disorders of People over the Age of Fifty*. Rev. ed. Garden City, N.Y.: Random House, 1999.

Marieb, Elaine N. *Essentials of Human Anatomy and Physiology*. 10th ed. San Francisco: Pearson/Benjamin Cummings, 2012.

"NINDS Peripheral Neuropathy Information Page." *National Institute of Neurological Disorders and Stroke*, Sept. 19, 2012.

Parker, James N., and Philip M. Parker, eds. *The Official Patient's Sourcebook on Peripheral Neuropathy*. San Diego, Calif.: Icon Health, 2002.

"Peripheral Nerve Disorders." *MedlinePlus*, May 9, 2013.

Senneff, John A. *Numb Toes and Other Woes: More on Peripheral Neuropathy*. San Antonio, Tex.: MedPress, 2001.

Stahl, Rebecca J., and Rimas Lukas. "Neuropathic Pain." *Health Library*, Mar. 15, 2013.

NEUROETHICS

Category: Ethics

Specialties and related fields: Bioethics, neuroscience, addiction research, social psychology

Definition: Two interrelated disciplines: the ethical, societal, and legal implications of neuroscience, and the cognitive basis for ethics and moral behavior.

Key terms:

brain-machine interface: direct communication between a living brain and a computer or other external device

neuroenhancement: drugs or therapies that improve or modify cognition

neuroimaging: a category of research techniques that produce images of brain anatomy and/or activity

psychopathy: a class of behavioral disorders characterized by a lack of remorse and empathy, antisocial behavior, and poor self-control

SCIENCE AND PROFESSION

The easiest definition of neuroethics is "the neuroscience of ethics, and the ethics of neuroscience." While this is perhaps too glib, it encapsulates the dual nature of the discipline-one that allows professionals from many disciplines to fit under the "neuroethics" umbrella. Neuroethicists range in profession from lawyers to policymakers, with concentrations in neuroscience and philosophy.

Legal teams often consult with neuroethicists about the use of neuroscience in the courtroom, especially as it pertains to personal responsibility. Some have argued that the neurological basis of morality should play a role in how offenders are prosecuted and treated. Using neuroimaging as a lie detector test has been widely debated, although it has been largely dismissed from American courts.

Neuroethicists also influence public policy about the ethical use of neuroscientific information and research, sitting on panels such as the Presidential Commission for the Study of Bioethical Issues.

Doctors and neuroscientists are frequently confronted with neuroethical questions. In the course of their research, scientists may discover unexpected health information, such as a predisposition to a progressive neurological disorder. They must then decide whether to disclose this information to the subject. Patients also regularly ask their physicians for prescriptions to drugs with off-label uses as neuroenhancers, including attention deficit hyperactivity disorder (ADHD) and narcolepsy medications.

A number of major universities now have departments exclusively dedicated to neuroethics. They generally grant masters and PhD's in the discipline. There are also two peer-reviewed neuroethics journals, Neuroethics and the American Journal of Bioethics-Neuroscience (AJOB-Neuro).

PERSPECTIVE AND PROSPECTS

Both neuroscience ethics and the cognitive basis for morality have a long tradition in medicine, as well as in law and philosophy. However, neuroethics as a defined field can be traced back to a Dana Foundation meeting called "Neuroethics: Mapping the Field." The proceedings of this meeting were published in a book that has become a widely-used reference guide.

Some neuroethics topics are simply bioethical issues that are specific to neuroscience. The idea of "brain doping," sometimes called cosmetic pharmacology, taps into the wider discussion of improving performance in healthy people, although there is the added dimension of personhood and morality. Because of these additional layers, neuroethics can diverge widely from traditional biomedical ethics to include issues of the self and identity.

For instance, some neuroethicists have discussed a "morality pill," a theoretical pill that could make a person more likely to adhere to a given set of ethics (i.e., giving a psychopath a treatment for empathy). Many mental illnesses or personality disorders might be treatable with direct intervention, but potential loss of memory or personality must be weighed against the benefits.

The use of brain scans in the courtroom is often a cause for controversy. Some data shows a correlation between psychopathy and specific patterns of brain activity or anatomy, rising to a discussion of biology versus responsibility. If a person is biologically incapable of controlling their impulses, are they still legally responsible for their actions?

The growing use of brain-machine interfaces is another ripe topic for discussion. Brain implants have been used to restore vision to the blind, while gamers can don special headsets to turn brainwaves into screen action. Each use of a brain-machine interface requires a risk-benefit analysis. Is the implant safe enough? Will "mind-reading" devices violate privacy? Neuroethicists have even been called on to discuss the use of mind reading in police or military interrogations.

Future neuroethical discussions will likely focus on access to and use of new, better neuroenhancement techniques, and privacy issues arising from the use of neuroscience in marketing, law, and medical treatment.

—*Caroline Taylor Ferguson*

See also Cognitive enhancement; Concussion; Neurology; Neuroscience; Traumatic brain injury

For Further Information:

The Center for Neuroscience and Society at the University of Pennsylvania. neuroethics.upenn.edu/. Up-to-the-minute information on neuroethics news and events, as well as educational resources and briefs on a number of neuroethics topics.

Churchland, Patricia. *Braintrust: What Neuroscience Tells Us about Morality*. Princeton, NJ: Princeton University Press, 2011. Written for a general audience, Churchland discusses the biological basis of empathy, cooperation, and other moral behaviors.

Farah, Martha J., ed. *Neuroethics: An Introduction with Readings*. Cambridge, MA: MIT Press, 2010. A primer packed with writings from prominent neuroethicists around the world, commonly used in classroom settings.

Gazzaniga, Michael. *The Ethical Brain*. New York: Dana Press, 2005. Written by the father of cognitive neuroscience, this compulsively readable book covers the biological basis of morality, personhood, and enhancement.

Glannon, Walter. *Bioethics and the Brain*. New York: Oxford University Press, 2006. Glannon focuses on the ethical implications of modern neuroscience technologies at a graduate school-level.

Illes, Judy, and Barbara J. Sahakian, eds. *Oxford Handbook of Neuroethics*. Oxford: Oxford University Press, 2011. Features 50 chapters that cover the majority of the field so far, written by a variety of the leading experts.

The International Neuroethics Society website, www.neuroethicssociety.org. Includes information on the annual meeting, links to books and blogs by members, and a calendar of neuroethics-related events.

Levy, Neil. *Neuroethics: Challenges for the 21st Century*. Cambridge: Cambridge University Press, 2007. This graduate school-level book delves into the philosophy underlying neuroethical studies.

Marcus, Steven J., ed. *Neuroethics: Mapping the Field*. New York: Dana Press, 2004. Proceedings of the 2002 Dana Foundation meeting that defined neuroethics as a discipline.

Sahakian, Barbara, and Jamie N. LaBuzetta. *Bad Moves: How Decision Making Goes Wrong and the Ethics of Smart Drugs*. New York: Oxford University Press, 2013. The authors discuss what scientists know about the biological underpinnings of decision making, and how that can be altered with drugs.

NEUROFIBROMATOSIS

Category: Disease/Disorder
Also known as: Von Recklinghausen disease
Anatomy or system affected: Bones, nervous system, skin
Specialties and related fields: Dermatology, genetics, neurology, orthopedics, plastic surgery
Definition: A genetic disease affecting the nervous system, skin, and bones that produces multiple nerve tumors (neurofibromas), deeply pigmented areas of skin (café-au-lait spots), and bone deformities.

CAUSES AND SYMPTOMS

Most infants born with neurofibromatosis, which is also known as Von Recklinghausen disease, have few symptoms until puberty. Disease progression and signs and symptoms vary from mild (in about one-third of affected children) to moderate and severe disfigurement and organ failure. The disease causes abnormal growths of nerve tissue along the peripheral nerve tracts of the head, neck, trunk, and extremities, usually involving the brain and spinal cord (the central nervous system) later. These so-called neurofibromas appear as multiple, visible growths lying beneath the skin. Also typical are the many areas of deeply pigmented skin, known as café-au-lait (coffee-and-milk) spots. In addition, severely disfiguring bone defects of the skull and spine can be caused by neurofibromas.

Some patients lead nearly normal lives, with only cosmetic problems from the café-au-lait spots and visible neurofibromas. Most patients, however, experience serious consequences from deep growths and skeletal deformities. Depending on the size and location of these tumors, they can cause blindness, deafness, developmental disorders, seizures, pain, and paralysis. Other organs, especially the kidneys and glands, are frequently damaged as well. The most feared complication is the transformation of these benign tumors into cancerous ones.

TREATMENT AND THERAPY
No cure exists for neurofibromatosis. Supportive therapy includes surgical removal of the neurofibromas

MRI image showing malignant peripheral nerve sheath tumor in the left tibia in neurofibromatosis type-1. Photo by Filip via Wikimedia Commons.

INFORMATION ON NEUROFIBROMATOSIS
Causes: Genetic factors
Symptoms: Multiple nerve tumors, deeply pigmented areas of skin (café-au-lait spots), bone deformities
Duration: Chronic
Treatments: Supportive therapy, including surgical removal of neurofibromas, reconstructive plastic surgery to correct disfigurement, counseling

and reconstructive plastic surgery for the sometimes severe disfigurement that can result from deep tumors and bone deformities. The skull, spine, and eye sockets are particularly affected. Social isolation and embarrassment are serious problems with neurofibromatosis, and counseling is essential. The prognosis is variable depending on the size and location of the tumors. Both cancer and organ failure can shorten the patient's life.

Because neurofibromatosis is genetic, occurring in one in three thousand births, genetic analysis of the parents is essential if there is a family history of the disease. Prenatal testing can determine if the fetus has inherited the defect. Research is now focusing on correcting the genetic error in the developing fetus.

—*Connie Rizzo, MD, PhD*

See also Bone disorders; Bones and the skeleton; Dermatology; Dermatopathology; Genetic diseases; Genetics and inheritance; Nervous system; Neuralgia, neuritis, and neuropathy; Neurology; Neurology, pediatric; Skin; Skin cancer; Skin disorders; Skin lesion removal; Tumor removal; Tumors.

For Further Information:
Ablon, Joan. *Living with Genetic Disorder: The Impact of Neurofibromatosis.* Westport, Conn.: Auburn House, 2001.
Children's Tumor Foundation. www.ctf.org.
Currey, John D. *Bones: Structures and Mechanics.* 2d ed. Princeton, N.J.: Princeton University Press, 2006.
Daube, Jasper R., ed. *Clinical Neurophysiology.* 3d ed. New York: Oxford University Press, 2009.
Korf, Bruce R., and Allan E. Rubenstein. *Neurofibromatosis: A Handbook for Patients, Families, and Health Care Professionals.* 2d ed. New York: Thieme Medical, 2005.
"Learning About Neurofibromatosis." *National Human Genome Research Institute,* September 16, 2012.
"Neurofibromatosis Fact Sheet." *National Institute of Neurological Disorders and Stroke,* January 13, 2012.
Nicholls, John G., A. Robert Martin, and Bruce G. Wallace. *From Neuron to Brain.* 4th ed. Sunderland, Mass.: Sinauer, 2007.
Rosenblum, Laurie. "Neurofibromatosis." *Health Library,* August 30, 2012.
Victor, Maurice, and Allan H. Ropper. *Adams and Victor's Principles of Neurology.* 9th ed. New York: McGraw-Hill, 2009.

NEUROIMAGING

Category: Procedure
Also known as: Neuroradiology
Anatomy or system affected: Back, blood vessels, brain, head, neck, nerves, nervous system, spine
Specialties and related fields: All
Definition: The art and science of photographing living brain or nervous system tissue.
Key terms:
cerebral angiography: X-ray photography of blood vessels inside the skull
computed tomography (CT): originally computed axial tomography (CAT) scan; any of several techniques, with or without contrast media, for creating images of internal body structures by means of the mathematical reconstruction of a large series of parallel sectional X rays
contrast medium: any substance or chemical that is inserted, ingested, or injected into the body to improve the visibility of certain parts seen by X-ray or other medical imaging technique
echoencephalography: a technique of using reflected ultrasound to create a graphic representation of brain structures
electroencephalography (EEG): electronic measurement and graphic depiction of brain waves
magnetic resonance imaging (MRI): a technique of creating images by resonating hydrogen nuclei inside the body
magnetoencephalography (MEG): a type of MRI, designed to measure brain activity directly rather than infer it from other data
positron emission tomography (PET): a type of CT using a short-lived radioactive isotope as a contrast medium
single photon emission computed tomography (SPECT): a type of CT using a gamma camera to record the pattern of gamma rays emitted from a radioactive drug given to the patient

INDICATIONS AND PROCEDURES

Images of the living brain or other part of the central nervous system are indicated for any disorder anywhere in the body that may have neurological involvement or complications. Psychiatrists may also order neurological images for their patients whose mental disorders may have physical causes. Typical indications for neuroradiologic diagnosis include cancer, stroke, and head trauma, especially closed head injury.

Depending on what tissue is involved and what condition is suspected, the physician may order any of dozens of neuroimaging methods. The most common in the early twenty-first century are computed tomography (CT), magnetic resonance imaging (MRI), posi-

tron emission tomography (PET), single photon emission computed tomography (SPECT), and magnetoencephalography (MEG). Additional methods include electroencephalography (EEG), near infrared spectroscopy (NIRS), diffuse optical imaging (DOI), and other techniques.

USES AND COMPLICATIONS

Besides clinical uses in diagnosing disease in individual patients, neuroimaging is also valuable as a research tool for studying Alzheimer's disease, Parkinson's disease, multiple sclerosis, epilepsy, and other degenerative and acute conditions that affect the central nervous system. It can also increase the understanding of drug effects on the brain, natural aging processes, brain function localization, autism, psychiatric disorders, and many other kinds of physiological events. Well-funded initiatives exist for "brain mapping" to create precise, molecular-level, function-specific atlases of the human brain, as well as the brains of mice, rats, and many other animals. The Laboratory of Neuro Imaging (LONI) at the University of California, Los Angeles (UCLA) is the world leader in this kind of research.

Risks are minimal for patients undergoing brain scans. Usually the worst that can happen is that the scan may provide inadequate diagnosis. The physical dangers are generally the same as for CT or MRI scans on other parts of the body. Occasionally, CT brain scans trigger seizures, especially in children. The chance of these inadvertent seizures is much less with MRI. Another safety advantage of MRI over CT is that MRI does not use radioactive materials. On the other hand, MRIs can be harmful if there is metal inside the body, such as from bone or joint repair, or a pacemaker; doctors must be notified of this ahead of time.

PERSPECTIVE AND PROSPECTS

Neuroimaging began almost immediately after German physicist Wilhelm Conrad Röntgen discovered x-rays in 1895. The limits of using plain film x-rays to diagnose nervous system diseases and other soft tissue disorders soon became apparent. Nevertheless, because of its simplicity and thanks to the pioneering work of Austrian neurologist Artur Schüller and Swedish radiologist Erik Lysholm, physicians until the early 1970s generally preferred plain film to the three other methods available for intracranial and spinal diagnosis: pneumography, radiopaque myelography, and cerebral angiography. These other three all involved using contrast media to improve the detail in the x-ray.

American physician Walter Dandy invented pneumography at Johns Hopkins University in 1918. After observing that x-rays show air as black, soft tissue as gray, and bone as white, Dandy developed techniques to inject air into the central nervous system to serve as a contrast medium. The resulting x-rays clearly highlighted abnormalities such as tumors, but the technique was very dangerous. French scientists Jean Athanase Sicard and Jacques Forestier developed radiopaque myelography, the use of contrast media in spinal x-rays, in the early 1920s.

In the 1920s, Portuguese physician António Egas Moniz developed cerebral angiography, a technique in which a rapid series of skull x-rays were taken immediately after injecting a radioactive contrast medium into both carotid arteries. This proved to be an excellent method of showing abnormalities and displacements caused by tumors, but was disfavored because of its significant danger to the patient and the ugly surgical scars left on the patient's neck.

British physicist Godfrey Newbold Hounsfield and his team of radiologists built the first practical clinical CT scanning machine in 1971. Between 1971 and 1977, several scientists developed practical MRI from facts about the magnetic properties of atomic nuclei that had been known since the 1950s. These two methods soon superseded both plain film and cerebral angiography as the preferred methods of neuroimaging. Today, there are a great variety of specialized MRI techniques geared toward different kinds of body imaging and diagnosis; an especially important one for brain imaging is functional MRI (fMRI), which can measure neural activity.

—*Eric v. d. Luft, PhD, MLS*

See also Angiography; Brain; Computed tomography (CT) scanning; Echocardiography; Imaging and radiology; Magnetic resonance imaging (MRI); Mammography; Nervous system; Noninvasive tests; Nuclear medicine; Nuclear radiology; Positron emission tomography (PET) scanning; Radiation sickness; Radiation therapy; Radiopharmaceuticals; Single photon emission computed tomograph (SPECT); Ultrasonography.

For Further Information:
Cabeza, Roberto, and Alan Kingstone, eds. *Handbook of Functional Neuroimaging of Cognition*. 2d ed. Cambridge, Mass.: MIT Press, 2006.
Carter, Rita, and Christopher D. Frith. *Mapping the Mind*. Rev. ed. Berkeley: University of California Press, 2010.
Clarke, Edwin, and Kenneth Dewhurst. *An Illustrated History of Brain Function: Imaging the Brain from Antiquity to the Present*. 2d rev. ed. San Francisco: Norman, 1996.
Damasio, Hanna. *Human Brain Anatomy in Computerized Images*. 2d ed. New York: Oxford University Press, 2005.
D'Esposito, Mark. *Functional MRI: Applications in Clinical Neurology and Psychiatry*. Boca Raton, Fla.: Taylor & Francis, 2006.
Dumit, Joseph. *Picturing Personhood: Brain Scans and Biomedical Identity*. Princeton, N.J.: Princeton University Press, 2004.
Mori, Susumu, et al. *MRI Atlas of Human White Matter*. Boston: Elsevier, 2005.
"Neuroimaging and Mental Illness: A Window into the Brain." *National Institutes of Mental Health*, 2013.
"Neurological Imaging." *National Institutes of Health*, March 29, 2013.
Taveras, Juan M. "Diamond Jubilee Lecture: Neuroradiology-Past, Present, and Future." *Radiology* 175 (1990): 593-602.
Toga, Arthur W., and John C. Mazziotta, eds. *Brain Mapping: The Methods*. 2d ed. Boston: Academic Press, 2002.
Toga, Arthur W., and John C. Mazziotta, eds. *Brain Mapping: The Systems*. San Diego, Calif.: Academic Press, 2000.
Toga, Arthur W., John C. Mazziotta, and Richard S. J. Frackowiak, eds. *Brain Mapping: The Disorders*. San Diego, Calif.: Academic Press, 2000.
Van Bruggen, Nick, and Timothy P. L. Roberts, eds. *Biomedical Imaging in Experimental Neuroscience*. Boca Raton, Fla.: CRC Press, 2003.

NEUROLOGY

Category: Specialty
Anatomy or system affected: Brain, ears, hands, head, muscles, musculoskeletal system, nerves, nervous system, psychic-emotional system, spine
Specialties and related fields: Audiology, endocrinology, genetics, physical therapy
Definition: The study of the structure and function of the nervous system.
Key terms:
axon: the cellular extension of the neuron that conducts electrical information, transmitting it to the dendrite of the next neuron through the synaptic gap between them
cellular automaton: a self-reproducing entity and mathematical model for complex systems, including animal nervous systems
dendrite: the extension of the neuron that receives electrical information from neurotransmitters moving across the synaptic gap from the axon of a preceding neuron
neuroglial cell: a supportive cell for neurons within the central nervous system of animals
neuron: the principal nervous system cell that conducts electrical information from its dendritic extensions, through its cell body, to its axonic extensions, and on to other cells
neurotransmitter: a chemical messenger or hormone that relays electrical information across a synapse from the axon of one neuron to the dendrite of another neuron
plasticity: a phenomenon of many animal nervous systems, particularly those in higher vertebrates, in which central nervous system neurons grow in patterns based upon input information

Schwann cell: a supportive cell for neurons in the peripheral nervous systems of vertebrate animals that wraps around and insulates axons using the protein myelin

synapse: the gap between the transmitting axon of one neuron and the receiving dendrite of another neuron

von Neumann machine: a cellular automaton or machine that can think and self-replicate; based on the attempts of the physicist John von Neumann to duplicate the human nervous system in computers

THE PHYSIOLOGY OF THE NERVOUS SYSTEM

Neurology is the study of the nervous system, an intricate arrangement of electrically conducting nerve cells that permeate the entire animal body. Nervous tissue, which represents a principal means of cell-to-cell communication within animals, is one of four adult tissues found within the organs of most animals. The remaining three adult tissues-epithelia, connective tissue, and muscle-rely heavily on nervous tissue for their proper functioning, particularly muscle tissue.

Nervous tissue is a primary characteristic of most animal species. Evolutionarily, nerve tissue arose from cells that primarily were endocrine in origin. Endocrine cells are hormone producers that secrete hormones for distribution through the organism via the organism's bodily fluids and circulatory systems. Hormones and closely related chemical messengers called neurotransmitters are molecules that are produced in one part of the organism (such as by an endocrine cell or gland), travel through the organism, and target cells in another part of the organism. Hormones or neurotransmitters usually are composed of proteins (long chains of amino acids, or polypeptides) or of fats such as steroids. These chemical messengers affect gene expression within their target cells. Hormones and neurotransmitters determine whether genes are active or inactive. In active genes, the deoxyribonucleic acid (DNA) of the gene encodes messenger ribonucleic acid (mRNA), which encodes protein. An inactive gene does not encode protein. All events within the target cell are influenced by the presence or absence of gene-encoded proteins.

Hormones are effective cell-to-cell communicative and control molecules within all organisms, including animals. In animals, however, hormones and neurotransmitters have become elaborated as parts of extensive nervous systems. The nervous systems of animals have developed according to the evolution of a specialized nervous cell type called a neuron.

The neuron, a specialized, electrically conducting cell, is the basic unit of the nervous system. A neuron is unlike many other cells because it can assume diverse shapes and can assume (relatively) great lengths, sometimes spanning many centimeters. A neuron consists of a cell body containing a nucleus, where the genetic information resides, and numerous organelles, including the energy-producing mitochondria and protein-synthesizing ribosomes. There may be a few or many cellular extensions of its cytoplasm and membrane that twist the neuron into a very distorted appearance. The two principal types of extensions are axons and dendrites.

A dendrite is an electrically receiving extension of a neuron; it receives electrical information from another neuron. An axon is an electrically transmitting extension of a neuron; it transmits electrical information to another neuron. An axon of one neuron transmits electrical information to the dendrite of another neuron. Yet the two neurons are not in direct contact; the axon does not touch the dendrite. A gap called a synapse separates the axon from the receiving dendrite.

Electrical information crosses the synapse via a special type of hormone called a neurotransmitter, a protein encoded by the genes and synthesized by the ribosomes of the neuron. Electrical information traveling along the axon of a neuron triggers the release of a specified quantity of neurotransmitter proteins at the synapse. The neurotransmitters diffuse across the synapse where, upon making contact with the dendritic membrane of the next neuron, they depolarize the dendrite and allow the electrical information transmission to continue unabated.

Actual electrical conduction in a neuron involves membrane depolarization and the influx of sodium ions and the efflux of potassium ions. Electrical conduction along a neuronal segment involves the depolarization of the membrane with the movement of sodium cations into the neuron. Electrical conduction for a particular neuronal segment ends with repolarization of the neuronal membrane as potassium cations move across the neuronal membrane and out of the neuron. The passing electrical action potential, which is measured in millivolts, involves simultaneous depolarization and repolarization in successive regions of the neuron. The initial depolarization is triggered by neurotransmitters contacting the dendritic membrane. Sodium and potassium ion pumps continue the successive stages of depolarization and repolarization along the dendrites, cell body, and axons of the neuron until neurotransmitters are released from a terminal axon across a synaptic gap to depolarize the membrane of the next neuron.

Within animal nervous systems, neurons are very plastic: they grow in specified patterns, much like crystals, in response to stimuli and contacts with other neurons. A neuron may have one or many axonic and dendritic extensions. A neuron with one dendrite and one axon is termed bipolar. A neuron with many dendrites and many axons is termed multipolar; such a neuron makes many contacts with other neurons for the transmission of electrical information along many different neural pathways.

Animal nervous systems usually consist of centralized, concentrated neurons that form the center of nervous control, called the central nervous system. In vertebrate animals, the central nervous system consists of the billions of neurons composing the brain and spinal cord. Additionally, peripheral neurons extend throughout the animal body, permeating virtually every cell and tissue region and thus forming the peripheral nervous system, composed of billions of dispersed neurons.

Functionally, neurons are of three principal types: sensory, motor, and internuncial neurons. Sensory neurons detect stimuli and transmit the electrical information from the stimulus toward the central nervous system. The sensory neurons are arranged one after another, transmitting the electrical action potential from axon to neurotransmitter to dendrite, and so on. The central nervous system processes this information, usually utilizing an intricate array of connected internuncial neurons and specialized neuronal regions devoted to specific bodily functions. Once the central nervous system has processed a response to the stimulus, the response is affected by motor neurons, which transmit electrical information back to the body. Motor neurons will transmit electrical information between each other in the same fashion as sensory neurons. The motor neurons, however, often will terminate at some effector tissue, usually a muscle. Neurotransmitters released from the last motor neuron will depolarize the muscle membranes and trigger the biochemical and physical contraction of muscle. The muscle responds to the stimulus.

The primary purpose of nervous systems in animals is to respond to stimuli, both internal and external. Sensory neurons detect stimuli and direct this information to the central nervous system, where internuncial neurons process the information to appropriate decision centers, which direct a response along a chain of motor neurons to a muscle or muscles that physically respond to the initial stimulus. This chain of nervous communication is called a reflex arc. Virtually every activity in the body requires reflex arcs involving central and peripheral nervous system sensory, internuncial, and motor neurons.

The neurons of vertebrate animal nervous systems are very plastic and make trillions of neuron-to-neuron interconnections for the accurate processing of information, the reception of stimuli information, and the direction of response information along reflex arcs. Within the central and peripheral nervous systems of the human body, millions of information transfer processes occur by reflex arcs every second along trillions of neuronal interconnections. The number of such electrical information transfers that must occur accurately every moment within the body is staggering, yet the human nervous system accomplishes these amazingly intricate tasks with ease. No supercomputer yet devised even comes close to the complexity and efficiency of the vertebrate animal nervous system.

SCIENCE AND PROFESSION

Neurologists attempt to understand the structure of the nervous system, including the functioning of the neuron, neuronal plasticity, supporting nerve cells (neuroglia and Schwann cells), neurotransmitters, neuronal patterning in learning, how vision and hearing occur, nerve disorders, and the embryological development of the nervous system.

Neurons are among the most flexibly specialized cells in animal tissues. Animal nerve tissue is derived from embryonic ectodermal tissue. The ectoderm is a tissue layer of cells formed very early in animal development. Very early in development following conception, all animals undergo a blastula stage, in which the embryo is a hollow sphere of roughly five hundred cells. A region of the blastula called the blastopore folds to form a channel of cells through the blastula, thus initiating the gastrula stage.

The gastrula has three embryonic tissues: ectoderm, mesoderm, and endoderm. The ectoderm and endoderm continue to divide and differentiate into epithelial cells. Mesodermal cells multiply and differentiate into muscle and connective tissue cells. Dorsal ectodermal cells (cells that will become the back side of the organism) fold inward to form a nerve cord. The neurons of this nerve cord multiply and differentiate into central and peripheral nervous tissue.

In humans, the dorsal nerve cord becomes the billions of centralized neurons composing the spinal cord. The neurons in the anterior region of the spinal cord will fold, multiply, and differentiate into the various brain regions. The complete, fully functional human brain has an estimated one hundred billion neurons that grow plastically and form trillions of interconnections for the accurate processing of electrical information.

The embryonic brain consists of three principal enfolded regions: the prosencephalon (forebrain), the mesencephalon (midbrain), and the rhombencephalon (hindbrain). Each of these three embryonic regions folds and differentiates further. The prosencephalon neurons multiply and differentiate to become the cerebrum, thalamus, and hypothalamus. The mesencephalon region becomes the corpora quadrigemina and cerebral peduncles, areas that connect other brain regions and coordinate sensory and motor impulses for basic reflexes. The rhombencephalon becomes the cerebellum, pons, and medulla oblongata; these are brain regions that control basic bodily processes such as coordination, prediction of movements, and maintenance of heart rate and respiration.

Furthermore, special regions of brain tissue develop into external sensory apparatuses: eyes for vision, ears for hearing and balance, and nasal and tongue chemoreceptors for smell and taste. Millions of sensory neurons flow from these special sense organs to highly complicated brain regions that analyze, interpret, learn from, and react to these sensory stimuli. Neurophysiologists attempt to decipher the mechanisms by which the brain processes information. For example, the hundreds of thousands of retinal neurons in the eye collect light images reflected from objects, convert these diverse stimuli into thousands of bits of electrical information, and combine this information along an optic nerve. The optic nerve then transmits the electrical information of vision to the posterior occipital region of the cerebrum within the brain, where millions of visual processing neurons position the inverted, reversed visual image and interpret it.

How the brain neurons process such information is not well understood and is the subject of intense study. While neurophysiologists have a fairly good understanding of nervous system structure, nervous system function represents a tremendous challenge to investigating scientists.

Structurally, neurons are supported by nerve cells called neuroglia in the central nervous system and Schwann cells in the peripheral nervous system. Neuroglia include four cell types: astrocytes, ependyma, microglia, and oligodendrocytes. Astrocytes stabilize neurons, ependyma allow cerebrospinal fluid exchange between brain ventricles and neurons, microglia clean up dead and foreign tissue, and oligodendrocytes insulate neurons by wrapping around them and secreting an electrically insulating protein called myelin. In the peripheral nervous system, Schwann cells behave much like oligodendrocytes; they wrap around axons and electrically insulate the axons with myelin for the efficient conduction of electrical information.

Specific neurological research is focused on neuronal plasticity in learning, the effects of various neurotransmitters upon neural activity, and diseases of the central nervous system. Various models of neuronal plasticity have been proposed to explain how learning occurs in higher vertebrates, including humans and other mammals. Most of these neuronal processing models involve the spatial patterning of neural bundles, which orient information in space and time. The plastic growth of these neurons in specified directions and locking patterns contributes to memory, learning, and intelligence in higher mammals such as primates (which include humans and chimpanzees) and cetaceans (dolphins and whales).

Neurotransmission can be affected by a variety of physical states and chemical influences. The extensive use and misuse of pharmaceuticals and drugs can have serious effects upon the nervous system. Furthermore, developmental errors of the nervous system and aging can contribute to various diseases and disorders.

PERSPECTIVE AND PROSPECTS

The nervous system of humans and higher vertebrate animals presents a tremendous variety of exciting research possibilities. The brain, the seat of human consciousness, represents a mystery to scientists even with the intense scientific scrutiny devoted to this organ. The brain is studied to understand how humans learn and how they might accelerate this exceptional ability. The intricate connections between billions of very plastic cerebral cortical neurons enable millions of electrical information impulses to direct millions of simultaneous activities every second. Brain structure, neural pathways, and techniques of learning and cognition are studied indirectly in human subjects and more directly in other intelligent mammals such as chimpanzees, gorillas, dolphins, and whales. These studies include analyses of the senses as well as poorly understood extrasensory perceptions that may be linked to exceptional nervous system activity.

Researchers in the field of artificial intelligence attempt to generate cellular automatons, machines that can think and self-replicate. Artificial intelligence research began with the work of the brilliant physicist and computer pioneer John von Neumann, who attempted to mimic the human nervous system within computer systems-systems that have been called von Neumann machines. Yet no true thinking machines have been developed. The best supercomputers yet devised by humans may process data far more rapidly than the human brain, but they are no match for the human brain's capacity to process millions of data items simultaneously.

While the basic physical and chemical mechanisms of neuronal function have been deciphered by neurological scientists, research into neurotransmission across synaptic gaps continues. One principal neurotransmitter at muscular junctions is acetylcholine, which triggers muscle contractions following a motor neural impulse. When acetylcholine is not needed, it is destroyed by a molecule called acetylcholines-terase. Two types of molecular poisons can affect neuromuscular activity: acetylcholine inhibitors, which compete with acetylcholine; and antiacetylcholines-terases, which inhibit acetylcholinesterase and, therefore, accelerate acetylcholine activity. Acetylcholine competitors (such as atropine, nicotine, caffeine, morphine, cocaine, and valium) block acetylcholine at neuromuscular junctions, thereby stopping muscular contractions and producing flaccid paralysis; death can result if the heart or respiratory muscles are affected. Antiacetylcholinesterases, such as the pesticides sevin and malathion, leave acetylcholine free to contract muscles endlessly, thereby causing convulsions.

Neurology also is devoted to understanding the biochemical and genetic basis for various neurological disorders, including Alzheimer's disease, parkinsonism, seizures, abnormal brain wave patterns, paralysis, and coma. Neurological research also is concerned with the nature of pain, the sense organs, and viral diseases of the nervous system, such as meningitis, encephalitis, herpes simplex virus 2, and shingles. The complexity of the human nervous system has inspired an enormous variety and quantity of research.

—*David Wason Hollar, Jr., PhD*

See also Alzheimer's disease; Amnesia; Anesthesia; Anesthesiology; Aneurysmectomy; Aneurysms; Aphasia and dysphasia; Apnea; Ataxia; Attention-deficit disorder (ADD); Audiology; Balance disorders; Batten's disease; Behçet's disease; Bell's palsy; Biofeedback; Biophysics; Botox; Brain; Brain damage; Brain disorders; Brain tumors; Carpal tunnel syndrome; Cerebral palsy; Chiari malformations; Cluster headaches; Concussion; Craniotomy; Creutzfeldt-Jakob disease (CJD); Critical care; Critical care, pediatric; Cysts; Dementias; Disk removal; Dizziness and fainting; Dyslexia; Ear infections and disorders; Ear surgery; Ears; Electrical shock; Electroencephalography (EEG); Electromyography; Emergency medicine; Encephalitis; Epilepsy; Fetal tissue transplantation; Ganglion removal; Grafts and grafting; Guillain-Barré syndrome; Hallucinations; Head and neck disorders; Headaches; Hearing loss; Hemiplegia; Huntington's disease; Hypothalamus; Intraventricular hemorrhage; Laminectomy and spinal fusion; Learning disabilities; Leukodystrophy; Lower extremities; Lumbar puncture; Memory loss; Ménière's disease; Meningitis; Migraine headaches; Motor neuron diseases; Motor skill development; Multiple sclerosis; Narcolepsy; Nervous system; Neuralgia, neuritis, and neuropathy; Neurofibromatosis; Neuroimaging; Neurology, pediatric; Neurosurgery; Numbness and tingling; Otorhinolaryngology; Palsy; Paralysis; Paraplegia; Parkinson's disease; Physical examination; Poliomyelitis; Porphyria; Prion diseases; Psychiatry; Psychiatry, child and adolescent; Psychiatry, geriatric; Quadriplegia; Rabies; Radiculopathy; Reflexes, primitive; Restless legs syndrome; Sciatica; Seizures; Sense organs; Shock therapy; Skin; Sleep disorders; Smell; Snakebites; Spina bifida; Spinal cord disorders; Spine, vertebrae, and disks; Strokes; Subdural hematoma; Sympathectomy; Taste; Tay-Sachs disease; Tetanus; Tics; Touch; Transient ischemic attacks (TIAs); Tremors; Unconsciousness; Upper extremities; Vagotomy; Vagus nerve.

For Further Information:

Alberts, Bruce, et al. *Molecular Biology of the Cell.* 5th ed. New York: Garland, 2008.

Bear, Mark F., Barry W. Connors, and Michael A. Paradiso. *Neuroscience: Exploring the Brain.* 3d ed. Philadelphia: Lippincott Williams & Wilkins, 2007.

Bloom, Floyd E., M. Flint Beal, and David J. Kupfer, eds. *The Dana Guide to Brain Health.* New York: Dana Press, 2006.

"Brain Basics: Know Your Brain." *National Institute of Neurological Disorders and Stroke,* 20 Mar. 2013.

Chiras, Daniel D. *Biology: The Web of Life.* St. Paul, Minn.: West, 1993.

Daube, Jasper R., ed. *Clinical Neurophysiology.* 3d ed. New York: Oxford University Press, 2009.

"Disorder Index." *National Institute of Neurological Disorders and Stroke,* 2013.

Lilly, John C. *Programming and Metaprogramming in the Human Biocomputer.* Rev. 4th ed. New York: Julian Press, 2000.

Marieb, Elaine N. *Essentials of Human Anatomy and Physiology.* 10th ed. San Francisco: Pearson/Benjamin Cummings, 2012.

Nicholls, John G., A. Robert Martin, and Bruce G. Wallace. *From Neuron to Brain.* 5th ed. Sunderland, Mass.: Sinauer, 2012.

"Neurologic Diseases." *MedlinePlus,* 13 Aug. 2013.

Snyder, Solomon H. "The Molecular Basis of Communication Between Cells." *Scientific American* 253, no. 4 (October, 1985): 132-141.

NEUROLOGY, PEDIATRIC

Category: Specialty

Anatomy or system affected: Brain, ears, hands, head, muscles, musculoskeletal system, nerves, nervous system, psychic-emotional system, spine

Specialties and related fields: Audiology, endocrinology, genetics, neonatology, pediatrics, perinatology, physical therapy

Definition: The treatment of nervous system disorders in infants and children.

Key terms:

autonomic nervous system: the body system that regulates involuntary vital functions and is divided into sympathetic and parasympathetic divisions

brain stem: the medulla oblongata, pons, and mesencephalon portions of the brain, which perform motor, sensory, and reflex functions and contain the corticospinal and reticulospinal tracts

cerebellum: section of the brain located between the cerebrum and brainstem that is responsible for balance in motor functions

cerebrum: the largest and uppermost section of the brain that integrates memory, speech, writing, and emotional response

chorea: irregular, involuntary movement disorder of any part of the extremities

dysarthria: motor speech disorder due to weakness or damage of muscle *lesion*: a visible local tissue abnormality such as a wound, sore, rash, or boil, which can be benign, cancerous, gross, occult, or primary

neoplasm: abnormal tissue growth that can be cancerous

neurologic: dealing with the nervous system and its disorders

paralysis: the loss of muscle function or sensation as a result of trauma or disease

pediatric: pertaining to neonates, infants, and children up to the age of twelve

tic: abrupt, involuntary, repetitive sounds or movements

SCIENCE AND PROFESSION

Neurologic illness and injury are principal causes of chronic disability when they occur in children because they result in the development of abnormal motor and mental behaviors and/or in the loss of previously existing capabilities, with a common problem in children being musculoskeletal dysfunction. Pediatric neurology involves the ongoing assessment of an infant's or child's neurologic function, which requires the pediatric neurologist to identify problems; set goals; use appropriate interventions, including physical therapy, teaching, and counseling; and evaluate the outcome of treatment.

The pediatric neurologist looks for certain positive or negative signs of dysfunction in the nervous system. Positive signs of neurologic dysfunction include the presence of sensory deficits; pain; involuntary motor events such as tremor, chorea, or convulsions; the display of bizarre behavior or mental confusion; and muscle weakness and difficulty controlling movement. Negative signs are those that represent loss of function, such as paralysis, imperception of external stimuli, lack of speaking ability, and/or loss of consciousness.

Neurologic disease can manifest in a variety of ways. There are disorders of motility, such as motor paralysis, abnormalities of movement and posture caused by extrapyramidal motor system dysfunction, cerebellum dysfunction, tremor, myoclonus, spasms, tics, and disorders of stance and gait. Pediatric neurological disorders may arise from nervous system malformations such as agenesis of the corpus callosum, central nervous system (CNS) vascular malformations, Dandy-Walker Syndrome, neural tube defects, and CNS cysts. There are disorders of neurocutaneous syndromes such as von Hippel-Lindau Disease, Tuberous Sclerosis, Neurofibromatosis, Sturge-Weber Syndrome, and Ataxia Telangiectasia. Pain and other disorders of somatic sensation, headache, and backache may occur, such as general pain and localized pain in the craniofacial area, back, neck, and extremities. There

are disorders of the special senses that can affect any of the cranial nerves, leading to changes in smell, taste, hearing, vision, ocular movement, and pupillary function, as well as dizziness and equilibrium disorders. Epilepsy and disorders of consciousness, such as seizures and related disorders, coma and related disorders, syncope, and sleep abnormalities also fall under the category of neurologic disease. Derangements of intellect, behavior, and language as a result of diffuse and focal cerebral disease—such as delirium and other confused states, dementia, and Korsakoff syndrome—fall under this category as well, as do lesions in the cerebrum and disorders of speech and language. Anxiety and disorders of energy, mood, emotion, and autonomic and endocrine functions are other signs of neurological disease, such as lassitude and fatigue, nervousness, irritability, anxiety, depression, disorders of the limbic lobes and autonomic nervous system, and hypothalamus and neuroendocrine dysfunction. Disorders can also manifest from intoxication such as from medication overdose, electrolyte abnormalities, and bacterial or viral infections. Depending on the acuity of these etiologies, the neurological sequelae may be reversible if treated in a timely manner. Risk factors such as genetics, neonatal or maternal complications, medical history, and the environment play a role in the pathogenesis of pediatric neurological disorders. In addition, many clinical manifestations of these disorders overlap, requiring the pediatric neurologist to conduct a thorough history and physical exam as well as order the appropriate labs and imaging to obtain an accurate diagnosis.

DIAGNOSTIC AND TREATMENT TECHNIQUES

The pediatric neurologist begins with a medical history of the infant or child to determine if the problem is congenital or acquired, chronic or episodic, focal or generalized, and static or progressive. The patient's age and order of symptom onset are important components in formulating an accurate diagnosis. Acute onset symptoms may be related to infection, medication or other forms of intoxications, and electrolyte imbalances whereas symptoms of chronic onset include differential diagnoses such as inborn metabolic disorders, neoplasms, and degenerative diseases. The focus of the pediatric neurologist in taking the patient's history is on genetic disorders, the medical history of family members, and perinatal events, with an emphasis on the mother's health, mother's age during conception, form of conception such as whether reproductive technology was used, nutrition, intrapartum complications, and medications, as well as tobacco, alcohol, or drug use during pregnancy. Birth records are also reviewed by the pediatric neurologist to acquire information on labor duration, assistive devices or medications during labor, the presence of meconium during delivery, the child's gestational age, appearance, pulse, grimace, activity, and respiration (APGAR) scores, birth weight, head circumference, and neonatal complications. Neonatal screening can also help the pediatric neurologist to gain more information about the presence of amino acid metabolism disorders, organic acid conditions, hemoglobin diseases, endocrine disorders, and fatty acid oxidation pathologies.

In regards to the medical history of family members, the pediatric neurologist will ask if other members have experienced similar symptoms as the child and can help the pediatric neurologist to see if there is a genetic basis to the child's clinical presentation. The disease may be autosomal dominant, in which the disorder is present in successive generations; it may also be autosomal recessive where although it may not present in successive generations, it may present in a sibling. X-linked recessive conditions will present in male family members and can help in narrowing down the differential diagnoses. Other diseases can be passed down through mitochondrial inheritance or through trinucleotide repeats where disease manifestation presents earlier in age and in increasing severity in the following generations. The pediatric neurologist will also inquire about the child's social history, identifying factors including poverty, bullying, violence, home environment, or negligence.

Considerable information about a child's or infant's behavior or neuromuscular function can be obtained by observation of the child's alertness and curiosity, trust or apprehension, facial and eye movements, limb function, and body posture and balance during simple motor activities. Observation of the child in speech can disclose abnormalities such as articulation issues, stuttering, dyspnea, and dysarthria. Abnormal facial and eye findings such as eye blinking or staring, head nodding, lip twitching, chorea, and tics further aids in formulating an accurate diagnosis. The child's behavior includes attention span, impulsivity, and caregiver-child interaction. The pediatric neurologist will inquire of any signs of developmental regression by asking if the child is no longer able to perform activities that the child was previously capable of participating in. If possible, the pediatric neurologist will ask the child about instances of weakness, numbness, headaches, pain, tremors, nervousness, irritability, drowsiness, loss of memory, confusion, hallucinations, and loss of consciousness. Headaches, abdominal pain, or reluctance to attend school may be associated with neurologic disturbances, with contributing factors including subtle developmental disabilities, specific learning disabilities, and depression. Disorders of

movement include tics, developmental clumsiness, ataxia, chorea, myoclonus, or dystonia.

A complete neurologic examination includes an evaluation of mental status, craniospinal inspection, cranial nerve testing, sensory testing, musculature evaluation, an assessment of coordination, and autonomic function testing. Mental status evaluation involves the assessment of orientation, memory, intellect, judgment, language, attention, maturity level, and affect. Craniospinal inspection includes the palpation, percussion, and auscultation of the cranium and spine. It involves inspection of any asymmetry, protuberances or indentations. In a newborn for example, the pediatric neurologist will evaluate the cranial sutures and fontanels, determining if there is any presence of bulging fontanels, asymmetrical head shapes, and any sutural separation. Cranial nerve testing assesses the motor and sensory function of the head and neck. Sensory testing measures peripheral sensations, including responses to pinprick, light touch, vibration, and fine movement of the joints. In musculature evaluation, weakness is associated with altered tendon reflexes, indicating lower motor neuron lesions, whereas exaggerated tendon reflexes are associated with an extensor response of the big toe following plantar stimulation (Babinski reflex). In coordination assessment, smooth fine and gross motor movements demand integrated function of the pyramidal and extrapyramidal systems, whereas hyperreflexia, increased muscle stiffness, and problems with muscle coordination reflect spasticity. The evaluation of autonomic function involves bowel and bladder function, emotional state, and symmetry of reflex activity, particularly resting muscle tone and positioning of the head. A head tilt may be related to pathologies within the cerebellum or brainstem where the tilt is on the same side as the affected side of the brain. Etiologies of head tilt include neoplasms that increase intracranial pressure by mass effect or cerebellar tonsillar herniation through the foramen magnum also increasing intracranial pressure. Cerebellar function can be tested through repetitive finger tapping such as from thumb to pinky, finger-to-nose, heel-to-knee-to-shin stroking, and gait. The pediatric neurologist will observe if the child's gait is narrow or wide and presence of asymmetry of the arm and legs.

Additional diagnostic aids include lumbar puncture (spinal tap), complete blood count (CBC), myelography, electroencephalography (EEG), ultrasound, magnetic resonance imaging (MRI), and computed tomography (CT) scanning. In the prenatal period, ultrasound is used to evaluate for pathologies such as hydrocephalus, intraventricular hemorrhage, and other abnormalities. In late infancy and onward, CT is used in the setting of conditions including trauma, stroke, or increased intracranial pressure. MRI is used when CT findings are uncertain and can aid in detection of white matter pathologies, CNS neoplasms, hemorrhages, and hypoxic-ischemic insults. Lumbar puncture is used to sample spinal fluid for CNS infection. However, lumbar puncture is avoided if there is suspicion of increased intracranial pressure, cardiorespiratory instability or coagulation disorders. Imaging of the brain can be performed prior to lumbar puncture testing to assess for any increased intracranial pressure. Pediatric neurologists use EEG to determine etiology of nonconvulsive seizures as well as identifying the cause of focal neurological deficits in children. There is ongoing research on the use of positron emission tomography (PET) in evaluating schizophrenia, epilepsy, language disorders, attention-deficit disorders, tuberous sclerosis, CNS neoplasms, and movement disorders.

PERSPECTIVE AND PROSPECTS

Pediatric neurologists have been greatly assisted in their recognition of neurologic disease in infants and children by brain-imaging techniques, such as CT scanning and MRI. Event-mediated evoked potentials are also used to assess the conduction and processing of information within specific sensory pathways. These advances have enabled an accurate evaluation of the integrity of the visual, auditory, and somatosensory pathways and the uncovering of single and multiple lesions within the brain stem and cerebrum. Particularly noteworthy are CT scanning and sonographic detection of clinically silent intracranial hemorrhages in premature infants. Genetic technologies such as exome sequencing have helped in identifying causes of intellectual disability and pave the way for formulating management strategies. The genetic complexity of epilepsy is another subject of ongoing research with great progress using exome sequencing. Studies have found rare variants that lead to the development of epilepsy. Stem cell therapy research is ongoing in helping patients regain neurological function. Genome-wide methylation testing is being conducted to look for etiologies of intellectual disability and have been exploring genetic mosaicism as a possible mechanism. Gene therapy trials have contributed greatly in neuromuscular disorders with the use of gene-editing in treating pathologies such as spinal muscular atrophy.

Late twentieth- and early twentieth-century success in assisting premature infants has produced a population of patients at risk for developing cerebral palsy, developmental disabilities, epilepsy, and various learning disorders. The higher incidence of neurologic disease in the pediatric age group likely results from the increased ability of medical science to detect nervous system disturbances and from the increased survival rate of premature infants. Neurologic patients are compromised in nearly every aspect of living and have a high incidence of psychiatric problems, and their recovery is often slow and unpredictable. Another challenge of studying these pathologies is the lack of appropriate animal models in learning the disease mechanism and testing medical treatments. Furthermore, many pediatric neurological diseases are rare and studies require multicenter recruitment and longer enrollment period to obtain an adequate sample size. There is also the challenge of generalizability in regards to gender, race, and age of the participants in the study as compared to the general population. Furthermore, because medical advances have resulted in an increased survival rate following serious neurological insult, more individuals are in need of long-term rehabilitation. The financial cost associated with this care presents an ongoing challenge to health care systems and to researchers examining effective means to restore function.

—Clara Abouelsaad, OMS-III

See also: Amnesia; Anesthesia; Anesthesiology; Aphasia and dysphasia; Apnea; Ataxia; Attention-deficit disorder (ADD); Audiology; Batten's disease; Biofeedback; Biophysics; Brain; Brain damage; Brain disorders; Brain tumors; Carpal tunnel syndrome; Cerebral palsy; Chiari malformations; Cluster headaches; Concussion; Craniotomy; Creutzfeldt-Jakob disease (CJD); Critical care, pediatric; Dizziness and fainting; Dyslexia; Ear infections and disorders; Ear surgery; Ears; Electrical shock; Electroencephalography (EEG); Emergency medicine; Encephalitis; Epilepsy; Ganglion removal; Grafts and grafting; Guillain-Barré syndrome; Hallucinations; Head and neck disorders; Headaches; Hearing loss; Huntington's disease; Hydrocephalus; Intraventricular hemorrhage; Laminectomy and spinal fusion; Learning disabilities; Leukodystrophy; Lower extremities; Lumbar puncture; Memory loss; Ménière's disease; Meningitis; Migraine headaches; Motor neuron diseases; Motor skill development; Multiple sclerosis; Narcolepsy; Nervous system; Neuralgia, neuritis, and neuropathy; Neurofibromatosis; Neuroimaging; Neurology; Neurosurgery; Numbness and tingling; Otorhinolaryngology; Palsy; Paralysis; Paraplegia; Pediatrics; Physical examination; Poliomyelitis; Porphyria; Prion diseases; Psychiatry, child and adolescent; Quadriplegia; Rabies; Reflexes, primitive; Seizures; Sense organs; Skin; Sleep disorders; Smell; Snakebites; Spina bifida; Spinal cord disorders; Spine, vertebrae, and disks; Sympathectomy; Taste; Tay-Sachs disease; Tetanus; Tics; Touch; Tremors; Unconsciousness; Upper extremities.

For Further Information:
Bonkowsky, Joshua L., et al. "Pediatric Neurology Research in the Twenty-First Century: Status, Challenges, and Future Directions Post-COVID-19." *Pediatric Neurology*, vol. 113, 2020, pp. 2-12, doi.org/10.1016/j.pediatrneurol.2020.08.012.
"Diseases and Conditions: Brain and Nervous System." *KidsHealth*. Nemours Foundation, 2013.
"Disorder Index." *National Institute of Neurological Disorders and Stroke*, 2013.

Fenichel, Gerald M. *Clinical Pediatric Neurology: A Signs and Symptoms Approach*. 6th ed., Saunders/Elsevier, 2009.

Hay, William W., Jr., et al., editors. *Current Diagnosis and Treatment in Pediatrics*. 21st ed., McGraw-Hill Medical, 2012.

"Head, Neck, and Nervous System." *HealthyChildren.org*. American Academy of Pediatrics, 2013.

Jankovic, Joseph, et al. *Bradley's Neurology in Clinical Practice*. Elsevier, 2021.

Kliegman Robert, et al., editors. *Nelson Textbook of Pediatrics*. 19th ed., Saunders/Elsevier, 2011.

Marshall, Randolph S., and Stephan A. Mayer. *On Call Neurology*. Elsevier, 2021.

Miller, Steven P., and Donna M. Ferriero. "Pediatric Neurology: Improved Care of the Developing Brain." *The Lancet Neurology*, vol. 12, no. 1, 2013, pp. 16-18, doi.org/10.1016/s1474-4422(12)70292-2.

"Neurologic Diseases." *MedlinePlus*, 13 Aug. 2013.

Scheffer, Ingrid E. "Lightning Progress in Child Neurology in the Past 20 Years." *The Lancet Neurology*, vol. 21, no. 2, 2022, pp. 111-113, doi.org/10.1016/s1474-4422(22)00002-3.

Swaiman, Kenneth F., et al. *Swaiman's Pediatric Neurology: Principles and Practice*. Elsevier, 2017.

Victor, Maurice, et al. *Adams and Victor's Principles of Neurology*. 9th ed., McGraw-Hill Medical, 2009.

Volpe, Joseph J. *Neurology of the Newborn*. 5th ed., Saunders/Elsevier, 2008.

NEUROPSYCHOLOGY

Category: Specialty
Anatomy or system affected: Brain
Specialties and related fields: Neurology, neuroscience, pharmacology, psychiatry, psychology, rehabilitation
Definition: The scientific study of the biological underpinnings of behavior such as emotion, awareness, memory, language, and cognition.
Key terms:
amnesia: a condition exhibited by memory problems
aphasia: a condition exhibited by language problems
neuropsychological tests: standardized assessments used to evaluate a person's strengths and weaknesses of cognitive functioning
occupational therapy: the use of treatment programs to help people learn or recover skills associated with activities of daily living or work
traumatic brain injury: injury to the brain that usually results from an accident

SCIENCE AND PROFESSION

Neuropsychology is an interdisciplinary field that emerges from the study of biological mechanisms underlying psychological phenomena such as emotion, language, memory, perception, movement, and consciousness. In contrast to the discipline of cognitive psychology, which explores the conceptual and theoretical processes of the mind, neuropsychology investigates the relationship between brain function and behavior.

Most neuropsychologists have earned doctorates, with degrees coming from programs specifically in the area of neuropsychology or a general experimental program that includes postdoctoral work in neuropsychology. Neuropsychologists work in academia (colleges and universities), in private industry, for federal and state government agencies, and in private practice. They should not be confused with neurologists and psychiatrists who are physicians with medical degrees (MD's). Those who study neuropsychology find that knowledge in the field opens up a variety of occupational choices, such as biomedicine, nursing, psychiatric health care, cognitive rehabilitation, occupational therapy, physical therapy, neurology, psychiatry, neuroscience, laboratory technician, and pharmacology.

Neuropsychology is typically broken down into two areas of inquiry: experimental neuropsychology (also known as cognitive neuroscience) and clinical neuropsychology (sometimes referred to as human neuropsychology). Experimental neuropsychologists most often work in university settings and conduct laboratory studies using either nonhuman animals (mice, rats, etc.) or humans who suffer from head trauma, neurological disease, or illness. A common goal of empirical research is to learn more about the basic neurological or neurophysiological mechanisms associated with specific behaviors, with an emphasis on understanding more about brain/behavior relationships. In contrast, clinical neuropsychologists usually work in health care settings (hospital, health clinic, rehabilitation center), where they assess and evaluate clinical populations such as those who suffer from traumatic brain injury, amnesia, aphasia, and other brain-based problems. More importantly, the clinical neuropsychologist wants to help patients by developing treatment protocols that will help them either improve or maintain their current level of functioning. The U.S. Department of Labor/Employment and Training Administration, which sponsors the Occupational Information Network (O*NET), lists some of the major tasks of neuropsychologists as follows:

- Conduct neuropsychological evaluations such as assessments of intelligence, academic ability, attention, concentration, sensory-motor function, language, learning, and memory.
- Write or prepare detailed clinical neuropsychological reports using data from psychological or neuropsych- ological tests, self-report measures, rating scales, direct observations, or interviews.

- Diagnose and treat conditions involving injury to the central nervous system such as cerebrovascular accidents, neoplasms, infectious or inflammatory diseases, degenerative diseases, head traumas, demyelinating diseases, and various forms of dementing illnesses.
- Interview patients to obtain comprehensive medical histories.
- Establish neurobehavioral baseline measures for monitoring progressive cerebral disease or recovery.
- Diagnose and treat psychiatric populations for conditions such as somatoform disorder, dementias, and psychoses.
- Distinguish between psychogenic and neurogenic syndromes, two or more suspected etiologies of cerebral dysfunction, or between disorders involving complex seizures.

One of the largest patient populations that a clinical neuropsychologist works with comprises those who suffer from a traumatic brain injury (TBI). The range of therapeutic needs for a TBI patient can vary greatly. A neuropsychologist will begin to assess cognitive and behavioral deficits by conducting a series of neuropsychological tests. Once an assessment has been completed, a treatment plan can then be developed to help the individual progress as far as they are capable. Since a brain injury can influence several systems in the body, it is common for a neuropsychologist to work in conjunction with an interdisciplinary team. A TBI patient can receive several supportive therapies such as cognitive therapy, sensory-motor therapy, occupational therapy, speech and language therapy, physical therapy, among others.

PERSPECTIVE AND PROSPECTS

Neuropsychology is a subspecialty of the discipline of psychology. It is difficult to pinpoint when scientists and physicians first began to study behavior as a method to explore brain functioning; however, by the late 1800s, definite evidence supporting localization theory began to emerge. This theory hypothesized the brain was composed of separate areas that were responsible for different functions. In competition with localization theory was the concept of equipotentiality, which held the belief that mental abilities depended on the whole brain rather than just a single localized area. Thus, when those who subscribed to equipotentiality encountered a brain injury, the amount of brain damage that occurred was more important than the specific area that was compromised.

In 1861, Paul Broca, a French surgeon, treated a patient who had been unable to speak for several decades. After the patient's death, Broca performed an autopsy and discovered a lesion in the left frontal lobe near the lateral fissure that demarcates the frontal lobe from the temporal lobe of the brain. After studying several additional cases of patients with a similar language disturbance, Broca published his results in 1865. This paper supported localization theory since language processes were localized to specific brain structures. This language disturbance is now known as Broca's aphasia.

The discipline of neuropsychology continued to gain acceptance as additional brain structures that mediated specific behaviors were discovered. The development of neuropsychological tests along with the introduction of functional brain imaging technologies (e.g., functional magnetic resonance imaging, positron emission tomography) were also pivotal in the growth of neuropsychology.

—*Bryan C. Auday, PhD, and Elaine Hong*

See also Concussion; Glasgow coma scale; Neurology; Neuroscience; Traumatic brain injury

For Further Information:
Brain Injury Association of America: www.biausa.org/.
Kalat, James W. *Biological Psychology.* 11th ed. Belmont, CA: Wadsworth, 2013.
Kolb, Bryan, and Ian Q. Whishaw. *Fundamentals of Human Neuropsychology.* 6th ed. New York: Worth Publishers, 2009.
Horton Jr, Arthur MacNeill, and Danny Wedding. *The Neuropsychology Handbook.* 3rd ed. New York: Springer Publishing Company, 2008.
Lambert, Kelly G., and Craig H. Kinsley. *Clinical Neuroscience: Psychopathology and the Brain.* 2nd ed. New York: Oxford University Press, 2011.
Zillmer, Eric A., Mary V. Spiers, and William C. Culbertson. *Principles of Neuropsychology.* 2nd ed. Belmont, CA: Thomson Wadsworth, 2008.

NEUROREHABILITATION

Category: Procedure
Anatomy or system affected: Brain
Specialties and related fields: Neurology, Neuroscience, Psychiatry, Psychology, Rehabilitation
Definition: The systematic use of structured activities designed to improve cognitive, emotional, and social functioning in a person recovering from an injury to the brain.
Key terms:
functional compensation: a process that allows for recovery of function by rerouting neural connections to alternate brain structures that will take over the processing demands of a damaged area
neural plasticity: the ability of the nervous system to change structurally or chemically in order to enhance its ability to adapt to environmental change

neuropsychologist: a doctoral-level professional with specialized training in brain-behavior relationships to assess and to develop treatment plans for patients who suffer from brain injury

traumatic brain injury: any wound to the brain that results from a blow to the head

OVERVIEW

Each year in the United States, approximately 1.7 million people sustain a traumatic brain injury. This does not include hundreds of thousands of people who are diagnosed with neurological diseases (e.g., stroke, Parkinson's disease, dementia) or illnesses (e.g., viral encephalitis). Any of these conditions can lead to permanent brain injury that can produce impairments in cognitive, behavioral, emotional, and psychosocial functioning. In many instances, these impairments require rehabilitation services designed to improve functional outcomes for patients.

Once a patient with a brain injury has attained a level of health where he/she does not require any immediate, life-sustaining medical treatment, a neuropsychologist, along with other rehabilitation specialists, such as physical therapists, occupational therapists, speech therapists, and sensory-motor therapists, will complete a comprehensive evaluation. This evaluation, which uses a set of standardized measures, will provide information about a patient's strengths and deficiencies in areas related to cognition, such as memory, language, and decision-making. In addition, social and emotional processing will be evaluated along with possible physical problems such as balance, gait, and other mobility issues.

After the comprehensive assessment is completed, it will be used to guide and construct a rehabilitation treatment plan that involves the implementation of therapies to address deficits caused by brain injury. Over the course of treatment, a neuropsychologist, in consultation with other specialists, will continue to assess functional outcomes in order to determine the effectiveness of the treatment plan.

MECHANISMS INVOLVED WITH NEUROREHABILITATION

Understanding how the brain is able to recover from an injury can help both patients and rehabilitation specialists. Both groups frequently need reminding that recovery tends to happen in a two-stage process. Acute recovery occurs over days and months and involves several structural and chemical processes. One of these processes includes the re-stabilization of neurochemical imbalances that can arise with neuropathways become damaged. Another acute recovery process involves the repairing of vascular structure in order for vital oxygen, glucose (the primary source of energy for brain cells), and nutrients to be delivered to surviving tissue. Long-term recovery occurs over years and can involve strengthening cerebral reorganization, which is a type of compensatory strategy to reinstate brain functionality. Typically, this involves rerouting connections from a damaged area to a healthy structure that then begins the task of processing neural signals that was previously performed by the damaged tissue. Another potential mechanism for recovery of function involves the regenerative sprouting or axonal regrowth of neurons that are able to create new connections with nearby healthy brain cells. This ability to create new connections among brain cells, which is referred to as synaptogenesis, can reestablish neuronal pathways that had been compromised by injury.

The various mechanisms just described allow the central nervous system to change both in terms of structure and function. This ability to change is referred to as neural plasticity. Plasticity is a central player in recovery from brain injury. Age is directly correlated with plasticity—in general, the younger the individual who suffers from brain injury, the better the long-term prognosis for recovery. In addition to age, cognitive reserve is another important factor related to neurorehabilitation. Individuals with higher levels of education are more resilient to the deleterious effects of brain injury. It is theorized that these individuals maintain more intricate neuroanatomical pathways. This affords them a redundancy of neural pathways which acts as a sort of back-up system if the primary neural networks become damaged. The additional pathways make it easier for the brain to establish functional compensation.

In general, recovery of function in the central nervous system is related to the size of the lesion and its location. Early recovery within the first week can be an excellent indicator for overall neurorehabilitation improvement.

—*Bryan C. Auday, PhD*

See also: Neurology, Neuroscience, Brain injury

For Further Information:
Ashley, Mark J. "Repairing the Injured Brain: Why Proper Rehabilitation is Essential to Recovering Function." *Cerebrum*, July, 2012.
Barisa, M.T., Dean, R.S., and Noggle, C.A. (Eds.). *NeuropsychologicalRehabilitation*. New York, NY: Springer Publication Company, 2013.
Kolb, B. and I.Q. Whishaw. *Fundamentals of Human Neuropsychology*. 6th ed. New York, NY: Worth Publishers, 2009.
Lambert, K.G. and C.H Kinsley. *Clinical Neuroscience: Psychopathology and the Brain*. 2nd ed. New York, NY: Oxford University Press, 2011.

NEUROSCIENCE

Category: Specialty
Anatomy or system affected: Brain, autonomic nervous system
Specialties and related fields: Neurology, psychiatry, pediatrics, pharmacology, geriatrics, toxicology, neuropsychology
Definition: The scientific study of nerves, the nervous system, and associated behaviors.
Key terms:

axon: the part of a neuron responsible for sending information to other neurons

dendrite: the part of a neuron responsible for receiving information from other neurons through the binding of neurotransmitters

electroencephalograph: a physiological instrument used to record electrical activity from the scalp

electrophysiology: the study of the electrical properties of cells

excitation: one consequence of the binding of neurotransmitters to the dendrite of a neuron; when the neuron receives enough excitation in its dendrite, the cell will release the neurotransmitter from its axon onto other cells

neuron: the basic cell of the nervous system; commonly referred to as a "brain cell"

neurotransmitter: any of a number of chemicals that facilitate communication between neurons

plasticity: a characteristic of brain cells that allows them to change as a result of stimulation and/or changes in activity

synapse: the space between the axon of one neuron and the dendrite of another where communication between cells takes place

SCIENCE AND PROFESSION

Neuroscience is a broad, interdisciplinary field that spans many disciplines, including medicine, psychology, biology, chemistry, physics, computer science, mathematics, economics, education, ethics, and law. The term neuroscience replaced several earlier labels for the field, including psychobiology, biopsychology, and biological psychology. Neuroscience is closely related to neurology and neurobiology, although the former focuses on clinical and medical phenomena and the latter is concerned more with biology than behavior. Most neuroscientists have earned PhD's, though some will also hold MD's (to contrast, all neurologists are physicians).

There are many subdisciplines within neuroscience, such as behavioral neuroscience (which examines the relationship between the brain and behavior using animal models), cellular and molecular neuroscience (explores chemical and electrical events at the cellular level), cognitive neuroscience (uses neuroimaging to study the brain's role in thinking, feeling, and behaving in humans), computational neuroscience (uses computer modeling to understand how neurons and neuronal networks work), and developmental neuroscience (examines how the nervous system changes over the course of a lifetime).

PERSPECTIVE AND PROSPECTS

Though the heart was seen as the seat of intellect in the ancient world, the Greek Hippocrates and later the Roman, Galen, theorized that it may be the brain that is responsible for complex behaviors. Despite the accuracy of these early thinkers, it would be hundreds of years before neuroscience advanced beyond the gross anatomical studies that existed during the middle ages and early Renaissance. It was only after several notable discoveries about the physics of electrical conduction that neuroscientific progress resumed, this time with advances in electrophysiology.

Around the turn of the twentieth century, the two great neuroanatomists, Camillo Golgi and Santiago Ramon y Cajal debated whether the structure of the nervous system was a "reticulum" (Golgi) or a discontinuous series of "connections" between neurons (Cajal). Though neither anatomist possessed a microscope powerful enough to determine who was correct at the time, over fifty years later Palade and Palay used electron microscopy to verify the existence of synapses and show that it was Cajal who was correct. This demonstration, along with the work of Nobel Laureates John Eccles and Bernard Katz, among others, solidified a modern understanding of the typical structure and workings of the nervous system: namely that though communication within individual neurons is electrical in nature, communication between neurons is chemical and occurs through the release of a neurotransmitter from an axon into the synapse. Once in the synapse, the neurotransmitter then binds to the dendrite of a different neuron, thus creating a change in the electrical potential within that neuron.

While neuroanatomists and neurophysiologists were unraveling where and how messages are sent in the nervous system, the Canadian psychologist, Donald Hebb, theorized about how information could be retained. In his 1949 book, On the Organization of Behavior, Hebb outlined the parameters via which the nervous system could be modified in response to activity, the phenomenon now known as "plasticity." His book, one of the most influential texts in all of neuroscience, laid the foundation for everything from development of the visual system to learning and memory.

Though prior to the 1950s, most neuroscientific research was conducted using animal models, the advent of modern neuroimaging techniques, such as functional magnetic resonance imaging, or fMRI, revolutionized the study of the brain and behavior in humans. Unlike brain wave recordings collected using an electroencephalograph (EEG), which had been used for decades, fMRI allowed neuroscientists to see exactly where within the brain activity was taking place when a human was thinking or behaving.

Continuing advances in technology now allow neuroscientists to peer into the brain with greater resolution and detail. Because of this enhanced ability to see what happens within the brain when a human engages in complex reasoning, these advances have facilitated the integration of neuroscience with seemingly unrelated fields such as economics and education.

—Jerome L. Rekart, PhD

See also Neuropsychology; Neurology; Psychiatry

For Further Information:
Carter, Rita. *Mapping the Mind.* Berkeley, CA: University of California Press, 2010.
Gazzaniga, Michael S. *The Cognitive Neurosciences.* Cambridge, MA: MIT Press, 2009.
Gross, Charles G. *A Hole in the Head: More Tales in the History of Neuroscience.* Cambridge, MA: MIT Press, 2012.
Hebb, Donald O. *The Organization of Behavior: A Neuropsychological Theory.* New York: Wiley, 1949.
Kalat, James W. *Biological Psychology.* 11th ed. Belmont, CA: Wadsworth, 2013.
Kandel, Eric, James Schwartz, Thomas Jessell, Steven Siegelbaum, and A.J. Hudspeth. *Principles of Neural Science.* 5th ed. New York: McGraw Hill Professional, 2012.
LeDoux, Joseph. *Synaptic Self: How Our Brains Become Who We Are.* 2nd ed. London: Penguin Books, 2003.
McGill University. *The Brain from Top to Bottom.* thebrain.mcgill.ca.
Satel, Sally, and Scott O. Lilienfield. *Brainwashed: The Seductive Appeal of Mindless Neuroscience.* New York: Basic Books, 2013.
Society for Neuroscience. BrainFacts.org. www.brainfacts.org.

NEUROSIS

Category: Disease/Disorder
Anatomy or system affected: Brain, nerves, nervous system, psychic-emotional system
Specialties and related fields: Ethics, family medicine, neurology, psychiatry, psychology, public health
Definition: A psychiatric disorder in which the patient continues to be rational and in touch with reality.
Key terms:
agoraphobia: the fear of being in crowds
anxiety disorder: an emotional state that ranges from mild concern to disabling fear

bipolar disorders: disorders characterized by periods of depressed and elevated mood
hysterical amnesia: a dissociative disorder in which patients, capable of reading and writing, cannot remember simple things like their names
obsessive-compulsive disorder: a condition characterized by the ritualistic performance of repetitive actions
somatization disorder: a persistent condition in which patients complain about physical problems for which no cause is apparent

CAUSES AND SYMPTOMS

The distinction between neurosis and psychosis is that those suffering from neuroses are in touch with reality and usually realize that they have a problem. In contrast, psychotics frequently lose touch with reality and do not recognize that they are sick and in need of immediate professional help.

The most common neurosis is depression. Those with major depression experience, for no overt reason, a persistent and overwhelming sadness coupled with an all-encompassing sense of despair. It is normal for people who suffer such ills as the death of a loved one, the loss of a job, or severe financial reverses to be depressed. In such cases, their depression is usually mitigated when the cause is removed or when they distance themselves from it. On the other hand, those who suffer from major depression cannot attribute their suffering to an immediate cause. They are frequently sad and usually do not know why. Depression is also a major component of bipolar disorders, in which episodes of major depression are followed by periods of mania, or elevated mood.

Other common forms of neurosis are obsessive-compulsive disorder (OCD), somatization disorder, hypochondria, various phobias or fears, anxiety disorders, psychosexual disorders, and hysterical amnesia. All these problems occur less frequently than major depression.

An example of obsessive-compulsive disorder may be the compulsion of its victims to wash their hands thirty or forty times a day. Those who have a somatization disorder complain of largely imagined illnesses for which no physical cause can be detected. Often termed hypochondria, this disorder is more frequent in women, especially middle-aged women, than in men.

Most people suffer from one or more phobias that do not disable them. Fear of heights (acrophobia) and abnormal fear of public or open areas (agoraphobia) are quite common, as are the fear of some living things such as spiders or scorpions (arachnophobia) or the fear of closed places (claustrophobia). Many of those suffering from such phobias can usually control

---

INFORMATION ON NEUROSIS

Causes: Psychological disorder
Symptoms: Distressing and unacceptable anxiety, impaired daily functioning, depression, abnormal fear
Duration: Often chronic; may involve acute episodes
Treatments: Counseling, psychoactive medications

---

them by confronting them rationally, although some phobias may be so intense that they result in panic.

Hysterical amnesia, a dissociative disorder, is relatively rare. Often it is connected with anxiety disorder. Victims tend to panic to the point that they suffer temporary memory loss. Although they remain in touch with reality, they may not be able to remember their names, addresses, telephone numbers, and other obvious bits of information.

Post-traumatic stress disorder (PTSD) has become increasingly common. In extreme cases, it may result in psychotic behavior, although it is more often neurotic in its manifestation. PTSD usually occurs in people who have been subjected to combat situations or to life-threatening natural disasters such as earthquakes, hurricanes, floods, and fires.

TREATMENT AND THERAPY

The usual treatment in persistent cases of neurosis is psychotherapy rendered by a clinical psychologist or psychiatrist, frequently over an extended period. Severe cases may require meetings with a professional three or four times a week in order to be effective. Mild cases can sometimes be dealt with in only two or three visits, especially if the patient is cooperative and committed to dealing with the problem.

Neuroses usually do not require such drastic treatment as electric shock therapy or brain surgery, although such treatment was sometimes prescribed in the past. Currently, more than twenty prescription drugs exist to treat such neuroses as bipolar and somatization disorders. Often, patients need to try several of these medications before finding the one that suits them best. Patients must be cautioned, however, not to expect immediate results. When they find a medication that works well for them, they are advised to continue taking it even after their initial symptoms disappear.

PERSPECTIVE AND PROSPECTS

Substantial biochemical advances during the early years of the twenty-first century have resulted in improved understanding of the relationship between body chemistry and both neuroses and psychoses.

Such advances have also been accompanied by changes in the way psychiatric therapy is delivered. Group therapy reduces the cost of treatment. In many situations, because it is so interactive, it proves superior to the one-on-one therapy that psychotherapy and psychoanalysis provide.

The public at large has become more sophisticated than past generations in dealing with neuroses. Nevertheless, the management of the most common neurosis, depression, remains challenging. Most suicides are committed by those suffering from the depths of depression, a condition that gives them a sense of hopelessness.

—*R. Baird Shuman, PhD*

See also Antianxiety drugs; Anxiety; Bipolar disorders; Depression; Hypochondriasis; Midlife crisis; Obsessive-compulsive disorder; Panic attacks; Paranoia; Phobias; Postpartum depression; Post-traumatic stress disorder; Psychiatric disorders; Psychiatry; Psychiatry, child and adolescent; Psychiatry, geriatric; Psychoanalysis; Psychosis; Psychosomatic disorders; Stress.

For Further Information:

American Psychiatric Association. *Diagnostic and Statistical Manual of Mental Disorders: DSM-5*. 5th ed. Washington, DC: American Psychiatric Association, 2013.

Craske, Michelle G. *Origins of Phobias and Anxiety Disorders: Why More Women than Men?* New York: Elsevier, 2003.

Frankl, Victor E. *On the Theory and Therapy of Mental Disorders: An Introduction to Logotherapy and Existential Analysis*. New York: Brunner-Routledge, 2004.

Gossop, Michael. *Theories of Neurosis*. New York: Springer, 1981.

Rapee, Ronald M., and David H. Barlow, eds. *Chronic Anxiety: Generalized Anxiety Disorder and Mixed Anxiety-Depression*. New York: Guilford Press, 1991.

Russon, John. *Human Experience: Philosophy, Neurosis, and Elements of Everyday Life*. Albany: State University of New York Press, 2003.

NEUROSURGERY

Category: Procedure
Anatomy or system affected: Bones, brain, glands, head, nerves, nervous system, psychic-emotional system, spine
Specialties and related fields: General surgery, neurology, psychiatry
Definition: Surgery involving the brain, spinal cord, or peripheral nerves, including craniotomy, lobotomy, laminectomy, and sympathectomy.
Key terms:
aneurysm: the swelling of a blood vessel, which occurs with the stretching of a weak place in the vessel wall
cannula: a tube or hypodermic needle implanted in the body to introduce or extract substances

commissurotomy: the severing of the corpus callosum, the fiber tract joining the two cerebral hemispheres

hematoma: a localized collection of clotted blood in an organ or tissue as a result of internal bleeding

lesion: a wound or tumor of the brain or spinal cord

lobectomy: the removal of a lobe of the brain, or a major part of a lobe

lobotomy: the separation of either an entire lobe or a major part of a lobe from the rest of the brain

trephination: the opening of a hole in the skull with an instrument called a trephine

INDICATIONS AND PROCEDURES

Neurosurgery refers to any surgery performed on a part of the nervous system. Brain surgery may be used to remove a tumor or foreign body, relieve the pressure caused by an intracranial hemorrhage, excise an abscess, treat parkinsonism, or relieve pain. In cases of severe mental depression or untreatable epilepsy, psychosurgery (such as lobotomy) may alleviate the worst symptoms, although these procedures are now rare. Surgery may be performed on the spine to correct a defect, remove a tumor, repair a ruptured intervertebral disk, or relieve pain. Surgery may be performed on nerves to remove a tumor, relieve pain, or reconnect a severed nerve.

Most brain operations share some common procedures. Bleeding from the numerous tiny blood vessels in the brain is controlled by use of an electric needle, a finely pointed instrument that shoots a minute electric current into the vessel and seals it. (This same instrument can be used as an electric knife for bloodless cutting.) Brain tissue is kept moist by continued washing with a dilute salt solution. The brain tissue itself is handled with damp cotton pads attached to the end of forceps.

If the brain is swollen, it may be treated by intravenous injections of urea. The resulting increase in the salt concentration of the blood draws the water away from the brain. In addition to drawing off excess water, the brain's size is temporarily reduced, giving the surgeon extra room to maneuver. To help reduce bleeding within the brain, the patient's blood pressure can be lowered by half temporarily through an injection of a drug into the blood. The patient's temperature is also reduced, which lowers the brain's need for oxygen and ensures that the reduced blood flow will not be deleterious.

An operation in which a hole is cut into the skull is called a craniotomy. If only a small hole is required, the procedure is called trepanation (or trephination) and uses an instrument called a trephine, resembling a corkscrew with a short, nail-like tip and a threaded cutting disk. The size of the opening that is made ranges from 1.5 centimeters (0.6 inches) to 3.8 centimeters

(1.5 inches) in diameter and, if necessary, may be enlarged with an instrument called a rongeur. This type of surgery is performed to insert needles or cannulas and to remove subdural hematomas. If too much of the bony skull has to be removed (or is fractured by accidental means), a substitute for the bone is inserted. The substitute is usually made of plastic, such as acrylic.

Brain surgery for advanced Parkinson's disease will not cure the disease but may help alleviate some of its symptoms. The major symptoms are tremor, stiffness, weakness, and slowed movements. For patients who do not respond well to medication, a form of neurosurgery called deep brain stimulation (DBS) can be used to reduce or stop the shaking, by implanting a small device called a brain pacemaker that emits electrical impulses to block abnormal activity in affected regions of the brain.

When pain becomes unbearable, such as the pain associated with cancer, the nerves carrying these pain messages can be interrupted anywhere between the brain and the cancerous region. The nerve to the affected organ can be severed, the nerve roots of the spinal cord can be cut, or the cut can be made within the spinal cord.

Hypophysectomy is the surgical removal of the pituitary gland. It is usually performed to slow the growth and spread of endocrine-dependent malignant tumors of the breast, ovary, or prostate gland. It may also be used to stop the deterioration of the retina that may come with diabetes mellitus or to remove a pituitary tumor. Hypophysectomy is considered only as a last resort when cryosurgery or radioactive implants fail to destroy the pituitary tissue. There are two ways to reach a diseased pituitary gland by surgery. One way is to go through the nose. The skull is entered through the sphenoid sinus, and the floor of the bony saddle of the middle of the skull is cut to reach the gland. The second means is by craniotomy. The skull is opened through an incision in the hairline above the forehead. A flap of bone, hinged at eyebrow level, is brought forward so that the surgeon can see the entire affected area clearly. The gland is completely excised.

Psychosurgery is now considered only as a last resort, when nothing else can possibly work. It is rarely undertaken because of the availability of so many drugs to control mental illnesses. In the cases when a lobotomy is performed, it can be done under local anesthesia through tiny holes drilled in the roof of the eyes' orbits. An instrument is then inserted to separate the lobes of the brain.

A laminectomy is performed to relieve compression of the spinal cord caused by injury (the displacement of a bone) or by the degeneration of a disk; it may also be used to find and remove a displaced intervertebral disk. A laminectomy is performed under general anesthesia. The surgeon makes an incision in the back, vertically over the tips of the vertebral bones. The large, thick muscles that lie on either side are peeled back from the surface of the bones. The lamina itself is the part of a vertebral bone that forms the back wall of the spinal canal. When the laminae are cut away, the spinal canal is opened so that the spinal cord covering can be cut. Once the cord is exposed, a particular condition can be treated. It may then be necessary to fuse the vertebrae. The removal of the laminae causes little interference with support or motion of the spine, although recovery from the surgery requires that the patient remain prone for several days to keep the spine in alignment.

Fusion of the vertebrae is the surgical joining of two or more spinal vertebrae to stabilize a segment of the spinal column following severe trauma, a herniated (ruptured) disk, or a degenerative disease. The surgery is performed under general anesthesia. The cartilage pads are removed from between the posterior portions of the affected vertebrae. Bone chips are cut from the vertebral ridges and inserted as a replacement for the removed cartilage. Postoperative motion must be limited until the articulating bones heal.

Severe pain that cannot be controlled by analgesics (painkillers) may be treated by surgery. One procedure, a cordotomy, removes a section of the spinal cord so that most of the nerve fibers that transmit pain messages to the brain are destroyed. At first, the patient does experience less pain, but after a few months, the pain can recur and become worse than before. The recurrence of pain is likely attributable to the reconstruction of some axons that carry ascending messages. Other painful conditions can be treated with surgery. Trigeminal neuralgia (or tic douloureux) is one such condition. These severe attacks of stabbing pain in the face may last a minute or more. The trigeminal nerve can be injected with a concentrated alcohol solution, which will prevent it from working for a year or two. This condition is usually treated surgically by drilling a burr hole in the temple and cutting across the lower two-thirds of the nerve trunk at the site.

Asympathectomy surgically interrupts a part of the sympathetic nerve pathways. It is used to relieve the pain of vascular disease. The surgery involves removing the sheath from around an artery. This sheath carries the sympathetic nerve fibers that control vasoconstriction. Once the sheath is removed, the vessel relaxes and expands so that more blood travels through it.

USES AND COMPLICATIONS

While neurosurgery offers the hope of recovery to people suffering with tumors, aneurysms, and brain injuries, it may result in complications that can bring disability, coma, or even death. Therefore, three issues must be taken into account before neurosurgery is performed. First, these surgeries involve higher risk than most other procedures. Second, diseases that necessitate neurosurgical treatment may render patients wholly or partially incompetent to understand the implications of their surgery. Third, sometimes matching the appropriate surgery to the patient's condition is an uncertain process. Even standard neurosurgical procedures have not been proven in every event.

Because the diagnosis of a brain tumor is often seen as fatal, many believe that surgery has little value as therapy, especially for malignant tumors. Others suggest, however, that the more radical the surgery, the greater the chance of survival for the patient. The problem arises when a tumor is found within the center area of the brain, where the primary sensory and motor cortices are situated. Surgical methods of the past tended to exacerbate the problems of the patient. The use of lasers and microscopy, however, may increase the chance of successful treatment. Using these tools, incisions of no longer than 2 centimeters can be made. Using the microscope, the surgeon can guide the laser to the tumor, which is gently melted and vaporized-all without disturbing the brain. This method is especially useful for reaching deep-seated tumors.

Stereotactic surgery is a means by which monitoring devices are inserted into the brain cortex. These devices can detect lesions, stimulate or record areas within the cortex, or in some other way study the brain. The two things necessary to perform this surgery are a stereotactic atlas (or map) of the brain and the instrumentation for the procedure. The atlas is a series of individual maps, each representing a slice of the brain. The stereotactic instrument consists of two parts: a head holder, which maintains the patient's head in a particular position and orientation, and an electrode holder, which holds the device that is to be inserted.

The purpose of the lesion method of stereotactic surgery is to remove, damage, or destroy a part of the brain in such a way that the behavior of the patient can be monitored to determine the functions of the affected area. Surgery to produce lesions is an extremely precise, and therefore dangerous, surgery. Structures within the brain are tiny, convoluted, and tightly packed, and any surgery performed on an area may therefore damage adjacent areas. There are four different methods of producing lesions.

Aspiration lesions are performed when the target site is in a more accessible area of the brain, where the surgeon can see it clearly and can use the proper instruments. The cortical tissue is aspirated by a handheld pipette, and then the tougher white matter layers are peeled away. Deeper lesions are created with high-frequency (radiofrequency) currents passed through carefully placed electrodes. The heat of the current destroys the tissue. The amount of tissue to be removed is regulated through control of the current's duration and intensity. In the third method, a nerve or tract to be removed can be cut with a scalpel. A tiny incision severing the nerve does not have to do damage to surrounding tissues, so the lesion is small.

The fourth method is cryogenic blockade. In this method, a coolant is pumped through the tip of an implanted cryoprobe to cool the area. When the tissue is cooled, the neurons do not fire. The temperature must remain above freezing, however, to prevent destruction of the tissue. Although the result is not a true lesion, since function returns, this cooled area acts as a lesion because the behavior that it governs is interrupted. Consequently, cryogenic blockade is said to produce a reversible lesion.

A commissurotomy, or severing the connection between the two cerebral hemispheres, may be performed in cases of severe epilepsy if no other treatment is successful. After the two halves are separated (the brain stem is left intact), each hemisphere maintains all the centers that mediate its functions, except that each cortex sees only half the world. For example, visual messages are crossed so that the opposite hemisphere is stimulated by only one eye's input. If both eyes and both hemispheres are working, however, vision should be unaffected. In fact, no real deficits should occur in these patients' behavior. They retain the same verbal intelligence, reasoning, perception, motor coordination, and personality, because of the brain's extraordinary ability to preserve unity, or oneness.

Commissurotomies were first performed in the hope of reducing the severity of convulsions and seizures associated with epilepsy. The rationale was that the severity of the convulsions would be reduced if discharges could be limited to the hemisphere from which they originated. The benefits far surpassed expectations; many patients never experience another convulsion.

PERSPECTIVE AND PROSPECTS
Archaeological evidence shows that people living in the Stone Age performed trepanation. This operation was likely performed to release evil spirits or demons: There is little evidence of fractures of the skulls that have been found, and the pieces of skulls that were excised were preserved and worn as talismans. Today, surgeons in some tribal cultures perform the same surgery; in some cases, some are done for ritual purposes, while others are performed for head injuries as well as headache, dizziness, and epilepsy. Trepanation laid the groundwork for brain surgery as it is still practiced.

Perhaps the most intriguing possibility for future research is transplanting brains or brain tissue. Brain transplants have come a long way from their portrayal in science fiction. In 1971, the first real evidence that transplanted tissue could survive was found. These successful attempts were made in rats. Further studies have shown that transplants have a higher survival rate in tissue richly vascularized with sufficient room to grow. It is hoped that neurotransplant surgery can be used to treat brain damage. One approach would be to develop procedures of implantation that would stimulate the regeneration of the patient's own tissue. A second approach would be to replace damaged tissue with healthy tissue of the same type.

The major question that will have to be answered before successful regeneration is accomplished is why neurons of the peripheral nervous system (PNS) regenerate but the neurons of the central nervous system (CNS) do not. One hypothesis would be that they are too structurally different. This theory is disputed by studies that show CNS neuron regeneration in the peripheral nervous system, while PNS neurons do not regenerate in the central nervous system. Other evidence to refute the hypothesis is that peripheral sensory neurons regenerate until they reach the spinal cord, then regeneration ceases. Therefore, perhaps there is an environmental factor within the central nervous system that prohibits regeneration, such as scar tissue that forms only in the area of CNS damage. Experiments to prove or disprove this theory are inconclusive. The other possibility is that the insulating cells wrapped around CNS neurons are different enough from the Schwann cells of PNS neurons that regeneration is discouraged.

Attempts to replace damaged tissue with healthy tissue have been most useful in treating Parkinson's disease (with its rigidity, tremors, and lack of spontaneous movement). One type of tissue used for replacement is fetal neural tissue. It not only survives but also innervates adjacent tissue, releases neurotransmitters (in this case dopamine), and alleviates the symptoms of parkinsonism. A possible substitute for neural tissue is autotransplantation with some of the patient's own adrenal medulla. This tissue could be used because it too releases dopamine. Investigations thus far have been controversial, but the operation is being performed worldwide.

—*Iona C. Baldridge*

See also Aneurysmectomy; Brain; Brain damage; Brain disorders; Brain tumors; Chiari malformations; Craniotomy; Cysts; Electroencephalography (EEG); Fetal tissue transplantation; Ganglion removal; Laminectomy and spinal fusion; Laser use in surgery; Lumbar puncture; Nervous system; Neuroimaging; Neurology; Neurology, pediatric; Pain; Pain management; Parkinson's disease; Positron emission tomography (PET) scanning; Psychiatric disorders; Psychiatry; Radiculopathy; Spina bifida; Spinal cord disorders; Spine, vertebrae, and disks; Stem cells; Subdural hematoma; Tics; Tumor removal; Tumors.

For Further Information:

Bear, Mark F., Barry W. Connors, and Michael A. Paradiso. *Neuroscience: Exploring the Brain*. 3d ed. Philadelphia: Lippincott Williams & Wilkins, 2007.

Bloom, Floyd E., M. Flint Beal, and David J. Kupfer, eds. *The Dana Guide to Brain Health*. New York: Dana Press, 2006.

Daube, Jasper R., ed. *Clinical Neurophysiology*. 3d ed. New York: Oxford University Press, 2009.

Pinel, John P. J. *Biopsychology*. 8th ed. Boston: Pearson Allyn & Bacon, 2011.

Post, Kalmon, et al., eds. *Acute, Chronic, and Terminal Care in Neurosurgery*. Springfield, Ill.: Charles C. Thomas, 1987.

"What Is Neurosurgery?" *Patient Education Institute*, April 2, 2009.

Zollinger, Robert M., Jr., E. Christopher Ellison, and Robert M. Zollinger, Sr. *Zollinger's Atlas of Surgical Operations*. 9th ed. New York: McGraw-Hill, 2011.

NEUTROPHIL

Category: Biology

Anatomy or system affected: immune system, circulatory system

Specialties and related fields: immunology, hematology, cytology

Definition: A neutrophil is a type of white blood cell that fights infection and is the most abundant of the white blood cell types.

Key terms:

white blood cells: White blood cells function in the immune system and are made in the bone marrow. There are many types of white blood cells, including granulocytes, monocytes, and lymphocytes.

polymorphonuclear leukocytes: Polymorphonuclear leukocyte, or PMN, is another term for neutrophil, based on the irregularly-shaped multi-lobed nuclei characteristic of this cell type.

granulocytes: Granulocytes are a type of white blood cell with granules which contain enzymes released during infection or other immune responses such as allergy. The different types of granulocytes include neutrophils, eosinophils, and basophils.

phagocytosis: A phagocyte is a cell that eats, 'phago' being derived from the Greek word 'for eat'.

STRUCTURE AND FUNCTIONS

Neutrophils play essential roles in the immune system. They are the most abundant white blood cell type and the first cells to arrive at the site of infection or injury. Neutrophils comprise about 55-75% of a normal white blood cell count, with normal cell counts ranging from 2-7 billion cells per liter of blood. Along with eosinophils and basophils, neutrophils comprise a type of white blood cell known as granulocytes, so named because they contain small 'granules' or grain-like shapes, within their cytoplasm. These granules store microbe-fighting enzymes. Neutrophils specialize in the capture, engulfment, and killing of microorganisms.

Neutrophils are produced in the bone marrow and are short-lived with lifespans measured in hours. In the bone marrow, it takes about one week for a neutrophil to develop from a progenitor cell into a mature neutrophil. The bone marrow produces about 100 billion neutrophils every day. Once produced, neutrophils live only about 4-10 hours in the blood stream or 1-2 days if they migrate into tissue. To prevent rapid depletion of neutrophils during an infection, the bone marrow stores a large number of granulocytes that can be mobilized quickly in response to infection. Newly formed cells have a round nucleus, but as cells mature, the nucleus become more irregular and lobular, which gives the appearance of having multiple nuclei. Because of their multi-lobed nuclei, these cells are often referred to as polymorphonuclear leukocytes. Neutrophils are characterized histologically by cytoplasmic granules, nuclear features, and staining characteristics and functionally by their role in immune responses against infectious microorganisms.

When an invasion of foreign organisms is detected by the body, the cells of the body send out chemical signals that recruit cells to the site of invasion. An important feature of the role of neutrophils in immune defense is their mobility; unlike some of the other white blood cells, neutrophils aren't limited to a specific area of circulation. They can move freely through the walls of veins and into tissues of the body to immediately attack antigen. The neutrophils are the first cells to respond and travel through the bloodstream to the site of infection. Once at the site of infection, neutrophils attach themselves to walls of blood vessels and enter surrounding tissue to attack invaders and prevent more organisms from entering the blood.

A primary function of neutrophils is phagocytosis and killing of microorganisms. Although neutrophils utilize an arsenal of antimicrobial weapons to destroy their target, phagocytosis, or 'cell-devouring' is one of their primary strategies. Neutrophils surround and engulf bacteria and other microorganisms, the granules of the neutrophil, which are filled with enzymes that can digest many types of cellular material, are released to destroy the organisms. At the same time, neutrophils can also release potent forms of reactive oxygen-based molecules-such as superoxide or hydrogen peroxide-that can destroy bacteria in a process known as 'oxidative burst'. Even in dying, neutrophils have developed a method to kill their targets. Under certain conditions, a neutrophil can undergo a process called NETosis, a form of cell death that releases a mesh-like network of fibers containing antimicrobial enzymes and chemicals. Scientists have termed these neutrophil extracellular traps (NET).

DISORDERS AND DISEASES
Normally, the body regulates production of neutrophils and other white blood cells to respond to infection or injury. Abnormal neutrophil counts may be caused by infection or another condition. Too many or too few neutrophils in the blood stream can indicate blood disorders with the potential to be serious conditions. Neutrophilia, a high number of neutrophils in the blood, can result from infection or reaction to medication. Neutrophilia is generally associated with acute inflammation, although it may result from certain diseases such as chronic myelogenous leukemia, which is a type of cancer of blood-forming tissues. More common is a disorder called neutropenia, which is an abnormally low number of neutrophils in the blood. Neutropenia is most often found in cancer patients undergoing chemotherapy but can also result from inherited disorders that affect the immune system as well as by a number of acquired diseases. Neutropenia significantly increases the risk of life-threatening bacterial infection.

PERSPECTIVE AND PROSPECTS
Neutrophils are critical in immune response, and are first responders to infection. In addition to direct uptake and destruction of invading pathogens, neutrophils also secrete chemicals that recruit reinforcements, including other specialized cell types, to the site of infection to assist with immune defense. Although neutrophils are the most abundant circulating leukocyte, their full spectrum of biological functions in the immune system is still emerging. Enhanced understanding of the full capabilities of neutrophils can hopefully lead to improved treatment options for diseases involving neutrophils.

—*Catherine J. Walsh, PhD*

For Further Information:
Bain, Barbara J. *Blood Cells: A Practical Guide*. 5th ed., Wiley Blackwell, 2015. A guide for identifying different blood cells and includes information on blood collection and clinical laboratory tests.
Gabrilovich, Dmitry, editor. *The Neutrophils: New Outlook for Old Cells*. 3rd ed., Imperial College P, 2013. Provides an overview of the biology of neutrophils, including role of neutrophil in cancer and ways to use neutrophils in treatment.
Territo, Mary. "Neutrophilic Leukocytosis." *Merck Manual*, www.merckmanuals.com/home/blood-disorders/white-blood-cell-disorders/neutrophilic-leukocytosis. Accessed 19 Jan. 2017. The information provided on this website focuses on neutrophilic leukocytosis, or high number of leukocytes, including possible diseases associated with the condition.
"Types of White Blood Cells." *New Health Advisor*, www.newhealthadvisor.com/Types-of-White-Blood-Cells.html. Accessed 21 Sept 2017. An informative website with general information about the types of white blood cells important in human health, including a short video explanation on white blood cell types.
"White Blood Cell Disorders." *Dana-Farber/Boston Children's Cancerand Blood Disorders Center*, www.danafarberboston childrens.org/conditions/blood-disorders/white-blood-cell-disorders.aspx. Accessed 19 Jan. 2017. A website that includes a brief description of some white blood cell disorders in children and possible treatments.

NIACIN

Category: Anatomy/Biology
Also known as: Vitamin B3; nicotinic acid
Anatomy or system affected: All
Specialties and related fields: Endocrinology; nutrition
Definition: A water-soluble vitamin that serves a key role in several body systems including the breakdown of fats, proteins, and carbohydrates into energy and the production of certain adrenal hormones.
Key terms:
adrenal: an endocrine gland located above each kidney; the inner part of each gland secretes epinephrine (adrenaline) and the outer part secretes hormones that help regulate blood pressure, blood sugar levels, and metabolism
cholesterol: a waxy substance made by the liver and also acquired through diet. High levels in the blood may increase the risk of cardiovascular disease
cirrhosis: chronic degenerative liver disease in which normal cells are replaced by fibrous tissue and normal liver function is disrupted
gout: a disease in which uric acid, a waste product that normally passes out of the body in urine, collects in the joints and the kidneys
plaque: a compound made up of fat, cholesterol, calcium, and other substances found in the blood. It can stick to the walls of arteries, partially or totally blocking blood flow
watersoluble: a compound that dissolves in water. Water-soluble vitamins are not stored in the body the way fat-soluble vitamins are, so the body needs a regular supply of water-soluble vitamins.

BACKGROUND

Niacin, also known as vitamin B3 or nicotinic acid, is a water-soluble vitamin that serves a key role in metabolism. The liver makes a small amount of niacin, but not enough for human health. Most niacin must be obtained from food. Niacin occurs naturally in many foods and is added to other foods. It is also added to over-the-counter multivitamins. Niacin supplements are available in high concentrations for people who need them for health reasons, but high-dose supplements require a physician's prescription. Although niacin occurs naturally and is important to several body systems, excessive amounts of niacin can have serious, and even life-threatening, side effects.

SOURCES OF NIACIN

Good natural sources of niacin include red meat, fish, and poultry. In 1938, the United States began fortifying flour with niacin, so today most flours, cereals, bread, and pasta contain niacin. These products are labeled "fortified" or "enriched." Because of the fortification program, most Americans get enough niacin from their diet without taking a dietary supplement. In addition, the liver can manufacture small amounts of niacin from the amino acid tryptophan, which occurs in many of the foods that contain niacin, as well as seeds, tofu, dairy products, lentils, and beans.

The niacin in supplements is synthesized in a laboratory either chemically or through microbial fermentation, a process by which bacteria or other microbes digest or process one substance to produce another.

BENEFITS

Niacin is necessary for healthy skin and proper nerve function. It helps in digestion and metabolism, the process by which the body breaks down protein, carbohydrates, and fats to generate energy. The presence of niacin helps the adrenal glands in the production of hormones and aids the liver in processing harmful chemicals and other substances so they can be removed from the body.

The circulatory system also benefits from the presence of niacin. Prescription-strength niacin may be used to regulate cholesterol levels in the blood, although this is less common now that statin drugs are available. Studies have shown that niacin can increase high-density lipoprotein (HDL)—"good cholesterol"—by as much as 30 percent. HDL collects and transports low density lipoprotein (LDL) to the liver, where it is removed from the blood stream. LDL is considered "bad cholesterol" because it clogs arteries and leads to the formation of plaque and cardiovascular disease. Niacin is known to help with migraine headaches and dizziness, both of which can be related to circulation issues. In addition, niacin's beneficial effects on the circulatory system can help some men with erectile dysfunction.

Niacin also has been shown to help some skin disorders. Acne patients who use a topical gel containing niacin have shown improvement in their condition. Nicotinamide, a form of niacin, has been shown to help prevent some forms of skin cancer, especially in patients who already have had skin cancer.

SIDE EFFECTS

Niacin is water soluble, so excessive amounts are generally excreted in the urine and not stored in the body. However, some people do experience side effects when taking niacin and can have serious problems if too much is consumed. The most notable and common side effect is known as niacin flush. Niacin flush can occur even with normal levels of the vitamin such as those found in a fortified cereal, especially if consumed close to the same time as a multivitamin or other source of the vitamin. A person experiencing niacin flush feels warmth and redness, itching, and/or tingling of the face, neck, and arms, which eventually subsides on its own. Niacin flush is not dangerous, but it can be uncomfortable or frightening, especially if the individual does not realize that it is caused by excess niacin and is not a symptom of a more serious condition. Consuming hot beverages or alcohol can worsen niacin flush and should be avoided at the time of taking a niacin supplement. For those who take prescription-strength niacin on a regular basis for a health problem, the issue of flushing may lessen with time.

Taking too much niacin for an extended period can cause liver damage, high blood glucose (sugar) levels, gout, stomach ulcers, and skin rashes. However, too little niacin can cause problems, too. Deficiencies are uncommon in developed countries but can result from alcoholism, prolonged diarrhea, and liver disorders such as cirrhosis. A deficiency can make the skin especially prone to damage from the sun.

NIACIN DEFICIENCY

The most severe result of niacin deficiency is pellagra, a disorder characterized by digestive problems including diarrhea, skin inflammations, and dementia or impairment of mental processes. Pellagra occurs often in poor populations that rely on corn as a food staple. Corn contains significant amounts of niacin but not in a form that can be absorbed through normal human digestion. The niacin does become digestible—or bioavailable—if the corn is first treated in an alkaline solution, such as the lime solution used for the preparation of corn tortillas in Mexico. The digestive issues caused by pellagra often lead to other nutritional deficits as well, and the condition can be fatal. Pellagra is treated through the administration of niacin and by supplementing nutrition to overcome other deficiencies caused by the condition.

SUPPLEMENTS

While niacin supplements are readily available, many physicians do not recommend taking them, especially without medical direction or supervision. As previously noted, deficiencies are uncommon in developed countries because sources of niacin are readily available through diet. Many physicians say that supplementation is not necessary and may cause uncomfortable side effects such as flushing, nausea, and stomach upset. It also can alter liver test results and lead to muscle breakdown.

—Janine Ungvarsky;
updated by Tish Davidson, MA

For Further Information:

Johnson, Larry. E. "Niacin." *Merck Manual-Consumer Version.* Merck Sharp & Dohme Corp. 2017. www.merckmanuals.com/home/disorders-of-nutrition/vitamins/niacin 25 (accessed July 31, 2017). An easy-to-understand source of information on niacin deficiency and toxicity.

Natural Standard. "Niacin." Mayo Clinic, 2017. www.mayoclinic.org/drugs-supplements/niacin—niacinamide/background/hrb-20059838 (accessed July 31, 2017). Comprehensive explanation of the role of niacin in human health.

"Niacin." *Linus Pauling Institute Micronutrient Information Center.* Oregon State University July 2012. lpi.oregonstate.edu/ mic/vitamins/niacin (accessed July 31, 2017). A somewhat technical but authoritative monograph on the function of niacin in the body.

"Vitamin B3." University of Maryland Medical Center August 6, 2015. www.umm.edu/health/medical/altmed/supplement/vitamin-b3-niacin (accessed July 31, 2017). Clear, direct overview of niacin and its role in the body.

U.S. National Library of Medicine. "Niacin." MedlinePlus, February 2, 2015.www.nlm.nih.gov/medlineplus/ency/article/002409.htm (accessed July 31, 2017). Easy to understand summary of the importance of niacin in health.

NICOTINE

Category: Treatment
Anatomy or system affected: Central nervous system, lungs
Specialties and related fields: Drug dependency, rehabilitation
Definition: an active ingredient in tobacco products that stimulates the central nervous system in low doses

Today's advertising for cigarettes must carry stern warnings concerning the dangers of smoking and even second-hand smoke from those irresponsible people who have no concern for their own health. Those who have "kicked the habit" are amused to see movie stars or athletes of another day proudly displaying snuff, pipes or a chaw. It is now widely accepted that tobacco is strongly addictive and dangerous to our health. Campaigns by government offices and private foundations, sales restrictions, and high rates of taxation have reduced usage, but smoking remains a major health concern.

While smoking has been found to fill the mouth, throat, and lungs with an astounding array of unhealthy chemicals it is still true that nicotine is the cause of what is undeniably an addiction. The sole beneficial use of this poisonous chemical has been in administering progressively smaller amounts to aid in overcoming one's dependency.

BRIEF HISTORY

The use of nicotine has a long history. There is evidence that humans who first migrated from Asia to the Americas at least 15,000 years ago imported a strong affinity for the use of psychoactive plants. It appears that their belief system centered on a spirit world. These plants provided hallucinations and a number of species that enhanced out-of-body experiences. At least one species, *Nicotiana rustica*, was partially domesticated. While initially, ingestion was by chewing sucking, drinking, or licking, smoking became the preferred method. This observation may have been related to the smoke that suggested its relation to the spirits.

There is a large amount of evidence that the use of tobacco was very wide spread among Native Americans when European explorers and missionaries arrived. In most cases the growing of the plants, curing of the leaves, and consumption of the product was a male activity. The sailors returning to Europe in the sixteenth century brought the fad with them. The English were smoking extensively and in 1595 produced the first book devoted to tobacco. That volume contains illustrations of Europeans smoking a pipe. Soon not only Europe, but also many remote parts of the world were described as "besotted with the herb".

These observations raise the question of why the civilized world adopted so readily a habit of those usually referred to as savages. A tempting suggestion points to the fact that the medical community almost universally endorsed smoking. The evidence shows that its use was recommended as efficacious, or even as a cure, for everything from flatulence to the bubonic plague. This rapid growth occurred in spite of the strong efforts of rulers to suppress its use. Smokers might be decapitated in China and Persians were threatened with loosing parts of their body nose, lips, or ears.

OVERVIEW

There appears to be little question that nicotine has harmful effects on the human body. The ingestion of this drug causes the heart to beat faster and blood pressure to rise. There is evidence that smokers are at significant risk of strokes and heart attacks. Pregnant women are strongly advised to refrain from smoking since nicotine seems to interfere with the transfer of oxygen and nutrition to the fetus. Research on possible links between nicotine and cancer continue and thus far they do not seem to be direct. On the other hand, it does appear to promote the growth of tumors.

In spite of huge efforts by the tobacco industry to suppress evidence of nicotine's harmful effects, the courts have acted against them since the early 1990's. Among the several efforts to promote "safer" methods of using tobacco, none have shown the promise of e-cigarettes. Numerous ads have claimed that such devices afford the pleasure of smoking while eliminating the health risks.

These devices create a solution of nicotine and flavoring in glycerol or the closely related propylene glycol and vaporize it with a heated coil. The vapor created, is inhaled as in traditional smoking. It has been shown that the mist inhaled does contain chemicals known to be undesirable. It has also been found that the smoker's lungs are exposed to tiny particles of metal that likely come off the metal coil or its solder joints. These bits of matter are so small that they can travel deep into the lungs. A variety of ailments can be made worse, for example, asthma, bronchitis, and emphysema. Studies of these potential concerns are facing several problems. No one has determined how much vapor users breathe in. Each study makes different assumptions. It is also true that we have yet to determine the products produced by the vaporization of glycol or propylene glycol.

On the legal front there is still no restriction on the contents and they do not have to be specified. It is also true that, unlike tobacco products, there are no age restrictions on the purchase of e-cigarettes. They are readily available through electronic media. It appears that it will be a while before serious studies reveal just how safe vaping really is.

It has also been suggested that the use of e-cigarettes is an ideal way to quit smoking. Once again the hard, scientific evidence is not available. Until carefully conducted studies are published it is impossible to answer this question. A government bureau recommends that the smoker wishing to quit, explore the available, proven, safe, and effective methods.

—*K. Thomas Finley, PhD*

See also: Addiction, Stimulants

For Further Information:

Balfour, David J. K. *The Neurobiology and Geneticsof Nicotineand Tobacco*. Cham: Springer, 2015.

Brick, John, and Carlton K. Erickson. *Drugs, the Brain, and Behavior: The Pharmacologyof Drug Use Disorders*. New York: Routledge, 2013.

Di Giovanni, G. *NicotineAddiction: Prevention, Health Effects, and Treatment Options*. Hauppauge: Nova Biomedical, 2012.

Dina, Fine Maron. "Smoke Screen: Are E-Cigarettes Safe?" *Scientific American* 310 (May 2014): 31-32.

Ferrence, Roberta, *et al. Nicotineand Public Health*. Washington DC: American Public Health Association, 2000.

Garrett, Bob. *Brain & Behavior: An Introduction to Biological Psychology*. Los Angeles: SAGE, 2015.

Kuhar, Michael J. *The Addicted Brain: Why We Abuse Drugs, Alcohol, and Nicotine*. Upper Saddle River: FT P, 2012.

Owens, Carlton L. *NicotineDependence, SmokingCessation and Effects of Secondhand Smoke*. Hauppauge: Nova, 2015.

Wand, Kelly. *Tobaccoand Smoking*. Detroit: Greenhaven, 2012.

NIEMANN-PICK DISEASE

Category: Disease/Disorder

Anatomy or system affected: Bones, brain, liver, lungs, nervous system, respiratory system, spleen

Specialties and related fields: Biochemistry, endocrinology, family medicine, genetics, hematology, internal medicine, neurology, pathology, pediatrics, public health

Definition: This lipid disease group, resulting from inactive sphingomyelinase and cholesterol-modifying enzymes, causes lipid buildup in the brain and other organs, mental and physical debilitation, and a short life span.

Key terms:

enzyme: a protein biocatalyst that speeds up a biochemical reaction

foam cell: a large, foamy-appearing, lipid-rich cell, usually a white blood cell

lipid: a fatlike substance

CAUSES AND SYMPTOMS

Niemann-Pick disease (NPD), which consists of several lipid storage diseases, is characterized by an enlarged liver and spleen and the accumulation of fatlike sphingomyelin and cholesterol. Many patients have enlarged spleens and livers soon after birth and develop severe mental damage. In others, symptoms lag; mental damage may not occur, or organ enlargement and mental damage may be postponed. The main forms, types A through C, are attributable to low levels of sphingomyelinase, which normally alters sphingomyelin for use and excretion.

Type A, or infantile NPD, is the most common type. The abdominal organs enlarge, and nervous system damage occurs in early infancy. The spleen and liver enlarge by the age of six months, motor function and intellectual capabilities are then lost, and death occurs by four years of age. Patients are emaciated, jaundiced, and have swollen abdomens and cherry-red spots in the macular region of the eye. Large histiocytes (foam cells) abound in the bone marrow, spleen, lymph nodes, adrenal glands, and lungs.

Type B, or juvenile nonneuropathic NPD, is also common. Enlarged abdominal organs develop as quickly as in type A, but no neurological impairment occurs. An enlarged spleen appears first, followed by liver enlargement. Lungs are often so damaged that frequent breathlessness occurs. Abdominal pain is caused by the huge size of the liver, and the patient is susceptible to respiratory infections. Nevertheless, patients with this type of disease reach adulthood in fair health.

Type C, a rarer chronic form, is asymptomatic for approximately two years. Symptoms then develop gradually, accompanied by lost speech and motor coordination and epilepsy. The liver and spleen are smaller than in types A and B. These patients die in their teens.

Type D, a very rare form, is similar to Type C and has only been found in French Canadians in Nova Scotia.

The pathology of Niemann-Pick disease includes abundant foam cells in the spleen, bone marrow, liver, lungs, and lymph nodes. Nervous tissue may be altered similarly. Foam cells contain brown lipofuscin pigment. This and blue to blue-green stained intracellular material leads to an alternate name, sea-blue histiocytes.

The spleen of a patient with NPD is large, pale, and filled with foam cells, though few hematologic changes occur except for anemia late in the disease. The liver of a type A patient is usually about 50 percent larger than normal, while the liver of a type B patient grows so large that it deforms and causes abdominal pain. Foam cells soon fill the liver, although it usually functions adequately. They also fill the lymph nodes, spleen, lungs, and bone marrow. Their number varies with NPD type and duration. In most types, the foam cell-filled adrenal glands, gonads, thyroid, pituitary, and pancreas function adequately. However, the brains of type A and C patients drop in weight by 25 to 50 percent and are severely damaged.

The predominant lipid accumulant is sphingomyelin, made of fatty acids joined to substances called sphingosine and phosphocholine. Sphingomyelin content in the spleens of type A, B, and C patients is twenty-five, eighteen, and two to twelve times normal, respectively. A thirtyfold increase of liver sphingomyelin occurs in types A and B. Smaller increases, approximately ten times normal, oc-

> **INFORMATION ON NIEMANN-PICK DISEASE**
>
> **Causes:** Genetic enzyme deficiency
> **Symptoms:** Liver and spleen enlargement; sometimes severe mental damage, loss of motor function, emaciation, jaundice, swollen abdomen, red spots in eyes, breathlessness
> **Duration:** Chronic and progressive
> **Treatments:** None; enzyme and genetic testing of prospective parents, symptom alleviation through spleen removal or antibiotics

cur in type C. Also, sphingomyelin levels increase threefold to sevenfold in the lymph nodes of all NPD patients. Cholesterol and other sphingolipids also increase in the tissues of NPD patients. It is believed that lipid increases are causative.

Sphingomyelinase deficiency is greatest in types A and C, in which 4 to 20 percent of normal levels occur. In type C, they are about 50 to 90 percent normal levels. The NPD defect is genetic alteration of sphingomyelinase, yielding mutant enzyme less able to break down sphingomyelin.

TREATMENT AND THERAPY
Niemann-Pick disease can be prevented only through the enzymatic and genetic testing of prospective parents. Members of at-risk ethnic groups can be tested for sphingomyelinase in their lymphocytes and muscle cells. Genetic counseling can also be used. The disease is transmitted through an autosomal recessive gene, so both parents must carry the gene to transmit disease. If both parents are carriers of a defective NPD gene, each of their children has a 25 percent chance of having the disease and a 50 percent chance of being an asymptomatic carrier.

There is no cure for Niemann-Pick disease. Therapeutic approaches include spleen removal, which diminishes abdominal pain, but it is not widely used. Patients with lung damage who experience frequent respiratory infections and pneumonia are treated with antibiotics, but long courses and high doses are required. Bone marrow transplantation has been done, with mildly encouraging results for patients with type B, but it is not a common treatment. Some children or teenagers with type C disease have been helped by low-cholesterol diets. However, the life expectancy of patients with NPD has not been prolonged much. Miglustat can help alleviate the nervous system symptoms of type C patients.

PERSPECTIVE AND PROSPECTS
In 1914, Albert Niemann, a German pediatrician, reported an eighteen-month-old Jewish child with huge

liver and spleen, swollen lymph glands, and jaundice. The child had poor motor control, could not suckle, and died before age two. Postmortem examination showed large lipid deposits in the liver, spleen, lymph nodes, kidneys, and adrenal glands. The overall symptoms and rapid death suggested a new illness. In the 1920s, Ludwig Pick studied other cases and named Niemann-Pick disease. NPD, seen in all ethnic groups, is most common in Ashkenazic Jews. Type B patients are often of Spanish ancestry. Type C, which is less common, occurs most in Nova Scotians.

It is believed that enzyme replacement therapy (mostly sphingomyelinase) may ease the lives of NPD victims when an effective methodology for the frequent delivery of purified enzymes is developed and the enzymes are available in sufficient amounts. Recombinant deoxyribonucleic acid (DNA) research should contribute greatly. However, such treatment of severe NPD (types A and C) will be difficult because of the need to deliver enzymes to the brain.

Another avenue is transplanting healthy livers and spleens, which is presently done to treat other diseases. The problems are scarce donated organs and difficulty placing them in debilitated NPD patients. Transplantation may prove more promising in the future. Also, researchers have identified animal models and genes that, when defective, contribute to NPD. Understanding these issues may produce successful NPD treatments.

—*Sanford S. Singer, PhD;*
updated by LeAnna DeAngelo, PhD

See also Brain damage; Enzyme therapy; Enzymes; Gaucher's disease; Genetic counseling; Genetic diseases; Glycogen storage diseases; Lipids; Metabolic disorders; Metabolism; Mucopolysaccharidosis (MPS); Screening; Tay-Sachs disease.

For Further Information:
Dugdale, David C. "Niemann-Pick Disease." *MedlinePlus*, December 7, 2012.
Lichtman, Marshall A., et al., eds. *Williams Hematology.* 8th ed. New York: McGraw-Hill, 2011.
National Institute of Neurological Disorders and Strokes. "Niemann-Pick Disease Information Page." *National Institute of Neurological Disorders and Stroke*, October 6, 2011.
National Niemann-Pick Disease Foundation. *NPD: National Niemann-Pick Disease Foundation Inc.*, May 21, 2013.
Parker, James, and Phillip Parker, eds. *Official Parent's Sourcebook on Niemann-Pick Disease.* San Diego, Calif.: Icon Health, 2007.
Raddidadi, Ali A., and Abdulazix Al Twaim. "Type A-Niemann-Pick Disease." *Journal of European Academy of Dermatology and Venereology* 14 (July, 2000): 301-303.

NONALCOHOLIC STEATOHEPATITIS (NASH)

Category: Disease/Disorder
Also known as: Fatty liver, nonalcoholic fatty liver disease (NAFLD)
Anatomy or system affected: Endocrine system, gastrointestinal system, liver
Specialties and related fields: Endocrinology, family medicine, gastroenterology, internal medicine, pediatrics
Definition: Fatty inflammation of the liver that is not caused by alcohol.
Key terms:
central obesity: excessive abdominal fat
hyperlipidemia: an excess of fat or lipids in the blood
insulin resistance syndrome: a condition characterized by the decreased sensitivity to insulin that is associated with central obesity, metabolic syndrome, and diabetes
metabolic syndrome: a condition defined by the presence of three or more of high blood pressure, abdominal obesity, high triglycerides, low high-density lipoproteins (HDL) cholesterol, and abnormal fasting blood sugar
nonsteroidal anti-inflammatory drugs (NSAIDs): a class of medications for inflammation that do not contain steroids; includes aspirin and ibuprofen

CAUSES AND SYMPTOMS

The liver is a complex organ located in the right upper abdomen. It plays a role in converting carbohydrates, fats, and proteins from food into usable forms for the body. It also manufactures cholesterol, stores sugar, and metabolizes certain medications and chemicals. Nonalcoholic steatohepatitis (NASH) is characterized by the storage of excess fat in the liver, with associated inflammation. The cause of this disorder is not completely understood. The accumulation of excess fat in the liver is related to the body's inability to use its own insulin, a common problem found in adults and children with central obesity. NASH is also found in individuals with other medical conditions, such as diabetes, metabolic syndrome, high blood pressure, and hyperlipidemia. Other causes of excess fat storage are certain medications, exposure to occupational toxins, and some surgical procedures. The excess fat causes damage to the cells of the liver that is similar to the damage caused by excess alcohol intake.

The majority of people with NASH have no symptoms, and the disorder is suspected from liver function tests. Studies have shown, however, that elevated liver enzymes do not always occur in individuals with NASH. If symptoms are present, then they may in-

> ## INFORMATION ON
> ## NONALCOHOLIC STEATOHEPATITIS (NASH)
>
> **Causes:** Accumulation of fat in the liver; related to diabetes, metabolic syndrome, high blood pressure, hyperlipidemia
> **Symptoms:** Often none, sometimes fatigue or mild abdominal discomfort; enlarged liver and severe liver disease may develop
> **Duration:** Chronic
> **Treatments:** Often none; treatment of associated conditions, liver transplantation if severe

clude fatigue or mild discomfort in the upper right side of the abdomen. The liver may be enlarged. Fatty liver may be identified on ultrasound, but a biopsy of the liver must be performed in order to determine the extent of the disorder. A liver biopsy is a minor surgical procedure that is performed by inserting a needle into the liver through a small incision and removing cells for evaluation under the microscope. The disorder may range from inflammation of the liver to cirrhosis, a chronic, progressive disease with extensive scarring of the liver that causes destruction of liver cells. If the destruction advances, then the liver loses the ability to function. Severe liver disease occurs in approximately 20 percent of those with NASH.

TREATMENT AND THERAPY
Treatment goals include the identification and treatment of associated conditions and the reduction of insulin resistance. Adopting a healthy lifestyle is the primary treatment for NASH. Those who are overweight are encouraged to lose weight gradually and to exercise. Triglyceride and cholesterol levels should be kept within normal limits. Strict blood sugar control is indicated for diabetics with NASH. A few studies have found that daily vitamin E reduces abnormal liver enzymes. Insulin-sensitizing drugs, normally used by diabetics, have also shown promise for the treatment of NASH and its associated insulin resistance. Lipid-lowering drug studies have also shown some improvement in blood liver function tests, but not in the follow-up biopsy tests for inflammation and damage.

It is generally recommended that individuals with NASH avoid alcohol and certain medications, such as acetaminophen, that may further damage the liver. If the individual develops severe cirrhosis, then a liver transplant may be necessary to avoid death.

PERSPECTIVE AND PROSPECTS
In 1958, fatty liver disease was first identified in a small group of obese individuals. In 1980, the term nonalcoholic steatohepatitis was coined to describe a small group of patients at the Mayo Clinic who had liver biopsy findings similar to those with alcoholic liver disease. Since 2000, pediatricians have reported the presence of NASH in obese children, as well as in children with other endocrine disorders. The increase in obesity and diabetes in the United States has been linked to the increasing numbers of individuals diagnosed with NASH.

Diagnosis is confirmed with a liver biopsy, or, less commonly, with a noninvasive diagnostic method. Ultrasound and abdominal computed tomography (CT) scans are sometimes used, as are newer x-ray techniques and laboratory blood analyses.

Drug therapy continues to be investigated after promising pilot studies. Further study is also needed in the area of the disease process and its potential for progression in some individuals.

—*Amy Webb Bull, DSN, APN*

See also Abdomen; Abdominal disorders; Alcoholism; Cholesterol; Cirrhosis; Diabetes mellitus; Gastroenterology; Gastroenterology, pediatric; Gastrointestinal disorders; Gastrointestinal system; Hypercholesterolemia; Hyperlipidemia; Inflammation; Insulin resistance syndrome; Internal medicine; Liver; Liver disorders; Liver transplantation; Metabolic syndrome; Metabolism; Obesity; Obesity, childhood; Transplantation.

For Further Information:
Adams, L. A., and P. Angulo. "Treatment of Non-alcoholic Fatty Liver Disease." *Postgraduate Medicine Journal*, 82 (May, 2006): 315-322.
Harrison, Stephen A., and Adrian M. Di Bisceglie. "Advances in the Understanding and Treatment of Nonalcoholic Fatty Liver Disease." *Drugs* 63, no. 22 (2003): 2379-2394.
Howson, Alexandra. "Nonalcoholic Fatty Liver Disease." *Health Library*, May 14, 2013.
"Liver Disease: Fat Inflames the Liver." *Harvard Health Letter* 26 (February, 2001): 4.
Nakajima, Kenichirou, et al. "Pediatric Nonalcoholic Steatohepatitis Associated with Hypopituitarism." *Journal of Gastroenterology* 40, no. 3 (March, 2005): 312-315.
"Nonalcoholic Fatty Liver Disease." *Mayo Clinic*, February 19, 2011.
Nonalcoholic Steatohepatitis." *National Digestive Diseases Information Clearinghouse*, April 30, 2012.
Porth, Carol M. "Disorders of Hepatobiliary and Exocrine Pancreas Function." In *Pathophysiology: Concepts of Altered Health States*. 8th ed. Philadelphia: Wolters Kluwer/Lippincott Williams & Wilkins, 2010.

NONBINARY GENDER

Category: Development
Also known as: Gender-nonconforming, agender, bigender, gender-fluid, multigender
Anatomy or system affected: Psychological and emotional functioning

Specialties and related fields: Genetics, pediatrics, psychiatry, psychology

Definition: A term that refers to people whose gender does not fall within the binary categories of man/boy and woman/girl.

Key terms:

agender: a term that refers to people who don't identify as a specific gender

cisgender: a person whose sense of personal identity and gender corresponds with their birth sex

gender dysphoria: a description in the *Diagnostic and Statistical Manual of Mental Disorders* (DSM) of the feeling of distress associated with the incongruence between one's gender and one's sex assigned at birth

gender expression: refers to how one behaves, dresses, acts, and speaks in relation to gender; descriptors could include feminine, masculine, or androgynous

gender identity: a personal sense of gender that may differ from that assigned biologically at birth

gender-nonconforming: term used to describe people who do not conform with the prescribed social expectations associated with a person's sex assigned at birth and typically refers to gender expression

genderqueer: a gender identity and/or sexual orientation adopted by some who do not align with heterosexual or homosexual norms

misgendering: using gendered language or pronouns that are inaccurate

BINARY VS. NONBINARY

Gender binary refers to the common idea that there are two genders only: man/boy and woman/girl. Those genders are generally considered to be opposites, with men behaving, dressing, and speaking in ways stereotypically considered masculine, and women behaving, dressing, and speaking in ways stereotypically considered feminine. In many cultures, despite evidence to the contrary, a gender binary is assumed to be the norm, and society has rigid expectations of those it labels man or woman.

Many people, however, do not fit into those categories and do not consider themselves to be exclusively men or women. These people are sometimes referred to as nonbinary—an umbrella term encompassing many alternative gender identities and acknowledging that gender exists on a spectrum. Several different experiences can fall under that umbrella: Some people, for example, do not feel as they adhere to any gender at all (agender or genderless), while others feel that their identity comprises multiple genders (bigender or pangender). Still others fluctuate (gender-fluid) or identify with an entirely different category, such as genderqueer, which highlights a sexual attraction to those who cannot be easily slotted into male or female roles.

It is important to distinguish between nonbinary people and those who identify as transgender, since most transgender people are not nonbinary and identify firmly as male or female, although their assigned sex at birth differs from their later gender identity. It is also important to avoid confusion between nonbinary and intersex people (those with anatomical features or genes that don't fit the usual physical characteristics of male or female), since nonbinary people are usually born with bodies that fit typical physical norms of male and female.

According to one recent study, an estimated 1.2 million adults aged eighteen to sixty identify as nonbinary in the United States alone.

GENDER EXPRESSION VS. GENDER IDENTITY

While the terms gender identity and gender expression are often used interchangeably, they mean different things. A gender identity refers to the ingrained personal sense of what one's gender is: man, woman, nonbinary, or gender-fluid, for example. Gender expression, on the other hand, includes how one acts. When we refer to someone dressing in a feminine way or like a "tomboy," we are discussing gender expression.

It is a mistake to assume that all nonbinary people dress and behave in an androgynous manner. Some exhibit typically masculine gender expression, while others might express themselves with the trappings of femininity or a combination of the two. Because gender identity is different from gender expression, it is impossible to "tell" another's identity just by looking at them.

It is also vital to keep in mind that sex and gender mean two very different things: sex refers to a person's external physical characteristics, such as having either a penis or vagina, while gender is a broader term associated with a person's own sense of themselves. A person's self-identified gender has little to do with the sex ascribed to them at birth because of their physical characteristics.

In addition to occurring on a spectrum, gender can be described as a journey of exploration—one that is not necessarily predictable or linear—for some people. Certain children might initially identify with the sex assigned to them at birth but later consider themselves nonbinary, or vice versa.

HISTORICAL PERSPECTIVE

Some observers, particularly those who stand in opposition to civil rights for the transgender and nonbinary communities, argue mistakenly that alternative gender identities are a recent phenomenon. In actuality, there is well-documented evidence that nonbinary people have existed for centuries.

The Hijras of South Asia provide one of the oldest examples of gender variance. Encompassing those who in the West would be defined as transgender, intersex, or eunuchs, the *hijras* were long thought to possess sacred powers and were called upon to deliver blessings at weddings or births. In 2014, the Supreme Court of India recognized hijras as a legally designated third gender.

Indigenous North Americans also have a long history of recognizing various gender identities. Navajo tribes, for example, recognized four genders roughly corresponding to cisgender and transgender men and women, with the terms *nadleehi* for those who adopt femininity and *dilbaa* for those who adopt masculinity. In another example, the Lakota tribe believed those they termed *winkte* (males who adopt the clothing, work, and mannerisms that Lakota culture usually considers feminine) had supernatural powers like those of India's hijras. In these and many other indigenous cultures, "two-spirit" people are respected and, in some cases, even revered.

Additionally, historians have pointed out that several paintings from eighteenth-century Italy depict *il femminiello*, those assigned male at birth who dressed and behaved like women and who were considered harbingers of good luck for their families.

MENTAL HEALTH CONSIDERATIONS

In the past, mental-health practitioners often pathologized gender-diverse individuals, and it was not uncommon for someone seeking help to be prescribed so-called conversion therapy, a pseudoscientific process aimed at "correcting" an individual's sexual orientation or gender identity. Besides being ineffective, the practice caused lasting psychological damage to many, and in 1997, the American Psychiatric Association issued a strong statement condemning it. Still, it was not until 2013 when the *Diagnostic and Statistical Manual of Mental Disorders* (DSM) eliminated the term "gender identity disorder" as a diagnosable sexual dysfunction and replaced it with "gender dysphoria," a general description of the severe psychological discomfort experienced by some whose physical traits do not align with their gender identity.

While attitudes have changed, nonbinary people often experience stigma among those in the general population, and common microaggressions include hearing that nonbinary people do not really exist, are attempting to be trendy, are mentally unbalanced, or are merely seeking attention. They are at high risk of rejection by family, discrimination at school or in the workplace, and denial of appropriate medical care.

Surveys have revealed that almost half of nonbinary people had suffered serious psychological distress or anxiety. Those circumstances have been tied clinically to higher rates of disease and physical-health problems.

GENDER-NEUTRAL LANGUAGE

It's always important to defer to a person's given gender identifier. Misgendering—being called by a former name or incorrect pronoun—is a source of great distress to many nonbinary people because it can be experienced as an attempt by the speaker to erase or negate the person's authentic identity. While some nonbinary people use binary pronouns, such as he/him/his or she/her/hers, others have a strong preference for such neutral terms as they/them/theirs or ze/zir/zirs. In 2019, *Merriam-Webster* announced that the definition of "they" had expanded to include reference to a single person whose gender identity is nonbinary. (Editors of the iconic dictionary pointed out that what is sometimes called the "singular they" actually has a long history of use in English despite falling out of favor in past decades.)

Other examples of the sensitive use of gender-neutral terms include person instead of man or woman, child instead of son or daughter, sibling instead of sister or brother, parent instead of mother or father, and partner or spouse instead of husband or wife.

—Mari Rich

For Further Information:

Cerretani, Jessica. "What It Means to Be Non-Binary: A Guide for Parents." Boston Children's Hospital, 4 Dec. 2019, answers.childrenshospital.org/non-binary-guide/. Accessed 15 Mar. 2022.

Matsuno, E., and S. L. Budge. "Non-Binary/Genderqueer Identities: A Critical Review of the Literature." *Current Sexual Health Reports*, vol. 9, no. 3, 2017, pp. 116-20.

Matsuno, E., A. Webb, H. Hashtpari, et al. "Nonbinary Fact Sheet." *Society for the Psychology of Sexual Orientation and Gender Diversity*, n.d., www.apadivisions.org/division-44/resources/nonbinary-fact-sheet.pdf. Accessed 15 Mar. 2022.

Tordoff, D. M., J. W. Wanta, A. Collin, et al. "Mental Health Outcomes in Transgender and Nonbinary Youths Receiving Gender-Affirming Care." *JAMA Network Open*, vol. 5, no. 2, 2022, p. e220978, doi:10.1001/jamanetworkopen.2022.0978.

"Transgender and Non-Binary People FAQ." Human Rights Campaign, n.d., www.hrc.org/resources/transgender-and-non-binary-faq. Accessed 15 Mar. 2022.

"Understanding Non-Binary People: How to Be Respectful and Supportive." *National Center for Transgender Equality*, 5 Oct. 2015, transequality.org/issues/resources/understanding-non-binary-people-how-to-be-respectful-and-supportive#:~:text=Non%2DBinary%20Defined&text=Some%20people%20don't%20identify,agender%2C%20bigender%2C%20and%20more. Accessed 15 Mar. 2022.

NONINVASIVE PRENATAL TESTING (NIPT)

Category: Prenatal

INDICATIONS AND PROCEDURES
Noninvasive prenatal test, NIPT, is a prenatal screening test. It assesses the risk of a fetus having certain chromosomal abnormalities and is available in over sixty countries. It is a maternal blood test, and analyses the cell-free deoxyribonucleic acid (DNA) (cfDNA), of maternal and fetal origin, that is found in the maternal blood.

Approximately 10 percent (3 percent to 20 percent) of the cfDNA in maternal circulation is of fetal origin, mostly from the placenta, with a considerably lesser contribution from the fetus. The cfDNA is found as small fragments of 150 to 200 base pairs.

The test is done via a peripheral sample of the expectant mother's blood. Usually, 8 to 10 cc is submitted to the performing laboratory for analysis for cfDNA.

By analyzing the cfDNA in the blood sample, the laboratory is looking to determine if the cfDNA from the fetus is in proportion to all the expected forty-six chromosomes, and consequently, to assess the likelihood that one or more of the chromosomes are in excess or absent. This is known as aneuploidy, the condition of having missing or extra chromosomes. At present, there are a variety of techniques used, often specific to the laboratory, to accomplish this test.

NIPT can be done at any time during the pregnancy, usually starting as early as nine to ten weeks gestational age. Results can be available in three to seven days, reported as positive, negative or indeterminate (no-call results).

USES AND COMPLICATIONS
Most fetuses with chromosomal aneuploidies are nonviable and lead to early miscarriage. Some of these fetuses have the potential to survive to the newborn period, only to have a high rate of mortality shortly after birth. Others survive longer, but are associated with significant morbidities. Can we detect the fetus that has a chromosomal aneuploidy?

NIPT as a prenatal screening test, was developed for the detection of certain chromosomal aneuploidies of the fetus, early in pregnancy. It has a better detection rate than previous screening tests that utilize maternal blood samples and/or sonogram.

NIPT allows for the screening of a number of chromosomal aneuploidies. Screening early in the pregnancy allows for the option of early diagnostic testing in the case of a positive screening result. Diagnostic

testing, via chorionic villi sampling or amniocentesis, could then be done to confirm or disprove the chromosomal abnormality. This would allow for the consideration of a termination early in the pregnancy if a chromosomal aneuploidy was confirmed.

There is no concern that the fetal cfDNA in the maternal blood is from a previous pregnancy. The half-life of fetal cfDNA is less than twenty minutes, and it is constantly being refreshed. It disappears from maternal circulation within a few hours postpartum. Therefore, NIPT only obtains fetal cfDNA from the present pregnancy.

NIPT assesses the fetal risk for the most common aneuploid conditions. It includes Trisomy 21 (T21, Down syndrome), which is the single most common cause of intellectual disabilities and the highest incidence at birth of any chromosomal abnormalities. It also tests for Trisomy 18 (T18, Edwards syndrome), and Trisomy 13 (T13, Patau syndrome).

With NIPT, using cfDNA in the maternal blood sample, the detection rate/false positive rate is: for Trisomy 21 (Down syndrome, T21), 99.7 percent/0.04 percent, for Trisomy 18 (Edwards syndrome, T18), 97.9 percent/0.04 percent, and for Trisomy 13 (Patau syndrome, T13), 99.0 percent/0.04 percent. NIPT is the recommended screening for these aneuploid chromosomal abnormalities.

In addition, NIPT can screen, with high detection rate, for the more common sex chromosome aneuploidies, which when taken together, have an overall prevalence of 1:500, They are therefore more common than major trisomies. The more common sex chromosome aneuploidies are: 45,X (Turner syndrome) detection rate 95.8 percent, 47,XXY and 48, XXYY (Klinefelter syndrome) detection rate 95 percent, 47,XYY (Jacobs syndrome) detection rate 95 percent, and 47, XXX (triple X syndrome) detection rate 95 percent. Though prenatal screening test have never been directly structured and addressed to the recognition of sex chromosome aneuploidies, they have a 95 percent sensitivity for these conditions, and a false-positive rate of percent.

It is important to be aware that screening tests are not definitive. They provide a risk assessment, that represents an expectant mother's chance of carrying a fetus with the chromosomal abnormality in question. With screening tests, there is no guarantee that the fetus does or does not have the chromosomal aneuploidies screened for.

A negative result indicates a considerable reduction in the risk for the chromosomal abnormalities being screened for. A positive result will be positive for a specific chromosomal or sub chromosomal abnormality, and indicates a considerably increased risk for that specific chromosomal abnormality in the fetus. By reviewing the results of the screening test, the clinician can determine whether to offer diagnostic testing, and the expectant mother can determine if she wishes to undergo one of the diagnostic tests.

Diagnosis relates to a process that determines the presence or absence of a disease state. Diagnostic results are communicated as "normal" or "abnormal". Amniocentesis and chorionic sampling are prenatal diagnostic tests, and are still the gold standard and provide definitive results. They are older tests, that were initially developed to test for chromosomal aneuploidies. However, they are invasive, and carry a risk of miscarriage.

Indeterminate or "no-call" results generally occur in 2 percent of samples. It is usually due to an inadequate fetal fraction, the proportion of fetal cfDNA in the total cfDNA, extracted from a maternal specimen. Multiple conditions can contribute to a low fetal fraction, such as maternal weight, fetal gestational age, maternal medical conditions and medications, unrecognized twin pregnancy, placental or maternal mosaicism, the fetal aneuploidy itself and in vitro fertilization with a donor egg. These are not direct contraindications to NIPT, but they must be considered when ordering these screens.

NIPT screens for only a limited number of chromosomal aneuploidies, identified above. Also, not every patient is screened for all conditions. The clinician decides which test(s) to order, from the selections the specific laboratory offers. Test manufactures offer optional add-ons, for rarer trisomies, copy number variants and microdeletions. But the add-ons, which for microdeletions alone number in the hundreds, only test for between five and seven microdeletions. This adds to the cost of the test, but add little value, as these tests are for much rarer conditions. And the rarer the condition, the higher false positive rates. This can give positive screening results that are incorrect about 85 percent of the time.

The American College of Obstetrics and Gynecology (ACOG) does not recommend using NIPT for these rarer conditions, due to a lack of evidence regarding validity.

HISTORY
- In 1947, Swaminathan and Butt documented the presence of cfDNA in the circulation in adult serum.
- In 1959, Lejeune and colleagues, demonstrated that Down syndrome is caused by an extra copy of chromosome 21 (trisomy 21, T21). This is of clinical importance, as Down syndrome is the single most common cause of intellectual disability. It has the highest incidence at birth of any chromosomal abnormality.
- In 1972, Bang and Northeved, from Denmark, was the first to report amniocentesis done with the guide of an ultrasound.
- In 1982, Simoni performed the first chorionic villus sampling.
- In 1997, Lo and colleagues, discovered the presence of cfDNA of fetal origin in maternal plasma, and that it could be reliably detected. Ten years later, they showed that analysis of cfDNA of fetal origin allowed for the detection of trisomy 21 (T21), or Down syndrome.
- In 1997 Lo and colleagues, reported the presence of cfDNA from the Y chromosome of male fetuses in the maternal plasma during pregnancy.

PERSPECTIVE AND PROSPECTS
NIPT using cfDNA screening was made available in the United States in November 2011, with the goal to make noninvasive screens more sensitive and lower their false-positive rate. It has rapidly expanded into clinical practice as a reliable, accurate, and popular prenatal screen. The American College of Obstetricians and Gynecologists (ACOG) and American College of Medical Genetics and Genomics (ACMG) have issued guidelines on how best to integrate this screening into clinical practice for the benefit of their patients. Their present recommendation is that all prenatal screens and tests should be made available to all women, regardless of age.

The present NIPT is a screening test. However, as the test accuracy improves, it has the potential of becoming a diagnostic test. It may also have the accuracy to test for several monogenic (single gene) diseases.

Another potential for prenatal testing would be the use of fetal cells found in maternal circulation. The presence of fetal cells in maternal circulation is much rarer compared to cfDNA. Usually well below 100 fetal cells can be successfully identified and isolated from 10 ml of maternal blood. However, fetal cells have the advantage of allowing for more accurate noninvasive analysis. At present it is not possible as a commercial prenatal test. It has a higher cost, a lower throughput, and a more complex clinical validations compared to cfDNA assays. The belief is that these challenges in fetal cell assay will be resolved in the not-too-distant future.

Future applications of cfDNA found in blood are being considered regarding malignancies. Research is looking to the future at clinical applications of cfDNA that involve screening, diagnosis and management of malignancies. And there may be more future uses for cfDNA, waiting to be uncovered.

—*Linda Roethel, MD*

For Further Information:

"Applying Guidelines in Practice: Noninvasive Prenatal Testing." *Omnia Education*. Supplement to *OBG Management*, Dec. 2020.

Errol R. Norwitz, and Brynn Levy. "Noninvasive Prenatal Testing: The Future Is Now." *Reviews in Obstetrics & Gynecology*, vol. 6, no. 2, 2013, pp. 48-62.

Luigi Carbone, Federica Cariati, Laura Sarno, et al. "Non-Invasive Prenatal Testing: Current Perspectives and Future Challenges." *Genes*, vol. 12, 2021, no. 15.

Monica A. Lutendorf, Katie A. Stoll, Dana M. Knutzen, and Lisa M. Foglia. "Noninvasive Prenatal Testing: Limitations and Unanswered Questions." *Genetics in Medicine*, 5 Sept. 2013, doi:10.1038/gim.2013.126.

Sarah Kliff, and Aatish Bhatia. "Tests Predicting Rare Disorders in Fetuses Are Usually Wrong." *New York Times*, 2 Jan. 2022.

Vardit Ravitsky, Marie-Christine Roy, Hazar Haidar, et al. "The Emergence and Global Spread of Noninvasive Prenatal Testing." *Annual Review of Genomics and Human Genetics*, vol. 22, 2021, pp. 309-18.

Noninvasive Tests

Category: Procedures

Anatomy or system affected: All

Specialties and related fields: Cardiology, emergency medicine, nuclear medicine, obstetrics, pathology, preventive medicine, radiology

Definition: Diagnostic techniques that do not involve the collection of tissue or fluid samples or the introduction of any instrument into the body; most noninvasive tests involve imaging or the measurement of electrical activity.

Key terms:

computed tomography (CT) scanning: a method of producing images of cross sections of the body

diagnosis: recognition of diseases based on physical examination, the microscopic and chemical results of laboratory findings, and an analysis of imaging results

Doppler shift: the increase in frequency of sound waves as the source of the waves approaches the observer or instrument; Doppler techniques are often used to assess blood flow in body channels such as veins

echocardiogram (EC): a graph of cardiac motion and heart valve closure produced by sending sound waves to the heart and recording their deflections

electrocardiogram (EKG or ECG): a diagnostic tool used to detect disturbances in the electrical activity of the heart

magnetic resonance imaging (MRI): a procedure using magnetic fields to determine blood vessel condition, fluid flow, and tissue contours and to detect abnormal masses

signal-averaged electrocardiogram (SAECG): a sophisticated EKG which detects subtle and potentially lethal cardiac conduction defects

sonography: the use of sound waves deflected from internal body organs to find growing masses (including fetuses) and abnormal lesions; also called ultrasound

X radiology: the use of ionizing radiation of short wavelength to detect abnormalities in primarily dense portions of the body

INDICATIONS AND PROCEDURES

Noninvasive tests are used in the initial diagnosis of a disease or abnormality and for the monitoring of certain conditions and body processes. Most such tests involve imaging techniques. Primary among them are x-radiology, computed tomography (CT) scanning, magnetic resonance imaging (MRI), electrocardiography (EKG or ECG), and ultrasound.

Diagnostic x-ray examinations are often the first step in complex technological solutions to medical diagnoses and health problems. New uses for diagnostic x-rays are constantly being devised. It is common practice for hospitals to require chest x-rays for all outpatients visiting x-ray departments, and hospital inpatients are usually given chest x-rays before admission or surgery.

Computed tomography (CT) scanning, also known as computed axial tomography (CAT) scanning, uses a computer to interpret multiple x-ray images in order to reconstruct a cross-sectional image of any area of the body. The inventors of the procedure for CT scanning were awarded a Nobel Prize in 1979.

After the patient is placed in the CT scanner, an x-ray source rapidly rotates around it, taking hundreds of pictures. The pictures are electronically recorded and stored by a computer. The computer then integrates the data into cross-sectional "slices." The CT scanner can assess the composition of internal structures, which it is able to discriminate from fat, fluid, and gas. The scanner can show the shape and size of various organs and lesions and has the capability of detecting abnormal lesions as small as one or two millimeters in diameter.

Magnetic resonance imaging (MRI), unlike CT scanning (which uses x-rays), uses magnetic fields passing through the body to detect details of anatomy and physiology.

MRI equipment consists of a tunnel-like magnet that creates a magnetic field around the patient. This magnetic field causes the hydrogen atoms found in the body-water has two hydrogen atoms and one oxygen atom in the molecule-to line up. At the same time, a radio frequency signal is quickly transmitted to upset the uniformity of the formation. When the radio frequency signal is turned off, the hydrogen atoms return to their proper lineup, and a small current is generated. By detecting the speed and volume with which the atoms return, the computer can display a diagnostic image on a monitor.

MRI is noninvasive, and no pain or radiation is involved. The procedure takes from fifteen to forty-five minutes, depending on the number of views needed. Diagnostic x-rays rely on variations of density on film, and areas of soft tissue, for example, produce little or no shadow and are difficult to distinguish in any detail. MRI images, on the other hand, allow tumors, muscles, arteries, and vertebrae to be seen with great clarity.

Monitoring and providing electrical support to the heart constitute other useful noninvasive techniques. A healthy heart generates electrical impulses rhythmically and spontaneously; this activity is controlled by the sinoatrial (S-A) node, the heart's natural pacemaker. From there, the impulses pass through specialized conduction tissues in the atria and into the atrioventricular (A-V) node. Then the electrical impulses enter the ventricular conduction system, the bundle of His, and the right and left bundle branches. From the bundle branches, the impulses spread into the ventricles through the network of Purkinje fibers. The spread of electrical stimulation through the atria and the ventricles is known as depolarization. The standard electrocardiogram (ECG or EKG) records this activity from twelve different angles. The EKG records the heart's electrical activity and provides vital information concerning its rate, rhythm, and conduction system status. Detecting changes in the EKG can help to diagnose ventricular conduction problems and ventricular hypertrophy.

The signal-averaged electrocardiogram (SAECG) is another noninvasive procedure that is a promising diagnostic tool for many cardiac patients. Unlike the standard twelve-lead EKG, the SAECG can detect conduction abnormalities that often precede sustained ventricular tachycardia-which is second only to myocardial infarction (heart attack) as the leading cause of sudden death. The SAECG records the heart's electrical activity via six electrodes applied to the frontal and posterior chest walls. The SAECG can often pick up repolarization delays that occur when ischemic (damaged) tissue impedes the passage of electrical impulses through a portion of the myocardium, a condition that can lead to ventricular tachycardia.

A valuable weapon in the battle against sudden cardiac death is the temporary pacemaker, which provides support for the heart's electrical conduction system. Such devices can provide vital support when there is no time to prepare for an invasive procedure and are also used when invasive procedures are contraindicated.

Another method for diagnosing heart problems is echocardiography, a technique for recording echoes of ultrasonic waves when these waves are directed at areas of the heart. The principle is similar to that used in the sonar detection of submarines and other underwater objects. In this very simple and painless procedure, the patient lies on a table while a small, high-frequency generator (transducer) is moved across the chest. The instrument projects ultrasonic waves and receives the returning echoes. As the waves pass through the heart, their behavior differs, depending on whether there is any calcification present, whether there is a blood clot or any other mass in the cavity of the heart, whether certain heart chambers are enlarged, whether the valves within the heart open and close in the proper fashion, and whether any part of the heart is thicker than it should be.

Sonography, or ultrasound, imaging and the images produced are unique: patients can hear their blood flowing through the carotid arteries of the neck, and physicians can see a braintumor or watch a human fetus suck its thumb. This simple and inexpensive imaging technique has aided in the development of fetal medicine as a subspecialty. Sonography uses sound waves to look within the body by using a piezoelectric crystal to convert electric pulses into vibrations that penetrate the body. These sound waves are reflected back to the crystal, which reconverts them into electric signals. Many doctors foresee much growth in the use of ultrasound as a noninvasive procedure.

USES AND COMPLICATIONS

Historically, diagnostic x-rays have been used for the detection of metal objects, cavities in teeth, and broken bones. Films of various parts of the body, such as the abdomen, skull, and chest, have been taken ever since x-rays were first discovered in the late nineteenth century. Dentists and orthodontists use x-rays to check for jaw fractures, tooth misalignment, gum disease, tartar deposits, impacted teeth, and bone cancer. Chronic illnesses that can be detected by x-rays include arthritis, tuberculosis, osteoporosis, emphysema, ulcers, pneumonia, and urinary tract infections.

The CT scanner uses a series of narrow, pencil-like x-ray beams to scan the section of the body under investigation. CT scans allow the rapid diagnosis of brain abnormalities, cysts, tumors, and blood clots. Newly developed body scanners assist in the early detection of cancers and other diseases of the internal organs.

Magnetic resonance imaging has undergone an explosive growth in applications. In 1982, there were only six machines in operation. Hospitals often used a portable MRI device, which can be driven from place to place with a tractor-trailer truck. As the cost for

MRI machines decreases, however, more hospitals are purchasing this equipment instead of sharing it.

The MRI machine is able to differentiate the brain's gray matter (nerve cells) from the brain's white matter (nerve fibers). Gray matter contains 87 percent water, and white matter contains 72 percent water. Thus, since MRI detects the protons in the hydrogen in water, a great difference in contrast between the two types of brain material is seen on the resulting scan. MRI is also useful in detecting and monitoring the progression of multiple sclerosis because the fatty tissue that normally exists around nerve fibers deteriorates, and these abnormal, fat-free areas can be clearly imaged.

MRI research seeks ways of analyzing the numerous chemical elements found in the body and aids in the study, diagnosis, treatment, and cure of a host of human diseases.

EKGs are useful in the detection of irregularities in the heart's electrical conduction system. This technology can also help in the diagnosis of ventricular hypertrophy, pulmonary emboli, and intraventricular conduction problems.

Echocardiograms, based on sound waves, are used to detect infarcts (areas of necrosis, or tissue death), valve closure between heart chambers, and abnormal thickening of myocardial muscle. Sonography is perhaps best known for its contribution to diagnostic medicine in the study of human fetal development. Determining the age of a developing embryo is now standard procedure, and clear images can be obtained at five weeks of gestation, when the embryo is only five millimeters long. Fetal weight can be determined by volume, and fetal anatomy can also be studied. Congenital heart defects can be spotted very early, and neural brain defects can be discovered as well.

The great advantage of ultrasound is that it emits no ionizing radiation and thus can be used on pregnant women without danger to the fetus. Ultrasound can also detect gallstones, kidney stones, and tumors and can monitor blood flow. Its applications have grown exponentially since its discovery.

Noninvasive tests such as x-rays, MRI, and CT scanning have become a crucial part of the detection and treatment of cancer. They are vital in determining the source and extent of the malignancy.

Mammography is a subset of x-ray imaging that is useful in detecting breast cancer. The equipment used in mammography is designed to image breast tissue, which is usually soft and of uniform density. Very small changes in density can be identified in fine detail, including small areas of calcification. Radiation doses must also be kept to a minimum. The film interpretation of mammograms is difficult, but early detection of breast cancer is often possible.

In the United States, the Public Health Service, in a memo dated June 1, 1993, delegated authority for implementing the Mammography Quality Standards Act (MQSA) of 1992 to the Food and Drug Administration (FDA). The MQSA is intended to ensure that mammography is reliable and safe. The act makes it unlawful for any facility to provide services unless it is accredited by an approved private nonprofit or state body and it has received federal certification indicating that it meets standards for quality. Each facility must also pass an annual inspection conducted by approved federal personnel. The law was enacted in response to the need for safe, early detection of breast cancer. Mammography is the most effective technique for early detection of this type of cancer.

Given a choice, most persons would prefer a noninvasive diagnostic tool. The earliest used diagnostic tool was the x-ray. X-rays were discovered in 1895 by a German professor named Wilhelm Conrad Röntgen. The first x-rays were produced in a Crookes tube, a pear-shaped glass tube in which two electrodes, the cathode (negative electrode) and anode (positive electrode), were placed at right angles to each other. The tube was then evacuated of gas. In Röntgen's first experiment, the cathode was "excited" with an electrical current, producing a beam of cathode rays, or electrons. These electrons were directed across the tube from the cathode and struck the glass, causing it to glow and, at the same time, producing x-rays, which excited a fluorescent screen. In a modern x-ray tube, the cathode ray strikes a target in the anode rather than the glass. Modern equipment also uses high-energy electricity in order to energize the tube at the high voltages necessary for producing x-rays.

Radiology has come far. From a medical discipline with a limited but vital function (that of aiding diagnosis), it has become interventional. It is a field that has moved into therapy-repairing a growing variety of abnormalities, averting surgery, and sometimes achieving results beyond the reach of surgery.

In addition to the simple x-ray, physicians now have more powerful diagnostic devices: MRI, CT scanning, and sonography. Cardiac conditions and abnormalities are quite easily analyzed via the ECG or echocardiogram. Where once the diagnosis of gallstones required a two-day x-ray test and twelve grams of diarrhea-causing pills, now ultrasound allows a diagnosis to be made painlessly and noninvasively, in ten to fifteen minutes.

The computer has been the core in the revolution in imaging. As more information becomes available and the density of information grows exponentially, larger and faster computers have been developed to assimilate this information. Computer visualization both interprets data and generates images from data in order to provide new insight into disease states through visual methods. Visualization and computation promise to play a key role in diagnostic medicine.

—Jane A. Slezak, PhD

See also Computed tomography (CT) scanning; Diagnosis; Echocardiography; Electrocardiography (ECG or EKG); Electroencephalography (EEG); Imaging and radiology; Magnetic resonance imaging (MRI); Mammography; Neuroimaging; Physical examination; Prognosis; Radiation therapy; Screening; Single photon emission computed tomography (SPECT); Ultrasonography; Urinalysis.

For Further Information:

A.D.A.M. Medical Encyclopedia. "Imaging and Radiology." *MedlinePlus*, March 22, 2012.
Chopra, Sanjiv. *The Liver Book: A Comprehensive Guide to Diagnosis, Treatment, and Recovery*. New York: Simon & Schuster, 2002.
Crawford, Michael, ed. *Current Diagnosis and Treatment-Cardiology*. 3d ed. New York: McGraw-Hill Medical, 2009.
Galton, Lawrence. *Med Tech*. New York: Harper & Row, 1985.
Griffith, H. Winter. *Complete Guide to Symptoms, Illness, and Surgery*. Revised and updated by Stephen Moore and Kenneth Yoder. 5th ed. New York: Perigee, 2006.
MedlinePlus. "Diagnostic Imaging." *MedlinePlus*, May 24, 2013.
Merva, Jean. "SAECG: A Closer Look at the Heart." *RN* 56 (May, 1993): 51-53.
National Institute of Biomedical Imaging and Bioengineering. "Image-Guided Interventions." *National Institutes of Health*, March 29, 2013.
Pagana, Kathleen Deska, and Timothy J. Pagana. *Mosby's Diagnostic and Laboratory Test Reference*. 9th ed. St. Louis, Mo.: Mosby/Elsevier, 2009.
Sochurek, Howard. *Medicine's New Vision*. Easton, Pa.: Mack, 1988.
Solomon, Jacqueline. "Take the EKG One Step Further." *RN* 55 (May, 1992): 56-60.
Wolbarst, Anthony Brinton. *Looking Within: How X-Ray, CT, MRI, Ultrasound, and Other Medical Images Are Created*. Berkeley: University of California Press, 1999.

NONSTEROIDAL ANTI-INFLAMMATORY DRUGS (NSAIDs)

Category: Class of Drug

Anatomy or system affected: Any area of inflammation or pain throughout the body

Specialties and related fields: Primary care, internal medicine, family medicine, orthopedic surgery, rheumatology, nurse practitioner, physician assistant

Key terms:

arachidonic acid: an omega-6 unsaturated fatty acid the body requires to function properly; when broken down in the body, prostaglandins are produced

COX-1 AND COX-2: cyclooxygenase 1 and 2 (COX-1 and COX-2) are important enzymes in the function of the human body; they both convert arachidonic acid to prostaglandins and are implicated in pain, inflammation, cell multiplication, and other key biologic responses

NSAIDs: nonsteroidal anti-inflammatory drugs (NSAIDs) are medications that are used to control pain and inflammation in the body

osteoarthritis: a progressive disorder of the joints caused by gradual loss of cartilage that can result in the development of bone spurs and cysts at the margins of joints

prostaglandins: one of several hormone-like substances that participate in a wide range of body functions such as the contraction and relaxation of smooth muscle, the dilation and constriction of blood vessels, control of blood pressure, and modulation of inflammation

Reye syndrome: a rare but serious disease that most often affects children ages 6 to 12 years old; can cause brain swelling and liver damage; may be related to using aspirin to treat viral infections

INDICATIONS

Prostaglandins are responsible for many functions in the body and can foster inflammation, pain, and fever. Enzymes known as COX-1 and COX-2 are produced by cells in the body. They are responsible for synthesizing prostaglandins from a fatty acid called arachidonic acid. The degradation of membrane phospholipids generates arachidonic acid by enzymes called phospholipases A2, activated when cells are damaged. Nonsteroidal anti-inflammatory drugs (NSAIDs) inhibit the activity of the COX-1 and COX-2 enzymes, which synthesize prostaglandins that cause pain and inflammation.

The most well-known NSAIDs are aspirin, ibuprofen, and naproxen. Still, there are many other NSAIDs, including the following generic drugs: ketoprofen, sulindac, fenoprofen, diclofenac, flurbiprofen, ketorolac, piroxicam, indomethacin, mefenamic acid, meloxicam, nabumetone, oxaprozin, famotidine, meclofenamate, tolmetin, and salsalate.

NSAIDs are used to reduce fever and inflammation and for pain control. They are among the most commonly prescribed medications used for inflammation and pain control, particularly for osteoarthritis, joint pain, or muscle strain.

NSAIDs are commonly indicated for use in the following conditions: joint pain and inflammation from osteoarthritis and rheumatoid arthritis; gout (build-up of uric acid causing pain in the extremities); headaches; pain after surgery; pain from an injury such as sprains or strained muscles; and pain from kidney stones.

Many NSAIDs also have an anti-clotting effect. Preventing clotting can prevent strokes and other cardiovascular issues. However, NSAIDs are not generally taken to prevent cardiovascular disease. A common side effect of NSAIDs is high blood pressure (hypertension), which offsets the anti-platelet action.

Coated 200 mg tablets of generic ibuprofen, a common NSAID. (Ragesoss via Wikimedia Commons)

However, low-dose aspirin (81 mg.) is often recommended to patients who have already been diagnosed with cardiovascular disease to reduce the chances of heart attack and stroke. Many people also take low-dose aspirin as a preventative measure. However, researchers are still unsure whether or not it is helpful for a healthy individual to take low-dose aspirin as a preventative treatment against heart attack or stroke.

USES AND COMPLICATIONS

Although NSAIDs are generally safe, it is reported that as many as 30-35% of individuals who take NSAIDs experience some side effects or adverse drug reactions. Various NSAIDs may affect individuals differently.

The most common reported side effects of NSAIDs are gastrointestinal problems. Usually, the reactions are mild, but sometimes they can result in more serious problems. Gastrointestinal side effects may include nausea, indigestion, excess gas, vomiting, stomach ulcers, or intestinal bleeding.

Many over-the-counter NSAIDs are produced with a special coating called an enteric coating to lessen the chance of gastrointestinal side effects. Unfortunately, to date, there is no evidence that coating the medication effectively reduces the possibility of digestive side effects.

NSAIDs carry an increased risk of cardiovascular disease. Some research implies that serious cardiovascular diseases such as heart attacks and stroke are twice as likely in people using NSAIDs, even if there is no pre-existing heart disease.

As mentioned in the Indications section, low-dose aspirin is an exception to this adverse reaction. It is often used to reduce the risk of further heart attack and stroke among those who have a pre-existing condition.

Kidney problems can also be a side effect of using NSAIDs, especially when combined with the use of other drugs such as those used to treat high blood pressure. Sometimes NSAIDs can also affect the kidneys' filtering ability, leading to water retention and high blood pressure. Recent studies have suggested that routine increased use of NSAIDs by athletes, for example, ultrarunners, to decrease pain from muscle soreness or stiffness and pain, may increase the chance of them developing acute kidney injury.

Suppose an individual using NSAIDs experiences pain in the kidneys, a reduction in the amount of urine produced, or changes in the urine color. In that case, they should let their healthcare provider know immediately.

NSAIDs have been linked to erectile dysfunction, but it is not understood why. Men—particularly middle-aged men—regularly taking NSAIDs are up to 2.4 times more likely to suffer from erectile dysfunction.

Less common side effects of taking NSAIDs may also include an allergic skin reaction to sunlight (rash).

A recent study at Fred Hutchinson Cancer Research Center in Seattle, Washington, concluded that NSAIDs improved survival for certain colorectal cancer patients. In the study, NSAIDs were associated with about a 25 percent reduction in all-cause mortality. However, a positive effect of NSAIDs is their ability to increase survival in people with colon cancer. However, the benefit versus increased risk of cardiovascular issues still needs to be determined.

Aspirin and other NSAIDs are also thought to prevent the growth of intestinal polyps that can precede the development of colorectal cancer. Aspirin and other NSAIDs activate cell suicide pathways found in intestinal stem cells that can carry a certain mutated gene known as *APC* and make the cells dysfunctional. According to a 2014 study at the Pittsburgh Cancer Institute (UPCI) and the School of Medicine, NSAIDs activate the early auto-destruction of cells that could lead to precancerous polyps and tumors.

PRECAUTIONS

NSAIDs are not recommended during pregnancy, especially in the last trimester of pregnancy. These drugs can affect the infant's developing heart and kidneys and contribute to premature birth and miscarriage. Also, NSAIDs should not be used in individuals with kidney disease, congestive heart failure, or liver cirrhosis to prevent the kidneys from failing (acute renal failure).

NSAIDs should not be given to an individual taking an anti-clotting medication (other than low-dose aspirin if prescribed by their healthcare provider) since this may increase the risk of bleeding.

Parents should not give children or teens aspirin for viral infections because of the risk of Reye's syndrome.

NSAIDs are not recommended for individuals with uncontrolled diabetes, active congestive heart failure, nasal polyps, phenylketonuria (an inherited disorder that prevents the disposal of the amino acid phenylalanine), ulcerative colitis, and gastroesophageal reflux disease (GERD).

Individuals need to tell their healthcare provider about any other medications they are taking since some drug combinations should not be used with

NSAIDs. When taken with some kidney and blood pressure medications, NSAIDs may cause them to work less effectively.

People should always discuss their NSAID use with their healthcare provider. Usually, treatment with higher doses of NSAIDs is used to control pain and reduce inflammation, e.g., in osteoarthritis, a sprain, etc. A prescription from a healthcare provider is needed for the higher doses to be taken at regular intervals throughout the day as prescribed. For temporary conditions to relieve pain, like back pain, for example, over-the-counter doses of NSAIDs are adequate.

The Federal Drug Administration (FDA) suggests individuals obtain medical attention right away if any of the following occur: chest pain, shortness of breath, trouble breathing, slurred speech, or weakness on one side or part of the body.

—*Joanne R. Gambosi, BSN, MA*

For Further Information:
Al-kaf, Ali, ed. *Nonsteroidal Anti-Inflammatory Drugs.* IntechOpen, 2017.
de Falla, Kathlee. "NSAIDs: Nonsteroidal Anti-Inflammatory Drugs." *Spine-Health*, 20 May 2019, www.spine-health.com/treatment/pain-medication/nsaids-non-steroidal-anti-inflammatory-drugs. Accessed 7 Apr. 2022.
Fookes, C. "Nonsteroidal anti-inflammatory drugs." Drugs.com, 22 Mar. 2018, www.drugs.com/drug-class/nonsteroidal-anti-inflammatory-agents.html. Accessed 7 Apr. 2022.
NSAIDs. National Health Service, 27 Feb. 2019, www.nhs.uk/conditions/nsaids/. Accessed 7 Apr. 2022.
NSAIDs (Non-Steroidal Anti-Inflammatory Drugs). American College of Rheumatology, Dec. 2020, www.rheumatology.org/I-Am-A/Patient-Caregiver/Treatments/NSAIDs. Accessed 7 Apr. 2022.
Patient Fact Sheet: NSAIDs (Non-Steroidal Anti-Inflammatory Drugs). American College of Rheumatology, Mar. 2019, www.rheumatology.org/Portals/0/Files/NSAIDs-Nonsteroidal-Anti-Inflammatory-Drugs-Fact-Sheet.pdf. Accessed 7 Apr. 2022.
Solomon, Daniel H. "Patient Education: Nonsteroidal Anti-inflammatory Drugs (NSAIDs) (Beyond the Basics)." *UpToDate*, 8 Mar. 2022, www.uptodate.com/contents/nonsteroidal-antiinflammatory-drugs-nsaids-beyond-the-basics. Accessed 7 Apr. 2022.

Noroviruses

Category: Disease/Disorder
Also known as: Norwalk-like viruses
Anatomy or system affected: Gastrointestinal system, immune system
Specialties and related fields: Gastroenterology, immunology, virology

Definition: A family of viruses that cause acute gastroenteritis.
Key terms:
gastroenteritis: an inflammation of the stomach and large intestines
Norwalk virus: a virus named for a 1968 outbreak of acute gastroenteritis in Norwalk, Ohio; it is the prototype strain for a group of single-stranded ribonucleic acid (RNA) viruses now called noroviruses

CAUSES AND SYMPTOMS

Noroviruses, also known as Norwalk-like viruses (NLV), are members of the family Caliciviridae and are the leading cause of nonbacterial acute gastroenteritis outbreaks in the United States. Noroviruses are suspected of causing over twenty million cases of acute gastroenteritis annually with an estimated 570-800 deaths, 56,000-71,000 hospitalizations, 400,000 emergency department visits, and 1.7-1.9 million outpatient visits each year. Often, norovirus-caused gastroenteritis is thought to be "stomach flu," but it is not related to influenza, a respiratory illness caused by the influenza virus. Norovirus infection is also commonly referred to as "food poisoning," although there are other numerous causes of food poisoning. Noroviruses are not related to bacteria or parasites that can cause gastroenteritis.

The illness associated with a norovirus infection lasts twelve to sixty hours and is characterized by a sudden onset of nausea, vomiting, abdominal cramps, and watery diarrhea. Vomiting is more prevalent among children, whereas adults tend to experience diarrhea. Additional symptoms, including headache, fever, chills, and myalgia (muscle pain), are also reported. Although NLV causes a self-limited acute gastroenteritis, the elderly, children, and those with severe underlying medical conditions are at increased risk for complications as a result of volume depletion, dehydration, and electrolyte disturbances. Although rare, severe dehydration caused by NLV gastroenteritis can be fatal. Hospitalization of otherwise healthy adults infected with NLV is rare.

The incubation period after exposure to a norovirus is 24 to 48 hours. The virus is transmitted by a fecal-hand-oral contamination route, directly from person to person, through contaminated food or water, or by direct contact with a contaminated surface. One of the main transmission sources is the diapers of infants with diarrhea. Aerosolized vomit has also been implicated as a transmission mode. Noroviruses are very contagious (less than 100 virus particles can establish an infection), and can spread rapidly throughout closely populated environments. Schools, hospitals, restaurants, amusement parks, fairgrounds, summer camps, and cruise ships are especially susceptible to mass infections. However, any place that food or drink is served, including the home environment, is susceptible to NLV infection. Because of high rates of infection and the persistence of noroviruses in the environment, transmission is difficult to control through routine sanitary procedures. People infected with NLV are contagious from the moment that they begin feeling symptoms to at least three days after recovery. In some cases, infected individuals have been contagious up to two weeks after recovery. Patients with compromised immune systems can shed viruses for months following infection.

Most people infected with noroviruses recover in twenty-four to forty-eight hours, with no long-term health effects related to their infection. No evidence suggests that infected persons can become long-term carriers of the virus, but it is essential for those recovering from an infection to use good hand-washing and other hygienic practices.

TREATMENT AND THERAPY

Outbreaks of norovirus gastroenteritis can occur in multiple settings. According to the Centers for Disease Control and Prevention, between 2010 and 2011, of the 1,518 confirmed norovirus outbreaks in the United States, a total of 14 percent was contracted in restaurants or at catered events; 63 percent in nursing homes, residential institutions, and hospitals; 4 percent in schools and day care centers; 4 percent in vacation settings, including camps and cruise ships; and the rest in other settings. While person-to-person spread of the disease extends NLV outbreaks, the initial event is often the contamination of a common source such as a surface or food or water. Thus, efforts to prevent an initial contamination and subsequent transmission help to prevent the occurrence and spread of norovirus gastroenteritis outbreaks.

Food contamination by food handlers is the most frequent transmission agent. Any food item has the potential to be infected with norovirus through fecal contamination, and certain foods show a higher concentration of infections. Shellfish tend to concentrate NLVs in their tissues if they live in contaminated waters in which fecal waste is either dumped overboard from ships or released from shoreline sewage systems. Ready-to-eat foods that require handling but no subsequent cooking also pose a risk. Noroviruses are relatively resistant to environmental change and can survive temperatures as high as 140 degrees Fahrenheit (60 degrees Celsius) and chlorine levels of up to 10 parts per million, which far exceeds chlorine levels in public water systems. NLV infection can occur from the ingestion of contaminated water, including municipal water, well water, stream water, commercial ice, lake water, and swimming pools.

> ### INFORMATION ON NOROVIRUSES
>
> **Causes:** Viral infection transmitted through contaminated food or water, fecal-hand-oral contamination, direct person-to-person contact, or direct contact with contaminated surface
>
> **Symptoms:** Sudden onset of nausea, vomiting, abdominal cramps, and watery diarrhea; may also include headache, fever, chills, and muscle pain
>
> **Duration:** Twelve to sixty hours
>
> **Treatments:** None; prevention through food safety measures (proper handing) and good hygiene (frequent hand-washing, germicides)

Noroviruses can be spread person-to-person by direct fecal-oral contact and airborne transmission. This is the most effective way that the virus spreads in populations in close proximity, such as people in nursing homes and on cruise ships. The most effective means of stopping the transmission of NLV is by frequent hand-washing with soap and hot water. Unfortunately, noroviruses are quite stable in the environment and resist temperatures up to 60°C (140°F), and freezing, and disinfection with alcohol or chlorine. Therefore, it is recommended that all surfaces be lathered with soap vigorously for ten seconds, then rinsed thoroughly under moving water. A mask should be worn by anyone cleaning areas contaminated with feces or vomitus. Soiled linen and clothes should be handled carefully and with a minimum of agitation. Soiled surfaces should be cleaned with a germicidal product containing at least 10 percent bleach.

Neither a specific antiviral treatment nor a vaccine has been developed for noroviruses, although the development of a vaccine is underway. NLV infection cannot be treated with antibiotics because it is not caused by bacteria. Because there are many different strains of norovirus, developing an individual long-lasting immunity is difficult. Consequently, NLV infections can recur throughout a person's lifetime. Because of genetic factors, some people are more likely than others to be infected and to develop severe symptoms.

—Randall L. Milstein, PhD;
updated by Michael A. Buratovich, PhD

See also: Childhood infectious diseases; Common cold; Diarrhea and dysentery; Epidemics and pandemics; Epidemiology; Fever; Food poisoning; Gastroenteritis; Gastroenterology; Gastroenterology, pediatric; Gastrointestinal disorders; Influenza; Nausea and vomiting; Rotavirus; Viral infections.

For Further Information:
Barclay, Leslie, et al. "Notes from the Field: Emergence of New Norovirus Strain GII.4 Sydney-United States." *Morbidity and MortalityWeekly Report* 62,03. (January 25, 2013): 55.

Centers for Disease Control and Prevention. "Outbreaks of Gastroenteritis Associated with Noroviruses on Cruise Ships- United States, 2002." *Morbidity and Mortality Weekly Report* 51 (2002): 1112-1115.

"'Cruise Ship Virus' Also Sickens One Million US Kids Yearly." *MedlinePlus/HealthDay*, March 20, 2013.

Dolan, Raphael. "Noroviruses-Challenges to Control." *New England Journal of Medicine* 357. (2007): 1072-1073.

Fankhauser, R. L., S. S. Monroe, J. S. Noel, et al. "Epidemiologic and Molecular Trends of 'Norwalk-Like Viruses" Associated with Outbreaks of Gastroenteritis in the United States." *Journal of Infectious Disease* 186. (2002): 1-7.

Hall, Aron J. et al. "Updated Norovirus Outbreak Management and Disease Prevention Guidelines." *Morbidity and Mortality Weekly Report* 60, RR03. (March 4, 2011): 1-15.

Meyers, H. "Norwalk Virus, Noroviruses, and Viral Gastroenteritis." *Public Health Bulletin, County of Orange Health Care Agency* 52, 2. (2003): 1-8.

"Norovirus Infection." *Mayo Clinic*, April 5, 2011. "Norovirus is Now the Leading Cause of Severe Gastroenteritis in US Children." *Centers for Disease Control and Prevention*, March 21, 2013.

Umesh, D. P., E. S. Wuiroz, A.W. Mounts, et al. "Norwalk-Like Viruses: Public Health Consequences and Outbreak Management." *Morbidity and Mortality Weekly Report* 50, RR-9. (2001): 1-13.

NUCLEAR MEDICINE

Category: Specialty

Anatomy or system affected: Bones, brain, gallbladder, glands, kidneys, heart, and musculoskeletal system

Specialties and related fields: Cardiology, endocrinology, internal medicine, nephrology, neurology, oncology, radiology, urology

Definition: The field of medicine that employs radioactivity for both diagnostic and therapeutic purposes; the former involves imaging techniques, while the latter uses large amounts of radioactive material to destroy cells.

Key terms:

cathode-ray tube: a display device used for the presentation of nuclear medicine data; it displays images in real time

collimator: a device used for restricting and directing gamma rays by passing them through a grid made of metal, which absorbs the rays

gamma radiation: electromagnetic radiation of a short wavelength that is emitted by the nucleus of a radionuclide during radioactive decay

half-life: a unique characteristic of a radionuclide defined by the time during which its initial activity is reduced by one-half; this period varies among radionucleotides from less than one-millionth of a second to millions of years

pharmacological stresstesting: a procedure wherein a pharmacological agent is administered to a patient to increase blood flow to the heart, thereby enabling coronary artery disease, if present, to manifest itself

radionuclide: a species of atom (of natural or artificial origin) that exhibits radioactivity

radiopharmaceutical: a sterile, radioactively tagged compound that is administered to a patient for diagnostic or therapeutic purposes

scintillation: the production of flashes emitted by luminescent substances when excited by high-energy radiation

tomography: the term that describes all types of body-section imaging techniques, in which a visual representation is restricted to a specified section or "cut" of tissue within an organ

tracer: a radioactive substance introduced into the body, the progress of which may be followed by means of an external radioactivity detector; it must not affect the process that it is used to measure

SCIENCE AND PROFESSION

Nuclear medicine is the branch of medicine that uses radioactive substances in the diagnosis and treatment of diseases. A discussion of such technology requires an understanding of the nature of radioactivity and the tools employed by specialists in this medical field.

Radioactivity is the spontaneous emission of particles from the nucleus of an atom. Several kinds of emissions are possible. Gamma-ray emission is the type with which nuclear medicine imaging is concerned. The activity of radionuclides is measured in terms of the number of atoms disintegrating per unit time. The basic unit of measurement is the curie. Radiopharmaceuticals that are administered are in the microcurie or millicurie range of activity. Most radionuclides used in nuclear medicine are produced from accelerators, reactors, or generators. Accelerators are devices that accelerate charged particles (ions) to bombard a target. Cyclotron-produced radionuclides that are used frequently in nuclear medicine include gallium 67, thallium 201, and indium 111. The core of a nuclear reactor consists of material undergoing nuclear fission. Nuclides of interest in nuclear medicine that are formed from reactors include molybdenum 99, iodine 131, and xenon 133.

In generator systems, a "parent" isotope decays spontaneously to a "daughter" isotope in which the half-life of the parent is longer than that of the daughter. The parent is used to generate a continuous supply of the relatively short-lived daughter radionuclides and is therefore called a generator. The most commonly used generator system is molybdenum 99 (with a half-life of sixty-seven hours) and technetium 99m (with a half-life of six hours). The daughter, technetium 99m, is the most widely used radioisotope in nuclear medicine. It is obtained from the generator in a physiologic sodium chloride solution as the pertechnetate ion. It can be used alone to image the thyroid, salivary glands, or gastric mucosa, or it can be labeled to a wide variety of complexes that are picked up physiologically by various organ systems.

The scintillation camera, or Anger camera (named for its inventor, Hal O. Anger), is the most commonly used static imaging device in nuclear medicine. The scintillation camera produces a picture on a cathode-ray tube of the distribution of an administered radionuclide within the target organ of a patient. It uses the gamma rays emitted by the nuclide and a collimator to create the image as a series of light flashes on a disk-shaped sodium iodide crystal. The system determines the location of each scintillation and then produces a finely focused dot of light on the face of the cathode-ray tube in a corresponding position. The complete picture is then produced on photographic film. The camera normally contains two parts, the head and the computer console. The head serves as the gamma-ray detector. It absorbs incoming gamma rays and generates electrical signals that correspond to the positions where the absorptions took place. These signals are sent to a computer to be processed and to produce a picture that can be displayed on film or stored on disk for video display.

The collimator normally consists of a large piece of lead with many small holes in it. There are many types of collimators; the most common being parallel-hole types. The holes are of equal, constant cross section, and their axes form a set of closely spaced, vertical, parallel lines. The materials between the holes are called septa. Once a radioisotope is injected or ingested, it travels to the target organ. Gamma-rays from the target organ are emitted in all directions. The collimator allows only those gamma rays traveling in a direction essentially parallel to the axis of its holes to pass through to the crystal. The crystal is made of sodium iodide, with a small amount of thallium impurity. The thallium is transparent and emits light photons whenever it absorbs a gamma ray. This action by the collimator causes the light flashes in the crystal to form an image of the nuclide distribution located below it. This image will preserve gray-scale information, since the number of gamma rays received by any given region of the crystal will be directly proportional to the amount of nuclide located directly below that region.

Single-photon emission computed tomography (SPECT) is a tomographic imaging technique employing scintillation cameras to display the information at a given depth in sharp focus, while blurring information above and below that depth. There are two distinct methods of SPECT, each based on the type of images produced. The first, longitudinal section tomography, provides images of planes parallel to the long axis of the body. The second method, transverse section tomography, is perpendicular to the long axis of the body. Transverse section tomography with a rotating gamma camera has received wide clinical acceptance, partly because of the information that it provides and its multiple-use capability, since these systems can perform routine planar imaging as well as SPECT imaging. In this system, the gamma camera is a device mounted to a gantry and capable of rotating 360 degrees around the patient. These systems must be interfaced with a computer. The orbit around the patient is circular, and from 32 to 180 equiangular images are acquired over a 360-degree arc. Image acquisition is by computer. The images are stored digitally, and image reconstruction is achieved by filtering each projection, with geometric correction for photon attenuation. Noise reduction is generally accomplished by the application of filters. The efficiency of rotating systems can be improved by incorporating additional detectors (most often two or three), which rotate around the patient. Virtually any organ in the body for which an appropriate radiopharmaceutical exists can be studied with SPECT techniques.

Positron emission tomography (PET) scanning utilizes positron-emitting radionuclides, such as carbon 11, nitrogen 13, oxygen 15, and fluorine 8 (a bioisosteric substitution for hydrogen), which are isotopes of elements that occur naturally in organic compounds. These tracers enter into the biochemical processes in the body so that blood flow; oxygen, glucose, and free fatty acid metabolism; amino acid transport; pH; and neuroreceptor densities can be measured. A positron is an antimatter electron. This positron-emitting radiopharmaceutical is distributed in a patient's system. As a positron is emitted, it travels several millimeters in tissue until it meets a free electron and annihilation occurs. Two gamma rays appear and are emitted 180 degrees apart from each other. A scintillation camera could be used to detect these gamma rays, but a collimator is not needed. Instead, the patient is surrounded by a ring of detectors. By electronically coupling opposing detectors to identify the pair of gamma rays simultaneously, the location where the annihilation event must have occurred (the coincidence) can be determined. The raw PET scan consists of a number of coincidence lines. Reconstruction could simply be the drawing of these lines as they would cross and superimpose wherever there is activity in the patient. In practice, the data set is reorganized into projections.

2084 • Nuclear medicine

DIAGNOSTIC AND TREATMENT TECHNIQUES

Nuclear medicine is widely used in the diagnosis and prognosis of coronary artery disease, especially in conjunction with either physical stress testing (treadmill or bicycle exercise) or pharmacological stress testing. The patient is instructed to exercise on the treadmill until his or her heart rate has significantly increased. At peak exercise, a radioisotope, usually thallium 201 or technetium 99m, is injected into a vein. Stress images are obtained. Because the injected tracer corresponds to the blood flow through the arteries that supply oxygen to the heart muscle, those vessels that have a blockage exhibit decreased flow, or decreased tracer delivered to that area of the heart. Rest images are also obtained. Rest and stress images are compared, and differences in the intensity of the tracer, analyzed by a computer, help to identify blocked arteries and the extent of the blockage. This technique is also used in follow-up of patients who have undergone bypass surgery or angioplasty to determine if blockage has recurred. Nuclear cardiology is also used to measure the ejection fraction (the amount of blood ejected by the left ventricle to all parts of the body) and motion of the heart. Patients with cardiomyopathy, coronary artery disease, or congenital heart disease often have decreased function of the heart. Certain medications used in cancer therapy can also damage the heart muscle. These patients are followed closely to determine if they are developing toxicity from their drug therapy. In these studies, commonly called MUGA scans, a small portion of the patient's blood is extracted. A radioactive tracer is tagged to this blood, which is then reinjected. The gamma camera takes motion pictures of the beating heart and, through the aid of computers, calculates the ejection fraction.

Nuclear medicine can be very helpful in locating primary or metastatic tumors throughout the body, and it is unique in its ability to assess the viability of a known lesion and its response to radiation or chemotherapy. Breast cancer, lymphomas (especially low-grade), differentiated thyroid cancer, and most sarcomas (both bone and soft tissue) are tumors that will metabolize the appropriate injected radiopharmaceutical. The resulting images will show increased localization in an active tumor but none in those masses that have been destroyed by treatment. By injecting a radioisotope that has been tagged by bone-seeking agents, doctors can view images of an entire skeleton. Multiple fractures, metastatic disease, osteomyelitis, osteoporosis, and Paget disease are but a few of the diseases that can be identified quickly and with minimal exposure of the patient to radiation.

Functional as well as anatomical information can be obtained by using nuclear medicine techniques to image the genitourinary tract, especially the kidneys. A perfusion study may be performed as the first phase of structural imaging. This study is done primarily to evaluate the vascularity (amount of blood vessels) of renal (kidney) masses. Cystic lesions and abscesses are usually avascular (having few or no blood vessels), and tumors are usually moderately or highly vascular. Uncommonly occurring arteriovenous (A-V) malformations show high vascularity. An evaluation of blood flow may also be important in patients who have received a kidney transplant. Anatomical renal imaging is performed to evaluate the position, size, and shape of the kidneys. Renal function studies have proven to be very sensitive in the diagnosis of both bilateral and unilateral kidney disease. By following specific tracers through the kidneys, doctors are able to evaluate the filtration by the glomeruli (capillary tufts) and the function of the tubules. Radionuclide cystography (imaging of the bladder), although not performed routinely, is extremely useful in diagnosing vesicoureteral reflux (urine reflux from the bladder back to the ureters), a relatively common problem in children.

Radionuclide imaging plays a significant role in the diagnosis of disease involving the gastrointestinal tract. Swallowing function, esophageal transit, gastroesophageal reflux, gastric emptying, gallbladder function, pulmonary aspiration of liver disease, and gastrointestinal bleeding can all be evaluated with nuclear medicine. The application of radioactive materials in the endocrine system provides historical benchmarks in the field of nuclear medicine with the use of radioiodine to assess the dynamic function of the thyroid gland. Radioiodine uptake testing is important and useful in the diagnosis of thyroid disease, specifically hyperthyroidism and hypothyroidism, thyroiditis, and goiters. Thyroid imaging is employed for the detection and functional evaluation of solitary or multiple thyroid nodules and the evaluation of aberrant thyroid tissue, metastases of thyroid cancer, and other tumors containing thyroid tissue. The therapeutic value of nuclear medicine is best demonstrated in its role in the treatment of Graves' disease, toxic adenoma, toxic multinodular goiter, and metastatic thyroid carcinoma. The purpose of the therapeutic application of radioiodine to hyperthyroidism (an overactive thyroid) is to control the disease and return the patient to a normal state. The accumulation and retention of radioiodine, with the subsequent radiation effects upon the thyroid cells, underlie the basic principle behind radionuclide therapy. The treatment of thyroid carcinoma with radioiodine is directed toward the control of metastatic foci and palliation of patients with thyroid carcinoma. Not all thyroid tumors localize radioiodine; therefore, care must be taken for proper patient selection by assuring a tumor's response to iodine.

Monoclonal antibody imaging has become important not only diagnostically but also therapeutically. Antibodies with perfect specificity for antigens of interest—in this case, malignancies—are produced. These antibodies are labeled with a large dose of radioactivity and injected into the patient. This "magic bullet" is then directed only to the antigen-producing areas. As in thyroid treatment, the radiation effect destroys only those cells to which the radioactivity is attached, leaving the noncancerous cells undamaged. Although this treatment is primarily a research protocol, the future role of radioactive monoclonal antibodies in the treatment of malignant disorders could be significant.

Clinical applications of PET scanning have focused on three areas: cardiology, oncology, and neurology/psychiatry. The principal clinical utility of PET in cardiology lies primarily in accurately differentiating infarcted, scarred tissue from myocardium, which is viable but not contracting because of a reduced blood supply. PET offers a noninvasive procedure to distinguish tissue viability, which allows more accurate patient selection for surgery and angioplasty than conventional approaches. In cancer cases, PET can determine cellular viability and the growth of tumor tissue and can directly measure the effectiveness of a given radiation or chemotherapy regimen on the metabolic process within the tumor. PET can differentiate tumor regrowth from radiation necrosis. Because of the unique ability of PET scanning to assess metabolic function, it can aid in the diagnosis of dementia and other psychoses as well as offer possible effective treatment of these disorders. PET is also helpful in detecting the origin of seizures in patients with complex epilepsy and can be used to locate the lesion prior to surgical intervention. PET can determine the viability of brain tissue after a stroke (one of the most common causes of death in the United States), permitting the clinician to select the most effective (and least invasive and expensive) form of treatment.

Nuclear imaging techniques are quite safe. Allergic reactions to isotopes are essentially nonexistent. In fact, the few that have been reported can be traced back to a contaminant in the injected dose. The radiation burden is far less than that of fluoroscopic radiographic examination and is equal to that of one chest x-ray, regardless of the picture produced.

Having said that, health concerns surround repeated CT scans of children. Epidemiological studies have established that children are significantly more sensitive to radiation than adults. Furthermore, children have a longer life expectancy than adults, which increases their opportunities to acquire and express radiation damage. Despite the advances in CT scanning technology that provide higher-quality images at lower doses of radiation, the settings of the CT machine must take into ac-

count the child's smaller size or the child will receive too much radiation. Also, multiple CT scans should be avoided in children when necessary.

PERSPECTIVE AND PROSPECTS

Natural radioactivity was discovered in the late nineteenth century. The first medical success with a radioisotope was Robert Abbe's treatment of an exophthalmic goiter with radon in 1904. In 1934, the Joliot-Curies produced artificial radioisotopes, specifically phosphorus 32. In 1938, Glenn T. Seaborg synthesized iodine 131. Phosphorus 32 was used to treat chronic leukemia and iodine 131 to treat thyroid cancer. Both treatments fell victim to radiation hysteria fueled by the aftermath of World War II. For a decade, nuclear medicine was equated with the "atomic cocktail" and was used only sporadically as a therapeutic modality. In 1949, the first gamma camera was introduced by Benjamin Cassen. It was called a tap scanner because as it measured radioactivity, it would tap ink on a piece of paper. The intensity of the ink mark was directly proportional to the radioactivity that was being scanned. The first nuclear medicine image was that of a thyroid gland.

Although discovered in the late 1930s, the imaging properties of the short-lived technetium 99m were not understood until the early 1960s. Its six-hour half-life and its chemical properties were ideally suited to imaging with the scintillation camera newly introduced in 1965. From that time on, nuclear medicine grew in its role as a diagnostic tool, with technetium agents becoming the primary radiopharmaceuticals employed in the detection of disease.

With the addition of computers and array processors to the technology, tomographic imaging became increasingly useful in the localization and quantification of disease states. Improved body attenuation correction and computerized three dimensional imaging enable physicians to quantify the size and extent of abnormalities quite accurately. When one examines the relative role and costs of transmission computed tomography (CT) scanning versus SPECT, a number of factors must be kept in mind. On the side of advantage of SPECT are the low costs compared to CT scanning. Additionally, no contrast is required in the SPECT study, which lessens the chance of adverse patient reaction. CT scanning is still primarily an anatomic diagnostic tool, while SPECT, by employing physiological radiopharmaceuticals, demonstrates the functional features of organs. By repeated imaging during the course of treatment, minute changes in the physiologic biochemical process can be detected and appropriately addressed.

Because of the physiologic nature of nuclear medicine, the development of radiopharmaceuticals to detect other disease states is essential for further growth in this field. It is interesting that much activity in this area is now centered on the treatment of diseases, primarily malignant ones. As PET scanning becomes more frequently used, new positron radiopharmaceuticals will be introduced. Theoretically, all biochemical reactions in the body can be imaged, if the proper radiopharmaceutical is produced.

—Lynne T. Roy;
updated by Michael A. Buratovich, PhD

See also: Biophysics; Imaging and radiology; Invasive tests; Magnetic resonance imaging (MRI); Noninvasive tests; Nuclear radiology; Positron emission tomography (PET) scanning; Radiation therapy; Radiopharmaceuticals; Single photon emission computed tomography (SPECT).

For Further Information:

Brown, G. I. *Invisible Rays: A History of Radioactivity.* Stroud, England: Sutton, 2002.
Brucer, Marshall. *A Chronology of Nuclear Medicine, 1600-1989.* St. Louis, Mo.: Heritage, 1990.
Christian, Paul E., Donald Bernier, and James K. Langan, eds. *Nuclear Medicine and PET: Technology and Techniques.* 5th ed. St. Louis, Mo.: Mosby, 2004.
Gupta, Tapan K. *Radiation, Ionization, and Detection in Nuclear Medicine.* London: Springer, 2013.
Iskandrian, Ami E., and Mario S. Verani, eds. *Nuclear Cardiac Imaging: Principles and Applications.* 4th ed. New York: Oxford University Press, 2008.
Iturralde, Mario P. *Dictionary and Handbook of Nuclear Medicine and Clinical Imaging.* 2d ed. Boca Raton, FL: CRC Press, 2002.
National CancerInstitute, "Radiation Risks and Pediatric Computed Tomography (CT): A Guide for Health Care Providers." www.cancer.gov/about-cancer/causes-prevention/risk/radiation/pediatric-ct-scans, June 7, 2012.
Powsner, Rachel A., Matthew R. Palmer, and Edward R. Powsner. *Essentials of Nuclear Medicine Physics and Instrumentation.* 3d ed. Malden: Wiley-Blackwell, 2013.
Taylor, Andrew, David M. Schuster, and Naomi P. Alazraki. *A Clinician's Guide to Nuclear Medicine.* 2d ed. Reston, Va.: Society of Nuclear Medicine, 2006.
Ziessman, Harvey, Janis O'Malley, and James Thrall. *Nuclear Medicine: The Requisites.* 4th ed. Philadelphia: Elsevier, 2014.

NUCLEAR RADIOLOGY

Category: Procedure
Also known as: Nuclear medicine
Anatomy or system affected: Bones, brain, glands, kidneys, musculoskeletal system, nervous system
Specialties and related fields: Nuclear medicine, radiology
Definition: The use of radiopharmaceuticals for the diagnosis of disease and the assessment of organ function.

Key terms:
collimator: a device that directs photons into a crystal for their detection
gamma camera: a system composed of a cesium-iodide crystal, collimator, and computer which is used to detect radioactivity and create an image of its distribution
radioisotope: a radioactive atom
radiopharmaceutical: the combined form of a pharmaceutical labeled with a radioisotope

INDICATIONS AND PROCEDURES

Nuclear radiology, also known as "nuclear medicine," is a subspecialty of radiology that uses radiotracers to look at various functions of the human body. Radiotracers are molecules that are tagged with a small amount of radioactive isotope. Depending on the radiotracers that is used, these radioactive molecules have affinities to certain parts of the body (such as bone, heart, kidney, thyroid, brain). The most common radiotracer is FDG (F-18 fluorodeoxyglucose), which is radioactive glucose. Glucose can be thought of as a source of sugar that the body turns into energy. Since cancer cells metabolize sugar for its accelerated cell division, FDG is used to identify lesions that are suspicious for cancer.

USES AND COMPLICATIONS

Positron emission tomography/Computed tomography (PET/CT) scans are used to locate possible cancer and metastasis. Metastasis is the process or ability of the primary cancer to spread to distant parts of the body.

Bone scintigraphy (also known as a "bone scan") can locate bone infection (e.g., osteomyelitis), bone cancers (both primary or metastases), or fractures.

Myocardial perfusion imaging can show the function of the heart muscle. The imaging is done at rest and then again after exercise. If the radiotracers are not picked up by a section of the heart after exercise, but was picked up by that same section of the heart at rest, it represents ischemia (i.e., a lack of oxygen to the heart muscles). This can help determine if cardiac surgery is indicated to revascularize the heart muscle.

Thyroid uptake scan is used to determine thyroid function. This can help evaluate nodules, goiters, or if the thyroid has hyperfunction (i.e., Graves' disease) or hypofunction (i.e., hypothyroidism).

An RNC Nuclear scan tags red blood cells (RBCs) with radiotracers to locate bleeding sites in the gastrointestinal tract (the stomach and intestines).

Risks of nuclear medicine include radiation risk and allergic reactions. A very small dose of radiotracers are used during these imaging and are considered a low radiation exposure that does not lead to known long-term adverse affects. Allergic reactions are rare and usually mild.

PERSPECTIVE AND PROSPECTS

Artificially produced radionuclides were thought to be discovered by Frederic Joliot-Curie and Irene Joliot-Curie (also known as Madame Curie) in 1934. In 1946, the first thyroid cancer was successfully treated with radioactive iodine. However, it was not until 1950s that nuclear medicine was widely used. Today, nuclear medicine is used for the diagnosis and treatment of many diseases. This field of medicine continues to advance. Recently, Florbetapir F18 became the first US Food and Drug Administration (FDA)-approved imaging agent that can be used to identify Alzheimer's disease. Prior to this, Alzheimer's disease was only confirmed through postmortem (i.e., after death) identification of neurofibrillary tangles in the brain.

—*Elizabeth Lynn, MD and Leonard Ong, MD*

See also: Biophysics; Imaging and radiology; Magnetic resonance imaging (MRI); Nuclear medicine; Positron emission tomography (PET) scanning; Radiation therapy; Radiopharmaceuticals.

For Further Information:

American College of Radiology and Radiological Society of North America. "Radiology Information for Patients." *RadiologyInfo.org for Patients*. General Nuclear Medicine, 2018, www.radiologyinfo.org/en/info/gennuclear. Accessed 10 Apr. 2022.

Freudenrich, C. *How Nuclear Medicine Works. HowStuffWorks*, science.howstuffworks.com/nuclear-medicine.htm. Accessed 10 Apr. 2022.

Society of Nuclear Medicine and Molecular Imaging. "Fact Sheet: What Is Nuclear Medicine and Molecular Imaging?" *SNMMI*. Accessed 10 Apr. 2022.

NUMBNESS AND TINGLING

Category: Disease/Disorder
Also known as: Paresthesias, dysesthesias, hypesthesias
Anatomy or system affected: Legs, muscles, musculoskeletal system, nerves, nervous system, skin
Specialties and related fields: Neurology, physical therapy
Definition: Abnormalities of sensation that are attributable to nerve damage or disorders.

Symptoms. Patients commonly report various sensory aberrations that are often described as "pins and needles," tingling, prickling, burning of varying severity, or sensations resembling electric shock. The accepted term for these symptoms is *paresthesias* or *dysesthesias*.

When severe enough to be painful, they can be referred to as painful paresthesias.

The other major sensory symptom is a reduction or loss of feeling in an area of skin. Most patients use the relatively unambiguous term *numbness*; however, the more formal medical term is *hypesthesia*. Paresthesias and hypesthesias are usually restricted to a part rather than all of the cutaneous territory of a damaged root or nerve.

The distribution of nonparesthetic pain is seldom as anatomically specific as the paresthesias themselves. Patients with carpal tunnel syndrome, for example, often have arm and shoulder pain that suggests compression of a cervical root rather than of the distal median nerve (a combined motor and sensory nerve). The paresthesias, by contrast, are usually localized to the tips of the fingers innervated by the median nerve. Similarly, in patients with cervical or lumbosacral radiculopathies (any diseased condition of the roots of spinal nerves), the distribution of pain in the upper or lower limbs often correlates poorly with the root involved. The paresthesias, however, are felt usually either along the entire area or, more commonly, in the distal part of the skin area innervated by the damaged root (the dermatome).

Examination. In attempting to localize the site of a lesion, the physician innervates major muscles from the spinal nerve roots (myotomes) through the plexuses, the individual peripheral nerves and their branches, and also the cutaneous areas supplied by each of these components of the peripheral nervous system. Traditionally, the site of the lesion can be deduced from which muscles and nerves are involved and from where the various branches of the peripheral nerves arise.

In motor examination, the muscles and tendon reflexes are examined first because weakness and reflex changes are often easier to elicit than are sensory signs. The muscles are first examined for atrophy. Since muscles become atrophic when denervated, the focal atrophy can sometimes identify accurately a nerve lesion. The lack of atrophy in a weak muscle either indicates an upper motor neuron lesion or raises the suspicion of spurious weakness. A systematic examination of individual muscles is then performed.

In sensory examination, the patient describes the area of sensory abnormality, which often tells as much as a formal examination. Testing light touch with the examiner's finger is frequently all that is required for confirmation. If this reveals no abnormality, retesting with a pin may disclose an area of sensory deficit. Pinpricks in normal and abnormal areas are compared.

It is important to examine the entire course of an affected nerve for bone, joint, or other abnormalities that may be causing the nerve damage. Local tender-

INFORMATION ON NUMBNESS AND TINGLING

Causes: May include neurological damage or disease, exposure to environmental toxins, infection, carpal tunnel syndrome, injury or trauma, metabolic disturbances

Symptoms: Prickling or burning sensations; pain and inflammation; impaired mobility

Duration: Acute to chronic

Treatments: Varies; may include physical therapy, use of ergonomic or corrective devices, surgery, drug therapy

ness of the nerve and/or a positive Tinel's sign (paresthesias produced in the area of the nerve when the nerve is tapped or palpated) may also help to identify the site. Many normal persons experience mild tingling when nerves such as the ulnar at the elbow or the median at the wrist are tapped lightly, so this finding is significant only when the nerve is very sensitive to light percussion. Conversely, a badly damaged nerve may be totally insensitive to percussion or palpation.

Nerve conduction studies and the electromyographic examination of muscles evaluate the function of large-diameter, rapidly conducting motor and sensory nerve fibers. These two complementary techniques are valuable tools in the accurate assessment of focal peripheral neuropathies, helping in the localization of the nerve lesion and the assessment of its severity.

Diagnosis. Peripheral nerves causing sensory symptoms may be damaged anywhere along their course from the spinal cord to the muscles and skin that they innervate. The site of a focal neuropathy (the focus of neurologic disease) may therefore be in the nerve roots, the spinal nerves, the ventral or dorsal rami (branches), the plexuses (network of nerves), the major nerve trunks, or their individual branches. The character, site, mode of onset, spread, and temporal profile of sensory symptoms must be established and precipitating or relieving factors identified. These features-and the presence of any associated symptoms-help identify the origin of sensory disturbances, as do the physical signs. Sensory symptoms or signs may conform to the territory of individual peripheral nerves or nerve roots. Involvement of one side of the body, or of one limb in its entirety, suggests a central lesion. Distal involvement of all four extremities suggests polyneuropathy (several neurologic disorders), a cervical cord or brain-stem lesion, or, when symptoms are transient, a metabolic disturbance such as hyperventilation syndrome. Short-lived sensory complaints may be indicative of sensory seizures or cerebral

ischemic phenomena (local and temporal deficiency of blood supply caused by obstruction of the circulation to a part) as well as metabolic disturbances. In patients with cord lesions, there may be a transverse sensory level. Dissociated sensory loss is characterized by the loss of some sensory modalities and the preservation of others. Such findings may be encountered in patients with either peripheral or central disease and must therefore be interpreted in the clinical context in which they are found.

The absence of sensory signs in patients with sensory symptoms does not mean that symptoms have a nonorganic basis. Symptoms are often troublesome before signs of sensory dysfunction have had time to develop.

—Genevieve Slomski, PhD

See also Carpal tunnel syndrome; Nervous system; Neuralgia, neuritis, and neuropathy; Neurology; Neurology, pediatric; Pain; Sense organs; Spinal cord disorders; Spine, vertebrae, and disks.

For Further Information:

Heller, Jacob L. "Numbness and Tingling." *MedlinePlus*, April 3, 2011.

Herkowitz, Harry N., et al. *Rothman-Simeone The Spine*. 5th ed. Philadelphia: Saunders/Elsevier, 2006.

Mathers, Lawrence H., Jr. *The Peripheral Nervous System: Structure, Function, and Clinical Correlations*. Menlo Park, Calif.: Addison-Wesley, 1985.

National Institute of Neurological Disorders and Stroke. "NINDS Paresthesia Information Page." *National Institute of Neurological Disorders and Stroke*, May 6, 2010.

Rosenbaum, Richard B., and José L. Ochoa. *Carpal Tunnel Syndrome and Other Disorders of the Median Nerve*. 2d ed. Boston: Butterworth-Heinemann, 2002.

Senneff, John A. *Numb Toes and Other Woes: More on Peripheral Neuropathy*. San Antonio, Tex.: MedPress, 2001.

Sutton, Amy L., ed. *Back and Neck Disorders Sourcebook*. 2d ed. Detroit, Mich.: Omnigraphics, 2004.

NURSING

Category: Specialty

Anatomy or system affected: All

Specialties and related fields: Critical care, emergency medicine, geriatrics and gerontology, neonatology, nutrition, oncology, occupational, primary care, informatics, midwifery, pediatrics, perinatology, preventive medicine, research, public health

Definition: A helping profession that focuses on the care of the sick and disabled and on the maintenance of the health and well-being of all individuals.

Key terms:

assessment: the systematic process of collecting, validating, and communicating patient data; these data will include information gathered from the patient's history and from physical examination and laboratory test results

healing: the restoration to a normal physical, mental, or spiritual condition

health: a condition in which all functions of the body, mind, and spirit are normally active

holistic: the philosophy that individuals function as complete units or integrated systems and are not understood merely through their parts

illness: the condition of being sick or diseased

nurture: the act or process of raising or promoting development and well-being

service: work done or duty performed for another or others

treatment: any specific procedure used for the cure or improvement of a disease or pathological condition

THE ROLE OF NURSING

It is difficult at times to distinguish nursing from medicine, since there are so many ways in which they interrelate. Whereas some people think that nursing began with Florence Nightingale (1820-1910), nursing is as old as medicine itself. Throughout history, there have been periods when the two fields functioned interdependently and times when they were practiced separately from each other. It seems likely that the role of the mother-nurse would have preceded the magician-priest or medicine-man. Even the seeds of medical knowledge were sown by the natural remedies used by the mother. Over the course of human history, the words *nurse* and *nursing* have had many meanings, and the connotations have changed as tribes became highly developed and sophisticated nations. The word *nurse* comes from the Latin *nutrix*, which means "nursing mother." The word *nursing* originated from the Latin *nutrire*, meaning "to nourish." The word *nurse* as a noun was first used in the English language in the thirteenth century, being spelled "norrice," then evolving to "nurice" or "nourice," and finally to the present "nurse." The word *nurse* as a verb meant to suckle and to nourish. The meanings of both the noun and the verb have expanded to include more and more functions related to the care of all human beings. In the sixteenth century, the meaning of the noun included "a person, but usually a woman, who waits upon or tends the sick." By the nineteenth century, the meaning of the verb included "the training of those who tend the sick and the carrying out of such duties under the supervision of a physician." With the origin of nursing as mother care came the idea that nursing was a woman's role. Suckling and nurturing were associated with maternal instincts. Ill or helpless children were also cared for by their mothers. The image of the nurse as a loving and caring mother remains popular.

The true spirit of nursing, however, has no gender barriers. History has seen both men and women respond to the needs of the sick. The role of the nurse has certainly expanded from that of the mother in the home, nourishing infants and caring for young children. Care of the sick, infirm, helpless, elderly, and handicapped and the promotion of health have become vital aspects of nursing as a whole. In history, the role of nursing developed with the culture and society of a given age. Tribal women practiced nursing as they cared for the members of their own tribes. As tribes developed into civilizations, nursing began to be practiced outside the home. As cultures developed, nursing care became more complex, and qualities other than a nurturing instinct were needed to do the work of a nurse. Members of religious orders, primarily those composed of women, responded by devoting their lives to study, service, and self-sacrifice in caring for the needs of the sick. These individuals were among the educated people of their time, and they helped set the stage for nursing to become an art and a science.

It was not until the nineteenth century that the basis of nursing as a profession was established. The beliefs and examples of Florence Nightingale laid that foundation. Nightingale was born in Italy in 1820, but she grew up in England. Unlike many of the children of her time, she was educated by governesses and by her father. Against the wishes of her family, she trained to be a nurse at the age of thirty-one. Amid enormous difficulties and prejudices, she organized and managed the nursing care for a military hospital in Turkey during the Crimean War. She returned to England after the war, where she established a school, the Nightingale Training School for Nurses, to train nurses. Again, she encountered great opposition, as nurses were considered little more than housemaids by the physicians of the time. Because of her efforts, the status of nurses was raised to a respected occupation, and the basis for professional nursing in general was established.

Nightingale's contributions are noteworthy. She recognized that nutrition is an important part of nursing care. She instituted occupational and recreational therapy for the sick and identified the personal needs of the patient and the role of the nurse in meeting those needs. Nightingale established standards for hospital management and a system of nursing education, making nursing a respected occupation for women. She recognized the two components of nursing: promoting health and treating illness. Nightingale believed that nursing is separate and distinct from medicine as a profession.

Nightingale's methods and the response of nursing to American Civil War casualties in the 1860s pointed out the need for nursing education in the United States. Schools of nursing were established, based on

Types of Nursing

Nurses may become involved in many areas of health care, including the administration of diagnostic tests, the performance of physical examinations, and assistance during surgical procedures. ©EBSCO

the values of Nightingale, but they operated more like apprenticeships than educational programs. The schools were also controlled by hospital administrators and physicians.

In 1896, nurses in the United States banded together to seek standardization of educational programs, to establish laws to ensure the competency of nurses, and to promote the general welfare of nurses. The outcome of their efforts was the American Nurses Association. In 1900, the first nursing journal, the *American Journal of Nursing*, was founded. The effects of World War II also made clear the need to base schools of nursing on educational objectives. Many women had responded to the need for nurses during the war. A great expansion in medical knowledge and technology had taken place, and the roles of nurses were expanding as well. Nursing programs developed in colleges and universities and offered degrees in nursing to both women and men. While there were im-

pressive changes in the expectations and styles with which nursing care has been delivered from ancient times into the twenty-first century, the role and function of the nurse have been and continue to be diverse. The nurse is a caregiver, providing care to patients based on knowledge and skill. Consideration is given to physical, emotional, psychological, socioeconomic, and spiritual needs. The role of the nurse-caregiver is holistic and integrated into all other roles that the nurse fulfills, thus maintaining and promoting health and well-being.

The nurse is a communicator. Using effective and therapeutic communication skills, the nurse strives to establish relationships to assist patients of all ages to manage and become responsible for their own health needs. In this way, the nurse is also a teacher who assists patients and families to meet their learning needs. Individualized teaching plans are developed and used to accomplish set goals.

The nurse is a leader. Based on the self-confidence gained from a nursing education and experience, the nurse is able to be assertive in meeting the needs of patients. The nurse facilitates change to improve care for patients, whether individually or in general. The nurse is also an advocate. Based on the belief that patients have a right to make their own decisions about health and life, the nurse strives to protect their human and legal rights in making those choices.

The nurse is a counselor. By effectively using communication skills, the nurse provides information, listens, facilitates problem-solving and decision-making abilities, and makes appropriate referrals for patients.

Finally, the nurse is a planner, a task that calls forth qualities far beyond nurturing and caring. In an age confronted with controversial topics such as abortion, organ transplants, the allocation of limited resources, and medical research, the role of nurses will continue to expand to meet these challenges in the spirit that allowed nursing to evolve and become a respected profession.

SCIENCE AND PROFESSION

While the nurse-mother of ancient times functioned within a very limited framework, the modern nurse has the choice of many careers within the nursing role. The knowledge explosion of the last century created many job specialties from which nurses can choose a career. The clinical nurse specialist is a nurse with experience, education, or an advanced degree in a specialized area of nursing. Some examples are enterostomal therapy, geriatrics, infection control, oncology, orthopedics, emergency room care, operating room care, intensive and coronary care, quality assurance, and community health. Nurses who function in such specialties carry out direct patient care; teach patients, families, and staff members; act as consultants; and sometimes conduct research to improve methods of care.

The nurse practitioner is a nurse with an advanced degree who is certified to work in a specific aspect of patient care. Nurse practitioners work in a variety of settings or in independent practice. They perform health assessments and give primary care to their patients.

The nurse anesthetist is a nurse who has also successfully completed a course of study in anesthesia. Nurse anesthetists make preoperative visits and assess patients prior to surgery, administer and monitor anesthesia during surgery, and evaluate the postoperative condition of patients.

The nurse midwife is a nurse who has successfully completed a midwifery program. The nurse midwife provides prenatal care to expectant mothers, delivers babies, and provides postnatal care after the birth.

The nurse administrator functions at various levels of management in the health care field. Depending on the position held, advanced education may be in business or hospital administration. The administrator is directly responsible for the operation and management of resources and is indirectly responsible for the personnel who give patient care. The nurse educator is a nurse, with a master's or doctoral degree, who teaches or instructs in clinical or educational settings. This nurse can teach both theory and clinical skills.

The nurse researcher usually has an advanced degree and conducts special studies that involve the collection and evaluation of data in order to report on and promote the improvement of nursing care and education.

DUTIES AND PROCEDURES

Creativity and education are the keys to keeping pace with continued changes and progress in the nursing profession. Nurses are expected to play many roles, function in a variety of settings, and strive for excellence in the performance of their duties. A service must be provided that contributes to the health and well-being of people. The following examples of nursing-an operating room nurse and a home health nurse-provide a limited portrait of how nurses function and what roles they play in health care.

Operating room nurses function both directly and indirectly in patient care and render services in a number of ways. Operating room nurses, usually known as circulating nurses, briefly interview patients upon their arrival at the operating room. They accompany patients to specific surgery rooms and assist in preparing them for surgical procedures. They are responsible for seeing that surgeons correctly identify patients prior to anesthesia. They are also directly attentive to patients when anesthesia is first administered.

Circulating nurses perform the presurgical scrub, which is a cleansing of the skin with a specified solution for a given number of minutes. It is their overall responsibility to monitor aseptic (sterile) techniques in certain areas of the operating room and to deal with the situation immediately if aseptic techniques are broken. They count the surgical sponges with surgical technologists before the first incision is made, throughout the procedure as necessary, and again before the incision is closed. They secure needed items requested by surgical technologists, surgeons, or anesthesia personnel: medications, blood, additional sterile instruments, or more sponges. At times, they prepare and assist with the operation of equipment used for surgeries, such as lasers, insufflators (used for laparoscopic surgery), and blood saver and reinfuser machines. They arrange for the transportation of specimens to the laboratory. They may also be instrumental in sending communications to waiting family members when the surgery takes longer than anticipated. When the surgery is completed, they accompany patients to the recovery room with the anesthesia personnel.

Home health nurses, on the other hand, function in a very different manner. This type of nurse usually works for a private home health services agency, or as part of an outreach program for home services through a hospital. Referrals come to the agency or program via the physician, through the physician's office, by way of the social services department in a hospital, or by an individual requesting skilled services through the physician.

The following scenario is an example of a patient whom a home health nurse may be requested to see: a seventy-six year-old man who was hospitalized with a recent diagnosis of diabetes mellitus, for which he is now insulin-dependent. He also has an open wound on his right ankle. The number of days allowed for hospitalization for his diagnosis has expired, but he still needs help using a glucometer to take his blood sugar readings and assistance with drawing up his insulin. He still has questions about how to manage his diabetes, especially the dietary parameters. He is unable to manage the wound care on his right ankle. His wife is willing to assist him, but she has no knowledge about diabetes or wound care. The home health nurse performs the following assessments on the initial visit: general physical condition, the patient's level of knowledge and understanding and his ability to manage his diabetic condition, all medications used, and the patient's understanding of the actions, side effects, and interactions of these medications. An assessment is made of the home setting in general: the patient's safety, the support system, and any special needs, such as assistive devices. If services such as physical therapy, occupational therapy, or speech therapy are needed, the nurse makes these referrals. If the patient requires additional in-home services, a referral to a medical social worker is made. Wound care is performed, and the nurse will then set up a plan of care, with the patient's input, for follow-up visits. Guidelines requested by the physician, as well as approval needed by health insurance companies covering the cost for home health services, will be taken into consideration when planning ongoing visits. If the home health agency has a nurse who is a diabetic specialist, the nurse can either consult with that specialist about the care of this patient or have the diabetic specialist make a home visit.

PERSPECTIVE AND PROSPECTS
From the beginning of time, nursing and the role of the nurse have been defined by the people and the society of a particular age. Nursing as it is known today is still influenced by what occurred over the centuries.

In primitive times, people believed that illness was supernatural, caused by evil gods. The roles of the physician and the nurse were separate and unrelated. The physician was a medicine man, sometimes called a shaman or a witch doctor, who treated disease by ritualistic chants, by fear or shock techniques, or by boring holes into a person's skull with a sharp stone to allow the evil spirit or demon an escape. The nurse, on the other hand, was usually the mother who tended to family members and provided for their physical needs, using herbal remedies when they were ill.

As tribes evolved, the centers for medical care were temples. Some tribes believed that illness was caused by sin and the displeasure of gods. The physician of this age was a priest and was held in high regard. The nurse was a woman, seen as a slave, who performed menial tasks ordered by the priest/physician. Living in the same era were Hebrew tribes who used the Ten Commandments and the Mosaic Health Code to develop standards for ethical human relationships, mental health treatment, and disease control. Nurses visited the sick in their homes, practiced as midwives, and provided for the physical and spiritual needs of family members who cared for the ill.

These nurses provided a family-centered approach to care. With the advent of Christianity, the value of the individual was emphasized, and the responsibility for recognizing the needs of each individual emerged. Nursing gained an elevated position in society. A spiritual foundation for nursing was established as well. The first organized visiting of the sick was done by deaconesses and Christian Roman matrons of the time. Members of male religious orders also cared for the sick and buried the dead.

During the time of the Crusades, there were both male and female nursing orders, and nursing at this time was a respected vocation. Men usually belonged to military nursing orders, who cared for the sick, on one hand, and defended the hospital when it was under attack, on the other. In medieval times, hospitals became a place to keep, not cure, patients. There were no methods of infection control. Nursing care was largely custodial, and the practice of accepting individuals of low character to supplement inadequate nursing staffs became common.

The worst era in nursing history was probably from 1500 to 1860. Nursing at this time was not a respected profession. Women who had committed a crime were sent into nursing as an alternative to serving a jail term. Nurses received poor wages and worked long hours under deplorable conditions. Changes in the Reformation and the Renaissance did little or nothing to improve the care of the sick. The attitude prevailed that nursing was a religious and not an intellectual occupation. Charles Dickens quite aptly portrayed the nurse and nursing conditions of the time through his caricatures of Sairey Gamp and Betsey Prig in *Martin Chuzzlewit* (1843- 1844).

It was not until the middle of the nineteenth century that this situation began to change. Through Nightingale's efforts, nursing became a respected occupation once more. The quality of nursing care improved tremendously, and the foundation was laid for modern nursing education. As innovations in health care have an impact on nursing, nurses' roles will continue to expand in the future. Nursing can also be a background from which both men and women begin to bridge gaps of service where other affiliations are needed: computer science, medical-legal issues, health insurance agencies, and bioethics, to name a few. The words of Florence Nightingale still echo as a challenge to the nursing profession:

> *May the methods by which every infant, every human being will have the best chance of health, the methods by which every sick person will have the best chance of recovery, be learned and practiced! Hospitals are only an intermediate state of civilization never intended, at all events, to take in the whole sick population.*

Nursing will continue to meet this challenge to improve the quality of health care around the world.

—*Karen A. Mattern and Mary Dietmann, EdD, APRN, CNS; updated by Geraldine Marrocco*

See also: Aging: Extended care; Allied health; Anesthesiology; Cardiac rehabilitation; Critical care; Critical care, pediatric; Emergency medicine; Geriatricsand gerontology; Holisticmedicine; Hospitals; Immunizationand vaccination; Intensive care unit(ICU); Neonatology; Nutrition; Pediatrics; Physical examination; Physician assistants; Preventive medicine; Surgical procedures; Surgical technologists; Terminally ill: Extended care.

For Further Information:
American Nurses Association. *NursingWorld*, 2013. Delaune, Sue C., and Patricia K. Ladner, eds.
Fundamentals of Nursing: Standards and Practices. 4th ed. Albany, N.Y.: Delmar Thomson Learning, 2011.
Dolan, Josephine A., M. Louise Fitzpatrick, and Eleanor K. Herrmann. *Nursingin Society: A Historical Perspective*. 15th ed. Philadelphia: W. B. Saunders, 1983.
Donahue, M. Patricia. *Nursing: The Finest Art*. 3d ed. Maryland Heights: Mosby Elsevier, 2011.
Kozier, Barbara, et al. *Fundamentals of Nursing: Concepts, Process, and Practice*. 2d ed. Harlow, England; NewYork: Pearson, 2012.
MedlinePlus. "Health Occupations." *MedlinePlus*, August 29, 2013.
Park, Melissa, et al. "Nurse Practitioners, Certified Nurse Midwives, and Physician Assistants in Physician Offices." *Centers for Disease Control and Prevention:NCHSDatabrief*, August 17, 2011.
United States Department of Labor. "Licensed Practical and Licensed Vocational Nurses." *Bureau of LaborStatistics: OccupationalOutlook Handbook*, March 29, 2012.
United States Department of Labor. "Registered Nurses." *Bureau of LaborStatistics: OccupationalOutlook Handbook*, March 29, 2012.
Vorvick, Linda J. "Types of Health Care Providers." *MedlinePlus*, August 14, 2012.

NUTRITION

Category: Biology
Anatomy or system affected: All
Specialties and related fields: Biochemistry, preventive medicine, public health
Definition: The science of food and beverage analysis, metabolism, physical needs for health and disease prevention.
Key terms:
calorie: a measure of the energy in food or of the energy used by the body
carbohydrate: one of three macronutrients; foods that provide carbohydrates are starches, sugars, fruit, vegetables, and milk products
fat: one of three macronutrients; foods that provide fat are oils, margarine, butter, meat, and dairy
macronutrient: carbohydrate, protein, or fat
minerals: inorganic substances that are essential for body processes; the major minerals include calcium, phosphorus, magnesium, sodium, chloride, and potassium
protein: one of three macronutrients; foods that provide protein are meat and dairy, with smaller amounts of protein found in starches
vitamins: organic (carbon-containing) substances found in plants and animals that are essential for body processes; examples include vitamins A, C, and D and the B vitamins

STRUCTURE AND FUNCTIONS

Nutrients are necessary for all aspects of living, including cellular metabolism, individual organ function, and multiple organ systems function. Breathing, moving, thinking, playing, and working all rely on the availability of nutrients. The study of nutrition has revolved around either healthy growth and development or nutrition in relation to the prevention and treatment of disease. Periods of noticeable growth, such as pregnancy, infancy, childhood, and adolescence, are particular areas of study in nutrition because nutrient needs change during these periods.

The amount of calories required to maintain a healthy weight during each stage of the life cycle depends upon the amount of energy expended. Higher caloric requirements are found when body mass is relatively large and energy output is relatively high, as seen in later adolescence and young adulthood. Because men generally have a larger body mass than women, they usually have a larger caloric requirement.

Macronutrients. Carbohydrates are an important source of energy. The recommended range of intake is 45 to 65 percent of the total caloric intake. Each gram of carbohydrate contributes 4 calories to the diet. Carbohydrates are found in starchy foods such as potatoes or corn, in vegetables and fruits, and in milk and yogurt. Carbohydrates are not found in meats or fats unless the food is a mixed dish, such as a hamburger casserole or a candy bar. Simple carbohydrates are those that require little digestion, such as sucrose or sugar. Complex carbohydrates include those that require more digestion, such as starches and fiber. General dietary guidelines suggest an increase in the higher fiber foods. The recommendation is to consume 25 to 35 grams of fiber each day; Americans generally consume 5 to 10 grams. In addition to fruits and vegetables, nuts and seeds, whole wheat bread, and cereal are higher fiber foods.

Dietary protein is required to supply essential amino acids so that the body can synthesize new proteins such as enzymes or hormones, or structural proteins to build muscle. Meats (including pork, beef, chicken, or turkey), fish, eggs, and nuts contain substantial amounts of protein. Protein is also found in dairy products such as milk, cheese, and yogurt. Some protein can be found in most foods, including starches and vegetables, the exception being those foods that are all fat, such as oil, or all simple carbohydrates, such as sugar. Each gram of protein contributes 4 calories to the diet. Protein requirements are closely related to caloric intake. With adequate or excess calories, protein is pared, meaning that less can be consumed while still meeting all body demands for protein. In these cases, protein does not need to be used for energy. With inadequate caloric intake, however, higher levels of protein are required to meet the body's needs because some protein will also be converted to calories for energy needs. The recommended intake assumes that adequate calorie needs are consumed. Protein requirements may be higher than the recommend levels in cases of stress. Although both psychological and physical stress can increase protein requirements, physical stress (including surgery and burns) usually causes a more substantial increase in requirements.

Dietary fat is a risk factor in the development of atherosclerosis or heart disease. Because of this, dietary fat intake recommendations are restricted both in total intake and type of fat ingested. Saturated fat is solid at room temperature and is derived from animals. Lard, shortening, and bacon fat are examples. Unsaturated fat can either have many unsaturated bonds (polyunsaturated) in the structure or one (monounsaturated). Polyunsaturated fat is liquid at room temperature and is derived from plants such as corn or soybeans. Monounsaturated fat is derived from plants such as canola or olive oil. Whereas recommendations had previously specified levels of intake for both polyunsaturated and monounsaturated fats, current recommendations reflect only a limited total fat intake with a restriction on transfats in particular. Transfat is an unsaturated fat that has been partially hydrogenated. This process causes a liquid fat to become more solid and is sometimes desirable in baked products. Transfats are linked to cardiovascular disease and should be limited. Foods that have higher values of transfat should be labeled as such and are most often processed baked goods, such as cookies, cakes, or pies, or snack foods, such as chips. Regardless of the type of fat, each gram of fat contributes 9 calories to the diet.

Minerals. The major minerals include calcium, phosphorus, magnesium, sodium, chloride, and potassium. These minerals are at times referred to as electrolytes, meaning that they can have a negative or positive charge, thus conducting electricity. In the body, these anions (negatively charged) and cations (positively charged) are important for the action potentials of cells, nerve conduction, and the excitation of muscles. The trace minerals are so called because only very small amounts are needed on a daily basis. One of the most common trace minerals is iron. The amounts of minerals in a particular food often vary depending on the soil in which a plant is grown or the feed that an animal consumes. Minerals are inorganic and cannot be destroyed with cooking or processing.

Calcium is required for normal growth and development of bone as well as nervous and muscular activity, enzyme regulation, and blood clotting. Food labels may designate a food as an excellent source (at least 200 milligrams of calcium) or a good source (100 to 199 milligrams of calcium). Poor intake of calcium is associated with the development of porous bones, or osteoporosis.

Most phosphorus is in bone as hydroxyapatite, although phosphorus also occurs as phospholipids in most cell membranes and is a component of nucleic acids. Phosphorus functions as an acid-base buffer, in enzymatic reactions, and in energy transfer. Phosphorus is found in nearly all foods, but good sources include meat, milk products, eggs, grains and legumes, and soft drinks.

About half of the body magnesium is found in bone, but magnesium is essential for hundreds of enzymatic reactions as well as muscle contraction. Green leafy vegetables, fruits, grains, and nuts as well as milk, meat, shellfish, and eggs are good sources of magnesium.

Potassium is found in many foods, including milk, meat, fruit, and vegetables. Together with sodium, potassium is involved with maintaining fluid balance. A diet high in sodium and low in potassium may be involved in the development of high blood pressure, or hypertension. The major source of sodium in the diet is salt, which is sodium chloride. Foods high in sodium include any food with visible salt (such as crackers and snack foods), pickled foods, processed foods such as lunch meat, canned soup, canned meat, and cured foods such as bacon and ham. A diet high in potassium and calcium and low in sodium is recommended to prevent hypertension.

Most of the body's iron is found in hemoglobin in red blood cells, where its function is to transport oxygen in the blood. Food sources of iron are either heme (from meat) or nonheme (from plant sources or iron-fortified foods). Very little iron is excreted from the body, with most of the iron from degraded hemoglobin being reabsorbed in the gastrointestinal tract. A deficiency of iron occurs gradually with chronic poor intake of iron-rich foods. Other causes of iron deficiency include excess blood loss and malabsorption. Chronic iron deficiency will cause anemia.

Vitamins. Vitamin A food sources include both animal sources (retinoids) and plant sources (carotenoids). Good animal food sources of vitamin A include liver, egg yolks, milk fat, and fish oils. Carotenoids can be converted to retinol in the intestinal mucosa and will then have the same metabolic role as retinoids from animal sources. The most common of these is beta carotene, but there are more than five hundred carotenoids. Vitamin A is required for optimal vision, with most of its effects found in the maintenance of night vision. Vitamin A also has a role in maintaining epithelial tissues, mucus production, and bone health. Vitamin A appears to have a role in fertility and in maintaining immune function as well.

Vitamin C is an important antioxidant with the biochemical ability to neutralize free radicals. Free radicals are metabolites of oxygen used in the cell and are believed to promote aging and several chronic diseases. Good sources of vitamin C include citrus fruits, broccoli, kiwi, potatoes, strawberries, and tomatoes, as well as most other fruits and vegetables. Heat, alkalinity, and exposure to air will destroy vitamin C. Therefore, certain cooking, processing, and storage practices can greatly reduce the vitamin C content of food.

Another antioxidant is vitamin E. Vitamin E is really a group of compounds, the most common of which is α-tocopherol. Good sources of vitamin E include vegetable oils, margarines, and nuts. Vitamin E is not destroyed by exposure to air, primarily because it is protected in dietary fat. Vitamin E can be destroyed by high temperatures such as in frying.

Vitamin D food sources are very limited. While milk is fortified with vitamin D, other dairy products, such as cheese and yogurt, generally are not. Some new products are being fortified with both calcium and vitamin D, such as yogurt, margarine, and juice. Exposure of the skin to sunlight converts a pre-vitamin D compounds to vitamin D_3 (cholecalciferol). Cholecalciferol will be hydroxylated in the liver and the kidney before it becomes active vitamin D. Vitamin D is required for calcium regulation and bone health, but emerging areas of research suggest that vitamin D may have a role in autoimmune diseases as well.

The B vitamins are water soluble and include thiamin, niacin, riboflavin, pantothenic acid, vitamin B_6, biotin, folate, and vitamin B_{12}. As a group, the B vitamins are essential for the metabolism of macronutrients, as well as cell growth and division and all organ functions. The B vitamins are found in a variety of foods, although vitamin B_{12} is primarily found in animal products. Once a concern for vegetarians, vitamin B_{12} is now fortified in many cereals and nonmeat breakfast foods.

DISORDERS AND DISEASES

Most chronic diseases result as a complex interaction between genetics and environmental factors. Diet is an important environmental factor that is potentially modifiable, and it has received much attention in the prevention of chronic disease. Most chronic disease prevention or treatment includes a nutritional component. The most prevalent chronic diseases in the United States are cancer, cardiovascular disease, diabetes, obesity, and osteoporosis.

Cancer. Although overall rates are declining in the United States, cancer continues to be a major cause of mortality. In general, cancer involves three phases: initiation, promotion, and progression. During the initiation step, there is a genetic alteration that may remain quiescent or continue though the second step of promotion. During promotion, cellular proliferation is stimulated and the abnormal cells begin to grow without regulation. The third phase is progression, when the neoplastic cells become invasive and spread or metastasize to other parts of the body. Dietary components may be involved in the initiation and promotion of certain cancers as well as their inhibition. The dietary components that have been linked to the development of cancer include dietary fat, total calories, and alcohol, as well as salted, cured foods and molds that may grow in certain foods.

Antioxidants have been investigated as inhibitors of cancer. Fruits and vegetables are rich sources of antioxidants, and high fruit and vegetable intake has been linked to a lower incidence of certain cancers. The results of many studies, however, are inconclusive. Although high intake of dietary fat and red meat has been associated with an increased risk of colon cancer, lower fat diets have not proved to be an effective intervention in decreasing colon cancer incidence. Nevertheless, a diet high in fruits and vegetables, at least five servings each day, and lower in fat and alcohol is recommended as a preventive measure against cancer. Some of the benefit of high fruit and vegetable intake may be attributable to the fiber content of these foods. Higher fiber diets increase fecal bulk, thereby diluting any carcinogens that enter the gastrointestinal tract. By increasing intestinal motility, fiber also decreases the amount of time that fecal material is in the gastrointestinal tract, thereby limiting exposure of the mucosa to potential toxins.

Cardiovascular disease. Cardiovascular diseases are the leading cause of death in the United States. They include arrhythmias, congestive heart failure, and valvular diseases, but most of the morbidity and mortality is related to coronary heart disease, or atherosclerosis. Hyperlipidemia is a risk factor for atherosclerosis, and dietary fat has influence on the level of blood lipids. According to the Center for Disease Control (CDC), the recommended intake of fat is 25 to 35 percent of total calories per day. Of that dietary fat, less than 7 percent of total calories should be saturated fat and less than 1 percent should be transfat. Lower fat meats and dairy are recommended, as well as replacement of some meat with vegetable alternatives. Sources of transfat should be limited. The effects of various levels of polyunsaturated and monounsaturated fats are debated. While limited intake of cholesterol is recommended, cholesterol intake has had less of an effect on blood lipids than total fat and transfat.

Eating fish, especially oily fish, is recommended as a source of omega-3 fatty acids, which are long-chain polyunsaturated fatty acids associated with a decreased risk of certain heart diseases. The two omega-3 fatty acids are eicosapentaenoic acid (EPA) and docosahexaenoic acid (DHA). Although fish may contain contaminants known to be hazardous to health, the benefits of eating it are believed to outweigh the risks for adults. Restricted intake may be recommended for children and pregnant women. Supplements of DHA and EPA are not recommended for the prevention of heart disease, although they may be prescribed as treatment under a physician's supervision.

Higher intakes of fruits, vegetables, and whole grains are recommended to prevent heart disease. In addition to fiber, these foods may contain antioxidants or other bioactive compounds that are beneficial to health. In addition, these foods may displace other, higher calorie foods from the diet, thus promoting a healthy weight. Limiting foods high in added sugars is recommended because of the association of these foods with weight gain and obesity. Obesity is a significant risk factor for cardiovascular disease, and achieving a healthy weight through diet and physical activity is important.

A healthy weight is also significant in the maintenance of optimal blood pressure. Because sodium intake is associated with increases in blood pressure on average, limiting sodium intake is also recommended for heart health. Limited amounts of alcohol, if alcohol is consumed at all, is also included as a healthy lifestyle measure for the prevention of heart disease. Moderate alcohol intake is generally considered to be two drinks for men and one drink for women each day.

Foods that are being investigated concerning their role in the prevention of cardiovascular disease include soy and plant stanols. Supplements of antioxidants and fish oils for their DHA and EPA are generally not recommended, but foods containing these compounds may be beneficial.

Diabetes. The incidence of diabetes continues to grow in parallel to the incidence of obesity. Diabetes mellitus has been categorized as either insulin-dependent diabetes mellitus (IDDM), which is also called type 1 diabetes, and non-insulin-dependent diabetes mellitus (NIDDM), also known as type 2 diabetes. Nutrition is an important component of both the prevention and treatment of diabetes, regardless of type.

Obesity enhances insulin resistance. Therefore, a main goal in type 2 diabetes is to prevent or reduce obesity. Weight loss in obese persons with type 2 diabetes improves glycemic control and blood lipid profile. Because carbohydrates are the main determinant of postprandial plasma glucose, the amount of carbohydrates and timing of foods eaten may need to be regulated. The total amount of carbohydrates in the diet or meal is more important than the type of carbohydrate, with certain exceptions. Liquid carbohydrates are more easily digested and absorbed than those from solid foods. Beverages such as milk and orange juice may cause a more rapid rise in blood glucose. Sucrose and sucrose-containing foods do not need to be eliminated, but these foods do need to be included in the total carbohydrates and calories consumed for meal planning and coverage with medication. Restriction of sucrose and sucrose-containing foods usually relates to the restriction of total calories. The glycemic response to carbohydrates depends on many components, including the type of carbohydrate, the cooking or processing, prior food intake, other macronutrients in the food, and glycemic control of the individual. Because dietary modifications need to be individualized, people with diabetes should receive individualized medical nutrition therapy, preferably by a registered dietitian or certified diabetes educator.

Obesity. Obesity occurs when caloric intake exceeds the needs of the individual and is therefore stored in adipose tissue. Although normal weight varies with age, gender, and height, for each group there are indicators of obesity. Usual indicators of obesity are based on the assumption that variations in weight at various heights are attributable to body fat and are often calculated as the body mass index (BMI). According to the CDC, a BMI of between 25 and 30 is considered overweight, and above 30 is considered obese. The optimal macronutrient distribution to facilitate weight loss is not known. Higher and lower amounts of protein, fat, and carbohydrates have been investigated, without clear conclusions. Consuming fewer calories while increasing the amount of calories used through physical activity remains the cornerstone of obesity prevention and treatment.

Osteoporosis. As with other chronic diseases, the incidence of osteoporosis continues to rise. Osteoporosis is asymptomatic until the condition produces deformity or contributes to fractures. While genetics play an important role in the development of osteoporosis, modifying risk factors include diet and physical activity. Optimal levels of calcium have been shown to be beneficial in maintaining high bone mineral density, which is critical in preventing osteoporosis. Most calcium is obtained from dairy products, although increasingly grain-based foods and juices are being fortified with calcium. Vitamin D plays a critical role in regulating calcium balance. Therefore, adequate vitamin D status is important in preventing osteoporosis. Vitamin D deficiency can be a contributing factor to osteoporosis in older individuals secondary to poor skin synthesis, lower hydroxylation of vitamin D in the kidneys, and inadequate nutritional intake. As with calcium, more food products are being fortified with vitamin D with an increasing awareness of osteoporosis.

PERSPECTIVE AND PROSPECTS

Although the science of nutrition began as a branch of biochemistry, early discoveries of the health properties of food date to the eighteenth century and the discovery that limes could prevent the painful bleeding disorder scurvy. Since then, the knowledge of nutrition has progressed beyond identifying deficiency diseases toward an understanding and appreciation of the complexity of nutrition in optimal health. In addition to further investigations into macronutrients, vitamins, and minerals, many bioactive substances in foods are being identified, such as bioflavinoids and probiotics. The interactions of these and more traditional nutrients are being investigated as potential modifiers of chronic disease and promoters of longevity.

—*Karen Chapman-Novakofski, RD, LDN, PhD*

See also Acid reflux disease; Aging: Extended care; Anorexia nervosa; Antioxidants; Appetite loss; Arteriosclerosis; Beriberi; Breast-feeding; Bulimia; Caffeine; Cancer; Carbohydrates; Carcinogens; Cholesterol; Diabetes mellitus; Dietary reference intakes (DRIs); Digestion; Eating disorders; Enzyme therapy; Enzymes; Failure to thrive; Fiber; Food biochemistry; Food Guide Pyramid; Gastroenterology; Gastroenterology, pediatric; Gastrointestinal system; Gastrostomy; Geriatrics and gerontology; Heart disease; Hirschsprung's disease; Hypercholesterolemia; Hyperlipidemia; Kwashiorkor; Lactose intolerance; Lipids; Macronutrients; Malabsorption; Malnutrition; Mercury poisoning; Metabolic disorders; Metabolism; Obesity; Obesity, childhood; Osteoporosis; Phenylketonuria (PKU); Phytochemicals; Pinworms; Protein; Roundworms; Scurvy; Sports medicine; Supplements; Tapeworms; Taste; Tropical medicine; Vitamins and minerals; Weaning; Weight loss and gain; Weight loss medications; Worms.

For Further Information:

American Diabetes Association. *American Diabetes Association Complete Guide to Diabetes.* 4th rev. ed. New York: Bantam Books, 2006.

"Defining Overweight and Obesity." *Centers for Disease Control.* July 17, 2013.

Duyff, Roberta Larson. *American Dietetic Association Complete Food and Nutrition Guide.* 3d ed. Hoboken, N.J.: John Wiley & Sons, 2007.

Lichtenstein, Alice H., et al. "Diet and Lifestyle Recommendations Revision 2006: A Scientific Statement from the American Heart Association Nutrition Committee." *Circulation* 114, no. 1 (July 4, 2006): 82-96.

"Nutrition for Everyone: Dietary Fat." *Center for Disease Control.* July 17, 2013.

"Nutrition for Everyone: Vitamins and Minerals." *Center for Disease Control.* July 17, 2013.

U.S. Department of Health and Human Services and U.S. Department of Agriculture. *Dietary Guidelines for Americans 2005.* 6th ed. Washington, DC: Government Printing Office, 2005.

O

OBESITY

Category: Disease/Disorder
Anatomy or system affected: Abdomen, blood vessels, circulatory system, endocrine system, gastrointestinal system, heart, intestines, joints, psychic-emotional system, respiratory system, stomach
Specialties and related fields: Endocrinology, family medicine, internal medicine, nutrition, psychiatry, psychology, public health
Definition: A condition in which the body carries abnormal or unhealthy amounts of fat tissue, leading the individual to weigh in excess of 20 percent more than his or her ideal weight.

Key terms:

adipose tissue: fat; a soft tissue of the body composed of cells (adipocytes) that contain triglyceride, a compound consisting of glycerol and fatty acids; in obesity, there may be increased numbers of adipocytes, and the cells may contain an increased amount of triglyceride

basal metabolic rate(BMR): the minimal energy expended for maintenance of the vegetative functions of the body (respiration, heat production, and so on), expressed as calories per hour per square meter of body surface

body mass index(BMI): weight in kilograms divided by height in meters, squared (kg/m2); since this value is relatively independent of height and sex, the same standard values can be used for all adults.

calorie: 1 kilocalorie, which is the amount of heat (energy) needed to raise the temperature of 1 kilogram of water by 1 degree Celsius

metabolism: the sum of the physical and chemical processes by which living matter is produced, maintained, and transformed

resting metabolic rate(RMR): similar to the BMR, but more easily measured (the subject is resting rather than in a truly basal state)

CAUSES AND SYMPTOMS

Obesity is a condition in which the body accumulates an abnormally large amount of adipose tissue, or fat. It is a multifactorial, chronic disease that is rapidly increasing and having devastating effects on health, especially in the United States. The disease has social, cultural, genetic, metabolic, behavioral, and

---

INFORMATION ON OBESITY

Causes: May include endocrine disorders, poor diet, lack of exercise, psychic-emotional disorders, genetic factors
Symptoms: Excessive weight possibly leading to such health problems as strain on weight-bearing body parts leading to arthritis, hypertension, arteriosclerosis, difficulty breathing, sleepiness from inadequate oxygen delivery to tissues
Duration: Often chronic
Treatments: Diet and lifestyle regulation, medications, surgery

---

psychological components. People who are obese also face stigma and discrimination in work and social settings. Obesity is the second leading cause of preventable deaths in the United States, resulting in an estimated 300,000 deaths each year.

Because it is not practical to measure body fat content directly but it is easy to measure weight and height, the body mass index (BMI), is the most widespread method to identify and quantify obesity. BMI also closely correlates with body fat Being overweight and being obese are not the same condition. A BMI of 25 to 29.9 is considered to be overweight, a BMI of 30 or more is obese, and a BMI of 40 or more is severely obese. In 2012 the National Center for Health Statistics reported that in 2009 to 2010 35.7 percent of adults in the United States were obese. In 2006, it was estimated that 64.5 percent of adults in the United States were overweight, 30.5 percent were obese, and 4.7 percent were severely obese. This latter figure increased from only 2.9 percent in a 1994 survey done by the National Health and Nutrition Examination Survey, which also found that 46.6 percent of adults were overweight and 14.4 percent were obese.

The Centers for Disease Control and Prevention cites a 2009 report in *Health Affairs*, which estimated that the annual cost of obesity in the United States was $147 billion in 2008 dollars. The National Institutes of Health funded approximately $836 million in obesity research for fiscal year 2012, and set funding estimates for fiscal year 2014 at about $843 million. The Patient Protection and Affordable Care Act of 2010 listed obesity screening and counseling among the preventative services that all new group health plans and individual market plans under the act are required to provide without patient cost sharing.

An important function of adipose tissue is to store energy. If the intake of energy in the form of food calories is greater than the expenditure of energy, then the excess calories are stored, mainly in the adipose tissue, with a resulting gain in weight. Expenditure of energy depends largely on the resting metabolic rate or resting energy expenditure, defined as the calories used each day to maintain normal body metabolism. Additional calories are expended by exercise or other activity, by the digestion and metabolism of food, and by other metabolic processes. Because of this simple relationship between energy intake, energy utilization, and energy storage, weight gain can occur only when there is increased caloric intake, decreased caloric expenditure, or both.

Genetic factors appear to be very important in determining the presence or absence of obesity. Body weight tends to be similar in close relatives, especially in identical twins, who share the same genetic makeup. The extent to which genetic factors affect food intake, activity level, or metabolic processes is not known.

One theory holds that each individual has a "set point" that determines body weight. When food intake is decreased, experiments have shown less weight loss than predicted by the caloric deficit, suggesting that the body has slowed its metabolic rate, thus minimizing the deviation from the original set point.

Many believe that physiologic regulation of body weight, which tends to maintain a preferred weight for each individual, explains some of the difficulty in treating obesity. The discovery and role of leptin in regulating weight helps to explain this apparent set point of weight for each individual. There are other causes of obesity as well. Lesions in the hypothalamus, a part of the brain, can make animals eat excessively and become obese, and rare cases of obesity in humans are attributable to disease of the hypothalamus. In hypothyroidism, a condition in which the thyroid gland produces too little thyroid hormone, the metabolic rate is slowed, which may cause a mild gain in weight. In Cushing's syndrome, which is caused by excessive amounts of the adrenal hormone cortisol or by drugs that act like cortisol, there is an accumulation of excessive fat in the face and trunk, which disappears when the disease is cured or the drug is stopped. Weight gain has also occurred with the use of other drugs, including some antidepressants and tranquilizers.

While most physicians and the public assume that the main factor causing obesity is excessive food intake in relation to physical activity, it has not been possible to prove that overweight people eat more than slender people do. This may be the case because it is very difficult to measure food intake under normal conditions, or perhaps because obese individuals tend to underestimate their food intake when dietary histories are taken. Some experts believe, however, that differences in metabolic efficiency and the physiologic set point for body weight are the principal causes of obesity in some people, rather than excessive food intake. The basal metabolic rate (BMR) varies fairly widely among persons of the same age, sex, and body size, and stud-

A "super obese" male with a BMI of 53 kg/m2: weight 182 kg (401 lb), height 185 cm (6 ft 1 in). He presents with stretch marks and enlarged breasts. Photo via Wikimedia Commons. [Public domain.]

ies have shown large differences in the daily caloric intake needed to maintain a constant body weight in normal people; these observations support the possibility that metabolic differences could contribute to obesity.

Many health problems are associated with obesity. The majority of people who develop non-insulin-dependent diabetes mellitus are overweight, and manifestations of the disease commonly improve or disappear if the individual succeeds in losing weight. Hypertension (high blood pressure) is more common with obesity, and weight loss may lower the blood pressure enough to lessen or avoid the need for medication. Arteriosclerosis, or "hardening of the arteries," is more prevalent in obese persons and causes an increased risk for heart attacks and strokes. Certain forms of cancer are more prevalent with obesity: cancer of the colon, rectum, and prostate in men and cancer of the uterus, gallbladder, ovary, and breast in women. Severe obesity can cause difficulties in breathing, namely obstructive sleep apnea, with sleepiness resulting from inadequate oxygen delivery to the tissues and sometimes from interruption of sleep at night. In addition, conditions such as arthritis may be worsened by the additional strain that obesity places on weight-bearing parts of the body.

The distribution of excess adipose tissue differs among individuals. Two main patterns have been described: android obesity (more commonly affecting men), in which fat accumulates mainly in the abdomen and upper body; and gynoid obesity (more common in women), in which fat accumulates mainly in the hips, thighs, and lower body. This distinction has received much attention because persons with android obesity are more likely to suffer from diabetes, hypertension, and cardiovascular disease. The closest association with these diseases is seen when sensitive measurements of abdominal visceral fat mass are made with computed tomography (CT) scanning. A simple measurement of the waist circumference compared with the hip circumference—the waist-to-hip ratio—can also be used to identify those obese individuals at greater risk for diabetes and cardiovascular disease.

TREATMENT AND THERAPY

Many obese people are highly motivated to lose weight because of the common perception that a slim body build is more attractive than an obese one. Many other overweight individuals desire to lose weight because of health problems related to obesity. As a result, the human and financial resources devoted to weight loss efforts are extensive. Unfortunately, the long-term results of the treatment of obesity are successful in only a minority of cases. The only measures useful in the treatment of obesity are those that decrease the intake

or absorption of calories or those that increase the expenditure of calories. The basis for any long-term weight reduction program is a low-calorie diet. The average daily calorie requirement in the United States is approximately 1,600 calories for women and 2,300 calories for men; decreasing an individual's intake, usually to between 800 and 1,500 calories, will result in weight loss, provided that energy expenditure does not decrease. A balanced diet, with 20 percent to 30 percent of the calories derived from fat (considerably less fat than is found in the typical American diet) is usually recommended. Many unbalanced diets, or "fad diets," have enjoyed periods of popularity. Rice diets, low carbohydrate diets, vegetable diets, and other special diets may produce rapid weight loss, but long-term persistence with an unbalanced diet is rare and the lost weight is often regained.

Many patients fail to lose weight with low-calorie diets. More severe calorie restriction can be achieved with very low-calorie diets that provide only 400 to 800 calories daily. This level of caloric restriction is unsafe unless a very high proportion of the diet consists of high-quality protein, with correct amounts of other nutrients such as vitamins and minerals. These requirements can be met with special formula diets under careful medical supervision. Such a program is recommended for severely obese patients who are otherwise healthy enough to tolerate this degree of caloric restriction. Because most people find it difficult to lower their calorie intake, behavioral management programs may be combined with dietary restrictions. Dieters can be taught techniques for self-monitoring of food intake, such as keeping a daily log of meals and exercise, which will increase the awareness of eating behavior as well as point out ways in which that behavior can be modified. There are techniques for reducing exposure to food and the stimuli associated with eating, such as keeping food out of sight, keeping food handling and preparation to a minimum, and eliminating the occasions when food is eaten out of habit or as part of a social routine. Ways can be sought to increase the social support of friends and family for weight-losing behavior and for reinforcement of compliance with dietary restrictions. Interestingly, the "diet merry-go round" which many mildly obese individuals experience—restricting their caloric intake until a weight goal is achieved, ending the diet only to resume overeating and regain the weight lost—often results in higher weight. Over time, such a pattern can "cycle" the individual to a dangerously high weight. Such individuals tend to experience more success if they can adjust their long-range eating behavior to moderate, rather than restrictive, intake of food. Many physicians would prefer to see their obese patients remain relatively stable in weight, reducing slowly over time, to avoid physical stress and ensure success. When establishing dietary weight loss programs, it is crucial to set realistic goals such as an initial goal of 5-7% of body weight loss. The Mediterranean diet, which involves high consumption of fruits, vegetables, grains, and legumes with limited dairy and meat intake, has been shown to have numerous health benefits including diabetes prevention and reduced risk of cardiovascular disease.

Because obesity is caused by an excess of calorie intake over calorie expenditure, another approach to weight loss is to increase energy utilization by increasing physical activity. Some studies have shown that overweight individuals are less active than their non-obese counterparts. This fact could contribute to their obesity, since less energy utilization results in more energy available for storage as fat. Decreased activity could also be a result of obesity, since a heavier person must do more work, by carrying more pounds, than a non-obese person who walks or climbs the same distance. Each pound of fat contains energy equal to about four thousand calories. If an obese person expends four hundred extra calories each day by walking briskly for one hour, it will take ten days for this activity to result in the loss of one pound. In a year, this increased calorie expenditure would result in a thirty-six-pound weight loss. More vigorous exercise, such as running, swimming, or calisthenics, would lead to more rapid weight loss, but might not be advisable for every person because of the increased prevalence of certain health problems in obese individuals, such as heart disease, hypertension, and musculoskeletal disorders. For this reason, any exercise program that involves vigorous physical activity should be undertaken with medical supervision.

Exercise as part of a weight-loss program has additional benefits. The function of the cardiovascular system may be improved, and muscles may be strengthened. Exercise will lead to loss of adipose tissue and gain in lean body mass as weight is lost, a change in body composition that is beneficial to overall health. Although some fear that physical activity will lead to an increase in appetite, studies show that any increase in food intake that occurs after exercise is usually not great enough to match the calories expended by the exercise. Medications that decrease appetite are occasionally used to help people comply with a low-calorie diet. Some appetite suppressants act like adrenaline and may cause such side effects as nervousness, irritability, and increased heart rate and blood pressure. Other drugs may stimulate serotonin, a chemical transmitter in the central nervous system that decreases appetite, and may cause drowsiness as a side effect. The use of these medications is controversial because of their side effects and their limited effectiveness in promoting weight loss. Several surgical procedures, collectively referred to as bariatric surgery, have been used to treat severe obesity that has impaired the patient's health and has resisted other treatment. There are stringent criteria for being a surgical candidate. Typically a patient has to have a BMI>40 or have a BMI between 35.0 to 39.9 with at least one serious comorbidity, which can include type 2 diabetes, hypertension, asthma or sleep apnea. Pre-operative counseling as well as psychological and cognitive assessments often takes place to ensure patients are realistic about goals post-surgery and are prepared to make serious lifestyle modifications.

Bariatric surgical procedures lead to weight loss through two basic mechanisms: malabsorption and restriction. Malabsorptive procedures decrease nutrient absorption through the removal of a portion of intestine. Restrictive procedures decrease caloric intake through restriction of stomach capacity anatomically. The most commonly performed bariatric procedures done today include the following:

Roux-en-Y gastricbypass: a combined restrictive and malabsorptive procedure wherein the stomach is divided and a new, smaller gastric pouch is created, and the small intestine is also divided with a limb created and connected to the gastric pouch to bypass the initial portion of the intestine

Sleeve gastrectomy: a restrictive procedure in which the majority of the stomach is removed. This is the most commonly performed procedure both globally and in the U.S.

Laparoscopic adjustable gastricbanding: a restrictive procedure where an adjustable band is placed around the entrance to the stomach. This procedure is being performed less in light of the aforementioned procedures which cause increased weight loss and improved comorbidity resolution.

Liposuction is not a suggested weight loss strategy as studies indicate it does not actually cause improvements in insulin sensitivity or cardiovascular risk factors.

PERSPECTIVE AND PROSPECTS

Fat has several important functions in the human body. It serves as a cushion for the body frame and internal organs, it provides insulation against heat loss, and it is a storage site for energy. Fat stores energy very efficiently since it contains approximately nine calories per gram, compared with approximately four calories per gram in protein and carbohydrate. The presence of reserve stores of energy in the form of fat is particularly important when regular food intake is interrupted and the body becomes dependent on its fat deposits to maintain a source of fuel for daily metabolism and physical activity. In affluent, culturally advanced societies, however, where food is abundant and modern conveniences greatly reduce the need for physical exertion, many people tend to accumulate excessive amounts of fat, since energy that is taken in but not utilized is stored in the adipose tissue. In the early twenty-first century, health officials were concerned by findings that showed one in every fifty Americans were "extremely obese," meaning their BMI measured at least 50 and they were at least one hundred pounds overweight. This number had quadrupled since the 1980s. Obesity is a critical public health problem because it increases the risk of diabetes, hypertension, cardiovascular disease, and other illnesses. Also, many overweight men and women are distressed by the effects of their weight on their social interactions and self-image, and, despite laws, face discrimination in workplace settings. Therefore, many obese individuals desire to lose weight. Childhood and adolescent obesity is also becoming a growing problem, with the prevalence of severe obesity increasing. Childhood obesity is more common among American Indian, Mexican-American and black children and is also more prevalent among lower-income communities. Childhood obesity increases the risk for comorbidities later in life including diabetes, hypertension, and heart disease.

Unfortunately, the results of weight-loss programs and countless individual efforts at dieting to achieve this goal have often been disappointing. Short-term weight loss can often be achieved; programs utilizing low-calorie diets, behavior modification, exercise, and sometimes appetite-suppressing drugs usually lead to a weight loss of ten to thirty pounds or more over a period of several weeks or months. The problem is that after a year or more, the great majority of these dieters have regained the lost weight. It appears that the maintenance of a low-calorie diet and an increase in physical activity require a degree of commitment and willingness to endure inconvenience, self-deprivation, and sometimes even physical discomfort that most people can accept for short periods of time but not indefinitely. There are exceptions—some people do succeed in maintaining long-term weight loss—but more commonly dieters return to or surpass their original weight. It is as if the body's set point can be overcome temporarily by intense effort, but not permanently. Because of the poor prognosis for long-term weight loss, some experts now question the extent to which efforts should be devoted to the treatment of obesity. Nevertheless, because one cannot predict which obese individuals will succeed in achieving long-term weight reduction and because of the important health benefits of maintaining a normal body weight, most physicians agree that serious efforts should be made to treat obesity. Overweight individuals should identify the modifications in their diet and

lifestyle that would be most beneficial and should attempt, with medical supervision, to initiate and maintain the behavior needed to bring about permanent weight loss.

Bariatric surgery has been enjoying increasing popularity as a weight loss strategy. According to the American Society of Metabolic and Bariatric Surgery, there were 196,000 bariatric surgery procedures done in 2015, compared to 158,000 in 2011. With the advent of laparoscopic, minimally-invasive surgery, patients now have improved recovery and diminished morbidity compared to open surgery. Expected weight loss at 2 years post surgery is 60% for sleeve gastrectomy and 70% for Roux-en-Y gastric bypass. Because of the rapid weight loss that takes place, patients often are counseled that they may have excess loose skin that will require plastic surgery for removal.

In 2006, in an effort to reduce the incidence rate of obesity in the United States, the Alliance for a Healthier Generation, the William J. Clinton Foundation, and the American Heart Association announced an agreement to fight childhood obesity. Five leading food manufacturers vowed to reformulate their products in order to provide more nutritious choices for children in schools. In 2010 President Barack Obama and First Lady Michelle Obama each announced initiatives to help prevent childhood obesity.

—E. Victor Adlin, MD and Karen E. Kalumuck, PhD; updated by LeAnna DeAngelo, PhD and Ananya Anand, MSc

See also: Arteriosclerosis; Bariatric surgery; Cholesterol; Cushing's syndrome; Diabetes mellitus; Eating disorders; Endocrine disorders; Endocrinology; Exercise physiology; Glands; Heart disease; Hormones; Hyperadiposis; Hypercholesterolemia; Hyperlipidemia; Hypertension; Malnutrition; Metabolic syndrome; Metabolism; Nutrition; Obesity, childhood; Prader-Willi syndrome; Sleep apnea; Thyroid disorders; Weight loss and gain; Weight loss medications.

For Further Information:
American Academy of Pediatrics. *A Parent's Guide to Childhood Obesity: A Roadmap to Health*. Edited by Sandra G. Hassink. Elk Grove Village, Ill.: Author, 2006.
American Obesity Treatment Association. *American Obesity*, n.d. Björntorp, Per, ed. *International Textbook of Obesity*. Chichester: Wiley, 2002.
Brownell, Kelly D., and Katherine Battle Horgen. *Food Fight: The Inside Story of America's ObesityCrisis and What We Can Do About It*. New York: McGraw-Hill, 2004.
Carson-DeWitt, Rosalyn. "Overweight in Adults." *Health Library*, June 24, 2013.
Centers for Disease Control and Prevention. "Overweight and Obesity." *Centers for Disease Control and Prevention*, April 27, 2012.
Finkelstein, Eric A., et al. "Annual Medical Spending Attributable to Obesity: Payer- and Service-Specific Estimates." *Health Affairs* 28, no. 5 (2009): w822-w831.

Koplan, Jeffrey P., Catharyn T. Liverman, and Vivica I. Kraak, eds. *Preventing Childhood Obesity: Health in the Balance*. Washington, DC: National Academies Press, 2005.

MedlinePlus. "Obesity." *MedlinePlus*, August 29, 2013.

National Heart, Lung, and Blood Institute. "What Are Overweight and Obesity?" *National Heart* Obesity Society. *Obesity.org*, 2010.

Ogden, C. L., et al. "Prevalence of Obesity in the United States, 2009-2010." *NCHS Data Brief* no. 82 (January, 2012).

Wadden, Thomas A., and Albert J. Stunkard, eds. *Handbook of Obesity Treatment*. Rev. ed. New York: Guilford Press, 2004.

OBESITY, CHILDHOOD

Category: Disease/Disorder

Anatomy or system affected: Abdomen, blood vessels, circulatory system, endocrine system, gastrointestinal system, heart, intestines, joints, psychic-emotional system, respiratory system, stomach

Specialties and related fields: Endocrinology, family medicine, internal medicine, nutrition, pediatrics, psychiatry, psychology, public health

Definition: Having a body mass index (BMI) at or above the 95th percentile for children of the same age and sex. Rapid changes from infancy through adolescence are part of normal and expected development, and the norm used to identify childhood obesity must be correct for that child's age and sex.

Key terms:

adipose tissue: a type of fat storage cell constellation that is also involved in energy regulation and hormone release

body mass index (BMI): a formula that estimates the percentage of body fat compared to overall weight; usually expressed in metrics, a person's weight in kilograms divided by height in meters, squared (kg/m2)

hormones: chemical signaling substances in the bloodstream that foster communication between individual organs and the rest of the body

metabolic syndrome: a cluster of traits that can include obesity, high blood pressure, abnormal lipid levels, and high insulin levels in blood; their presence often marks the first phase of more serious diseases

CAUSES AND SYMPTOMS

An imbalance between energy expended (how active one is) and energy ingested (how much one eats and drinks) will promote weight gain. When ingestion regularly exceeds expenditure, the unused energy is stored in adipose tissue, or body fat. In the past, animal species that developed the capacity to store fat had a better chance of surviving times of scarcity. However, in many developed countries chronic storage of excessive energy is less necessary for survival and produces its own physical pathology. Almost every person who eats and drinks more than he or she uses in energy (usually calculated in calories) will produce adipose tissue to store the excess energy.

Peptide hormones such as leptin and adiponectin regulate and balance the energy expended with energy ingested. Studies have shown that when leptin is absent (leptin deficiency), massive obesity is present. Adiponectin, increases sensitivity to insulin and is an anti-inflammatory signaler. Together, leptin and adiponectin, along with other peptide hormones, initiate a series of signaling processes that eventually lead to hormones that balance hunger, energy expenditure, and body weight.

It is important to note that in addition to the underlying genetic and physiologic causes of obesity, there are several behavioral, economic, and sociocultural factors that contribute to childhood obesity as well. In 2011-14, among children and adolescents aged two to nineteen years, the prevalence of obesity decreased as the head of household's level of education increased. Obesity prevalence was also lower in higher income groups for non-Hispanic Asian boys, Hispanic boys, non-Hispanic white girls, non-Hispanic Asian girls, and Hispanic girls. Obesity prevalence did not differ by income among non-Hispanic black girls.

The formal definition of obesity in children is a body mass index (BMI) greater than or equal to the 95th percentile. Children between the 85th and 95th percentiles are at risk for obesity; those less than the 85th percentile are generally considered to have normal weight when correlated with their height.

Childhood obesity has many detrimental effects and comorbidities (other diseases and disorders) that often extend into adolescence and adulthood. It is simplistic to say that obese children will become obese adults. Still, childhood obesity often produces a metabolic syndrome that continues into adolescence and adulthood. This syndrome has serious implications for quality of life and life expectancy. Metabolic syndrome is a combination of high insulin levels (hyperinsulinemia), obesity, high blood pressure (hypertension), and abnormal lipid levels (dyslipidemia). Together, these produce aortic and coronary atherosclerosis (hardening of

---

INFORMATION ON CHILDHOOD OBESITY

Causes: May include poor diet, lack of exercise, genetic factors

Symptoms: Excessive weight relative to age and height, possibly leading to health problems and adult obesity

Duration: Often chronic

Treatments: Improved diet and increased activity

the arteries) and clogging of the arteries by fatty deposits in the blood.

The psychosocial impact of childhood obesity are no less serious than physical symptoms, leading to poor body image, low self-confidence, social isolation, recurrent anger, early forms of eating disorders, clinical depression, and negatively acting-out in school and other social settings. Promoting physical activity is an important intervention to lessen the psychological harm of obesity as much as is controlling the amount and type of food and drink.

TREATMENT AND THERAPY

The most effective treatment for child obesity is prevention, and it can begin shortly after birth. Research shows that breast-fed children have significantly lower rates of obesity in later years. As infants become toddlers and toddlers become children, the difference between healthy weight gains and weight gains that suggest the onset of obesity often require the expert eye of a pediatrician or family physician. A healthy five-pound weight gain in one ten-year-old child may not be healthy in another child of the same age.

It is not until adolescence that children play a significant role in choosing and purchasing food. Until then, whatever children eat is most likely what adults have purchased or provided. Preventing obesity and correcting it when it occurs requires thoughtful selection of food and beverage items at home and school. Fast and take-out foods are always an easy solution to busy, hectic family schedules, but they are almost always obesity-promoting. Junk food snacks, also a quick solution to the transient hunger pangs of youth, are similarly harmful.

Prevention and treatment are almost one and the same in dealing with child obesity. Parents control the food world of children, and making available a variety of healthy choices becomes an important part of achieving and maintaining healthy bodies that have modest amounts of adipose tissue, as children with a BMI of less than 20 are also unhealthy. Obesity is much less likely to occur in families and schools that support healthy lifestyles: balanced nutritional consumption, physical activity and exercise, and sufficient sleep. (As a group, children who consistently get less sleep than they need are more likely to be obese than are children who sleep enough. The specific number of hours any child might need is a function of several factors, including age.)

Successful school-based interventions in the management of obesity include a prioritization of physical education classes, healthy choices on the student menu and in vending machines, proportional servings, encouraging water as the main beverage, and the ready availability of after-school activities that involve physi-

Children with varying levels of body fat. Photo by Walter Siegmund, via Wikimedia Commons.

cal activity, such as intramural sports. When these elements are not present, effective obesity management for school-age children is difficult.

The key to successful long-term obesity prevention and treatment involves awareness of and respect for the individual child's personal preferences and enjoyments-nothing will enhance motivation more. Decreasing sitting time and the active encouragement of free play is far more effective than mandates to exercise or reduce food intake. Even in families where genetics play a major role in obesity, a healthy lifestyle will decrease the negative impact that obesity can have on the children's overall health.

PERSPECTIVE AND PROSPECTS

In 2019, the Centers for Disease Control and Prevention (CDC) reported that data from the 2017-18 National Health and Nutrition Examination Survey showed that about 19.3 percent of US children and adolescents from ages two to nineteen are obese. Although a national study by the CDC showed that obesity among low-income preschoolers declined in nineteen states between 2008 and 2011, childhood obesity remains an epidemic that has achieved the status of a public health crisis. Obesity has profound impacts on children's long-term physical and psychological health and, more often than not, leads to serious comorbidities in adulthood that are costly to treat and difficult to control. Focused strategies on modifying behavior and the slow but steady acquisition of healthy habits are the only ways that children will reliably manage the balance between calories consumed and calories burned. Adult habits, good and bad, are usually fostered during childhood. They reflect the level of care, attention, and perseverance of caregivers. Childhood obesity can be a problem of adults' mismanagement much more than it is a problem of children's choices. Parents and teachers make a major contribution to children when they provide a health-oriented environment in which children are more likely to acquire the habits that promote wellness throughout their lives.

On February 9, 2010 President Barack Obama created the Task Force on Childhood Obesity, which was charged with reviewing existing programs and formulating a national plan of action, and First Lady Michelle Obama announced the start of her own campaign to end childhood obesity, Let's Move.

—*Rachelle G. Ford, MD*

See also: Bariatric surgery; Cholesterol; Diabetes mellitus; Eating disorders; Endocrine disorders; Endocrinology; Exercise physiology; Glands; Heart disease; Hormones; Hyperadiposis; Hypercholesterolemia; Hyperlipidemia; Hypertension; Malnutrition; Metabolic syndrome; Metabolism; Nutrition; Obesity; Thyroid disorders; Weight loss and gain; Weight loss medications.

For Further Information:
American Academy of Pediatrics. "Obesity." *American Academy of Pediatrics*. Accessed 14 Mar. 2022.
Centers for Disease Control and Prevention. "Childhood Overweight and Obesity." *Centers for Disease Control and Prevention*. Accessed 14 Mar. 2020.
———. "Obesity Among Low-Income Preschoolers Declines in Many States." *CDC Newsroom*, 6 Aug. 2013.
Jones, Pamela. "Obesity—Children and Teens." *Health Library*, 18 Mar. 2013.
MedlinePlus. "Obesity in Children." *MedlinePlus*, 22 Aug. 2022.
Ogden, Cynthia, and Margaret Carroll. "NCHS Health E-Stat: Prevalence of Obesity among Children and Adolescents: United States Trends 1963-1965 through 2007-2008." *Centers for Disease Control and Prevention*, 4 June 2010.
Okie, Susan. *Fed Up! Winning the War Against Childhood Obesity*. National Academies Press, 2005.

OBSESSIVE-COMPULSIVE DISORDER

Category: Disease/Disorder
Anatomy or system affected: Psychic-emotional system
Specialties and related fields: Psychiatry, psychology

Definition: An anxiety disorder characterized by intrusive and unwanted but uncontrollable thoughts, by the need to perform ritualized behavior patterns, or both; the obsessions and/or compulsions cause severe stress, consume an excessive amount of time, and greatly interfere with a person's normal routine, activities, or relationships.

Key terms:
anal stage: the stage of psychosexual development in which a child derives pleasure from activities associated with elimination
anxiety: an unpleasant feeling of fear and apprehension
biogenic model: the theory that every mental disorder is based on a physical or physiological problem
major affective disorder: a personality disorder characterized by mood disturbances
monoamine oxidase inhibitors: antidepressant compounds used to restore the balance of normal neurotransmitters in the brain
phobia: a strong, persistent, and unwarranted fear of a specific object or situation
selective serotonin reuptake inhibitors (SSRIs): primary medications used for obsessive-compulsive disorder
Tourette's syndrome: a childhood disorder characterized by several motor and verbal tics that may develop into the compulsion to shout obscenities
tricyclics: medications used to relieve the symptoms of depression

CAUSES AND SYMPTOMS

Obsessive-compulsive disorder (OCD) is an anxiety disorder characterized by intrusive and uncontrollable thoughts and/or by the need to perform specific acts repeatedly. Obsessive-compulsive behavior is highly distressing because one's behavior or thoughts are no longer voluntarily controlled. The more frequently these uncontrolled alien and perhaps unacceptable thoughts or actions are performed, the more distress is induced. A disturbed individual may have either obsessions (which are thought-related) or compulsions (which are action-related), or both. At various stages of the disorder, one of the symptoms may replace the other.

OCD affects 1 to 2 percent of the population; most of those afflicted begin suffering from the disorder in early adulthood, and it is often preceded by a particularly stressful event such as pregnancy, childbirth, or family conflict. It may be closely associated with depression, with the disorder developing soon after a bout of depression or the depression developing as a result of the disorder. OCD affects men and women equally.

Obsessions generally fall into one of five recognized categories. Obsessive doubts are persistent doubts that a task has been completed; the individual is unwilling to accept and believe that the work is done satisfactorily. Obsessive thinking is an almost infinite chain of thought, targeting future events. Obsessive impulses are very strong urges to perform certain actions, whether they be trivial or serious, that would likely be harmful to the obsessive person or someone else and that are socially unacceptable. Obsessive fears are thoughts that the person has lost control and will act in some way that will cause public embarrassment. Obsessive images are continued visual pictures of either a real or an imagined event.

Four factors are commonly associated with obsessive characteristics, not only in people with OCD but in the general population as well. First, obsessive individuals are unable to control their mental processes completely. Practically, this means the loss of control over thinking processes, such as intrusive thoughts of a loved one dying or worries about hurting someone unintentionally. Second, there may be thoughts and worries over the potential loss of motor control, perhaps causing impulses such as shouting obscenities in church or school or performing inappropriate sexual acts. Third, many obsessive individuals may be afraid of contamination and suffer irrational fear and worry over exposure to germs, dirt, or diseases. The last factor is checking behavior, or backtracking previous actions to ensure that the behavior was done properly, such as checking that doors and windows are shut, faucets are turned off, and so on. Some common obsessions are fear of having decaying teeth or food particles between the teeth, worry about whether the sufferer has touched germs, and fear of contracting a sexually transmitted disease.

Compulsions may be either mild or severe and debilitating. Mild compulsions might be superstitions, such as refusing to walk under a ladder or throwing salt over one's shoulder. Severe compulsions become fixed, unvaried ritualized behaviors; if they are not practiced precisely in a particular manner or a prescribed number of times, then intense anxiety may result. These strange behaviors may be rooted in superstition; many of those suffering from the disorder believe that performing the behavior may ward off danger. Compulsive acts are not ends in themselves but are "necessary" to produce or prevent a future event from occurring. Although the enactment of the ritual may assuage tension, the act does not give the compulsive pleasure.

Several kinds of rituals are typically enacted. A common ritual is repeating; these sufferers must do everything by numbers. Checking is another compulsive act; a compulsive checker believes that it is necessary to check and recheck that everything is in order. Cleaning is a behavior in which many compulsives

---

> ### INFORMATION ON
> ### OBSESSIVE-COMPULSIVE DISORDER
>
> **Causes:** Psychological factors; may involve physical defects, genetics, or biochemical disorders
> **Symptoms:** Excessive repetitive behavior, anxiety, depression, intrusive and uncontrollable thoughts, irrational fears, checking behavior
> **Duration:** Often chronic with acute episodes
> **Treatments:** Psychotherapy, drug therapy

must engage; they may wash and scrub repeatedly, especially if they think that they have touched something dirty. A fourth common compulsive action is avoidance; for certain superstitious or magical reasons, certain objects must be avoided. Some individuals with compulsions experience compelling urges for perfection in even the most trivial of tasks; often the task is repeated to ensure that it has been done correctly. Some determine that objects must be in a particular arrangement; these individuals are considered "meticulous." A few sufferers are hoarders; they are unable to throw away trash or rubbish. All these individuals have a constant need for reassurance; for example, they want to be told repeatedly that they have not been contaminated.

No single cause for OCD has been isolated. Several theories provide some examples of attempts to explain the basis of OCD psychologically. They involve guilt, anxiety, and superstition. Sigmund Freud first proposed that obsessive thoughts are a replacement for more disturbing thoughts or actions that induce guilt in the sufferer. These thoughts or behaviors, according to Freud, are usually sexual in nature. Freud based his ideas on the cases of some of his young patients. In the case of a teenage girl, for example, he determined that she exchanged obsessive thoughts of stealing for the act of masturbation. The thoughts of stealing produced far fewer guilt feelings than masturbation did. Replacing guilt feelings with less threatening thoughts prevents one's personal defenses from being overwhelmed. Other defense mechanisms may be parlayed into OCD. Undoing, one of these behaviors, is obliterating guilt-producing urges by undergoing repetitive rituals, such as handwashing. Since the forbidden urges continue to recur, the behavior to replace those urges must continue. These behaviors are then negatively reinforced because anxiety decreases when the behavior is performed, thereby maintaining the behavior. Another mechanism is reaction formation. When an unacceptable thought or urge is present, the sufferer replaces it with an exactly opposite behavior. Many theorists believe that both obsessive and compulsive behaviors arise as a consequence of overly harsh toilet training. Thus the person is fixated at the anal stage and, by reaction formation, resists the urge to soil by becoming overly neat and clean. A third mechanism is isolation, the separation of a thought or action from its effect. Detachment or aloofness may isolate an individual from aggressive or sexual thoughts.

The superstition hypothesis proposes a connection between a chance association and a reinforcer that induces a continuation of the behavior. Many theorists believe that the same sequence is involved in the formation of many superstitions. A particular obsessive-compulsive ritual may be reinforced when a positive outcome follows the behavior; anxiety results when the ritual is interrupted. An example would be a student who only uses one special pencil or pen to take exams, based on a previous good grade. In actuality, there is seldom a real relationship between the behavior and the outcome. This hypothesis, too, fails to explain the development of obsessions.

Another theory is accepted by those who believe that mental disorders are the result of something physically or physiologically amiss in the sufferer, employing data from brain structure studies, genetics, and biochemistry. Indeed, brain activity is altered in those suffering from OCD, and they experience increased metabolic activity. Whether the activity is a cause or an effect, however, is unclear. Studies of genetics in families, at least in twins, reinforce the idea that genetics may play a small role in OCD because there appears to be a higher incidence of the disorder in identical twins than in other siblings. Yet these results may be misleading: Because all the studies were carried out on twins who were reared together, environment must also be considered as a contributing cause. It should be noted, however, that relatives of OCD sufferers are twice as likely as unrelated individuals to develop the same disorder, indicating that the tendency for the behavior could be heritable.

TREATMENT AND THERAPY
Obsessional symptoms are not uncommon in the general population. While many people have been diagnosed with OCD, others are too horrified to admit to their symptoms, or they do not realize that their behavior is abnormal and do not seek treatment.

Diagnostic techniques evaluating OCD usually involve psychological evaluation. It is important to determine whether an individual is actually suffering from OCD or other potential problems such as schizophrenia or a mood disorder. Additionally, it is important to determine whether more than one disorder is present. OCD may occur in conjunction with other disorders, such as substance use disorders, eating disorders, and mood disorders. When this occurs, treatment

must be adjusted. For example, when depression is also noted, both disorders must be treated.

In cases when differentiation is required between OCD and schizophrenia, the concern is to understand the nature of the dysfunctional thoughts and behaviors. For instance, a distinction can be made by determining the motive behind the ritualized behavior. Stereotyped behaviors are symptomatic of both disorders. In the person with schizophrenia, however, the behavior is triggered by delusions rather than by true compulsions. People suffering from true delusions cannot be shaken from them. They do not resist the ideas inundating their minds, and ritualized behavior does not necessarily decrease the feelings associated with the intrusive ideas. On the other hand, obsessive people usually experience decreases in anxiety when they perform their rituals and may be absolutely certain of the need to perform their rituals, though other aspects of their thinking and logic are perfectly clear. They generally resist the ideas that enter their minds and realize the absurdity or abnormality of the thoughts to some extent. As thoughts and images intrude into the obsessive person's mind, the person may sometimes appear to have symptoms that mimic schizophrenia.

Other problems having symptoms in common with OCD are Tourette syndrome and stimulant use. What seems to separate the symptoms of these disorders from those experienced with OCD is that the former are organically induced. Thus, the actions of a sufferer from Tourette syndrome may be mechanical since they are not intellectually dictated or purposely enacted. In the case of the stimulant user, the acts may bring pleasure and are not resisted, but reinforced by the drug effects.

"Normal" people also have obsessive thoughts; in fact, the obsessions of normal individuals are not significantly different from the obsessions of those with OCD. The major difference is that those with the disorder have longer-lasting, more intense, and less easily dismissed obsessive thoughts. The importance of this overlap is that mere symptoms are not a reliable tool to diagnose OCD, since some of the same symptoms are experienced by the general population.

Assessment of OCD separates the obsessive from the compulsive components so that each can be examined. Obsession assessment should determine the triggering fears of the disorder, both internal and external, including thoughts of unpleasant consequences. The amount of anxiety that these obsessions produce should be monitored. The compulsive behaviors then should be examined in the same light.

The greatest chance for successful treatment occurs with individuals who experience mild symptoms that are usually obsessive but not compulsive in nature, who seek help soon after the onset of symptoms, and who had few problems before the disorder began. While OCD can be challenging to treat, many valuable and successful treatment strategies are available. Types of treatment fall into four categories: psychotherapy, behavioral therapy, drug therapy, and psychosurgery. The treatments of choice tend to be behavioral and drug therapies.

When psychotherapy is attempted, it usually begins with some type of analysis. The degree of dysfunction, the stressor triggering the symptoms, and the psychological makeup of the individual often determine whether the analysis will be successful. The major goal of a more psychoanalytical approach is to find and then remove an assumed repression so that the individual can deal with whatever they fear in an open and honest fashion. Some analysts believe that focusing on the present is most beneficial, since delving into the past may strengthen the defensive mechanism (the compulsive behavior). If the patient attempts to "return" to the mitigating event, then the analyst usually intervenes directly and actively and brings the individual back to the present by encouraging, pressuring, and guiding him or her.

The most effective treatment for controlling OCD is the behavioral approach. Behavioral therapy focuses on breaking the connection between the stimulus (what induces the compulsion or obsession) and the compulsions and obsessions. Response prevention involves two stages. First, the individual is subject to flooding, the act of exposing the individual to the real and/or imagined stimuli that cause anxiety. This process begins with brief exposure to the stressors while the therapist assesses the individuals's thoughts, feelings, and behaviors during the stimulus period. In the second stage, the individual is flooded with the stimuli but restrained from acting on those stressors. Although flooding may produce intense discomfort at first, patients are gradually desensitized to the stimuli, causing the resulting anxiety to decrease. The therapist must expend considerable time preventing the response, discussing the anxiety as it appears, and supporting the person as the anxiety abates. To be more effective, treatment may also occur in the home with the guidance and support of family members who have been informed about how best to interact with the person needing treatment. Therapists may also help the person break the connection between triggers and responses by aiding the individual in replacing the symptoms of the obsession or compulsion with healthier preventive or replacement actions. Similarly, aversive methods may be used to break the chain of behavior. They might include a nonvocal, internal shout of "Stop!" The action of snapping a rubber band on the wrist when the obsessive thoughts enter the mind or physically restraining oneself if the compul-

sive action begins may also be helpful. This latter approach may be so uncomfortable and disconcerting to the patient that it may work only under the supervision supplied by a hospital. With any of these approaches, however, if the individual is also depressed or has other complicating conditions, then successful treatment will require additional steps.

Drugs commonly used to treat OCD that have met with some success include selective serotonin reuptake inhibitors (SSRIs), antidepressants, tricyclics, monoamine oxidase inhibitors, LSD, and tryptophan. SSRIs often have remarkable effects on OCD, helping individuals to experience a change in their thinking and behavior, as well as relief. They are usually the first line of treatment in addressing OCD through drug therapy. Psychiatrists also may prescribe tranquilizers to reduce the client's anxiety; however, these drugs are usually not adequate to depress the frequent obsessive thoughts or compulsive actions and so are not a treatment of choice. More general antidepressants may benefit those suffering from depression as well as OCD. It has also been observed that as depression lifts, some of the compulsive behavior may also decrease. Monoamine oxidase inhibitors (MAOIs), another form of antidepressants, are used in treating OCD associated with panic attacks, phobias, and severe anxiety. When medication is halted, however, the patient often relapses into the previous obsessive-compulsive state, so these too are not necessarily a treatment of choice. Drugs such as tryptophan may provide some relief through its affects on melatonin. Similarly, LSD and other hallucinogenic drugs have been tested as potential treatments for this condition because of their effects on serotonin receptors; however, their status as illicit drugs and the significant side effects from other aspects of the actions of these substances do not make them practically useful.

Some psychosurgeons may resort to psychosurgery to relieve a patient's symptoms. The improvement noted after surgery may simply be attributable to the loss of emotion and dulling of behavioral patterns found in any patient who has undergone a lobotomy. Because such surgery may result in a change in the patient's intellect and emotional response, it should be considered only in extreme, debilitating cases. Newer surgical techniques do not destroy as much of the cerebral cortex. These procedures separate the frontal cortex from lower brain areas in only an 8-centimeter square area.

PERSPECTIVE AND PROSPECTS

Descriptions of OCD-like behavior go back to medieval times; a young man who could not control his urge to stick out his tongue or blurt out obscenities during prayer was reported in the fifteenth century.

Medical accounts of the disorder and the term "obsessive-compulsive" originated in the mid-nineteenth century. At that time, obsessions were believed to occur when mental energy ran low. Later, Freud stated that OCD is accompanied by stubbornness, stinginess, and tidiness. He attributed the characteristics to a regression to early childhood, when there are perhaps strong urges to be violent and/or to dirty and mess one's surroundings. To avoid acting on these tendencies, he theorized, an avoidance mechanism is employed, and the symptoms of obsession and/or compulsion appear. Other features related to this regression are ambivalence, magical thinking, and a harsh, punitive conscience.

An unpleasant consequence of OCD behavior is the effect that the behavior has on the people who interact with the sufferer. The relationships with an obsessive person's family, schoolmates, or coworkers all suffer when a person with OCD takes up time with uncontrollable and lengthy rituals. These people may feel not only a justifiable concern but also resentment. Some may feel guilt over the resentful feelings because they know the obsessive-compulsive cannot control these actions. An obsessive-compulsive observing these conflicting feelings in others may respond by developing depression or other anxious feelings, which may cause further alienation.

Although not totally disabling, OCD behaviors can be strongly incapacitating. A famous figure who suffered from OCD was millionaire and aviator Howard Hughes (1905-1976). A recluse after 1950, he became so withdrawn from the public that he communicated only via telephone and intermediaries. His obsession-compulsion was the irrational fear of germs and contamination. It began with his refusal to shake hands with people. If he had to hold a glass or open a door, he covered his hand with a tissue. He would not abide any of his aides eating foods that gave them bad breath. He disallowed air conditioners, believing that they collected germs. Because Hughes acted on his obsessions, they became compulsions.

Most parents will agree that children commonly have rituals to which they must adhere or compulsive actions they carry out. A particular bedtime story may be read every night for months on end, and children's games involve counting or checking rituals. It is also not atypical for adults without psychiatric disorders to experience some mild obsessive thoughts or compulsive actions, as seen in an overly tidy person or in group rituals performed in some religious sects. Excessively stressful events may trigger obsessions as well.

Further research into the biopsychosocial causes of OCD will be important in developing future treatment approaches. Such causes and treatment may also be useful for understanding other behaviors that have

compulsive features, such as problems related to substance use, gambling, eating, and sexual behavior.

—Iona C. Baldridge;
updated by Nancy A. Piotrowski, PhD

See also Addiction; Anorexia nervosa; Antianxiety drugs; Anxiety; Bipolar disorders; Bulimia; Depression; Eating disorders; Grief and guilt; Neurosis; Panic attacks; Paranoia; Phobias; Post-traumatic stress disorder; Psychiatric disorders; Psychiatry; Psychiatry, child and adolescent; Psychiatry, geriatric; Psychoanalysis; Schizophrenia; Stress; Tics.

For Further Information:
American Psychiatric Association. *Diagnostic and Statistical Manual of Mental Disorders: DSM-5*. 5th ed. Arlington, Va.: Author, 2013.
Barlow, David H. *Anxiety and Its Disorders*. 2d ed. New York: Guilford Press, 2004.
Barlow, David H., ed. *Clinical Handbook of Psychological Disorders*. 4th ed. New York: Guilford Press, 2008.
Kring, Ann M., et al. *Abnormal Psychology*. 12th ed. Hoboken, N.J.: John Wiley & Sons, 2012.
McCoy, Krisha, and Michael Woods. "Obsessive-Compulsive Personality Disorder." *Health Library*, Sept. 30, 2012.
Menzies, Ross, and Padmal de Silva, eds. *Obsessive Compulsive Disorder: Theory, Research, and Treatment*. New York: Wiley, 2003.
"Obsessive-Compulsive Disorder." *MedlinePlus*, Apr. 11, 2013.
"Obsessive-Compulsive Disorder: When Unwanted Thoughts Take Over." *National Institute of Mental Health*, 2010.
Oltmanns, Thomas F., et al. *Case Studies in Abnormal Psychology*. 9th ed. Hoboken, N.J.: John Wiley & Sons, 2012.
Scholten, Amy, and Brian Randall. "Obsessive-Compulsive Disorder." *Health Library*, Sept. 10, 2012.
"What You Need to Know about Obsessive-Compulsive Disorder." *International OCD Foundation*, 2012.

OBSTETRICS

Category: Specialty
Anatomy or system affected: Reproductive system, uterus
Specialties and related fields: Embryology, genetics, gynecology, neonatology, perinatology
Definition: The medical science dealing with pregnancy and childbirth, including the health of both mother and unborn infant and the delivery of the child and the placenta at the time of birth.
Key terms:
amniocentesis: a technique by which a fine needle is inserted through a pregnant woman's abdomen and into the uterus and amniotic sac in order to collect fetal amniotic cells for biochemical and genetic analysis
birth defect: a genetic or developmental abnormality which occurs in utero that leads to anatomic or

functional problems after birth; the defect can be serious, with potentially significant consequences for the fetus or mother, or the defect can be minor

cesarean section: a surgical procedure whereby the infant is delivered through an incision on the mother's abdomen

forceps: curved metal blades that are carefully placed around the fetal head through the vagina to facilitate delivery

gestation: the period from conception to birth, in which the fetus reaches full development in order to survive outside the mother's body

placenta: an organ in the uterus through which the fetus receives its oxygen and nutrients and removes its waste products; it serves as a blood barrier between the mother's circulatory system and the fetal circulatory system

Rh0(D) immune globulin: also known as RhoGAM; a type of gamma globulin protein injected into Rh-negative mothers who may have an Rh-positive fetus to protect the fetus from an immune reaction called isoimmunization

trimester: one of three periods of time in pregnancy, each period lasting three months; the first trimester is zero to twelve weeks of gestational age, the second trimester is thirteen to twenty-four weeks of gestational age, and the third trimester is twenty-five to thirty-seven weeks of gestational age

ultrasonography: an imaging modality in which sound waves penetrate bodily tissues in order to generate an image; in obstetrics, this technique is commonly used to assess the fetus, amniotic fluid, and uterus and ovaries

vacuum: a device with a suction cup that is applied to the fetal head through the vagina to assist in delivery of the infant

SCIENCE AND PROFESSION

Obstetrics is the branch of medical science dealing with pregnancy and childbirth in women. Once conception has occurred and a woman is pregnant, major physiological changes occur within her body as well as within the body of the developing embryo or fetus. Obstetrics deals with these changes leading up to and including childbirth. As such, obstetrics is a critical branch of medicine, for it involves the complex physiological events by which every person comes into existence.

The professional obstetrician is a licensed medical doctor whose area of expertise is pregnancy and childbirth. Often, the obstetrician is also a specialist in the closely related science of gynecology, the study of diseases and conditions that specifically affect women, particularly nonpregnant women. The obstetrician is especially knowledgeable in female anatomy and physiology, including the major bodily changes that occur during and following pregnancies. Obstetricians also have a detailed understanding of the necessary diagnostic procedures for monitoring fetal and maternal health, and they are educated in the latest technologies for facilitating a successful pregnancy and childbirth with minimal complications. Obstetrical care is also provided by certified nurse midwives (CNMs) and by nurse practitioners, particularly those with certification in women's health (women's health care nurse practitioners).

Broadly, the diseases and conditions managed by the clinicians in this field include preconception counseling, normal prenatal care, and the management of pregnancy-specific problems such as preeclampsia, gestational diabetes, premature labor, premature rupture of membranes, multiple gestations, fetal growth problems, and isoimmunization. In addition, obstetricians manage medical problems that can occur in any woman but that take on special importance in pregnancy, such as thyroid disorders or infections. Obstetricians make assessments and decisions regarding when a baby is best delivered, particularly if there are in utero conditions that make it safer for the baby to be born immediately, even if prematurely. Obstetricians manage both normal and abnormal labors. They are able to assess the progress and position of the infant as it makes its way down the birth canal. They are knowledgeable about pain control options during labor and make decisions regarding when a cesarean section is indicated. Obstetricians assist with normal vaginal deliveries, either spontaneous or induced, and sometimes use special instruments such as forceps or vacuum-suction devices. They also perform cesarean sections. Obstetricians are trained in appropriate postpartum care for the mother and infant.

In natural, spontaneous fertilization, pregnancy begins with the fertilization of a woman's egg by a man's sperm following sexual intercourse, the chances of which are highest if intercourse takes place during a two-day period following ovulation. Ovulation is the release of an unfertilized egg from the woman's ovarian follicle, which occurs roughly halfway between successive periods during her menstrual cycle. Fertilization usually occurs in the upper one-third of one of the woman's fallopian tubes connecting the ovary to the uterus; upon entering the woman's vagina, sperm must travel through her cervix to the uterus and up the fallopian tubes, only one of which contains a released egg following ovulation.

Once fertilization has occurred, the first cell of the new individual, called a zygote, is slowly pushed by cilia down the fallopian tube and into the uterus. Along the way, the zygote undergoes several mitotic cellular divisions to begin the newly formed embryo, which at this point is a bundle of undifferentiated cells. Upon reaching the uterus, the embryo implants in the lining of the uterus. Hormonal changes occur in the woman's body to maintain the pregnancy. One of these hormones is human chorionic gonadotropin, which is the chemical detected by most pregnancy tests. Failure of the embryo to be implanted in the endometrium and subsequent lack of hormone production (specifically the hormone progesterone) will cause release of the endometrium as a bloody discharge; the woman will menstruate, and there will be no pregnancy. Therefore, menstrual cycles do not occur during a pregnancy.

The embryo will grow and develop over the next nine to ten months of gestation. The heart forms and begins beating at roughly five and one-half weeks following conception. Over the next several weeks and months, major organ systems begin to organize and develop. By the end of the first three months of the pregnancy, the developing human is considered to be a fetus. All the major organ systems have formed, although not all systems can function yet. The fetus is surrounded by a watery amniotic fluid within an amniotic sac. The fetus receives oxygen and nutrients from the mother and excretes waste products into the maternal circulation through the placenta. The fetus is connected to the placenta via the umbilical cord. During the second and third trimesters, full organ system development; massive cell divisions of certain tissues such as nervous, circulatory, and skeletal tissue; and preparation of the fetus for survival as an independent organism occur. The fetus cannot survive outside the mother's body, however, until the third trimester.

Changes also occur in the mother. Increased levels of the female steroid hormone estrogen create increased skin vascularization (that is, more blood vessels near the skin) and the deposition of fat throughout her body, especially in the breasts and the buttocks. The growing fetus and stretching uterus press on surrounding abdominal muscles, often creating abdominal and back discomfort. Reasonable exercise is important for the mother to stay healthy and to deliver the baby with relative ease. A balanced diet also is important for the nourishment of her body and that of the fetus.

Late in the pregnancy, the protein hormones prolactin and oxytocin will be produced by the woman's pituitary gland. Prolactin activates milk production in the breasts. Oxytocin causes muscular contractions, particularly in the breasts and in the uterus during labor. Near the time of birth, drastically elevated levels of the hormones estrogen and oxytocin will cause progressively stronger contractions (labor pains) until the baby is forced through the vagina and out of the woman's body to begin its independent physical existence. The placenta, or afterbirth, is discharged shortly thereafter.

DIAGNOSTIC AND TREATMENT TECHNIQUES
The role of the obstetrician is to monitor the health of the mother and unborn fetus during the course of the pregnancy and to deliver the baby successfully at the time of birth. Once the fact of the pregnancy is established, the obstetrician is trained to identify specific developmental changes in the fetus over time in order to ensure that the pregnancy is proceeding smoothly.

The mainstay of diagnosis is the physical examination during prenatal visits. Early in the pregnancy, prenatal visits occur monthly, but they become more frequent as the pregnancy progresses. During these visits, the woman may receive counseling regarding a balanced diet, folic acid and iron supplementation, and substances or foods to avoid that may pose a risk to the pregnancy. The woman's growing uterus is measured to confirm proper growth, and, if indicated, a vaginal or cervical examination may be performed. After ten weeks of gestational age, fetal heart tones are also assessed at every prenatal visit using a simplified ultrasonic technique, to ensure that they are within the normal number of beats per minute. Fetal heart tones that are abnormally slow may indicate a fetus in jeopardy.

The other main component of diagnosis is through laboratory tests. Early in the pregnancy, the woman will receive a Pap test to screen for cervical cancer. Blood tests will be ordered to determine whether the mother is a carrier of the human immunodeficiency virus (HIV) or hepatitis B or C viruses, which can be transmitted to the fetus. In addition, the mother is checked for anemia, and the blood type of the mother is assessed. If the mother's blood type indicates that she is Rh negative, she will receive RhoGAM in the third trimester to prevent the development of a disease called isoimmunization, a condition that could be fatal to the fetus. An additional diagnostic test performed routinely during pregnancy is a screening test for diabetes, which pregnant women are at increased risk for.

Another important method of diagnosis in obstetrics is ultrasonography. Ultrasonography early in pregnancy can determine the gestational age of a pregnancy in cases in which a woman's last menstrual period is unverified. The correct development of the fetus and the presence of any birth defects can be assessed using this procedure. Ultrasound can also determine whether the placenta is growing in a safe location and whether the proper amount of amniotic fluid is found in the amniotic sac. Toward the end of pregnancy, ultrasound is an invaluable diagnostic tool for determining fetal well-being and the position of the infant in the uterus in preparation for delivery. Ultrasound is also a useful tool in guiding diagnostic procedures. For instance, amniocentesis can be extremely safe when performed under ultrasound guidance. Finally, one of the main methods of diagnosis in the third trimester is fetal heart monitoring. This technique involves following the heartbeat of the infant while in utero.

The heart rate of the infant is typically followed for twenty to thirty minutes. Any concerning dips in the heart rate may be indicative of a poor fetal state and a cause for increased monitoring or, in extreme cases, delivery of the infant.

Obstetricians have at their disposal a variety of treatment modalities. They are trained to turn manually fetuses that are in a breech (feet-first) position, a procedure called external cephalic version. In cases where the artificial induction of labor is desirable, the obstetrician may employ mechanical or hormonal means of cervical dilation, followed by infusions of a hormone called pitocin to stimulate contractions or the artificial rupture of the amniotic sac to promote natural contractions. When immediate delivery of the infant is needed and the chances of it emerging via the vaginal route are remote, then the obstetrician may perform a cesarean section. Common indications for cesarean section include fetal distress and lack of progress in labor.

Other treatments commonly used by obstetricians include the use of medications such as magnesium to relax the uterus in cases of premature labor and maternal steroid injections to induce fetal lung maturity when the fetus is premature but delivery is anticipated. When a woman experiences difficulty in the final stages of labor and the fetal head has descended almost to the vaginal opening, the obstetrician may employ forceps or vacuum devices to facilitate the delivery, particularly in cases of fetal distress. Obstetricians also treat the complications associated with childbirth, including postsurgical care after a cesarean section and repair of any lacerations of the vagina, cervix, or rectum after vaginal delivery.

PERSPECTIVE AND PROSPECTS

Obstetrics is central to medicine because it deals with the very process by which all humans come to exist. The health of the fetus and its mother in pregnancy is of primary concern to these doctors. The field of obstetrics has blossomed as a sophisticated specialty, more likely to be practiced by obstetricians, certified nurse midwives, and specially trained and certified nurse practitioners, rather than the general practitioners who used to provide this care.

Advances in medical technology have enabled more precise analysis and monitoring of the fetus inside the mother's uterus, and obstetrics has therefore become a complex specialty in its own right. Technology such as ultrasonography and fetal heart rate monitoring, among other techniques, allows the obstetrician to collect a much larger supply of fetal data than was available to the general practitioner of the 1960s. Increased data availability enables the obstetrician to monitor the pregnancy closely and to identify any problems earlier.

New advances in product development continue to improve the diagnostic ability of obstetricians. One example is the development of a test for fetal fibronection, which enables obstetricians to predict which patients are at low risk of premature delivery. This test involves a simple swab of the upper vagina. When negative, this test is highly reliable and allows the pregnant patient to leave the hospital and avoid prolonged and unnecessary hospitalization.

Advances in prenatal diagnosis and basic science have made it possible for parents to obtain information about their fetuses down to the molecular level. Through techniques such as amniocentesis and chorionic villus sampling (in which a small sample of placental cells is obtained early in pregnancy), genetic analysis has enabled the detection of chromosomal defects responsible for intellectual disabilities and single-gene defects responsible for inherited diseases (such as cystic fibrosis). Amniocentesis has also made it possible to detect biochemical changes that may be indicative of major structural defects in the fetus, as well as to assess the developmental maturity of organs such as the lungs.

Advances in medical practice have dramatically decreased the morbidity and mortality of premature birth. For instance, with the introduction and widespread use of maternal steroid injections, the severity of serious diseases of prematurity, such as respiratory distress syndrome, has been dramatically reduced. The development of drugs against HIV has prevented the transmission of the virus from mother to infant in many cases.

The medical science of obstetrics continues to advance. There is ongoing research into the physiology and basic science of preeclampsia and eclampsia, common and potentially dangerous diseases peculiar to pregnancy. Fetal surgery programs at academic centers open the possibility that serious birth defects may be correctable while the fetus is in utero. Although many controversies currently exist in the field of obstetrics, an increased push toward medical practice grounded in scientific evidence promises many exciting advances in the future. It is hoped that many of these advances will result in improved outcomes and quality of life for patients.

—David Wason Hollar, Jr., PhD;
updated by Anne Lynn S. Chang, MD

See also Amniocentesis; Assisted reproductive technologies; Birth defects; Breast-feeding; Breasts, female; Cesarean section; Childbirth; Childbirth complications; Chorionic villus sampling; Conception; Congenital disorders; Critical care; Down syndrome; Ectopic pregnancy; Embryology; Emergency medicine; Episiotomy; Family medicine; Fetal alcohol syndrome; Fetal surgery; Gamete intrafallopian transfer (GIFT); Genetic counseling; Genetic diseases; Genital disorders, female; Gestational diabetes; Gonorrhea; Growth; Gynecology; In vitro fertilization; Incontinence; Miscarriage; Multiple births; Neonatology; Ovaries; Pap test; Perinatology; Placenta; Postpartum depression; Preeclampsia and eclampsia; Pregnancy and gestation; Premature birth; Reproductive system; Rh factor; Rubella; Spina bifida; Stillbirth; Teratogens; Toxoplasmosis; Ultrasonography; Urology; Uterus; Women's health.

For Further Information:

American College of Obstetricians and Gynecologists. *American College of Obstetricians and Gynecologists*, 2013.

Cohen, Barbara J. *Memmler's The Human Body in Health and Disease*. 11th ed. Philadelphia: Wolters Kluwer Health/Lippincott Williams & Wilkins, 2009.

Doyle, Kathryn. "Midwife-Led Care Linked to Fewer Premature Births." Reuters Health Information. *MedlinePlus*, August 28, 2013.

Gabbe, Steven G., Jennifer R. Niebyl, and Joe Leigh Simpson, eds. *Obstetrics: Normal and Problem Pregnancies*. 6th ed. Philadelphia: Saunders, 2012.

Gaudin, Anthony J., and Kenneth C. Jones. *Human Anatomy and Physiology*. New York: Harcourt Brace Jovanovich, 1997.

Harkness, Gail, ed. *Medical-Surgical Nursing: Total Patient Care*. 10th ed. St. Louis, Mo.: Mosby, 1999.

Limmer, Daniel, et al. *Emergency Care*. 12th ed. Boston: Brady, 2012.

MedlinePlus. "Childbirth." *MedlinePlus*, August 13, 2013.

MedlinePlus. "Pregnancy." *MedlinePlus*, August 29, 2013.

Vorvick, Linda J. "Certified Nurse-Midwife." *MedlinePlus*, September 12, 2011.

Vorvick, Linda J. "Choosing the Right Health Care Provider for Pregnancy and Childbirth." *MedlinePlus*, August 23, 2012.

Wallace, Robert A., Gerald P. Sanders, and Robert J. Ferl. *Biology: The Science of Life*. 4th ed. New York: HarperCollins, 1996.

OCCUPATIONAL HEALTH

Category: Specialty

Anatomy or system affected: All

Specialties and related fields: Environmental health, epidemiology, internal medicine, preventive medicine, psychology, public health, pulmonary medicine, toxicology

Definition: The application of health care that focuses on injury and illness prevention and the treatment of injuries that can occur in the workplace or that result from a person's employment.

SCIENCE AND PROFESSION

The discovery that eighteenth-century chimney sweeps were prone to developing testicular cancer is often cited as the first example of an acknowledged occupational illness. In fact, physicians and other health care professionals had been aware for many centuries that certain jobs were linked to particular medical disorders: millers developed coughs, and hatmakers became mentally unbalanced. Textbooks urged physicians to consider a patient's occupation both in diagnosing and in treating illness. The emergence of occupational health as a distinct specialty within the medical professions is, however, a relatively recent phenomenon.

The Industrial Revolution brought with it not only the separation of one's home life from one's work life but also an increased risk of injury from factory machinery. Spinning jennies, power looms, mill wheels and belts, and early assembly line processes all carried the risk of accidental amputations, mangled limbs, and other permanently crippling injuries. Not surprisingly, much of the early emphasis of occupational health focused on safety. While company doctors treated the injured workers, engineers sought ways to reduce the job hazards.

By the twentieth century, several different but related specialties had evolved that focused on different aspects of occupational health. Industrial hygienists combine training in engineering and public health and attempt to improve safety in the workplace by providing education and training for workers and by redesigning the work area to eliminate hazards. Doctors of occupational medicine are employed by both government and industry to diagnose and to treat occupational illnesses and work-related disabilities. In addition to diagnosing and treating work-related injuries and illnesses, occupational health care providers may provide preemployment physical examinations, health screenings, and health promotion education and risk management programs based on occupational hazards and outcomes of trends of injuries or risks identified in the workplace. Public awareness of occupational health issues has led to the passage of legislation creating such agencies as the United States Occupational Safety and Health Administration (OSHA). All occupational health specialists in the United States must work within guidelines established by OSHA. There is a high cost to society from such disabilities as the black lung disease suffered by coal miners and the toxic or radioactive exposure experienced by workers ranging from hospital laboratory technicians to pipefitters and welders. As a result, occupational health has become an ever-expanding, complex, and important medical specialty.

DIAGNOSTIC AND TREATMENT TECHNIQUES

Because occupational health problems can affect any part of the human anatomy, their diagnostic and treatment techniques are drawn from all areas of medical science. If a worker is injured on the job or suffers from an easily recognizable problem, such as a repetitive motion disorder, diagnosis and treatment can be quite straightforward. In the case of repetitive motion, problems such as carpal tunnel syndrome, which is sometimes experienced by word processing operators, might be treated by advising patients to change their work posture, providing them with splints to align the wrists and hands properly, employing corrective surgery to alleviate pain, and redesigning the work site to prevent future problems. The treatment for many on-the-job injuries will also include an extensive course of physical and rehabilitative therapy to allow the worker to return to work eventually, either at the old job or at a new one.

Many occupational health problems, however, are not as readily diagnosed as carpal tunnel syndrome. The industrial hygienist and the doctor of occupational medicine often must rely on the expertise of epidemiologists and toxicologists to determine the substances to which occupational exposure may be responsible for a worker's ill health. In cases in which workers complain of vague symptoms such as chronic fatigue, nausea, or neuropathy (loss of nerve function), an accurate diagnosis can prove elusive. The medical literature contains numerous examples of occupational illnesses that mimicked other common disorders. For example, doctors misdiagnosed a cosmetologist as suffering from multiple sclerosis (a degenerative disease of the central nervous system) when she was actually experiencing nerve damage caused by many years of exposure to the chemical solvents used to apply and remove artificial fingernails. Because many occupational illnesses can take years or even decades to appear, in some cases an accurate diagnosis may never be achieved. Once a diagnosis is made, treatment for an occupational illness caused by exposure to chemicals, for example, can be as simple as assigning the worker to tasks that eliminate exposure or as technologically sophisticated as using dialysis or chemical chelation to remove toxins from a patient's blood.

PERSPECTIVE AND PROSPECTS

Occupational health is one of the most challenging specialties in modern medicine. Practitioners must combine skills and knowledge gleaned from a wide spectrum of related skills. The proliferation of technologically complex methods and materials in the workplace has resulted in occupational exposures and illnesses that were unknown until the twentieth century.

At the time that occupational health first emerged as a distinct concern in the medical community, industrial hygiene focused almost exclusively on safety in the workplace. If the factory could be designed so that workers did not risk losing a limb whenever they operated machinery, the hygienist could feel a sense of accomplishment.

Workplace safety remains a concern in occupational health, but obvious hazards such as poorly lit work areas or exposed moving parts on machines have been joined by a host of subtler threats to workers' well-being. Epidemiologists and toxicologists have linked on-the-job exposure to dust, heavy metals, radiation, solvents and other chemicals, and even blood-borne pathogens to a host of cancers, disabling diseases, reproductive problems, and other concerns. Yet, not only must the industrial hygienist and doctor of occupational medicine worry about protecting workers from these physical hazards, but the modern occupational health specialist must also be concerned with the long-term effects of repetitive motions, noise exposures, and even emotional stress. As the influence of workers' jobs on those workers' health and on the health of their families is recognized as a major factor in a family's overall well-being, the importance of the occupational health specialist becomes increasingly obvious within modern society. Occupational health specialists employed in government, industry, and private practice, each approaching the question of worker wellness from a slightly different perspective, all fill a vital and expanding niche in modern medical practice.

The regulatory agency OSHA was created by Congress in 1970 to ensure safe work environments free of hazards that could cause death or serious physical harm to employees. It has the authority to fine or charge employers who do not follow safety regulations. The National Institute of Occupational Safety and Health (NIOSH), also created in 1970, conducts research and advise OSHA on issues related to hazards in the workplace.

—*Nancy Farm Mannikko, PhD;*
updated by Sharon W. Stark, RN, APRN, DNSc

See also Allied health; Altitude sickness; Asbestos exposure; Asphyxiation; Biofeedback; Carcinogens; Cardiac rehabilitation; Carpal tunnel syndrome; Chronic obstructive pulmonary disease (COPD); Environmental diseases; Environmental health; Hearing loss; Interstitial pulmonary fibrosis (IPF); Law and medicine; Lead poisoning; Lung cancer; Lungs; Mesothelioma; Multiple chemical sensitivity syndrome; Nasopharyngeal disorders; Preventive medicine; Pulmonary diseases; Pulmonary medicine; Pulmonary medicine, pediatric; Radiation sickness; Skin disorders; Stress; Stress reduction; Tendon disorders; Tendon repair; Teratogens; Toxicology.

For Further Information:

Caplan, Robert D., et al. *Job Demands and Worker Health: Main Effects and Occupational Differences.* Ann Arbor: University of Michigan Press, 1980.

Cralley, Lester V., and Patrick R. Atkins, eds. *Industrial Environmental Health: The Worker and the Community.* 2d ed. New York: Academic Press, 1975.

Gatchel, Robert J., and Izabela Z. Schultz. *Handbook of Occupational Health and Wellness.* New York: Springer, 2012.

Guzik, Arlene. *Essentials for Occupational Health Nursing.* Malden: Wiley-Blackwell, 2013.

Koren, Herman. *Illustrated Dictionary and Resource Directory of Environmental and Occupational Health.* 2d ed. Boca Raton, Fla.: CRC Press, 2005.

Levy, Barry S., et al., eds. *Occupational Health: Recognizing and Preventing Disease and Injury.* 5th ed. Philadelphia: Lippincott Williams & Wilkins, 2006.

Morgan, Monroe T. *Environmental Health.* 3d ed. Belmont, Calif.: Thomson/Wadsworth, 2003.

Sadhra, Steven S., and Krishna G. Rampal, eds. *Occupational Health: Risk Assessment and Management.* Malden, Mass.: Blackwell Scientific, 1999.

Sellers, Christopher C. *Hazards of the Job: From Industrial Disease to Environmental Health Science.* Chapel Hill: University of North Carolina Press, 1999..

Smedley, Julia, et al., eds. *Oxford Handbook of Occupational Health.* 2d ed. Oxford: Oxford University Press, 2012.

World Health Organization. "Occupational Health." www.who.int/occupational_health/en.

ONCOLOGY

Category: Specialty

Anatomy or system affected: All

Specialties and related fields: Critical care, cytology, general surgery, genetics, immunology, pathology, pharmacology, radiology

Definition: The study of cancer—its causes, its possible spread throughout and destruction of the body, and its medical treatment.

Key terms:

cancer: a tumorous growth of abnormal cells that invade other tissues, choke off available resources, and eventually destroy major organs and the organism

carcinogen: a chemical or radiation mutagen that causes changes in genes, leading to the cancerous state in a cell

cellular transformation: the process in which a cell becomes cancerous, which begins with abnormal changes in gene expression and cell differentiation

hormone: a chemical messenger, usually composed of protein or steroid, that controls the gene expression within target cells and thereby affects cellular development

mutagen: a chemical or an ionizing radiation that causes a change in the nucleotide sequence of the deoxyribonucleic acid (DNA) of a gene, possibly affecting the gene's normal expression

mutation: a change in the nucleotide sequence of the DNA (i.e., the genetic information) of a gene

oncogene: a gene within the chromosomes of all the cells of an individual organism that triggers cancerous cellular transformation when it is expressed incorrectly

protein kinase: an enzyme type that often is encoded by oncogenes; this enzyme attaches phosphate molecules to certain amino acids on specifically targeted proteins

tumor: an uncontrollable growth of cells within a tissue region that may be benign (noninvasive) or malignant (invasive cancer)

virus: an obligate intracellular parasite, composed of nucleic acid protected by a protein capsid, which reproduces inside cells

SCIENCE AND PROFESSION

Oncology is the scientific study and treatment of cancers, tumors, and other abnormal tissue growths. This field is an important part of medical science because of the prevalence of cancer within the human population, particularly in the progressively older populations of Western societies, in which people enjoy life-prolonging medical advances. Cancer ranks second only to heart disease as a killer of people in Western nations. Its victims number in the hundreds of thousands each year.

The study of cancer and its various physiological manifestations involves an understanding of several diverse biological disciplines, including genetics, developmental biology, embryology, neurology, endocrinology, and general physiology. The oncologist must synthesize information from these scientific fields in diagnosing, monitoring, and treating the disease. The oncologist works closely with the cancer patient's other physicians, surgeons, laboratory technicians, radiation therapists and chemotherapists, and pharmacists in treating cancerous tumors.

A tumor is an abnormal growth of cells within a specific tissue or organ beyond that tissue or organ's normal developmental pattern. Tumors may be either benign or malignant. Benign tumors are noninvasive; benign tumor cells multiply more rapidly than normal cells within a single, localized region that grows larger and larger. A benign tumor does not spread to other body regions. A malignant tumor, however, is invasive; it grows rapidly and uncontrollably. A malignant tumor is a cancer that consists of grotesquely aberrant cells that can break off and be carried through the affected individual's bloodstream and/or lymphatic system to other body regions, where they lodge and overcrowd or outcompete normal body cells.

Cells function normally as a result of the hormonal control of thousands of protein-encoding genes located on twenty-three pairs of chromosomes. The order of nucleotide nitrogen bases on a gene's deoxyribonucleic acid (DNA) polynucleotide chain serves as the genetic code. A change in the nucleotide sequence of DNA is called a "mutation." A substance causing a mutation, which is called a "mutagen," may be ionizing radiation (e.g., ultraviolet light, X-rays, or gamma radiation) or a chemical. The DNA of a gene encodes ribonucleic acid (RNA), which encodes protein. Thus, an alteration in the nucleotide sequence of DNA, such as the replacement of a cytosine by an adenine nitrogen base, affects the messenger RNA nucleotide information sequence and, subsequently, the protein amino acid sequence. Proteins serve important structural, enzymatic, and hormonal roles within and between cells. A mutation within the DNA nucleotide sequence of a particular cellular gene affects the resulting protein encoded by that gene. Consequently, a variety of cellular functions are affected in sequence. In some cases, the cell is transformed into a cancerous state.

Mutagens that alter certain genes and then trigger cellular transformation into a cancerous state are called "carcinogens." Only certain mutagens are carcinogens. An altered gene encodes a protein that has an incorrect amino acid sequence, thereby altering the normal functioning of the protein. An aberrant protein enzymatically or hormonally alters the functioning of other molecules within the cell, thereby directing the cell into the cancerous state.

The precise genes and proteins that are affected in transformed cells have not been identified completely. It appears that certain cancer-causing genes called "oncogenes" are involved, as well as certain oncogene-encoded enzymes called "protein kinases." Protein kinases attach phosphate molecules to certain amino acids on certain cellular proteins, thereby altering the functioning of the proteins and triggering developmental changes within the cell. Certain viruses can also trigger these changes by activating oncogenes and protein kinases. The cell becomes cancerous as a result of these influences.

DIAGNOSTIC AND TREATMENT TECHNIQUES
Oncologists must confront a variety of cancers that affect many different tissues. Common cancers affecting women include breast, colon, lung, uterine, ovarian, and lymphatic cancers, while common cancers affecting men include prostate, lung, colon, bladder, and lymphatic cancers. Oncologists must identify and treat these tumors as rapidly and as efficiently as possible.

The successful treatment of cancer begins with its early detection. The classic seven warning signs of cancer are a sore that does not heal, a lump on the body, a persistent cough, difficulty in swallowing, unusual bleeding, a change in a wart or mole, and a change in

bladder or bowel movements. The presence of cancer in a patient can be identified by an oncologist by means of several techniques, including cytological (cellular) analysis, biopsy, and direct observation. Cytological techniques employ the microscopic examination of discarded cells from the suspected cancerous region. Biopsy involves the surgical removal of suspected cancerous tissue from an individual and the subsequent chemical and microscopic analysis of the removed tissue cells. Cancer cells are morphologically and chemically distinct from normal body cells.

Cancerous cell masses can be directly observed within the body by means of probing tubes that contain fiber-optic imaging devices and that can be inserted into body cavities. Such medical technology can visualize directly the trachea, bronchi, and larger bronchioles of the lungs; the esophagus and stomach; the colon and rectum; and the reproductive organ passageways, such as the vagina and cervix. Cancerous tumors also can be located via more elaborate techniques, such as computed tomography, magnetic resonance imaging, mammography, radioactive isotopes, X-rays, and ultrasound.

Computed tomography (CT) scanning is an enhanced X-ray survey of selected regions of the patient's body. The patient lies within the device, which rotates andX-rays around the patient, thereby generating a three-dimensional, computer-enhanced image of the tumor. Conventional X-rays can identify many tumors; however, computed tomography can penetrate deeper tissues with greater sensitivity. Mammography is an example of a regular X-ray treatment that utilizes low-energy X-rays beamed at a woman's breasts. Per the US Preventive Services Task Force (USPSTF), mammography is recommended every two years for women of age fifty or older with an average risk for breast cancer.

Similarly, the ingestion of certain radioactive isotopes such as iodine can be used to localize tumors. Certain elemental isotopes concentrate in specific body tissues and organs. The radioactive isotope concentrates in a particular tissue that is imaged, and any abnormal growths can be detected. Magnetic resonance imaging and ultrasound use magnetic fields and sound waves, respectively, to image interior tissues and detect abnormalities in tissue growth.

Once the presence of cancer and the type of cancer have been established, prompt treatment should ensue. The oncologist must determine the appropriate course of treatment. The three main types of cancer management include surgery, radiotherapy, and systemic therapy (including hormonal therapy, chemotherapy, and immunotherapy). Surgery and radiotherapy are commonly known as "local therapy" given they target only a specific local region that contains the cancer. In contrast, systemic therapy can target the whole body or "system." Depending on the specific cancer and its location, each management may be given alone or in combination with the other managements. Accessible cancers, such as skin cancers, may be removed surgically. Radiotherapy and systemic therapy are used because cancer cells are more sensitive to these treatments than are normal body cells, thus are more easily killed. Radiotherapy, or radiation therapy, involves the killing of the cancerous tumor through the use of a concentrated beam of ionizing radiation such as X-rays or gamma rays or an ingested or injected radioactive isotope (such as radioactive iodine for certain thyroid cancers) that will concentrate in the target cancerous tissue. Hormonal therapy uses medications that either decreases or increases the level of a specific hormone in the patient, depending on whether their cancer cells thrives in the presence or absence of it, respectively. Chemotherapy involves the internal administration of cytotoxic (cell-killing) chemicals to the patient; cancer cells are particularly susceptible to these chemicals. Immunotherapy utilizes a patient's own immune system to destroy cancer cells, and is an ongoing field of research.

There are possible side effects associated with any cancer treatment, mainly because normal cells are damaged as well as cancerous cells in the treatment. The side effect of surgery is mainly local to where the cancerous tissue is located, given surgery is done to cut out the cancer and the surrounding normal cells may be affected during the procedure. The side effect of radiotherapy is also mainly local given radiotherapy is aimed at the cancerous tissue at a specific region, so the surrounding normal cells is also affected. The side effect of systemic therapy may be "systemic," meaning affecting the whole body, given the therapy can travel throughout the body, with possible side effects including weakness, nausea, vomiting, diarrhea, loss of hair, and anemia.

In cases of certain tissue tumors and cancers, such as leukemia and bone cancer, tissue transplants from carefully matched individuals have been very effective in saving the lives of these cancer patients. The advent of molecular cloning and the use of tissue-specific viral gene vectors provide another avenue by which the oncologist will treat cancer in the future.

The oncologist's goals are to remove or kill the cancerous growth and to arrest its spread (metastasis) to other body tissues. The prevention of metastatic spreading is of critical importance, because the establishment of tumors in multiple body regions makes treatment much more difficult and patient death much more likely. Also, the oncologist must help the patient to cope psychologically with the disease and the possibility of dying. Sometimes, the cancer may have pro-

gressed enough that it cannot be safely eliminated. In such cases, some patients may die from the cancer or its complications, while other patients may die with the cancer from another cause. In all cases, it is paramount that the oncologists work with the patients to determine the optimal management approach that balance the quantity (or length) and the quality of life.

Oncological research and the treatment of neoplastic (cancerous) tissues represent formidable tasks for medical science. Cancer is the number-two killer of Americans, and tumors are responsible for countless other ailments and millions of dollars of medical expenses. The use of surgery, systemic agents (including hormonal therapy, chemotherapy, and immunotherapy), and radiotherapy to destroy or remove cancers has proven to be effective in saving thousands of lives.

PERSPECTIVE AND PROSPECTS
Cancer is an increasing problem in Western societies, where medical science is increasing longevity and where industry and business place extraordinary levels of stress upon individuals. Most theories of aging maintain that accumulated genetic mutations in somatic cells during organismal development contribute to the breakdown of body systems, particularly the immune system. Although cancer can occur at any age, its probability of occurrence accelerates with aging.

Cancer cells are present in the bodies of all humans. Out of approximately 1,000 trillion cells within the human body, it is inevitable that mistakes will occur frequently within the gene regulation mechanisms of certain cells. Humans and other life-forms are exposed continuously to radiation and carcinogenic chemicals of varying types. A critical gene within a critical cell eventually will mutate so that the cell follows a cancerous pathway.

A healthy person with a strong immune system, however, quickly will destroy these mutated, transformed cancers. Individuals having weakened immune systems as a result of stress, aging, illness, and so forth are more susceptible to cancer because the mutated cells have the opportunity to multiply and spread rapidly throughout the body before the person's immune system can respond. Many scientists are beginning to identify aging and stress as diseases, and cancer as a symptom of these diseases.

As the body ages, more and more mutations accumulate, thereby increasing the probability that cancer cells will develop, survive, and multiply. At the same time, the aging immune system cannot respond to abnormal cells and infections as rapidly. Consequently, cancer cells elude the victim's immune system and spread to other body regions.

Evidence is implicating stress as a contributor to incidences of disease, illness, cancer, aging, and premature death in the human population. Stress causes abnormal elevations in nerve and endocrine (hormonal) systems that affect a tremendous variety of cellular and tissue-specific processes within the human body. Elevated levels of hormones for prolonged periods of time can permanently alter the gene expression of certain body tissues, causing these tissues to develop abnormally. Stress is a major problem in fast-paced, technological societies, and it is probably no coincidence that heart disease and cancer are the two principal killers of people in such societies.

Additionally, certain cancers may be infectious. In 1910, Peyton Rous determined that the Rous sarcoma virus, which infects chickens, can trigger cancerous tumors. Subsequent investigators corroborated Rous's findings, and nearly two dozen viruses have been identified that are capable of initiating cellular transformation in animals. Such oncogenic viruses either carry an oncogene or activate oncogenes in their host cells when they infect cells. All viruses must infect cells in order to reproduce. Some viruses can insert their genetic material into the host cell's DNA, thereby affecting the expression of host-cell genes at the viral insertion point; this may be one method of oncogenic viral cellular transformation into cancer. Among the oncogenic viruses that infect humans are hepatitis B; the papillomavirus, which also causes warts; and the Epstein-Barr virus. The Epstein-Barr virus usually causes infectious mononucleosis. In a region of western central Africa, however, humans develop a deadly lymph node cancer called "Burkitt lymphoma" when exposed to the virus—a phenomenon that has baffled oncologists.

Genetic damage caused by chemicals and radiation to which humans are exposed to has a substantial effect upon the incidences of tumors and cancer. The link between ionizing radiation (e.g., ultraviolet light or gamma radiation) and cancer has been established. The links between various chemicals and cancer are more difficult to sustain, however, often leading to controversies over the banning of certain substances and the health risks associated with contact with such substances (e.g., saccharin or motor oil). The Ames test for chemical mutagens is a very effective assessment of whether a chemical is mutagenic; it was developed by biochemist Bruce Ames and his colleagues at the University of California, Berkeley, in the 1970s.

The problems posed by cancer are immense and will require decades of intense medical research. Advances in oncological research are saving many lives each year. Understanding gene regulation within living cells and developing more effective diagnostic techniques and cancer-inhibiting treatments are important steps in conquering this disease.

—*Kristin Hsieh, MD*

See also: Amputation; Anal cancer; Biopsy; Bladder cancer; Bladder removal; Blood testing; Bone cancer; Bone grafting; Bone marrow transplantation; Breast biopsy; Breast cancer; Breasts, female; Burkitt's lymphoma; Cancer; Carcinogens; Carcinoma; Cells; Cervical, ovarian, and uterine cancers; Chemotherapy; Colorectal cancer; Colorectal polyp removal; Cytology; Cytopathology; Dermatology; Dermatopathology; Endometrial biopsy; Gallbladder cancer; Gene therapy; Genital disorders, female; Genital disorders, male; Gynecology; Hematology; Histology; Hodgkin's disease; Hysterectomy; Imaging and radiology; Immunology; Immunopathology; Kaposi's sarcoma; Kidney cancer; Laboratory tests; Laryngectomy; Liver cancer; Lung cancer; Lymphadenopathy and lymphoma; Malignancy and metastasis; Mammography; Mastectomy and lumpectomy; Melanoma; Mouth and throat cancer; National Cancer Institute (NCI); Nephrectomy; Parathyroidectomy; Pathology; Plastic surgery; Proctology; Prostate cancer; Prostate gland removal; Radiation therapy; Sarcoma; Screening; Serology; Skin cancer; Skin lesion removal; Stomach, intestinal, and pancreatic cancers; Stress; Terminally ill: Extended care; Testicular cancer; Thyroidectomy; Tumor removal; Tumors.

For Further Information:

Alberts, Bruce, et al. *Molecular Biology of the Cell*. 5th ed., Garland, 2008.

Berger, Ann, et al., editors. *Principles and Practice of Palliative Care and Supportive Oncology*. 4th ed., Lippincott Williams & Wilkins, 2012.

Dark, Graham G. *Oncology at a Glance*. Wiley-Blackwell, 2013.

DeVita, Vincent T., et al., editors. *Cancer: Principles and Practice of Oncology*. Lippincott Williams & Wilkins, 2011.

Dollinger, Malin, et al. *Everyone's Guide to Cancer Therapy*. 5th ed., Andrews McMeel, 2008.

Eyre, Harmon J., Dianne Partie Lange, and Lois B. Morris. *Informed Decisions: The Complete Book of Cancer Diagnosis, Treatment, and Recovery*. 2nd ed., American Cancer Society, 2002.

Harnett, Paul, John Cartmill, and Paul Glare, editors. *Oncology: A Case-Based Manual*. Oxford UP, 1999.

Joesten, Melvin D., Mary E. Castellion, and John L. Hogg. *The World of Chemistry: Essentials*. 4th ed., Brooks Cole, 2007.

Jorde, Lynn B., et al. *Medical Genetics*. 3rd ed., Mosby/Elsevier, 2006.

OPHTHALMOLOGY

Category: Specialty

Anatomy or system affected: Eyes

Specialties and related fields: General surgery, optometry

Definition: The study of the anatomy and physiology of the eye, as well as treatment of vision problems or diseases, ranging from corrective lenses to delicate surgery.

Key terms:

ciliary body: a ring of tissue that surrounds the eye; the uveal portion of this tissue contains the ciliary muscle that adjusts the degree of curvature of the lens *cornea*: the transparent portion of the first layer of the eye

keratitis: a state of inflammation of the cornea that may cause partial or total opacity, leading to loss of vision

retina: the key sensory element located in the eye's inner layer

sclera: the opaque portion of the outer layer of the eye; commonly referred to as the "white of the eye"

SCIENCE AND PROFESSION

Among the sense organs and functions in the body, probably the most complex are the eye and the process of vision that it supports. Ophthalmologists study both the anatomy and the physiology of the eye in order to understand and treat common and rare eye diseases.

The principal anatomical element of vision is the eyeball, or eye globe, located in the right and left orbital openings of the skull. It is embedded in a complex system of tissues surrounded by ocular muscles that control its movement. Adjacent to the eye and also within the bony orbit is the lacrimal gland, which is responsible for keeping the eye moist. Only the front third of the globe is exposed. This exposed area is made up of the central transparent portion, the cornea, and a surrounding white portion, which is only part of the sclera, the main component mass of the globe itself. The sclera is a very dense collagenous (protein-rich) structure which has two large openings (the anterior and posterior scleral foramina) and a number of smaller apertures that allow for the passage of nerves and blood vessels into the eye. It is through the posterior scleral foramen that three main components sustaining the eye's functions pass: the optic nerve, the central retinal vein, and the central retinal artery.

The eye has three main layers, within which are further specialized divisions. The outer layer consists essentially of the transparent cornea and opaque sclera. The middle layer, called the uvea, is made up of the choroid, which is the outer coating of the layer; the ciliary body, which contains key eye muscles that affect the degree of curvature in the lens; and the iris, which, with the lens located immediately behind it, separates the anterior from the posterior chambers of the eye. This iris itself has two layers, the stroma and the epithelium. The latter is immediately recognizable to the layperson, since its cells are markedly pigmented, giving to each individual a characteristic eye color.

It is the opening in the iris, called the pupil, that allows the passage of light into the inner layer of the eye, which contains the key sensory portion of the organ, the retina. Before light reaches the inner layer and the retina, it passes through the lens of the eye, located immediately behind the iris (which it supports), and through the largest area of open space within the eye, the vitreous cavity. This posterior cavity, like the smaller forward cavity of the eye, is filled with a transparent hydrogel called aqueous humor, made up mainly of water (about 95 percent of its total mass) in a collagenous framework within which the main component is hyaluronic acid. The aqueous humor is very similar to plasma but lacks its protein concentration. The pupil of the eye serves a purpose similar to the diaphragm (or f-stop) on a camera; it opens wider (dilates) or closes (contracts) according to the intensity of light striking the eye. (This reaction explains why, after a few minutes in an apparently totally dark room, the eye adjusts at least in part to the lower intensity of light.) For purposes of examining the internal structures of the eye, ophthalmologists sometimes place special drops in the eye to cause the pupil to dilate.

The lens of the eye, which is held in place behind the pupil by zonular fibers, consists of onionlike lens fibers. These are the product of epithelial cells that "migrate" from their place of origin in a germinative zone next to the edges of the lens to the anterior portion of the concentric structure of the lens. The central or internal layers of lens fibers, called the embryonic nucleus, represent the earliest cell specialization processes before birth. By contrast, the anterior and posterior lens fibers are constantly renewed at the surface.

As light passes through the transparent lens fibers, the phenomenon of refraction results, in the simplest possible explanation, both from the concentric shape of the lens itself and from a differential in the index of refraction occurring in the "younger" outside layers of lens fibers and that of the "older" central layers; the latter have a greater index of refraction than the former. Another phenomenon that increases the refractive power of the lens occurs when the zonular fibers that hold it in place relax under the influence of the ciliary muscle, making the lens more spherical in shape. The resultant increase in refractive power is called accommodation.

It is the retina, located in the last layer of the eye, that receives the light images passing through the lens and transmits them to the brain via the optic nerve. Physiologists consider the nerve-related function of the retina to be comparable in many details with all other sensory phenomena in the body, including touch and smell. The retina itself consists of a very thin outer layer, called the retinal pigment epithelium, and an inner layer, the sensory retina. On the surface of the retina, one finds a layer of photoreceptor cells. Once affected by the absorption of light rays reaching them from the lens, these cells form synapses with an intermediate layer of modulator cells. A synaptic relationship may be defined as an excitatory functional contact between two nerve cells, causing either a chemical or an electrical response. The modulator cells-referred to as neurons when their function is to receive synaptic transmissions from receptor cells-in turn pass the "message" of light to ganglion cells forming the innermost cellular layer of the retina. These cells transmit electrical discharges through the optic nerve to the brain, where they are registered as images.

DIAGNOSTIC AND TREATMENT TECHNIQUES

Ophthalmologists must deal with a wide variety of problems affecting the eyes, ranging from injuries to the diagnosis of vision problems that can be corrected with eyeglasses or contact lenses. Perhaps the most important area of applied ophthalmology, however, involves treating the diseases that may occur in several areas of the eye.

An entire category of diseases can appear in the conjunctiva, the thin mucous membrane that lines the inner portion of the eyelid and covers the exterior of the sclera. Conjunctivitis refers to inflammatory conditions that may attack this membrane. Some conditions cause mere irritation, while others may lead to serious infections. In acute catarrhal, or mucopurulent, conjunctivitis, the conjunctival blood vessels become congested with mucus and then with pus, which accumulates on the margins of the eyelids. If untreated, this form of contagious, easily transmitted infection begins to affect the cornea, by causing prismatic distortions and eventually abrasions that may infect the cornea itself. A more serious form of conjunctivitis is referred to as purulent conjunctivitis; it is sometimes associated with complications of the sexually transmitted disease gonorrhea.

Inflammation of the cornea, or keratitis, usually comes from the passage of virulent organisms from the conjunctival sac, which, although exposed to the external environment, may not itself react to the presence of bacteria. There are many different types of keratitis. Individuals may be vulnerable to infections in the cornea as a result of abrasions (one of the main reasons that all ophthalmologists recommend against rubbing the eye to remove irritating particles) or because of abnormal conditions affecting the surface of the cornea. Among the latter, ophthalmologists list excessive dryness in the eye and the side effects of malnutrition leading to a condition called keratomalacia, which is common in underdeveloped countries.

Bacteria such as pneumococci (the primary contributor to pneumonia in the lungs) may cause infections that result in corneal ulceration, the most common form of keratitis. In such cases, the area affected by the ulceration may increase considerably as epithelial tissue in the cornea attaches itself to the ulcer. Corneal ulcers may be removed by surgery, although the effect of remaining scar tissue may reduce the level of vision.

The prospect of success in corneal transplant operations has not eliminated the need for ulcer removal surgery, since transplants depend on the availability of "fresh" cornea donors.

Another form of corneal infection, herpes zoster (a form of skin rash also called shingles), is caused by the virus that causes chickenpox; it is common among aged patients whose cellular immunity systems suffer from decreased efficiency. In herpes zoster ophthalmicus, an infection that begins in the eye spreads via the nasociliary branch of the ophthalmic nerves and appears as red blotches on the surface of the skin (usually near the eye orbits on the side of the infection only). Zoster attacks are accompanied by rather severe pain. Ophthalmologists use several key drugs to treat this condition, including Distalgesic, Fortral, or Pethidine. Resultant depression in the patient may be relieved by prescribing amitriptyline.

Inflammation and possible infection of other regions of the eye also occur. Some zones, such as the sclera, tend to be more resistant to invasion because of the density of their fibrous tissues. Superficial inflammation of the sclera, called episcleritis, may be transitory but recurrent. Ophthalmologists will prescribe the anti-inflammatory drug Tandearil in the form of drops. More serious but much less common is the condition called scleritis, which extends much deeper into the tissue of the sclera and may affect the cornea and the uveal tract in the middle layer of the eye. Treatment of scleritis involves the use of steroid therapy, such as the corticosteroid drug prednisolone, often supplemented with Tandearil.

Uveitis is a term that applies to inflammations that occur in the uveal tract. The name suggests that such complications are not limited to one or another of the parts of the uveal zone (the iris or the ciliary body): All are affected and must be treated simultaneously.

The most common vision problem is myopia (nearsightedness). While most people still choose to correct nearsightedness with contact lenses or glasses, laser techniques such as photorefractive keratectomy (PRK) and laser in situ keratomileusis (LASIK) have shown some promise in treating myopia. Early enthusiasm for radial keratotomy has waned because of erratic results.

The most widely known eye disorders are probably glaucoma and cataracts. Glaucoma occurs when pressure caused by an excessive amount of aqueous humor increases inside the eyeball, specifically in the area of the retina. Impairment of vision may be slight, occurring at first in the peripheral area of sight. Further deterioration, however, may lead to blindness in the eye. Regular treatment with drugs that reduce the production of aqueous humor is necessary in patients suffering from chronic glaucoma. Acute glaucoma, which is very sudden, represents only about one-tenth of recorded cases. It must be treated within less than a week to avert permanent blindness.

Cataracts occur when there is a loss of full transparency in the lens of the eye. Cataracts occurring among children are congenital or hereditary in origin. Cataract-like damage to the lens of the eye may also result from exposure to the sun's rays (which is especially dangerous when one views the sun without protection during eclipses), extreme heat, x-rays, or nuclear radiation. Most characteristically, however, cataracts (from slight to advanced stages) are associated with the aging process. Formerly, cataract surgery was difficult and the recovery period slow, so patients were advised to wait as long as possible to have cataracts removed. Improvements in surgical techniques and materials mean that patients no longer need to wait until their vision is severely impaired to have this surgery. Most cataract extractions are combined with implantation of an intraocular lens, so that patients do not need to wear specially prescribed contact lenses or thick glasses following surgery.

Ophthalmologists make use of laser surgery for an increasing number of eye disorders. Lasers are used to treat eye problems caused by diabetes and hypertension, to treat or prevent some types of glaucoma, and to treat other, rarer eye conditions. Macular degeneration, an important cause of decreased central vision, may be arrested by laser therapy, but the technique does not repair existing damage.

Microsurgical techniques have further revolutionized eye care and have led to more effective management of conditions (such as retinal detachment) that formerly caused blindness.

PERSPECTIVE AND PROSPECTS

Knowledge of the anatomy and physiology of the eye evolved gradually through history and then spectacularly in the latter half of the twentieth century. The most extraordinary advances in the later period were made in the field of eye surgery. For an understanding of how vision itself worked, it took centuries for surprisingly unscientific views to cede to the first modern theories and then, with the advance of anatomical dissection, the practical possibility of examining both normal and abnormal conditions of the organ in the laboratory.

An early but not widespread theory of how the eye sees, held into the Middle Ages, depended on what now seems to be the fantastic conception of *eidola*, or "skins." Those who believed this theory held (in part correctly) that something must be leaving the objects that one perceives through the eyes. This "something" was thought to be a skinlike picture that, once detached from the object in question, actually entered the eye (after an unexplainable physical contraction) through the pupil, the aperture in the eye that is visible in many different animals. Another widespread theory was a prescientific version not of light rays but of "visual rays" that were thought to leave the interior of the eye, returning to record the colors and shapes of objects encountered.

Historians generally agree that the tenth-century Arab scientist Ibn al-Haytham, known in the West as Alhazen, was the first to suggest that rays of light entered the eye to stimulate what he called the "sensorium." Although Alhazen's theory predated a scientific explanation of the nature of light itself, he based his views on the phenomenon of the lingering image on the eye's "sensorium" of strong light, particularly that of the sun, even after the eyelids closed out the object emitting light. He even proposed a basic theory of refraction of light inside the eye. According to his theory, the sensorium recorded images according to an exact formula that reconstituted both the "shape" and the "order" in which rays are received by the eye, depending on the angle at which they strike the spherical surface of the cornea. Alhazen even warned that although the eye's sensorium always duplicated this formula exactly, the observer (actually, the observer's brain) could be "tricked" by the reproduction of certain ray patterns that might resemble something that was not "real"-the optical illusion.

Alhazen's views would be examined and extended during the late sixteenth and mid-seventeenth centuries in the West by the scientific pioneers of optics, specifically the Italian Francesco Maurolico (died 1575) and the famous German astronomer Johannes Kepler (1571-1630). Kepler's best-known work complemented that of his Italian contemporary Galileo Galilei (1564-1642), marking a breakthrough in the science of optics and the use of lenses to make telescopes in order to explore the skies. Only in later generations, however, did the ophthalmological relevance of some of his findings concerning the measurement of light reflected off the objects "seen" by a lens become clear.

As specialized interest in the eye progressed along with the constant advance of science in the eighteenth and nineteenth centuries, exact observation of the internal features of the organ of vision hinged on both the historical progress of anatomical dissection and the development of instruments to look into the living eye. One of the principal figures who contributed to the latter field was the Swedish ophthalmologist Allvar Gullstrand (1862-1930). Gullstrand received the Nobel Prize in Physiology or Medicine in 1911 for his application of physical mathematics to the study of refraction of light in the eye. He gained additional worldwide attention for his research on astigmatism (the failure of rays to be focused by the lens accurately on a single central point) and for devising the so-called slit lamp for viewing the interior of the eye through the use of an intense beam of light.

In the area of eye surgery, a major landmark was achieved in the 1960s when the Spanish ophthalmologist Ramón Castroviejo began to develop a method for surgical transplant of fully transparent corneas from deceased donors to replace damaged corneas in eye patients.

—*Byron D. Cannon, PhD;*
updated by Rebecca Lovell Scott, PhD, PA-C

See also Aging: Extended care; Albinos; Astigmatism; Biophysics; Blindness; Blurred vision; Cataract surgery; Cataracts; Color blindness; Conjunctivitis; Corneal transplantation; Eye infections and disorders; Eye surgery; Eyes; Geriatrics and gerontology; Glaucoma; Keratitis; Laser use in surgery; Macular degeneration; Microscopy, slitlamp; Myopia; Optometry; Sense organs; Trachoma; Vision; Vision disorders.

For Further Information:
Buettner, Helmut, ed. *Mayo Clinic on Vision and Eye Health: Practical Answers on Glaucoma, Cataracts, Macular Degeneration, and Other Conditions.* Rochester, Minn.: Mayo Foundation for Medical Education and Research, 2002.
Kaufman, Paul L., and Albert Alm. *Adler's Physiology of the Eye: Clinical Application.* 10th ed. St. Louis, Mo.: Mosby, 2003.
Museum of Vision. "Healthy Eyes, Healthy Body." *Foundation of the American Academy of Ophthalmology,* 2011.
Newell, Frank W. *Ophthalmology.* 8th ed. St. Louis, Mo.: Mosby, 1996.
Palay, David A., and Jay H. Krachmer, eds. *Primary Care Ophthalmology.* 2d ed. Philadelphia: Mosby/Elsevier, 2006.
Remington, Lee Ann. *Clinical Anatomy of the Visual System.* New York: Butterworth-Heinemann/Elsevier, 2012.
Riordan-Eva, Paul, and John P. Whitcher. *Vaughan and Asbury's General Ophthalmology.* 17th ed. New York: Lange Medical Books/McGraw-Hill, 2007.
Ronchi, Vasco. *Optics: The Science of Vision.* Translated and revised by Edward Rosen. Rev. ed. New York: Dover, 1991.
Spalton, David J., Roger A. Hitchings, and Paul A. Hunter, eds. *Atlas of Clinical Ophthalmology.* 3d ed. Oxford: Mosby/Elsevier, 2013.
Sutton, Amy L., ed. *Eye Care Sourcebook: Basic Consumer Health Information About Eye Care and Eye Disorders.* 3d ed. Detroit, Mich.: Omnigraphics, 2008..
Yanoff, Myron, and Jay S. Duker, eds. *Ophthalmology.* 3d ed. St. Louis, Mo.: Mosby/Elsevier, 2009.

OPPORTUNISTIC INFECTIONS

Category: Disease/Disorder
Anatomy or system affected: All
Specialties and related fields: Bacteriology, immunology, internal medicine, microbiology, virology

Definition: Potentially life-threatening diseases occurring in people with weakened immune systems by microorganisms that typically do not cause severe illnesses in otherwise healthy people.

Key terms:
CD4: a type of white blood cell (specifically a type of T cell) that is affected by the human immunodeficiency virus (HIV)
encephalitis: inflammation of the brain
immunocompromised: the state of having a weakened immune system
lumbar puncture: also known as a spinal tap; a procedure that involves insertion of a needle into the lumbar spinal column
pneumonia: infection of the lung
prophylaxis: a method of preventing a disease

CAUSES AND SYMPTOMS

Opportunistic infections can be caused by various microorganisms, including viruses, bacteria, fungi, and protozoa. While they are capable of infecting healthy persons, the infection is either without symptoms or the disease is mild. It is in those who lack a healthy immune system that these organisms cause disastrous infections. Acquired immunodeficiency syndrome (AIDS), resulting from human immunodeficiency virus (HIV), is a widely known disease that weakens the immune system. There are other situations, however, in which the immune system can be compromised and become susceptible to opportunistic infections, such as being on chronic glucocorticoid therapy, taking immunosuppressive medications after organ transplantation, undergoing chemotherapy for cancer, being malnourished, or having a genetic predisposition.

Pneumocystis jirovecii is a fungus capable of causing life-threatening pneumonia in the immunocompromised. In those with HIV, the majority of *Pneumocystis* pneumonia develops in those with a very low CD4 cell count. Common symptoms include fever, cough, progressive difficulty breathing (especially with exertion), fatigue, chills, chest pain, and weight loss.

Toxoplasmosis is a ubiquitous infection caused by the intracellular protozoan parasite *Toxoplasma gondii*, which makes cats their hosts. Transmission is via ingestion of contaminated soil or undercooked meats that contain the protozoan oocyte. Infection in the healthy person is usually asymptomatic, but the organism can remain dormant in the host indefinitely. In immunocompromised patients such as those with very low CD4 cells, the organism reactivates and causes active infection. The central nervous system is the principal site of involvement. *T. gondii* can cause encephalitis and masses within the brain. Symptoms may include confusion, fever, seizures, and headache. *T. gondii* can also cause pneumonia accompanied by difficulty breathing, fever, and cough. Other organs such as the intestines, liver, bone marrow, bladder, spinal cord, testes, pancreas, eyes, heart, and liver can be infected, although this is less common. Pregnant women who have an active infection can pass it to their offspring, leading to infantile neurological deficits, intellectual disabilities, and eye infections.

Mycobacterium avium complex (MAC) usually causes widespread disease in the immunocompromised and is due to two nontuberculous species, *M. avium* or *M. intracellulare*. These organisms are ubiquitous in the environment such as in soil, with transmission typically through inhalation or ingestion. Acquisition of infection typically takes place when the CD4 count is extreme low. Symptoms include fever, night sweats, abdominal pain, diarrhea, weight loss, weakness, and wasting.

Cytomegalovirus (CMV) is a herpes virus found worldwide. It is commonly transmitted via feces, saliva, breast milk, urine, and genital secretions. In immunocompetent individuals, the virus remains latent and usually does not cause any severe disease. In the immunocompromised, however, the dormant virus reactivates and infection occurs. Symptoms generally include fever, night sweats, chills, fatigue, and muscle and joint aches. Other symptoms depend on the organ system affected: Gastrointestinal involvement typically produces symptoms of colitis (inflammation of the colon), such as abdominal pain and bloody diarrhea; lung involvement produces a pneumonitis (inflammation of the lung) with cough and difficulty breathing; and eye involvement (retinitis) can lead to blindness. The adrenal gland and the nervous system can also be affected.

Another opportunistic fungus associated with immunocompromised hosts is *Cryptococcus neoformans*, which causes cryptococcosis. The organism is normally found in soil contaminated with pigeon droppings, and transmission is usually through inhalation. The initial site of infection is in the lungs where it subsequently spreads to the brain, causing what is known as meningoencephalitis (inflammation of the brain and its surrounding protective tissues). Meningoencephalitis is the most common clinical syndrome in immunocompromised patients, developing slowly over one to two weeks with fever, malaise, headache, stiff neck, photophobia (aversion to bright lights), and vomiting. Disseminated rash is another symptom occurring in those with a weakened immune system.

There are many other causes of opportunistic infections, including the viruses *Varicella* and herpes simplex; the bacteria *Nocardia*, *Listeria*, and the less

> ### INFORMATION ON OPPORTUNISTIC INFECTIONS
> **Causes:** Viruses, bacteria, fungi, protozoa
> **Symptoms:** Fever, weakness, lack of appetite, rash, cough, difficulty breathing, confusion, headache, blurry vision, chest pain, weight loss, night sweats
> **Duration:** Acute to chronic
> **Treatments:** Antibiotics, antiviral medications, antifungal medications, antiprotozoan medications

common *Mycobacterium* species; the protozoans *Cryptosporidium*, *Isospora*, *Microsporidia*, and *Cyclospora*; and the fungi *Coccidioides*, *Candida*, *Histoplasma*, and *Aspergillus*. While all these organisms are capable of causing disease in the healthy, their impact on the immunocompromised is much more severe.

TREATMENT AND THERAPY

Treatment of specific infections is important in addressing the disease, but what is more important is to correct the underlying deficit, which is the weakened immune system. In some cases, this may not be possible, such as in those who require immunosuppressive therapy after organ transplantation or those undergoing chemotherapy for cancer. However, advances in HIV therapy with the implementation of highly active antiretroviral therapy (HAART) as well as institution of prophylaxis against opportunistic infections have dramatically decreased the mortality rate in these patients.

Treatment of *Pneumocystis* pneumonia requires the demonstration of organisms from respiratory specimens. Treatment is with anti-Pneumocystis regimens typically for twenty-one days, with or without corticosteroids. The latter is used in severe cases when oxygenation becomes problematic. Symptoms typically worsen after two to three days of therapy as a result of increased inflammation in response to dying microorganisms. After initial therapy, prophylactic therapy against future infections is instituted.

Treatment of toxoplasmosis requires antiprotozoan medications for at least six weeks. Prophylaxis against future infection is also required, which is the same medication as that used for *Pneumocystis* prophylaxis. In high-risk persons, as a means of prevention it is important to avoid undercooked meats and cat litter boxes. Treatment of MAC involves combination antibiotics for at least twelve months, with subsequent prophylaxis.

CMV infection is treated with antiviral agents. Immunoglobulin may be used to reduce the risk of infection in certain transplant recipients. If the eye is involved, then a pellet that releases an antiviral agent may be implanted into the eye with surgery. While not curative, this treatment may hinder the progression of the eye disease.

The treatment of cryptococcosis is with antifungal agents, initially with combination medications for what is known as induction therapy, followed by consolidation therapy, and finally maintenance therapy. Because the disease can also cause an increased pressure surrounding the brain, frequent lumbar punctures are sometimes required to relieve this pressure, or if severe enough, a drain placed in the spinal cord may be necessary to continuously relieve the pressure.

While prophylactic therapy is needed when the CD4 cell count is low, it may be withdrawn when the CD4 cells improve.

PERSPECTIVE AND PROSPECTS

Pneumocystis was originally identified by the Brazilian physician Carlos Chagas in 1909. Chagas was also the discoverer of the protozoan *Trypanosoma cruzi*, the organism that causes trypanosomiasis, or Chagas' disease. Initially, he mistakenly thought that the *Pneumocystis* cysts from the lungs of rats were part of the *Trypanosoma* life cycle. It was in 1910 that the Italian physician Antonio Carini discovered that these cysts were also present in lungs without *T. cruzi* infection, and he thus concluded that these cysts were a different type of infection. In 1912, Pierre and Marie Delanoe at the Pasteur Institute also confirmed that these cysts were present in the absence of *T. cruzi* infection, and they subsequently named these cystlike organisms *Pneumocystis carinii*, after Carini. Because these infections appeared to affect only rats, however, the organism did not become a major issue at that time.

It was not until the 1940s that *P. carinii* was found to cause pneumonia in human infants and adults. However, these patients all had some type of immune system compromise, such as malnutrition, genetic immune deficiency, or immunosuppressive medications. Before the AIDS epidemic, there were fewer than one hundred confirmed cases per year in the United States. It was later determined that there were several species of *Pneumocystis*, one of which causes disease in rats and another in humans. It was in 1999 when the term *P. jirovecii* (named after the Czech parasitologist Otto Jiroveci) was officially coined to refer to the disease occurring in humans. *P. carinii* still refers to the disease in rats. It was also in 1999 that *Pneumocystis* was recognized as a fungus rather than a protozoan, as previously thought.

In late 1980 to early 1981, the Centers for Disease Control and Prevention (CDC) described a cluster of five cases of *Pneumocystis* pneumonia in young gay men. Since then, the cases of *Pneumocystis* pneumonia

increased, as did the cases of Kaposi's sarcoma (rare HIV-related skin cancer). It was soon realized that both of these illnesses were not exclusive to gay males; they also affected heterosexuals, intravenous drug users, and others who were immunocompromised. In 1982, the CDC officially coined the term "acquired immunodeficiency syndrome," or AIDS, for this syndrome. In 1983, Luc Montagnier and his team from the Pasteur Institute isolated a virus that was thought to be the causative agent of AIDS, which they termed lymphadenopathy-associated virus. In 1984, Robert Gallo and his team from the United States also isolated a virus presumptive to cause

AIDS; they named it human T lymphotropic virus type III (HTLV-III). Later, it was recognized that both viruses were the same, and the virus was officially termed human immunodeficiency virus (HIV) in 1986.

In the beginning of the AIDS epidemic, death was certain. Treatment of HIV did not begin until 1986, when the Food and Drug Administration (FDA) approved the first antiviral agent, zidovudine, a nucleoside reverse transcriptase inhibitor (NRTI)-an agent that inhibits viral replication. However, single agent therapy did not prove to be as effective due to drug resistance. In 1995, newer classes of antiviral medications were approved-non-nucleoside reverse transcriptase inhibitor (NNRTI) and protease inhibitors (PI)-and began the trend of combination therapy of what is now known as highly active antiretroviral therapy (HAART). The thought behind combination therapy is that if the virus develops a genetic mutation and becomes resistant to one drug, the other two would still be active against it. However, while successful, even this powerful combination of drugs is still not adequate enough to achieve a complete cure since the virus is capable of remaining dormant inside cells and becoming resistant to medications even after a brief episode of missed doses.

In 2007, the FDA approved two new classes of antiretroviral therapy, integrase inhibitors and CCR5 co-receptor antagonists, which are used for advanced stages of HIV infection.

As of 2013, there are currently no available vaccines effective against HIV, although there are vaccines in various stages of clinical trial. A report in 2009 of a study of healthy volunteers with an experimental HIV vaccine in Thailand showed only a modest success rate (about 31 percent) in the prevention of HIV. In 2013, however, a two-year-old child was declared "functionally cured" of HIV infection, but further research will be conducted to determine if the results can be replicated in clinical trials involving other HIV-infected children.

While there are still obstacles to conquer in the fight against HIV, the battle against opportunistic infections has made great strides with the introduction of HAART and prophylactic medications.

—Andrew Ren, MD

See also Acquired immunodeficiency syndrome (AIDS); Bacterial infections; Fungal infections; Human immunodeficiency virus (HIV); Immune system; Immunodeficiency disorders; Immunology; Kaposi's sarcoma; Protozoan diseases; Terminally ill: Extended care; Viral infections.

For Further Information:
Fauci, Anthony, eds. *Harrison's Principles of Internal Medicine.* 17th ed. New York: McGraw-Hill, 2008.
Mandell, Gerald, et al., eds. *Mandell, Douglas, and Bennett's Principles and Practice of Infectious Diseases.* 7th ed. Philadelphia: Churchill Livingstone/Elsevier, 2010.
Mathis, Diane J., and Alexander Y. Rudensky, eds. *Immune Tolerance.* Cold Spring Harbor, N.Y.: Cold Spring Harbor Laboratory Press, 2013.
"Opportunistic Infections and Their Relationship to HIV/AIDS." *AIDS.gov,* November 16, 2011.
Rubin, Robert, eds. *Clinical Approach to Infection in the Compromised Host.* 4th ed. New York: Kluwer Academic, 2002.
St. Georgiev, Vassil. *Opportunistic Infections: Treatment and Prophylaxis.* Totowa, N.J.: Humana Press, 2003.
Stine, Gerald James. *AIDS Update 2013: An Annual Overview of Acquired Immune Deficiency Syndrome.* New York: McGraw-Hill, 2013.
"Surveillance for Norovirus Outbreaks." *Centers for Disease Control and Prevention,* January 28, 2013.
"Toddler 'Functionally Cured' of HIV Infection, NIH-Supported Investigators Report." *National Institutes of Health,* March 4, 2013.

OPTOGENETICS

Category: Cellular
Key terms:
biosensors: a device that monitors and transmits data about life processes
genetically encoded calcium indicators (GECIs): a key signal molecule measuring calcium involved with cell functions in the cardiorespiratory system, neurotransmission, and immune system function
opsins: light sensitive proteins found in retinal photoreceptor cells
optogenetics: neuroscience technique using genes for light-sensitive proteins that are introduced into specific types of cells in order to monitor and/or control cellular activity using light signals
photostimulation: the use of light to activate biological compounds in cells or tissues

OVERVIEW

Optogenetics includes techniques that control cells with light or use light to record cellular activity. Target cells can have enzymes or proteins that are light

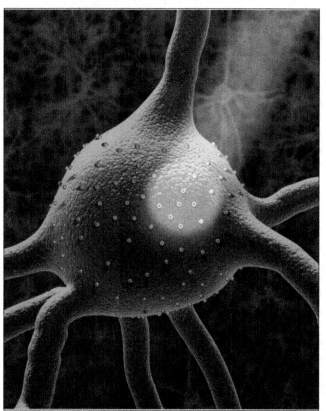

A neuron expressing the protein channelrhodopsin is activated by light. Image by McGovern Institute for Brain Research at MIT/statenews website/hayadan website, via Wikimedia Commons.

activated or genetically modified molecules are used in target cells to monitor or control cellular activity. The use of certain wavelengths of light in combination with various biosensors allows for real time recording of cellular biological activity in living organisms.

Genetically encoded biosensors include genetically encoded calcium indicators (GECIs), which fuse green fluorescent protein, peptides, and other compounds. These GECIs can be used to monitor neuronal activity and other cellular functions. Many light sensitive protein optogenetic activators have been formulated and are used in the optogenetic toolbox, including various opsins like channelrhodopsin (ChR) and archaerhodopsin (Arch).

INDICATIONS AND PROCEDURES

Optogenetics is an innovative technology enabling optical modulation of cells within a variety of living and functioning tissues. Natural or genetically engineered proteins containing a photoreceptive property are coupled to various biological functions. The optogenetic toolbox has been significantly expanded in the last several years, providing protein properties needed for therapeutic responses including optogenetic vision restoration. Optogenetics uses a combination of genetic manipulation and a scientific use of the behavior of light. Optogenetics can be used for studies of brain functioning and provides tools for the specific control of groups of neurons and other cells tagged with genetically encoded biosensors. Optical monitoring of cellular functioning is noninvasive, allows for spatial resolution, and can provide information about groups of cells acting together for an action.

Multiple neuronal circuits and billions of interconnected neurons exist in a functioning brain. Observing neuronal circuits and neuron activity concurrently while observing behavioral aspects enables a better understanding of brain functioning. Optogenetic photostimulation of presynaptic neurons creates a response in postsynaptic neurons that can be measured in high resolution both spatially and temporally. These types of studies can lead to a deeper understanding of the brain's functional organization. Brain anatomy is well known, but real time functionality needs more study. Optogenetic technology can be used to control or monitor the activity of genetically tagged neurons with light sensing technology. Cells are genetically engineered to contain a light-sensitive opsin. These molecules can be an ion channel, membrane pump, or a cellular protein receptor. Engineered cells are illuminated with light frequencies that stimulate the genetically targeted cells. The opsin-bound tagged cells undergo a structural change that can lead to pump activation, channel opening, cell depolarization or cell hyperpolarization. Neural silencing or activation can occur and this activity can be recorded. Since the introduction of optogenetics many opsin variations have been discovered or formulated. Neuronal activity can now be inhibited or stimulated on various timescales and/or intracellular pathways can be modulated on fast or slow timescales with a many different light wavelengths.

USES AND COMPLICATIONS

Optogenetics presents great potential to control tissue/cellular functioning with the delivery of light to target cells that have been genetically modified. Light-sensitive proteins (various opsins) are placed into cells, including neurons, which enables the optical control of cellular functioning. Human trials testing optogenetic techniques and procedures date from 2016. This technology has potential for medical treatments or therapies of retinitis pigmentosa, neurological problems such as Parkinson's disease, psychiatric disorders such as schizophrenia, autism, depression, addiction and vision restoration. Ethical issues include how, where, and on whom optogenetics is used—which diseases, which populations—and there are possibilities that these new techniques could be used for memory modification.

Reportedly, a blind person with retinitis pigmentosa has been treated with optogenetics and visual function was partially recovered, demonstrating the great potential of this technology. However, the associated research and clinical trials of this optogenetic technology has raised ethical and safety concerns. General guidelines on what risks gene therapy patients should receive have been developed, focusing on tissue changes, cancer risk, and gene transfer, among other concerns. Although these risks have been studied and are unlikely to occur, unknown impacts of the treatments can be a concern with novel therapies.

PERSPECTIVE AND PROSPECTS

Optogenetics has improved neuroscience by enabling in vivo real time analyses of the activity of neurons and behavior. Expanding optogenetic toolboxes and techniques enable the study and research of neuronal activity and the functioning of neuronal circuits in living tissue. Also, improvement of microscopic techniques has advanced the investigation of brain function, particularly by allowing whole-brain optical approaches. Optogenetics has enhanced understanding of the neural circuits and neural circuit dysfunction associated with mood disorders, Parkinson's disease, and addiction. Blindness from retinitis pigmentosa and potentially other diseases could be treated effectively treated with this new technology. Optogenetics probes the specific underlying roles of explicit neural circuit components. Study and research using optogenetic tools and procedures has the potential to contribute more significant knowledge and understanding of neural circuits involved with behavior and behavioral activity.

—*Richard P. Capriccioso, MD*

For Further Information:
Duebel, J., K. Marazova, and J. A. Sahel. "Optogenetics." *Current Opinion in Ophthalmology*, vol. 26, no. 3, 2015, pp. 226-32, doi.org/10.1097/ICU.0000000000000140. Discusses developments in optogenetics and potential applications in ophthalmology to restore vision in retinal diseases.

Harris, A. R., and F. Gilbert. "Restoring Vision Using Optogenetics Without Being Blind to the Risks." *Graefe's Archive for Clinical and Experimental Ophthalmology = Albrecht von Graefes Archiv fur klinische und experimentelle Ophthalmologie*, vol. 260, no. 1, 2022, pp. 41-45, doi.org/10.1007/s00417-021-05477-6. Discussion of optogenetics in general and in specific with retinitis pigmentosum, including ethical considerations.

Huang Cao, Zhen Fang, Denis Burdakov, and Zoltan Sarnyai. "Optogenetics: Potentials for Addiction Research." *Addiction Biology*, vol. 16, 2011, pp. 519-31, doi.org/10.1111/j.1369-1600.2011.00386.x. Using optogenetic techniques to better understand neurological pathways and the biological process of addiction.

Huang F., B. Tan, and H. Jiang. "Optogenetic Investigation of Neuropsychiatric Diseases." *International Journal of Neuroscience*, vol. 123, no. 1, Jan. 2013, pp. 7-16, doi:10.3109/00207454.2012.728651. PMID: 23002710. Using optogenetic techniques and procedures to better understand neurological pathways and the biological process of neuropsychiatric diseases.

Xu, X., T. Mee, and X. Jia. "New Era of Optogenetics: From the Central to Peripheral Nervous System." *Critical Reviews in Biochemistry and Molecular Biology*, vol. 55, no. 1, 2020, pp. 1-16, doi.org/10.1080/10409238.2020.1726279. Expansion of optogenetic techniques from the central nervous system to the peripheral nervous system.

OPTOMETRY

Category: Specialty
Anatomy or system affected: Eyes
Specialties and related fields: Ophthalmology
Definition: A field involving the provision of eye exams, the prescription of corrective lenses, and the diagnosis and treatment of eye disease, but not eye surgery.

Key terms:

clinical refraction: the determination of appropriate optical powers and related parameters to promote optimal visual acuity

contact lens: a small, shell-like glass or plastic lens that rests directly on the external surface of the eye to serve as a new anterior surface and thus correct refractive error as an alternative to spectacles, to protect the eye, or to serve as a prosthetic device promoting a more normal appearance of a disfigured eye

ophthalmologist: a physician who specializes in the comprehensive care of the eyes and the visual system; ophthalmologists provide visual, medical, and surgical eye care and diagnose general diseases of the body

prism: an optical element or component that, by virtue of two nonparallel plane faces, deviates the path of a beam of light

spectacles: a pair of ophthalmic lenses held together with a frame or mounting; also called glasses

SCIENCE AND PROFESSION

Optometry has been defined as "the art and science of vision care" by Monroe J. Hirsch and Ralph E. Wick in *The Optometric Profession* (1968). The American Optometric Association has stated that "Doctors of Optometry are independent primary health care providers who specialize in the examination, diagnosis, treatment and management of diseases and disorders of the visual system." Optometrists examine eyes and the visual system. They prescribe spectacles and contact lenses, optimize binocularity (the manner in which the two eyes work together), and improve visual function. Optometrists are trained to detect, treat, and manage disorders and diseases of the eyes and related structures.

Optometry is one of the youngest of the learned professions, which were originally restricted to law, medicine, and theology. Following the earlier lead of organized medicine, optometrists successfully organized and passed the first optometry practice law in 1901. Optometrists today complete a university education and then spend four additional years in a specialized school or college of optometry to receive the OD (doctor of optometry) degree. Many optometrists spend an additional year training in special-interest residency programs after graduation. Optometrists practice independently in private offices, although increasing numbers of optometrists also work in groups, the military, public health agencies, and university and hospital environments.

Distinctions are made between optometrists, ophthalmologists, and opticians. Ophthalmologists are physicians who diagnose and treat eye diseases and who perform eye surgery. They complete a premedical university education, four years of medical school, one year of internship, and three or more years of specialized training in ophthalmology. Many ophthalmologists also complete one or more years of fellowship subspecialty training. Opticians are technicians trained in the manufacture and dispensing of optical aids.

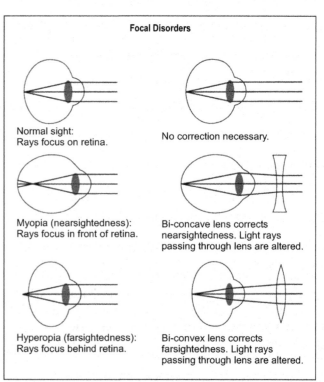

Focal Disorders

Normal sight: Rays focus on retina.

No correction necessary.

Myopia (nearsightedness): Rays focus in front of retina.

Bi-concave lens corrects nearsightedness. Light rays passing through lens are altered.

Hyperopia (farsightedness): Rays focus behind retina.

Bi-convex lens corrects farsightedness. Light rays passing through lens are altered.

©EBSCO

A device called a phoropter, which is used to evaluate a patient's vision. Photo via Wikimedia Commons. [Public domain.]

DIAGNOSTIC AND TREATMENT TECHNIQUES

A portion of the eye examination performed by optometrists is called clinical refraction. To the physicist, refraction is the bending of light as it passes through an interface separating two differing media (such as water and air). Refraction, however, has also come to mean the clinical evaluation of the human visual system. Clinical refraction generally results in a spectacle prescription; such a prescription will contain the spherical optical power, and the astigmatic optical power and its axis when appropriate, that are necessary to provide optimally focused light on the retina for each eye.

A clinical refraction also includes an assessment of binocularity, which is the way in which both eyes are used simultaneously such that each retinal image contributes to the final visual percept. (The retina is the inner nerve layer of the eye upon which the optics of the eye focuses the image of the outside world.) Much effort is made, during a refraction, to attain maximum visual comfort by optimizing binocularity. Occasionally, it is necessary to utilize a prismatic element in the spectacle prescription as well as optical powers to this

end. In other cases, the clinician may suggest a course of eye exercises to assist the patient in achieving improved binocularity without, or in supplement to, spectacles. Some patients may be found to suffer from severe binocular dysfunction and are referred for surgical consideration.

Near vision is tested during a refraction, especially for those people more than forty years of age who might require optical assistance for near work. The cornea is the clear, circular "window" in the front of the eye through which the colored iris is seen. Behind the iris is a crystalline lens. The cornea and the lens act together to focus light on the retina. The cornea provides most of the refractive power of the eye, and the lens serves to fine-tune the image in a process called accommodation. As one ages, however, the ability to accommodate deteriorates. Some form of near correction, either with two pairs of spectacles or with some form of bifocal, is then necessary. Only minimal optical power is needed at first, but as the aging process continues, the need for stronger near correction increases.

For a given patient, an analysis of binocularity, the determination of near vision requirements, and a consideration of additional occupational or avocational tasks (such as sports) make up his or her "functional vision." For some patients, the data gleaned in a standard refraction will provide the optometrist with all the information necessary to recommend comfortable visual correction for all tasks. For other patients, some additional thought and consideration may be required. For example, a very tall, fifty-year-old patient may not require as strong a reading correction as another shorter individual of the same age because the former has longer arms and is more used to holding reading material at a greater distance than the latter. In addition, providing visual care to patients using computers and video display terminals has become a rapidly growing subarea in functional vision.

No clinical refraction would be complete without an assessment of ocular health. This examination consists of observation of the eyes and related structures, as well as a testing of function. Good visual acuity, in and of itself, is fairly good evidence that the function of the eye is normal. Some ocular diseases, however, may occur and-at least initially-leave central vision intact. The structures of the eye are inspected with the assistance of instruments such as a clinical biomicroscope, or slitlamp microscope, to examine the outer ocular structures, and an ophthalmoscope, which allows inspection of the structures of the inner eye. Pupillary dilation with pharmaceutical agents in the form of drops allows inspection of the peripheral retina. The pressure in the eye should be tested, a process called tonometry, and the field of vision evaluated. Many optometrists also bear the responsibility for the treatment of certain ocular diseases.

As is true for all professionals, when the management of a specific problem is beyond one doctor's training, interest, or licensure, referral is made to another, more appropriate, doctor. For example, a patient with an age-related cataract (clouding of the crystalline lens) may be referred to an ophthalmologist for surgery, and an optometrist who suspects multiple sclerosis will refer the patient to a neurologist.

There are subspecialty areas in optometry, such as the prescription of appropriate visual aids for patients with particularly poor vision, known as low vision rehabilitation. Other subspecialty areas include industrial vision, developmental vision and vision therapy, and ocular disease. Contact lens care has become a large subspecialty in optometry. In fitting contact lenses, the curvature of the cornea, the quality of the patient's tears, and the health of the ocular surface and associated structures (such as eyelids) are all important considerations. Contact lenses are usually intended as devices to provide vision as an alternative to spectacles (although there are occasions when contact lenses may be used as prosthetics, to cover a damaged eye, or as

therapy for a specific disease). The clinician must modify the original refractive findings to adjust for the placement of the lens because it will rest directly on the ocular surface instead of being attached to a frame half an inch from the eye. The contact lens must be designed so that the surface of the eye is not compromised by its presence. The proper contact lens care system is vitally important for the initial and continued success of a contact lens fitting. Continuing professional supervision is essential in maintaining optimal vision and safe contact lens wear.

PERSPECTIVE AND PROSPECTS

Evidence suggests that spectacles were first used to assist human vision in Europe at about the end of the thirteenth century. Organizations of spectacle makers were formed in Europe in the fourteenth and fifteenth centuries. These guilds policed the quality of spectacles and the working conditions under which their manufacture occurred. Spectacles were sold to the public in stores and by peddlers. Individuals self-selected the lens or lenses that seemed most appropriate to them for their visual tasks. Retailers selling spectacles eventually began to assist their clientele in making an informed selection. Over time, spectacle vendors evolved into opticians. Some "refracting" opticians tested vision to provide what they believed to be the most appropriate correcting lenses for a particular person. Physicians at that time did not recommend or examine the eyes for spectacles, preferring the use of medication for eye difficulties.

The impetus for optometry's modern development and legal recognition in the United States began with a confrontation between optometry and ophthalmology. A New York refracting optician named Charles Prentice referred a patient to Henry D. Noyes, an ophthalmologist, in 1892. Noyes wrote Prentice a thank-you note for the referral but suggested that Prentice should not have charged a fee (of three dollars) for his services-such being the right reserved to professionals such as physicians. Prentice responded, defending his practice of charging for his services. Noyes sent Prentice's letters to another ophthalmologist, D. B. St. John Roosa, who expressed his opinion that Prentice was in violation of the law by charging a fee for his services. By 1895, Roosa had announced that he would seek legislation to prevent opticians from practicing, and Prentice responded by organizing the Optical Society of the State of New York. This society eventually introduced a bill to the New York legislature to regulate the "practice of optometry." Optometry was defined as refraction, dispensing (that is, selling) spectacles, and related services.

This bill was quite controversial and never came to a vote. Later, however, another New York optometrist, Andrew J. Cross, while visiting Minnesota to teach a program in optics, scoffed at the notion that Minnesota could pass an optometry practice act before New York. Thus inspired, the Minnesotans passed their law, which included a regulatory board, in 1901. Arguing that optometry was separate and distinct from medicine, optometrists proceeded to obtain practice acts in all the states over the next twenty-three years.

Optometrists sought to be professionals rather than businesspeople and developed an agenda that included the formation of organizations: both the American Optometric Association (AOA) and the American Academy of Optometry were established early in the twentieth century. Efforts were made both to reduce the commercial aspects of practice and to improve educational standards. A code of ethics and stringent rules of conduct were adopted by the AOA.

The first American optometric schools were extensions of apprenticeships and offered short courses (one to two weeks) in refraction. Eventually, private schools were established to train both physicians and nonphysicians. Academic programs developed from these independent schools, such as the Southern California College of Optometry and the Illinois College of Optometry. A milestone two-year optometry course began at Columbia University in New York in 1910; Cross and Prentice were instrumental in preparing the curriculum. Ohio State University began a four-year program in 1915, and the University of California, Berkeley, established an optometry course in 1923. By the late twentieth century, seventeen schools and colleges of optometry trained optometrists in the United States; many of the university programs also provided academic postgraduate studies. Similar programs were created in England, Australia, Canada, Europe, Asia, Africa, and South America.

Optometrist and lawyer John G. Classe credits the major change in the way optometry developed in the latter half of the twentieth century to contact lenses and modern tonometry. Prior to technical improvements in contact lenses and tonometry, the practice of optometry was limited and nonmedical. The commercial success of contact lenses brought about research in physiology, which in turn expanded biological knowledge and improved contact lenses. The ability to use a tonometer without drops to test for increased intraocular pressure (a condition called glaucoma) gave optometrists additional responsibility in ocular disease management. Unfortunately, the subsequent changes in practice placed optometry in even greater direct conflict with ophthalmology.

In a meeting held in January 1968, many of the leaders of the schools and colleges of optometry, the chair of the AOA's Council on Optometric Education, and the editor of the *Journal of the American Optometric Association* unofficially discussed the future of the profession. Court decisions had ruled that optometrists had the legal responsibility to detect, diagnose, and refer ocular disease, and many optometrists were frustrated by the limited scope of their practice. This group believed that optometry should discard its original concept of being a drugless profession dedicated solely to ocular function. They argued that optometric education should be expanded in the fields of ocular pharmacology, anatomy, physiology, and pathology so that optometrists would become primary entry points into the health care system for patients. Finally, it was concluded that the state laws that govern the practice of optometry should be updated to allow the optometrist to practice what he or she was taught, including the appropriate use of pharmaceutical agents.

In 1971, Rhode Island became the first state to amend its optometry law to permit the use of diagnostic pharmaceutical drugs. Despite continued opposition from ophthalmology, all fifty states followed over the next twenty years. In 1976, West Virginia became the first state to permit the use of therapeutic drugs, and thirty-two states had enacted similar laws by 1993.

—Barry A. Weissman, OD, PhD

See also Aging: Extended care; Astigmatism; Biophysics; Blurred vision; Cataracts; Eye infections and disorders; Eyes; Geriatrics and gerontology; Glaucoma; Myopia; Ophthalmology; Optometry, pediatric; Sense organs; Strabismus; Trachoma; Vision; Vision disorders.

For Further Information:
Buettner, Helmut, ed. *Mayo Clinic on Vision and Eye Health: Practical Answers on Glaucoma, Cataracts, Macular Degeneration, and Other Conditions.* Rochester, Minn.: Mayo Foundation for Medical Education and Research, 2002.
Classe, John G. "Optometry: A Legal History." *Journal of the American Optometric Association* 59, no. 8 (1988): 641-50.
Eger, Milton J. "Now It Can and Should Be Told." *Journal of the American Optometric Association* 60, no. 4 (1989): 323-26.
Gregg, James R. *History of the American Academy of Optometry.* Washington, DC: American Academy of Optometry, 1987.
Millodot, Michel. *Dictionary of Optometry and Visual Science.* 7th ed. New York: Butterworth-Heinemann/Elsevier, 2009.
Museum of Vision. "Healthy Eyes, Healthy Body." *Foundation of the American Academy of Ophthalmology,* 2011.
Remington, Lee Ann. *Clinical Anatomy of the Visual System.* New York: Butterworth-Heinemann/Elsevier, 2012.
Sutton, Amy L., ed. *Eye Care Sourcebook: Basic Consumer Health Information About Eye Care and Eye Disorders.* 3d ed. Detroit, Mich.: Omnigraphics, 2008.
"What Is a Doctor of Optometry?" *American Optometric Association,* June 2012.

ORAL AND MAXILLOFACIAL SURGERY

Category: Specialty
Anatomy or system affected: Gums, head, mouth, teeth
Specialties and related fields: Anesthesiology, dentistry, oncology, otorhinolaryngology, plastic surgery
Definition: A specialty of dentistry that deals with the diagnosis and management of diseases or conditions of the mouth, teeth, jaws, and face.

Key terms:

mandible: the lower bone of the jaw

maxilla: two fused bones that make up the upper jaw and the mid-portion of the facial skeleton

nitrous oxide: a chemical compound that at room temperature forms a colorless gas, also known as laughing gas, used to produce anesthesia and analgesia during surgery

obstructive sleep apnea: periods of interrupted breathing during sleep caused by airway obstruction in the nose or throat

orthgnathic surgery: surgical procedures of the jaws to correct structural deformity caused by congenital or growth defects

temporomandibular joint: the hinged joint that attaches the head of the mandible to the skull

SCIENCE AND PROFESSION

The specialist in oral and maxillofacial surgery deals with the anatomical region of the head that includes the oral cavity and the hard and soft tissues that compose that part of the facial skeleton formed by the mandible and the maxilla. The mandible is the bone that forms the lower jaw, and the maxilla is the fusion of the two bones that form the middle part of the face, or the upper jaw.

The maxilla forms the roof of the mouth, the lateral walls and floor of the nose, and the floor of the eye cavities. The maxilla contains the maxillary sinuses and holds the upper teeth. The mandible holds the lower teeth and attaches to the temporal bone of the skull at the temporomandibular joint (TMJ).

The diseases and conditions treated by oral and maxillofacial surgeons are numerous and diverse. They may include extraction of impacted teeth, dental implants, benign and malignant lesions of the oral cavity, TMJ disorders, management of facial pain syndromes, facial fractures, obstructive sleep apnea, and surgical correction of congenital deformities. Oral and maxillofacial surgeons will treat infections of the jaws, oral cavities, and salivary glands and may perform facial cosmetic procedures.

Most oral and maxillofacial surgeons begin their training after dental school. Increasingly, medical doctors are being integrated into the specialty through additional dentistry training and subsequent entry into an oral and maxillofacial training program. The oral and maxillofacial surgical residency includes general surgery, plastic surgery, medicine, and anesthesia. A four-year residency program grants a degree that makes these surgeons board eligible in oral and maxillofacial surgery. Some American oral and maxillofacial surgeons complete a six-year residency program that grants a medical degree as well. Graduates of the residency program may elect to pursue additional fellowship training in head and neck cancer, cosmetic facial surgery, pediatric maxillofacial surgery, or maxillofacial trauma.

Oral and maxillofacial surgery is recognized as a dental specialty. The American Board of Oral and Maxillofacial Surgery is responsible for certifying oral and maxillofacial surgeons in the United States. The board is recognized and approved by the Council on Dental Education of the American Dental Association. In order to become board certified, a typical applicant will have completed four years of undergraduate studies and four years of dental school, followed by an approved training program. Candidates must present letters of recommendation from board-certified oral and maxillofacial surgeons and then pass a written and oral examination. After completion of these qualifications, applicants are granted the title of diplomat of the American Board of Oral and Maxillofacial Surgery. The board requires that its diplomats be recertified every ten years.

DIAGNOSTIC AND TREATMENT TECHNIQUES

Oral and maxillofacial surgeons take careful and detailed histories of present and past medical conditions, including family history, medication history, and allergy history. Examination of the oral and maxillofacial area includes a complete examination of the oral cavity and the use of radiologic techniques to visualize the soft tissues and bone structure of the jaw and the mid-face. Many oral and maxillofacial surgeons perform conventional radiographs (x-rays) and panoramic radiographs of the upper and lower jaw in their office. The diagnosis of oral and maxillofacial conditions is further aided by the use of diagnostic images from computed tomography (CT) scans and magnetic resonance imaging (MRI).

Oral and maxillofacial surgeons perform surgical procedures both at the hospital and in the office. Because many biopsies and dental procedures are done in the office, these specialists must be proficient in administering oral sedation, local anesthetics, nitrous oxide, intravenous sedation, and general anesthesia. Patients who come to oral and maxillofacial surgeons come from all age groups. They may have multiple medical conditions and require a broad range of medical and surgical care. The oral and maxillofacial surgeon must be part medical doctor, part general surgeon, and part dentist.

Some of the more common treatment techniques in oral and maxillofacial surgery include dental procedures for removal of impacted teeth or teeth that cannot be restored. These surgeons may work along with restorative dentists to reconstruct bone for placement of dental implants. In the event of facial trauma, oral and maxillofacial surgeons may be called upon to repair routine and complex fractures, repair lacerations, and reconstruct damaged nerves and blood vessels. Oral and maxillofacial surgeons may diagnose and treat benign cysts and growths in the oral cavity, including cysts that form in the salivary glands. Head and neck cancer diagnosis and treatment may include malignant lesions of the jaws, lips, or oral cavity.

A major component of the specialty involves reconstructive and orthognathic surgery to correct congenital deformities such as facial asymmetry, bite deformities, and cleft lip or palate. Obstructive sleep apnea is being increasingly recognized; severe cases may be life threatening and may be an indication for surgical intervention by an oral and maxillofacial specialist. Maxillomandibular advancement surgery may be performed in selected cases. The procedure involves moving the upper and lower jaws forward. The bones are surgically separated and advanced to increase the opening of the airway. The procedure is done in the hospital under general anesthesia and may take three to four hours to complete. In cases of severe obstructive sleep apnea that do not respond to conservative treatments, this type of orthognatic surgery may be the treatment of choice.

Chronic facial pain disorders that oral and maxillofacial surgeons deal with include TMJ disease and neurogenic pain syndromes. TMJ disorders may cause pain in the ear, headache, or pain when moving the jaw. The oral and maxillofacial surgeon may treat this condition conservatively with medication or splint therapy. In more severe cases, open or arthroscopic joint surgery may be indicated. The most common craniofacial pain syndrome is trigeminal neuralgia. If medications are not effective, then the oral and maxillofacial surgeon may treat this condition with local nerve block, surgical destruction of the nerve, or microvascular decompression of the trigeminal nerve root.

Because of their surgical training, their familiarity with the soft tissue and structural anatomy of the face, and their experience with office-based surgery and anesthesia, oral maxillofacial surgeons are uniquely qualified and positioned to take advantage of recent developments in facial cosmetic surgery. Facial cosmetic surgery may be indicated for birth defects, deformity resulting from injury, or aging process reversal. Facial plastic surgery that may be performed by the oral and maxillofacial surgeon includes cheekbone implants, chin augmentation, facial and neck liposuction, lip enhancement, and face lift surgery. These specialists may also use the surgical laser to remove outer layers of damaged skin, inject collagen to fill wrinkles, and use Botox injections to reduce muscle activity that causes wrinkles.

PERSPECTIVE AND PROSPECTS

Hesy-Re, an Egyptian scribe who lived around 2600 BCE, is credited as the first dentist. The Greek physician Hippocrates, who lived between 500 and 300 BCE, described treatments of diseased teeth and gums, including the use of forceps to extract teeth and wires to stabilize fractured jaws. During the early part of the Middle Ages, most oral surgery was performed by monks; after the popes forbade monks from practicing medicine, barbers became responsible for extracting teeth and draining dental abscesses. In 1723, the French surgeon Pierre Fauchard described the practice of dentistry, including oral anatomy and operative and restorative procedures; he is credited with being the founder of modern dentistry. The American Revolutionary War figure Paul Revere advertised himself as a dentist, in addition to being a fine silversmith. The first dental school was established in 1840 as the Baltimore College of Dental Surgery, and in 1867 the Harvard Dental School became the first university-affiliated dental school. In 1844, the Connecticut dentist Horace Wells performed the first dental extractions done using nitrous oxide as an anesthetic.

Simon P. Hullihen of Wheeling, West Virginia, both a medical doctor and a dentist, is considered to be the founder of oral surgery. He specialized in operations on defects of the mouth and head and performed hundreds of operations for cleft lip, cleft palate, and other abnormalities of the mouth and jaw.

Another contributing factor to the development of the specialty of oral and maxillofacial surgery was the devastating injuries suffered by soldiers during the great wars of the twentieth century. It became clear to battlefield surgeons that dentists were needed to help align dental occlusion in facial injuries and fractured jaws. Dentists became valued members of the surgical team, and today dentistry is still the field from which most oral and maxillofacial surgeons come.

In 1945, a committee was authorized to establish an American Board of Oral Surgery (ABOS). In 1947, the ABOS was approved by the American Dental Association. The name of the board was changed to the American Board of Oral and Maxillofacial Surgery in 1978 to reflect the complete scope of the specialty.

Advancements in cosmetic and reconstructive surgery put the oral and maxillofacial surgery specialist at the cutting edge of medical innovation. An example is the French oral and maxillofacial surgeon Bernard Devauchelle, who along with his colleagues at the University Hospital Center of Amiens, France, performed the first human face transplant. In November 2005, Devauchelle and his team transplanted the central and lower face of a thirty-eight-year-old woman whose nose, lips, and chin had been lost as a result of a dog bite. Their success was reported around the world and hailed as a milestone in surgical history. Today, the specialty of oral maxillofacial surgery is a dynamic field that attracts both medical and dental school graduates. Although the residency program is long and arduous, the rewards of the specialty are great.

—Chris Iliades, MD

See also Anesthesia; Anesthesiology; Birth defects; Cleft lip and palate; Cleft lip and palate repair; Dental diseases; Dentistry; Dentistry, pediatric; Facial transplantation; Fracture repair; Head and neck disorders; Jaw wiring; Orthodontics; Periodontal surgery; Periodontitis; Plastic surgery; Root canal treatment; Surgery, general; Teeth; Temporomandibular joint (TMJ) syndrome; Tooth extraction; Toothache; Wisdom teeth.

For Further Information:
Coulthard, Paul, et al. *Oral and Maxillofacial Surgery, Radiology, Pathology, and Oral Medicine*. 3d ed. London: Elsevier, 2013.
Ellis, Edward, et al. *Contemporary Oral and Maxillofacial Surgery*. 6th ed. St. Louis: Mosby/Elsevier, 2013.
Meneghini, Fabio, and Paolo Biondi. *Clinical Facial Analysis: Elements, Principles, and Techniques*. London: Springer, 2012.
Miloro, Michael, et al. *Peterson's Principles of Oral and Maxillofacial Surgery*. 2d ed. Philadelphia: BC Decker, 2004.
Mitchell, David A. *An Introduction to Oral and Maxillofacial Surgery*. New York: Oxford University Press, 2006.
White, R. L. "Oral and Maxillofacial Surgery: Defining Our Present, Shaping Our Future." *Journal of the American College of Dentistry* 76, no. 1. (Spring, 2009): 36-39.

ORCHIECTOMY

Category: Procedure
Anatomy or system affected: Reproductive system
Specialties and related fields: Urology
Also known as: Testicle removal
Definition: Excision of a testicle, usually performed as part of cancer therapy.
Key terms:
electrocautery: a needle charged with electricity that is heated and placed on the tissue; often used to remove warts and polyps

lymphadenectomy: the removal of lymph nodes, one or more in a group
seminoma: the most common cancer of the testes

INDICATIONS AND PROCEDURES
Orchiectomy is usually performed for benign or malignant conditions. For metastatic carcinoma of the prostate, bilateral orchiectomy (removal of both testicles) is often utilized. For primary tumors of the testes that are malignant, radical orchiectomy is performed for the best result.

During simple orchiectomy, the patient's genitalia are prepared in a sterile manner. An incision is made in the scrotum, and the testis is withdrawn from its sac. The spermatic cord is clamped during the procedure, and then cut.

When it comes to radical orchiectomy, the genitalia and the inguinal region (the upper groin and lower lateral abdominal region) are prepared in a sterile manner, and an inguinal skin incision is made. Then the spermatic cord is freed and clamped Next, the testis is pulled up from the scrotum. A radical orchiectomy would typically be necessary in the case of suspected testicular cancer. Once the tumor is verified, either by gross analysis or by a frozen section, the cord is doubly clamped and then cut.

It is important for patients undergoing an orchiectomy to have blood drawn and a urine sample collected and to stop any aspirins that they may be taking a week before the procedure. Also, all nonsteroidal anti-inflammatory drugs (NSAIDs) should be discontinued two days before the procedure.

Orchiectomy can also be a part of gender reassignment surgery and is mostly done in clinics that specialize in it. It is considered genital reconstruction. Prior to the genital reconstruction, patients usually undergo hormone therapy for several months or as long as a year before going through the surgery. The patient must be sure that he wants to live life as a woman with real-life experiences as a female with all the social implications.

USES AND COMPLICATIONS
Orchiectomy can be used to treat testicular cancer. Seminoma is a type of testicular cancer that, if the tumors are localized, in 98 percent of the patients is curable with orchiectomy and low doses of adjuvant radiotherapy. Advanced cancer at stage II is curable with orchiectomy and radiation therapy to the involved areas for 85 to 90 percent of patients. In metastatic diseases, stage III or localized advanced disease is primarily curable in 90 percent of the patients if combined with chemotherapy. Nonseminoma germ cell tumors (NSGCTs) seem to resist radiation therapy

and are more likely to travel to the lungs, brain, bones, and liver.

Both seminoma and nonseminoma are highly curable if caught early enough, even if the cancer has spread beyond the testes to other body parts and tissues, as compared to other cancers. When it comes to relapse of the disease, the risk is lowered with retroperitoneal lymphadenectomy followed by chemotherapy, but this protocol does not improve survival. It is also possible that removing the lymph nodes may cause infertility.

Patients who have undergone orchiectomy may go to work the next day, if they desire. However, some patients may need a day or two before they feel ready. It is important to drink fluids and to abstain from alcoholic beverages. Sometimes, the patient may feel nauseated if the procedure was performed because of cancer. Some pain and swelling may develop, which is normal, and the physician may prescribe medications to counteract them.

One of the major risks of orchiectomy is a sudden hormone change, and side effects may occur, such as loss of muscle mass, brittle bones, weight gain, fatigue, erection problems, loss of sexual desire, hot flashes, enlargement and tenderness in the breasts, and sterility.

Undergoing orchiectomy for male-to-female genital reconstruction requires a diagnosis from a psychiatrist, as well as letters from mental health counselors in support of this procedure.

PERSPECTIVE AND PROSPECTS

In 1941, orchiectomy was first used on a patient suffering from advanced prostate cancer. Indications from this therapy showed no apparent improvement of survival from it. In 1967, the Veterans Administration Cooperative Urological Research Group or (VACURG), presented information on more than two thousand patients who had received different types of therapies, including orchiectomy.

From 1984 through 1993, a study was performed on seventy-two patients with stage C and stage D prostate cancer whereby forty-four out of sixty-one patients had a partial response, and a good response on the tumor markers.

—*Marvin Morris, LAc, MPA*

See also Genital disorders, male; Glands; Hydroceles; Men's health; Orchitis; Reproductive system; Surgery, general; Testicles, undescended; Testicular cancer; Testicular surgery; Testicular torsion; Urology; Urology, pediatric; Vascular system.

For Further Information:

Dawson, C. "Testicular Cancer: Seek Advice Early." *Journal of Family Health Care* 12 (2002): 3.

Geldart, T. R., P. D. Simmonds, and G. M. Mead. "Orchiectomy After Chemotherapy for Patients with Metastatic Testicular Germ Cell Cancer." *BJU International* 90 (September, 2002): 451-455.

Incrocci, L., et al. " Treatment Outcome, Body Image, and Sexual Functioning After Orchiectomy and Radiotherapy for Stage I-II Testicular Seminoma." *International Journal of Radiation Oncology, Biology, Physics* 53 (August 1, 2002): 1165-1173.

Khatri, Vijay P., and Juan A. Asensio. *Khatri: Operative Surgery Manual*. Philadelphia: Saunders, 2003.

Neff, Deanna M. "Orchiectomy." *Health Library*, September 26, 2012.

"Testicular Cancer Treatments: The Inguinal Orchiectomy." *Testicular Cancer Resource Center*, December 9, 2012.

ORCHITIS

Category: Disease/Disorder
Also known as: Epididymoorchitis
Anatomy or system affected: Genitals, reproductive system
Specialties and related fields: Family medicine, virology
Definition: An inflammation of one or both testicles.

CAUSES AND SYMPTOMS

Orchitis is usually a consequence of epididymitis, an inflammation of the tube that connects the vas deferens and the testicles. It can also result from prostate infections. The source of inflammation can be either bacterial or viral organisms. The disease is typically caused by a generalized infection, such as mumps, scarlet fever, or typhoid fever. Chronic cases of orchitis can be produced by syphilis, gonorrhea, chlamydia, tuberculosis, and parasitic infections. In most cases of orchitis, only one testis is infected.

The most frequent cause of orchitis is the mumps, a viral infection. About one-third of males with the mumps develop orchitis at some stage of the illness, usually within four to six days after it begins. In prepubertal boys, about 20 percent develop mumps-induced orchitis. It is much rarer for males who are past puberty.

Symptoms of orchitis include nausea, fever, fatigue, and tenderness and significant swelling of the affected testis. Other effects may include groin pain, pain during urination, discharge from the penis, pain associated with intercourse and ejaculation, and blood in the semen.

TREATMENT AND THERAPY

If orchitis is produced by a bacterial infection, then antibiotics are the most effective treatment. Anti-inflammatory drugs are also commonly prescribed. If the source of infection is viral, then orchitis can be treated only with proper bed rest, elevation and support of the testes, and pain-relieving drugs. The application of ice packs periodically to the infected area helps reduce the pain. If acute pain occurs in the scrotum or testicles, then immediate medical attention is necessary.

When orchitis is properly treated and the cause is bacterial, normal function of the testis is typically preserved. If mumps is the source of orchitis, then shrinking of the testicles often occurs. Sterility may also occur, though it is very rare in cases of unilateral (one-sided) orchitis. Immunization against mumps is the best preventive treatment to avoid the possible complications of orchitis, although there have been a few cases of mumps-induced orchitis developing subsequent to a mumps-measles-rubella (MMR) vaccine. Spread of bacteria associated with sexually transmitted diseases (STDs) that can cause epididymo-orchitis in sexually active men can be minimized through monogamy and the use of condoms.

PERSPECTIVE AND PROSPECTS

The first recorded description of orchitis goes back to Hippocrates in the fifth century BCE. Physical examination often reveals a tender, enlarged testicle on the affected side. Tender, enlarged lymph nodes in the groin area may also indicate the presence of orchitis.

Doppler ultrasound of the groin area can be used to confirm a diagnosis of orchitis by showing increased blood flow to the affected region, as well as tissue textures that are associated with infection. This test can also reveal any presence of scrotal abscesses. Nuclear magnetic resonance (NMR) imaging may also be used to help diagnose the presence of orchitis.

—*Alvin K. Benson, PhD*

See also Antibiotics; Bacterial infections; Chlamydia; Gonorrhea; Men's health; Mumps; Parasitic diseases; Prostate

gland; Reproductive system; Scarlet fever; Sexually transmitted diseases (STDs); Syphilis; Testicles, undescended; Testicular cancer; Testicular surgery; Testicular torsion; Typhoid fever; Tuberculosis; Viral infections.

For Further Information:
Kliegman, Robert M., et al., eds. *Nelson Textbook of Pediatrics.* 19th ed. Philadelphia: Elsevier/Saunders, 2011.
"Orchitis." *Mayo Clinic*, October 7, 2011.
Rosenfeld, Isadore. *Symptoms.* New York: Bantam Books, 1994.
Standring, Susan, et al., eds. *Gray's Anatomy: The Anatomical Basis of Clinical Practice.* 40th ed. New York: Churchill Livingstone/Elsevier, 2008.
Taguchi, Yosh. *Private Parts: An Owner's Guide to the Male Anatomy*, edited by Merrily Weisbord. 3d ed. Toronto: McClelland & Stewart, 2003.
Van De Graaff, Kent M. *Human Anatomy.* 6th ed. New York: McGraw-Hill, 2002.
Vorvick, Linda J., Louis S. Liou, and David Zieve. "Orchitis." *MedlinePlus*, October 9, 2012.

ORGANS. SEE SYSTEMS AND ORGANS.

ORTHODONTICS

Category: Specialty
Anatomy or system affected: Gums, mouth, teeth
Specialties and related fields: Dentistry
Definition: A dental specialty in which the teeth are straightened and moved into positions in the jaws that yield a correct and attractive arrangement.
Key terms:
analgesic: a medication (such as aspirin) that reduces or eliminates pain
dental arch: the arched bony part of the upper and lower jaws, in which the teeth are found
lingual: related to the tongue; in orthodontics, the inner sides or faces of the teeth
malocclusion: an incorrect fit of the upper and lower teeth when they are brought together
mastication: the act of chewing food
occlusion: the fit of the upper and lower teeth when they are brought together

SCIENCE AND PROFESSION

The term "orthodontics" comes from the Greek words meaning "straight teeth." It is practiced by a dental specialist called an orthodontist. Orthodontists graduate from dental school and then specialize in orthodontics. To explore orthodontics as a field, one must first consider teeth and the mouth. Ideally, thirty-two human teeth are arranged in appropriate orientations in the dental arches of each jaw. Four incisors are located in the center of each arch; on either side of them are a cuspid or canine tooth, followed by two bicuspids (premolars) and three molars.

The first molar on the side of each jaw is viewed as particularly important to orthodontics. Appropriate tooth development within the jaw and correct tooth eruption enable proper dental health, which keeps teeth in the mouth for most of an individual's life. They also ensure appropriate mastication of food and good digestive health, as well as self-confidence with an attractive smile.

Teeth are rarely optimally placed in the jaws. One important reason for this is heredity. This facet of orthodontics relates to the teeth and to jaws. The genes that control the size and shape of human teeth and jaws vary considerably. In addition, the genes for teeth and jaws are highly individualized and often poorly related to one another. Hence, it is likely that orthodontic problems caused by tooth-jaw mismatch will occur.

Other aspects of the development of irregular tooth positioning arise from living. In some cases, teeth are damaged by decay, oral diseases, or injury. In others, poor oral habits such as thumb sucking move them out of appropriate positions. In many cases, minor problems may be handled by restorative dentistry, such as filling dental caries (cavities) or placing crowns. Most treatment of poorly positioned teeth, however, is carried out by orthodontists on nearly 5 million Americans per year. The majority of these patients are children, but many adults are presently undergoing orthodontic treatment.

There are several main goals of orthodontic treatment involving the bones of the jaws and the teeth. First, occlusion is improved so that all teeth engage one another properly for chewing and swallowing. Speech patterns are also improved, because almost twenty letter sounds involve interactions between tooth, tongue, and jaw movements. Another goal is increased resistance to decay and periodontal disease, which cause havoc in mouths where teeth are too close together or misaligned in other ways. The final orthodontic goal is improved appearance, which is for many individuals the primary reason for undergoing treatment.

Most orthodontic problems are termed malocclusions and are caused by defects of teeth and/or the jaws. Malocclusions are often classified according to the system developed by Edward H. Angle, the originator of modern orthodontics. He developed three classes of occlusion, defined by relationships between the upper and lower first molars.

In normal occlusion (class I), the lower first molars are seen slightly farther forward than their upper counterparts when the mouth is closed. This relationship positions the rest of the teeth for optimum chewing. When the arch length of either jaw is too small for all the teeth to be in appropriate positions, they become crowded. Also, in some individuals bimaxillary protrusion occurs, in which the front teeth of the jaws flare outward. These occurrences are unattractive and lead both to tooth decay and to periodontal disease.

Classes II and III are malocclusions that can be considered together. They are caused by improper positioning in the closed mouth of the lower first molars, either very far back or very far forward. In the first case (class II), the position of the first molars produces buck teeth because of the protrusion of the upper jaw in the closed mouth. The resulting problems are uncosmetic appearance and the ease with which buck teeth can be knocked out. Class II malocclusion is most often attributable to a hereditary size mismatch of the jawbones. Class III malocclusion is often termed crossbite. It causes the lower jaw to be positioned so that the lower front incisors are in front of the upper ones. In some cases, this problem is treated by orthodontics; in others, surgery is required.

The Angle classification system does not include faulty vertical relationships of the jaws, which produce other problems. Examples are overbite, which hides the lower teeth entirely in the closed jaw, and open bite, which leaves a gap between the upper and lower front teeth in the closed mouth. These situations may be asymmetric and make closures lopsided.

Functional malocclusions are also caused by thumb sucking, chewing of the lower lip, or tongue thrusting. With thumb sucking, class II malocclusion may result or be enhanced, or open bite may occur. Chewing the lower lip will cause the upper front teeth to flare outward, and tongue thrusting (often a consequence of mouth breathing because of asthma) may cause open bite, crossbite, or class II malocclusion.

Defects of the teeth themselves occur as well. They are caused by overretention or underretention of the baby teeth and missing or lost permanent teeth. These conditions cause the remaining teeth to drift in the mouth and should be corrected as soon as possible in order to preclude occlusion problems.

DIAGNOSTIC AND TREATMENT TECHNIQUES
The first stage of orthodontic treatment is an extensive diagnostic procedure that requires several office visits. First, the orthodontist compiles a complete dental and medical history. Then, the patient's mouth and teeth are examined thoroughly. This effort, accomplished in one visit, leads to a preliminary treatment plan. During the next visit, complete x-rays of the jaws are taken to show their relationship to each other, dental impressions of the teeth and jaws are made, and color photographs of the face and mouth are taken.

On the third visit, the patient is given a comprehensive diagnosis, and a treatment plan is described. At this point, the patient is informed about the problems to be treated, the probable consequences if they are left untreated, the steps to be used and their duration, the results that are expected, and any possible treatment complications. The overall cost of the treatment is also discussed. After agreement is reached, treatment begins and may require up to several years of visits at varied intervals. The process begins with the use of orthodontic appliances worn to move the teeth to new positions. After this, a simpler appliance called a retainer is worn until the bone of the tooth sockets, remodeled by the earlier treatment, is able to maintain the new dental arrangement.

Patient compliance with treatment instructions is crucial. Short-term noncompliance can lengthen the treatment period greatly; extreme noncompliance may completely destroy the endeavor. Most aspects of modern orthodontic treatment are relatively painless. If soreness occurs, it may usually be relieved quickly by combining saltwater gargles, temporary soft diets, and mild analgesics. Soreness caused by the rubbing of metal appliance parts against the inside of the cheeks or lips may be prevented by application of a wax supplied by the orthodontist. Pain that lasts for more than several days should be reported; it can usually be alleviated by an office visit where the orthodontist adjusts the offending portion of the appliance.

Throughout the course of orthodontic treatment, it is recommended that patients keep careful written records of orthodontic instructions and a complete daily record of use of the orthodontic appliance prescribed. The orthodontic appliances also need to be kept clean, stored carefully if removable, and guarded carefully during sports or other physical activities. The teeth must also be kept clean to prevent tooth decay. In addition, hard or sticky foods must be avoided.

The mechanical devices used by orthodontists vary widely. Their purposes are to direct jaw growth, to move selected teeth, to alter the behavior of the jaw muscles, and to maintain the position of the teeth once they have been moved. These appliances operate on two main principles. First, bone growth slows when pressure is applied against it and accelerates when the bone is kept in traction. This is how desired facial bone growth is attained. Second, when pressure is applied to the bone in tooth sockets, bone growth slows on the side to which the pressure is applied. Conversely, the growth of bone is stimulated on the other side of the tooth. This is the principle that generates tooth movement in the mouth. Applied properly, the combination of jaw and tooth treatment achieves results that can be fine-tuned over the treatment period. A lengthy treatment period ensures the

minimum amount of pain while this movement occurs.

There are two main categories among the many orthodontic appliances used: fixed and removable appliances. Each category has numerous subcategories, and there are variants within each subcategory. Fixed appliances are firmly affixed in the mouth for the duration of treatment. They are made of metal cylinders shaped to fit snugly around individual teeth and cemented in position. The main fixed appliance types are bracketed appliances, lingual arch wires, habit control appliances, and space retainers.

Bracketed appliances, usually called braces, move teeth and direct growth of bone in the dental arches. Although braces are often disliked by patients on aesthetic grounds, orthodontists view them as an unrivaled means to cause precise tooth movement and directed bone growth. They are made up of several components. First, bands (metal cylinders) are applied around chosen anchor teeth. Then, metal or sturdy synthetic polymer brackets are cemented to each tooth in positions that determine the direction of the force to be applied to it. Next, arch wires are passed across each bracket to the anchor teeth, where they are attached to the bands. Elastic or wire ligatures keep the arch wires in the brackets at all times.

Much of the pressure that engenders tooth movement comes from the shape of the arch wires and their composition. Elastic bands are also used to provide special treatment to a given tooth or tooth group. These bands must be removed before eating and replaced daily. When necessary, external headgear is used to apply pressure to teeth and/or jaws, either pulling them forward or pushing them backward.

Lingual bracketed appliances, a newer device often called "invisible braces," are fixed appliances attached to the teeth on the inside of the dental arch. They are not externally visible except for the bands on the anchor teeth. Thus, they are advantageous aesthetically. They do not function as well as standard braces, however, and often interfere with normal speech. Other fixed appliances include lingual arch wires, habit control devices, and space retainers.

A wide variety of removable appliances may also be used. They are either entirely or partly removable by wearers. Removable appliances are most effective when worn constantly, but they can be removed at meals and on special occasions. Their use gives much less precise results than fixed appliances, however, and requires the continuous, unflagging cooperation of patients. Active, partly removable appliances put pressure on teeth and jaws. Functional appliances, which are completely removable, alter the pressure created by the muscles of the mouth and so act on the teeth and bones (for example, lip bumpers, which keep lips away from teeth).

Removable habit control appliances and space retainers are used, respectively, to prevent activities such as thumb sucking and to maintain desired spaces between teeth until the new dental arrangements have stabilized. They are specially designed bands, acrylic plates, and/or combinations. Space retainers exert enough pressure on teeth to keep them in place but not to move them. Special headgear may also be used as an auxiliary to in-the-mouth appliances. In some cases, diseased or extra teeth must be extracted as part of the treatment regimen.

PERSPECTIVE AND PROSPECTS

Orthodontics has changed markedly since its inception. The changes include efforts at making braces more appealing and a changing clientele, evolving from one in which most patients were children to a population having many adult customers. The new direction in producing more cosmetic bracketed appliances arises from several factors.

First is the development of stronger and better synthetic polymer and ceramic replacements for metals, allowing the creation of materials that are less visible and that still produce the unrivaled therapeutic capabilities of bracketed appliances. A second factor is the interest of adults in orthodontic treatment. This discriminating population wishes to appear as attractive as possible, even in braces, and has both the independence of judgment and the monetary power to drive trends toward the use of such materials.

The adult move toward orthodontics in the United States is founded partly on the funding of orthodontic work by entities as diverse as Medicaid for welfare recipients and third-party group dental insurance plans. In addition, the adult public is being made more aware that it is not necessary to live out life with an unattractive smile simply because orthodontic treatment was not attempted in childhood or adolescence.

Considerable research has been carried out in the treatment of problems associated with orthodontics, including the root tip resorption that often halts such treatment. It is hoped that a combination of these endeavors and factors will continue to improve orthodontics.

—*Sanford S. Singer, PhD*

See also Bones and the skeleton; Braces, orthodontic; Dentistry; Jaw wiring; Orthodontics; Periodontal surgery; Teeth; Tooth extraction.

For Further Information:

Doundoulakis, James, and Warren Strugatch. *The Perfect Smile: The Complete Guide to Cosmetic Dentistry.* Long Island, N.Y.: Hatherleigh Press, 2003.

Gluck, George M., and Warren M. Morganstein, eds. *Jong's Community Dental Health.* 5th ed. St. Louis, Mo.: Mosby, 2003.

Houston, W. J. B., C. D. Stephens, and W. J. Tulley. *A Textbook of Orthodontics.* 2d ed. Boston: Wright, 1992.

Klatell, Jack, Andrew Kaplan, and Gray Williams, Jr., eds. *The Mount Sinai Medical Center Family Guide to Dental Health.* New York: Macmillan, 1991.

"Malocclusion of Teeth." *MedlinePlus*, February 22, 2012.

Mitchell, Laura. *An Introduction to Orthodontics.* 4th ed. New York: Oxford University Press, 2013.

"Orthodontics: Braces and More." *Columbia University College of Dental Medicine*, May 5, 2010.

Smith, Rebecca W. *The Columbia University School of Dental and Oral Surgery's Guide to Family Dental Care.* New York: W. W. Norton, 1997.

ORTHOPEDIC BRACES. SEE BRACES, ORTHOPEDIC.

ORTHOPEDIC SURGERY

Category: Procedure

Anatomy or system affected: Bones, feet, hands, hips, joints, knees, legs, ligaments, muscles, musculoskeletal system, nervous system, spine, tendons

Specialties and related fields: General surgery, orthopedics, physical therapy, podiatry, rheumatology, sports medicine

Definition: Surgical procedures involving the bones or joints.

Key terms:

polymethylmethacrylate: a material used in the fixation of bones

valgus: a musculoskeletal deformity in which a limb is twisted outward from the body

varus: a musculoskeletal deformity in which a limb is twisted toward the body

INDICATIONS AND PROCEDURES

Orthopedic surgery encompasses a number of different procedures carried out to repair injuries affecting the skeletal system and joints or to repair tissues associated with these structures. Such surgery may also attempt to correct associated neurological injury. In addition, orthopedic surgery is used to correct musculoskeletal problems that may be congenital in origin.

Among the congenital conditions for which orthopedic surgery may be warranted are bowlegs (valgus knees) and knock-knees (varus knees). In the case of bowlegs caused by a congenital malformation, one or both legs are bent outward at the knee. In knock-knees caused by congenital conditions, the knees are curved inward, causing the lower legs to twist away from the body.

Treatment begins with a thorough evaluation of the problem. Based on x-ray analysis, an orthopedic surgeon may make a decision as to whether surgery can be used in the correction of the problem. During the surgical procedure itself, the affected limbs are properly aligned; they are splinted upon completion of the surgery. The chances of success are greatest in younger children. In an analogous situation, if a limb is twisted during fetal development, the child may exhibit misalignment of the structure following birth. Since bone at this stage of life is only beginning its growth, maintaining the limb in a splint may correct the problem. If necessary, the surgeon may decide to realign the limb at the joint through orthopedic surgery.

Tumors that originate in bone are uncommon. If they occur, such growths must be removed as quickly as possible because of the speed with which they spread to adjacent and distant structures in the body if the tumor is cancerous. The first signs of bone cancer include pain and swelling in the affected region. Spontaneous fractures may occur. X-ray and biopsy analyses are necessary to confirm the diagnosis of cancer. If the tumor is benign, it may be removed through surgery. Osteomas, which are tumors that arise from connective tissue within the bone, may require radiation or chemotherapy in addition to surgical removal.

Commonly, orthopedic surgery is used to correct fractures or dislocations. As with any procedure, a thorough evaluation is necessary prior to a final decision. This evaluation often includes x-ray and computed tomography (CT) analyses. If the injury involves the spine, treatment must both correct the problem and prevent secondary injury to the spinal cord. Fractures to the vertebral column may produce fragments that pose a threat to the spinal cord. Under these conditions, orthopedic surgery is used to immobilize or straighten the spinal column; this may involve external braces or an internal brace such as a Harrington distraction rod. The patient may be immobilized for weeks to months, depending on the extent of the injury and the course of treatment.

USES AND COMPLICATIONS

One of the most common applications of orthopedic surgery is the repair of trauma or fractures to bones. For example, a blow to the face, either intentional or accidental, may result in fractures to the nose or facial bones. Injuries to other skeletal structures, including the spine, may also result from the incident. This is particularly true if the source of the injury was an automobile accident. Upon clinical examination by a physician, it may be apparent that facial bones have been fractured. X-ray analysis may be used to confirm the

initial diagnosis. Proper repair and restoration of features will be the primary concern of the orthopedic surgeon, assuming that the injuries are not life-threatening. In the event of facial injuries, damage to teeth and other periodontal regions will also be a consideration. In many cases, wire fixation may be a sufficient course of treatment. If more severe, the fracture may require screw-plate fixation, particularly in complicated fractures.

If uneventful or uncomplicated, the healing of such injuries usually requires about six weeks of immobilization. The procedure and immobilization, however, are inherently uncomfortable. If a muscle tear is severe or significant, resulting in a pull to the bone or joint, an associated fracture may heal improperly because of the dislocation of tissue. Proper evaluation of surgical options, including the use of metallic plates, can limit any such complications.

Although cancers originating in bone tissue are uncommon, they nevertheless present problems for the orthopedic surgeon. Fractures related to tumor development are generally treated in much the same way as uncomplicated breaks. If damage to the bone, either through the tumor itself or as a result of therapy, is severe, even surgical repair may not be sufficient to heal the structure and allow mobility or normal function. If the fracture is near the joint, the bone may require realignment or resection, resulting in a shortening of the structure. In some cases, internal fixation with polymethylmethacrylate bone cement may be used to augment repair.

PERSPECTIVE AND PROSPECTS

The introduction of computed tomography (CT) scanning technology in the 1970s allowed for much more detailed evaluation of bone and joint injuries. Much of the technology is best applicable in a post-traumatic situation, evaluating the result of injury rather than its cause. Magnetic resonance imaging (MRI) is based on different technology but produces results that are similar to CT scans.

The destruction of bone as a function of aging or of disease is not well understood. Degenerative bone disease as a result of arthritis is among the most common of arthritic conditions, affecting nearly half of middle-aged adults in some manner. Such conditions, particularly among the elderly, remain to be fully addressed.

The ability to carry out bone transplants, developed extensively in the latter half of the twentieth century, allowed for at least partial replacement of damaged bone. Replacement structures may come from the patient's own body or from a cadaver. In addition, orthopedic technology has resulted in prostheses for the replacement of most joints in the body.

Joint replacements are dramatic. Individuals with crippling deformities can have nearly normal function restored through replaced joints. The most commonly replaced joints include hips and knees. Other joints can also be replaced. Individuals who have their hips and knees replaced usually start walking on the replaced joint in the first or second postoperative day. Complete rehabilitation requires several months.

—Richard Adler, PhD;
updated by L. Fleming Fallon, Jr., MD, PhD, MPH

See also Amputation; Arthroplasty; Arthroscopy; Bone grafting; Bowlegs; Bunions; Casts and splints; Disk removal; Fracture repair; Hammertoe correction; Hammertoes; Heel spur removal; Hip fracture repair; Hip replacement; Jaw wiring; Joints; Kneecap removal; Knock-knees; Laminectomy and spinal fusion; Orthopedics; Orthopedics, pediatric; Physical rehabilitation; Prostheses; Rotator cuff surgery.

For Further Information:
Bentley, George, and Robert B. Greer, eds. *Orthopaedics.* 4th ed. Oxford, England: Linacre House, 1993.
Brotzman, S. Brent, and Kevin E. Wilk. *Clinical Orthopaedic Rehabilitation.* 2d ed. Philadelphia: Mosby, 2003.
Callaghan, John J., Aaron Rosenberg, and Harry E. Rubash, eds. *The Adult Hip.* 2d ed. Philadelphia: Lippincott Williams & Wilkins, 2007.
Doherty, Gerard M., and Lawrence W. Way, eds. *Current Surgical Diagnosis and Treatment.* 13th ed. New York: Lange Medical Books/McGraw-Hill, 2010.
Griffith, H. Winter. *Complete Guide to Symptoms, Illness, and Surgery.* 6th ed. New York: Perigee, 2012.
Mulholland, Michael W., et al., eds. *Greenfield's Surgery: Scientific Principles and Practice.* 5th ed. Philadelphia: Lippincott Williams & Wilkins, 2011.
Tapley, Donald F., et al., eds. *The Columbia University College of Physicians and Surgeons Complete Home Medical Guide.* Rev. 3d ed. New York: Crown, 1995.
McPhee, Stephen J., and Maxine A. Papadakis, eds. *Current Medical Diagnosis and Treatment.* Los Altos, Calif.: Lange Medical, 2011.
Zollinger, Robert M., Jr., E. Christopher Ellison, and Robert M. Zollinger, Sr. *Zollinger's Atlas of Surgical Operations.* 9th ed. New York: McGraw-Hill, 2011.

ORTHOPEDICS

Category: Specialty
Anatomy or system affected: Bones, feet, hands, hips, joints, knees, legs, ligaments, muscles, musculoskeletal system, nervous system, spine, tendons
Specialties and related fields: Physical therapy, podiatry, rheumatology, sports medicine
Definition: The field of medicine concerned with the prevention and treatment of disorders, either developmental or caused by injury or disease, that are associated with the skeleton, joints, muscles, and connective tissues.

Key terms:
articulation: a joint between two bones of the skeleton; also called an arthrosis
bursa: a connective tissue sac filled with fluid that reduces friction at joints
collagen: a fibrous protein found in skin, bone, ligaments, tendons, and cartilage
inflammation: the reaction of tissue to injury, with its corresponding redness, heat, swelling, and pain
ligament: a structure of tough connective tissue that attaches one bone to another bone
synovial: referring to the lubricating fluid in the joints or the membrane surrounding the joints
tendon: a structure of tough connective tissue that attaches a muscle to a bone

SCIENCE AND PROFESSION

Orthopedics is the branch of medicine primarily concerned with the movement of the human body and its parts, as well as disorders that affect its function. Such activities as maintaining posture, walking, doing manual work, and exercising involve a complex relationship between the nervous system, muscular system, and skeletal system. While orthopedists must be familiar with the nervous system, they focus primarily on the prevention and treatment of disorders of the skeleton and muscles. They also have expertise in the proper development of these systems in childhood and the changes that occur as a result of aging.

When a person decides to make a movement, the brain sends signals to the muscles. The muscles contract and, by pulling on the bones to which they are attached, cause that part of the body to move. The anchor point for the muscle is the origin, and the attachment point to the bone that is being moved is the insertion. Muscles work in groups to perform a movement. The principal muscle involved is the prime mover, or agonist. The muscles that help the prime mover are called synergists. When a prime mover contracts, the muscle on the opposite side of the bone, termed the antagonist, must relax. An illustration of this would be the muscle and bone interaction involved in the flexing of the arm. The biceps muscle, anchored to bone in the shoulder, contracts, pulling on the bone in the lower arm to which it is attached by a tendon. Its synergist, the brachialis, also contracts. On the back of the upper arm, its antagonist, the triceps muscle, relaxes to allow the arm to bend. When the arm is extended, the triceps becomes the prime mover for that action, and the biceps is the antagonist.

The skeletal system is made of bone and cartilage. Bone cells, called osteocytes, take in nutrients from the blood and constantly renew the bony matrix. The chemical composition of bone includes calcium and phosphorus salts, which provide stiffness. The fibrous protein collagen gives bones some flexibility. Cartilage cells, called chondrocytes, manufacture cartilage, which is a mass of collagen and elastic fibers embedded in a gelatin-like substance. The nature of this structure gives cartilage more flexibility than bone, which makes it an ideal substitute for bone in certain areas. The ribs, for example, are attached by cartilage to the sternum, or breastbone. This arrangement allows for the expansion of the chest during breathing.

Tendons, ligaments, and bursas are also part of the skeletal and muscular systems. Tendons attach muscles to bones. They are made of fibrous tissue so strong that, under stress, the muscle will tear or the bone will break before the tendon will be damaged. Ligaments, which are also made of fibrous tissue, attach bones to other bones and provide stability at the joints. Bursas are fluid-filled connective tissue sacs that lie between muscle and bone, tendon and bone, or other areas around joints. They reduce the damage that occurs to the softer tissue as it rubs against bone with each movement. Because of their close interdependence, the skeleton, attached muscles, and other associated structures are often referred to as the musculoskeletal system.

The health of the musculoskeletal system during childhood is of primary importance to an individual in attaining full growth and physical function as an adult. In the early developmental stages of the embryo and fetus, a skeleton of cartilage is formed. This structure is replaced with bone in a process called ossification that continues for years after birth. Good nutrition is vital to this process. In particular, the body requires adequate amounts of protein, calcium, and vitamin D. The ends of a long bone are separated from the shaft of the bone by cartilage until the child reaches full growth. Care should be taken when participating in sports, since damage to these areas could affect the growth of that limb. Hormonal production influences the development of the skeleton. Adequate amounts of growth hormone are needed to ensure that proper growth is attained. At puberty, sex hormones, especially testosterone, stimulate the final growth spurts and completion of the adult skeleton.

Young adults have attained their full growth, but the skeleton must renew itself continually to remain strong and maintain its ability to repair injury. A woman of childbearing age must eat a healthy diet if she is to nourish a fetus that, in turn, is developing its own skeleton. Both men and women must take care to exercise, since the stress of activity not only builds muscle but also sends messages to the bone to maintain its strength. Calcium and vitamin D intake must continue, or the bones may begin to dissolve some of their calcium matrix. Automobile accidents, work injuries, and sports injuries are more likely to occur at this stage of life.

As adults age, metabolic and other cellular processes become less efficient, and care must be taken to maintain functions and prevent further losses. At one time, disorders such as osteoarthritis and osteoporosis were considered an inevitable part of the aging process. While heredity is certainly a risk factor in these conditions, a substantial body of evidence has been accumulated showing that some degenerative processes can be traced to lifestyle and diet. Osteoarthritis is the type of joint tissue degeneration that is associated with wear and tear on the joints. A person who is obese puts excessive pressure on the skeletal system, especially the hips, knees, and ankles. This pressure increases the damage to the joints. A person who fails to exercise begins to lose flexibility in the joints, and muscles become weaker.

Osteoporosis occurs as bones become porous and brittle. As osteocytes age, they become less efficient at calcium absorption and renewal of the bony matrix. At a time in life when more calcium is needed to make up for this inefficiency, most people consume fewer dairy products, either because of lactose intolerance or because of the ingestion of other beverages. Older women are at particular risk because their bones are lighter than those of men. After the menopause, women lose some of the protection that estrogen provided by stimulating the absorption of calcium and thus bone renewal. If older people lose the ability to move as surely as before and their reflexes slow down, then injuries are more likely to occur as a result of falls. These injuries are much more serious if the bones are brittle. Even if osteoporosis is not a factor, fractures and other injuries in an older individual do not heal as quickly as they would in a younger person.

Because of their knowledge of developmental processes, orthopedists, as well as pediatricians, are able to advise parents concerned about their growing children and the appropriate precautions for sports activities. Recommendations are made by orthopedists with regard to the design and utilization of safety equipment to prevent or reduce injury. Advice on nutrition and exercise for adults may also be given by physicians in an effort to reduce the incidence of problems as a person ages, allowing continuation of an active, independent life.

DIAGNOSTIC AND TREATMENT TECHNIQUES

In nonemergency situations, patients with some pain or disorder of the muscles, bones, or joints are usually referred to an orthopedic surgeon. The first office visit begins with a review of the condition, during which the physician will take a general medical history and obtain a history of the current complaint. This history will include the time frame from onset, any action that may have initiated the condition, and a description of any difficulty in movement that the patient is having. A physician will then perform a physical examination to determine the specific areas affected and observe range-of-motion exercises to determine if function has been lost.

X-rays or other imaging methods are ordered to see whether any structural defect can be seen. Blood tests may be ordered if a disease process is suspected. Once a diagnosis has been made, a physician may prescribe medication, order physical therapy or home exercises, schedule surgery, or take other therapeutic measures to correct the condition. The types of abnormalities treated by orthopedists generally fall into one of three categories: injuries caused by accidents, repetitive motion disorders, and diseases affecting the skeleton, skeletal muscles, or joints.

The most common situation in which a patient sees an orthopedist is after an accidental injury. If the injury is severe, the patient may be transported to a hospital emergency room, with care taken to keep the injury site immobilized until a physician can see the patient. The type of treatment needed will be determined by the type and severity of the injury. In a closed or simple fracture, the skin is unbroken; the bones are manipulated back in line and then immobilized with a plaster cast or brace. An open or compound fracture occurs when the ends or fragments of the bone protrude through the skin. In this case, or if surgery is needed to align the bones properly, there is a higher risk of infection. In some cases, pins or wires must be used to hold the bone in position. Fractures of the skull or vertebrae are of special concern because of the possibility of permanent damage to the brain or spinal cord; a neurologist (a physician with specialty training in the nervous system) is usually called to assist an orthopedic surgeon.

Because of twisting movements, injuries that affect one or more joints are common. A dislocation occurs when the bones at a joint are separated. An orthopedist must realign the bones as closely as possible to the original positions and immobilize the joint to allow healing to occur. A sprain results from severe twisting of a joint without dislocation. The severity of joint injury and recovery time depend on the extent of the damage to surrounding ligaments, tendons, cartilage, and other tissues. A special procedure called arthroscopy may be scheduled since damage to soft tissue may not be revealed in an x-ray. An orthopedic surgeon inserts a flexible tube, called an arthroscope, into the injury site. This tube, combined with lights and a camera, allows the surgeon to view the joint cavity to see if any abnormality is present, and, if possible, to repair it.

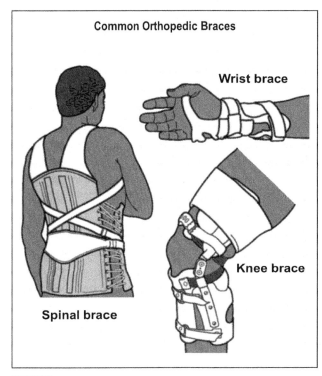

Common Orthopedic Braces

Wrist brace

Knee brace

Spinal brace

©EBSCO

Some damage to the musculoskeletal system is not the result of a single accident but of actions that are repeated over a long period of time as a part of work duties or recreational activities. These are termed repetitive motion disorders. For example, bursitis, or inflammation of the bursas, may arise in a baseball pitcher's shoulder or a tennis player's elbow. Because the same motion is repeated over and over, the rub of the bursa and other soft tissue over bone causes irritation and inflammation, resulting in pain each time the movement is attempted. Treatment consists of reducing the inflammation by using cortisone or other similar drugs, usually by injection at the affected site, coupled with rest. Resumption of the activity may occur following recommendations from an orthopedist or therapist on a change in technique aimed at reducing the trauma. In some cases, the condition becomes chronic, and the patient may have to discontinue the activity altogether.

Many occupations arising in the mid-twentieth century involved relatively small movements of the hands and wrists. A worker on an assembly line who installs a specific part and an employee who uses a computer keyboard all day are examples of people at high risk for repetitive motion disorders. An understanding of the structure of the wrist leads to better understanding of the problem involved. The median nerve leads from the spinal cord through a tunnel in the carpal bones of the wrist and then branches out to the fingers. It is encircled, together with tendons leading to the fingers, by the transverse carpal ligament. When constant friction causes swelling of the tendons and tissues adjacent to the nerve, the nerve is pinched, resulting in pain, tingling, and weakness in the hand and fingers. This condition is termed carpal tunnel syndrome. Therapy may include changing work positions, wearing a splint to hold the wrist straight, using medications to reduce inflammation, and injecting cortisone at the injury site. If the problem continues, surgery may be needed. In this procedure, the orthopedic surgeon makes an incision in the wrist and cuts the transverse carpal ligament, thus releasing the pressure on the nerve and tendons. If the motion or activity that initially caused carpal tunnel syndrome is not stopped, the condition is likely to recur.

Diseases can affect the bones and joints. Congenital defects and inheritance may result in deformities that can be treated by orthopedic devices or surgery. Hormone therapy may be used by a physician to help a child attain full growth. Nutritional disorders, such as rickets, may cause the softening of the bones, with the corresponding bowed-leg deformity. Caused by a vitamin D deficiency, rickets must be treated not only with vitamin therapy but also with braces to keep the legs straight while the bones harden. Multiple myeloma is a form of cancer that invades the bone and bone marrow and must be treated with chemotherapy as well as surgery to remove the tumor. Infections such as gangrene affect the limbs and, if not treated in time, may necessitate amputation by the orthopedic surgeon.

Of all the diseases of the musculoskeletal system, arthritis and related disorders are the most common. "Arthritis" is a general term referring to inflammation of a joint. Osteoarthritis is a degenerative disease that results to some extent from the aging process, although it can be exacerbated by obesity, lifestyle, or injury. Arthritis can also be caused by infection or by deposits of uric acid crystals, a condition called gout. The most serious form of joint disease is rheumatoid arthritis, a term that is sometimes used to encompass a group of related disorders. These diseases are classified as autoimmune conditions because the body is making antibodies against itself-in this case, against the tissues associated with the joints. The disease process itself is often treated by a specialist called a rheumatologist, who tries various medications to alleviate the condition. An orthopedic surgeon may be called upon to help correct the deformities resulting from the disease or to replace defective joints with artificial ones. Special care must be taken in cases of juvenile rheumatoid arthritis, since the growth process may also be affected. Systemic lupus erythematosus (SLE), ankylosing spondylitis, and scleroderma are some of the other autoimmune diseases that affect the musculoskeletal system.

PERSPECTIVE AND PROSPECTS

In the study of prehistoric humans, a major source of information is their skeletal remains. Archaeologists have found evidence of broken bones that were set and healed, indicating some rudimentary attempts at the treatment of injuries. Examination of hieroglyphs shows that ancient Egyptians set bones and used wooden splints held in place by the same gum and bandages that were used to wrap mummies. There were no medical specialties, and the treatment of wounds and fractures was part of the duties of any medical practitioner.

The branch of medicine known as orthopedics had its start in the eighteenth century. A physician named Jean André Venel (1740-91) opened an institute in Switzerland with the purpose of correcting skeletal deformities in children. The term "orthopedics" is actually a combination of two Greek words: *orthos*, meaning "straight" or "correct," and *pais*, meaning "child." Treatment of congenital deformities such as clubfoot and defects caused by rickets or injury was the primary function of this type of clinic.

In the nineteenth century, the development of quick-setting plaster for casts aided physicians in the immobilization of broken bones after they were set. The development of anesthesia and antiseptic techniques to prevent infection allowed the practice of orthopedic surgery to expand. Research using the microscope added to the understanding of the structure and function of bone as a living tissue.

In 1895, Wilhelm Conrad Röntgen (1845-1923) discovered that radiation from a cathode-ray tube would produce a photographic image of the bones of his hand. By the early twentieth century, the medical x-ray came into widespread use, providing an invaluable diagnostic tool for orthopedists. In the 1940s and 1950s, better understanding of radioactive phenomena allowed the development of safer x-ray equipment and techniques. In the 1970s and 1980s, other imaging techniques, such as computed tomography (CT) scanning and magnetic resonance imaging (MRI), increased the ability of orthopedic surgeons to diagnose and treat musculoskeletal disorders.

One of the greatest orthopedic surgical advances has been in the ability to treat badly damaged limbs. At one time, the best the orthopedic surgeon could do for some patients was to amputate the limb to prevent the spread of infection and the development of gangrene, then help the patient cope with the amputations by use of artificial limbs. More sophisticated techniques, incorporating the use of the microscope with computer-directed surgical instruments, allow the reattachment of limbs in many cases by enabling the surgeon to connect even the smallest blood vessels and nerves.

If amputation is necessary, artificial limbs, or prostheses, have also become more sophisticated. Artificial hands have become functional as a result of computer technology that enables the patient to direct the movement of the fingers by contracting and relaxing arm muscles. New plastics and other materials are being developed and used for synthetic joint replacements which increase the mobility of, and decrease the pain for, arthritic patients.

Joints are now routinely replaced. The most common replacements are hip and knee joints, although techniques have been developed to replace other joints in the body. The surgery is performed in a hospital. Recipients are encouraged to begin to use their replaced joints within twenty-four to forty-eight hours after surgery. Complete rehabilitation requires several months of increasingly intense physical activity and exercise. Contemporary materials have an expected useful life of twenty or more years.

A better understanding of the natural healing process at the cellular level has also allowed advances in the treatment of fractures. It has been found that attaching a device that generates a weak electric current can increase the rate of healing in some patients. This current stimulates the multiplication of osteocytes and the growth of new bone in the area.

As the understanding of disease and of degenerative processes increases, better treatments can also be devised. Osteoporosis, for example, is known to be a preventable condition when a correct diet and sufficient physical exercise are maintained throughout life. After the menopause in women, treatment with estrogen replacement therapy gives further protection against osteoporosis. New imaging devices allow osteoporosis to be detected at an earlier stage and more aggressive treatment measures to be applied. The genetic factor in diseases and conditions that trigger autoimmune disorders are other areas of research that are being pursued. While accidents will always occur, orthopedic research into the injury process can help devise methods of prevention, as well as new treatments for the orthopedic problems that do arise.

—*Edith K. Wallace, PhD;*
updated by L. Fleming Fallon, Jr., MD, PhD, MPH

See also Amputation; Arthritis; Arthroplasty; Arthroscopy; Bone cancer; Bone disorders; Bone grafting; Bones and the skeleton; Bowlegs; Bunions; Bursitis; Cancer; Cartilage; Casts and splints; Chiropractic; Collagen; Craniosynostosis; Disk removal; Dwarfism; Ewing's sarcoma; Feet; Flat feet; Foot disorders; Fracture and dislocation; Fracture repair; Geriatrics and gerontology; Growth; Hammertoe correction; Hammertoes; Heel spur removal; Hip fracture repair; Hip replacement; Jaw wiring; Joints; Kinesiology; Kneecap removal; Knock-knees; Laminectomy and spinal fusion; Ligaments; Lower extremities; Muscle sprains, spasms, and disorders; Muscles; Neurofibromatosis; Orthopedic surgery;

Orthopedics, pediatric; Osgood-Schlatter disease; Osteoarthritis; Osteochondritis juvenilis; Osteogenesis imperfecta; Osteomyelitis; Osteonecrosis; Osteopathic medicine; Osteoporosis; Paget's disease; Physical examination; Physical rehabilitation; Pigeon toes; Podiatry; Prostheses; Rheumatoid arthritis; Rheumatology; Rickets; Rotator cuff surgery; Scleroderma; Scoliosis; Slipped disk; Spina bifida; Spinal cord disorders; Spine, vertebrae, and disks; Spondylitis; Sports medicine; Systemic lupus erythematosus (SLE); Tendon disorders; Tendon repair; Upper extremities.

For Further Information:
American Academy of Orthopaedic Surgeons. www.aaos.org.
Cash, Mel. *Pocket Atlas of the Moving Body*. New York: Crown, 2000.
Currey, John D. *Bones: Structures and Mechanics*. 2d ed. Princeton, N.J.: Princeton University Press, 2006.
Delforge, Gary. *Musculoskeletal Trauma: Implications for Sport Injury Management*. Champaign, Ill.: Human Kinetics, 2002.
Marcus, Robert, David Feldman, and Jennifer Kelsey, eds. *Osteoporosis*. 3d ed. Boston: Academic Press/Elsevier, 2008.
Marieb, Elaine N., and Katja Hoehn. *Human Anatomy and Physiology*. 9th ed. San Francisco: Pearson/Benjamin Cummings, 2013.
"Orthopedic Services." *MedlinePlus*, March 1, 2012.
Rosen, Clifford J., Julie Glowacki, and John P. Bilezikian. *The Aging Skeleton*. San Diego, Calif.: Academic Press, 1999.
Salter, Robert Bruce. *Textbook of Disorders and Injuries of the Musculoskeletal System*. 3d ed. Baltimore: Williams & Wilkins, 1999.
Tortora, Gerard J., and Bryan Derrickson. *Principles of Anatomy and Physiology*. 13th ed. Hoboken, N.J.: John Wiley & Sons, 2012.

ORTHOREXIA NERVOSA

Category: Disease/Disorder
Anatomy or system affected: All
Specialties and related fields: Nutrition, health
Definition: Orthorexia nervosa is an obsession focused on the optimal healthfulness of an individual's diet and an obsession with eating "clean" or "pure" food.
Key terms:
cognitive behavioral therapy: a type of psychotherapy in which people learn to recognize and change negative and self-defeating patterns of thinking and behavior
Diagnostic and Statistical Manual of Mental Disorders: the handbook the American Psychiatric Society uses to categorize and diagnose mental disorders

BACKGROUND

As more information about nutritional research is released to the public, it generally results in a healthier population. However, some individuals take this information as absolute fact, without understanding that research is a work in progress. They develop an unhealthy obsession with applying the knowledge at a level that most in the population do not. This obsession is most commonly focused on types of foods purported to be best for perfect health, how they should be prepared, and when and how much should be eaten.

The term orthorexia nervosa was coined by Steven Bratman, an American physician, in 1997. The term means "correct diet," and denotes an unhealthy fixation with eating food that is optimally healthy, "clean," "pure," and "correct." This obsession goes well beyond the desire to eat a healthy diet and extends to rituals involving eating the exact amount of "correctly" prepared food at the specific times during the day or allowing certain foods to be eaten only during certain seasons. This obsession can interfere with social relationships (e.g., the refusal to eat at friends' houses or in restaurants) and may result in nutritional deficits.

Orthorexia nervosa is not considered an official psychiatric disorder like anorexia nervosa or bulimia. It does not have an official diagnosis in the *Diagnostic and Statistical Manual of Mental Disorders*; however, it shares many characteristics with obsessive-compulsive disorders and anorexia nervosa. Ursula Philpot, chair of the British Dietetic Association, stated that individuals who have this condition are only concerned about the quality of food they consume, and only eat what they perceive to be "pure" food. When these individuals experience intense feelings of hunger and cravings, they punish themselves for being weak. The deprivation can be so severe that it results in death.

Physicians and eating disorder specialists often fail to distinguish between orthorexia nervosa and anorexia nervosa. It is important to understand the difference; anorexia nervosa is an eating disorder that results from the fear of being overweight, whereas in orthorexia nervosa, the goal is to achieve perfect health by controlling diet, not necessarily to lose weight. Still, both disorders can lead to malnutrition and health problems.

Even though increased attention is being given to better understanding the risk factors, behavior, and outcomes of therapy, there remains much to be learned. As of 2015, only one study has addressed the overlap of orthorexia, or other obsessive-compulsive disorders, with another type of eating disorder, including bulimia and anorexia. It appears that the longer a person is preoccupied with healthy eating, the higher the likelihood that he or she will develop a clinical eating disorder (up to 53 percent three years after diagnosis). Orthorexia can also develop in an individual recovering from another eating disorder.

OVERVIEW
Individuals with orthorexia nervosa are preoccupied with eating healthy foods, and avoid those high in fat,

preservatives, animal products, or pesticides. Many of these individuals become malnourished because they avoid sources of necessary nutrition in favor of a small number of "safe" foods. One example of dietary restriction is the raw food diet. Individuals who follow this and similarly restrictive diets (i.e., veganism or fruitarianism) have an elevated risk of becoming emaciated, and can develop nutritional deficiencies if they do not sufficiently vary their diet to ensure adequate intake of vitamins, minerals, proteins, fiber, and other nutritional requirements found in food.

Orthorexia disorders are similar to and potentially overlap other psychiatric disorders such as obsessive-compulsive disorders, somatic symptom disorder, hypochondria, and psychotic spectrum disorders. One interesting overlap between orthorexia and other eating disorders is the displeasure with eating and the trading of control over one's life for control over diet.

It is not clear what demographic group is more susceptible to developing the disorder. In one 2008 study in Germany, nutrition students were investigated for developing the disorder because of their in-depth knowledge of nutrition and how to achieve optimal health. It was found that nutrition students did not have higher orthorexic tendencies than non-nutrition students. In a similar study in Portugal, it was found that orthorexic tendencies measured by a diagnostic questionnaire decreased as a nutrition student progressed through their education. The orthorexia questionnaire measured eating behaviors and attitudes toward nutrition. The students did have higher scores in regard to having more restrictive eating behaviors than non-nutrition students, but this is unsurprising given their education about healthy eating; however, it did not indicate that these students had unhealthy attitudes towards eating.

Symptoms of orthorexia nervosa include obsessive concern about one's diet, spending excessive amounts of time analyzing the source of a food for pesticides, worrying about whether milk or meat contains growth hormones or antibiotics, worrying about the safety of genetically modified foods (GMOs), overcooking food (thus losing nutrition) or eating only raw food, and avoiding packaged food. These individuals spend a lot of time planning menus, measuring portions, and obsessing about health and diet. Orthorexic individuals develop nutritional deficiencies because they tend to omit entire food groups. Nutritional deficiencies can lead to medical complications such as anemia, osteopenia, and metabolic, hormonal, and blood deficiencies.

Diagnosis of orthorexia nervosa is performed using a fifteen-point questionnaire, called ORTO-15. This questionnaire assesses the beliefs of patients about their perception of eating healthy, food selection attitudes, food consumption habits, and the extent that food concerns affect daily life. Responses are scored using a four-point scale; a score below 40 is considered diagnostic of orthorexia whereas a score higher than 40 indicates a healthy view of eating. In addition, blood samples are drawn to assess for nutritional deficiencies.

Treatment for orthorexia nervosa has not been standardized. After a diagnosis has been made, the patient is referred to psychotherapists and dietitians, and sometimes prescribed medication (often antidepressants) and behavioral therapy. Psychotherapists focus their therapy according to the patient's needs. Among the varied approaches, patients undergo cognitive behavioral therapy to restructure their thoughts and reprogram their minds to avoid obsessive behavior and attitudes toward their diet. It appears that patients who undergo these therapies have some success in changing their attitudes towards food, with correct education about nutrition.

—*Mandy M. McBroom, MPH;*
updated by Tish Davidson, MA

See also: Anorexia nervosa, Nutrition

For Further Information:

Bratman, Steven. "The Authorized Orthorexia Self-Test." www.orthorexia.com (accessed August 1, 2017). An extensive description of orthorexia and how to determine if one has it by the doctor who coined the term.
Brytek-Matera, Anna, et al. "Predictors of Orthorexic Behaviours in Patients with Eating Disorders: A Preliminary Study." *BMC Psychiatry* 15. (2015): 1-8. bmcpsychiatry.biomedcentral. com/articles/10.1186/s12888-015-0628-1 (accessed August 1, 2017). A scholarly article examining the traits that predict orthorexia.
Kratina, Karin. "Orthorexia Nervosa." National Eating Disorders Association. www.nationaleatingdisorders.org/orthorexia-nervosa (accessed August 1, 2017). Easy-to-understand discussion about where orthorexia nervosa fits into the general picture of eating disorders.
Reddy, Sumathi. "When Healthy Eating Calls for Treatment." *Wall Street Journal - Eastern Edition* 11 Nov. 2014: D1+. www.wsj.com/articles/when-healthy-eating-calls-for-treatment-1415654737 (accessed August 1, 2017). Newspaper article discussing whether and when orthorexia rises to the level of needing to be treated.

OSGOOD-SCHLATTER DISEASE

Category: Disease/Disorder
Anatomy or system affected: Knees, musculoskeletal system, tendons
Specialties and related fields: Orthopedics, pediatrics
Definition: Pain caused by the patellar (kneecap) tendon pulling away from the tibia (shin bone).

> **INFORMATION ON OSGOOD-SCHLATTER DISEASE**
>
> **Causes:** Rapid skeletal growth, repetitive motion associated with sports
> **Symptoms:** Pain below kneecap; swollen, bony bump
> **Duration:** Chronic during childhood
> **Treatments:** Usually self-resolving; alleviation of symptoms with rest, ice, elastic bandages, leg elevation, pain medications, brace or cast in severe cases

CAUSES AND SYMPTOMS

Osgood-Schlatter disease is most frequently found in young athletes during their years of rapid growth. It is more common in boys, who are typically affected between the ages of thirteen and fourteen. Girls usually are affected at younger ages, ten to eleven. However, children are at risk between the ages of ten and eighteen, especially during their rapid skeletal growth years. Children who play sports that involve running or repetitive jumping have the highest risk.

The most common symptom of Osgood-Schlatter disease is pain below the kneecap. There is usually a swollen, bony bump in that area. Pain is often felt when the bump is touched or when the knee is bent or fully extended in activities such as running, jumping, kneeling, squatting, or lifting weights. As the child matures, Osgood-Schlatter disease will usually go away. When children stop growing, the patellar tendon is stronger and the pain and swelling disappear. Very seldom does the disease continue after rapid growth stops.

If the pain persists, then the child should see a pediatrician or orthopedist. The physician will examine the knee area and the location of pain in order to make a diagnosis. If the source of the pain is unclear, then an x-ray will be taken of the knee to verify Osgood-Schlatter disease.

TREATMENT AND THERAPY

The best treatment for Osgood-Schlatter disease is simply rest. Depending on the severity of the condition, the child may have to decrease activity levels or stop playing sports for several months. Deep knee bending and jumping should be minimized, and running may need to be limited. To treat the pain, the knee should get more rest, and ice should be applied for twenty minutes three times per day. Elastic bandages should be used to compress the knee area, and the leg should be elevated when possible.

Over-the-counter pain relievers can be taken. In extreme cases, a brace or cast may be used.

After recovery from the pain, the child can slowly return to previous activity levels. Additionally, a physical therapist can prescribe exercises that will help strengthen the leg muscles around the knee to minimize the chances of a recurrence.

There is no surgical procedure for Osgood-Schlatter disease unless the patellar tendon is fully torn from the tibia. This should not happen if the patient gets proper rest, in which case Osgood-Schlatter disease will resolve itself.

—*Bradley R. A. Wilson, PhD*

See also Bone disorders; Bones and the skeleton; Growth; Orthopedic surgery; Orthopedics; Orthopedics, pediatric; Physical rehabilitation; Sports medicine; Tendon disorders; Tendon repair.

For Further Information:

Dunn, J. F., Jr. "Osgood-Schlatter Disease." *American Family Physician* 41, no. 4 (1990): 173.

Globus, S. "Osgood-Schlatter: More than Growing Pains." *Current Health 2* 28, no. 4 (2002): 20.

Kaneshiro, Neil K. "Osgood-Schlatter Disease." *MedlinePlus*, November 12, 2012.

Lackey, E., and R. Sutton. "Rest Is Best for Common Knee Swelling." *GP: General Practitioner* 1c (2003): 75.

Parker, James N., and Philip M. Parker, eds. *The Official Patient's Sourcebook on Osgood-Schlatter Disease*. San Diego, Calif.: Icon Health, 2002.

Woodward, A. H. "Osgood-Schlatter Disease." *Pediatrics for Parents* 11, no. 1 (1990): 11.

OSTEOARTHRITIS

Category: Disease/Disorder

Anatomy or system affected: Bones, hands, hips, immune system, joints, knees, legs, musculoskeletal system

Specialties and related fields: Internal medicine, orthopedics, physical therapy, rheumatology

Definition: A group of more than one hundred inflammatory diseases that damage joints and their surrounding structures, resulting in symptomatic pain, disability, and systemwide inflammation.

Key terms:

anti-inflammatory drugs: drugs to counter the effects of inflammation locally or throughout the body; these drugs can be applied locally or introduced by electric currents (in a process called "iontophoresis"), by injections into the joint or into the muscles, or by mouth; the three classes of these drugs are steroidal, immunosuppressant, and nonsteroidal

cartilage: material covering the ends of bones; it does not have a blood supply or nerve supply but may swell or break down

inflammation: the body's defensive and protective responses to trauma or foreign substances by dilution, cellular efforts at destruction, and the walling-off of irritants; characterized by pain, heat, redness, swelling, and loss of function mediated through a chemical breakdown

physical modalities: the physical means of addressing a disease, which include heat, cold, electricity, exercises, braces, assistive devices, and biofeedback

rehabilitation: a physician-led program to evaluate, treat, and educate patients and their families about the sequelae of congenital disabilities, trauma, disease, and degenerative conditions, with the goals of alleviating pain, preventing complications, correcting deformities, improving function, and reintegrating individuals into the family and society

synovium: the cellular lining of a joint, having a blood supply and a nerve supply; the synovium secretes fluid for lubrication and protects against injury and injurious agents

CAUSES AND SYMPTOMS

Approximately one in six people (more than 15 percent) suffers from one of approximately one hundred varieties of arthritis, and 2.6 percent of the population suffers from arthritis that limits their activities. Although many people over seventy-five years of age experience arthritis, the disease can occur in the young due to infections, rheumatic conditions, or congenital disabilities. Young and middle-aged adults experience the disease due to trauma, infections, and rheumatic or immune reactions. Arthritis may be located in joints, joint capsules, the surrounding muscles, or diffusely throughout the body. Inflammation of the joint lining (synovium) can similarly afflict the linings of other organs: the skin, colon, eyes, heart, and urinary passage. Those suffering from the disease may therefore suffer from psoriasis and rashes, spastic colitis and diarrhea, dryness of the eyes, inflammations of the conjunctiva or iris, frequent urination, discharge, and burning upon urination, and other symptoms.

The collagen-type arthritic diseases involve the binding materials in the body or connective tissues. They may be rheumatologic, generally more diffuse, in the distal joints (as in juvenile rheumatoid arthritis and rheumatic fever) or the skin and muscles (dermatomyositis). Psoriatic arthritis causes severe punched-out defects in the joints. Reiter's and Sjögren's syndromes involve the eyes and the joints. Genetic conditions, such as Gaucher's disease, frequently run in families. Metabolic disturbances, such as gout can leave uric acid deposits in the skin and the joints. Gout sufferers experience very painful, hot, tender, and swollen joints—often in the large toe. Immunologically mediated arthritides may be associated with infections, liver diseases, bowel disturbances, and immune deficiencies. Localized infections may be bacterial, viral, or fungal. "Miscellaneous disorders," a basket category, include conditions that do not fit into any above categories: Psychogenic disorders and arthritis associated with cystic disorders are examples. Arthritis may also be associated with tumors that grow from cartilage cells, blood vessels, synovial tissue, and nerve tissue. Blood abnormalities may give rise to hemorrhages into joints (a side effect of sickle cell disease and hemophilia). They can be disabling and very painful, sometimes requiring surgery. Traumatic and mechanical derangements—sports and occupational injuries, leg-length disparity, and obesity—may elicit acute synovial inflammation with subsequent degenerative arthritis. Finally, wear-and-tear degeneration can occur in joints after years of trauma, repetitive use, and (especially in the obese) weight-bearing. The most common types of arthritis are rheumatoid arthritis (also called "atrophic or proliferative arthritis"), osteoarthritis, hypertrophic arthritis, and degenerative arthritis.

The inflammatory reactions in response to injury or disease consist of fluid changes—the dilation of blood vessels accompanied by an increase in the permeability of the blood vessel walls and outflow of fluids and proteins. Harmful substances are immobilized with immune reactions and removed by the cellular responses of phagocytosis and digestion of foreign materials, resulting in the proliferation of fibrous cells to wall off the damaging substances, leading to scar formation and deformities. The chemical reactions to injury commence with the degradation of phospholipids when enzymes are released by injured tissue. Phospholipids—fatty material that is normally present—break down into arachidonic acid, which is further broken down by other enzymes, lipoxygenase, and cyclooxygenase, re-

sulting in prostaglandins and eicosanoic acids. Most anti-inflammatory medications attempt to interfere with the enzymatic degradation process of phospholipids. They could damage the liver and kidneys and the body's blood-clotting ability.

The physician bases the diagnosis of arthritic disease on the patient's medical history and a physical examination. The history will elicit the onset of pain and its relation to the time of day and difficulties performing the activities of daily living. Specific procedures such as joint aspiration, laboratory studies, and X-ray or magnetic resonance imaging (MRI) may help establish the diagnosis and the treatment. Functional classification has evolved that is similar to the cardiac functional classification: Class 1 patients perform all usual activities without a handicap; class 2 patients perform normal activities adequately with occasional symptoms and signs in one or more joints but still do not need to limit their activities; class 3 patients find that they must limit some activities and may require assistive devices; class 4 patients are unable to perform activities, are largely or wholly incapacitated, and are bedridden or confined to a wheelchair, requiring assistance in self-care.

A person's medical history or surgical conditions and medications can influence the physician's diagnosis and prescription for treatment. Patients may present a gross picture of the body to the physician showing the joints involved in their symmetry (whether distal or proximal, and whether weight-bearing or posttraumatic in distribution). Physicians may ask (verbally or by questionnaire) for a history of other system complaints, which they can check more thoroughly. The physician will check the joints, skin, eyes, abdomen, heart, and urinary tract during a physical examination. The neuromuscular evaluation may reveal localized tenderness of the joints or muscles, swelling, wasting, weakness, and abnormal motions. Joints may have weakened ligamentous, muscle, and tendon supports that could give rise to instability or grinding of joints, with subsequent roughening of cartilage surfaces. The arthritides are frequently associated with muscular pains called "fibrositis" and "myofascial pain syndromes."

Fibrositis is a diffuse muscular pain syndrome with tenderness in the muscles, no muscle spasms, and no limitations in motion; all laboratory tests are within normal limits. It is frequent in postmenopausal women who have a history of migraines, cold extremities, spastic colitis, softening of the bone matrix accompanied by loss of minerals, and irritability. Myofascial trigger points can be found in men and women with acutely tender nodules, or cords felt in muscles. The pain of these trigger points is referred to more distal areas of the muscles that may not be tender to touch.

Normal knee vs. one affected by Osteoarthritis. Image by Bruce Blaus, via Wikimedia Commons

Physicians may frequently miss the acutely tender trigger points. Tests will show whether the pain occurs when muscles are contracted with motion when muscles are contracted without motion, or when motion is carried out passively by the examiner without muscular effort by the patient.

Joint pathology is generally associated with some limitation in the range of motion. Sensation testing, muscle strength, and reflex changes may also indicate nerve tissue damage. Nerves occasionally pass close to joints and may be pinched when the joint swelling encroaches upon the passage opening. This condition may result in carpal tunnel syndrome. The median nerve at the wrist becomes pinched, causing pain, numbness, and weakness in the hand. Pinched nerves may also be associated with tarsal tunnel syndrome. The nerve at the inner side of the ankle joint may be compressed and cause similar complaints in the feet. Other nerves may be constricted when exiting the spine and passing through muscles undergoing spasms.

The medications used to treat arthritis can involve the nervous system. An evaluation and estimation of the severity of the disease can be obtained by electrical testing, as in electroneuromyography. The nerves are stimulated, and their rate of transmitting the stimulus is measured. The normal transmission rate for nerves is forty-five meters per second. Neurologists can determine delays at areas of impingement by measuring the transmission rate of a stimulus from different points along the nerve paths. Abnormal or damaged muscles will cause muscle fibers to contract spontaneously or fibrillate. Arthritis may limit chest expansion during inspiration and after expiration because of arthritis in the spine or lung pathology. Involvement of the spine can also be measured by the posture, the ability to move the neck, and the ability to move the lower back.

Arthritis of the spine leads to a progressive loss in motion. The amount lost can be measured by comparing the normal motion with the restricted motion of the patient. Arthritis may limit the neck movement in all directions, rotation of the head to the sides can restrict the driving view, and the head may gradually tilt forward. The lower back may also exhibit restriction in all directions; for example, it may be limited in forward bending because of spasms in the muscles in the back. Tilting backward of the trunk may be limited and painful when the vertebral body overgrowth of osteoarthritis or degenerative arthritis restricts the space for the spinal cord. The nerves pinched in their passage from the vertebrae may thus cause radiculitis, irritation of the nerves as they exit from the spine, leading to pain and muscle involvement. Circumferential measurements of the involved joints and the structures above and below can confirm swelling, atrophy from disuse or inaction, or atrophy from a damaged nerve supply. When measurements are repeated, they can indicate improvement or deterioration. One type of arthritis that most often affects the spine is ankylosing spondylitis. It occurs predominantly in males in their late teenage and early adult years.

Testing of blood for cells, chemicals, or enzymes is helpful. The simplest test—the sedimentation (or "sed") test—measures how blood cells settle out of the plasma. Normally, women have a more rapid rate of sedimentation than men. When this rate exceeds the normal range, active inflammation in the body is indicated. Comparisons of sed tests performed at different stages can reveal the disease's rate of progression or improvement. The chemicals tested may include uric acid for gout and sugar for diabetes. Blood tests for immune substances and antibodies are also possible. However, the American College of Rheumatology recommends avoiding comprehensive testing of antibodies. The joint fluid can be aspirated and analyzed, particularly for appearance, density, number of blood cells, and sugar levels. Cloudy fluid, the tendency to form clots, a high cell count, and lower-than-normal sugar levels in the joint fluid (compared to the overall blood sugar level) indicate abnormalities. With inflammatory arthritides, the X-rays will show the results of synovial fluid and cellular overabundance. Clumps of pannus break off and may destroy the cartilage and bone. Because of increased vascularity and blood flow, Bones in these joints have fewer minerals. They will appear less dense, a condition known as osteoporosis.

Deformities in inflammatory arthritis may result from unequal muscle pulls or the destruction or scarring of tissues; such deformities can occasionally be prevented by using resting splints, which are most important for the hands.

Degenerative and posttraumatic arthritis show joint narrowing, thinning of the cartilage layer, hardening of the underlying bone (called "eburnation"), and marginal overgrowth of the underlying bone (called "osteophytes"), resulting in osteoarthritis. Osteophytes, or marginal lipping in the back, may enhance symptoms of lower back pain. The cushions between the vertebrae, called "discs," are more than 80 percent water, which diminishes with aging, bringing the joints in the back (the facets) closer together and compressing the facet joints between the vertebrae. Irritation and arthritis of these joints are the results. Other organ structures may be involved as well.

A diagnosis of rheumatoid arthritis should include two to four of the following criteria: morning stiffness, three or more joints involved symmetrically (especially the hands), six weeks or longer in duration, rheumatoid nodules that can be felt under the skin, blood tests showing a serum rheumatoid factor, and the radiographic evidence described above.

TREATMENT AND THERAPY

Treating arthritis may vary from home treatment to outpatient treatment to hospitalization for acute, surgical, and rehabilitative care. Educating patients about their condition, prognosis, treatment goals, and treatment methods are necessary. Patients must be aware of warning signs of progression, drug effects, local and systemic side effects of drug therapy, and diet associated with relieving pain, stiffness, and inflammation. Suppose surgery is contemplated for joint replacement or other reasons. In that case, the surgeon should fully inform patients about expectations and the rate of functional activities. Postoperative restrictions in the range of motion must be given; hip bending should not exceed ninety degrees for hip replacement. Patients must limit the rotation and overlapping of their legs initially after surgery.

Some physicians provide a questionnaire that outlines the activities of daily living and recommends how a patient should perform such activities and how much time should be spent at rest. The goals generally are to maintain function, alleviate pain, limit the progression of deformities, prevent complications, and treat associated and secondary disease states. In patients with degenerative arthritis—most often the elderly, who are at risk for other organ failures—arthritides associated with systemic diseases and other organ involvements may require care. Patients with rheumatoid arthritis, for example, frequently are anemic. Anti-inflammatory drugs, normally used to treat arthritis, may cause blood loss through the gastrointestinal tract and even ulcerations. The physician may therefore prescribe alternative therapies.

Other therapies can include assistive devices, counseling patients and their families regarding home management, medicinal regimen and compliance, behavior modification, sexual advice, and biofeedback. The aim is to reduce the need for and frequency of medical care by balancing rest and activity and between effective drug dose, toxicity, and physical modalities. The patient may need various braces and assistive devices to protect joints and allow function. Scarring of a wrist joint can be alleviated by avoiding positions that inhibit function. Shoulders should not be left with arms close to the body since frozen shoulders aggravate neck and arm problems.

Physicians may offer physical therapy, occupational therapy, assistive devices for self-care, ambulation, or home and automobile modifications. Assistive devices may include reachers, an elongated shoehorn handle, thickened handles for utensils, walkers, canes, crutches, and wheelchairs. Homes may require ramps for easier access, widened doors to allow wheelchair passage, grab bars in bathtubs, or raised toilet seats for easier transference from a wheelchair.

INFORMATION ON OSTEOARTHRITIS

Causes: Traumatic injuries, joint overuse, obesity, genetic or metabolic diseases

Symptoms: Joint pain (commonly in hands, hips, knees, spine); stiffness in morning or after long periods of immobility; development of nodes

Duration: Chronic and progressive

Treatments: Occupational therapy; physical therapy; moderate exercise; heat therapy (warm soaks, paraffin, mud treatments); pain medications such as topical analgesic ointments, acetaminophen, NSAIDs (ibuprofen, naproxyn); COX-2 inhibitors; glucosamine; chondroitin; injections of cortisone or hyaluronic acid; surgery in severe cases

---

Heat therapy may reduce the pain, loosening and liquefying tightened tissues. Somewhat like gelatin, tissue liquefies when heated and solidifies when cooled. Patients frequently will be stiffer after protracted rest periods (for example, on waking) and feel better after some activity and exercise. Heated pools offer an excellent heating and exercise modality. The type of heat modality used will depend upon the depth of heating desired. Hot packs and infrared lamps will predominantly heat the skin surface areas and some underlying muscles. Diathermy units heat the muscular layers, and ultrasound treatments heat the deepest bony layers. Ultrasound (but not diathermy) can even be used in patients with metallic implants such as joint replacements.

Transcutaneous electrical nerve stimulation can be used to alleviate pain. The units can regulate the frequency of electrical impulses. The usual starting rate is 100 cycles, which can alleviate pain in a few minutes; this rate is later changed to 4 cycles, which will give hours of relief even when discontinued. The intensity can also be varied. The sensation desired is a slight tingle. The effect described induces an increase in the release of beta-endorphin, a substance naturally produced by the body with effects similar to morphine. Endorphin is produced by other physical therapy procedures, including hypnosis, acupuncture, suggestion, and stress, among others.

Patients in chronic pain may show a reduced level of beta-endorphin, and an increase in substance P. They may find no relief of pain with physical therapy. Substance P is a small peptide that increases the nerves' sensitivity to stimuli, producing greater pain. Patients with chronic pain may show depression, hysteria, and hypochondriasis on the Minnesota Multiphasic Personality Inventory and may require antidepressants. Exercise programs can help to increase endorphin levels. These exercises may range from simple movements performed by a therapist (the patient remaining passive) to active exertion against loads for strength. Stretching or gentle, intermittent traction may gradually decrease contractures. Still, neck traction should not be used in patients with rheumatoid arthritis of the neck.

Surgery may occasionally be necessary to alleviate pain, replace joints, or alleviate contractures. Isometric or static exercises can mobilize muscles without joint movement and maintain muscle viability during joint pain. Individuals can, however, be trained to perform activities more efficiently and effectively, thus saving energy. Posture training may alleviate postural muscle fatigue. In acute stages of inflammation, the treatment choices are rest, ice, compression, proper positioning, and medicines for pain and inflammation. Heat modalities should not be used in acute cases since the speed of chemical reactions increases on heating; the chemical enzyme activity of collagenase that destroys cartilage could increase the rate and extent of the damage. The simplest way to prepare cold applications is to fill a plastic container with water and refrigerate it. Physicians may also use fluoromethane or other refrigerant sprays. The hot packs sold in pharmacies can similarly be soaked in water and placed in the refrigerator to create an ice pack.

The medicinal approach utilizes nonsteroidal anti-inflammatory drugs (NSAIDs), such as aspirin, indomethacin, ibuprofen, naproxen, piroxicam, nabumetone, and other drugs as necessary. NSAIDs effectively treat osteoarthritis pain, but they can cause gastrointestinal, renal, and cardiovascular side effects, especially in older adults, and should not be used long-term. When possible, consider topical NSAIDs for knee or hand pain instead of oral NSAIDs since topical agents have fewer adverse effects than oral medications. COX-2 selective NSAIDs, such as celecoxib, inhibit inflammation-induced cyclooxygenase and neither interfere with platelet function nor cause gastrointestinal toxicity. However, although celecoxib may increase the risk of clots in small blood vessels, its cardiovascular safety profile at commonly prescribed dosages is about the same as naproxen and ibuprofen. Acetaminophen is generally less effective than NSAIDs but is better tolerated at doses of four g/day. Above doses of four g/day, acetaminophen causes severe hepatotoxicity.

Other medications for osteoarthritis include the serotonin and norepinephrine reuptake inhibitor duloxetine. While duloxetine is also Food and Drug Administration (FDA)-approved for anxiety, it is also approved for neuropathic and osteoarthritic pain. Duloxetine, however, is only modestly effective. Additionally, it has side effects that include headache, nausea, sleepiness, insomnia, dry mouth, constipation, diarrhea, decreased appetite, excessive sweating, and elevated blood pressure.

Opioids, such as tramadol relieve osteoarthritis pain. Surprisingly, opioids only provide slightly more relief than placebos in clinical trials. Furthermore, continued use of opioids can lead to dependence and tolerance to their effects. Opioids should not be considered first-line treatments for osteoarthritis pain but reserved as last resort medications for patients with intractable osteoarthritis pain.

Corticosteroid injections (methylprednisolone or triamcinolone) into the joint capsules are generally safe and effective for the local treatment of osteoarthritis. Such treatments provide pain relief that diminishes two months after administration. Still, most clinicians wait at least three months between injections. These treatments can accelerate cartilage destruction in affected joints.

Injections of commercially available hyaluronic acid preparations into the joint space may increase the viscosity and elasticity of synovial fluid. Increased joint lubrication may, in turn, prevent the degradation of articular cartilage. The FDA has approved intra-articular injections of hyaluronic acid for osteoarthritis of the knee. However, it has only modest beneficial effects. No reliable data shows that hyaluronic acid injections slow the progression of osteoarthritis.

PERSPECTIVE AND PROSPECTS

Historically, arthritis was treated with electric eels (as the source of electric shocks) and warm baths or sands. Some experimental treatments presently being tried include electric current to joints to reduce intra-articular pressures and the fluid and cellular content in joints. Acupuncture seems to increase beta-endorphin levels and relieve pain. Unfortunately, extensive reviews of controlled clinical trials have shown that acupuncture has little or no impact on arthritis. Topical use of capsaicin, an extract from peppers, is reported to counteract substance P. One group is attempting the experimental procedure of washing out inflamed joints with a saline-type solution. Though widely promoted for pain relief and joint mobility, turmeric has not been approved by the FDA for any indication. Exercises maintain and improve strength, agility, range of motion, and endurance. Good health habits-including adequate rest, good nutrition, and nutritional supplements, can be beneficial.

—*Michael A. Buratovich, PhD*

For Further Information:
For Patients and Caregivers. American College of Rheumatology, n.d., www.rheumatology.org/I-Am-A/Patient-Caregiver. Accessed 10 Apr. 2022.
Osteoarthritis. American College of Rheumatology, *Dec. 2021,* www.rheumatology.org/I-Am-A/Patient-Caregiver/Diseases-Conditions/Osteoarthritis. *Accessed 10 Apr. 2022.*

Osteoarthritis. Arthritis Foundation, n.d., www.arthritis.org/diseases/osteoarthritis. Accessed 10 Apr. 2022.

Osteoarthritis. Cleveland Clinic, n.d., my.clevelandclinic.org/health/diseases/5599-osteoarthritis. Accessed 10 Apr. 2022.

Osteoarthritis. Mayo Clinic, 16 Jun. 2021, www.mayoclinic.org/diseases-conditions/osteoarthritis/symptoms-causes/syc-20351925. Accessed 10 Apr. 2022.

Osteoarthritis. The National Institute of Arthritis and Musculoskeletal and Skin Diseases, Oct. 2019, www.niams.nih.gov/health-topics/osteoarthritis. Accessed 10 Apr. 2022.

Osteoarthritis (OA). The Centers for Disease Control and Prevention, 27 Jul. 2020, www.cdc.gov/arthritis/basics/osteoarthritis.htm. Accessed 10 Apr. 2022.

What is Arthritis? Versus Arthritis, n.d., www.versusarthritis.org/about-arthritis/conditions/osteoarthritis/. Accessed 10 Apr. 2022.

OSTEOCHONDRITIS JUVENILIS

Category: Disease/Disorder
Also known as: Legg-Calvé-Perthes disease, coxa plana, pseudocoxalgia
Anatomy or system affected: Bones, circulatory system, hips, joints, musculoskeletal system
Specialties and related fields: Orthopedics, vascular medicine
Definition: The disturbance of the blood supply to the tops of the thigh bones, resulting in their destruction.

CAUSES AND SYMPTOMS
Osteochondritis juvenilis may be the result of trauma and damage to the blood vessels that serve the thigh bone (femur) in children, aged approximately two to twelve years. The patient, who in the majority of cases is male, usually experiences tenderness in the hip joint area during the early stages of the disease, accompanied by limping, pain in the thigh or knee, and limited movement of the leg. Usually it is difficult to rotate the leg or move it sideways. In 90 percent of cases, only one leg is affected. In such cases, one leg may be shorter than the other, and the child favors the affected leg. If the disease is not treated, atrophy of the thigh muscle results.

TREATMENT AND THERAPY
Most cases of osteochondritis juvenilis do not require treatment beyond observation, particularly with children under the age of six who have a small amount of damage. For children over six with most of the joint affected, a more aggressive therapy is needed, and older children with the disease are at greater risk for osteoarthritis later in live.

Physical therapy, coupled with braces and crutches or bed rest with traction, is used in the most severe

---

INFORMATION ON OSTEOCHONDRITIS JUVENILIS

Causes: Trauma and damage to blood vessels that serve thigh bone
Symptoms: In early stages, tenderness in hip joint, limping, pain in thigh or knee, limited leg movement
Duration: Chronic
Treatments: Physical therapy, braces and crutches, bed rest with traction

---

cases. For most children, a Scottish Rite brace is used. Such a brace is belted around the waist and wrapped around the thighs, with a bar holding the knees apart so that the legs are held at a slight angle away from the body. The child wears the brace until the bone heals, usually in about six months.

If the child is more than eight years old, if the brace is too restrictive for an active child, or if the brace must be worn more than six months, surgical correction may be recommended. In these cases, the end of the affected bone is reshaped and the tip of the femur placed back into its socket. Occasionally, the hip socket must be reshaped instead.

—*Rose Secrest*

See also Blood vessels; Bone disorders; Bones and the skeleton; Braces; Circulation; Joints; Lower extremities; Orthopedics; Orthopedics, pediatric; Osteonecrosis; Vascular system.

For Further Information:
Currey, John D. *Bones: Structures and Mechanics.* 2d ed. Princeton, N.J.: Princeton University Press, 2006.
Kellicker, Patricia Griffin. "Legg-Calve-Perthes Disease." *Health Library,* May 7, 2013.
Kliegman, Robert M., and Waldo E. Nelson, eds. *Nelson Textbook of Pediatrics.* 19th ed. Philadelphia: Saunders/Elsevier, 2011.
Perthes Association. www.perthes.org.uk/.
Shapiro, Frederic. *Pediatric Orthopedic Deformities: Basic Science, Diagnosis, and Treatment.* San Diego, Calif.: Academic Press, 2001.
Staheli, Lynn T. *Fundamentals of Pediatric Orthopedics.* 4th ed. Philadelphia: Wolters Kluwer/Lippincott Williams & Wilkins, 2008.
Wenger, Dennis R., and Mercer Rang. *The Art and Practice of Children's Orthopaedics.* New York: Raven Press, 1993.

OSTEOCLAST

Category: Biology
Anatomy or system affected: Bone marrow, bones, cells
Specialties and related fields: Endocrinology, geriatrics, hematology/oncology, orthopedics, pathology, pediatrics

Definition: Large, specialized multinucleated cells that breaks down extracellular bone matrix and reabsorbs its tissue components

Key terms:

acidity: condition of having a low pH, or more than the normal number of protons (H⁺s), which can destroy adjacent tissue

apoptosis: controlled process by which cells systematically shrink and self-destruct in response to a particular signal, in a programmed cell suicide

hydrolysis: the process of breaking down a compound, such as a protein or other complex structure, by inserting an H_2O molecule to break a covalent bond

lacuna: the small pit, or 'lake,' that an osteoclast forms over a section of bone about to be resorbed

macrophage: the general term for the large polymorphonuclear immune cells, found in numerous locations in the body, that work primarily by phagocytosing, or 'eating,' extracellular tissues

osteoblast: specialized mononucleate cell that produces the extracellular component of bone

osteoid: the extracellular substance that makes up about half the volume and mass of bone and becomes mature bone once mineralized, primarily with calcium and phosphate

protease: an enzyme that catalyzes the breakdown of proteins

STRUCTURE AND FUNCTIONS

Like all the dynamic, non-static tissues in the body, bone is a living substance that must be continuously broken down and resynthesized in order to function. Bone turnover happens at the cellular level and is controlled primarily by two cell types: osteoblasts and osteoclasts. Whereas osteoblasts are anabolic cells that synthesize new bone, making complex proteins from amino acids, sugars, and minerals, osteoclasts are catabolic cells that break down these materials—particularly type 1 collagen—into their basic components, such as calcium, phosphate, collagen, and water. Normal osteoclast function is necessary for ongoing remodeling of bone throughout the human lifespan, and either overactivity or underactivity of osteoclasts can lead to disease, such as osteoporosis, osteopetrosis, Paget's disease of bone, or nonunion of a fracture. Osteoclastic activity is also necessary for dissolving small bone fragments that get broken down and reabsorbed after a fracture, and for helping bones in children to remodel into their adult size and shape. The word *osteoclast* comes from the Greek for "bone," *osteon*, and "broken," *klastos*.

Bone is a type of connective tissue and, as such, is derived from mesoderm, the middle layer of the developing human embryo. In a healthy adult, bone marrow is responsible for producing most of the blood cells in the body, including platelets, red blood cells, and white blood cells. Macrophages, a destructive type of white blood cell, are the most numerous cell type in the body, and they have different names and specialized functions depending on their location in the body. For example, Kupffer cells are macrophages that reside in the liver; microglia are macrophages that migrate to the brain and spinal cord; histiocytes are activated macrophages in the lymph system; and epithelioid cells are activated macrophages involved in a foreign body reaction. Osteoclast is the name for the specialized macrophages that resorb mature bone. Unlike the aforementioned types, however, these macrophage derivatives return from the bloodstream into bones after differentiating, then fusing together to form giant, multinucleate cells. Osteoclasts may have anywhere from 5 to 200 nuclei.

Most types of macrophages destroy tissues through phagocytosis, in which they reach out multiple projections and 'eat,' or phagocytose, foreign cells or substances. Since extracellular bone forms a highly reinforced, intricate structure, osteoclasts must adopt a different strategy in order to break it down. After receiving its activation signal, an osteoclast forms a sealed pit, also called a lacuna, over a section of mature bone. *Lacuna* is actually Latin for "lake," and they are so called because when viewed under a microscope, they appear to form small lakes within the areas of bone being resorbed. Because it is sealed at its edges, the use of a pit protects nearby bone from incidental destruction by the catalytic chemical processes generated by the osteoclast.

After forming a lacuna, an osteoclast degrades bone matrix through several different methods. The most important of these are acidity, enzymatic reactions, and reactive oxygen species. Acidity refers to the generation of a low pH, which directly damages the extracellular bone matrix in the same way that acidity of the stomach breaks down food. Osteoclasts achieve this through ion channels, which pump charged hydrogen atoms, i.e. protons, directly into the sealed pit they have created. Enzymatic reactions destroy bone tissue through catalysis, in which special enzymes such as proteases break down proteins. Hydrolysis is the most notable way that proteases achieve this. Finally, osteoclasts also degrade bone matrix through the generation of reactive oxygen species. Reactive oxygen species refer to any oxygen-containing molecule in which an oxygen atom has an unpaired electron, also known as a free radical. Free radicals are highly chemically unstable and contribute significantly to the breakdown of molecules both in the setting of osteoclasts and also elsewhere in the body.

Type 1 collagen is the primary structural component of extracellular bone. After breakdown by osteoclasts, it reverts to individual amino acids and short chains of amino acids, namely lysine, proline, and especially glycine, which makes up more than a third of collagen. Other components of extracellular bone include minerals such as calcium and phosphate, and a large amount of water. After reabsorption, building blocks can then diffuse to other tissues in the body or remain in the bone for reuse by osteoblasts.

Numerous hormonal signals are known to influence osteoclasts. Chief among these is parathyroid hormone, also called PTH, which is made by the four small parathyroid glands in the neck and primarily regulates the concentration of calcium in the bloodstream. Parathyroid hormone release is triggered by a drop in blood calcium levels. In response, one of its actions is to indirectly stimulate osteoclasts, which will then increase the amount of bone they resorb in order to release calcium from mature bone and make it available for use in the bloodstream. Of note, low-level, pulsed increases in parathyroid hormone have actually been observed to have the opposite effect, stimulating osteoblasts and inhibiting osteoclasts. Thus, a synthetic form of parathyroid hormone called teriparatide has actually been approved as a last-resort treatment for osteoporosis. Estrogen is the other major hormone known to act on osteoclasts, which has an opposite effect in that it induces apoptosis, or programmed cell-death, of osteoclasts, and thereby decreases bone resorption.

DISORDERS AND DISEASES

Osteoclast dysfunction occurs primarily in one of two ways: overactivity, resulting in excess resorption of bone, or underactivity, resulting in pathologic hardening and stiffening of bone. Bone remodeling is homeostatic and requires an equal balance between formation by osteoblasts and turnover by osteoclasts. Disease can therefore occur anytime there is continued imbalance between these two forces.

Osteoporosis is an example of bone thinning and decreased density due to imbalance between osteoblasts and osteoclasts. Although its specific biochemical mechanisms are still under research, it is hypothesized to occur both from under stimulation of osteoblasts and from overstimulation of osteoclasts. Osteoporosis is a chronic process, however, and does not result in increased blood calcium and phosphate levels, unlike osteoclast stimulation by high levels of parathyroid hormone. Osteopetrosis represents the opposite end of the spectrum and is a disorder of osteoclast dysfunction. It occurs from loss of function mutations in the enzymes that generate the acidity in the resorption pit, such as carbonic anhydrase II.

Paget's disease of bone, so-called to distinguish it from Paget's disease of breast, is also known as osteitis deformans and represents a more complex example of osteoclast pathology. Paget disease is a dynamic disorder seen primarily in adults that proceeds through four phases, called the lytic, mixed, sclerotic, and quiescent phases. In the lytic phase, osteoclast overactivity predominates, and affected bones subsequently become thinner and weaker. In the mixed phase, osteoclasts and osteoblasts are both overactive and result in a disordered destruction and formation of bone. In the sclerotic phase, the osteoclast activity declines, and osteoblasts cause affected bones to become dense and brittle. Finally, in the quiescent phase, both cell types decline in activity, leaving behind an overly dense, poorly formed bone mass. It can be treated with bisphosphonates such as alendronate, arrest the disease in the early stages by inhibiting osteoclast activity.

Osteoclast dysfunction is also associated with masses and tumors. *Osteitis fibrosa cystica* is Latin for "disease process of the bone consisting of fibers and fluid-filled sacs" and is one such disease process involving osteoclasts. Although its root cause is typically due to primary hyperparathyroidism, it results in cystic masses of osteoclasts. Young adults can also develop tumors of osteoclasts, which are called giant cell tumors or osteoclastomas and usually seen at the ends of the long bones of the leg, i.e. the tibia or femur.

PERSPECTIVE AND PROSPECTS

Teriparatide is a relatively novel therapy for osteoporosis that was approved for use in the U.S. in 2002. Although parathyroid hormone is typically thought of as decreasing bone mass through its indirect action on osteoclasts, the pathway for stimulation osteoclasts begins with a signal upstream, from osteoblasts. Thus, in the same way that pulsating gonadotropic hormone causes normal gonad physiology, but continuous high-dose gonadotropic hormone suppresses gonadal activity, teriparatide, as a recombinant parathyroid hormone analog, stimulates osteoblasts without triggering osteoclasts if given in pulsating low doses daily.

Pharmaceutical treatment with bisophosphonates is the mainstay for osteopetrosis, which is primarily a disease of osteoclasts. But bisphosphonates are not curative, and thus can only forestall progression of this disease. Since osteoclasts are derived from bone marrow macrophages, bone marrow transplant can offer a more definitive treatment for osteopetrosis. However, bone marrow transplant for osteopetrosis may cause a pathologic increase in blood calcium levels as a side effect, which carries the risk of significant cardiac dysfunction.

—*Walter Klyce, BA and Derek T. Nhan, BS*

See also: Anabolism; Bone Marrow; Bones; Calcium; Catabolism; Enzyme; Macrophage; Osteoblast; Osteopetrosis; Osteoporosis; Paget's disease of bone; Parathyroid gland; Parathyroid hormone; Phosphate; Tumor; Vitamin D

For Further Information:
"Bone Cells." ASBMR Bone Curriculum, depts.washington.edu/bonebio/ASBMRed/cells.html.
"Major Progress in Understanding Osteoclast Function." Mayo Clinic, www.mayoclinic.org/medical-professionals/ clinical-updates/endocrinology/research-explores-mechanisms- regulate-bone-resorption-formation.
"Skeleton: Bone Growth." BBC. www.bbc.co.uk/science/ humanbody/body/factfiles/bonegrowth/femur.shtml.
"Your Bones." KidsHealth, The Nemours Foundation, kids health.org/en/kids/bones.html.

INFORMATION ON OSTEOGENESIS IMPERFECTA

Causes: Genetic disorder
Symptoms: Imperfect bone formation, multiple and recurrent fractures, bluish sclera of eyes, thin skin that bleeds easily, frequent nosebleeds, elevated body temperatures
Duration: Chronic
Treatments: Hormonal therapy, exercise

OSTEOGENESIS IMPERFECTA

Category: Disease/Disorder
Also known as: Brittle bone disease
Anatomy or system affected: Auditory, cardiovascular, dental, musculoskeletal, pulmonary, visual
Specialties and related fields: Cardiology, dentistry, ophthalmology, orthopedics, otolaryngology
Definition: A type 1 collagen defect leading to increased bony fragility and reduced bone mass, causing increased risk for fracture and extremity deformities. Also manifests systemically with heart valve abnormalities, pulmonary compromise, hearing loss, and dental abnormalities due to altered quantity or quality of collagen.

Key terms:
osteoblasts: cells responsible for the production of bone
osteoclasts: macrophage-like cells in bone marrow that degrade bone to recycle, remodel, and heal it.
type 1 collagen: a connective tissue protein involved in the structure of bone, tendons, and ligaments

CAUSES AND SYMPTOMS

Osteogenesis imperfecta (OI) is an inherited bone disease characterized by an overall low bone mass and increased skeletal fragility, leading to an increased risk for fractures and growth impairment. The disorder is transmitted autosomally—meaning on the 22 non-sex chromosomes—and, depending on the subtype, inherited in an either autosomal dominant or recessive pattern. It has an overall incidence of about 1 case for every 15,000 to 20,000 children.

The defect in OI occurs in the synthesis pathway for collagen, a vital structural component of connective tissue, and more specifically in the type 1 complex, which is the building block that provides the strength and stiffness for bones, tendons, and ligaments. Collagen is composed of a sequence of amino acids, the basic element of proteins, which combine to form subunits that are wound around one another to create a triple helix. These helices pack together in an organized fashion to form the fibrils capable of withstanding the significant forces necessary in bone. In OI, mutations occur in the structural genes that code for collagen synthesis (specifically COL1A1 and COL1A2), causing osteoblasts either to secrete severely abnormal collagen or an inadequate amount of collagen. Alternatively, OI is also caused by mutations in genes that cause: (1) defects in collagen modification (*CRTAP, LEPRE1, PPIB, TMEM38B*); (2) abnormalities in collagen folding and cross-linking (*SERPINH1, FKBP10, PLOD2*); (3) ossification or mineralization defects (*IFITM5, SERPINF1*); and (4) defects in osteoblast development combined with collagen insufficiencies (*WNT1, CREB3L1, SP7*).

Weakened bony architecture causes patients with OI to be particularly susceptible to skeletal deformities and ultimately fractures without obvious trauma. Fractures can occur anywhere in the body, but are most commonly seen in the ribs and long bones such as arms and legs. Many patients with OI will present immediately at birth with numerous broken bones because of trauma endured during the birthing process. Others may present during childhood, at which point OI can sometimes be difficult to distinguish from non-accidental sources of trauma, such as child abuse.

While the hallmark of OI involves increased bony fragility, contributing to various orthopedic manifestations such as fractures, scoliosis, and long-bone deformities, type 1 collagen is prevalent in numerous tissues, and, thus, can affect nearly every system in the body. Hearing loss is present in more than 50% of patients and typically develops between ages 20-40. This occurs because of the thinning and fracture of the bones in the ear, which are necessary for transmission of sound. Patients with OI also frequently have dental abnormalities because of the abnormal collagen in dentin, the substantive component of teeth. Defective tooth collagen causes a condition called *dentinogenesis imperfecta* characterized by abnormal pulp and a grey-to-yellow discoloration of the teeth. Other involvements in OI include thinning of the sclerae in the eye, which causes a blue color due to visualization of the underlying veins. However, of these extra-skeletal features, the most severe are the involvements in the cardiovascular and pulmonary systems. Cardiac involvement includes increased stiffness of the heart valves leading to poor pump function of the heart.

The pulmonary complications such as respiratory distress and pneumonias are typically the most devastating for patients with OI and usually occur in combination with scoliosis and rib fractures.

Given the wide spectrum of clinical features, David Sillence, an Australian physician, developed a classification scheme based originally on 4 distinct groups of OI. Types 1 and 4 have autosomal dominant inheritance, while types 2 and 3 are inherited recessively. Type 1 is considered the mildest variant and describes a triad of hearing loss, blue sclera, and fractures that occur primarily in childhood and decrease after puberty. Patients with type 2 are typically stillborn or die within the first few weeks of life secondary to fractures of the thoracic cavity that lead to respiratory failure and frequent lung infections. Types 3 and 4 are in the spectrum between types 1 and 2. Type 3 is characterized as the most severe, non-lethal form with a large multitude of fractures that continue beyond puberty with severe scoliosis. Type 4 is associated with a moderate set of symptoms between types 1 and 3. Since the original classification, four additional discrete categories have been identified, creating a total of 8 distinct groups.

TREATMENT AND THERAPY

Given that a cure has not yet been developed for OI, treatment is largely symptomatic. From a musculoskeletal perspective, treatment is focused on a combination of physical therapy, orthopedic surgery, and medications. Patients with OI have been shown to benefit from exercise programs that help to improve muscle strength and stretching for mobility. These therapies are started from the infant stage in collaboration with the parent, to teach them how to manage an unusually fragile baby. Surgery is frequently the primary modality for management of the high fracture potential in OI. The major procedures are insertion of rods described as "telescoping" which elongate as the patient grows are usually paired with osteotomies to cut and realign a misshapen bone. For OI scoliosis, bracing has been shown to have limited potential due to the fragility of the ribs. As a result, patients with OI frequently undergo fusion procedures of the spine to provide corrective alignment. Pharmacologically, bisphosphonates are the mainstay, with the idea that reducing the breakdown of bone by osteoclasts helps to increase the bony matrix to be more resistant to fractures. The improvement expected with bisphosphonates usually peaks within 2-4 years. Patients are also typically started on calcium and vitamin D, if their diet is not sufficiently fortified. Growth hormone is another medication usually started not because of abnormalities in the hormonal axis, but to improve overall bone remodeling by recruiting

Jordanne Whiley was born with osteogenesis imperfecta and at aged 14, she became Britain's youngest ever national women's singles champion in wheelchair tennis. Photo by Fernando Frazão/Agência Brasil, via Wikimedia Commons.

osteoblasts to increase bone formation and limiting bone resorption by osteoclasts.

Extra-skeletal screening is also an important adjunct to therapy for OI, specifically regular hearing screens and dental check-ups. In addition, evaluation with echocardiography is essential to evaluate for cardiac abnormalities, especially in the setting of an audible murmur or in patients with scoliosis or a history of rib fractures. Ultimately, a multidisciplinary team is vital for providing coordinated care to help patients with OI improve their mobility and daily functioning while keeping the comorbidities at bay.

PERSPECTIVE AND PROSPECTS

Although the molecular basis for OI has been identified for 40 years, research is still in the early stages of developing a targeted gene-based therapy to selectively increase or correct the mutation in type 1 collagen synthesis. Preliminary studies have focused on harnessing the potential of mesenchymal stem cells from bone marrow or fetal liver that can differentiate into osteoblasts as a potential mechanism for improving the bony structure in patients afflicted with OI. Several clinical trials have shown that such stem cell treatments are safe, and that implanted stem cells engraft into bone and improve bone density and quality. Patients in these trials were still required to take prescribed bisphosphonates. Thus, management involves a multi-modal approach to effectively treat the manifestations of OI.

—*Derek T. Nhan, BS and Walter Klyce, BA*

For Further Information:

Chan, Jerry, K. Y., and Cecilia Götherström. "Prenatal transplantation of mesenchymal stem cells to treat osteogenesis imperfecta." *Frontiers in Pharmacology* 2014; 5: 223.

"Osteogenesis Imperfecta Facts." *FastFacts — OsteogenesisImperfecta Foundation | OIF.org*, Osteogenesis Imperfecta Foundation, 2015.

"Osteogenesis Imperfecta - Genetics Home Reference." *U.S. National Library of Medicine*, National Institutes of Health, 5 Sept. 2017.

"Osteogenesis Imperfecta." *NORD (National Organization for Rare Disorders)*, National Organization for Rare Disorders, 2017.

OSTEOMYELITIS

Category: Disease/Disorder
Anatomy or system affected: Bones, joints, musculoskeletal system, blood
Specialties and related fields: Bacteriology, orthopedics, infectious diseases, vascular surgery, pathology
Definition: A secondary bacterial infection of the bone and bone marrow.

CAUSES AND SYMPTOMS

Osteomyelitis is an infection of the bone with various organisms including bacteria and fungi. Since the advent of penicillin in the early twentieth century and subsequent antibiotics, the severity and mortality rate of the infection has significantly decreased.

Bones become infected when they are introduced to bacteria from events such as from trauma or foreign bodies. Most commonly the bacteria is *Staphylococcus aureus*. Bone can be infected via the hematogenous route, bacteria travel from another source in the body via blood. Hematogenous osteomyelitis in children affects the long bones whereas hematogenous spread in adults usually infects the vertebrae. The infection can be from contiguous spread, which is more likely in a trauma or surgery setting when the bone has been ma-

---

INFORMATION ON OSTEOMYELITIS

Causes: Bacterial infection
Symptoms: Fever, drowsiness, dehydration, bone pain, localized swelling and redness
Duration: Several days to weeks
Treatments: Hospitalization, intravenous antibiotics, surgery

---

nipulated. Foreign bodies, including prosthetics such as hips and knees, can also be associated with osteomyelitis.

In children, bacteria usually enter the body via an infection of the mucous membranes in the throat or an infected wound in the skin. In the case of a heel puncture, a bacterium that breeds in old athletic shoes, *Pseudomonas aeruginosa* can be the culprit. In the elderly or debilitated adults, infections can spread to the bone from skin ulcers that are found on points of constant pressure such as hips and buttocks.

Symptoms of osteomyelitis usually include fever, bone pain, swelling, and redness of the affected area. Other general symptoms may also occur such as fatigue, malaise, or abnormal lab results. When a joint near the infected area is flexed, severe pain and tenderness can result. With a heel puncture, the heel tends to hurt and swell, but there is often no fever. Over time, the bacteria form pus and can eventually start to have a foul odor.

TREATMENT AND THERAPY

Some patients may undergo radiologic evaluation with magnetic resonance imaging (MRI) or computed tomography (CT) imaging or have a bone biopsy to assess the infection and guide treatment plans. If osteomyelitis is discovered early, antibiotics can be administered for four to six weeks but may need to be given for longer periods of time. Initial treatment is usually given intravenously and patients are hospitalized. Once lab results and temperature return to normal, and blood cultures and sensitivities are obtained, the antibiotic regimen can be tailored to the specific organism or organisms causing the infection. The patient then has an option of continuing treatment outside the hospital with antibiotic administration via a peripherally inserted central catheter (PICC) line. During this time, the affected bones should not be exposed to undue stress until easy, pain-free movement is achieved. The injured area may be immobilized. Risks during the time of treatment include fracture and the development of osteoporosis.

In severe cases—cases in which the infection was not discovered early—surgery that removes the infected bone or bone marrow may be necessary. If the osteomyelitis is not treated, the infection enters the bloodstream and the disease becomes chronic. Extensive bone damage, arthritis, abscesses, or necrosis can occur. Treatment may involve debridement or, in extreme cases, amputation of the infected bone.

Some patients are at an increased risk for longer recovery times due to various comorbidities that delay bone and wound healing such as diabetes mellitus or arterial disease. Thus, treatment may also include vascular surgery. if the patient has extensive vascular disease that could potentially impair the healing process. Patients who choose to enhance recovery time may be a candidate for hyperbaric oxygen therapy that delivers extra oxygen to the body in hopes of enhancing nutrients required for the healing process. This is in adjunct to antibiotic therapy.

—*Nhi Nai, MD*

See also: Amputation; Antibiotics; Arthritis; Bacterial infections; Bone disorders; Bone marrow transplantation; Bones and the skeleton; Infectious Diseases; Joints; Orthopedics; Orthopedics, pediatric; Osteonecrosis; Pathology; Vascular surgery; Wound care.

For Further Information:
A.D.A.M. Medical Encyclopedia. "Osteomyelitis." *MedlinePlus*, 30 May 2012.
Badash, Michelle, and Rosalyn Carson-DeWitt. "Osteomyelitis." *Health Library*, Sept. 2011.
Biddle, Wayne. *A Field Guide to Germs*. 3rd ed., Anchor Books, 2010.
Currey, John D. *Bones: Structures and Mechanics*. 2nd ed., Princeton UP, 2006.
Norden, Carl W., editor. *Osteomyelitis*. W. B. Saunders, 1990.
"Osteomyelitis." *Mayo Foundation for Medical Education and Research*, 30 Nov. 2012.
Osteomyelitis: A Medical Dictionary, Bibliography, and Annotated Research Guide to Internet References. Icon Health, 2004.
Schmitt, S. K. "Osteomyelitis." *Infectious Disease Clinics of North America*, June, 2017.
Wilson, Michael, Brian Henderson, and Rod McNab. *Bacterial Disease Mechanisms: An Introduction to Cellular Microbiology*. Cambridge UP, 2002.

OSTEONECROSIS

Category: Disease/Disorder
Also known as: Aseptic necrosis, avascular necrosis, ischemic necrosis
Anatomy or system affected: Bones, hips, joints, knees, musculoskeletal system
Specialties and related fields: Orthopedics, rheumatology
Definition: A disorder that occurs when the blood supply to bone is cut off, causing the death of bone tissue and leading to the collapse of joints in the affected areas.

INFORMATION ON OSTEONECROSIS

Causes: Interruption of blood supply to bone; may result from trauma, corticosteroid use, excessive alcohol consumption, bone disorders, cancer treatment
Symptoms: Joint pain and loss, death of bone tissue
Duration: Chronic and progressive
Treatments: Nonsteroidal anti-inflammatory drugs (NSAIDs), anticoagulants, statins, exercises, electrical stimulation, surgery (core decompression, bone grafting, osteotomy, joint replacement)

CAUSES AND SYMPTOMS

Osteonecrosis-from *osteo*, meaning "bone," and *necro*, meaning "death"-may be either posttraumatic or nontraumatic, in some cases with risk factors identified and in others with no known cause (idiopathic). Approximately twenty thousand new cases are diagnosed each year in the United States, most commonly between the ages of twenty and fifty, with the average age of onset at thirty-eight. Osteonecrosis is of equal prevalence in men and women.

Some risk factors seem to predispose people to osteonecrosis, including the use of corticosteroids (to treat inflammatory conditions) as well as excessive alcohol ingestion. Both steroid and alcohol use may lead to a buildup of lipids in the blood vessels, decreasing blood flow to bones. Injury to a bone or joint (such as a fracture) may damage the blood vessels, decreasing the blood supply and causing bone death. Medical conditions which affect the bone (gout, osteoarthritis, osteoporosis) may predispose someone to osteonecrosis. Cancer treatments (radiation and chemotherapy) and organ transplantation also increase the risk of osteonecrosis, as do other medical conditions including sickle cell disease and acquired immunodeficiency syndrome (AIDS). The medication Fosamax, a bisphosphenate used to treat osteoporosis, has been linked to osteonecrosis of the jaw.

Often, few symptoms occur in early stages of the disease. Preliminary symptoms include pain in the affected joint, followed by collapse of joint surfaces and increased pain. Pain occurs initially only when the joint is in use and later even at rest. The bones most commonly affected are the ends of the femur, the upper arm bone, and the knees, shoulders, and ankles. Within months to two years from the onset of symptoms, individuals may lose range of motion and suffer severe disability. Appropriate treatment must be undertaken to prevent the breakdown of joints, Therefore, immediate diagnosis is important. X-rays, magnetic resonance imaging (MRI), computed tomography (CT) scan, and bone scans serve as diagnostic tools when an individual is symptomatic.

TREATMENT AND THERAPY

Once the condition has been diagnosed, treatment should begin immediately. To decide on most effective treatments, physicians consider the age of the patient, the progression of the disease, the location of the bones involved, and the underlying cause. Treatment can be either medical or surgical. Medical treatments include the use of nonsteroidal anti-inflammatory drugs (NSAIDs) to decrease pain, anticoagulants (blood thinners) to improve blood supply to bone, and statins (cholesterol-lowering medications) to decrease lipid buildup in blood vessels, allowing improved blood flow to bone. Other medical treatments involve range of motion exercises, electrical stimulation to induce bone growth, and decreased weight-bearing on affected joints.

Surgical techniques used to treat osteonecrosis include core decompression, bone grafting, osteotomy, and joint replacement. In core decompression, the inner core of the bone is removed, thus reducing pressure within the bone. Core decompression is often followed by bone grafting to the decompressed area to support the joint. Osteotomy is a surgical reshaping of the bone to decrease stress on affected areas. Joint replacement is the surgical treatment of choice in advanced cases. Treatment may be an ongoing process that continues for years, as the disease progresses. Adequate treatment allows afflicted individuals to continue to live reasonably normal lives.

—*Robin Kamienny Montvilo, RN, PhD*

See also Alcoholism; Arthritis; Bone disorders; Bones and the skeleton; Circulation; Corticosteroids; Gout; Grafts and grafting; Joints; Necrosis; Orthopedics; Osteoarthritis, Osteoporosis; Steroids; Vascular medicine; Vascular system.

For Further Information:
Bianchi, Giancarlo I., and Pascual C. Giordano. *Osteonecrosis: Diagnosis, Treatment, and Management.* New York: Nova Science, 2013.
Icon Health. *Osteonecrosis: A Medical Dictionary, Bibliography, and Annotated Research Guide to Internet References.* San Diego, Calif.: Author, 2004.
Mont, Michael A., et al. *Osteonecrosis of the Hip.* New York: Springer, 2010.
National Institute of Arthritis and Musculoskeletal and Skin Diseases. *Osteonecrosis: Questions and Answers About Osteonecrosis (Avascular Necrosis).* Bethesda, Md.: US Department of Health and Human Services, 2011.
National Osteonecrosis Foundation. www.nonf.org.
Soucacos, Panayotis N., and James R. Urbaniak, eds. *Osteonecrosis of the Human Skeleton.* Philadelphia: W. B. Saunders, 2004.
Urbaniak, James R., and John Paul Jones, eds. *Osteonecrosis: Etiology, Diagnosis, and Treatment.* Rosemont, Ill.: American Academy of Orthopaedic Surgeons, 1997.

OSTEOPATHIC MEDICINE

Category: Specialty
Anatomy or system affected: Bones, muscles, musculoskeletal system
Specialties and related fields: Critical care, emergency medicine, family medicine, geriatrics and gerontology, internal medicine, physical therapy, preventive medicine, public health
Definition: The practice of medicine as dictated by the philosophy of treating the individual instead of merely the disease, by the belief that the musculoskeletal system is crucial to the health of the entire body, and by an emphasis on the interrelatedness of all bodily systems.

Key terms:

allopathic medicine: the traditional course of study leading to a doctorate in medicine; most practicing physicians are allopathic physicians

family medicine: the practice of medicine in which the physician cares for the basic needs of the family and emphasizes preventive health care, as well as the importance of the patient's environment

immune system: the system of the body that is responsible for the maintenance of health; includes the spleen, the thymus, bone marrow, and the lymphatic system

Medical College Admission Test (MCAT): a test of problem-solving skills taken by all candidates for medical school in the United States; used to predict which students will be successful

musculoskeletal system: the system of the body consisting of the muscles and skeleton particularly in relation to their role in the maintenance of health

obstetrics/gynecology: the practice of medicine which deals with the health of the female reproductive system; includes care of the pregnant woman and delivery of her baby, as well as care for infertile couples who need assistance in becoming pregnant

osteopathy: philosophy of medicine which emphasizes the treatment of the whole person, rather than only the disease; from the Greek *osteo*, meaning bone, and *pathos*, meaning to suffer or be in sympathy with

THE HISTORY OF OSTEOPATHY

Osteopathy is a medical philosophy that treats disease in the context of the whole person, taking into consideration the functions and interrelationships of all body systems as well as such factors as nutrition, environment, and psychology. The first college of osteopathic medicine was founded in Kirksville, Missouri, in 1892, by Andrew Taylor Still (1828-1917), a frontier physician and Civil War surgeon. By the opening decades of the twenty-first century, there were more than thirty colleges of osteopathic medicine across the United States.

Still was the son of the Reverend Abraham Still, a doctor as well as a minister. As a youth, Andrew often accompanied his father on house calls, where he helped with basic medical procedures. His study of medicine led to a doctorate of medicine (MD), and he was licensed in the state of Missouri.

During the Civil War and in his practice as a frontier doctor, Still became frustrated by his inability to cure patients using the available techniques. The suffering of his patients was difficult for him to tolerate. The lack of knowledge about diseases and their treatment drove him to reconsider ways to improve the lot of the ill and injured. He also suffered a great personal loss when an epidemic of spinal meningitis spread through Kansas. Three of his children died of the disease, and three others died shortly after they were born. These tragedies nearly caused Still to abandon his career, but, in spite of the fact that the practice of modern medicine was in its infancy, he was determined to find the answers that would help him conquer disease and improve the health of his patients.

After the war ended, Still spent his life studying, observing, comparing, and experimenting in the treatment of disease. His observations closely paralleled the theories that the Greek physician Hippocrates proposed two thousand years earlier. Both Still and Hippocrates encouraged the physician to concentrate on the patient, not the disease.

Still wanted to establish the first school of osteopathy at Baker University in Baldwin, Kansas. He was refused permission to do so, however, because his philosophy of medicine did not conform to the accepted medical practice of the day. He was ostracized in Kansas, and in 1874, he moved to Missouri, where he was still licensed as a doctor and was legally able to practice medicine. As an itinerant doctor, he gained fame throughout the area and was affectionately known as the "bonesetter." It was during this time that he perfected his practice of osteopathy. Still's reputation and popularity spread, and he soon required assistance in treating the patients who sought him out. He established the first school of osteopathic medicine in Kirksville, Missouri, as the American School of Osteopathy under the law governing scientific institutions in 1892.

In 1894, he received a new charter from the state of Missouri for an educational institution. By the authority of the charter, the school could have awarded an MD degree, but Still wanted his degree to be different and chose to award a doctor of osteopathy (DO) degree instead. During the next few years, osteopathic colleges became a trend, and at one time, thirty-seven of them existed, many of which were correspondence or diploma schools.

The American School of Osteopathy taught the art of manipulative therapy. Still and his followers believed that if they could regulate and correct malfunctions of musculoskeletal function, they could return the body to a healthful state. When possible, they also eliminated the use of drugs to treat disease. Although this approach now sounds extreme, at that time few, if any, drugs were on the market, and most had severe side effects.

At the time that Still was establishing the roots of osteopathy, many significant advances were made in medical knowledge and techniques, including germ theory, the development of antiseptic surgery, the development of anesthesia, and the reorganization of medical education. The emphasis of Still on the treatment of the entire person has taken on more importance in modern times with the development of the fields of holistic medicine and preventive care.

SCIENCE AND PROFESSION

The philosophy of osteopathic medicine suggests that a human being is an ecologically and biologically unified whole. Among its tenets are that the various body systems are joined through the nervous, endocrine, and circulatory systems and that if one region of the body is diseased, the entire body is diseased.

There are five basic premises of osteopathy. First, the unity of all body parts is a benefit that assists in the maintenance of health and the resistance to disease. Second, when the body is properly nourished and structural relationships are normal, the body is able to adapt to physiological changes that might otherwise put the body out of balance. Third, a healthy body depends on a healthy circulatory system and a nervous system that is able to conduct information to all areas of the body. Fourth, the musculoskeletal system does more than simply provide a framework for the body, and its normal function is critical to a healthy body. Fifth, it is not in the patient's best interest for the physician to treat only one aspect of the disease; the physician must treat the entire body and mind if the patient is to be cured. In modern times, the osteopathic physician uses manipulative therapy-in which rhythmic stretching and thrusting movements are used to realign joints and muscles properly-as one of many tools to cure the patient.

Osteopathic physicians and allopathic physicians have much in common. Both are members of the health care community who are fully trained physicians, who have taken a prescribed amount of undergraduate work, and who have received four years of training in a medical school. After completing medical school, osteopathic physicians take a one-year rotating internship in hospitals with approved intern training programs. They may then enter a medical specialty program which may require a three- to four-year residency program.

Both allopathic and osteopathic medical programs use scientifically accepted methods of diagnosis and treatment. In the United States, the graduates of these programs are licensed by the same state medical boards and can practice in all phases of medicine in all states.

Admission to a college of osteopathic medicine in the United States requires a minimum of three years of preprofessional education in an accredited college or university. Virtually all students in osteopathic school, however, have been awarded undergraduate degrees. Many osteopathic students were science majors in undergraduate school, but all areas of study are represented. Most schools require a minimum of two semesters of study in biology, physics, and inorganic and organic chemistry. Students are also required to take the Medical College Admission Test (MCAT), submit letters of recommendation, and demonstrate an understanding of osteopathic medicine.

During the first two years in a college of osteopathic medicine, students receive basic science and preclinical instruction in a classroom or laboratory environment. Students are required to take courses in anatomy, biochemistry, physiology, pharmacology, pathology, and microbiology.

Schools are organized along one of two lines. They teach either by discipline or by system. In a discipline curriculum, the student concentrates on one subject at a time, such as biochemistry or physiology. In those programs with a curriculum that is organized by system, the student will study one organ system from the perspective of various basic science disciplines. For example, when studying the circulatory system, the student would concentrate on the anatomy, biochemistry, physiology, and pathology of the blood vessels and heart before moving on to another system.

Most students of osteopathy are required to take the first part of an examination prepared by the National Board of Osteopathic Medical Examiners near the end of their second year. At the end of the second year or in the third year, the student concentrates on clinical instruction. Students of osteopathy may do clinical rotations in teaching hospitals, community hospitals, or physicians' offices in both urban and rural areas. Clinical instruction is designed to give the student experience in the diagnosis and treatment of a patient's symptoms. Students also attend seminars and conferences that are more specialized and that emphasize the disease process and the healing process.

The second part of the national boards is taken during the last year, and the third part is taken after the student has received the DO degree. After completion of the degree, the student participates in a one-year rotating internship in an approved hospital prior to selection of a residency program. Approximately 70 percent of all doctors of osteopathy enter one of the primary care specialties, including general practice, general internal medicine, obstetrics/gynecology, and pediatrics.

DIAGNOSTIC AND TREATMENT TECHNIQUES

Osteopathic medicine stresses the interdependence of structure and function. The application of manipulative therapy, and in particular joint mobilization, has been a hallmark of osteopathic medicine since its inception. Osteopathic physicians recognize human beings as complex biomechanical, biophysical, and biochemical organisms. They believe that structural disturbances can have wide-ranging effects that may spread to interconnecting systems. The biologic foundations of osteopathic medicine are based in the concepts of holism, homeostasis, unity of the body, environmental influences, and health-versus-disease.

Holism suggests that humans are whole beings that are not resolvable into component parts and that each "whole" is more than the sum of its parts. This premise can also be extended to mean that people are not isolated units-they are a part of their surroundings and thus are a part of their environment and the universe. The increased tendency toward specialization in health care would seem to be in conflict with this principle. Osteopathic medicine suggests a need to increase the number of generalists or primary care physicians to ensure adequate care of the whole person. It further requires time to know and understand the patient as a person in his or her own environment.

The concept of body unity suggests that the normal healthy body contains all the elements necessary to maintain optimum function. Osteopathic physicians would argue that when disease alters body function, there is adequate flexibility within the system to compensate for change and to return the body to a state of wellness. This concept is similar to the principle of general physiology known as homeostasis.

Homeostasis recognizes the fact that essential body functions such as acidity of the blood, body temperature, and blood pressure are maintained within relatively narrow limits. It is not unusual for these parameters to drift slightly from the norm, but they must be quickly and efficiently returned to normal if the body is to survive. Deviations that cannot be readjusted quickly lead to poor body function and even death. Therefore, the body expends much time and energy in maintaining homeostasis, which prevents changes in the environment from having a significant effect on body function.

The philosophy of osteopathic medicine presents the position that musculoskeletal function is important in the maintenance of homeostasis. If this system is "out of line" or in any way unhealthy, the body will have a more difficult time maintaining homeostasis. It further argues that a healthy musculoskeletal system is necessary for a healthy immune system and that an unhealthy immune system can interfere with homeostasis.

The osteopathic physician emphasizes the role of the environment in health. There is general agreement that a healthy environment contributes to a healthy body. However, a healthy environment here refers not only to the working and living environment of the patient, but also to all associates and family members who are directly involved with the patient.

The concept of health-versus-disease is central to the philosophy of osteopathic medicine. The osteopathic physician is not as concerned with the treatment of the disease as with the cause of the disease and the methods that can be used to prevent its continuation or recurrence. The concept of health implies that all components of the body are functioning as a unit and that all are contributing to the maintenance of homeostasis. Consequently, properly functioning circulatory, nervous, and endocrine systems are required. Disease, on the other hand, is present when cells do not receive appropriate circulation and/or nervous or endocrine regulation, causing a breakdown in the immune system or impairment of the adaptative mechanisms.

Although there are many similarities between allopathic and osteopathic physicians, some distinctions can be made. While the allopathic physician's philosophy emphasizes the value of the type of intervention used, the osteopathic physician stresses the importance of the body's ability to heal itself. Osteopathic medicine recognizes the musculoskeletal system as an important factor in the body's efforts to resist and overcome illness and disease. The major factor that separates osteopathic medicine from allopathic medicine is manipulative treatment, which is often called biomechanics. Osteopathic manipulative treatment is used in conjunction with other practices to provide the body with the means to cure itself.

PERSPECTIVE AND PROSPECTS
In 1894, when Andrew Taylor Still opened the first osteopathic medical school in Kirksville, Missouri, the medical community was skeptical of the methods of the osteopathic physician. Although Missouri was the first state to recognize an osteopathic medical school, there was resistance to licensing the graduates. In 1896, Vermont was the first state to enact legislation legalizing the licensing of osteopathy. Licensing in Missouri followed in 1897. By 1924, thirty-eight states had legally recognized osteopathy. In 1897, the American Osteopathic Association was formed to establish

professional standards of practice. Its objectives were to promote the public health and to maintain high standards of medical education in osteopathic colleges.

Members of the American Medical Association (AMA) were not as accepting of osteopathic physicians as was the general public. When World War I broke out, some allopathic physicians claimed that the osteopaths were insufficiently trained for military service. Although there was widespread disagreement across the country, these allopathic physicians were successful, and the osteopathic physicians were kept at home. This situation ultimately proved to be to the benefit of osteopathy: While allopaths were serving in foreign countries, health care in the United States was left to osteopaths.

In 1923, the AMA continued its efforts to limit the practice of osteopathic physicians by declaring that it was unethical for MDs to consult with DOs. In 1938, MDs were forbidden to engage in any professional relationship with DOs.

Acceptance of osteopathic physicians finally came in 1967, when the AMA voted to negotiate for the merger of the two professions. The American Osteopathic Association was not interested in such a merger, but allopaths and osteopaths were allowed to work side by side in hospitals, community health clinics, and offices throughout the United States.

In the United States in 2012, there were more than 82,000 osteopathic physicians across the nation, constituting almost 10 percent of practicing physicians. The education of osteopathic physicians is expected to have an increasingly important role in the United States as people continue to emphasize preventive and family medicine. In efforts to cut costs and to improve the availability of health care, the government and health care insurance providers have stressed the need for primary care-an area that has always been important to the osteopathic physician.

Two monthly journals are available in libraries throughout the United States: the *Journal of the American Osteopathic Association* and *The DO* These journals contain research studies from osteopathic physicians as well as articles regarding the profession and the education of its students.

—*Annette O'Connor, PhD*

See also Alternative medicine; Bones and the skeleton; Exercise physiology; Family medicine; Holistic medicine; Massage; Muscle sprains, spasms, and disorders; Muscles; Nutrition; Physical rehabilitation; Preventive medicine.

For Further Information:
American Association of Colleges of Osteopathic Medicine. *The Education of the Osteopathic Physician*. Rev. ed. Rockville, Md.: Author, 1990.

"About Osteopathic Medicine." *American Osteopathic Association*, 2013.

Chila, Anthony G., ed. *Foundations of Osteopathic Medicine*. 3d ed. Philadelphia: Wolters Kluwer Health, 2011.

Lederman, Eyal. *Fundamentals of Manual Therapy: Physiology, Neurology, and Psychology*. New York: Churchill Livingstone, 1997.

McKone, Walter Llewellyn. *Osteopathic Medicine: Philosophy, Principles and Practice*. Malden, Mass.: Blackwell Scientific, 2001.

Nicholas, Alexander S., and Evan A. Nichols. *Atlas of Osteopathic Techniques*. 2d ed. Philadelphia: Wolters Kluwer Health, 2012.

Still, Andrew T. *Philosophy of Osteopathy*. Kirksville, Mo.: Author, 1899.

OSTEOPETROSIS

Category: Disease/Disorder

Also known as: Marble bone disease, Albers-Schonberg disease

Anatomy or system affected: Hematologic, immunologic, musculoskeletal, neurologic, visual

Specialties and related fields: Hematology/oncology, neurology, neurosurgery, ophthalmology, orthopaedics

Definition: Defect in osteoclast function leading to impaired bone resorption, with increased density of bone but overall weaker bony structure and reduced bone marrow volume. Patients are thus more susceptible to fractures, bony deformities, and cranial nerve compression.

Key terms:

osteoblasts: Cells responsible for the synthesis of bony matrix

osteoclasts: Cells responsible for the resorption and digestion of the bony matrix

hematopoietic stem cells: Precursor cells for the production of various blood cell components, including red blood cells and white blood cells

CAUSES AND SYMPTOMS

Osteopetrosis describes a group of three inherited bone disorders that cause thickening and hardening of bone due to a defect in a type of cell called an osteoclast. The incidence of this condition ranges from 1 in 20,000 for the autosomal dominant inherited form, to 1 in every 250,000 live births, for the recessive subtype.

The bony architecture is dynamic and occurs via interactions between two cells—osteoblasts and osteoclasts, which both arise from bone marrow stem cells. Osteoblasts are responsible for synthesizing and secreting the bony matrix, laying the foundation for the ultimate development of bony structure. On the other hand, osteoclasts serve as their counterpart, working to remodel bone and calcified cartilage via reabsorption of bony tissue. This process of resorption occurs via the secretion of acidic compounds that break down the matrix and allow for the creation of various bony shapes as an individual grows.

Osteopetrosis occurs when mutations develop in the pathway for secreting these acidic molecules, thereby leading to unopposed action of osteoblasts, proliferation of the bony matrix, and increased density of bone. However, the primary bone matrix and calcified cartilage, which are not resorbed in osteopetrosis, are weaker than normal bone and thereby more fragile and susceptible to fractures.

Classification of osteopetrosis is based primarily on the severity of its clinical features and occurrence at different ages. In increasing severity, the three types include benign, intermediate, and malignant/infantile types. The benign or autosomal dominant variant, also known as osteopetrosis tarda, typically manifests in adulthood and is associated with increased fractures, scoliosis, hip osteoarthritis, and long bone deformities due to stress applied on the weaker bone. In addition, thickening of the skull can lead to narrowing around the cranial nerves including the optic nerve causing blindness. The other two subtypes—the intermediate and malignant variants—are inherited in an autosomal recessive fashion and are regarded as more severe.

The intermediate form usually appears within the first few years of life with an increased frequency of fractures and compression of the cranial nerves. Of the three types, these patients are most commonly affected by osteomyelitis, or an infection of bone, within the jaw.

The malignant, or infantile, form usually occurs within months of birth. It is the rarest type of osteopetrosis, but also the most severe. Its lethal nature occurs due to the bony overgrowth that narrows the bone marrow located at the center of bones. Marrow normally houses the stem cells vital for proliferation of blood cells, but it can be severely reduced in the malignant form of osteopetrosis, causing anemia and increased susceptibility to infections. Most infants with this type of osteopetrosis generally do not survive past the age of two and succumb as a result of severe bleeding or infection.

TREATMENT AND THERAPY

Various modalities are implemented, both surgical and non-surgical, to control the deficient resorption of bone that is central to osteopetrosis. Inteferon-gamma is an immune system modulator frequently prescribed because of its ability to increase the breakdown of bone, similar to osteoclasts. Other medications that have shown benefit include the steroid prednisone, which reduces the clearance of red and white blood cells. This both prevents anemia and reduces the risk of infection. In addition, a medication called Calcitriol—the precursor to the active form of Vitamin D—can help increase osteoclast production, and it has been shown to help reduce the frequency of fractures in osteopetrosis.

Surgical options may also be implemented for osteopetrosis. One option involves preventatively inserting nails into the medullary cavity of bones to fortify their structure in the setting of the increased fracture risk. However, caution must be taken, given that osteopetrotic bones are already weaker than normal bones and thus more likely to be damaged by an intramedullary nail than healthy bone would be. For patients with end-stage osteoarthritis, total hip and knee replacements have also been shown to be beneficial, since they allow for improved mobility.

PERSPECTIVE AND PROSPECTS

While 70% of cases of osteopetrosis fall into one of the three forms described above, the genetic underpinnings behind the remaining 30% have yet to be explained. Whole exome sequencing will likely play a role in this process to identify the key mutations in the osteoclast function that lead to this disorder. Further research into the mechanism of acid production by osteoclasts and the pathway for resorption of bone will also aid in the development of targeted interventions for treatment of osteopetrosis.

—*Derek T. Nhan, BS and Walter Klyce, BA*

For Further Information:

"Osteopetrosis - Genetics Home Reference." *U.S. National Library of Medicine*, National Institutes of Health, 2017.
Favus MJ, ed. Primer on the Metabolic Bone Diseases and Disorders of Mineral Metabolism, 3rd. ed. Lippincott-Raven; 1996:363-6.
"Osteopetrosis." *NORD (National Organization for Rare Disorders)*, NORD, 2015.

OSTEOPOROSIS

Category: Disease/Disorder
Anatomy or system affected: Bones
Specialties and related fields: Primary care, endocrinology, geriatrics, nutrition, physical medicine and rehabilitation, sports medicine, orthopedics
Definition: Decreased bone density caused by an imbalance of bone resorption relative to new bone formation, which decreases the number of interconnections in the bone and increases risk of fracture.
Key terms:
cytokine: proteins involved in cell signaling

fragility fracture: a fracture sustained after a fall from standing or when associated with a low bone mineral density
resorption: breakdown of bone elements
trabecular bone: also known as cancellous bone, the internal structural component of bone with a high surface area
T-score: standard deviations from average bone mineral density

CAUSES AND SYMPTOMS

Osteoporosis is a disease of the endocrine system. Multiple redundant mechanisms exist to maintain calcium and phosphorus in plasma circulation verses combining with collagen to form the inorganic component of bone. Part of bone homeostasis involves an equilibrium between calcium influx and efflux from the bone. Factors are summarized in figure 1.

Osteoporosis is a pathological state of bone demineralization causing weak trabecula, the structural component of the bone. Osteoclasts are specialized cells that breakdown bone; osteoblasts synthesize bone matrix by taking calcium and phosphorous from the blood. It is a dynamic process that alternates between breakdown and reconstruction of bone matrix, otherwise known as "resorption" and "formation," respectively. This constant remodeling uses multiple redundant mechanisms that are dependent on hormones, minerals, and cytokines, to establish an equilibrium. When bone resorption outweighs formation, bones become porous or less dense, and susceptible to fracture with minor trauma. Osteoporosis is a disease defined by decreased bone mineralization density. The World Health Organization (WHO) further operationalized this definition to be bone mineral density is 2.5 standard deviations lower than an average healthy woman, also known as a T-score of -2.5.

There are several mechanisms that disrupt bone homeostasis. Age and estrogen deficiency are the main contributors to bone loss, and several pathological

---

INFORMATION ON OSTEOPOROSIS

Causes: Aging, disease (e.g., hyperparathyroidism, multiple myeloma), amenorrhea, anorexia nervosa, physical inactivity

Symptoms: Increased bone fractures, severe and localized back pain, reduced height

Duration: Chronic

Treatments: Hormonal therapy (estrogens, calcitonin); drug therapy (bisphosphonates, teriparatide, slow-release sodium fluoride, calcitriol, raloxifene), calcium supplements

Figure 1. Factors Involved in Bone Homeostasis			
	Action	**Stimulated by**	**Inhibited by**
Osteoblasts	Lay down bone matrix (collagen, proteins)	PTH, estrogen, Romosozumab	–
Osteoclasts	Dissolves bone	Osteoblasts, RANK-L	Bisphosphonates, estrogens, Calcitonin, Denosumab
Parathyroid hormone (PTH)	Activates both osteoblasts and osteoclasts, activates vitamin D_3, increases calcium reabsorption in kidney	Low serum calcium	High serum calcium, Calcimimetics
Calcitonin	Inhibits osteoclasts, activates osteoblasts, increases calciuresis	High serum calcium	–
Vitamin D_3	Increases calcium uptake from the gut	PTH	Antiepileptics
Estrogens	Inhibits osteoclasts, activates osteoblasts	[genes x environment]	Aromatase inhibitors, androgen-deprivation therapy
Cytokines (e.g., RANK-L)	Activates osteoclasts	[genes x environment]	Denosumab

states that contribute to secondary osteoporosis. Estrogen inhibits osteoclast formation and induces apoptosis, leading to net bone formation; a lack of estrogen leads to an imbalance favoring bone resorption. Vitamin D deficiency leads to decreased serum calcium, causing a lack of building materials for bone formation. Cytokines are needed to signal osteoclasts maturity, and certain inflammatory states such as rheumatoid arthritis can cause a shift towards resorption. Cigarette smoking is a known risk factor for osteoporosis and is an area of active research to determine the exact mechanism for its association with decreased bone mineral density. Increased alcohol consumption causes a hypogonadism state and estrogen deficiency in men and women, as well as malnutrition and malabsorption.

Glucocorticoids have a multifactorial effect in the osteoporosis pathophysiology: inducing continuous parathyroid hormone (PTH) secretion which decreases bone formation and increases bone resorption, decreasing sex steroids which causes a relative estrogen deficiency, and inhibiting vitamin D metabolism. Some chemotherapy drugs (e.g., anastrozole, leuprolide) cause an estrogen deficiency state, some antiepileptic medications (e.g., phenytoin, valproic acid) interfere with vitamin D metabolism. Further research is needed to determine the exact mechanism for known determinants of decreased bone mass such as genetic factors, cigarette smoking, and other pharmaceuticals (e.g., proton pump inhibitor, lithium, heparin, and selective serotonin reuptake inhibitors).

Osteoporosis is a silent disease until a person suffers a fracture with minor trauma, such as a fall from standing. Although fragility fractures can occur at any skeletal site (excluding the face, skull, digits), the most notable fractures are vertebra and hip. Vertebral fractures have a range of presentations from asymptomatic or loss of height, to severe back pain that limits mobility and leads to deconditioning and isolation. Hip fractures often present with acute pain and deformities, requiring urgent surgical and medical intervention.

DIAGNOSIS AND TREATMENT

Asymptomatic diseases such as osteoporosis depend on routine screening by primary care physicians to diagnose and treat. The National Osteoporosis Foundation (NOF) as set forth recommendations for screening certain populations as outlined in figure 2.

Figure 2. NOF Recommendations for Screening	
Females ≥ 65yo Men ≥ 70yo	Postmenopausal females and males ages fifty to sixty-nine with risk factors
Adults > 50yo with a fracture	Adults with a condition (rheumatoid arthritis) or taking a medication associated with bone loss
	5 mg prednisone/day (or equivalent) for three months

A diagnostic workup for osteoporosis includes lab work and imaging with a Dual-energy X-ray Absorptiometry, or DEXA scan. 25-OH Vitamin D and serum calcium are the principal labs of interest, because deficiency could be corrected with supplementation. Low calcium would be indicative of vitamin D deficiency or malabsorption. High calcium would be indicative of hyperparathyroidism or malignancy, prompting further lab assessment of PTH and kidney function. A DEXA scan uses radiation to visualize and assess bone mineral density, which is reported according to standard deviations from normal, also known as a T-score.

The FRAX calculator is an online tool that uses patient demographics such as age, gender, body-mass index, smoking status, glucocorticoid use, alcohol use, and an optional entry for T-score at the femoral neck to estimate fracture risk. The WHO determined that risk is considered significant if there is a >20 percent chance of major osteoporotic fracture or >3 percent chance of hip fracture within the next ten years. It should be noted that secondary osteoporosis is an area of active research, and the FRAX calculator does not account for all known risk factors (chronic vitamin D deficiency, people living with human immunodeficiency virus (HIV), patients undergoing androgen deprivation therapy, physical inactivity). Nevertheless, the NOF has concluded that the following demographics are eligible for treatment of osteoporosis:

- T-score <-2.5
- History of fragility fracture
- Patients with an estimated ten-year risk of >20 percent major osteoporotic fracture or >3 percent hip fracture

After initiating treatment to correct any vitamin D deficiency, first-line treatment is with bisphosphonates (Alendronate, Risedronate, Zoledronic Acid,) which binds to and inhibits osteoclasts to decrease rate of bone reabsorption. Common adverse effects of bisphosphonates are esophageal irritation (with oral formulations), nephrotoxicity, hypocalcemia, osteonecrosis of the jaw, and atypical femoral fractures.

Raloxifene is a Selective Estrogen Receptor Modulator (SERM), which inhibits osteoclasts and activates osteoblasts. SERMs can only be used in women, and are contraindicated in patients with a history of venous thromboembolism, due to increased risk from the medication. Raloxifene and Tamoxifen for prevention of ER+ breast cancers, but Tamoxifen is not used for treatment of osteoporosis due to increased risk of endometrial cancer, whereas Raloxifene has no increased risk.

Cases of severe osteoporosis (T-score <-3.5) or refractory to first-line therapies are indications to consider Teriparatide, a PTH analog which stimulates osteoblasts with intermittent (daily) dosing. Teriparatide has high efficacy and an additional indication for glucocorticoid-induced osteoporosis, but it requires daily subcutaneous injections and carries a high economic cost.

Denosumab is a RANK-L inhibitor, which blocks osteoclast maturation. In addition to indications of severe osteoporosis or first-line treatment failure, Denosumab is indicated for androgen-deprivation therapy-induced bone loss and aromatase inhibitor-induced bone loss. The medication is not renally excreted and therefore it is often used for patients with chronic kidney disease. Upon discontinuation of Denosumab, there is a rebound decrease in bone density, therefore treatment is continued indefinitely once started. Although this medication also carries a high cost, injections are only given once every six months.

Romosozumab is a newer therapy, which is a monoclonal antibody that stimulates osteoblast metabolism, but has a US-black box warning for increased risk of myocardial infarction and stroke.

Among the lesser efficacy medications, calcitonin has a notable indication for an analgesic effect in acute fracture pain. Estrogens have a United States Preventive Services Taskforce (USPSTF) grade D recommendation for treatment, due to increased incidence of venous thrombus embolism.

Ongoing research is being undertaken to evaluate the optimal treatment length and screening intervals. Currently, recommendations are to repeat DEXA scans every two years or if considering drug holidays.

PERSPECTIVE AND PROSPECTS

According to the National Health and Nutrition Examination Survey III, approximately 9.9 million Americans carry the diagnosis of osteoporosis and 43.1 million Americans have low bone density. Females are disproportionately more affected than males, with one out of two females suffering a fragility fracture in their lifetime compared to one out of five males.

Fractures, especially in the elderly population, are a major source of pain, impaired mobility, loss of independence, and mortality. Studies have shown that hip fractures have a 2.5-fold increase in future fractures, and 8 to 36 percent increase in mortality within one year. Approximately 20 percent of hip fracture patients require long term rehabilitation care, and only 40 percent of patients regain their prefracture level of independence. Chronic pain and impaired mobility often contribute to decreased activity, social isolation, depression, and deconditioning which are compounding factors in morbidity.

In addition to screening for patients at risk for osteoporosis and fragility fractures, clinicians can undertake a risk reduction assessment to evaluate risk factors for falling such as low visual acuity, medications that cause orthostatic hypotension or sedation, deconditioning, lack of assistive devices, and urgent urinary incontinence. Glucocorticoids should be prescribed at the lowest dose and not be used for longer than necessary. Cigarette smoking and excessive alcohol use should be strongly discouraged. Patients with malabsorption, low body mass index, ovarian insufficiency, or undergoing androgen-deprivation therapy for prostate cancer should be screened and evaluated at an earlier age.

Vitamin D insufficiency is an independent risk factor for falls, and also indirectly increases risk of fracture due to decreased calcium absorption from the gut. Recommended daily allowances for vitamin D are 600 to 800 IU for all men and women under age sixty-five, and 1000 IU daily for women sixty-five and older. Serum 25-OH vitamin D levels less than 12 ng/dL should be corrected with 50,000 IU weekly, and then supplemented with 800 IU daily. Recommended calcium intake is 1,200 mg for women greater than age fifty and men greater than seventy, otherwise 1,000 mg daily for all other age groups.

Physical activity has a moderate effect in preventing bone loss but no substantial effect in gaining bone mass. Exercise has the added benefit of improving coordinating and balance, decreasing risk of falls.

Since a complete list of risk factors for has yet to be determined, clinicians should utilize shared decision-making to consider screening patients at risk for osteoporosis.

—*Shanelle Raugh, DO*

See also: Vitamin D deficiency, osteomalacia, hyperparathyroidism, estrogen deficiency, cigarette smoking, alcoholism; USPSTF guidelines.

For Further Information:
Cosman, F., et al. "Clinicians Guide to Prevention and Treatment of Osteoporosis." *Osteoporosis International*, vol. 15 Aug. 2014, pp. 2359-81doi.org/10.1007/s00198-014-2794-2.
"FRAX Fracture Risk Assessment Tool." *FRAX*, Centre for Metabolic Bone Diseases, University of Sheffield UK, www.sheffield.ac.uk/FRAX/tool.aspx?country=9.
Jameson, J. L., A. S. Fauci, D. L. Kasper, et al. "Osteoporosis." *Harrison's Principles of Internal Medicine*. Vol. 1, McGraw-Hill Education, 2018, pp. 2942-59.
Jeremiah, M. P., B. K. Unwin, M. H. Greenawald, and V. E. Casiano. "Diagnosis and Management of Osteoporosis." *American Family Physician*, vol. 92, no. 4, 15 Aug. 2015, pp. 261-68. PMID: 26280231.

OTOPLASTY

Category: Procedure
Anatomy or system affected: Ears, skin
Specialties and related fields: Audiology, family medicine, general surgery, pediatrics, plastic surgery
Definition: Cosmetic or reconstructive surgery performed on the outer ear.

INDICATIONS AND PROCEDURES
Otoplasty is performed to improve the appearance of the outer ear, typically to flatten protruding ears or to repair or reconstruct a missing or badly damaged ear. Since the ears have reached 90 percent of their adult size by the time a child reaches age five, the surgery can be performed either at this early age or later.

The first step in flattening protruding ears is to remove a flap of skin from the back of each ear. The underlying cartilage is then remolded, and the two edges of the wound are stitched together, bringing the ear closer to the head. Dressings are applied to the ears and left for a few days, when they are replaced by a headband that is worn for several weeks. The stitches are removed approximately one week after the surgery.

The reconstruction of a missing or badly damaged ear is a complex procedure that typically involves more than one operation, and long healing intervals are necessary between operations. The first step is to remove a piece of cartilage from a rib and sculpt it to resemble a normal ear. The cartilage is then transferred to a fold of skin where the ear will be located. A skin graft may be necessary. Dressings are applied to the ear for up to two weeks, and the stitches are then removed. In many cases, hearing in the reconstructed ear may not be normal. As long as hearing is normal in the other ear, however, no attempt is usually made to improve hearing in the reconstructed ear.

USES AND COMPLICATIONS
Possible complications associated with otoplasty operations include sensitivity of the ear to cold weather, especially during the first year after surgery, and skin graft failure. On rare occasions, excessive bleeding or infection of the surgical wounds may arise. For minor pain, the patient can take acetaminophen or ibuprofen. As the ear heals, a hard ridge usually forms along the incision, but it will gradually recede. The scar will be hidden in the crease between the scalp and the ear.

—*Alvin K. Benson, PhD*

See also Ear infections and disorders; Ears; Hearing loss; Plastic surgery; Surgery, pediatric.

For Further Information:
Converse, J. M. *Reconstructive Plastic Surgery*. 2d ed. Philadelphia: W. B. Saunders, 1977.
Davis, Jack. *Otoplasty: Aesthetic and Reconstructive Techniques*. 2d ed. New York: Springer, 1997.
"Otoplasty." *Mayo Clinic*, August 23, 2012.
Stedman, Thomas Lathrop. *Stedman's Plastic Surgery/ENT/Dentistry Words*. 5th ed. Philadelphia: Wolters Kluwer Health/Lippincott Williams & Wilkins, 2008.
Townsend, Courtney M., Jr., et al., eds. *Sabiston Textbook of Surgery*. 19th ed. Philadelphia: Saunders/Elsevier, 2012.

OTORHINOLARYNGOLOGY

Category: Specialty
Anatomy or system affected: Ears, nose, respiratory system, throat
Specialties and related fields: Audiology, neurology, pediatrics, plastic surgery
Definition: The study of the diseases and disorders of the ears, nose, and throat.

Key terms:

audiometer: an electronic device, often used in combination with a computer, that measures a patient's range of hearing

fenestration: the surgical opening of a passage in a closed or narrowing ear canal through which sound can pass

mastoidectomy: the surgical removal of the temporal or mastoid bone, which is located behind the ear

maxillofacial surgery: surgery of the face and neck, a form of cosmetic and reconstructive surgery

otologist: a medical doctor who specializes in diseases and disorders of the ear

stapedectomy: the surgical removal of all or part of the stapes or innermost ossicle of the ear

tomography: an X ray used in combination with sophisticated computers to create an image of a specific organ, blotting out everything in front or behind

SCIENCE AND PROFESSION

Otorhinolaryngology-whose practitioners are often referred to simply as otolaryngologists or ear, nose, and throat (ENT) doctors-is a medical specialty that requires a doctor of medicine degree followed by a hospital or medical center residency ranging from four to five years, depending on the institution in which it is served. Many physicians in this field develop subspecialties, for which additional training is requisite. Among the most common subspecialties are oncology of the head and neck, ear surgery, pediatric otolaryngology, and maxillofacial surgery.

The scope of the otorhinolaryngologist's job is broad and overlaps several other medical specialties, notably general surgery, neurosurgery, plastic surgery, pediatrics, ophthalmology, and oncology. The otorhinolaryngologist treats all diseases and lesions that occur above the clavicle or collarbone except for those belonging to two categories: diseases and disorders of the eyes, which fall into the province of ophthalmology, and brain lesions, which are usually treated by neurosurgeons.

Otorhinolaryngology has existed as a specialty since the late nineteenth century. The need for it was great because ear, nose, and throat problems had, through the centuries, been among the most persistent killers of human beings. The areas affected have much to do with the ability to take in food and air. They also are directly connected with speech, smell, taste, hearing, and balance. Dysfunction of the ears, nose, or throat can profoundly affect a person's well-being physically, emotionally, and socially.

Among the medical conditions and diseases that most frequently come under the purview of otorhinolaryngology are the following: cleft lip and palate deformities (which are often treated as well by plastic surgeons); thyroid tumors (which are also treated by oncological surgeons); skin cancers (which also fall within the practices of plastic surgeons and oncological surgeons); face lifts, the treatment of facial lacerations, and other reconstructive surgery (which plastic surgeons also handle); lumps on the salivary glands (which are sometimes treated by oncological surgeons); and jaw injuries, including fractures (which are treated by maxillofacial surgeons, many of them board-certified in otorhinolaryngology).

Some of the surgery once done by otorhinolaryngologists is now virtually unnecessary because of the development of antibiotics. For example, drugs can combat effectively the kinds of infections that used to result in mastoiditis (inflammation of the mastoid bone), which frequently required a mastoidectomy. The flexible fiber-optic endoscope permits doctors to look into areas that previously could be exposed only through surgery. Advances in research have revealed that nasal polyps, which had a high rate of recurrence and were removed on a continuous basis, can usually be treated effectively with antibiotics, making such surgery unnecessary.

Until the mid-twentieth century, the most serious operation performed by otorhinolaryngologists was the laryngectomy (removal of the larynx, or voice box). By the end of the century, however, many practitioners in this specialty were routinely performing surgeries on tongue cancers and thyroid tumors because otorhinolaryngologists are often the ones who initially discover these conditions during head and neck examinations.

Because otorhinolaryngologists have long dealt with the grafting of bone and skin and the surgical management of skin flaps, much reconstructive and cosmetic surgery now falls into their specialty. Removal of tumors from the base of the skull, the interior ear canal, or the posterior cranial depression by means of modified craniotomies can be done by otorhinolaryngologists, who sometimes work in tandem with neurosurgeons in such cases.

DIAGNOSTIC AND TREATMENT TECHNIQUES

The illnesses treated by otorhinolaryngologists have plagued the human race throughout history but could not be treated effectively until technology was developed that enabled physicians to look into the crowded crevices deep inside the body that were the source of many illnesses. In 1854, Manuel Garcia invented a concave mirror with a hole in its center through which doctors, attaching the implement to their heads, could peer as light from the mirror illuminated a patient's ears, nose, and throat. Doctors discovered that, using the reflecting head mirror in combination with an angled mirror held as far back as possible in the throat, they could illuminate the laryngeal area and the pharynx as well as the area behind the nose, all previously unavailable for visual inspection. Eventually, rather than examining affected areas with the bare eye, physicians had available to them, imbedded in the eyepiece of a hollow instrument with a light at the end, a magnifying telescope through which they could examine remote cavities with considerable ease and in great detail.

Modern otorhinolaryngologists can also examine patients under mild local anesthetic with sophisticated endoscopes, flexible devices that can easily be inserted into the nose, mouth, or ear of the patient. Such procedures are usually carried out in the doctor's office or in a hospital on an outpatient basis. These endoscopes, originally lighted with bulbs that heated up and burned out quickly, now carry light through light-bearing fiber-optic strands. In combination with small magnifying devices and cameras designed for this purpose, physicians can examine almost any area of the ears, nose, and throat and create color images, which can be invaluable in determining the presence of disease and in making an accurate diagnosis.

Modern technology has also made available to otorhinolaryngologists laser scalpels that permit extremely intricate surgery and accurate electronic audiometers. Audiometers eliminate the subjectivity of past tests of hearing acuity: In the nineteenth century, doctors either whispered into patients' ears, increasing the volume until their whispers could be heard, or used tuning forks to determine how much their patients could hear.

Treatment of disorders and diseases of the ear, nose, and throat have changed rapidly with the introduction of increasingly sophisticated surgical equipment and with the development of new drugs to control many conditions that once could be managed only by surgery. Computers have also been a valuable tool in diagnosing many of the problems that fall within this specialty.

All the anatomical areas with which otorhinolaryngologists must deal are interconnected; therefore a disease that begins in the ears can affect the nose and the throat, and vice versa. The most common diseases of the ears include deafness and Ménière's disease, an ill-

The Anatomy of the Nose and Throat

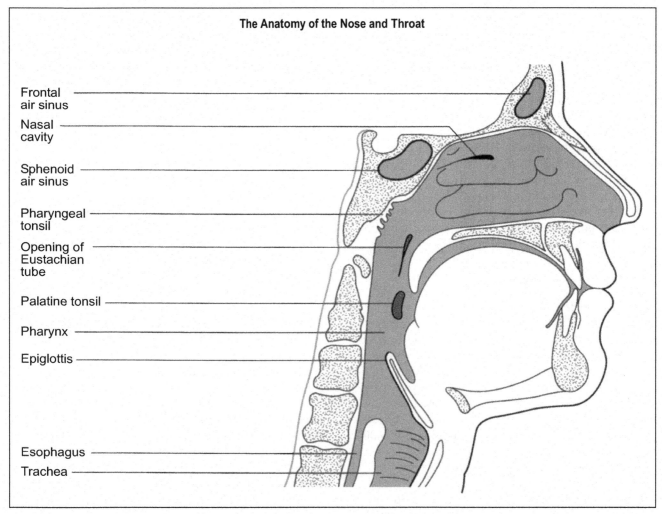

Frontal air sinus
Nasal cavity
Sphenoid air sinus
Pharyngeal tonsil
Opening of Eustachian tube
Palatine tonsil
Pharynx
Epiglottis
Esophagus
Trachea

ness caused by an accumulation of fluid in the ear's labyrinth that results in loss of balance. Both of these disorders are most common among people over fifty, although they can afflict people at any age. One out of every ten thousand babies born in the United States has some hearing deficit, and many-particularly those whose mothers contracted rubella (German measles) during pregnancy-are almost totally deaf.

Otologists (physicians who treat diseases and disorders of the ear) have made considerable headway in treating some forms of deafness, particularly conductive deafness, which results from a narrowing of the ear canal to the point of closure. Shortly before 1920, it was discovered that considerable hearing can be restored through fenestration-that is, through making a small surgical opening in the eardrum through which sound can pass. The complications associated with this procedure have been largely overcome with stapedectomy (the removal of all or part of the stapes, one of the bones of the middle ear) and the insertion of a prosthetic device, which is made of wire or Teflon and used in combination with a gelatin sponge or the patient's own veins, connective tissue, and fat. Although fenestration is highly successful in cases in which deafness is conductive, it does not alleviate deafness whose cause is sensorineural, so-called nerve deafness, which is often treated palliatively with hearing aids. These devices are constantly improving, however, as they are decreasing in size and increasing in effectiveness.

Tumors of the inner ear can now be successfully removed through a translabyrinthine approach. The ear canal is entered with tiny, well-illuminated laser instruments to which magnifying devices are attached. Such surgery is often performed by otologists, although many undertake it collaboratively with a neurologist. Pituitary tumors, once the responsibility almost solely of neurosurgeons who performed craniotomies to reach the diseased area of the brain, are often treated by otorhinolaryngologists, who approach the tumor through the nose. Thus the tumor can be removed without the need for debilitating surgery.

From the earliest beginnings of otorhinolaryngology, the larynx has been among the parts of the anatomy most often treated by its practitioners. The laryngectomy, with its radical side effect of rendering the patient unable to speak, was once the treatment of choice for malignant laryngeal tumors. Such tumors can now be treated successfully with radiation, obviating the need for more drastic treatment. Teflon injections have been used to treat patients whose vocal cords have been compromised by surgery or by radiation. Because the larynx is in the area of the thyroid glands, otorhinolaryngologists also possess expert knowledge of thyroid disorders and may perform a thyroidectomy (removal of the thyroid), a procedure that is now emphasized in their residencies.

Two of the most frequent surgical procedures of the field in the mid-twentieth century were the removal of the tonsils (tonsillectomy) and of the adenoids, the masses of lymphoid tissue in the lining at the back of the tongue that produce white blood cells, which fight disease. Tonsils and adenoids were once removed routinely if children suffered from frequent colds. Now this surgery is discouraged because it has been discovered that the tonsils and adenoids help children develop a resistance to infection. When these tissues become inflamed, they can be treated conservatively and successfully through medication.

Otorhinolaryngologists regularly work in concert with physicians in other specialties, particularly neurosurgery. An internist treating a patient who suffers from loss of balance usually refers that patient to an otologist, who orders diagnostic tests to check for fluid in the inner ear, which would suggest Ménière's disease. If such tests fail to reveal a buildup of fluid in the inner ear, the otologist usually refers the patient to a neurologist or neurosurgeon to check for other causes, including a tumor or a disorder in the central nervous system.

Otologists sometimes perform plastic surgery on ears that are abnormally protrusive. This reduction is a form of cosmetic surgery. By the end of the twentieth century in the United States, it was common for otorhinolaryngologists to perform most cosmetic and reconstructive surgeries related to these areas of the body. Consequently, residencies in this specialty offer considerable training in plastic surgery, especially in the procedures that otorhinolaryngologists have come to perform routinely in connection with thyroid, nasal, and other surgeries. They are often the physicians of choice in cases of cleft lip and cleft palate, the treatment of which normally falls largely within the province of reconstructive surgery. Because much cosmetic and reconstructive surgery involves the face, maxillofacial surgeons are often otorhinolaryngologists.

The common cold, although usually treated by an internist or family doctor if it is referred to a physician at all, sometimes involves complications such as bronchitis, pneumonia, or ancillary infections of the ears and sinuses. In such cases, an otorhinolaryngologist may be consulted for treatment. Dealing with the common cold is merely a waiting game: colds generally go away after a week or ten days. Colds afflict the average adult about four times a year and the average child twice that often (because young children have not yet built up the immunity that prevents infection).

PERSPECTIVE AND PROSPECTS

Many of the illnesses that fall within the purview of otorhinolaryngology became more threatening and more frequent when the Industrial Revolution of the eighteenth century caused the relocation of large numbers of people from rural to urban settings. Cities grew as factories opened. Living conditions were often deplorable and, at best, overcrowded. Added to this situation was the pollution of the air by the waste products expelled by smokestack industries. Wherever pollution is prevalent, diseases of the upper respiratory tract are endemic.

The eighteenth century spawned conditions that compromised the environment and severely affected humans, but until physicians had a way of examining the body's more remote crevices, the diagnosis and treatment of ear, nose, and throat problems were difficult. Such treatments as bleeding frequently killed rather than cured patients. Surgery was a treatment of last resort because the major anesthetic was whiskey. Patients sometimes died of shock from the unbearable pain that they suffered during surgical procedures.

Once physicians had reliable means of seeing into the body by using such equipment as reflective mirrors, endoscopes, x-rays, tomography, and ultrasonography, they could treat many illnesses nonsurgically. It is hoped that in the future even less invasive surgery will be done in all fields of medicine, including otorhinolaryngology.

Even when surgery is indicated, in the field of otorhinolaryngology it can often be performed without an incision by entering the body through the ear canal, nose, or throat. Advanced technology has produced surgical instruments that, in combination with computer imaging, work precisely and with less trauma. In cases where incisions are necessary, the opening is often so small that it is almost undetectable a year after the procedure.

—*R. Baird Shuman, PhD*

See also Antihistamines; Aromatherapy; Audiology; Cleft lip and palate; Cleft lip and palate repair; Common cold; Deafness; Decongestants; Ear infections and disorders; Ear surgery; Ears; Earwax; Esophagus; Epiglottitis; Halitosis; Hearing; Hearing loss; Hearing tests; Laryngectomy; Laryngitis; Ménière's disease; Motion sickness; Mouth and throat cancer; Myringotomy; Nasal polyp removal; Nasopharyngeal disorders; Nosebleeds; Otoplasty; Pharyngitis; Pharynx; Plastic surgery; Quinsy; Rhinoplasty and submucous resection; Sense organs; Sinusitis; Sjögren's syndrome; Smell; Sneezing; Sore throat; Strep throat; Taste; Tonsillectomy and adenoid removal; Tonsillitis; Tonsils; Voice and vocal cord disorders.

For Further Information:
American Academy of Otolaryngology-Head and Neck Surgery. "What Is an Otolaryngologist?" *American Academy of Otolaryngology-Head and Neck Surgery*, January, 2011.
Benjamin, Bruce, et al. *A Color Atlas of Otorhino- laryngology.* Edited by Michael Hawke. Philadelphia: J. B. Lippincott, 1995.
Chasnoff, Ira J., Jeffrey W. Ellis, and Zachary S. Fainman, eds. Rev. ed. *The New Illustrated Family Medical and Health Guide.* Lincolnwood, Ill.: Publications International, 1994.
Crumley, Roger L. "Otolaryngology-Head and Neck Surgery." In *Planning Your Medical Career: Traditional and Alternative Opportunities*, edited by T. Donald Rucker and Martin D. Keller et al. Garrett Park, Md.: Garrett Park Press, 1986.
Ferrari, Mario. *PDxMD Ear, Nose, and Throat Disorders.* Philadelphia: PDxMD, 2003.
Gulya, Aina J., and William R. Wilson. *An Atlas of Ear, Nose, and Throat Diagnosis and Treatment.* New York: Parthenon, 1999.
Kennedy, David W., and Marilyn Olsen. *Living with Chronic Sinusitis: A Patient's Guide to Sinusitis, Nasal Allergies, Polyps, and Their Treatment Options.* Long Island, N.Y.: Hatherleigh Press, 2007.
Vorvick, Linda J. "Types of Health Care Providers." *MedlinePlus*, August 14, 2012.
Woodson, Gayle E. *Ear, Nose, and Throat Disorders in Primary Care.* Philadelphia: W. B. Saunders, 2001.

Ovarian cancer. See Cervical, ovarian, and uterine cancers.

OVARIAN CYSTS

Category: Disease/Disorder
Anatomy or system affected: Reproductive system
Specialties and related fields: Gynecology
Definition: Benign growths that develop in the ovaries.

CAUSES AND SYMPTOMS

Ovarian cysts may occur at any age, individually or in numbers, on one or both ovaries. The cyst consists of a thin, transparent outer wall enclosing one or more chambers filled with clear fluids or old blood that presents as thick brownish or jellylike material; in some cases tissue material may be present as well. Such cysts range in size from that of a raisin to that of a large orange. The normal ovary measures 3 centimeters by 2 centimeters; the cystic ovary requiring investigation is one which is enlarged to more than twice its normal size. Large cysts may cause a feeling of fullness in the abdominal area, cramping pain with various levels of severity, or pain during vaginal intercourse. Often, however, there are no apparent symptoms, and the cyst is discovered only during a routine gynecologic examination when the clinician, on bimanual examination, discovers that one ovary is considerably enlarged. At this point, it is important to rule out malignancy, because ovarian cancers in their early stages also have no warning symptoms and can occur at any age.

Polycystic ovaries (ovaries containing multiple cysts) causing significant enlargement occur in a variety of conditions. For example, polycystic ovaries can result from an enzyme deficiency in the ovaries that interferes with the normal biosynthesis of hormones, resulting in the release of an abnormal amount of androgen (a substance producing or stimulating the development of male characteristics).

More than half of all ovarian cysts are functional; that is, they arise out of the normal functions of the ovary during the menstrual cycle. These cysts are relatively common. A cyst can form when a follicle (a small, spherical, secretory structure in the ovary) has grown in preparation for ovulation but fails to rupture and release an egg; this type is called a follicular cyst. Sometimes the structure formed from the follicle after ovulation, the corpus luteum, fails to shrink and forms a cyst; this is called a corpus luteum cyst.

Another type of ovarian cyst, most often found in younger women, is the dermoid cyst, which contains particles of teeth, hair, or calcium-containing tissue that are thought to be an embryologic (developmental) remnant; such cysts usually do not cause menstrual irregularity and are very common. Dermoids are bilateral in 25 percent of cases, making careful examination of both ovaries mandatory. The cyst has a thickened, white, opaque wall and is more buoyant than other types of cysts.

Ovarian cysts cause problems when they become very large, when they rupture and cause severe internal bleeding, or when a cyst's pedicle (a tail-like ap-

---

INFORMATION ON OVARIAN CYSTS

Causes: Depends on type; may include functional disorders involving follicles or corpus luteum, hormonal imbalance, embryological remnants

Symptoms: Often asymptomatic; with large cysts, may include feeling of fullness in abdomen, pain with intercourse, compromised fertility; if rupture occurs, severe internal bleeding and intense lower abdominal pain; if cyst becomes twisted, severe pain and possibly gangrene

Duration: Acute to chronic

Treatments: Oral contraceptives, surgery

---

pendage) suddenly twists and cuts off its blood supply, creating severe pain and possibly gangrene. Rupture of a cyst is followed by the acute onset of severe lower abdominal pain radiating to the vagina and lower back. The most severe symptoms of pain and collapse are associated with rupture of a dermoid cyst, as the cyst contents are extremely irritating.

Torsion (twisting) of a cyst may occur at any age but most often in the twenties; it may be associated with pregnancy. A twisted dermoid cyst is the most common, probably because of its increased weight. The onset of pain often occurs in the umbilical region and radiates to one or the other side of the pelvis. Pain on the right is frequently confused with appendicitis. Hemorrhage may sometimes occur from a vessel in the wall of the cyst or within the capsule.

TREATMENT AND THERAPY

The diagnosis of an ovarian cyst is made with consideration of the patient's age, medical and family history, symptoms, and the size of the enlarged ovary. In women under the age of thirty, clinicians, after a manual examination, will usually wait to see if the ovary will return to its normal size. If it does not, and pregnancy has been ruled out, a pelvic X-ray or a sonogram (the use of sound to produce an image or photograph of an organ or tissue), or both, can determine the exact size of the ovaries and distinguish between a cyst and a solid tumor. In women age forty and older, X-rays and sonograms may be done sooner. If uncertainty still exists, the physician may recommend laparoscopy, the visual examination of the abdominal cavity using a device consisting of a tube and optical system inserted through a small incision. The physician may also suggest the option of a larger incision and a biopsy.

In the case of the functional ovarian cyst, if no severe pain or swelling is present, the clinician may adopt "watchful waiting" for one or two more menstrual cycles, during the course of which this type of

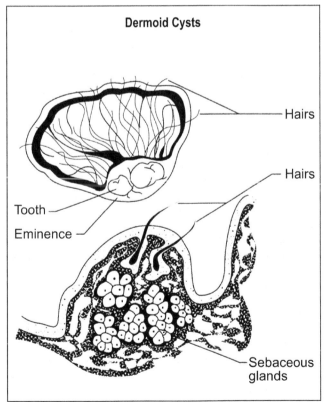

Dermoid Cysts

Hairs

Hairs

Tooth

Eminence

Sebaceous glands

Dermoid cysts are a relatively common form of ovarian cyst often found in younger women. ©EBSCO cyst frequently disappears on its own accord. Sometimes this process is hastened by administering oral contraceptives for several months, which establishes a regular menstrual cycle. Women already taking oral contraceptives rarely develop ovarian cysts.

In the case of torsion or rupture, surgical treatment is indicated, preferably the removal of the cyst only and preservation of as much of the normal ovarian tissue as possible. Sometimes, with a very large cyst, the ovary cannot be saved and must be removed, a procedure called oophorectomy or ovariectomy.

—*Genevieve Slomski, PhD*

See also Biopsy; Cyst removal; Cysts; Genital disorders, female; Infertility, female; Laparoscopy; Ovaries; Polycystic ovary syndrome; Women's health.

For Further Information:
Altcheck, Albert, Liane Deligdisch, and Nathan Kase, eds. *Diagnosis and Management of Ovarian Disorders.* 2d ed. San Diego, Calif.: Academic Press, 2003.
Ammer, Christine, et al. *The New A to Z of Women's Health: A Concise Encyclopedia.* 6th ed. New York: Checkmark Books, 2009.
Berek, Jonathan S., ed. *Berek and Novak's Gynecology.* 14th ed. Philadelphia: Lippincott Williams & Wilkins, 2007.
Kovacs, Gabor T., and Robert Norman, eds. *Polycystic Ovary Syndrome.* 2d ed. New York: Cambridge University Press, 2012.
Leung, Peter C. K., and Eli Y. Adashi, eds. *The Ovary.* 2d ed. San Diego, Calif.: Academic Press, 2004.
Mahajan, Damodar K., ed. *Polycystic Ovarian Disease.* Philadelphia: W. B. Saunders, 1988.
"Ovarian Cyst." *Family Doctor,* August 2010.
Rosenblum, Laurie. "Ovarian Cyst." *Health Library,* September 10, 2012.
Vorvick, Linda J., Susan Storck, and David Zieve. "Ovarian Cysts." *Medline Plus,* February 26, 2012.

OVARIES

Category: Anatomy
Anatomy or system affected: All
Specialties and related fields: Biochemistry, embryology, endocrinology, genetics, gynecology, obstetrics
Definition: The ovaries produce eggs and sex hormones in females.
Key terms:
atresia: the programmed process of cell death
corpus luteum: the structure that develops from an emptied ovarian follicle after ovulation
Fallopian tubes or oviducts: tubular structures attached at their lower ends to the uterus; the passageways for ova following ovulation
follicle: a structure composed of an oocyte and surrounding granulosa cells

hormone: a chemical messenger secreted by one cell type and acting on another to cause a predictable response
oocyte: a female germ cell that differentiates to become a mature ova
ovum (pl. ova): an egg cell

STRUCTURE AND FUNCTIONS
Ovaries develop from undifferentiated gonadal tissue in the absence of a Y chromosome. They are ductless glands located in the female pelvis, attached on either side of the uterus by the ovarian ligaments. Each is a flattened lumpy oval about 5 centimeters (cm) in length, 2.5 cm wide, and less than 1 cm in thickness. They are often described as being about the size and shape of an almond. There are three regions to each ovary: An outer cortex contains the developing oocytes, an inner medulla produces steroid hormones, and the hilum serves as the point of attachment and entry of blood vessels and nerves.

A principal function of the ovaries is gametogenesis, the production of ova through meiosis. This process begins during fetal life, and about 1 to 2 million immature oocytes are present in the cortex of the ovaries at birth. By puberty, this number has been reduced to about 300,000 through the process of atresia, and only about 400 mature ova are actually ovulated during life. The number of lifetime ovulated oocytes are reduced if oral contraceptives are used.

Recent research has found that it may be possible to increase oocyte numbers during life through the implantation of stem cells that are capable of mitosis. These stem cells can be isolated from the ovaries of reproductive age women. Studies done on mice have isolated germline stem cells from ovaries that can actively divide and produce oocytes when implanted in a human body.

Within the mature ovarian cortex are many follicles, each containing an oocyte. At any given time, there are oocytes in all stages of development, and only a small percentage of available oocytes ever undergo ovulation; the rest undergo atresia and are recycled by the body. This occurs because groups of oocytes are activated during ovulation, and only one makes it to the luteal stage, while the others undergo atresia.

Immature oocytes remain dormant until puberty. During this time, the hypothalamus region of the brain releases a surge of hormone, the Ganadotropin-releasing hormone, that initiates the release of hormones from the pituitary, which will drive the process of ovulation. During puberty, eggs mature successively, and one breaks through the ovarian wall each cycle in the process of ovulation. This continues until menopause, or cessation of reproductive functioning in the female. After release from the ovary, the ovum passes through the Fallopian tube and into the uterus. If the ovum is fertilized, then pregnancy ensues and the ovum (now a blastocyst) implants in the uterine lining.

Following ovulation, the empty follicle left in the ovary becomes the corpus luteum. It appears as a yellow body (because of lipid droplets in the cells) on the surface of the ovary and secretes progesterone to prepare the uterine lining for implantation. The corpus luteum deteriorates after ten to twelve days if conception does not occur, and the decrease in progesterone allows deterioration of the uterine lining, and thus, menstruation begins.

The ovarian medulla is also responsible for hormonogenesis. The primary steroids produced here are estradiol (estrogen) and progesterone. Androgens (particularly androstenedione and testosterone) are also secreted, but most of them are converted to estradiol within the ovary. Estrogens are essential for the development of ova and female body characteristics (including breasts, body shape, fat deposition, and body hair distribution) and for implantation and pregnancy maintenance. They also initiate mammary gland maturation and contribute to bone mineralization. Progesterone prepares the uterine lining for implantation and pregnancy, regulates the release of luteinizing hormone (LH) from the pituitary, and contributes to the maturation of mammary gland alveoli.

In addition to the steroid hormones, peptide hormones are produced by the ovaries. Relaxin is secreted from the corpus luteum and induces relaxation of the pelvic bones and ligaments, inhibits myometrial motility, softens the cervix, and induces uterine growth. Activins stimulate the release of follicle stimulating hormone (FSH) from the pituitary, and inhibin causes decreasing FSH output, although the mechanism is not yet understood. The ovary has been found to produce a variety of neuropeptides such as b-endorphin, adrenocorticotropin, α-melanocyte-stimulating hormone, vasopressin, and oxytocin. The physiologic roles that these peptides may play in the ovary are uncertain.

Human ovaries display a regular cycle in reproductively mature females. This cycle, known as menstruation, includes a follicular phase, during which FSH promotes growth and maturation of the granulosa cells, partial maturation of oocytes, synthesis of proteins, and estrogen secretion. Next is the ovulatory phase, during which one mature oocyte and the surrounding cells are discharged. Lastly is the luteal phase, in which progesterone is secreted. The average ovarian cycle is twenty-eight days, with a normal range between twenty-four and thirty-two days in length.

DISORDERS AND DISEASES

Polycystic ovary syndrome (PCOS), or Stein-Leventhal syndrome, is the most common ovarian disorder, affecting 6 to 10 percent of all women. The ovarian stroma becomes enlarged and produces excessive amounts of androgens. Atretic follicles accumulate and large numbers of cysts (fluid-filled sacs) may form; most are harmless and require no treatment. Ovarian follicle development is incomplete, and menstrual cycles are usually irregular. Symptoms can be alleviated with combination contraceptives and antiandrogens. Ovulation can sometimes be induced by clomiphene.

Ovulatory dysfunction is one of the causes of infertility. Most often this is hormonal in nature, and many cases of infertility can be overcome by hormone treatments.

Ovarian cancer is a major cause of death in females and comes in a variety of forms. The lifetime risk is about 1.6 percent, but it increases with age and in women with relatives who have had reproductive cancers. In women with an altered BRCA1 or BRCA2 gene, the risk is 25 to 60 percent, depending on the specific mutation. Pregnancy decreases the overall risk, as do oral contraceptives. Surgery is the treatment of choice, often followed by chemotherapy. Prognosis is poor overall, mostly due to the lack of clear symptoms that would lead to early diagnosis.

PERSPECTIVE AND PROSPECTS

The human ovary was first described by Renier De Graaf in 1672. In 1701, the first surgery to remove an ovarian tumor was performed by Robert Houston, and in 1809 the first known ovary removal (ovariectomy or oophorectomy) was performed by Ephraim McDowell. Throughout the nineteenth and early twentieth centuries, study of the ovaries centered on their anatomy and physiology, while during the latter part of the twentieth century studies turned to their endocrine functions.

Many postulated ovarian hormones are still being searched and studied for their effects. They include transforming growth factor beta (TGF-β), anti-Mullerian hormone (AMH), folliculostatins, and many other peptides involved in the control of growth and differentiation. Gonadotropin surge attenuating factor (GnSAF) has also been hypothesized to be physiologically involved in the control of LH secretion during the menstrual cycle.

—*Kerry L. Cheesman, PhD; updated by Catherine Avelar*

See also Amenorrhea; Assisted reproductive technologies; Cervical, ovarian, and uterine cancers; Contraception; Endometrial biopsy; Endometriosis; Gamete intrafallopian transfer (GIFT); Genital disorders, female; Gynecology; Hormone therapy; Hormones; Hot flashes; Hysterectomy; In vitro fertilization; Infertility, female; Menopause;

Menorrhagia; Menstruation; Obstetrics; Ovarian cysts; Pap test; Pelvic inflammatory disease (PID); Polycystic ovary syndrome; Pregnancy and gestation; Premenstrual syndrome (PMS); Puberty and adolescence; Reproductive system; Sterilization; Tubuligation; Uterus; Women's health

For Further Information:

Futterweit, Walter, and George Ryan. *A Patient's Guide to PCOS: Understanding-and Reversing-Polycystic Ovary Syndrome.* New York: Holt, 2006.

Johnson, J., J. Canning, T. Kaneko, J.K. Pru, and J.L. Tilly. "Germline Stem Cells and Follicular Renewal in the Postnatal Mammalian Ovary." *Nature* 428, no. 6979 (2004): 145-150.

Kaipia, Antti, and Aaron Hsueh. "Regulation of Ovarian Follicle Atresia." *Annual Review of Physiology* 59 (1997): 349-363.

Moore, K.L., T.V.N. Persaud, M.G. Torchia, and T.V.N. Persaud. *The Developing Human: Clinically Oriented Embryology.* Philadelphia: Saunders/Elsevier, 2008.

Plourde, Elizabeth. *Your Guide to Hysterectomy, Ovary Removal, and Hormone Replacement: What All Women Need to Know.* Ashland, OH: New Voice/ Atlas Books, 2002.

OVER-THE-COUNTER MEDICATIONS

Category: Treatment
Anatomy or system affected: All
Specialties and related fields: Family medicine, pharmacology, preventive medicine
Definition: Pills, capsules, tablets, or syrups that can be purchased without prescription for the self-treatment of common illnesses, such as colds, fever, and headache.

Key terms:

brand name: the name under which a drug is marketed by a pharmaceutical company

excipients: fillers, coloring, or coatings added to pills, tablets, capsules, or syrups

generic name: the unique name of a drug, typically the active chemical ingredient; a drug may be marketed under the generic name or the brand name

self-diagnosis: a determination of medical condition or illness without the benefit of a physician's input

self-prescription: the selection of over-the-counter medications without consulting a physician

self-treatment: the self-administration of one or more over-the-counter medications

INDICATIONS AND PROCEDURES

Drugs or medications that can be purchased directly, without a prescription, are called over-the-counter (OTC) medications or drugs. These medications may be suggested by physicians or simply purchased for consumption as a result of self-diagnosis and self-prescription. Most of the common OTC medications are used to treat common ailments such as cold and fever symptoms, headache, coughs, and similar complaints. Such self-treatment may be initiated at will and discontinued at any time.

Dozens of pharmaceutical companies produce and market hundreds of drugs for sale as over-the-counter medications, but they fall into only a few categories. The basic types of OTC medications, along with some brand examples, include analgesics (Advil, Tylenol), antacids (Milk of Magnesia), antidiarrheal medications (Imodium), antifungal agents (Tinactin), antihistamines (Benadryl), antiacne treatments (Clearasil), anti-inflammatory drugs (Motrin), decongestants (Sudafed), motion sickness (Meclizine), laxatives (Metamucil, Dulcolax), dandruff treatments (Selsun Blue), expectorants (Robitussin), hair growth formulas (Rogaine), and sleep aids (L-Tryptophan).

The most frequently used category of OTC medications is analgesics, which are more popularly known as painkillers. Analgesics include a diverse group of drugs that are used to relieve soreness, general body pain, and headaches. Probably the most common analgesic is aspirin, which is part of a group of medications termed nonsteroidal anti-inflammatory drugs (NSAIDs) that chemically affect the central and possibly the peripheral nervous system by leading to a decrease in prostaglandin production. Many analgesics are used in combination with other drugs such as vasoconstriction drugs that contain pseudoephedrine, which is especially important for the relief of sinus congestion, and in combination with antihistamine drugs, which relieve the worst symptoms of allergy.

Decongestants must certainly rank as the second most common category of OTC medications. Generally, decongestants are taken to relieve nasal congestion and allied symptoms of colds and flu by acting to reduce swelling of the mucous membranes of the nasal passageways. A recurring problem with most nasal decongestants is that they increase hypertension, but this effect is lessened by including one or more antihistamines in the preparation. The brand name drug Dimetapp, for example, is both an antihistamine and a decongestant, while various Tylenol products may contain drugs that collectively work to soothe sore throat, relieve nasal congestion, or suppress coughing.

Despite the fact that over-the-counter drugs are available to everyone, their marketing and use is restricted by the Food and Drug Administration (FDA) in the United States and similar agencies with regulatory powers in many other countries. The FDA mandates ingredients and labeling of OTC drugs and specifies rigid testing and safety standards that must be met prior to marketing. Pharmaceutical companies must apply to the New Drug Agency (NDA) for the approval of drugs. The NDA specifies testing requirements prior to issuing a license for the sales and marketing of the proposed new drug. Following approval, the FDA regularly reviews and maintains the right to remove or restrict marketing and sales of OTC drugs that create adverse side affects or are potentially addictive.

Following discovery, testing, and FDA approval of a new drug, it is given a unique trade name or brand name. The pharmaceutical company is awarded an exclusive patent to manufacture and market the drug for a specified period of time, usually seventeen years in the United States but of variable length in other countries. At the end of this time, the company no longer has proprietary rights to the drug, which may then be manufactured and marketed by other pharmaceutical companies. These drug companies may choose to market the drug under a new brand name of their choosing but not under the original label, which may still be manufactured by the original pharmaceutical company that designed and patented the drug. Spin-off products of these companies must still pass rigid FDA quality control standards which demonstrate that their product contains sufficient amounts of the active ingredients to promote bioequivalency before it can be marketed as an OTC medication-that is, the new drug has to be the therapeutic equal of the original drug.

Drugs manufactured by other pharmaceutical companies following patent expiration are typically called generic drugs and are strictly regulated by the U.S. Drug Price Competition and Patent Term Restoration Act (also known as the Hatch-Waxman Act), which was enacted in 1984. Tylenol, for example, is the exclusive brand name of an analgesic over-the-counter medication that contains the active chemical ingredient acetaminophen. Following the release of its patent, many other pharmaceutical companies started marketing pain relief drugs containing products for pain relief under the their own trade name or brand name. These copies are considered generic drugs and provide the consumer with a wide choice of the most popular drugs, usually at greatly reduced cost.

Manufacture and marketing of a generic drug by new companies usually means that their product costs considerably less, partly because of competition but mostly because the new drug companies did not bear the initial costs of development, marketing, and promotion that were part of the original financial investment of the parent company. Furthermore, manufacturers of generic drugs enjoy all the benefits of prior marketing, public acceptance, and possibly dependence on the most popular OTC medications. Generally, however, the parent company enjoys a certain competitive advantage of brand name recognition that promotes continued use of their marketed product, thereby reducing the impact of cheaper competition.

Over-the-counter medications may take the form of packets, tablets, capsules, pills, drops or droplets, ointments, inhalants, lotions, creams, suppositories, or syrups. Except for creams and topical ointments, OTC medications are administered orally, in contrast to drugs that are taken by injection. This mode of delivery places natural limits on their therapeutic effectiveness in several ways.

After being swallowed, OTC medications pass down the esophagus, through the stomach, and into the small intestine, where they are digested and absorbed. This mode of delivery requires a certain time interval between oral intake of the drug and its arrival in the bloodstream that transports it to target cells, tissues, and organs, thus delaying the effects of the drug. Tablets or capsules sometimes get stuck in the back of the mouth or on the lining of the esophagus, where they start to dissolve. When this happens, the ingredients may cause irritation, nausea, and sometimes vomiting, and the therapeutic value is lost. Furthermore, a certain amount of each key ingredient will be destroyed by the digestive enzymes of the gastrointestinal system, may be metabolized by cells of the intestinal epithelia, or may simply pass through the gut without being absorbed. Even following absorption into the blood, a certain amount of the drug may be lost because liver and other body cells set about removing foreign substances in the blood almost as soon as they are detected, generally by metabolizing the ingredient into a harmless chemical that will be excreted into the bile or be removed by the kidneys. This process explains why all drugs, including OTC medications, must be taken in repeated doses at regularly prescribed intervals in order to obtain maximum therapeutic value.

A final factor complicating delivery efficiency and thus the therapeutic value of OTC medications involves their packaging. Capsules, tablets, and pills in particular all contain substances in addition to the chemical ingredient, such as coatings, fillers, stabilizers, and often color additives. These substances, called excipients, do not contribute to the actual working of the drug itself, but they often modify both the rate and the extent of dissolution of the drug as it travels the gastrointestinal tract. While most excipients ultimately reduce the overall degree of delivery, some have important functions of permitting them to transit through the stomach, which has limited absorption ability, and into the small intestine, where chemical dissolution and absorption occurs at an optimum rate. For some drugs, the natural limits placed on delivery efficiency by gastrointestinal processes and excipient components can be sharply reduced by placing the capsule or tablet directly under the tongue, thus entirely bypassing the alimentary tract.

USES AND COMPLICATIONS
Primarily because of liability issues, all OTC medications include labels that are sometimes extensive. Label components typically consist of a list of one or more symptoms addressed by the medication, active ingredients contained in the drug, warnings, directions for use, and the date after which the medication should be discarded. For example, the label on a common OTC medication used to treat severe colds notes that it is to be used to relieve symptoms of nasal congestion, cough, sore throat, runny nose, headache and body ache, and fever. Directions for use are specific as to number of times a day, hours between use, and factors involving taking the medication, such as with or without glasses of water prior to or following administration and limits regarding food intake.

Most labels also carry prominent warnings regarding use with respect to age, alcohol consumption, sedatives or tranquilizers, and combinations of medications. Most over-the-counter medications also state that use should be continued only for a specified time and that, if symptoms persist, the user should stop taking the medication and consult a physician. Finally, the user is usually cautioned to stop taking the OTC medication immediately if headache, rash, nausea, or similar symptoms appear. Despite these warnings, even commonly used OTC medications pose certain health hazards, and the user is advised to take these medications with full recognition of potential problems.

In the United States, while the FDA periodically issues warnings regarding OTC medications, their actual use by consumers normally is not regulated, documented, or monitored. This has led to a number of concerns regarding real and potential overuse of OTC drugs, particularly for reasons unrelated to their medicinal intent. It has also led directly to the modification of certain OTC medications to engineer drugs that are highly addictive.

Because their use is unregulated-or, more correctly, cannot be regulated-over-the-counter medications can be deliberately abused. Overdosing with certain types of painkillers, for example, has become a frequent method of suicide attempt. The use of Tylenol in suicide attempts is increasing. Tylenol overdosing causes the destruction of liver cells that synthesize blood coagulants. Loss of these blood coagulants results in uncontrolled bleeding, most evidently through the eyes, nose, and mouth but also internally. Internal bleeding continues until death occurs, usually within a few days following onset.

Perhaps the most egregious misuse of OTC medications is to induce or achieve temporary "highs" that parallel those obtained by use of street or hard drugs. Cough suppressants that contain the drug dextromethorphan, for example, affect the central nervous system and can be used as mood-altering drugs that cause brain damage and even death at high doses. An even more serious abuse is the cooking of common drugs to obtain the highly addictive drug methamphetamine, popularly called meth. Also known as ice or speed, meth is a highly addictive drug that is often devastating and sometimes deadly. In some regions of the United States, it ranks with heroin and cocaine as the popular drug of choice. Record growth in use and the ability to cook meth from readily obtained OTC drugs has led to the creation of National Methamphetamine Awareness Day to draw attention at all levels to this problem.

This cooking process involves the conversion of certain OTC medications into meth. Some other sources for cooking meth include diet aids, tincture of iodine or other iodine solutions, and household cleaning solutions. In response to the widespread home manufacture of meth, a national federal law was enacted to require pharmacies to check photo identification and keep records of over-the-counter sales of cold medications that contain pseudoephedrine and ephedrine, which are the two popular ingredients in many cold medications. By-products of in-home meth cooking labs are garbage cans filled with Sudafed packages and a distinct odor of cat urine. The cooking process itself releases potentially harmful toxic chemicals that can pose serious health hazards to lungs and the respiratory system and also poses the risk of fire.

PERSPECTIVE AND PROSPECTS
Originally, OTC medications were available for purchase only at pharmacies, along with physician-prescribed drugs. Today, a varied selection of OTC medications is available at many retail outlets, including supermarkets, food stores, and even convenience stores, although pharmacies still continue to offer the greatest selection. This can lead to a confusion of terms, as such medications or drugs are often no longer sold "over the counter" but instead can be found on shelves alongside other items for sale.

To complicate matters, certain drugs are offered as OTC medications at low dosages but must be obtained by prescription at higher dosages. For example, the popular analgesic ibuprofen (Advil, Motrin) can be purchased as an OTC medication at dosages of less than 200 milligrams, but higher dosages can be obtained only via prescription. Similarly, the antidiarrheal medication Imodium, an opiate, is available as an OTC medication in liquid form, while tablets of Imodium are available only by prescription.

The status of over-the-counter medications may change over time, depending on effectiveness and safety issues. While some OTC drugs are removed from the general market following various concerns regarding safety, other drugs are transferred from prescription drugs to OTC medications. Examples include the antihistamine drug Benadryl, which is used to relieve symptoms of allergy and guard against allergic reactions, and the painkiller ibuprofen, both of which were, until recently, sold as prescription drugs only but are now available as OTC medications.

While the distribution and sale of over-the-counter medications is strictly regulated by state and federal laws in the United States, certain drugs that are deemed harmless may be offered for sale as medical cures for many ailments and thereby compete with OTC medications. These so-called miracle drugs have become increasingly popular because of the Web, which opens the door to purchases without prescription. Media promotions also sometimes offer these medications, complete with testimonials that dramatically describe their success as a cure-all for ailments. These types of medications are often labeled "quack" drugs. They pose a threat to users of prescription and OTC medications in several ways. First, they are generally useless, offering a nonexistent cure for health problems. Second, they are manufactured without regard to quality control measures that legitimate drug manufacturers must follow. Third, time may be lost in using the quack drug, especially if the condition is chronic and the symptoms need to be treated immediately. Finally, while some may be harmless, other quack drugs contain chemical ingredients that are potentially dangerous when used in combination with genuine over-the-counter medications.

—*Dwight G. Smith, PhD*

See also Aging: Extended care; Antihistamines; Anti-inflammatory drugs; Aphrodisiacs; Clinical trials; Decongestants; Digestion; Food and Drug Administration (FDA); Herbal medicine; Homeopathy; Metabolism; Pain management; Pharmacology; Pharmacy; Polypharmacy; Sports medicine; Veterinary medicine.

For Further Information:
"Careful: Acetaminophen in pain relief medicines can cause liver damage." *fda.gov*, January 13, 2011.
Griffith, H. Winter, and Stephen Moore. *Complete Guide to Prescription and Non-Prescription Drugs*. Rev. ed. New York: Penguin Group, 2010.
Litin, Scott C., ed. *Mayo Clinic Family Health Book*. 4th ed. New York: HarperResource, 2009.
"Over-the-Counter Medicines." *MedlinePlus*, June 24, 2013.
Prescription and Over-the-Counter Drugs. Rev. ed. Pleasant View, N.Y.: Reader's Digest, 2001.
Sanberg, Paul, and Richard M. T. Krema. *Over-the-Counter Drugs: Harmless or Hazardous?* New York: Chelsea House, 1986.
"Use Caution with Over-the-Counter Creams, Ointments." *fda.gov*, April 1, 2008.

OVERTRAINING SYNDROME

Category: Disease/Disorder
Anatomy or system affected: Endocrine system, lymphatic system, muscles, nervous system, psychic-emotional system
Specialties and related fields: Exercise physiology, psychology, sports medicine
Definition: Perceptible and lasting decrease in athletic performance, often coupled with mood changes, which does not quickly resolve following a normal period of rest.

CAUSES AND SYMPTOMS
To achieve peak athletic performance, increased effort in training, sometimes to the point of overexertion, is required. Initial periods of overexertion followed by a brief decrease in performance are often referred to as overreaching, which is distinguishable from overtraining syndrome by the desired increase in performance following a brief period of rest. Overtraining syndrome appears to develop from an overload of training, psychosocial stressors, and performance without adequate recovery or rest periods.

Diagnosing this syndrome can be complicated because a single diagnostic test or tool has yet to be developed. Symptoms may vary depending on the individual athlete or the sport, so other possible causes for a long-term decrease in performance, such as diet or disease, should be ruled out first. More than eighty-four symptoms or markers have been attributed to overtraining syndrome. Most often noted in diagnosis are impaired performance, variations in heart rate, variations in blood pressure, loss of coordination, elevated basal metabolic rate, decreased body fat, weight loss, chronic fatigue, sleep disturbances, increased thirst, headaches, nausea, elevated C-reactive protein (CRP), hormone changes, excessive production of cytokines, mood changes, depression, increased susceptibility to colds, difficulty concentrating, restlessness, increased aches and pains, and muscle soreness. Sport-specific stress tests conducted to the point of exhaustion may aid in the diagnosis.

TREATMENT AND THERAPY
Rest from training, performance, and/or competition is needed. The recovery period may take anywhere from several weeks to years. As the rest period needed to fully recover from overtraining syndrome may vary greatly from one athlete to the next, prevention is seen as the better option. To reduce the risk of developing this condition, a training schedule that alternates high and low training intensities with at least one day of rest is suggested. Other possible preventive measures

---

INFORMATION ON OVERTRAINING SYNDROME

Causes: Training overload, stress, inadequate recovery or rest periods
Symptoms: Impaired performance, loss of coordination, elevated metabolism, body fat loss, chronic fatigue, sleep disturbances, increased thirst, headaches, nausea, depression, muscle soreness
Duration: Chronic
Treatments: None; prevention through rest periods, stress management

---

include managing stress and maintaining a log to track training intensities, diet, and sleep.

PERSPECTIVE AND PROSPECTS

Research on the characteristics of overtraining syndrome, such as how it affects men and women differently or athletes from various sports, continues to offer new insight. More research, especially longitudinal research, is needed to better understand the condition including its diagnosis, prevention, and treatment. A number of physiological tests to aid in detecting overtraining syndrome, including hormone levels, enzyme levels, and blood plasma changes, have been implemented, but none thus far have proved to be a valid measure for diagnosing this condition.

—*Susan E. Thomas, MLS*

See also Ergogenic aids; Exercise physiology; Fatigue; Kinesiology; Metabolism; Muscle sprains, spasms, and disorders; Muscles; Nutrition; Physical rehabilitation; Physiology; Preventive medicine; Sports medicine; Stress; Stress reduction.

For Further Information:
Brooks, K. A., and J. G. Carter. "Overtraining, Exercise, and Adrenal Insufficiency." *Journal of Novel Physiotherapies* 3,125. (2013).
Hausswirth, Christophe. *Recovery for Performance in Sport.* Champaign, Ill.: 2013.
Kerksick, Chad M. *Nutrient Timing: Metabolic Optimization for Health, Performance, and Recovery.* Boca Raton, Fla.: 2012
Kreider, Richard B., Andrew C. Fry, and Mary L. O'Toole, eds. *Overtraining in Sport.* Champaign, Ill.: Human Kinetics, 1998.
McDuff, David R. *Sports Psychiatry: Strategies for Life Balance and Peak Performance.* Arlington, Va.: American Psychiatric Publishing, 2012.
Romain, Meeusen, et al. "Prevention, Diagnosis, and Treatment of the Overtraining Syndrome." *European Journal of Sport Science* 6, 1. (2006): 1-14.
Urhausen, Axel, and Wilfried Kindermann. "Diagnosis of Overtraining: What Tools Do We Have?" *Sports Medicine* 32, 2. (2002): 95-102.
Wyatt, Frank B., Alissa Donaldson, and Elise Brown. "The Overtraining Syndrome: A Meta-Analytic Review." *Journal of Exercise Physiology* 16, 2. (April 2013): 12-23.

OXYGEN THERAPY

Category: Treatment
Anatomy or system affected: Chest, circulatory system, heart, lungs, respiratory system
Specialties and related fields: Anesthesiology, cardiology, critical care, emergency medicine, preventive medicine, pulmonary medicine
Definition: Giving air enhanced by added oxygen to persons suffering from hypoxia, lack of sufficient oxygen in the tissues.

INDICATIONS AND PROCEDURES

The major indication for oxygen therapy is cyanosis, in which the skin assumes a bluish tint as a result of hypoxia, a reduced arterial saturation of oxygen to the tissues. In cases of extreme breathlessness, which may be caused by extreme physical exertion, hypoxia may occur, but the condition in most cases reverses itself within minutes if the affected person rests.

In older people whose circulatory systems have been compromised by such conditions as arteriosclerosis (narrowing of the arteries), hypoxia may be chronic. Asthmatics often require immediate oxygen therapy during severe attacks. People suffering from influenza or pneumonia may have accumulated secretions in their airways that limit the amount of oxygen that can reach their tissues. Such people are usually given oxygen administered through either a nasal catheter or a face mask.

In instances where respiratory difficulties persist, as in emphysema or chronic bronchitis, patients often receive prescriptions for oxygen cylinders for home use. They may also benefit from the home installation of an oxygen concentrator, a machine that removes oxygen from the atmosphere and remixes it in high concentrations with air. Such machines can supply oxygen-enhanced air to various rooms within a house so that ambulatory patients can breathe it for prolonged periods without being confined to one location. Some patients must breathe oxygen-enhanced air for up to fifteen hours a day.

USES AND COMPLICATIONS

Oxygen therapy is routinely used by anesthesiologists during many surgical procedures, but very high oxygen concentrations are usually avoided. Warm, humidified oxygen is preferred in surgical situations to prevent condensation and inordinate cooling, which can lead to complications. Such therapy is often administered through a catheter and used postoperatively for up to five days to prevent hypoxemia (reduced oxygen in the blood). In emergency rooms, pure oxygen is frequently given to patients in acute distress.

In some situations, physicians must use medications such as naftidrofuryl to reduce the brain's requirement for oxygen where hypoxemia is present, and brain damage may result if this complication is not addressed immediately. A thrombus (blood clot) may reduce blood flow substantially and reduce to dangerous levels the supply of oxygen to the brain and tissues. In such situations, anticoagulants such as heparin or warfarin often reduce or eliminate the thrombus and restore the body's circulation of oxygen.

—*R. Baird Shuman, PhD*

See also Alternative medicine; Altitude sickness; Asbestos exposure; Asthma; Brain damage; Bronchitis; Chronic obstructive pulmonary disease (COPD); Circulation; Drowning; Ergogenic aids; Exercise physiology; Hyperbaric oxygen therapy; Hypoxia; Influenza; Lungs; Pneumonia; Pulmonary diseases; Pulmonary hypertension; Pulmonary medicine; Pulmonary medicine, pediatric; Respiration; Sports medicine; Thrombosis and thrombus; Vascular medicine; Vascular system; Wheezing.

For Further Information:
Perry, Anne Griffin, and Patricia A. Potter, eds. *Clinical Nursing Skills and Techniques.* 6th ed. St. Louis, Mo.: Mosby/Elsevier, 2006.
Rosdahl, Caroline Bunker, and Mary Kowalski, eds. *Textbook of Basic Nursing.* 9th ed. Philadelphia: Lippincott Williams & Wilkins, 2008.
Sheldon, Lisa Kennedy. *Oxygenation.* 2d ed. Sudbury, Mass.: Jones and Bartlett, 2008.
Tallis, Raymond C., and Howard M. Fillit, eds. *Brocklehurst's Textbook of Geriatric Medicine and Gerontology.* 7th ed. Philadelphia: Saunders/Elsevier, 2010.

OXYTOCIN

Category: Biology
Anatomy or system affected: reproductive
Specialties and related fields: endocrinology, gynecology
Definition: a peptide hormone primarily synthesized by the hypothalamus and stored in the pituitary that stimulates uterine contractions during childbirth and milk ejection during breast feeding
Key terms:
autismspectrum disorders: a group of developmental disorders that includes autism, and Asperger syndrome among other disorders
placenta: an organ that develops during pregnancy that allows for an exchange of gases, nutrients and wastes between the mother and developing fetus
hypothalamus: the part of the brain the synthesizes oxytocin and vasopressin, links the nervous system with the endocrine system and has a myriad of physiological effects

milkejection/letdown effect: the process by which upon stimulation of the nipple, oxytocin is released and stimulates the contraction of alveoli of the mammary glands expelling milk towards the nipple

STRUCTURE AND FUNCTION
Oxytocin is a nine amino acid peptide hormone primarily synthesized by the hypothalamus and stored in the pituitary until released. Oxytocin is released late in pregnancy when the uterus and cervix become stretched. Oxytocin causes contractions of the uterus facilitating birth. The name oxytocin is derived from Greek and means "quick birth," a reference to the fact that the body produces increased amounts of oxytocin causing uterine contractions during childbirth. Oxytocin is often administered to induce labor. Oxytocin is also involved with breast feeding by playing a role in the milk ejection/letdown effect, which occurs when an infant sucks at the mother's nipple, producing nerve impulses that are communicated to the hypothalamus in the mother's brain, which then causes the pituitary gland to begin producing oxytocin. The oxytocin stimulates the contractions of the mammary sinuses expelling milk towards the nipple. Oxytocin may also be responsible for bonding enhancement that encourages the mother to continue nursing for as long as the infant is hungry, a clear evolutionary advantage, as it avoids the problem of undernourished babies of mothers who might otherwise curtail nursing. It is also thought that the oxytocin produced during nursing stimulates contractions of the uterus that help the mother heal the location at which the placenta was attached during pregnancy.

In popular culture it has gained recognition under a variety of monikers: "the social hormone," "the romantic hormone," "the intimacy drug," and so on. This is because one of oxytocin's effects appears to be the enhancement of empathy and of deep emotional bonds and the development of trust or romantic affiliation between adults. The evolutionary advantages that social bonding, affection, and love may offer are believed to support larger populations, which are more likely to survive. A number of studies have also suggested that oxytocin may play a significant role in human sexual arousal, orgasm, and fertilization. Oxytocin has been shown to be released during hugging and sexual intercourse where it may stimulate contraction for the uterus aiding the transport of sperm Since males do not give birth or breast feed, the role of oxytocin in males is not completely understood. Males and females respond somewhat differently to oxytocin.

PERSPECTIVE AND PROSPECTS
Scientists have been studying oxytocin since the early part of the twentieth century. The neuropeptide was

discovered in 1906 by Henry Hallett Dale, an English physiologist. Research, distinct from that involving childbirth and nursing, has to do with oxytocin's ability to assist the body in recovering from injuries. Folk wisdom has asserted that people are better able to overcome sickness and injury when they are attended by people with whom they share an affectional bond. This can even extend to animals, as indicated by the frequent use of "therapy dogs" to help patients cope with their illnesses by offering comfort and companionship. Scientists now believe there is evidence to support the observation that some types of wounds appear to heal more quickly and more completely when oxytocin is produced by the patient. This suggests a direct connection between the presence of supportive social bonds and improved patient outcomes, because having loved ones nearby during treatment causes the patient's body to produce greater amounts of oxytocin, which in turn augment the body's ability to heal itself.

A growing number of physicians believe that oxytocin may offer a number of profoundly important benefits to public health. One such benefit might be realized by those suffering from autism spectrum disorders. One aspect of autism common to many of those afflicted with the syndrome is a difficulty making connections with other people, or an impaired ability to understand or even take notice of the emotional states of others. This can give rise to the social awkwardness that is often associated with autism spectrum disorders. Those with such disorders frequently fail to respond appropriately to social cues because they are either unaware of the cues and their meaning, or they fail to notice them altogether. Some research has established a relationship between autism and the oxytocin gene. Research in progress seeks to determine whether those with autism spectrum disorders might experience a greater ability to empathize with others if they were to receive increased doses of oxytocin. The hope is that whatever mechanisms underlie oxytocin's ability to increase empathy and interpersonal bonding are the same mechanisms operating in autistic persons at an impaired level. If this research bears fruit, then there may be a host of related disorders such as social anxiety disorder and related anxiety-based syndromes worth exploring for treatment with oxytocin. The main challenge scientists face is to discover ways in which people can benefit from oxytocin in a more controlled, deliberate way, while finding ways to prevent the cynical and unethical misuse of the drug's properties.

—Scott Zimmer, MLS, MS;
updated by Charles L. Vigue, PhD

See also: Reproductive system

For Further Information:
Baron-Cohen, Simon, Helen Tager-Flusberg, and Michael V. Lombardo. *Understanding Other Minds: Perspectives from Developmental Social Neuroscience*. Oxford: Oxford UP, 2013.
Breuning, Loretta G. *Habits of a Happy Brain: Retrain Your Brain to Boost Your Serotonin, Dopamine, Oxytocin, &... Endorphin Levels*. Fort Collins: Adams, 2015.
Choleris, Elena, Donald W. Pfaff, and Martin Kavaliers. *Oxytocin, Vasopressin, and Related Peptides in the Regulation of Behavior*. Cambridge: Cambridge UP, 2013.
MacGill, Markus. Oxytocin: The love hormone? Medical News Today. September 4, 2017. www.medicalnewstoday.com/articles/275795.php
Mikulincer, Mario, and Phillip R. Shaver. *Mechanisms of Social Connection: From Brain to Group*. Washington, DC: American Psychological Assoc., 2014.
Moberg, Kerstin U. *The Hormone of Closeness: The Role of Oxytocin in Relationships*. London: Pinter, 2013.
Stoller, K. P. *Oxytocin: The Hormone of Healing and Hope*. Santa Fe: Dream Treader, 2012.
Takahashi, Toku, Irena Gribovskaja-Rupp, and Reji Babygirija. *Physiology of Love: Role of Oxytocin in Human Relationships, Stress Response and Health*. New York: Nova, 2013.

P

PACEMAKER IMPLANTATION

Category: Procedure

Anatomy or system affected: Chest, circulatory system, heart

Specialties and related fields: Biotechnology, cardiology

Definition: The introduction into the heart of a permanent instrument that uses electrical pulses to regulate its rhythm.

Key terms:

atrium: one of the two upper chambers of the heart; the right atrium receives blood returning through the veins; the left atrium receives oxygenated blood from the lungs

catheter: a thin tube that can be inserted into blood vessels, such as a vein leading into the heart, to carry electrical wires or optical fibers

circus movement: electrical impulses in the heart that continue firing instead of reaching a normal resting phase, causing heart flutter and fibrillation

electrocardiogram (ECG or EKG): a recording of electrical signals generated by the heart that are detected by electrodes placed on the chest, arms, and legs; used to diagnose heart abnormalities

fibrillations: rapid and chaotic contractions of the heart muscle that are usually fatal when they occur in the ventricles because of insufficient blood flow

heart block: a delay or blockage of the electrical signal traveling through the heart muscle, which upsets the synchronization between contractions of the upper and lower chambers

sinoatrial (S-A) node: a cluster of cells above the right atrium that emit electrical signals which initiate contractions of the heart; also called natural pacemaker cells

ventricles: the two lower chambers of the heart; the right ventricle pumps blood to the lungs, and the left ventricle pumps oxygenated blood to the body

INDICATIONS AND PROCEDURES

The first human-made pacemaker, which used electronic pulses to stimulate a regular heart rhythm, was built in the 1950s. Since then, the device has evolved into a sophisticated and reliable instrument. It was miniaturized so that it could be implanted under the skin of the patient. Tiny batteries that would last from five to fifteen years were developed. A microprocessor that can sense the need for different heart rates during sleep or strenuous exercise has become a standard component. Most recently, a small automatic defibrillator has been incorporated into some pacemakers to supply several large jolts of electrical energy in case of heart stoppage or other emergencies.

The normal rhythm of a healthy heart is regulated by natural pacemaker cells. These unique cells are located at the sinoatrial (S-A) node near the top interior of the heart, where blood empties from the veins into the right atrium. Electrical impulses originating at the S-A node travel to the atrioventricular (A-V) node, which is located where the four chambers of the heart come together. From there, the signal is relayed to the ventricles, causing the muscle fibers to contract. This pumping action forces blood to flow from the two ventricles to the lungs and the body arteries.

If the natural pacemaker cells or the nerve pathways in the heart do not function properly, the heart may beat too rapidly, too slowly, irregularly, or not at all. For example, the condition called heart block interrupts or delays the electrical signal at the A-V node. It can happen that only every second or third pacemaker signal triggers a contraction. Sometimes, the ventricles will start a contraction on their own, but it will not be synchronized with the blood flow from the atrium. An artificial electronic pacemaker can be used to overcome heart block.

The electrical activity of the heart is observed in an electrocardiogram (ECG or EKG). Metal electrodes are placed in contact with a patient's left arm, right arm, left leg, and sometimes chest. After suitable amplification, the signal can be displayed on a video screen or recorded by an ink pen on moving paper.

For a healthy heart, the normal ECG pattern starts with a small pulse (the P wave), which is followed by a group of three closely spaced pulses (the QRS complex) and a final small pulse (the T wave). This pattern is repeated approximately seventy-two times per minute for a person sitting at rest.

In brief, the P wave indicates contraction of the atrium, the QRS complex shows contraction of the ventricles, and the T wave represents the muscles' return to the resting state. If the heart "skips a beat" because of a heart block at the A-V node, the ECG will show a missing or delayed pulsation in the otherwise

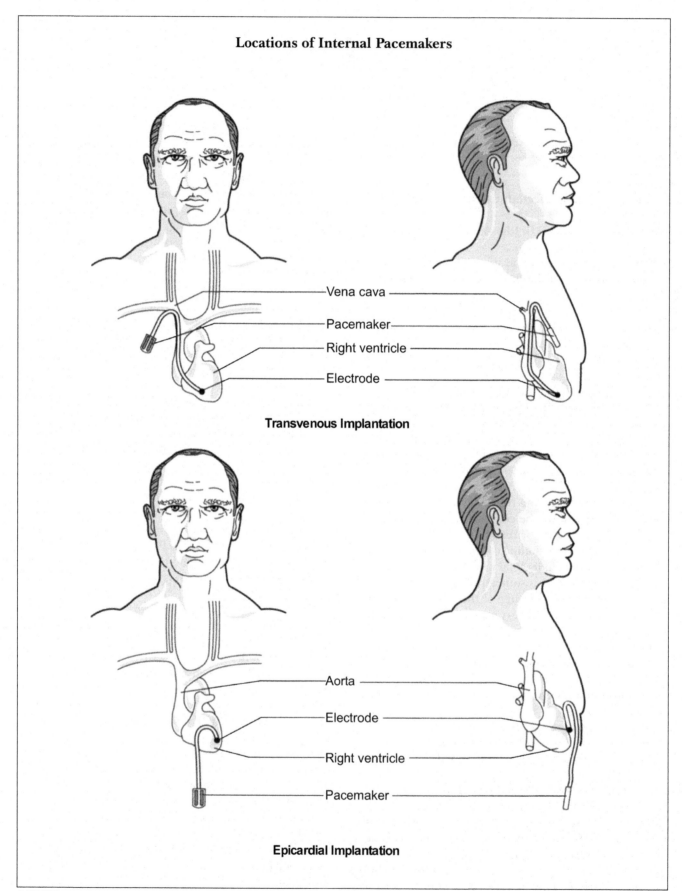

Locations of Internal Pacemakers

Vena cava
Pacemaker
Right ventricle
Electrode

Transvenous Implantation

Aorta
Electrode
Right ventricle
Pacemaker

Epicardial Implantation

regular pattern. If this happens in a sustained fashion, electronic stimulation is needed.

Two other serious malfunctions of the heart's electrical system are flutter and fibrillation. Flutter is a very rapid but still constant rhythm that may produce 200 to 300 beats per minute. Fibrillations are much more serious, causing chaotic, random contractions that can occur as often as 500 times per minute. There is insufficient time between contractions for blood to fill the ventricles. Pumping action becomes very inefficient, and death is likely to occur if the fibrillations continue.

To restore normal heart rhythm, a defibrillator is used to send a strong electric shock through the ventricular muscle fibers, which deactivates the heart's electrical system for several seconds. An electronic pacemaker may then replace the natural pacemaker cells to prevent the recurrence of fibrillations.

The cause of flutter and fibrillation is a process called "circus movement." Suppose the electrical impulses are diverted from their normal pathway by thickened or dead heart tissue. In such a case, the timing may be thrown off so that the ventricles are re-stimulated to contract again without waiting for the pacemaker's signal. Therefore, the heart is unable to reach its resting state.

In the ECG pattern, flutter shows up as a rapid pulsation with an indistinct QRS complex. Fibrillation is indicated by irregularly spaced pulses of random size that have no pattern at all. It is something like electrical noise coming from the heart, with no synchronization. Heart cells at many locations fire at random, producing ripples similar to those made by a handful of pebbles thrown into a lake.

The first artificial pacemaker was developed by Paul Zoll in 1952. When a patient suffering from heart block went into heart failure during surgery, Zoll inserted a needle electrode into the man's chest and applied regular voltage pulses from an external circuit. After two days, the man's heart resumed beating on its own, and the circuit was disconnected.

A portable artificial pacemaker was developed in 1957 by C. W. Lillehei and Earl Bakken. The electrode was inserted directly against the outer surface of the heart, and a battery pack and timer circuit were worn around the patient's waist. Three years later, the pacemaker was miniaturized sufficiently to be implanted under the skin of the patient's chest. This had the advantage of reducing the risk of infection.

The next major improvement was to redesign the fixed-rate pacemaker so that it could respond to variable demand during exercise or sleep. The demand pacemaker has a built-in sensor that monitors the heart's electrical system. An electronic microprocessor is programmed to recognize abnormal ECG pulses. Generally, the demand pacemaker is set to deliver a trigger pulse only when the heart rate falls below a certain point.

For people with a potential for unpredictable heart stoppage or fibrillation, a device called an implantable cardioverter defibrillator (ICD) has been developed. This unit, which is comparable to the external defibrillators used by emergency medical technicians but much smaller, can deliver several large jolts directly to the heart. Since implanted batteries are quite small, the circuit requires some time to recharge between shocks. The circuit is quite similar to the flash attachment of a camera, with its "slow charge, fast discharge" process.

USES AND COMPLICATIONS

The implantation of a pacemaker may become necessary as a result of a coronary artery disease, in which a buildup of plaque leads to irregularities in the heart's rhythm. Coronary artery disease is the main form of heart disease, which is the leading cause of death in the United States. Heart disease claimed nearly 600,000 American lives in 2010; it afflicts 11 percent of the US population. It is primarily a disease of modern, industrial society and is less frequently found in more rural, underdeveloped countries. In the United States, the death rate from heart attacks increased sharply after 1920, reached a peak in the mid-1960s, and has declined substantially since then.

A heart attack is usually caused by an oxygen deficiency in the heart muscle. The attack may come suddenly and without warning, but most often there is previous tissue damage that has weakened the heart over a period of time. A buildup of plaque in the arteries, called atherosclerosis, can reduce the rate of blood flow to a dangerously low level. The heart muscle tries to compensate for its reduced pumping power and may develop rhythmic irregularities, or arrhythmia. Eventually, heart block or ventricular fibrillations can ensue, leading to heart failure and death.

The famous Framingham Heart Study, initiated in 1948 in Framingham, Massachusetts, has been following the medical histories of approximately 5,000 men and women in order to identify the most important risk factors for heart disease. For example, the rate of heart disease among male smokers in this study was three times as high as that among nonsmokers. (This result is in addition to the much higher rate of lung cancer among smokers.) Other risk factors are excessive alcohol consumption, lack of exercise, high blood cholesterol, emotional or physical stress, and excess weight. Some unalterable risk factors are age, sex, and a family history of heart disease. The decline in heart attack deaths in recent years has been attributed to widespread changes of lifestyle to reduce the risk fac-

2186   •   Pacemaker implantation

tors, as well as to improvements in medical diagnosis and treatment.

Modern pacemakers are remarkably reliable and safe. One of the few precautions for pacemaker wearers is to avoid standing near high-level microwave sources (although household microwave ovens are harmless). The problem is that the metal wire going into the heart acts like an antenna; it can pick up stray microwave radiation, which can disrupt the electronics in the sensitive pacemaker circuit. Also, the battery in a pacemaker must be changed at five- to ten-year intervals to ensure proper operation.

Thousands of people receive implanted pacemakers each year. The procedure has become so routine that even small community hospitals are equipped to handle it. Many patients with heart block and irregular rhythm, especially elderly patients, have benefited greatly from this technological development.

PERSPECTIVE AND PROSPECTS

The creation of effective electronic pacemakers depends on an understanding of the structure and function of the human heart. Also, instruments such as x-ray machines and electrocardiographs are indispensable for monitoring an individual patient's response. This section will review the progress of the medical ideas and instruments that were the essential prerequisites for modern pacemakers. Good starting points are the pioneering studies of human anatomy made by Leonardo da Vinci (1452-1519) and Andreas Vesalius (1514-1564).

Leonardo dissected and studied the human body and made anatomical sketches in his notebooks. He recognized that the heart had four chambers, and he also drew the heart valves in detail. His interest in anatomy was that of an artist rather than that of a physician.

Vesalius was a professor of medicine at the University of Padua, in Italy. He taught anatomy and wrote a famous seven-volume treatise on the structure of the human body that had many excellent illustrations. His knowledge of anatomy came from the dissection of animals and of human cadavers obtained at night from paupers' graves. Some of his anatomical investigations contradicted traditional medical doctrine and brought him into conflict with the Catholic Church. Like Galileo, he believed that experimental information was superior to ancient textbooks.

William Harvey, a British physician, received his medical degree from the University of Padua in 1602. He is known for formulating the first accurate description of the circulation of the blood through the body. He showed that the volume of blood is fairly constant, so the function of the heart is to act as a recirculating pump. He had a clear understanding of the way in

which the right ventricle pushes blood through the lungs and the left one circulates it to the rest of the body. There was, however, one missing link in Harvey's theory: How did the blood get from the arteries to the veins for its return flow? The invention of the microscope in the 1670s made it possible to see the tiny, previously invisible capillaries, thus providing final confirmation of the circulation process.

The scientific investigation of electricity began in the eighteenth century. Benjamin Franklin studied lightning rods, and scientists learned how to build a friction machine that produced electricity in the laboratory. Taking an electric shock became an amusing, although somewhat dangerous, entertainment at parties.

About 1790, the Italian anatomist Luigi Galvani made an important, though accidental, discovery. A metal scalpel lying near an electrostatic machine came into contact with the leg of a recently dissected frog, causing a sudden twitching of the muscle. Evidently, there was a connection between the electric shock and the muscle contraction.

The modern pacemaker that stimulates the heart muscle works in the same way that Galvani's scalpel worked; however, a major evolution in physiological knowledge and medical practice had to take place before the pacemaker could be developed.

Wilhelm Conrad Röntgen was experimenting with high voltages in his laboratory in 1896 when he observed a mysterious new type of radiation, which he called x-rays. Unlike light, x-rays were able to pass through black paper, wood, and even thin metal sheets. They could cause certain paints to glow in the dark and could expose photographic film that was still in its light-tight box. For the medical profession, the discovery of x-rays was a major breakthrough.

X-ray technology has been improved in recent years. Electronic image intensifiers were developed in the 1950s in order to brighten the dim pictures on a fluorescent screen. A major breakthrough in the 1970s was the invention of computed tomography (CT) scanning. Instead of using film or a fluoroscope, a computer generates images of the heart and other internal organs on a video screen. For pacemaker implantation, x-ray apparatus is indispensable in order to observe the electrode's precise placement into the interior of the heart.

The electrodes of most pacemakers are installed with a catheter that is inserted through a vein, through the right atrium, through the valve, and finally touches the inside of the right ventricle. The first human heart catheterization is credited to Werner Forssmann in 1929, when he was a young intern at a hospital in Berlin, Germany. He requested permission to try the procedure on a patient, but his supervisor refused. Forssmann then decided to try it on himself. He anesthetized his left elbow, opened a vein, and inserted the catheter tube. As he pushed it up the arm, he watched its progress on an x-ray fluoroscope, which he had to view by reflection in a mirror held by a nurse. When the catheter had gone in 65 centimeters, Forssmann asked an x-ray technician to record it on film to prove that it had entered his heart. During the next two years, he repeated the procedure several times, but criticism by his medical colleagues forced him to discontinue it. He became a small-town doctor and was amazed to learn in 1956 that he had been awarded the Nobel Prize for Medicine.

Accumulated knowledge about the structure of the heart, improvements in surgery, the development of new drugs, and the availability of modern instrumentation have all contributed to a substantial improvement in the medical treatment of heart ailments in modern times. The development of artificial heart valves, the heart-lung machine, the success of heart bypass surgery, the use of laser beams for surgery, and the use of drugs to control high blood pressure are recent developments.

An important contribution from the field of electronics was the development of the transistor in the early 1950s. It made possible the whole technology of miniaturized electronics, replacing the bulky vacuum tubes that were used in old radio circuits. Implantable pacemakers and microprocessor sensors would not have been possible without transistors.

Human ingenuity no doubt will continue to develop new instruments for cardiac diagnosis and rehabilitation, building on the accomplishments of the innovators of the past.

—Hans G. Graetzer, PhD

See also Arrhythmias; Cardiac arrest; Cardiac rehabilitation; Cardiac surgery; Cardiology; Cardiology, pediatric; Cardiopulmonary resuscitation (CPR); Circulation; Echocardiography; Electrocardiography (ECG or EKG); Exercise physiology; Heart; Heart attack; Heart disease; Heart valve replacement; Vascular medicine; Vascular system.

For Further Information:
Corona, Gyl Garren. "Pacemakers: Keeping the Beat Today." *RN* 62, no. 12 (December, 1999): 50-52.
Crawford, Michael, ed. *Current Diagnosis and Treatment: Cardiology.* 3d ed. New York: McGraw-Hill Medical, 2009.
Davis, Goode P., Jr., and Edwards Park. *The Heart: The Living Pump.* Washington, DC: U.S. News Books, 1981.
Eagle, Kim A., and Ragavendra R. Baliga, eds. *Practical Cardiology: Evaluation and Treatment of Common Cardiovascular Disorders.* 2d ed. Philadelphia: Lippincott Williams & Wilkins, 2008.
Gersh, Bernard J., ed. *The Mayo Clinic Heart Book.* 2d ed. New York: William Morrow, 2000.
Jeffrey, Kirk. *Machines in Our Hearts: The Cardiac Pacemaker, the Implantable Defibrillator, and American Health Care.* Baltimore: Johns Hopkins University Press, 2001.
"Pacemaker." *Mayo Clinic,* April 17, 2013.
"Pacemaker Insertion." *Health Library,* November 26, 2012.
Sonnenberg, David, Michael Birnbaum, and Emil A. Naclerio. *Understanding Pacemakers.* New York: Michael Kesend, 1982.
Urone, Paul Peter. *Physics with Health Science Applications.* New York: John Wiley & Sons, 1986.
"What Is a Pacemaker?" *National Heart, Lung, and Blood Institute,* February 28, 2012.

PAGET'S DISEASE

Category: Disease/Disorder
Also known as: Osteitis deformans, Paget's disease of bone
Anatomy or system affected: Bones, head, hips, legs, musculoskeletal system, spine
Specialties and related fields: Genetics, orthopedics, rheumatology, virology
Definition: A chronic disorder resulting in enlarged and deformed bones.

CAUSES AND SYMPTOMS

Paget's disease of bone is a disorder characterized by excessive and abnormal formation of bone, most commonly in the spine, skull, pelvis, thighs, and lower legs. (Paget's disease of the nipple is a different disorder related to breast cancer.) The cause of this disease is under investigation. Genetic factors are a major component. Between 15 and 40 percent of all patients with Paget's disease have a positive family history of the disease, and the risk of developing Paget's disease is seven to ten times higher in relatives of those who have Paget's disease compared with relatives of those who do not have this disease. Several genes are known to regulate the cells that remodel bone, and mutations in some of these genes seem to be the main cause of Paget's disease in some patients.

In adult, nongrowing bone, the structure of bone is the result of the interplay between two types of cells-one

---

INFORMATION ON PAGET'S DISEASE

Causes: Unknown; possibly viral infection and genetic factors
Symptoms: Excessive and abnormal formation of bone (commonly in spine, skull, pelvis, thighs, lower legs); increased risk of fractures; curving of spine or legs; bone and joint pain
Duration: Chronic and progressive
Treatments: Bisphosphonates (pamidronate, alendronate, risedronate, tiludronate); pain medications (acetaminophen, NSAIDs); exercise; adequate intake of calcium and vitamin D; surgery

that deposits bone, the osteoblast, and another that resorbs bone, a multinucleate cell called the osteoclast. A signaling system called the RANK-RANKL-OPG system regulates osteoclast recruitment. RANK is a receptor on the surface of osteoclast precursor cells. RANKL is the ligand, or molecule, that binds to RANK to activate it. RANKL is secreted by bone marrow cells; when RANKL binds to the RANK molecules on the surface of osteoclast precursor cells, it activates an internal protein called p62. The activation of p62 pushes osteoclast precursor cells toward becoming mature, bone-resorbing osteoclasts. Osteoblasts, however, also secrete OPG, a soluble receptor that competitively binds RANKL and prevents osteoclast recruitment (see figure on page 2244). Mutations in the genes that encode RANK, OPG, or p62 cause various inherited forms of Paget's disease with varying severities and times when the disease manifests itself. Not all individuals who harbor these mutations, however, suffer from full-blown Paget's disease.

Paget's disease might also result from viral infections. Experimental infection of mouse osteoblasts with measles virus can cause Paget's disease in mice. Furthermore, osteoblasts from human patients with Paget's disease sometimes harbor measles virus or other closely related viruses. It is possible that the presence of mutations in genes that increase osteoclast activity in combination with chronic infection of osteoclasts by measles virus or similar viruses create an environment that nurtures the development of clinical Paget's disease.

Paget's disease is more common in people over the age of forty. The disease usually starts without any symptoms. It is often diagnosed when a person has radiographs taken for other reasons or has a higher-than-normal level of alkaline phosphatase in the blood. As the disease progresses, the patient may develop an enlarging skull, sometimes accompanied by headaches; increased risk of fractures; curving of the spine or legs; and bone and joint pain. Rarely, Paget's disease may lead to kidney stones, loose teeth when bones of the face are involved, and loss of hearing and vision when the enlarging skull compresses nerves to the eye and ear. People with severe Paget's disease may have heart problems such as congestive heart failure or abnormal heart rhythms. Less than 1 percent of people with Paget's disease will develop bone cancer.

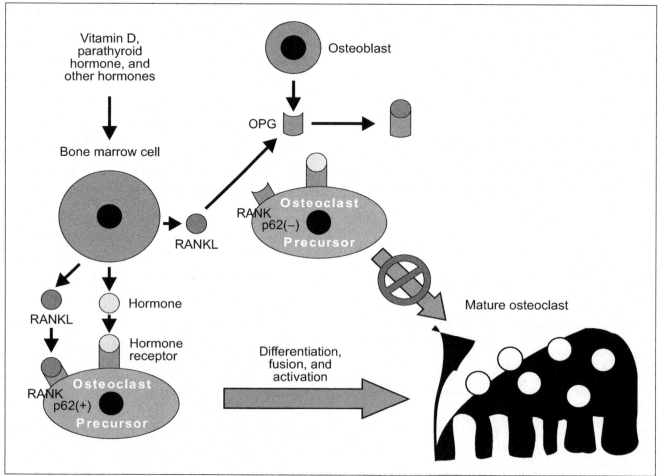

TREATMENT AND THERAPY

Bisphosphonates (such as etidronate, pamidronate, alendronate, risedronate, or tiludronate) are the main treatment for Paget's disease. Subcutaneous injections of salmon calcitonin successfully reverse the symptoms of Paget's disease, but 50 percent of all patients who receive this treatment develop an immune response against calcitonin and 10 to 20 percent of all patients become resistant to it. In patients with severe symptoms who do not respond to these more typical treatments, the antibiotic mithramycin has been used successfully, but the toxicity of this drug militates against its use for anything but worst-case scenarios.

Treatment is given when patients experience pain, deformities, nerve compression, or other symptoms or to prevent the risk of future complications when the skull, spine, legs, and/or pelvis are involved. Therapy is given until the levels of alkaline phosphatase in the blood return to normal, and it may need to be repeated if that level increases again. Acetaminophen or nonsteroidal anti-inflammatory drugs (NSAIDs) may be used to treat pain. Exercise and adequate intake of calcium and vitamin D are also recommended. Surgery may be needed to stabilize fractures, replace joints affected with severe pain from arthritis, or decompress nerves.

PERSPECTIVE AND PROSPECTS

Paget's disease likely has been around for many centuries, as it has been observed in a grossly thickened Egyptian skull dating from about 1000 BCE. The disorder is named after a British surgeon, Sir James Paget, who was the first to describe this condition in 1876. He noted five patients with thickened bones that were prone to fracture and deformity. Paget thought that the disorder resulted from chronic inflammation and named it osteitis deformans. Subsequently, researchers have shown that Paget's disease of bone arises from the overproduction of poor-quality bone, rather than from chronic inflammation.

Identification of mutations in candidate genes in patients who have active Paget's disease, coupled with the expression of these mutant genes in transgenic mice in which the endogenous copy of the same gene has been eliminated (so-called knockout mice), represents one of the most powerful techniques for studying the cause and pathology of Paget's disease. Combining Paget's disease-specific mutations in transgenic mice whose osteoblasts have been chronically infected with measles virus or respiratory syncytial virus has also greatly elucidated the nongenetic causes of this disease.

—*Meika A. Fang, MD;*
updated by Michael A. Buratovich, PhD

See also Bone disorders; Bones and the skeleton; Fracture and dislocation; Orthopedic surgery; Orthopedics; Orthopedics, pediatric.

For Further Information:
Daroszewska, Anna, and Stuart H. Ralston. "Genetics of Paget's Disease of Bone." *Clinical Science* 109, 3. (September, 2005): 257-263.
DeGroot, Leslie J., J. Larry Jameson, et al. *Endocrinology: Adult and Pediatric.* Philadelphia: Saunders/Elsevier, 2010.
Delmas, Pierre D., and P. J. Meunier. "Drug Therapy: The Management of Paget's Disease of Bone." *New England Journal of Medicine* 336, 8. (February 20, 1997): 558-566.
Kanis, John A. *Pathophysiology and Treatment of Paget's Disease of Bone.* 2d ed. London: Martin Dunitz, 1998.
Klippel, John H., ed. *Primer on the Rheumatic Diseases.* 13th ed. New York: Springer, 2008.
Litin, Scott C., ed. *Mayo Clinic Family Health Book.* 4th ed. New York: HarperResource, 2009.
McDermott, Michael T. *Endocrine Secrets.* Philadelphia: Elsevier, 2013.
"Paget's Disease of Bone." *MedlinePlus*, May 9, 2013.
Ralston, Stuart H. "Paget's Disease of Bone." *New England Journal of Medicine* 368.7. (2013): 644-650.
Roodman, David G., and Jolene J. Windle. "Paget Disease of Bone." *Journal of Clinical Investigation* 115, 2 (February, 2005): 200-208.

PAIN

Category: Disease/Disorder
Anatomy or system affected: All
Specialties and related fields: Most, especially anesthesiology, general surgery, genetics, internal medicine, neurology, oncology, physical therapy, psychiatry, rheumatology, sports medicine
Definition: An unpleasant, subjective experience of physical or mental suffering, a symptom of a real or potential underlying cause, condition, or injury.
Key terms:
acute pain: sudden, extreme pain that is short-term; serves as a warning of damage or disease
analgesic: a drug or medication that alleviates pain by blocking pain receptors
chronic pain: a deeper, aching pain that comes on slowly and lasts longer than the normal course for a specific injury or condition; may be constant or intermittent
cutaneous pain: caused by injuries to the skin or superficial tissues; brief and localized
endorphins: brain chemicals released by the body that act as natural painkillers
nociception: the process of transmitting pain messages to the brain through the spinal cord by sensitive nerve endings in skin and tissues
referred pain: pain experienced at a site other than the site of origin

substance P: a peptide found in nerve cells in the body, which serves as a chemical messenger (neurotransmitter) that carries pain messages along pathways to the brain

visceral pain: throbbing or aching pain that originates in the deeper body tissues and organs; of longer duration than cutaneous pain

CAUSES AND SYMPTOMS

Not all causes of pain are known or understood, but some basic causes of the most commonly reported pain include inflammation, as in arthritis, rheumatism, and infection; work-related and sports-related injuries; stress and tension; nerve pain, as from shingles, diabetic neuropathy, and sciatica; and pain related to such diseases as osteoporosis and cancer.

People have similar pain thresholds but different levels of pain tolerance, or how much pain they can bear. One congenital anomaly actually inhibits or eliminates the perception of pain. Pain tolerance is therefore subjective and can be influenced by socioeconomic status, cultural background, and socialization, with disparities noted in who suffers pain, what type of pain a person suffers, and how pain is perceived by the individual.

The most commonly reported types of pain are associated with the lower back, with severe or migraine headache, and with joint pain, particularly in the knees. Physiological pain is a response of the body associated with tissue damage or inflammation, or as a warning system to alert the body to potential physical harm. Although pain may be produced without a defined stimulus, such as with emotional or psychological pain, physiological pain is transmitted through stimulation of nerve pathways, a process called nociception. Nociceptors are free, sensitive nerve endings located outside the spinal column; they are found in skin and on internal surfaces, such as on the joints. Nociceptors, when stimulated, send signals through sensory neurons to the posterior horn of the spinal cord that are then transmitted to other nerve fibers, which travel upward through the brain stem to the thalamus, the gateway to conscious action in the brain. There, information is coordinated and localized and then sent to the cerebral cortex, where a conscious reaction to the stimulus is produced.

Pain is said to be referred when it is experienced at a location other than its site of origin. This occurs when nerve fibers carrying pain messages enter the spinal cord at the same place as other nerve fibers from other parts of the body using the same pathways. The other nerve fibers may become stimulated and result in painful perceptions in healthy areas of the body, such as referred pain from the heart to the neck, arm, and stomach.

INFORMATION ON PAIN

Causes: Infection, trauma, disease
Symptoms: Sensation may range from mild to severe
Duration: Acute to chronic
Treatments: Wide ranging; may include drug therapy, surgery, physical therapy, alternative medicine

---

Among theories of pain transmission, the gate control theory of Ronald Malzack and Patrick Wall helps to explain the differing degrees of pain that people may suffer. It is related to the amount of substance P, a peptide found in nerve cells throughout the body, that actually reaches the brain. The transmission of neurons is generally very rapid, as when touching a hot stove produces immediate action to protect the body from damage. Messages carried by substance P, however, travel more slowly, since they must pass through a special gateway in the spinal cord. At the same time, pain signals are also prompting the brain to release chemical endorphins, the body's natural painkillers, which must also pass downward through the same gate. Thus, there is some competition for passage, and the fewer receptors for substance P that actually arrive in the brain and attach to nerve cells there, the lower the pain perception. With healing, the gate closes, but when chronic pain occurs, it remains open even after healing or without an identified underlying cause.

The two basic types of pain are chronic and acute. Acute pain comes on suddenly and, although extreme, is generally brief in duration. Acute pain is a warning to the body about damage or disease, is localized, and is more easily treated. Chronic pain, however, occurs daily and lasts longer than would be common for a specific injury. It no longer serves to warn, and it is much more difficult to treat, although most sufferers can be helped. Chronic pain may last beyond resolution of an underlying cause, or it may grow out of an acute condition. In this case, it may become a learned response that no longer has a purpose but continues to hurt. Chronic pain may also occur without any apparent cause, creating disability, depression, and suffering.

Pain may be medically classified as either superficial or deep. Superficial pain, also called fast or cutaneous pain, is carried by nerve fibers on the skin and outer linings of the organs. These nerve fibers are plentiful in the intestines, cornea, and nose, for example, and pain messages are quickly delivered to the brain, such as when one is cut or burned. Also termed somatic pain, it is experienced as intense, or burning. Kidney stones or acid reflux from the stomach may create waves of this burning pain. Deep pain, on the other hand, also referred to as slow or visceral pain, comes

Referred Pain

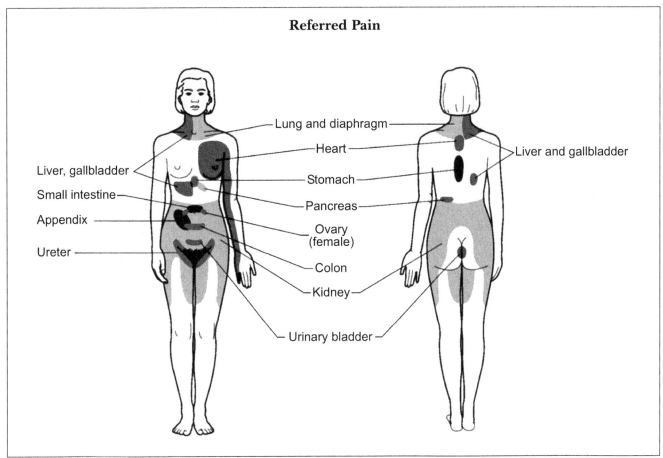

Liver, gallbladder

Small intestine

Appendix

Ureter

Lung and diaphragm

Heart

Stomach

Pancreas

Ovary
(female)

Colon

Kidney

Urinary bladder

Liver and gallbladder

Internal organs do not have the same type of neural sensors found in surface tissues; as a result, damage to internal organs may manifest itself in areas of the body away from the organ's location. ©EBSCO

from nerve fibers located in muscles, bones, and tissues of the internal organs, and it travels more slowly, taking longer to reach the brain. It may be experienced as dull aching or throbbing pain. The two types of pain may also occur at the same time.

TREATMENT AND THERAPY

The major treatment for pain in the United States has been analgesic medications, or drug therapy, with sufferers spending over an estimated $18 billion a year for relief in the form of both prescription and over-the-counter medications. There are no standard guidelines for the use of analgesics, since the degree of relief varies from one patient to another. These medications are classified as narcotic, such as morphine or opium-based addictive drugs, and nonnarcotic, such as aspirin, ibuprofen, and acetaminophen. Since patients respond differently, and many of the analgesics can carry significant side effects with cardiovascular, renal, and gastrointestinal toxicity, the lowest dose of the preferred medication is usually recommended to start. Painkillers must also often be administered with other medications directed to the underlying cause of the pain and must therefore be compatible.

One subcategory of nonnarcotic analgesics is made up of nonsteroidal anti-inflammatory drugs (NSAIDs). Another alternative, acetaminophen, addresses pain but has no effect on inflammation. Another nonnarcotic class of drugs, known as COX-2 inhibitors, suppress the COX-2 enzyme, which triggers inflammation. Although these drugs are seemingly well tolerated and effective, it was found that many of them endanger the heart, and several were withdrawn from the market.

Narcotic analgesics are the most effective, but long-term use can create dependency, and these drugs are stringently protected in the United States by state and federal laws. Doctors have therefore been hesitant to use them for severe chronic pain, even in patients dying from cancer or other painful diseases, when other medications are not working. This situation appears to be changing.

Nondrug therapies include such techniques as transcutaneous electrical nerve stimulation (TENS), massage therapy, neurosurgery, physical therapy and exercise, and mind-body therapies such as guided imagery, meditation, relaxation, and hypnosis. These therapies attempt to alleviate chronic pain in various ways by stimulating blood circulation, blocking nerve pain messengers, and enlisting the help of the brain, where pain messages are processed.

A combination of biomedical and nonbiomedical therapies also utilizes a number of alternative therapies for pain. Acupuncture and acupressure, the foundation of Chinese medicine, are thought to stimulate blood circulation and possibly the autonomic nervous system through insertion of very fine needles at crucial points in the body. Herbal medicine uses substances that are derived from plants with therapeutic or pharmacologic properties and benefits. Many of today's medicines have ingredients that originated in plants and can be synthesized in the laboratory. Guided imagery, aromatherapy, creative arts therapy, magnet therapy, and therapeutic touch are often used as adjuncts to dealing with pain, but most have not been proven. Like analgesics, these therapies address the control and management of pain rather than offering a cure.

Although many of these complementary therapies are not biomedically sanctioned or recognized, many sufferers of chronic pain try some form of complementary medicine. Little or no research has been done on many of these therapies, but their popularity relates to the fact that chronic pain is closely connected with the brain, affecting emotions, attitudes, and psychological stability, which are not addressed by conventional medicine and treatment. Some of these therapies may work through the placebo effect-meaning that if one expects the therapy to alleviate pain, then it will. Some approaches are backed by positive evidence, while others may have been shown to have no effect. Very little evidence exists about how or why many of these therapies are successful, but combination therapies are vital in alleviating pain, however they may work.

PERSPECTIVE AND PROSPECTS

The development of pain medicine and pain clinics devoted solely to the study and alleviation of pain is a fairly recent occurrence. Since pain was traditionally seen as a symptom rather than as a disease or condition in itself, the medical profession has generally focused on treating the cause, considering pain to be purely a diagnostic tool. The discovery and development of anesthetics for surgical procedures in the latter nineteenth century, however, was a huge advance in medical care and treatment and was a precondition for the later development of pain medicine. Anesthesiologists not only had to address traumatic and postoperative pain but also worked to refine techniques and developed expertise in management relating to other types of pain.

Anesthesiology progressed rapidly during World War II, with improved use of nerve blocking and anal-

gesics. Anesthesiologist John Bonica contributed significantly to this development of pain medicine. He was faced with extreme, intractable, complex, and phantom limb pain (the sensation of pain felt in a limb no longer there) in the injured during wartime and lacked knowledge or methods to treat them. As pain persisted and when physiological causes could not be identified, it became necessary to look elsewhere for the source of the pain. It became obvious that numerous specialists, including psychologists and psychiatrists, needed to consult and discuss their varied findings and opinions.

Practitioners of pain medicine mostly come from other medical fields most closely related to pain, such as neurology, anesthesiology, and rehabilitation. As defined by the American Academy of Pain Medicine, the specialty is concerned with the study, prevention, evaluation, treatment, and rehabilitation of people in pain. Many are certified as pain specialists through the American Board of Anesthesiology. While some pain clinics focus on specific types of pain, such as bone and joint, others address a broader spectrum of suffering and tend to use a variety of methods and treatments, including alternative therapies, to find whatever works. Some pain cannot be eliminated but can be minimized or controlled to allow the patient to function.

The need to study and understand the causes and alleviation of pain have become more urgent. According to the National Center for Health Statistics, one in four adults in the United States reported suffering pain lasting for at least twenty-four hours during the previous month, and one in ten reported pain lasting a year or more. Pain is usually seen as a result of another physical condition, but considering the costs that accompany pain and resulting disability in terms of dollars and loss of individual function reflected in absenteeism in the workplace, pain places an increasing burden on the American health care system. The general cost of pain and pain-related items is estimated to top $100 billion each year.

Research is being conducted into the origins and mechanics of pain in an attempt to identify new and more effective therapies. A study funded by the National Institutes of Health found that the perception of pain (the extent to which one feels pain) is inherited through a gene with a specific variant. This gene variant affects sensitivity to acute pain as well as the risk of developing chronic pain. Other genes may also play a role. This study opens up pathways for developing new treatments and approaches to pain.

Such professional organizations as the American Academy of Pain Medicine, the American Pain Foundation, the American Pain Society, and the International Association for the Study of Pain represent only a few of the growing number of resources for the study of pain and pain management. Alternative approaches are represented through organizations for specific therapies and the National Center for Complementary and Alternative Medicine.

—*Martha Oehmke Loustaunau, PhD*

See also Acupressure; Acupuncture; Alternative medicine; Amputation; Anesthesia; Anesthesiology; Arthritis; Back pain; Bruises; Burns and scalds; Cancer; Fibromyalgia; Headaches; Healing; Hypnosis; Local anesthesia; Massage; Meditation; Narcotics; Nervous system; Neuralgia, neuritis, and neuropathy; Neurology; Over-the-counter medications; Pain management; Physical rehabilitation; Prescription drug abuse; Self-medication; Skin; Stress; Stress reduction; Substance abuse; Toothache; Touch; Wounds.

For Further Information:
Baszanger, Isabelle. *Inventing Pain Medicine: From the Laboratory to the Clinic.* New Brunswick, N.J.: Rutgers University Press, 1998.
Bellenir, Karen, ed. *Pain Sourcebook: Basic Consumer Health Information About Specific Forms of Acute and Chronic Pain.* 2d ed. Detroit, Mich.: Omnigraphics, 2002.
Coakley, Sarah, and Kay Kaufman Shelemay, eds. *Pain and Its Transformations: The Interface of Biology and Culture.* Cambridge, Mass.: Harvard University Press, 2008..
Fishman, Scott M. *Bonica's Management of Pain.* 4th ed. Philadelphia: Lippincott Williams & Wilkins, 2012.
Vertosick, Frank T., Jr. *Why We Hurt: The Natural History of Pain.* New York: Harcourt, 2000.
Waldman, Steven D. *Atlas of Uncommon Pain Syndromes.* Philadelphia: Elsevier, 2014.
Wall, Patrick David. *Pain: The Science of Suffering.* New York: Columbia University Press, 2013.

PAIN MANAGEMENT

Category: Treatment
Anatomy or system affected: All
Specialties and related fields: Alternative medicine, anesthesiology, critical care, emergency medicine, geriatrics and gerontology, oncology, pharmacology, physical therapy, psychiatry, psychology
Definition: Any treatment or management technique to lessen or eliminate pain or make it more tolerable.

INDICATIONS AND PROCEDURES

Pain is experienced as an unpleasant reaction to either an external stimulus (e.g., a burn) or an internal process (e.g., a disease). The initial evaluation of pain is aimed at determining the cause. A good description by the patient aids diagnosis. The person experiencing the pain must be able to communicate the intensity, location, pattern (throbbing, steady, or intermittent) and type (crushing, burning, sharp, or dull). In addition, factors that make the pain better or worse must be known and communicated. Duration is important; recent onset is called "acute" pain while long-standing pain or pain that returns periodically is called "chronic."

Generally, the best way to treat pain is to prevent its occurrence. Failing that, a number of different interventions should be used together. Whatever treatment is used, the therapy must be tailored both to the patient and to the nature and severity of the pain. When medications are used, review of some important principles is essential, such as the pharmacology, duration of effectiveness, and optimal dose of a certain medication. Even the route of administration must be considered in every case.

Treatment may include combinations of simple analgesics, narcotics, and other treatments. Combinations take advantage of the additive pain relief while sparing the patient potential side effects. When choosing pain medications, a stepwise approach is often used. It starts with the simple analgesics: aspirin, acetaminophen, and nonsteroidal anti-inflammatory drugs (NSAIDs). These medications are generally well tolerated, although aspirin and NSAIDs can produce gastrointestinal distress ranging from mild heartburn to bleeding ulcers. Additionally, adjuncts to these types of medications might be icing or heat, depending on the nature of the problem.

For more severe pain, the second step often includes a narcotic analgesic with or without the simple analgesics. Narcotics are very potent and have a potential for addiction. Furthermore, they may produce problems such as confusion, nausea and vomiting, constipation, and drowsiness. If the pain has a significant inflammation component that does not resolve easily with milder analgesic approaches or with narcotics, then corticosteroids may be used to alleviate the pain. This approach does not lend itself well to longer-term pain management, however, because of side effects such as fluid retention, stomach irritation, thrush, muscle weakness, weight gain, bone loss, suppressed adrenal function, and increased risk of infections, among others.

The third step in pain control involves alternative methods of pain control. Treatments here include physical therapy, nerve-blocking injections, transcutaneous electrical nerve stimulation (TENS), and behavioral approaches. The latter method seeks to identify the causes of preventable pain (physical or mental) and takes steps to minimize pain.

Medical research is leading to interesting discoveries about the management of pain. In 2002, researchers announced that they had identified a key protein that controls severe pain, a discovery that could lead to better pain management for patients who suffer from chronic pain or pain associated with terminal cancer. The protein, known by the acronym DREAM (Downstream Regulatory Element Antagonistic Modulator), protects the neural reflex critical to survival, allowing individuals to feel pain and quickly pull away from its source, but over time, DREAM seems to help sharp pain fade as the protein becomes disabled. Moreover, while there are many types of pain, disabling the DREAM protein appears to reduce the severity of all of them. The next step in research will be to examine ways to disable the protein, a task that scientists deem difficult because of its location deep within individual cells. Additional research in this area recognizes that pain has different causes and that it may be more productive to examine mechanisms of pain rather than taking a disease-based approach.

—*Misa Hyakutake, MD*

See also: Acupressure; Acupuncture; Alternative medicine; Anesthesia; Anesthesiology; Biofeedback; Chiropractic; Hypnosis; Local anesthesia; Marijuana; Meditation; Narcotics; Over-the-counter medications; Pain; Palliative medicine; Pharmacology; Prescription drug abuse; Self-medication; Substance abuse.

For Further Information:
Cousins, Michael J., and P. O. Bridenbaugh, editors. *Cousins and Bridenbaugh's Neural Blockade in Clinical Anesthesia and Management of Pain*. 4th ed., Lippincott Williams & Wilkins, 2009.
Dillard, James M. *The Chronic Pain Solution: The Comprehensive, Step-by-Step Guide to Choosing the Best of Alternative and Conventional Medicine*. Bantam Books, 2002.
"DREAM Repression & Dynorphin Expression." *Qiagen.com*, 2013.
Ferrari, Lynne R., editor. *Anesthesia and Pain Management for the Pediatrician*. Johns Hopkins UP, 1999.
Ferrer-Brechner, Theresa. *Common Problems in Pain Management*. Year Book Medical, 1990.
Fishman, Scott, with Lisa Berger. *The War on Pain: How Breakthroughs in the New Field of Pain Medicine Are Turning the Tide Against Suffering*. HarperCollins, 2001.
Loeser, John D., editor. *Bonica's Management of Pain*. 4th ed., Lippincott Williams & Wilkins, 2010.
"Pain Management." *Nih.gov*, 29 Mar. 2013.
"Pain Management Facts." *Lls.org*, May 2013.
"Pain Management Programs." *Theacpa.org*, 2009.
Raj, Prithvi, and Lee Ann Paradise, editors. *Pain Medicine: A Comprehensive Review*. 2nd ed., Mosby, 2003.
Rosenfeld, Arthur. *The Truth About Chronic Pain: Patients and Professionals on How to Face It, Understand It, Overcome It*. Rev. ed., Basic Books, 2005.

PALLIATIVE CARE

Category: Specialty
Anatomy or system affected: All

Specialties and related fields: Most, especially critical care, internal medicine, geriatrics, oncology, pain medicine, cardiology, pulmonary, hematology, nephrology, psychology, radiology, nursing and ethics

Definition: Palliative care is a medical specialty which aims to maximize quality of life in people with life-threatening illnesses. Palliative care focuses on symptom control, pain management, and psychosocial support for patients and their families.

Key terms:

multidisciplinary care: A comprehensive care provided by professionals from different disciplines, including doctors, nurses, pharmacists, social workers, and many others.

pain management: A treatment to control pain and reduce suffering using pharmacological and/or non-pharmacological methods. The goal is to improve quality of life.

hospice: End-of-life medical care for people who are terminally ill. Similar to palliative care, the focuses are also symptom control, pain management and psychosocial support.

OVERVIEW

Palliative care is a multidisciplinary medical care approach for people with serious or life-threatening illnesses. These patients often suffer from severe pain, shortness of breath, fatigue, difficulty sleeping, or other distressing physical symptoms. They and their families may also experience stress or even depression while trying to cope with the patients' illnesses. The goal of palliative care is to maximize quality of life through pain management, symptom control as well as psychosocial support. Receiving palliative care does not mean that the patient has to stop the primary curative treatment. Instead, palliative care is like another layer of support on top of the original medical treatment plan. Palliative program not only cares for the patient, but also his or her family. It designs individualized plan of care taking into consideration the patient and the family's needs, values, beliefs, and goals.

Palliative care should not be confused with hospice, which focuses on end-of-life care and comfort. Patients in hospice programs usually have stopped the curative treatments; instead, emphasis is on pain and symptom relief and how to make the most out of the last days or months of life.

Individuals who may consider palliative care includes anyone who has severe illnesses and suffers from uncontrolled pain or other distressing physical or psychological symptoms. Examples of some devastating diseases include cancer, heart disease, lung disease, kidney failure, Human immunodeficiency virus

Palliative Care versus Hospice		
	Palliative Care	**Hospice**
Similarities	• Improve quality of life for people with severe illness—pain management, symptom control, psychosocial support • Patient and family-centered care • Team approach	
Differences — Timing	• During any stage of illness, doesn't need to be terminal	• Terminal stage of illness or with limited life expectancy (generally < 6 months, varies by different hospice programs)
Location	• Hospital • Extended care facility • Nursing home • Home	• Home • Extended care facility • Nursing home
Curative or life-prolonging treatment	• Continue	• Usually stopped
Insurance coverage	• Medicare • Medicaid • Most private insurance	• Medicare • Medicaid • Most private insurance

©EBSCO

infection / acquired immunodeficiency syndrome (HIV/AIDS). Lupus, Alzheimer's, and many others. People do not need to wait until the terminal stage of his or her illness to receive palliative care. It can be started during any stage of the illness to enhance quality of life. Applying for palliative care is not difficult. Patients and families with potential needs should talk to their doctors and ask for a referral for palliative care. Palliative care often starts in the hospital, but can be provided in various nursing facilities, outpatient clinics, hospices, or even at patients' home.

TREATMENT AND THERAPY
Palliative care is all about making the life more comfortable and meaningful for the patient and his or her loved ones. It is accomplished using a team approach. A palliative care team consists of professionals from different disciplines, including doctors, nurses, pharmacists, social workers, chaplains, nutritionists, counselors, and others. The team closely works with the patient and the family to assess their needs, values, beliefs, and goals. Patient education and counseling are also provided to help the patient better understand his or her health condition and how to more effectively cope with it. The palliative care team also works collaboratively with patient's primary health care providers to design a comprehensive and individualized treatment plan to maximize physical and emotional comfort.

The length of palliative care depends on the individual's health condition and family goals and needs. The financial aspect of the care is almost always a concern for patients and their families. The good news is

that Medicare, Medicaid, and most private insurance covers all or part of palliative treatment. In instances when palliative care is not fully covered by Medicare, Medicaid, or private insurance, there may be funds available within the community or through the state to subsidize the cost.

—*Zhongqi Weng*

See also Hospice, death and dying, end of life, euthanasia, oncology, pain, psychiatry, terminally ill, ethics

For Further Information:
Mayo Clinic. (2013). *Palliative Care: Symptom Relief During Illness.* Retrieved October 12, 2013, from www.mayoclinic.com/health/palliative-care/ MY01051.
National Caregivers Library. (2013). *Hospice vs. Palliative Care.* Retrieved October 13, 2013, from www.caregiverslibrary.org/caregivers-resources/grp-end-of-life-issues/hsgrp-hospice/hospice-vs-palliative-care-article.aspx.
National Hospice and Palliative Care Organization. (2013). *Palliative Care.* Retrieved October 12, 2013, from www.nhpco.org/palliative-care-0.
National Institute of Health, National Institute of Nursing Research. (2009). *Palliative Care.* Retrieved October 12, 2013, from www.ninr.nih.gov/newsandinformation/publications/palliative-care-brochure.

PALLIATIVE MEDICINE

Category: Specialty
Anatomy or system affected: All
Specialties and related fields: Anesthesiology, emergency medicine, family medicine, internal medicine,

obstetrics and gynecology, pediatrics, physical medicine and rehabilitation, psychiatry and neurology, radiology and surgery

Definition: The World Health Organization (WHO) defines palliative care as: An approach that improves the quality of life of patients and their families facing the problem associated with life-threatening illness, through the prevention and relief of suffering by means of early identification and impeccable assessment and treatment of pain and other problems, physical, psychosocial, and spiritual.

Key terms:

multidisciplinary: involving several medical specialties, requiring health care practitioners from various perspectives to work closely together to meet the needs of the patient

opioid medications: pain medications derived from opiates, such as morphine, oxycodone, codeine, and fentanyl; intended to control severe pain

SCIENCE AND PROFESSION

While in the United States, The National Hospice and Palliative Care Organization (NHPCO) defines palliative care as: Treatment that enhances comfort and improves the quality of an individual's life during the last phase of life. No specific therapy is excluded from consideration. The test of palliative care lies in the agreement between the individual, physician(s), primary caregiver, and the hospice team that the expected outcome is relief from distressing symptoms, the easing of pain, and/or enhancing the quality of life. The decision to intervene with active palliative care is based on an ability to meet stated goals rather than affect the underlying disease. An individual's needs must continue to be assessed and all treatment options explored and evaluated in the context of the individual's values and symptoms. The individual's choices and decisions regarding care are paramount and must be followed.

Palliative medicine is a specialty that spans disciplines. The goal is to comfort and support patients as they face life-threatening illnesses, not only relieving their suffering but also addressing their emotional and spiritual needs. Although palliative medicine is typically associated with the final stages of life-threatening conditions, patients may also benefit from specialized care while they are still undergoing active treatment. In that case, symptom relief and other interventions to improve their quality of life help improve their strength and stamina to endure additional cycles of therapy.

Palliative care may be provided in a long-term care facility, a hospital, or the patient's home. Care is provided by a team consisting of primary care physicians, specialists in the patient's condition (for example, oncologists, cardiologists, or pulmonologists), palliative medicine specialist, nurses, social workers, mental health specialists (psychologists, psychiatrists, or counselors), nutritionists, and clergy. The level and type of care provided are guided by the wishes and needs of the patient. Pain management is often the greatest need, but the patient may also require relief of other symptoms associated with the condition or its treatment, such as nausea, vomiting, decreased appetite, inability to eat, dehydration, constipation or diarrhea, shortness of breath, malaise, fatigue, anxiety, depression, and altered consciousness.

Palliative medicine is recognized as a basic human right in the International Bill of Human Rights of the United Nations. The document declares that all people have the right to adequate health and medical care, and further states that patients with chronic and terminal illnesses have the right to avoid pain and die with dignity. Following these principles, Canada decreed that every citizen has the right to palliative care. The European Committee of Ministers and the South African Department of Health declared that palliative care is a right of all citizens. Palliative medicine is formally recognized as a specialty in Australia, France, Germany, Hong Kong, Ireland, New Zealand, Poland, Romania, Slovakia, Taiwan, the United States, and the United Kingdom.

Palliative medicine is an essential component of care for patients suffering from any chronic, life-threatening illness, but the specialty has taken on an added significance in the field of oncology. In the United States, the Institute of Medicine stated in 1997 that any comprehensive cancer care plan should include palliative care. A 2005 resolution of the 58th World Health Assembly to improve cancer care placed palliative medicine on equal footing with surgery, radiation, and medical oncology.

Although recognized as a medical specialty, palliative medicine relies on the unique contributions of numerous disciplines. Education in palliative techniques begins at the undergraduate level and is incorporated into the training of a number of medical specialties, such as oncology and gerontology. Continuing education programs focus on educating health care professionals in quality palliative care techniques. Other projects build on these efforts, using other health care professionals, such as nurse practitioners and physician assistants, to develop quality palliative medicine programs in their institutions.

The American Society for Clinical Oncology (ASCO) actively promotes continuing education in palliative medicine. Palliative care is incorporated into educational materials and programs developed by ASCO. The society published an educational curriculum for continuing medical education on palliative medicine, and it has a study program devoted to supportive care. Palliative medicine is included in the training for internists, as adopted by the American Board of Internal Medicine.

The National Consensus Project for Quality Palliative Care issued guidelines for palliative care to establish continuity of care across institutions. The clinical practice guidelines have been incorporated into the hospital accreditation standards of The Joint Commission (formerly the Joint Commission for the Accreditation of Hospitals). Institutions are assessed on the eight domains of palliative care: structure and process, physical aspects, psychological and psychiatric aspects, spiritual and religious aspects, cultural aspects, care of the imminently dying patient, the ethical aspects of care, and the legal aspects of care. Additionally, the Center for the Advancement of Palliative Care developed the State-by-State Report Card on Access to Palliative Care in Our Nation's Hospitals. The report card measures patient access to palliative care and to palliative medicine specialists, access of medical students to training in palliative care, and access of physicians to specialty training in palliative care. The report card emphasizes the importance of a multidisciplinary approach to palliative medicine.

DIAGNOSTIC AND TREATMENT TECHNIQUES

Patient care is traditionally disease-oriented. Specialists in particular tend to focus narrowly on a specific organ or body system. Palliative care, however, takes a holistic, patient-centered approach. The emphasis is on communicating with the patient and family to assess the patient's specific needs and desires.

Palliative care can be divided into primary and secondary teams. The primary team, as defined by Medicare, is comprised by four core members (physician, nurse, social worker and spiritual counselor) and is responsible for assessing and managing symptoms, providing expertise regarding psychosocial services as well as communicating with the patient and family while involving the shared decision making model of care If, however, the patient's condition worsens and the primary team can no longer manage the symptoms, a palliative medicine specialist in the patient's condition is called. The palliative medicine specialist may be consulted on specific issues as needed or become a core member until the patient's death.

The whole-patient assessment begins with the patient's description of symptoms and level of function. Diagnostic tests may be used to evaluate symptom severity, but diagnosis is not the purpose. The emphasis is always on symptom relief.

Pain is a significant issue that must be managed properly. Inadequately controlled pain may reduce the effectiveness of treatment and wear the patient down psychologically. Proper pain management involves communication with and education of the patient and family members as well as continuous assessment of the effectiveness of pain medications. The World Health Organization (WHO) has developed an approach to pain for cancer patients, beginning with nonsteroidal anti-inflammatory drugs (NSAIDs), such as ibuprofen, and progressing through acetaminophen combined with an opioid medication, such as acetaminophen with codeine, and lastly to opioid medications such as morphine or oxycodone. The goal is to relieve pain while keeping the patient alert and in control.

The effect of the condition on the emotions and cognitive functioning of the patient is an important aspect of the palliative medicine assessment. Patients are facing serious issues while they battle their illnesses. They must cope with imminent death and the grief of their loved ones along with the fear of loss of control and dignity. Patients must be evaluated for depression and anxiety. Practical needs, such as relationship issues, legal affairs, and financial management, also need attention. The patient's spiritual needs should also be addressed. Spiritual counseling can be traditional religious advisement from a clergyperson or an informal discussion of personal beliefs, according to the desires of the patient.

Depression and anxiety are common among patients coping with life-threatening conditions. Feelings of sadness and depression are to be expected and should be managed appropriately even when they are not expected to be permanent. The members of the primary team who are in closest contact with the patient need to be alert for symptoms of depression that surpass the normal grieving process. Signs of major depression include persistent feelings of worthlessness, hopelessness, helplessness, and loss of self-esteem. Physical symptoms may include weight loss or changes in sleep habits, although these symptoms may also be attributed to the patient's underlying condition. Thoughts of suicide or requests by the patient to hasten death are not part of the coping process and are a sign of major depression. If the signs of depression fail to resolve after a few weeks, then the mental health specialists on the team are consulted and the depression should be treated.

Similarly, anxiety is an understandable and natural emotion as patients juggle financial concerns, family issues, medical concerns, and preparations for their own death. Anxiety may be managed through counseling or, if it is severe, with antianxiety medications.

The role of the palliative care team is not limited to the patient. The team assists family members in accepting the patient's condition, managing financial and insurance matters, and coping with grief. The health care

team can advise family members on what to expect as
the patient's condition deteriorates. Breathing difficulties, delirium or dementia, wasting, and incontinence
can be upsetting for family members to experience if
they are not properly prepared. After the patient's
death, the palliative care team assists family members
through the grieving process. The team follows up with
the family through phone calls and home visits, providing grief counseling or referral to caregiver support
groups or other mental health professionals when
needed. Bereavement services often last for several
months to a year after the patient's death.

PERSPECTIVE AND PROSPECTS
In the span of two decades, palliative medicine progressed from haphazard training through chance experiences to a recognized specialty. A 1998 member
survey by ASCO revealed 90 percent of the oncologists
who responded had no formal training in palliative
medicine. Rather, they indicated they learned through
"trial and error." Alarmingly, more than one-third
claimed that their education in palliative medicine was
from a "traumatic experience" with a patient. Most
had little training in how to discuss a poor prognosis
with patients and their families, and only 10 percent
had completed clinical training in palliative care.

Since that survey, ASCO and other professional societies have incorporated palliative medicine into their
continuing education curricula. More important, national and international groups have formally recognized the importance of palliative medicine in preserving the dignity and well-being of patients nearing the
end of their lives. In recent years, palliative medicine
has been incorporated as a routine part of comprehensive cancer care plans in the United States.

Despite these advances, much work remains. The
need for palliative medicine is increasing. The population is growing older while the prevalence of cancer is
rising. Cancer treatments are becoming more effective.
Although cancer death rates are declining, more people are living longer with the disease, resulting in
growing numbers of people who will benefit from palliative medicine.

To meet the growing need, health care practitioners
must be educated in palliative medicine. Fellowships in
palliative medicine (currently 93 in the United States),
continuing education, and readily available educational resources are needed now more than ever. Formal certifications and national guidelines and standards of practice have been adopted to ensure
consistency in the quality of palliative medicine across
states and individual institutions. The concept of palliative medicine continues to be incorporated into care
plans across medical disciplines. In 2006 the American
Board of Medical Specialties approved the creation of

Hospice and Palliative Medicine as a subspecialty to 10
medical disciplines, and after 2013, only those who
have completed an accredited fellowship program will
be able to be certified and practice this discipline.

Improving end-of-life care requires more than educational and quality control initiatives; it also requires
political will. Unless palliative medicine is viewed as a
priority by administrators and policy makers, quality
care cannot be ensured.

Pain management is an integral piece of palliative
medicine. Unfortunately, misconceptions remain
among health care practitioners as well as the general
public regarding the use of opioid medications. The
fear of addiction frequently results in less than optimal
pain control and patient suffering. The need for
higher doses of pain medications does not indicate addiction; it is more likely a sign the pain is inadequately
controlled or the condition is progressing. The United
Nations elevated effective pain control to a fundamental human right. In a formal statement, the UN
equated inadequate pain control with "cruel, inhuman,
and degrading treatment" and called for nations to
supply adequate pain medications to patients.

Collectively, the United Nations, individual countries, and medical societies are striving to ensure that
all patients suffering from terminal illnesses receive
compassionate and comprehensive care. The strength
of palliative medicine is in considering the patient as a
whole rather than focusing exclusively on a particular
diagnosis. Palliative medicine breaks from traditional
medical practice and creates a multidisciplinary team
to care for the patient. The direction of care is dictated
by the wishes of the patient and encompasses physical,
emotional, and the spiritual needs of the patient and
their families.

—Cheryl Pokalo Jones;
updated by Felix Rivera, MD

See also Aging; Cancer; Death and dying; Depression; Ethics; Euthanasia; Grief and guilt; Hospice; Narcotics; Pain;
Pain management; Phobias; Psychiatry; Psychiatry, child and
adolescent; Psychiatry, geriatric; Stress; Suicide; Terminally
ill: Extended care

For Further Information:
Chochinov, Harvey M., and William Breitbart. *Handbook of
Psychiatry in Palliative Medicine.* New York: Oxford
University Press, 2000. Discussion of the role of psychiatry
in palliative medicine.
Doyle, Derek, et al., eds. *Oxford Textbook of Palliative Medicine.*
New York: Oxford University Press, 2005. Comprehensive
text on palliative medicine, including the role of different
medical specialties in patient care.
Field, Marilyn J., and Cathleen K. Cassel, eds. *Approaching
Death: Improving Care at the End of Life.* Washington, DC:
National Academies Press, 1997. The documents from the
Institute of Medicine establishing the role of palliative
medicine in comprehensive cancer care.

National Hospice and Palliative Care Organization website: www.nhpco.org.

Woodruff, Roger. *Palliative Medicine: Evidence-Based Symptomatic and Supportive Care for Patients with Advanced Cancer.* 4th ed. New York: Oxford University Press, 2004. Review of recent research in the principles of palliative medicine and related ethical issues.

World Health Organization website on palliative care: www.who.int/cancer/palliative/en

PALPITATIONS

Category: Disease/Disorder
Also known as: Skipping beats, irregular heartbeat
Anatomy or system affected: Chest, circulatory system, heart, muscles
Specialties and related fields: Cardiology
Definition: A perceived irregularity of the normal heartbeat.

CAUSES AND SYMPTOMS

Individuals experiencing palpitations often describe a slight discomfort and uneasiness accompanied by a flutter or sudden change in heart rate. Palpitations are often a symptom of an abnormal heart rhythm known as an arrhythmia. Arrhythmias involve a change in the electrical activity of the heart resulting in a chaotic or irregular contraction of the heart muscle. The location of these arrhythmias within the heart muscle determines the type, duration, and intensity of the palpitations.

Palpitations are common among many people, regardless of age or gender. They are often diagnosed by cardiologists using several techniques aimed at measuring the electrical activity of the heart. Such tests include electrocardiograms (ECGs), Holter monitoring, and stress tests. Most palpitations do not indicate the presence of a serious cardiac problem. Instead, they are often the result of one cause or a combination of several causes. Several underlying causes of heart palpitations include a high caffeine intake, alcohol and tobacco use, fatigue, extreme physical exertion, stress and anxiety, and a poor diet.

Palpitations have not been shown to cause any damage to the heart muscle. Extended palpitations, however, may lead to decreased blood flow to areas of the brain, heart, or other parts of the body. This decreased blood flow can create oxygen deficits in these areas, leading to dizziness, loss of consciousness, chest pain, or shortness of breath. Palpitations accompanied by such symptoms may be a sign of other structural problems of the heart muscle or surrounding blood vessels and may be diagnosed with the use of an echocardiogram (an ultrasound technique) or invasive catheterization.

INFORMATION ON PALPITATIONS

Causes: Abnormal heart rhythm, high caffeine intake, alcohol or tobacco use, fatigue, extreme physical exertion, stress and anxiety, poor diet
Symptoms: Flutter or sudden change in heart rate, slight discomfort and uneasiness; in severe cases, decreased blood flow leading to dizziness, loss of consciousness, chest pain, shortness of breath
Duration: Brief, sometimes recurrent
Treatments: Removal of underlying cause; in severe cases, medications (beta-blockers, calcium-channel blockers), surgery (implantable defibrillator)

TREATMENT AND THERAPY

Most palpitations are treated by removing the underlying causes. Decreasing intake of caffeine, alcohol, and tobacco products often succeeds in lowering the frequency and severity of palpitations. Reducing levels of physical and emotional stress while maintaining proper diet and sleep patterns has also been successful in treating palpitations. Medications such as beta-blockers or calcium-channel blockers or other methods such as surgery or implantable defibrillators may be used to treat palpitations in more severe cases.

PERSPECTIVE AND PROSPECTS

Advances in medical technology have shown heart palpitations to be much more common than once thought. Today, heartbeat irregularities perceived as palpitations are rarely considered to be a sign of serious disease and are often easily treated or prevented.

—*Paul J. Frisch*

See also Addiction; Alcoholism; Anxiety; Arrhythmias; Caffeine; Cardiology; Cardiology, pediatric; Echocardiography; Electrocardiography (ECG or EKG); Exercise physiology; Heart; Nicotine; Panic attacks; Smoking; Stress; Stress reduction.

For Further Information:

American Medical Association. *American Medical Association Family Medical Guide.* 4th rev. ed. Hoboken, N.J.: John Wiley & Sons, 2004.

Berne, Robert M., and Matthew N. Levy. *Cardiovascular Physiology.* 8th ed. St. Louis, Mo.: Mosby, 2001.

Everett, Russell J., Mary N. Sheppard, and David C. Lefroy. "Chest Pain and Palpitations Taking a Closer Look." *Circulation* 128, no. 3 (September, 2013): 271-277. Print.

Icon Health. *Heart Palpitations: A Medical Dictionary, Bibliography, and Annotated Research Guide to Internet References.* San Diego, Calif.: Author, 2004.

Jonsb, Egil, et al. "Illness Perception Among Patients with Chest Pain and Palpitations Before and After Negative Cardiac Evaluation." *BioPsychoSocial Medicine* 6, no. 1 (2012): 19-26.

Larson, Lyle W. "Grad Students with Palpitations." *Clinicial Reviews* 23, no. 7 (July, 2013): 18-48.

Litin, Scott C., ed. *Mayo Clinic Family Health Book*. 4th ed. New York: HarperResource, 2009.

Zaret, Barry L., Marvin Moser, and Lawrence S. Cohen, eds. *Yale University School of Medicine Heart Book*. New York: William Morrow, 1992.

PALSY

Category: Disease/Disorder

Anatomy or system affected: Muscles, musculoskeletal system, nerves, nervous system

Specialties and related fields: Neurology, physical therapy

Definition: A paralysis or partial paralysis that is usually accompanied or followed by muscle weakness and muscle wasting over the affected area; in some cases, there may be residual electrical activity present, but the amount is usually small and the activity cannot be controlled.

Key terms:

Bell's palsy: paralysis of the seventh cranial nerve (facial nerve)

cerebral palsy: a palsy arising prenatally, at birth, or early in life within the central nervous system, affecting large portions of the cerebral hemispheres, with extensive paralysis of many major muscles

hemiplegia: paralysis involving an arm and a leg on the same side of the body

palsy: a paralysis or partial paralysis involving loss of motor control, usually accompanied or followed by muscle weakness and muscle wasting over the affected area

Parkinson's disease: also called shaking palsy; a degenerative paralysis resulting from destruction of certain cells in the substantia nigra, a structure near the base of the cerebral hemispheres

quadriplegia: paralysis involving all four extremities more or less equally

spastic: characterized by uncontrollable spasms

substantia nigra: a clump of cells located near the base of the cerebral hemispheres that secrete the neurotransmitter dopamine

CAUSES AND SYMPTOMS

In general, the term "palsy" describes any type of dysfunction of the motor nerves that impairs or reduces the conscious control of muscles. The paralysis or loss of motor control is usually accompanied or followed by weakness and wasting of the muscles in the affected area.

The most common type of palsy is Bell's palsy, a paralysis of the seventh cranial nerve, or facial nerve, often accompanied by pain over part or all of the affected area. The number of muscles involved varies. The paralysis usually occurs on one side of the face at a time, with the result that the undamaged muscles of the opposite side pull the facial skin to that side. Typically, the eye on the affected side remains open all the time because the muscles that close it have been affected; attempts by the patient to close the eye merely result in the eyeball rotating upward. The rest of the face on the affected side generally droops but remains flat; the brow fails to wrinkle, and the cheeks never thicken. Smiles and other facial expressions are asymmetrically contorted.

Thorough neurological testing is needed to assess how much damage has been done and which branches of the facial nerve have been affected. If the damage affects either hearing or taste, this finding indicates that the damage is closer to the root of the facial nerve, and the patient's chances for recovery are correspondingly much lower. If only a few muscles are involved, it indicates that the damage is farther from the root of the nerve, which usually forecasts a better chance of recovery. In most cases, Bell's palsy is thought to arise from a reduced blood supply to the affected nerves. Viral infection by herpes simplex or herpes zoster (shingles) is also a frequent cause; the viral infections are believed to cause demyelination (deterioration of the myelin sheath that insulates nerves) of the affected parts of the facial nerve. Other causes include injuries to the area just below or in front of the external ear resulting from blows to the head, surgery in this region, or other types of trauma.

Another common type of palsy is cerebral palsy, an impairment of movement and posture caused in most cases by injury, malformation, or other damage to the immature brain. Cerebral palsy is actually a group of paralytic disorders that begin during intrauterine development, at birth, or in early infancy. The extent of the paralysis may vary, often involving large groups of muscles while sparing others. Those muscles that are not totally paralyzed are often uncoordinated in their movements or poorly controlled; this is especially true of large muscle movements such as those of the limbs. In many cases, the patient exhibits a "scissors gait" in which the lower limbs are crossed and the one behind must be swung sideways before it is placed in front of the other limb. In addition to the lack of muscular control of the limbs, other symptoms variously include spasms, athetoid (slow, rhythmic, and wormlike) movements, or muscular rigidity. Speech is in many cases difficult or unclear if the muscles used in speaking are affected.

Mental deterioration may occur in some cases but not in others: Some patients with cerebral palsy are intellectually disabled, while others have managed to display brilliant artistic or literary talents with the use of whatever muscles still function in their bodies. Some cerebral palsy patients also suffer from seizure disorders such as epilepsy. Almost all cases of cerebral palsy are accompanied by some other type of neurological impairment, the nature of which varies greatly. In general, cerebral palsy is a nonprogressive type of disease; that is, it does not continually worsen. Afflicted individuals generally experience a normal life span, though with impaired motor functions.

The most common types of cerebral palsy are those that occur in infancy or earlier. Of this group, injuries received at birth (during forceps delivery, for example) form one of the largest and most well defined groups. Cerebral hemorrhage, a cause of many cerebral palsies, may occur either during intrauterine life or at birth. Cerebral palsy may also result from embryonic malformations, from injuries received during intrauterine life, or from injuries or other damage during the first two years of life. In addition to birth trauma, many other factors may contribute to a risk of cerebral palsy: premature delivery, breech delivery, toxemia of pregnancy, impairment of the baby's oxygen supply, maternal infection (especially rubella, also called German measles), premature detachment of the placenta during the birth process, and incompatibility between the Rh blood types of mother and child. Brain injuries caused by low oxygen levels (anoxia or hypoxia) can arise before, during, or after birth and can result from damage to the blood vessels, birth trauma, or infectious diseases such as meningitis or encephalitis.

Cerebral palsies are classified into two general types: pyramidal (or spastic) and extrapyramidal (or nonspastic). The pyramidal or spastic types show muscular spasms and other symptoms that persist with age and hardly vary with changes in emotion, tension, movement, or sleep. The pyramidal tracts of the brain stem are damaged in these forms of cerebral palsy. The extrapyramidal or nonspastic types are more variable and are subdivided into several subtypes according to the types of movement exhibited: none (rigid type), weak (dystonic type), rhythmic and wormlike (athetoid type), or uncoordinated shaking (ataxic type). The extrapyramidal tracts of the brain stem are damaged in all these forms of the disease. Most forms of cerebral palsy can also be described as hemiplegia (involving both extremities on one side of the body only), diplegia (involving both legs more than the arms), bilateral hemiplegia (involving the arms more than the legs), or quadriplegia (involving all four extremities more or less equally). Attempts to group the various forms of cerebral palsy by their causes have generally resulted in a lack of agreement among experts. One scheme divides the causes into

> **INFORMATION ON PALSY**
>
> **Causes:** May include genetic and environmental factors, birth defects, trauma during childbirth, reduced blood flow to affected nerves, viral infection, injury in front of ear (trauma, surgery)
> **Symptoms:** May include paralysis (partial or complete); muscle weakness, wasting, or rigidity; awkward gait; impaired facial movement; impaired speech; mental impairment; seizure disorders
> **Duration:** Acute to chronic
> **Treatments:** Drug therapy (vasodilators drugs such as cortisone, antiviral drugs such as acyclovir); surgery; application of warmth and avoidance of cold drafts

subependymal hemorrhage among premature infants, damage from oxygen deprivation to the growing brain (the vast majority of cases), and developmental abnormalities of the nervous system.

The most common form of cerebral palsy is infantile spastic hemiplegia, which accounts for about one-third of all cerebral palsies. Most cases of spastic hemiplegia (about 65 percent) are thought to result from birth trauma, either from forceps delivery or from the difficult passage of a very large head through the mother's pelvic girdle. Another 30 percent arise after birth, during the first year of life, either from head injury or from infections such as meningitis and encephalitis. Only 5 percent of spastic hemiplegias arise before birth from embryonic malformations or from toxemia of pregnancy. The rate at which cerebral palsy occurs is higher for babies born prematurely than for those born at term. It is also higher for large babies that may suffer injury during a difficult passage through the birth canal. In the United States, there is a somewhat higher incidence rate among Caucasians than among African Americans.

Parkinson's disease (also called paralysis agitans or shaking palsy) is a progressive or degenerative type of palsy. The disease usually produces a tremor that includes a distinctive "pill-rolling" movement of the thumb and forefinger; this tremor usually stops if a voluntary movement of some other kind is begun. Muscle weakness, stiffness, and muscular rigidity are common but with intermittent symptoms that come and go; movements generally become slow and difficult. The muscles involved in chewing and swallowing are often affected in Parkinson's disease, so patients are often advised to eat high-calorie, semisoft foods that require no chewing and are more easily swallowed than liquids. Involvement of the muscles of facial expression results in a masklike expression that does not alter with changes in emotion. Patients suffering from Parkinson's disease often have difficulty in initiating voluntary movements; this difficulty is often described by patients as a feeling of "being frozen in place."

The walking gait of Parkinson's disease patients is also very characteristic: The body above the waist leans forward, the head and shoulders droop, the feet shuffle slowly (and are barely lifted from the ground), and the arms are generally held slightly flexed and motionless rather than swinging. Many patients break into a trot or a run when they attempt to walk; as a result, patients often fall, most often forward. To prevent such falls, they frequently shuffle forward in very small steps. The shuffling gait is believed to result from a partial paralysis of the extrapyramidal motor system of neurons, which is generally responsible for controlling posture and coordinating motor activities.

Parkinson's disease is known to result from a disorder in the production of dopamine, a neurotransmitter chemical normally secreted by certain parts of the brain. The affected parts of the brain are the basal ganglia deep within the cerebral hemispheres, and especially the substantia nigra, a deeper structure that sends dopamine-secreting nerve fibers to the basal ganglia. In patients with Parkinson's disease, cells of the substantia nigra are often degenerate and pale from the loss of normal pigments, but this may be a result, rather than a cause, of the primary defect: an impairment of the brain's ability to convert dopa (dihydroxyphenylalanine) into the neurotransmitter dopamine.

The chemical n-methyyl-4-phenyl-1,2,3,4-tetrahydro-pyridine has been found to produce in experimental animals a disease very similar to Parkinson's disease. For this reason, many researchers suspect that the disease has an environmental cause that leads to the production of a related toxic chemical, one that presumably interferes with the production of dopamine.

Parkinson's disease is uncommon before the age of forty, but it becomes so common in people over sixty that it is the leading neurological disorder in this age group. In the United States, the incidence rate is about 130 per 100,000 in the general population and is roughly the same in all races and ethnic groups. About 10 to 15 percent of patients show mental deterioration (dementia) as the disease progresses. Patients often experience depression, social withdrawal, and generalized apathy.

Other, less common palsies include brachial birth palsy, Erb's palsy, Klumpke's palsy, true or progressive bulbar palsy, pseudobulbar palsy, Féréol-Graux palsy, posticus palsy, lead palsy, scrivener's palsy, pressure palsy, compression palsy, and creeping or wasting palsy.

Brachial birth palsy is a paralysis of the infant's arm resulting from an injury received at birth, involving the whole arm, the upper arm only (Erb's palsy), or the lower arm only (Klumpke's palsy). Erb's palsy, a brachial birth palsy of the upper arm, is caused by an injury at birth to the brachial plexus or the posterior roots of the fifth and sixth cervical nerves; the muscles involved generally include the deltoideus, biceps brachii, and brachialis, impairing the raising of the upper arm, flexion of the elbow, or supination movements involving the forearm. In Klumpke's palsy, which results from an injury at birth, the muscles of the forearm and the small muscles of the hand undergo atrophy; this form is often accompanied by paralysis of the cervical sympathetic nerves.

True or progressive bulbar palsy, a palsy and progressive atrophy of the muscles of the tongue, lips, palate, pharynx, and larynx, often occurs late in life and is caused by degeneration of the motor neurons leading to these muscles. Twitching or atrophy of the tongue and other affected muscles causes drooling, difficulties in swallowing, and ultimately a respiratory paralysis that results in death. Many experts consider true bulbar palsy to be a manifestation of the same disease that causes amyotrophic lateral sclerosis (ALS), which is popularly known as Lou Gehrig's disease.

Pseudobulbar palsy ("laughing sickness") is a paralysis of the lips and tongue that mimics true or progressive bulbar palsy, but it arises in the brain itself and is accompanied by difficulties in swallowing and by spasmodic laughter at inappropriate times. Féréol-Graux palsy, a one-sided (unilateral) paralysis of the motor nucleus of the lateral rectus muscle of one eye and the medial rectus muscle of the other eye, results from damage to the medial longitudinal fasciculus and impairs the ability to direct either eye toward the affected side. Posticus palsy is a paralysis of the posterior cricoarytenoideus muscle (cricoarytenoideus posticus), resulting in the vocal cords being held close to the midline.

Lead palsy is a paralysis of the extensor muscles of the wrist resulting from lead poisoning, while scrivener's palsy ("writer's cramp") is a repetitive motion disorder resulting in damage to the nerve controlling the small muscles of the hand. Pressure palsy is a paralysis caused by repeated or persistent compression of a nerve or nerve trunk. Compression palsy results from nerve compression, especially of the arm, caused by pressure from the use of a crutch (crutch palsy) or from compression of a nerve during sleep. Creeping palsy and wasting palsy are general terms for progressive muscle atrophy, such as that associated with ALS.

TREATMENT AND THERAPY

Bell's palsy is treated by various methods, including the application of warmth, the avoidance of cold drafts, or the administration of vasodilating drugs such as cortisone or antiviral drugs such as acyclovir. In unusual cases, surgery is performed to enlarge the passages through which the facial nerve passes, thus relieving compression on the nerve. In past generations, physicians often recommended treating eyes that could not be closed by taping them shut, especially in sleep. This treatment is no longer recommended. Instead, physicians usually advise patients who cannot close an affected eye to wear dark glasses during the day.

Many patients with Bell's palsy recover spontaneously on their own. The chances that a particular individual will spontaneously recover depend on the location of the damage and the extent of muscle involvement; the cases with the most favorable outcomes are those in which the damage is more peripheral and fewer muscles are involved. Frequent, repeated testing of each small group of facial muscles is needed to assess the extent of damage and the extent of any recovery.

Diagnosis of cerebral palsy is best made by a trained neurologist through observation of the patient's spontaneous motor movements and reflex actions. Infants who exhibit any reflex that persists beyond its appropriate age range, or any voluntary motor pattern that fails to develop at the appropriate age, should be examined more carefully for signs of nerve damage. For example, most babies can lift their heads by one month of age and their chests by two months. By three months of age, most babies can raise themselves up on their elbows, and by four months on their wrists. Newborn babies exhibit reflexes such as the Moro reflex, a flexion and "embracing" reflex in reaction to a sudden noise or other sudden stimulus or "startle"; however, the persistence of this reflex beyond six months of age (or its asymmetrical performance) may be indicative of some form of cerebral palsy. Another reflex often used in diagnosis is the "fencer" reflex, or asymmetric tonic neck reflex: Turning the baby's head toward one side usually causes extension movements in both the arm and leg on the side toward which the chin faces, while flexion movements usually take place on the opposite side of the body. This reflex is present at birth and disappears in a few months; its persistence after six months of age should be considered suspicious.

There is no cure for cerebral palsy. Treatment generally consists of physical rehabilitation and training the patient to use whatever muscles are still capable of being consciously controlled. This is a difficult form of therapy that must be tailored to the needs of each patient because individuals experience unique combinations of motor abilities and disabilities. Few patients with cerebral palsy are capable of walking on their own. Depending on the extent of impairment of muscle movements, some patients may require crutches or braces, while others use motorized wheelchairs. In cases in which there is speech impairment, speech therapy may also be needed to teach the patient to speak more clearly. Most types of cerebral palsy are already present during infancy; therapy for these types is always rather difficult because the patient is learning the necessary motor skills (such as walking or speaking) for the first time. Palsies that arise during adolescence or adulthood respond differently to therapy because the patient is relearning skills that had already been mastered.

Treatment for Parkinson's disease includes the administration of a number of drugs that are chemically related to dopamine, the missing neurotransmitter. The drug most often used is levodopa, or L-dopa, a derivative of a naturally occurring amino acid in the brain. The drug carbidopa is also given to help deliver most of the levodopa into the brain. Dopamine agonists (enhancers) such as bromocriptine and pergolide are frequently given. The antiviral drug amantadine has also been shown to have effects that counter the disease.

PERSPECTIVE AND PROSPECTS

The various palsies were identified in the nineteenth century. Bell's palsy was first described by Sir Charles Bell (1774-1842), a renowned Scottish anatomist. Parkinsonism was first described by James Parkinson (1755-1824), who called it "shaking palsy"; the understanding of the neurotransmitter dopamine and the use of L-dopa in the treatment of Parkinson's disease were development of the late twentieth century. Cerebral palsy was first described in 1861 by a London physician, William J. Little; the famous psychoanalyst Sigmund Freud (1856-1939) published an account of this disease in 1883. The most thorough early work on this disease was published in 1889 by the distinguished Canadian physician Sir William Osler (1849-1919), who coined the term "cerebral palsies" to describe the several types of the disease.

Several types of cerebral palsy that were more common in the early twentieth century, such as those caused by the use of obstetrical forceps during delivery, have decreased in incidence as a result of improved medical procedures. For larger babies that formerly faced a greater risk of cerebral hemorrhage and other brain injury from passage through the mother's pelvic girdle at birth, the increased frequency of cesarean sections has greatly reduced the rates of cerebral palsy arising at birth.

—Eli C. Minkoff, PhD

See also Amyotrophic lateral sclerosis; Bell's palsy; Cerebral palsy; Hemiplegia; Herpes; Motor neuron diseases; Nervous system; Neuralgia, neuritis, and neuropathy; Neurology; Neurology, pediatric; Paralysis; Paraplegia; Parkinson's disease; Physical rehabilitation; Quadriplegia; Shingles; Tremors.

For Further Information:
Bloom, Floyd E., M. Flint Beal, and David J. Kupfer, eds. *The Dana Guide to Brain Health*. New York: Dana Press, 2006.

Carson-DeWitt, Rosalyn. "Parkinson's Disease." *Health Library*, September 10, 2012.

Chipps, Esther, Norma J. Clanin, and Victor G. Campbell. *Neurologic Disorders*. St. Louis, Mo.: Mosby Year Book, 1992.

Daube, Jasper R., ed. *Clinical Neurophysiology*. 3d ed. New York: Oxford University Press, 2009.

Kliegman, Robert M., and Waldo E. Nelson, eds. *Nelson Textbook of Pediatrics*. 19th ed. Philadelphia: Saunders/Elsevier, 2011.

Iansek, Robert, and Meg. E. Morris, eds. *Rehabilitation in Movement Disorders*. Cambridge: Cambridge University Press, 2013.

Stanley, Fiona J., Eva Alberman, and Eva Blair. *Cerebral Palsies: Epidemiology and Causal Pathways*. New York: Cambridge University Press, 2000.

Stanton, Marion. *The Cerebral Palsy Handbook*. London: Vermilion, 2002.

United Cerebral Palsy. www.ucp.org.

Victor, Maurice, and Allan H. Ropper. *Adams and Victor's Principles of Neurology*. 9th ed. New York: McGraw-Hill, 2009.

Waxman, Stephen G. *Correlative Neuroanatomy*. 25th ed. New York: Lange Medical Books/McGraw-Hill, 2002.

Weiner, William J., Lisa M. Shulman, and Anthony E. Lang. *Parkinson's Disease: A Complete Guide for Patients and Families*, 3d ed. Baltimore, Md.: Johns Hopkins University Press, 2013.

PANCREAS

Category: Anatomy

Anatomy or system affected: Abdomen, endocrine system, gastrointestinal system, glands, immune system

Specialties and related fields: Endocrinology, gastroenterology, immunology, internal medicine

Definition: A vital organ that produces enzymes used in the digestive process and hormones such as insulin, which regulates blood sugar levels.

Key terms:

autoimmunity: a disorder in which the immune system starts to attack the body's cells as foreign matter

autosomal recessive disease: a disease caused by a gene (other than the X or Y chromosome) that must be on both chromosomes to be expressed

concordance: the inheritance of the same trait by both twins

duodenum: the initial part of the small intestine, where most of the digestion of food occurs

endocrine glands: ductless glands that secrete hormones directly into the bloodstream; these glands help to maintain homeostasis

exocrine glands: glands that excrete their products into tubes or ducts

STRUCTURE AND FUNCTIONS

The pancreas is an organ about 15 to 18 centimeters long and weighing 100 grams that is located in the abdominal cavity. The head of the organ is situated in the loop of the small intestine that forms at the site where the small intestine joins the stomach. The pancreas is enclosed in a thin connective tissue capsule. As an accessory gland of the digestive system, the pancreas is an exocrine gland. Scattered within the tissue of this exocrine gland, however, are small distinct regions known as the islets of Langerhans, which are a part of the endocrine system. The exocrine portion composes by far the greatest mass of tissue. In the guinea pig, for example, about 82 percent of pancreatic cells are exocrine cells, while the endocrine portion is about 2 percent. The remaining cells are associated with the duct system and the blood vessels.

The exocrine pancreas is an arrangement of tubules that continue to branch until they form very fine ducts called the intercalated ducts. Along the edges of the intercalated ducts are the acinar cells. These cells produce the pancreatic juices that aid in the digestion of food in the small intestine and help neutralize the contents of the small intestine. The products drain from the ducts into the main collecting duct, which joins the common bile duct and empties into the duodenum.

The islets of Langerhans, as is the case with all endocrine glands, have a well-developed blood supply. The hormones produced by these endocrine cells are emptied into the surrounding capillaries. The hormones flow into the general circulation where they are distributed to target cells throughout the body. Since the two portions of the pancreas are anatomically as well as functionally different, they will be considered independently.

The exocrine portion of the pancreas produces about 1 liter of aqueous fluid per day that is delivered directly to the duodenum. The two major components of the pancreatic juices are ions, which are used to neutralize the stomach contents as they enter the small intestine, and enzymes, which metabolize intestinal contents for absorption.

The various ions that are secreted include sodium, potassium, chloride, and bicarbonate ions. The sodium, potassium, and chloride are present in concentrations similar to their concentrations in the bloodstream. The bicarbonate ions act as the major buffer of the body. With only a few exceptions, the bloodstream and the contents of the body must be maintained at a pH of 7.4. Bicarbonate ions ensure that there is no change in pH.

The stomach is one of the areas of the body in which the pH varies. It may be as low as pH 1, which is highly acidic. The contents of the stomach empty directly into the duodenum, and while the cells of the stomach are capable of withstanding an acid environment, the cells of the small intestine are not. The acid must be rapidly neutralized in order to protect these cells. In addition, the enzymes that help to digest the food reaching the small intestine work optimally at about pH 7. If the pH varies significantly, the food will not be properly digested and vital nutrients will not be absorbed by the intestinal cells.

The production of bicarbonate by the duct cells is controlled by a hormone called secretin. The contents of the small intestine become acidic as food moves into the area from the stomach. When the pH is lowered, the cells of the small intestine release secretin, which in turn stimulates the pancreas to produce more bicarbonate. As bicarbonate enters the small intestine, it neutralizes the acid, and the stimulus to produce secretin is removed.

The pancreas also produces a variety of enzymes that digest proteins, sugars, lipids, and nucleic acids. In order for protein to be absorbed by the cells of the small intestine, it must be broken down into its building blocks, amino acids. This breakdown is an enzymatic process that occurs only when the appropriate enzymes are present and at a pH near neutrality. The enzymes that digest proteins include trypsin, chymotrypsin, and carboxypeptidase. Like protein, sugars, nucleic acids, and lipids must be digested to their subunits if they are to be absorbed. Sugars are metabolized by amylase, nucleic acids by either ribonuclease or deoxyribonuclease, and fats by lipase, phospholipase, or cholesterol esterase.

The secretion of enzymes by the pancreas is controlled by the hormone cholecystokinin. As the content of protein and fat increases in the lumen of the duodenum, the duodenal cells release cholecystokinin, which acts on the acinar cells of the pancreas to release the enzymes. As the food is digested, the level of cholecystokinin decreases and the release of enzymes from the pancreas also decreases.

The islets of Langerhans have four different cell types and produce four different hormones. The alpha and beta cells produce glucagon and insulin, respectively. The delta cells produce somatostatin, which inhibits the secretion of hormones by the alpha and beta cells. The F cells produce pancreatic polypeptide, the function of which is not yet understood.

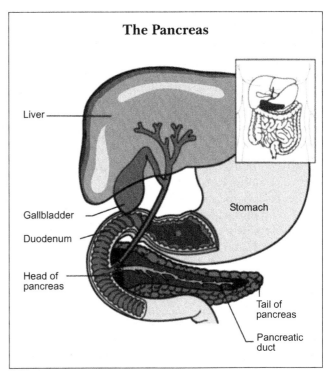

The Pancreas

The pancreas is an unusual gland that contains both endocrine tissue and exocrine tissue; the inset shows the location of the pancreas within the gastrointestinal system. ©EBSCO

Insulin secretion is stimulated or inhibited by a large number of factors. Blood glucose levels are the most important factor in the release of insulin from the beta cells. If blood glucose increases, insulin is released until glucose levels return to normal. When insulin is released into the bloodstream, it stimulates the uptake of glucose by target cells. Although insulin is best known for its action on glucose, it also stimulates the uptake of amino acids and fatty acids from the bloodstream during periods of adequate nutrition. Glucagon is an antagonist of insulin. It is released in response to low levels of glucose and acts on cells to release glucose, amino acids, and fatty acids into the circulatory system.

DISORDERS AND DISEASES
Diseases of the pancreas can be divided into two basic categories: diseases of the exocrine cells of the organ and those diseases that effect the function of the endocrine portion, the islets of Langerhans. The exocrine cells of the pancreas can be affected by various conditions, including acute pancreatitis, chronic pancreatitis, cystic fibrosis, and carcinoma of the pancreas. Also, because the pancreas is a gland and glandular organs typically have a large blood supply, it is at risk of injury any time that circulation is impaired. The islets of Langerhans may be affected by diabetes mellitus.

Inflammation of the pancreas (pancreatitis) can be either acute or chronic. While some cases are mild, it is considered a serious disease and has a high mortality rate. Although the acute form is more serious, patients with chronic pancreatitis may suffer from acute episodes.

Acute pancreatitis may result from obstruction of the pancreatic duct (possibly by gallstones from the gallbladder or by mucous plugs, as in cystic fibrosis), bile reflux, acute intoxication by alcohol, shock, infection by the mumps virus, hypothermia, or trauma. The diagnosis, pathology, and prognosis are the same regardless of the cause.

The onset of the disease is usually quite sudden, with severe pain in the abdomen, nausea, and vomiting. Diagnosis is made by the presence of amylase in the blood serum. Amylase is an enzyme produced by the pancreas that is used to digest carbohydrates in the small intestine. The presence of elevated levels of the enzyme is an indication that it is not reaching the small intestine and is spilling over into the bloodstream.

The powerful enzymes produced by the pancreas are used to digest proteins, carbohydrates, and fats. If for any reason these substances are not released from the pancreas, they will digest the cells of the pancreas and destroy them. As pancreatitis progresses, it will cause tissue inflammation and will lead to swelling of the organ. In addition, the enzymes may start to digest the cells of the blood vessels in the immediate area, causing bleeding into the tissue. The inflammation, combined with the bleeding, may lead to greater swelling and further inflammation.

Acute pancreatitis can lead to complications in other tissue as well, such as fat necrosis leading to the release of fatty acids from adipose tissue. The fatty acids bind to circulating calcium and may cause tetanus of the skeletal muscle as a result of calcium deficiency. If the enzymes released from the exocrine cells destroy the endocrine cells, the resulting loss of hormone production will lead to hyperglycemia and the complications that stem from it. Cysts or abscesses may also result from acute pancreatitis. Although this disease is usually self-limiting, in many cases it will lead to death.

Chronic pancreatitis is a recurring disease that may also demonstrate acute episodes. It has generally been associated with chronic alcoholism, which seems to be the major cause. Chronic pancreatitis is primarily a disease of middle age and occurs more frequently in men than in women. The patient generally complains of abdominal or back pain, often after a large meal or excessive alcohol consumption. Because of the lack of enzymes for lipid digestion, patients often excrete large quantities of undigested lipids. Without fat absorption, many fat-soluble substances such as vitamins A, D, E, and K will not be absorbed.

Because the patient with chronic pancreatitis is often malnourished from inadequate digestion and absorp-

tion of food and from vitamin deficiencies, there is associated weight loss and muscular wasting. The exocrine portion of the pancreas is gradually replaced by scar tissue, but the endocrine cells remain unaffected.

Disease of the pancreas can also be caused by cystic fibrosis. Cystic fibrosis, also known as mucoviscidosis, is an autosomal recessive disease of the exocrine glands. It occurs in about 1 in 2,500 live births of Caucasians but rarely occurs in African Americans or Asians. Cystic fibrosis affects the mucus-secreting glands in the body and leads to the production of abnormally thick mucus. About 80 percent of these patients have involvement of the pancreas. The onset and severity of the disease vary widely, but most infants born with cystic fibrosis have a pancreas that appears to be normal. As the abnormal mucus is produced, however, it may block the ducts of the exocrine glands and lead to the destruction of the exocrine tissue. The glandular tissue is progressively replaced by fibrous or adipose tissue or by cysts. The loss of pancreatic activity may lead to malabsorption of nutrients and vitamins. Although the islets of Langerhans are not affected by the disease in its early stages, eventually they also may be destroyed.

Tumors of the pancreas are primary tumors; there is almost no incidence of tumors metastasizing to the pancreas from other locations in the body. The exocrine tumors are generally adenocarcinomas, a type of cancer that is increasing in frequency throughout the world. An association with cigarette smoking and diabetes mellitus has been established. The tumors most commonly occur in the area of the gland where the major ducts leave the pancreas. As the tumors enlarge, they may put excessive pressure on the common bile duct, which is located in the same region. This pressure leads to the backup of bile in the liver known as obstructive jaundice; this is one of the earliest signs of pathology. Tumors located at other sites will not be detected until much later because they do not produce symptoms. Metastases of these tumors may be to the liver or surrounding lymph nodes. Because diagnosis is usually after the disease has progressed, the prognosis is poor even in operable cases.

The most common disease of the endocrine portion of the pancreas is diabetes mellitus. In 2009, over 68,000 individuals died of diabetes in the United States. Diabetes is a chronic disorder affecting carbohydrate, fat, and protein metabolism. It may be further classified as insulin-dependent or juvenile diabetes (type 1), non-insulin-dependent or adult-onset diabetes (type 2), or secondary diabetes. All forms of diabetes have a common pattern in which insulin is present in insufficient quantities, is absent, or does not function normally-all of which lead to hyperglycemia. Both type 1 and type 2 diabetes are inherited. In identical twins, there is a 50 percent concordance rate for type 1 and a 90 percent concordance for type 2. The latter figure indicates that heredity plays a more important role in type 2 diabetes.

Patients with type 1 diabetes are insulin-dependent. The disease starts at an early age and is sometimes referred to as juvenile diabetes. The decrease in insulin supply is caused by a decrease in functional beta cells in the islets of Langerhans. Evidence indicates that the beta cells are damaged or destroyed by an autoimmune reaction, which may follow a viral infection. Type 1 diabetics often have other endocrine disorders that are a result of autoimmunity. Type 2 diabetics produce some insulin, but not sufficient quantities. It appears that the tissues of these patients are resistant to insulin. The symptoms are less severe than those associated with type 1. Secondary diabetes is a result of some other disease that causes injury or destruction of beta cells. Diseases such as chronic pancreatitis or carcinoma of the pancreas can interfere with insulin production. The severity of the three forms of the disease varies widely, as does the treatment. The type 1 diabetic requires insulin for survival, while in many type 2 diabetics the disease may be controlled by diet and exercise.

Although the presence of insulin has several effects on the body, the lack of insulin has the most pronounced effect on serum glucose levels. If insulin supply is diminished or if the cells do not respond to the insulin produced, there is a rise in blood glucose levels exceeding the amount that the kidney can retain. As a result, glucose is excreted in the urine along with large quantities of water. The loss of glucose and water may lead to hypoglycemia and dehydration. The problem is further complicated if there is inadequate glucose available, which causes the cells to metabolize fats. One of the by-products of fat metabolism is the production of chemicals known as ketones, which are acids. Thus the dehydration may be accompanied by a more acidic serum.

The symptoms described above are acute and demand immediate attention. In addition to these symptoms, many abnormalities may appear in patients who have diabetes for ten or more years. The cardiovascular system is highly vulnerable to the disease, and the cause of death in about 80 percent of diabetics is a cardiovascular abnormality.

PERSPECTIVE AND PROSPECTS

Since the pancreas is a vital organ, any disease or injury to it will have serious consequences. Problems with the pancreas may be magnified because the diseases associated with the exocrine portion of the gland are not easily detected. In acute cases of pancreatitis, the onset is sudden and requires immediate treatment to control the extent of the disease. Even when the disease is treated early, many patients die. Surgery is complicated by the inflammation and hemorrhaging that may have previously occurred.

Chronic pancreatitis and cancer of the pancreas are even more difficult to diagnose since many of the symptoms are common to other ailments and may not even be present until the disease has progressed to an acute stage. The chronic condition is complicated because the body cannot absorb nutrients and vitamins. By the time that the diagnosis has occurred, the patient is weakened by the loss of weight and muscular wasting from malnutrition.

Diabetes presents its own unique set of problems. In type 1 diabetes, the patient is often unable to follow the prescribed diet and must continually monitor his or her glucose levels to ensure that the insulin doses are appropriate. Assuming that the patient is able to follow the diet and takes the medication as prescribed, there will still be complications-particularly of the cardiovascular system-that may include renal damage.

Pancreas transplants provide type 1 diabetics with hope when all other standard treatments have failed and they are faced with serious and often life-threatening complications. Pancreatic transplants are often performed in conjunction with a kidney transplant since the majority of patients are in the end states of renal failure, but the procedure is rarely performed on individuals suffering from pancreatic cancer because that form of cancer is highly malignant and the probability of it returning and attacking the new pancreas is very high.

Pancreatic transplants usually involve implanting a healthy (and insulin producing) organ into a patient while leaving the original pancreas in place since it is still able to produce essential digestive enzymes. Following surgery, many patients are able to maintain normal blood glucose levels, and diabetes-related nerve damage is often stabilized and sometimes repaired following transplantation. The risks involved in the surgery, however, are significant and should be taken into consideration: In addition to the potential for blood clots, infection, and inflammation of the new pancreas, rejection of the new organ is of great concern and can occur immediately following the surgery or at any time during the recipient's life. Because of this threat, the patient must take powerful immunosuppressive drugs for the remainder of his or her life, and these drugs come with their own set of potential side effects such as thinning of the bones, high cholesterol and blood pressure, weight gain, and acne and excessive hair growth over the body.

New procedures have been employed that involve the transplantation of only the beta cells of the islets of Langerhans rather than of the entire organ. Similar side effects and risks, such as blood clots and the necessity of immunosuppressive drugs, are also associated with this procedure.

It is likely that there will be significant progress with the treatment of diabetes as more becomes known about somatic gene therapy, cell transplants, immunosuppression, and the control of insulin receptors.

—Annette O'Connor, PhD

See also Abdomen; Abscess drainage; Abscesses; Diabetes mellitus; Digestion; Endocrine glands; Endocrinology; Endocrinology, pediatric; Enzymes; Fetal tissue transplantation; Food biochemistry; Gastroenterology; Gastroenterology, pediatric; Gastrointestinal disorders; Gastrointestinal system; Glands; Hormones; Internal medicine; Metabolic syndrome; Metabolism; Pancreatitis; Stomach, intestinal, and pancreatic cancers; Systems and organs; Transplantation.

For Further Information:

Calvagna, Mary. "Pancreatitis." *HealthLibrary*, October 31, 2012.

Goodman, H. Maurice. *Basic Medical Endocrinology*. 4th ed. Boston: Academic Press/Elsevier, 2009.

Howard, John M., and Walter Hess. *History of the Pancreas: Mysteries of a Hidden Organ*. New York: Kluwer Academic, 2002.

Marieb, Elaine N. *Essentials of Human Anatomy and Physiology*. 10th ed. San Francisco: Benjamin Cummings, 2010.

O'Reilly, Eileen, and Joanne Frankel Kelvin. *One Hundred Questions and Answers About Pancreatic Cancer*. 2d ed. Sudbury, Mass.: Jones and Bartlett Publishers, 2010.

"Pancreas Transplantation." *American Diabetes Association*, July 25, 2013.

"Pancreatic Islet Transplantation." *National Diabetes Information Clearinghouse*, August 1, 2012.

Pizer, H. F. *Organ Transplants: A Patient's Guide*. Cambridge, Mass.: Harvard University Press, 1991.

Valenzuela, Jorge E., Howard A. Reber, and André Ribet, eds. *Medical and Surgical Diseases of the Pancreas*. New York: Igaku-Shoin Medical, 1991.

PANCREATIC CANCER. SEE STOMACH, INTESTINAL, AND PANCREATIC CANCERS.

PANCREATITIS

Category: Disease/Disorder

Anatomy or system affected: Abdomen, endocrine system, gastrointestinal system, pancreas

Specialties and related fields: Endocrinology, gastroenterology, internal medicine

Definition: Inflammation of the pancreas, which may be acute or chronic.

INFORMATION ON PANCREATITIS

Causes: Sometimes unknown; often alcoholism and biliary tract disease; possibly trauma, certain medications, viral infections, hyperlipidemia, structural abnormalities in pancreas, hereditary disease

Symptoms: Pain, inflammation

Duration: Acute or chronic

Treatments: Pain medications, intravenous hydration, antibiotics, surgery, intensive care

---

CAUSES AND SYMPTOMS

Linked to the small intestines by the pancreatic duct, the pancreas contributes enzymes necessary to digestion. When the pancreas is damaged or its duct is blocked, the enzymes may begin to digest the pancreatic tissue itself, a process called autodigestion. Inflammation ensues, resulting in acute pancreatitis. Although there may be complications, most cases are self-correcting once the damaging agent is eliminated, and the pancreatitis does not recur. With continuing damage to the pancreas, however, the disease may become self-perpetuating and either break out periodically in attacks that mimic the acute form or cause few symptoms until much of the pancreas has been destroyed, a chronic form of pancreatitis that is difficult to treat. Either form can be fatal. Acute pancreatitis causes death in less than 5 percent of cases and generally does so because of complications, such as extensive tissue destruction and hemorrhage or infection. Complications from chronic pancreatitis can be fatal in as many as 50 percent of cases.

Although a variety of damaging agents are known to lead to pancreatitis, in as much as 15 percent of cases no clear cause is detectable; doctors call these cases idiopathic pancreatitis. Of detectable causes, alcoholism and biliary tract disease account for about 80 percent of both acute and chronic cases in the United States and Europe (the percentages vary widely in other parts of the world). Alcohol is the most common toxic agent causing pancreatitis, although susceptibility varies and only a minority of heavy drinkers develop acute pancreatitis; however, a long history of steady drinking is by far the most common cause of chronic pancreatitis. Gallstones in the common bile duct, or any other stricture or obstruction that backs up bile into the pancreatic duct, can trigger acute pancreatitis. Because surgeons can correct this problem by removing the obstruction, it seldom leads to chronic pancreatitis. Other, rarer causes include traumatic injury (especially the damage done by the steering wheel or seat belt during an automobile accident), damage incurred during abdominal surgery or endoscopic procedures in the small intestine, reactions to some medicines, viral infections, very high levels of fats in the blood (hyperlipidemia), structural abnormalities in the pancreas, or hereditary disease.

Despite the variety in causes, patients present a fairly limited set of symptoms, at least during an acute episode. Usually (but not always), they initially complain of steady pain in the upper abdomen that in severe cases seems to bore into them and radiate to the back. They may also have an enlarged abdomen, run a fever, experience nausea, and vomit. The physician is likely to find the abdomen distended, while the patient feels tenderness when it is touched. In severe cases, the patient may develop signs of shock, unstoppable hiccuping, jaundice, discoloration around the navel, fluid buildup in the peritoneal cavity, and impaired bowel function. While abdominal pain is a prominent feature of chronic pancreatitis as well, the most common associated symptoms are diarrhea, fatty stool, weight loss

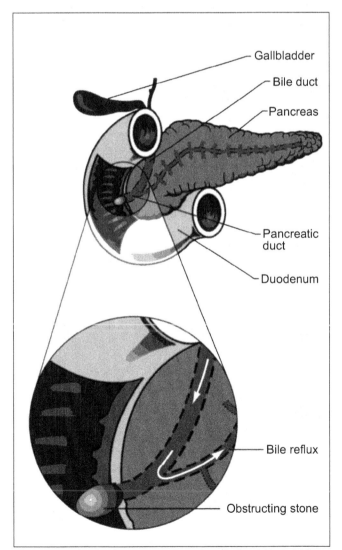

The pancreas, showing the pancreatic duct; when this duct is blocked, bile may reflux, leading to "autodigestion" of the pancreas. ©EBSCO

from poor digestion, and the development of diabetes mellitus.

Because none of these symptoms belongs exclusively to pancreatitis, physicians must conduct tests to establish the diagnosis; however, no single test is conclusive. Only by carefully showing that other possible diseases, such as pancreatic cancer, are not responsible for the symptoms can doctors be sure that pancreatitis is the culprit. Blood tests that detect elevated levels of amylase and lipase (pancreatic digestive enzymes) support the diagnosis. X-rays, ultrasonography, computed tomography (CT) scanning, and endoscopic inspection of the pancreas and common bile duct can identify both causes and complications of pancreatitis.

TREATMENT AND THERAPY
The treatment for pancreatitis depends on its cause. If the problem is abuse of alcohol or other drugs, physicians usually let an attack of acute pancreatitis run its course while the patient abstains from the offending substance. Nevertheless, even mild attacks frequently require hospitalization, because painkillers and intravenous hydration therapy are needed. If gallstones are thought to be the problem, plans are made to remove them by surgery. Patients with severe acute pancreatitis are sent to the hospital's intensive care unit, since they urgently need supportive treatment to stay alive. There, doctors insert a tube through the patient's nose and into the stomach to suck out excess gastric fluids and relieve pressure on the pancreas. They may give antibiotics if there is evidence of infection. Extra oxygen or mechanical assistance may be needed to support breathing. Occasionally, surgery may be called for even in pancreatitis not caused by gallstones, in order to cut away dead, infected tissue or drain fluid accumulations known as pseudocysts. Following an attack and treatment, a patient may require intravenous nourishment for weeks before the pancreas is ready to resume its full function.

Continued alcohol abuse will generally spur recurrent bouts of pancreatitis. Sometimes, however, the alcohol (or, rarely, slowly developing biliary tract disease) causes more subtle, gradual impairment of pancreatic function with few symptoms; in fact, some patients do not go to the doctor until the damage has become extensive and permanently disabling. Others have intense, continual upper abdominal pain that painkillers cannot reduce easily. (In fact, drug addiction from high dosages of painkillers often becomes a problem.) The doctor's first step is to stop the patient's alcohol intake. If gallstones or other obstructions are present, clearing the bile duct with surgery or an endoscopic procedure will decrease pain. Sometimes, high doses of pancreatic enzymes may be helpful in relieving pain.

In cases of uncontrollable pain, however, surgery may be needed to block the sympathetic nerves or even to remove all or part of the pancreas. If pancreatic function is sufficiently impaired by this procedure, or by the progress of the disease, chronic pancreatitis patients will digest food poorly and may require enzyme supplements to avoid continued weight loss. Since insulin is made in the pancreas, such patients may also develop diabetes. All chronic pancreatitis patients will need professional advice about appropriate diet and lifestyle changes.

—Roger Smith, PhD

See also Alcoholism; Diabetes mellitus; Endocrine disorders; Endocrinology; Endocrinology, pediatric; Enzymes; Gallbladders; Gallbladder diseases; Hypoglycemia; Obstruction; Pancreas; Stomach, intestinal, and pancreatic cancers; Stone removal; Stones.

For Further Information:
Büchler, M. W., et al., eds. *Acute Pancreatitis: Novel Concepts in Biology and Therapy*. Boston: Blackwell Science, 1999.
Calvagna, Mary. "Pancreatitis." *Health Library*, October 31, 2012.
Feldman, Mark, Lawrence S. Friedman, and Lawrence J. Brandt, eds. *Sleisenger and Fordtran's Gastrointestinal and Liver Disease: Pathophysiology, Diagnosis, Management*. 2 vols. Philadelphia: Saunders/Elsevier, 2010.
Levine, Joel S., ed. *Decision Making in Gastroenterology*. 2d ed. Philadelphia: B. C. Decker, 1992.
Melmed, Schlomo, et al., eds. *Williams Textbook of Endocrinology*. 12th ed. Philadelphia: Saunders/Elsevier, 2011.
Munoz, Abilio, and David A. Katerndahl. "Diagnosis and Management of Acute Pancreatitis." *American Family Physician* 62, no. 1 (July 1, 2000): 164-174.
"Pancreatitis." *Mayo Clinic*, January 15, 2011.
"Pancreatitis." *National Digestive Diseases Information Clearinghouse*, August 16, 2012.
Pancreatitis Supporters' Network. www.pancreatitis.org.uk.
Parker, James N., and Philip M. Parker, eds. *The Official Patient's Sourcebook on Pancreatitis*. San Diego, Calif.: Icon Health, 2002.

PANIC ATTACKS. SEE ANXIETY.

PAP TEST

Category: Procedure
Also known as: Pap sampling, Pap smear
Anatomy or system affected: Genitals, reproductive system, uterus
Specialties and related fields: Gynecology, oncology
Definition: A sampling of cells from the cervix or vagina used to screen for dysplasia (precancer) and cancer.

INDICATIONS AND PROCEDURES
Pap testing guidelines have recently changed. Formerly, the procedure was recommended for all women over the age of eighteen or for women who are sexually active. Revised guidelines have been issued by the American Cancer Society, the American College of Obstetricians and Gynecologists, and the Preventive Services Task Force, part of the US Department of Health and Human Services. These updated guidelines all stipulate that Pap tests should begin in women aged twenty-one and older. Updated guidelines have been issued as well for human papillomavirus (HPV) testing, which frequently accompanies the procedure; it is now recommended that HPV testing be done in women aged thirty and older because HPV in younger women is usually a transient infection that will clear without need for intervention.

The guidelines also recommend less frequent Pap testing for women who have had three consecutive negative tests; the guidelines also call for a cutoff to Pap testing in older women without abnormalities. Pap testing guidelines for women who have had a hysterectomy (with sampling of the vaginal cuff) vary depending on whether the hysterectomy was done for benign or malignant causes. The guidelines recommend that only women who have had malignant disease continue Pap testing.

A Pap test is performed easily in an office visit. Generally, the patient lies on her back with legs flexed and knees apart, although alternative positions can be utilized for women with limited mobility or with disabilities. A speculum is then carefully inserted into the vagina, and the cervix is visualized. A spatula is used to gently scrape off cells from the transition zone of the cervix. A cytobrush samples cells from the cervical canal. These cells are then placed in a preservative and sent to a pathology laboratory for analysis. The term "Pap smear" derives from the fact that before the advent of liquid preservative methods of collecting samples, samples were "smeared" on a glass slide and then sent to a laboratory for analysis.

USES AND COMPLICATIONS
The main use of Pap testing is to identify asymptomatic cases of dysplasia (abnormal growth) of the cervix and vagina. With early treatment of dysplasia, the incidence of and number of deaths from cervical cancer have decreased dramatically. Although cancer screening is the primary purpose and use of Pap testing, incidental findings may include vaginal infections of bacteria, fungi, or parasites. In rare cases, Pap tests may also detect abnormal cells shed from the endometrium.

There are no serious risks from the procedure. Women may see a small amount of spotting after the procedure as a result of abrasions from the spatula or cytobrush.

PERSPECTIVE AND PROSPECTS

The Pap test was introduced in 1943 by George N. Papanicolaou and Herbert F. Traut. Since then, the incidence of invasive cervical cancer has dramatically, although cervical cancer remains the second most prevalent malignancy among women worldwide, according to the World Health Organization.

A screening test analogous to cervical Pap sampling, called the anal cytology, or "anal Pap test," has been developed to screen for anal dysplasia and cancer. It has been used primarily on high-risk patients, such as those with human immunodeficiency virus (HIV), women who have had cervical or vulvar cancer, and HIV-negative men who have sex with men.

—Clair Kaplan, APRN/MSN;
additional material by Anne Lynn S. Chang, MD

See also Biopsy; Cervical, ovarian, and uterine cancers; Cervical procedures; Genital disorders, female; Gynecology; Reproductive system; Screening; Women's health.

For Further Information:

A.D.A.M. Medical Encyclopedia. "Pap Smear." *MedlinePlus*, February 26, 2012.

"Cervical Cancer Screening." *Centers for Disease Control and Prevention*, June 13, 2013.

Kumar, Vinay, et al., eds. *Robbins Basic Pathology*. 9th ed. Philadelphia: Saunders/Elsevier, 2013.

Lentz, Gretchen M., et al. *Comprehensive Gynecology*. 6th ed. Philadelphia: Mosby/Elsevier, 2012.

National Cancer Institute. "Cervical Cancer Screening." *National Institutes of Health, US Department of Health and Human Services*, July 19, 2012.

"Pap Test." *Health Library*, March 15, 2013.

Wright, Thomas C., Jr., et al. "2001 Consensus Guidelines for the Management of Women with Cervical Cytological Abnormalities." *Journal of the American Medical Association* 287, no. 16 (April, 2002): 2120-2129.

PARALYSIS

Category: Disease/Disorder
Anatomy or system affected: Legs, muscles, musculoskeletal system, neck, nerves, nervous system, spine
Specialties and related fields: Neurology, physical therapy
Definition: Pronounced weakness or the inability to produce movement in a part of the body resulting from a variety of causes.

Key terms:

brain cortex: the outer layer of the brain, or gray matter; divided into many areas, each with a different function, such as motion (the motor cortex) or sensation (the sensory cortex)

central nervous system: a system consisting of the brain, the brain stem, the cerebellum, and the spinal cord

hemiplegia: paralysis of one side of the body

motor: referring to parts of the nervous system having to do with movement production

nerve cell: the type of cells that make up the brain, spinal cord, and all the nerves; some initiate nerve impulses, some transmit impulses from one nerve cell to another, some transmit impulses from nerve cells to muscle cells, and some function to regulate other impulses

nerve impulse: a weak, localized electrical current generated by the movement of charged particles across and along a nerve cell membrane

nerves: bands of nervous tissue that carry both motor and sensory nerve impulses between the central nervous system and the rest of the body

neurotransmitters: chemical substances, such as acetylcholine, that are released by nerve cells into synapses when the nerve is stimulated; they stimulate the next nerve cell to fire in turn, thus passing the impulse from cell to cell

paraplegia: paralysis of the legs and lower trunk

peripheral nervous system: a system consisting of the nerves not located in the central nervous system; these nerves carry impulses from the central nervous system to the target muscles and relay sensory impulses from the rest of the body to the central nervous system

quadriplegia: paralysis of all four limbs

spinal cord: a large collection of nerve cells that relay impulses between the brain and the rest of the body; sometimes the spinal cord initiates nerve impulses of its own, such as reflexes

NERVOUS SYSTEM FUNCTIONS

To understand the causes of paralysis-weakness or the inability to move a part of the body-it is necessary to review briefly the motor nervous system and muscles. Following an action from initiation to completion through the motor nervous system may clarify this process. One may begin, for example, with a voluntary movement. An alarm clock rings early one morning. A sleeper hears the noise and decides to hit the snooze button. This decision is made in the cerebral cortex, which sends impulses to the nerves in the arm via the spinal cord.

The actual microscopic actions that result in a nerve impulse traveling from the motor cortex all the way to individual muscles will be briefly reviewed. An individual nerve cell, or neuron, comprises three parts: the dendrites, the cell body, and the axon. The cell body conducts the metabolism for the cell and otherwise keeps things in running order, but it has little direct involvement with the transmission of nerve impulses.

Dendrites are similar in appearance to the roots of plants. They are numerous and relatively short. Their function is to pick up impulses received either from sensory organs or from other cells. They do this when the receptors on their surface become activated by certain chemical signals released by neighboring nerve cells. Once these receptors are activated, they initiate a process known as depolarization.

In the most basic description, depolarization refers to the generation of a minute electrical charge on nerve cell membranes. It occurs through the motion of charged molecules, or ions, across the cell membrane. The specific ions involved include potassium, sodium, and calcium. Depolarization progresses down the length of the nerve cell. It passes through the dendrite to the cell body of the nerve cell and then to the axon. The axon is long and thin, some axons reaching lengths of three or more feet. Depending on its type and function, the axon may split into small filaments that go to several nerve or muscle cells, or it may remain single.

The sending axons do not touch the receiving cells when passing an impulse. Instead, they come close to the receiving cell's dendrites but leave a small gap (the synapse). Once a nerve impulse reaches the end of an axon, the axon releases chemical compounds called neurotransmitters.

Synthesized by the nerve cell, the neurotransmitter is collected and stored in small packets resting at the end of the axon. In response to depolarization, the small packets of neurotransmitter are released into the synapse, and the original electrical nerve impulse is converted into a chemical impulse. When the neurotransmitter is released, it diffuses across the gap and contacts specific receptors on the dendrite of the receiving nerve cell. The receiving nerve cell's receptors then depolarize the receiving nerve cell, converting the chemical impulse back into an electrical one.

The receiving nerve cell is forced to continue depolarizing until the neurotransmitter is no longer in contact with the receptor, or until the nerve cell itself becomes exhausted and cannot depolarize again. To allow the receiving nerve cell to stop firing and to prepare itself for another signal, the neurotransmitter must be removed rather quickly from the receptor. This can be done by the axon of the sending cell, which takes it back in, or by enzymes located within the synapse that actually destroy the neurotransmitter. The most common neurotransmitter is acetylcholine, and the most frequently encountered form of enzyme that destroys neurotransmitters is called acetylcholinesterase.

INFORMATION ON PARALYSIS

Causes: May include injury; infection, exposure to toxins, stroke, central nervous system disorders

Symptoms: Range from muscle weakness to complete immobility

Duration: Acute or chronic, depending on cause

Treatments: Depend on cause; may include surgery, physical therapy, spinal alignment and stabilization, drug therapy, toxin removal, hormonal therapy

---

The transmission of the nerve impulses signaling the hand to press the alarm clock's snooze button involves passing the impulses through several nerves. The impulses form synapses on nerve cells in the spinal cord before those cells pass the impulse down the spinal cord toward the arm to cause the desired action.

The spinal cord is protected inside the vertebral column, a hollow column of bone. This column is made up of a stack of vertebrae supported by solid bone in the front and a hollow ring of thinner bone in the back through which the spinal cord runs. The vertebrae are anchored to one another by bony connections; the facets and vertebral spines; fibrous ligaments to the front, back, and side; and the intervertebral disks. Disks are made up of soft, gelatinous material surrounded by fibrous tissue. The disks and joints in the vertebral column allow the spine to flex and turn, while the bony column surrounding the spinal cord provides protection.

When the nerve leaves the spinal cord, it travels in what is called the motor ramus, or "root." The ramus passes through an opening in the vertebral column called a foramen. While passing through the foramen, the ramus passes near the intervertebral disk. The motor nerve fibers (and consequently the nerve impulses sent out to turn off the alarm clock) in the motor ramus join with the sensory nerve fibers in the sensory ramus just outside the vertebral column, and together they form the spinal nerves. These spinal nerves regroup to form peripheral nerves.

A peripheral nerve is the part of the nervous system that finally contacts the muscles that turn off the alarm clock. Peripheral nerves carry both sensory and motor information in the same nerve. They are the only locations in which sensory and motor nerve fibers are so completely joined. Peripheral nerves must sometimes pass through relatively tight or exposed locations. An example of an exposed nerve is the "funny bone," the ulnar nerve, which causes an unpleasant sensation when struck. Nerves that pass through tight spaces may suffer entrapment syndromes. A common nerve entrapment syndrome is carpal tunnel syndrome, in which the median nerve is squeezed in the fibrous band around the wrist.

Finally, the arm muscles themselves become involved in the process of turning off the alarm. The muscles are made up of numerous muscle fibers, and each muscle fiber is made up of numerous muscle cells. Inside each muscle cell are two active protein filaments, actin and myosin, which pull together when activated, causing the muscle cell to shorten. When the majority of muscle cells "fire" at once, the whole muscle contracts. The signal from nerve to muscle cell is transmitted across a synapse. The snooze button is pushed, and the alarm ends. Finally, the signals to the arm end, and the filaments slide back to their initial positions, relaxing the muscle cells.

For actin and myosin to move well, there must be adequate blood flow and adequate concentrations of substances such as oxygen, glucose, potassium, sodium, and calcium. Many other substances are needed indirectly to keep muscle cells functioning optimally, including thyroid hormone and cortisone.

TYPES OF PARALYSIS
True paralysis is the inability to produce movement of a part of the body. Paralysis may result from problems at many locations in the body, such as the motor cortex of the brain, the spinal cord, the nerves in the arms or legs, the blood, or the muscle cells themselves. Doctors must determine the specific cause of paralysis or weakness since the treatment of each disease is different. The first task is to determine whether the weakness or paralysis is caused by a disease of the nervous system, the muscle cells, or one of the substances that interferes with nerve conduction or muscular contraction. Some characteristics of specific problems are helpful in this diagnosis.

Disease of the nervous system is most often associated with complete paralysis. Diseases affecting the muscle cells or the factors controlling them are usually associated with a partial rather than complete paralysis-there is weakness rather than a lack of movement. When weakness is severe, however, it may be mistaken for complete paralysis. The fact that diseases of the nervous system cause paralysis of one side of the body (hemiplegia) or one part of the body is helpful in diagnosis. Paralyzing conditions that affect muscle cells tend to result in whole-body weakness, although some muscles may be more severely affected than others. Another aid in differentiation is that neurologic diseases are almost always associated with some degree of impairment in sensation, while muscular causes are never associated with sensory loss.

Damage to the central nervous system and to the peripheral nervous system can be differentiated by features of the dysfunction. Central nervous system problems affect either half of the body or one region of the body, while peripheral damage affects only the muscles controlled by the damaged nerve or nerves. Central nervous system damage leaves pronounced reflexes, while damage to peripheral nerves results in an affected area without any reflexes. There is some muscle wasting with either type of paralysis, but the wasting seen after a peripheral nerve disease appears more quickly and more severely. When central nervous system damage occurs, the muscles involved are generally tight (spastic paralysis). Conversely, in patients with peripheral nervous system damage, muscles are usually loose. Through attention to these differentiating features, the source of paralysis can usually be discovered.

In adults, the most common cause of paralysis is stroke. A stroke results from interruption of the blood supply to a part of the brain. After being cut off from blood flow, the affected area dies. Brain tumors may also cause paralysis. Unlike strokes, however, which cause most of their damage as soon as the blood supply is interrupted, the damage produced by tumors tends to increase slowly as the tumor grows. An interesting feature of brain tumors is that they are surrounded by an area of swelling called edema. The edema, not the tumor itself, causes most of the neurologic changes. This distinction is important because edema is usually responsive to medical treatment.

Subdural hematomas are collections of blood that are outside the brain but inside the skull. They are seen most frequently in older people and alcoholics. To form a subdural hematoma, a small blood vessel becomes injured in such a way that blood slowly oozes from it, accumulates, and clots. Interestingly, the trauma may be so slight as to not be remembered by the patient. This clot may cause pressure on the motor cortex that results in paralysis. Generally, subdural hematomas are slow in onset.

Multiple sclerosis, a disease affecting the nervous system, causes scattered, multiple small areas of destruction virtually anywhere in the brain or spinal cord. The extent of paralysis depends on the sites and extent of the damaged areas. Patients often have impairments in vision, speaking, sensation, and coordination.

If the spinal cord is the cause, the extent and location of the paralysis and numbness depend on the size, location, and level of the lesion. Spinal cord paralysis may result from trauma, tumors, interruption of blood flow, blood clots, or infections such as abscesses. These disorders are similar, except for location, in most respects to the previously described conditions in the brain. One of the conditions, however-trauma of the spinal cord-is very different from trauma of the brain.

Significant trauma may result in fracture of the vertebral column. Spinal fractures may be classified as stable or unstable. Unstable fractures, unlike stable ones, are often associated with paralysis because unstable fractures allow subluxation to occur. Subluxation is a dislocation of the vertebral column that compresses the spinal cord. If it occurs in the neck, quadriplegia (paralysis of all four limbs) results. If it occurs lower down the spine, paraplegia (paralysis of both lower limbs) is seen. On occasion, through inadvertent or excessive movement, overenthusiastic rescuers cause permanent paralysis by converting a nonsubluxated fracture to a subluxated one during rescue attempts.

Another unique type of spinal cord trauma is the rupture of an intervertebral disk, which allows the gelatinous material to press on the spinal cord or on the rami leaving the spinal cord. In addition to causing severe pain, an intervertebral disk rupture may cause weakness or paralysis. It usually affects only one or two rami and spares the spinal cord itself. Trauma to the spinal cord is particularly dangerous to individuals with conditions that weaken the bony spine. These conditions include osteoporosis of all types and rheumatoid arthritis.

Peripheral nerve damage can occur through a number of conditions that may result in nerve degeneration, including diabetes mellitus, vitamin deficiencies, use or abuse of certain medications, and poisoning by toxins such as alcohol and lead. Sometimes, a temporary nerve degeneration called Guillain-Barré syndrome follows upper respiratory tract infections and may be quite serious if the respiratory muscles are affected. A peripheral nerves may also be damaged by direct trauma, or by pressure as it passes through a narrow compartment, as happens in carpal tunnel syndrome. Peripheral nerve conditions are accompanied by numbness, tingling, and weakness or paralysis of only the area served by the affected nerve.

Paralysis may complicate diseases affecting muscles, although in these cases the patients usually demonstrate weakness rather than paralysis. In muscular diseases, the paralysis (or weakness) tends to affect all the muscles of the body, although some may be more affected than others. The most frequent causes of paralysis in children are inherited diseases such as muscular dystrophy. In adults, muscular diseases are mainly attributable to hormonal imbalances caused by problems such as an underactive thyroid gland or an overactive adrenal gland.

Paralysis may result if the concentration of certain substances in the body is significantly altered, although weakness is a much more common occurrence. The concentration of potassium, sodium, calcium, glucose, and specific hormones may dramatically affect muscle strength. A specific, though uncommon, disease of this type is periodic hypokalemic paralysis, a condition that runs in families. In this disorder, the amount of potassium in the blood can be dramatically reduced for short periods of time, resulting in brief periods of severe weakness or paralysis. These episodes rarely have serious consequences.

Weakness or paralysis may result if the body is unable to produce adequate amounts of acetylcholine, or if this neurotransmitter is destroyed in the synapse before it can pass on its message. Myasthenia gravis is the most common example of this type of disorder. Affected patients initially have adequate strength, but they develop weakness and paralysis in muscles during periods of use because acetylcholine stores become depleted. The weakness in this condition tends to become more prominent as the day wears on. The most frequently used muscles are the most affected. This type of paralysis temporarily improves after rest or medication.

Another unique type of paralysis, called Todd's paralysis, may follow a generalized epileptic seizure. It happens only when the seizure has been so extensive and prolonged that the nerve cells in the brain are literally exhausted and no longer able to initiate the nerve impulses needed to generate movements. This paralysis is temporary.

Paralysis may be caused by a variety of psychiatric disorders, including hysteria, catatonic psychosis, conversion disorder, factitious disorder, and somatization disorder. In psychological paralysis, the patient's inability to move parts of the body is psychological. This paralysis is particularly common during periods of high stress such as combat. Psychological paralysis should be differentiated from malingering. In a psychological paralysis, the patients genuinely believe that they are paralyzed, whereas malingerers, though they deny it, know that they are not paralyzed. Malingering is usually seen when some benefit resulting from the paralysis is anticipated.

PERSPECTIVE AND PROSPECTS

Once a nerve cell has been destroyed, it cannot be repaired. This is the main reason that the outlook is quite poor when most types of paralysis occur. The only thing that doctors can do is to try to limit the extent of the paralysis. Improvements can be made only by training the neighboring cells to take over the functions of the lost cells.

After suffering a paralyzing event, a patient begins rehabilitation using a number of exercises. These activities are usually carried out with the help of physical therapists, occupational therapists, or kinesiotherapists. Unfortunately, progress is rather limited, and most patients are not able to resume their old lifestyle after suffering extensive paralysis.

It is very important to take seriously paralysis or weakness that is localized to a single muscle or single group of muscles. Doctors need to find out the cause of this weakness as soon as possible and take steps to minimize or reverse the damage prior to complete destruction of the nerve cells. Initial and subsequent stroke prevention, tumor treatments, hematoma evacuation, spinal alignment and stabilization, intervertebral disk surgery, toxin removal, hormonal manipulation, and ion correction are all currently available methods of dealing with paralysis.

Because of the poor prognosis for overcoming paralysis, research has focused on understanding how nerve cells grow. Some lower animals possess an ability to regenerate nerve cells when they are damaged. It is well known that a lobster which has lost one of its claws can regenerate that claw, as well as the nerves that control the claw's functioning. A lower animal nerve growth factor has been identified and is being examined by a number of researchers. It is likely that drugs which could aid regeneration of damaged nerve cells in higher animals will be discovered. Once available, these drugs will improve the outlook for recovery of patients with paralysis. These medications may also help with other conditions associated with nerve cell damage, such as Alzheimer's disease and Parkinson's disease.

Progress in medical treatment and an increased health awareness by the public will reduce the incidence of diseases such as diabetes mellitus and the intake of toxins, such as alcohol, that may cause paralysis. Seat belt laws and motorcycle helmet laws may reduce the incidence of paralysis by reducing the severity of injuries in motor vehicle accidents.

Progress in neurosurgery should also improve a patient's hope for recovery in trauma cases. Although dead nerve cells cannot regenerate, cut nerve filaments may be able to regenerate and reattach, which is why surgeons have been able to reattach severed limbs. With progressively finer techniques and equipment, the success rate should improve further. Future progress in neurosurgery may also benefit patients whose paralysis is attributable to causes other than trauma. Progress in genetic research may allow scientists to isolate the genes responsible for diseases causing paralysis. Diseases such as myasthenia gravis and muscular dystrophy could respond to treatment if genetic therapies are found.

—*Ronald C. Hamdy, MD, Mark R. Doman, MD, and Katherine Hoffman Doman*

See also Amyotrophic lateral sclerosis; Ataxia; Bell's palsy; Botox; Brain; Brain damage; Brain disorders; Brain tumors; Cerebral palsy; Epilepsy; Fracture and dislocation; Guillain-Barré syndrome; Hemiplegia; Motor neuron diseases; Multiple sclerosis; Muscular dystrophy; Nervous system; Neuralgia, neuritis, and neuropathy; Neuroimaging; Neurology; Neurology, pediatric; Neurosurgery; Numbness and tingling; Palsy; Paraplegia; Parkinson's disease; Quadriplegia; Seizures; Spinal cord disorders; Spine, vertebrae, and disks; Strokes.

For Further Information:

Bear, Mark F., Barry W. Connors, and Michael A. Paradiso. *Neuroscience: Exploring the Brain*. 3d ed. Philadelphia: Lippincott Williams & Wilkins, 2009.

Christopher and Dana Reeve Foundation, Paralysis Resource Center. www.christopherreeve.org.

Cure Paralysis Now. www.cureparalysisnow.org.

Goroll, Allan H., and Albert G. Mulley, eds. *Primary Care Medicine*. 5th ed. Philadelphia: Lippincott Williams & Wilkins, 2006.

Kandel, Eric R., James H. Schwartz, and Thomas M. Jessell. *Principles of Neural Science*. 5th ed. New York: McGraw-Hill Medical, 2013.

Lukas, Rimas. "Quadriplegia and Paraplegia." *Health Library*, March 15, 2013.

MedlinePlus. "Paralysis." *MedlinePlus*, August 9, 2013.

Nicholls, John G., A. Robert Martin, and Bruce G. Wallace. *From Neuron to Brain*. 5th ed. Sunderland, Mass.: Sinauer Associates, 2012.

"Progress for the Paralyzed." *MedlinePlus Magazine* 8, no. 1 (Spring, 2013): 10.

Tortora, Gerard J. *Principles of Anatomy and Physiology*. 14th ed. [S.I.]: John Wiley & Sons, 2013.

PARAMEDICS

Category: Specialty

Anatomy or system affected: All

Specialties and related fields: Cardiology, critical care, emergency medicine, geriatrics and gerontology, pulmonary medicine

Definition: Trained professional emergency medical technicians (EMTs) who provide sophisticated advanced life support in the field, especially intravenous therapy, cardiac monitoring, drug administration, cardiac defibrillation, and advanced airway management.

Key terms:

advanced life support (ALS): procedures such as intravenous therapy, pharmacology, cardiac monitoring, and defibrillation

basic life support (BLS): simple emergency lifesaving procedures that can aid a person in respiratory or circulatory failure

cardiopulmonary resuscitation (CPR): the artificial establishment of circulation of the blood and movement of air into and out of the lungs in a pulseless, nonbreathing patient

certification: the formal notice of certain privileges and abilities after completion of specified training and testing *defibrillation*: the termination of atrial or ventricular fibrillation (irregular heart muscle contractions), with restoration of the normal rhythm

emergency medical services (EMS): the combined efforts of several professionals and agencies to provide prehospital emergency care to the sick and injured

intravenous therapy: the introduction of medication into a vein with a special needle

intubation: the introduction of a tube into a body cavity, as into the larynx

SCIENCE AND PROFESSION

Emergency medical technician-paramedics (EMT-Ps) provide hospital emergency care in the field under medical command authority to acutely ill and/or injured patients and then transport those patients to the hospital by ambulance or other appropriate vehicle. The clinical knowledge possessed by the EMT-P includes the following systems and areas: the cardiovascular system, including the recognition of arrhythmias, myocardial ischemia, and congestive heart failure; the respiratory system, including acute airway obstruction, pneumothorax, chronic obstructive pulmonary disease (COPD), and respiratory distress; trauma to the head, neck, chest, spine, abdomen, pelvis, and extremities;

medical emergencies, including acute abdominal infections, diabetes mellitus, and allergic reactions; the central nervous system, including strokes, seizures, and alterations in levels of consciousness; obstetrical emergencies such as eclampsia; pediatric cases, including croup, epiglottitis, dehydration, child abuse, and care of the newborn; psychiatric emergencies, including problems with individuals who are suicidal, assaultive, destructive, resistant, anxious, confused, amnesiac, or paranoid; drug-related problems, including alcoholism, drug addiction, or overdoses; sexual assault and abuse; and various special situations, such as carbon monoxide and other noxious inhalations, poisoning, near drownings, overexposure to heat and cold, electrocution, burns, and exposure to hazardous materials.

The EMT-P must be able to fulfill many roles. First, paramedics must recognize a medical emergency, assess the situation, manage emergency care, and, if needed, extricate the patient. They must also coordinate their efforts with those of other agencies that may be involved in the care and transport of the patient. Paramedics should establish a good rapport with patients and their significant others in order to decrease their state of anxiety.

Paramedics administer emergency care in the field to sick or injured patients; among their primary tools are portable monitoring devices, such as an electrocardiograph (ECG or EKG) machine to check the electrical activity of the heart. ©EBSCO

The next step is to assign priorities to emergency treatment data for the designated medical control authority. Emergency treatment priorities must be assigned in cases where the medical direction is interrupted by communication failure or in cases of immediate, life-threatening conditions. Paramedics must record and communicate pertinent information to the designated medical command authority.

Meanwhile, they must initiate and continue emergency medical care under medical control, including the recognition of presenting conditions and the initiation of appropriate treatments. Such conditions include traumatic and medical emergencies, airway and ventilation problems, cardiac arrhythmias or standstill, and psychological crises. Paramedics must also assess the response of patients to treatment, modifying the medical therapy as directed by the medical control authority. EMT-Ps exercise personal judgment; provide such emergency medical care as has been specifically authorized in advance; direct and coordinate the transport of the patient by selecting the best available methods in concert with the medical command authority; record, in writing, the details related to the patient's emergency care and the incident; and direct the maintenance and preparation of emergency care equipment and supplies.

EMT-Ps must have a good working knowledge of human anatomy and must be familiar with its topographical language. Even though paramedics are not expected to diagnose every injury or illness, they can aid emergency department personnel by conveying correct information using medical terminology. Such information is gathered after examination of a patient at the scene of an accident or sudden illness.

The most important functions of the paramedic are to identify and treat any life-threatening conditions first and then to assess the patient carefully for other complaints or findings that may require emergency treatment or transportation to a hospital setting. Paramedics must distinguish between signs (measured information such as pulse, respiration, and temperature) and symptoms (patient complaints). They must be able to take complete patient histories, document all medications, and transfer this information to medical control.

The vital role of the respiratory system is stressed in all paramedical training courses. The function of the respiratory system is to provide the body with oxygen and to eliminate carbon dioxide. Paramedics must fully understand the breathing process, including gas exchange and the role and anatomic position of the air passages and lungs. They must understand the mechanics of breathing-how the diaphragm and intercostal muscles contract and relax during inspiration and expiration-and must realize that breathing is con-

trolled by the brain's response to levels of carbon dioxide and oxygen present in the arterial blood. Of special concern to the paramedic is the patient with COPD, who needs specialized oxygen support and careful watching.

Basic life support (BLS), formerly called cardiopulmonary resuscitation (CPR), is a series of emergency lifesaving procedures that are carried out in order to treat respiratory arrest, cardiac arrest, or both. CPR is a method of providing artificial ventilation and circulation. Its effectiveness depends on the prompt recognition of respiratory and/or cardiac arrest and the immediate start of treatment. Very often, the paramedic is able to defibrillate the patient immediately after cardiac arrest and restart the heart. Knowledge of how to provide BLS to the laryngectomy patient is part of paramedic education; in such cases, ventilation is often given via a stoma (opening) in the neck of the patient. Basic life support procedures must be modified for infants and children, since their respiration and pulse rates are higher than those of adults and require more rapid delivery of ventilatory and cardiac assistance.

Although breathing and heart rate are the primary interests of the paramedic, serious bleeding can also be life-threatening. Hence, paramedics must be well versed in blood circulation routes, control of bleeding, and the pressure points that can help in the control of serious hemorrhage. Serious bleeding often brings on a type of shock that is termed hypovolemic (meaning low blood volume). Paramedics must be alert to signs of impending shock and deal with this condition as soon as possible. Medical antishock trousers (MAST) are often used by paramedics to autotransfuse volumes of blood from the patient's lower extremities to the heart, lungs, and brain. These trousers are also used to control severe hemorrhage or the complications of pelvic fractures. The paramedic must be aware of the contraindications to the use of these devices as well; for example, persons with head injuries should not have the MAST device applied to them.

Paramedics need to identify the many types of shock. Anaphylactic shock is caused by an unusual or exaggerated allergic reaction of a person to a foreign protein. Psychogenic shock (fainting) is often self-correcting. Septic shock is caused by severe bacterial infections, while metabolic shock may arise from severe, untreated illnesses. Cardiogenic shock arises from an underlying cardiac condition and inefficient blood flow. In each case, the paramedic must be alert to the signs of each type of shock and be prepared to treat it, either with drugs delivered under medical control or with equipment present on the paramedic ambulance.

The more common types of injuries encountered by the paramedic are soft tissue injuries, caused by falls or accidents. The skin is the largest single organ of the body. It protects the body from the environment, regulates the body temperature, and transmits information from the environment to the brain. Soft tissue injuries can cause breaks in the skin, leaving the body vulnerable to infection and bleeding. Paramedic training includes treatment for massive traumatic wounds, such as gunshot or knife wounds.

Dealing with fractures is another part of paramedic training. While most fractures are not life-threatening, they can be painful and bring on patient shock; hence, paramedics need to deal with them quickly. Knowledge of the body's musculoskeletal system is vital to the performance of a paramedic.

Head injuries are a very challenging part of paramedic treatment, since the scalp contains many blood vessels and bleeding from head injuries is often profuse. The more serious head injury is often bloodless externally, but internal bleeding brings on pressure buildup in the skull and sudden coma. Such injuries are life-threatening and often require rapid treatment and transport.

Other medical emergencies include strokes (cerebrovascular accidents), diabetic coma or insulin shock, acute abdominal infections, and seizures. Prompt recognition and treatment by the paramedic are essential. Finally, treating the pediatric patient can be one of the most difficult emergencies, but saving a child's life or rescuing a child from permanent, disabling injury is very rewarding. The broad range of knowledge required of paramedics makes them a very special part of the health care team.

DIAGNOSTIC AND TREATMENT TECHNIQUES
Three technologies that distinguish the paramedic from the basic EMT are intravenous therapy, advanced airway management, and defibrillation.

Intravenous (IV) therapy may be an important procedure during the resuscitation of a patient who is suffering from hypovolemia, burn injury, blood loss, heatstroke, shock, electrolyte imbalance, or many other medical and surgical conditions. IV therapy is also important in providing an avenue of medication delivery in many medical situations, such as cardiac arrest, seizures, and asthma attacks. IV therapy is an invasive procedure that requires extensive training in its use in order for the paramedic to maintain the necessary skill level. In addition, paramedics must be aware of the indication for the use of IV therapy, the maintenance of such therapy, and possible complications.

IV therapy works via the infusion of fluid other than blood or blood products into the vascular system. This technique is used to establish and maintain direct access to the circulation or to provide fluids in order to maintain an adequate circulating blood volume. Fluids used for IVs are often referred to as electrolyte solutions, because the chemical compounds they contain are electrolytes. The most common electrolyte solutions used are sodium chloride solutions; for example, NS is a normal saline solution containing 0.9 percent sodium chloride. Occasionally, paramedics use plasma expanders or colloids, including Dextran. A common intravenous fluid is D5W, which is a 5-percent dextrose solution. The procedure for starting an IV includes preparing the solution, selecting the proper catheter size, selecting and preparing the site, and performing the venipuncture (insertion of a needle into a vein). Local complications to IV therapy may include some pain from the needlestick, hematoma formation at failed IV sites, infection, accidental arterial puncture, nerve damage, and thrombophlebitis. Environmental complications include cold climates, which cause IV solutions to freeze, and the danger of a needlestick to medical personnel during disposal. Proper precautions and periodic retraining keep paramedics up to date in their skills.

Advanced airway management means placing a tube into the patient's airway to maintain an open passage, to prevent aspiration of foreign bodies and stomach contents, and to allow the delivery of oxygen-enriched air. Three types of devices are employed in advanced airway management to achieve these objectives: the endotracheal tube (ENT), the esophageal obturator airway (EOA), and the pharyngeotracheal airway. The use of any of these devices by paramedics requires the consent of a medical director and adherence to written protocols. These devices require skill and instruction for proper insertion and use.

The ENT is placed through a patient's mouth or nose and directly through the larynx between the vocal cords. The tube may be placed blindly through the vocal cords using sounds of labored respirations as a guide, or it may be placed by feel through the cords. After placement, a soft balloon cuff near the end of the tube is then inflated with approximately 10 cubic centimeters of air to seal the trachea and anchor the tube, so that air can be blown directly into the lungs. The ENT prevents aspiration and gastric distension. It facilitates airway suctioning and enables the delivery of high volumes of oxygen at higher-than-normal pressures. In addition, certain medications may be given down the tube. ENT placement and use are difficult skills to master, requiring considerable practice and expert initial instruction. Direct visualization of the vocal cords is an important skill to have in order to prevent tracheal damage. If intubation takes too long, the resulting delay in oxygenation may lead to brain damage. Constant monitoring of lung sounds is needed to ensure that the tube stays in place.

The EOA has been in use since 1973 to facilitate airway management in cardiopulmonary resuscitation. The EOA is a plastic, semirigid tube approximately 30 centimeters long and 13 millimeters in diameter. The lower end of the tube is smooth, rounded, and closed. The upper third of the EOA is designed to function as an airway. It has sixteen holes in its wall at the junction of the middle and upper sections; when properly inserted, these holes will lie at the level of the pharynx and provide free passage of oxygen-enriched air to the lungs. The lower two-thirds of the EOA should lie in the esophagus. The balloon surrounding the end of the tube is normally inflated to block the esophagus and prevent the regurgitation of stomach contents backward into the airway. The face mask that comes with the EOA is designed to fit snugly about the patient's nose and mouth and must provide a tight seal. The EOA is used only for short-term airway management. It should be removed when the unconscious patient awakens and is able to protect the airway or when ENT placement has been performed over the EOA. At the time that the balloon is deflated and the EOA is removed, there is a high risk of vomiting and/or regurgitation of gastric contents. The EOA is not to be used on patients who are awake, on small children, or on patients with known esophageal disease.

The pharyngeotracheal airway is designed to provide lung ventilation when placed in either the trachea or the esophagus. This device is designed to be inserted blindly into the oropharynx and esophagus by paramedics who have received training and are authorized to use it. A pharyngeotracheal airway is contraindicated in conscious or semiconscious patients with a gag reflex. It should not be used with children under the age of fourteen or with adults under five feet tall.

With the use of any of these airway devices, the patient may regain consciousness while intubated. Such patients will usually gag, choke, and grasp at the device in an attempt to remove it, often resulting in injury to the airway. The patient's hands must be immediately restrained while the airway device is removed.

Defibrillation is the delivery of an electric current through a person's chest wall and heart for the purpose of ending ventricular fibrillation. The device used for this procedure is called a defibrillator (also automated external defibrillator or AED); it is typically a portable, battery-powered instrument that is used to record cardiac rhythm and to generate and deliver an electrical charge. Defibrillation can be a lifesaving measure in the treatment of sudden cardiac arrest in which the heart is in an arrhythmia known as ventricular fibrillation or ventricular tachycardia (VT). These two conditions occur when cardiac muscle becomes oxygen deficient or is injured or dies, causing the electrical system of the heart to be disturbed. Sometimes, the injured area of the heart begins to fire off uncoordinated electrical impulses. These irregular impulses can initiate abnormal beats called premature ventricular contractions (PVCs). If several of the PVCs occur close together, they produce the rhythm called ventricular tachycardia. If VT does not spontaneously convert back to a normal heart rhythm, it rapidly degenerates into ventricular fibrillation. The heart in VT beats faster and faster until its oxygen supply is depleted, at which point tissue injury begins and electrical impulses become completely uncoordinated and are fired at random.

If a defibrillator is applied to the patient and an electrical shock is given to the heart during the time of ventricular fibrillation, there is a good chance of restoring more normal electrical activity. This electrical countershock is thought to depolarize the cardiac muscle and conducting tissues instantaneously, thus resetting the electrical energies to the depolarized state. The patient's heart can then begin its normal conduction and contractions without having to contend with randomly generated electrical impulses. The electrical current delivered by defibrillators is measured in units called joules. In most protocols, the first shock is 200 joules, the second is between 200 and 300 joules, and the third and subsequent shocks are at the full 360-joule level. Paramedics using defibrillators need frequent continuing education in order to emphasize the practical skills of proper attachment of the electrodes, proper device operation, and recognition of cardiac arrhythmias.

PERSPECTIVE AND PROSPECTS

Emergency medical services (EMS) in the United States had its beginnings in 1966. In that year, the Committees on Trauma and Shock of the National Academy of Sciences National Research Council jointly published *Accidental Death and Disability: The Neglected Disease of Modern Society*. This joint report brought public attention to the inadequate emergency medical care being provided to the injured and sick in many parts of the United States. Two federal agencies initiated reform measures: The Department of Transportation (DOT) initiated the Highway Safety Act in 1966, and the Department of Health, Education, and Welfare enacted the Emergency Medical Services Act in 1973. Both created funding sources to develop prehospital emergency care in an effort to eliminate the majority of prehospital deaths. Local EMS systems were established in the early 1970s. In the 1980s, practitioners took a hard look at what had been done in the past, and the focus changed from establishing EMS systems to developing educational programs to provide consistent levels of quality care to the sick and injured.

The EMS system is made up of various components that work together to provide the sick and injured with the best possible emergency care in the shortest possible time. The EMS system represents the combined efforts of the first responder, the EMT with basic life support skills, the EMT-paramedic with advanced life support skills, emergency department personnel, physicians, allied health personnel, hospital administrators, EMS system administrators, and the overseeing governmental agencies.

Emergency medical technology is an exciting field of study. Few areas offer more direct application of theory and skills. All the information received in an EMT class will be important when it comes to saving lives and lessening human suffering. Emergency medical technology combines theoretical information, practical skills, and common sense. Above all, the EMS person dealing with a patient must possess great compassion and understanding.

The certification of an EMT-paramedic is formal notice of certain privileges and abilities after the completion of specific training and testing. The possession of a certificate obligates the individual to conform to the standard of care of other certified emergency medical care personnel. Nearly every state exempts emergency medical care from the licensure requirements of the Medical Practices Act for nonmedical personnel. (Because many emergency medical care procedures may be construed by the public to be the performance of a medical act, the EMT must be protected legally in those situations.) The need for prehospital care providers is ongoing, and recruiting people to enter this field continues to be a challenge to the agencies that oversee this work.

—*Jane A. Slezak, PhD*

See also Accidents; Arrhythmias; Burns and scalds; Cardiac arrest; Cardiopulmonary resuscitation (CPR); Choking; Critical care; Critical care, pediatric; Drowning; Electrocardiography (ECG or EKG); Emergency medicine; First aid; Fracture and dislocation; Heart attack; Heat exhaustion and heatstroke; Intravenous (IV) therapy; Respiration; Resuscitation; Shock; Strokes; Tracheostomy; Wounds.

For Further Information:

American Academy of Orthopaedic Surgeons. *Emergency Care and Transportation of the Sick and Injured.* Edited by Benjamin Gulli, Les Chatelain, and Chris Stratford. 10th ed. Sudbury, Mass.: Jones and Bartlett, 2011.
"EMTs and Paramedics." *Occupational Outlook Handbook.* Bureau of Labor Statistics, March 29, 2012.
Hamilton, Glenn C., et al. *Emergency Medicine: An Approach to Clinical Problem-Solving.* 2d ed. New York: W. B. Saunders, 2003.
Limmer, Daniel, et al. *Emergency Care.* 12th ed. Upper Saddle River, N.J.: Pearson/Prentice Hall Health, 2012.
Markovchick, Vincent J., and Peter T. Pons, eds. *Emergency Medicine Secrets.* 5th ed. Philadelphia: Mosby/Elsevier, 2011.
Rella, Francis J. *Manhattan Medics: The Gripping Story of the Men and Women of Emergency Medical Services Who Make the Streets of the City Their Career.* Hightstown, N.J.: Princeton Book Company, 2003.
Sanders, Mick J. *Mosby's Paramedic Textbook.* 4th ed. St. Louis, Mo.: Mosby/Elsevier, 2012.
Shapiro, Paul D., and Mary B. Shapiro. *Paramedic: The True Story of a New York Paramedic's Battles with Life and Death.* New York: Bantam Books, 1991.
Tangherlini, Timothy R. *Talking Trauma: Paramedics and Their Stories.* Jackson: University Press of Mississippi, 1998.

PARANOIA

Category: Disease/Disorder
Anatomy or system affected: Psychic-emotional system
Specialties and related fields: Psychiatry, psychology
Definition: Pervasive distrust and suspiciousness of others and a tendency to interpret others' motives as malevolent.

CAUSES AND SYMPTOMS

Paranoia is characterized by suspiciousness, heightened self-awareness, self-reference, projection of one's ideas onto others, expectations of persecution, and blaming of others for one's difficulties. Conversely, though paranoia can be problematic, it can also be adaptive. In threatening or dangerous situations, paranoia might instigate proactive protective behavior, allowing an individual to negotiate a situation without harm. Thus, paranoia must be assessed in context for it to be understood fully.

Paranoia can be experienced at varying levels of intensity in both normal and highly disordered individuals. As a medical problem, paranoia may take the face of a symptom, personality problem, or chronic mental disorder. As a symptom, it may be evidenced as a fleeting problem; an individual might have paranoid feelings that dissipate in a relatively brief period of time once an acute medical or situational problem is rectified.

As a personality problem, paranoia creates significant impairment and distress as a result of inflexible, maladaptive, and persistent use of paranoid coping strategies. Paranoid individuals often have preoccupations about loyalties, overinterpret situations, maintain expectations of exploitation or deceit, rarely confide in others, bear grudges, perceive attacks that are not apparent to others, and maintain unjustified suspicions about their relationship partner's potential for betrayal. They are prone to angry outbursts, aloof, and controlling, and they may demonstrate a tendency toward vengeful fantasies or actual revenge.

Finally, paranoia may be evidenced as a chronic mental disorder, most notably as the paranoid type of schizophrenia. In paranoid schizophrenia, there is a tendency toward delusions (faulty beliefs involving misinterpretations of events) and auditory hallucinations. Additionally, everyday behavior, speech, and emotional responsiveness are not as disturbed as in other variants of schizophrenia. Typically, individuals suffering from paranoia are seen by others as anxious, angry, and aloof. Their delusions usually reflect fears of persecution or hopes for greatness, resulting in jealousies, odd religious beliefs (such as persecution by God, thinking they are Jesus Christ), or preoccupations with their own health (such as the fear of being poisoned or of having a medical disorder of mysterious origin).

Paranoia may best be understood as being determined by a combination of biological, psychological, and environmental factors. It is likely, for example, that certain basic psychological tendencies must be present for an individual to display paranoid feelings and behavior when under stress, as opposed to other feelings such as depression. Additionally, it is likely that certain physical predispositions must be present for stressors to provoke a psychophysiological response.

Biologically, there are myriad physical and mental health conditions that may trigger acute and more chronic paranoid reactions. High levels of situational stress, drug intoxication (such as with amphetamines or marijuana), drug withdrawal, depression, head injuries, organic brain syndromes, pernicious anemia, B vitamin deficiencies, and Klinefelter syndrome may be related to acute paranoia. Similarly, certain cancers, insidious organic brain syndromes, and hyperparathyroidism have been related to recurrent or chronic episodes of paranoia.

In terms of the etiology of chronic paranoid conditions, such as paranoid schizophrenia and paranoid personality disorder, no clear causes have been identified. Some evidence points to a genetic component; the results of studies on twins and the greater prevalence of these disorders in some families support this view. More psychological theories highlight the family environment and emotional expression, childhood abuse, and stress. In general, these theories point to conditions contributing toward making a person feel insecure, tense, hungry for recognition, and hypervigilant. Additionally, the impact of social, cultural, and economic conditions contributing to the expression of paranoia is important. Paranoia cannot be interpreted out of context. Biological, psychological, and environmental factors must be considered in the development and maintenance of paranoia.

INFORMATION ON PARANOIA

Causes: May include psychological disorder (depression, schizophrenia), situational stress, drug intoxication or withdrawal, head injury, organic brain syndromes, pernicious anemia, B vitamin deficiencies, Klinefelter syndrome
Symptoms: Pervasive distrust and suspiciousness of others, tendency to interpret others' motives as malevolent, aloofness, heightened self-awareness, self-reference, blaming of others for one's difficulties, angry outbursts, controlling behavior
Duration: Acute to chronic
Treatments: Drug therapy, community-based therapy, cognitive and behavioral therapies

TREATMENT AND THERAPY

Three major types of therapies are available to treat paranoia: pharmacotherapies, community-based therapies, and cognitive-behavioral therapies. For acute paranoia problems and the management of more chronic, schizophrenia-related paranoia, pharmacotherapy (the use of drugs) is the treatment of choice. Drugs that serve to tranquilize the individual and reduce disorganized thinking, such as antipsychotics, phenothiazines and other neuroleptics, are commonly used. With elderly people who cannot tolerate such drugs, electroconvulsive therapy (ECT) has been used for treatment.

Community-based treatment, such as day treatment or inpatient treatment, is also useful for treating chronic paranoid conditions. Developing corrective and instructional social experiences, decreasing situational stress, and helping individuals to feel safe in a treatment environment are primary goals.

Finally, cognitive-behavioral therapies focused on identifying irrational beliefs contributing to paranoia-related problems have demonstrated some utility. Skillful therapists help to identify maladaptive thinking while unearthing concerns but not agreeing with the individual's delusional ideas.

PERSPECTIVE AND PROSPECTS

Certain life phases and social and cultural contexts influence behaviors that could be labeled as paranoid. Membership in certain minority or ethnic groups, immigrant or political refugee status, and, more generally, language and other cultural barriers may account for behavior that appears to be guarded or paranoid. As such, one can make few assumptions about paranoia without a thorough assessment.

Clinically significant paranoia is notable across cultures, with prevalence rates at any point in time ranging from 0.5 to 2.5 percent of the population. It is a problem manifested by diverse etiological courses requiring equally diverse treatments. Increased knowledge about the relationship among paranoia, depression and other mood disorders, schizophrenia, and the increased prevalence of paranoid disorders in some families will be critical. As the general population ages, a better understanding of more acute paranoid disorders related to medical problems will also be necessary. Better understanding will facilitate the development of more effective pharmacological and nonpharmacological treatments that can be tolerated by the elderly and others suffering from compromising medical problems.

—*Nancy A. Piotrowski, PhD*

See also Antianxiety drugs; Anxiety; Delusions; Hallucinations; Post-traumatic stress disorder; Psychiatric disorders; Psychiatry; Psychiatry, child and adolescent; Psychiatry, geriatric; Psychoanalysis; Schizophrenia; Shock therapy; Stress.

For Further Information:

Anderson F., and D. Freeman. "Socioeconomic Status and Paranoia: The Role of Life Hassles, Self-Mastery, and Striving to Avoid Inferiority." *The Journal of Nervous and Mental Disorders* 201, no. 8 (August, 2013): 698-702.

Barlow, David H., ed. *Clinical Handbook of Psychological Disorders.* 4th ed. New York: Guilford Press, 2008.

Bloom, Floyd E., M. Flint Beal, and David J. Kupfer, eds. *The Dana Guide to Brain Health.* New York: Dana Press, 2006.

Ellett, L. "Mindfulness for Paranoid Beliefs: Evidence From Two Case Studies." *Behavioural and Cognitive Psychotherapy* 41, no. 2 (2013): 238-242.

Graham, George. *The Disordered Mind: An Introduction to Philosophy of Mind and Mental Illness.* New York: Routledge, 2013.

Kring, Ann M., et al. *Abnormal Psychology.* 11th ed. Hoboken: John Wiley & Sons, 2010.

Munro, Alistair. *Delusional Disorder: Paranoia and Related Illnesses.* New York: Cambridge University Press, 1999.

Robbins, Michael. *Experiences of Schizophrenia: An Integration of the Personal, Scientific, and Therapeutic.* New York: Guilford Press, 1993.

Siegel, Ronald K. *Whispers: The Voices of Paranoia.* New York: Simon & Schuster, 1996.

Venter, Bruce. *Paranoid Schizophrenia My Label, My Life: How I Escaped the Strait Jacket of Serious Mental Illness.* Bloomington: AuthorHouse, 2012.

PARAPLEGIA

Category: Disease/Disorder
Anatomy or system affected: Legs, nervous system, spine
Specialties and related fields: Neurology
Definition: A motor or sensory loss in the lower extremities, with or without involvement of the abdominal and back muscles.

CAUSES AND SYMPTOMS

Paraplegia, the loss of motor and sensory function in the lower body, results in paralysis that may be complete or incomplete, spastic or flaccid, symmetric or asymmetric, and permanent or temporary. Almost half of the 10,000 to 12,000 spinal cord injuries reported each year result in paraplegia. This condition occurs twice as often in men as in women, and the incidence is highest between ages sixteen and thirty-five. Most spinal cord injuries result from trauma, especially automobile, motorcycle, and sporting accidents; gunshot wounds and falls also contribute. Less common causes are nontraumatic lesions, such as spina bifida, scoliosis, and chordoma.

In many patients, the onset of total or partial paralysis is immediate, resulting in loss of motion, sensation, and reflexes below the level of the lesion, with urinary retention and absence of perspiration in the paralyzed parts. In some patients, careful questioning and gentle examination are necessary to determine the extent of motor or sensory loss. Spinal cord injuries with motor and sensory loss may result in bowel, bladder, and sexual dysfunctions, depending on the level of the lesion and whether damage to the cord is complete or incomplete. In an incomplete spinal cord injury, perianal sensation, voluntary toe flexion, or sphincter control is still present. In a complete spinal cord injury, lack of sensation or voluntary muscle control is apparent and persists for twenty-four hours. Any return of functional muscle power distal to the injury is unlikely.

Diagnosis requires a clinical history, neurologic examination, and computed tomography (CT) scans. A lumbar puncture may rule out blocked cerebrospinal fluid circulation. Laboratory studies include a complete blood count (CBC), prothrombin time, electrolytes, twenty-four-hour urine for creatinine clearance, serum creatinine, and urinalysis. Weekly urine samples for culture and sensitivity are advisable during the entire rehabilitation period.

INFORMATION ON PARAPLEGIA

Causes: Spinal cord injuries, usually resulting from vehicle or sporting accidents, gunshot wounds, falls
Symptoms: Total or partial paralysis with loss of motion, sensation, and reflexes below lesion; urinary retention; absence of perspiration in paralyzed parts
Duration: Permanent or temporary
Treatments: Spinal alignment and stabilization, laminectomy, drug therapy (nitrofurantoin, vitamin C, analgesics and narcotics)

TREATMENT AND THERAPY

The four goals of treatment for any spinal cord injury are restoration of normal alignment for the spine, early assurance of complete stability of the injured spinal area, decompression of compressed neurologic structures, and early rehabilitation to an active and productive life.

Treatment begins at the scene of the accident by not moving the patient until the spine and head have been stabilized through strapping the patient to a board. Even after reaching the hospital, the patient is not removed from the board but placed on a stretcher while still strapped to it. Such stabilization helps prevent reversible damage from becoming permanent through additional injury to the neuraxis. Supportive treatment corrects systemic shock and controls local hemorrhage. Insertion of a Foley catheter ensures uninterrupted urine drainage.

Whenever possible, the care of spinal cord injuries emphasizes conservative treatment, such as closed reduction of fractures. However, unstable fractures and fracture dislocations require fusion following reduction, combined with recumbent immobilization until healing occurs. Bone fragments pressing on the spinal cord may require laminectomy (surgical removal of the vertebral arch). Drug therapy may include nitrofurantoin to prevent bladder infection; large doses of vitamin C to enhance utilization of protein and help minimize infection by acidifying the urine; diazepam, baclofen, or dantrolene sodium to relieve skeletal muscle spasms from upper motor neuron disorders; and, sparingly, analgesics and narcotics to relieve pain. The extent of paralysis cannot be accurately assessed until a year after the spinal cord injury.

—*Jane C. Norman, PhD, RN, CNE*

See also Accidents; Emergency medicine; Hemiplegia; Laminectomy and spinal fusion; Nervous system; Neuralgia, neuritis, and neuropathy; Neuroimaging; Neurology; Neurology, pediatric; Paralysis; Physical rehabilitation; Quadriplegia; Spinal cord disorders; Spine, vertebrae, and disks.

For Further Information:

Asbury, Arthur K., et al., eds. *Diseases of the Nervous System: Clinical Neuroscience and Therapeutic Principles.* 3d ed. New York: Cambridge University Press, 2002.

Bromley, Ida. *Tetraplegia and Paraplegia: A Guide for Physiotherapists.* 6th ed. New York: Churchill Livingstone/Elsevier, 2006.

Fehlings, Michael G. *Essentials of Spinal Cord Injury: Basic Research to Clinical Practice.* New York: Stuttgart, 2013.

Iansek, Robert, and Meg. E. Morris, eds. *Rehabilitation in Movement Disorders.* Cambridge: Cambridge University Press, 2013.

Kohnle, Diana. "Paraplegia." *Health Library,* November 28, 2012.

Victor, Maurice, and Allan H. Ropper. *Adams and Victor's Principles of Neurology.* 9th ed. New York: McGraw-Hill, 2009.

PARASITIC DISEASES

Category: Disease/Disorder
Anatomy or system affected: All
Specialties and related fields: Environmental health, epidemiology, family medicine, internal medicine, public health, virology
Definition: Diseases borne by parasites, or organisms that live within "host" organisms; parasites travel to their hosts via vectors that may include fleas, mosquitoes, rats, and other animals.

Key terms:

commensalism: a relationship in which one symbiont, the commensal, benefits from a host symbiont, but the host neither benefits nor is harmed by the commensal

host: a living plant or animal harboring or affording subsistence to a parasite

hyperparasitism: a relationship in which parasites act as hosts to other parasites

mutualism: a relationship between symbionts in which both members benefit from the association

parasitism: a relationship in which one symbiont, a parasite, harms its host symbiont or in some way lives at the expense of the host

phoresis: when two symbionts "travel together" but neither is physiologically dependent on the other

symbiont: any organism involved in a symbiotic relationship with another organism

symbiosis: a relationship in which two symbionts live in close association with each other; commonly, one symbiont lives in or on the body of the other

TYPES OF PARASITES

Parasites are organisms that take up residence, temporarily or permanently, on or within other living organisms for the purpose of procuring food. They include plants such as bacteria and fungi; animals such as protozoa, helminths (worms), and arthropods; and forms such as spirochetes and microscopic viruses.

The study of parasitism is a study of symbiosis. Symbiosis occurs when two organisms, known as symbionts, live in close association with each other, usually with one organism living in or on the body of the other. Such a living arrangement is called a symbiotic relationship. In a symbiotic relationship, the symbionts are usually, but not always, of different species, and the relationship need not be beneficial or damaging to either organism.

Often, two symbionts will exist together merely as traveling companions. Such a symbiotic relationship is called phoresis. In such cases, neither partner is physiologically dependent on the other, but the smaller of the two organisms has simply attached itself for the

> ### Information on Parasitic Diseases
> **Causes:** Infection with parasites, often through vectors
> **Symptoms:** Wide ranging; may include fever, malaise, vomiting, inflammation, joint pain, muscle aches, diarrhea
> **Duration:** Acute to chronic
> **Treatments:** Drug therapy, supportive care

ride. Examples of phoresis are bacteria carried on the legs of a cockroach and fungus spores on the feet of ants and beetles.

If a situation exists in which both symbionts benefit from an association, the partnership is referred to as a mutual relationship. In most cases, mutualism is obligatory because both symbionts have evolved to a point at which they are physiologically dependent on each other and the survival of both symbionts requires a continuous interrelationship. Such a relationship exists between termites and the protozoan fauna that live in their guts. Termites are unable to digest cellulose fibers, because their bodies cannot produce the proper enzyme, but protozoa that live in a termite's gut synthesize the ingested cellulose fibers and excrete a fermented product that nourishes the host termite. The protozoa benefit by living in a stable, secure environment, with a constant supply of food, and the termite is supplied with sustenance.

Another form of mutualism that is not obligatory is called cleaning symbiosis. In this instance, certain animals, called cleaners, remove other parasites, injured tissues, fungi, or invading organisms from a cooperating host. Examples of cleaning relationships include birds that groom the skins of rhinoceroses and the mouths of crocodiles, and tiny shrimp that remove parasites from the body surfaces of fish.

When one symbiont benefits from its relationship with its host but the host neither benefits nor is harmed, the condition is called commensalism. Examples of commensals are pilot fish and remoras, which attach themselves to turtles or other fish, using their hosts as transportation and scavenging food left over when the hosts eat; in no way, however, do they harm their hosts or rob them of food. Another example of commensalism exists between humans and the amoeba *Entamoeba gingivalis*. This amoeba lives in the human mouth, feeding on bacteria, food particles, and dead epithelial cells, but it never harms its human host. The amoeba is transmitted from person to person by direct contact and cannot exist outside the human mouth.

When one member of a symbiotic relationship actually harms its host or in some way lives at the expense of the host, it is then a parasite. The word *parasite* is derived from the Greek *parasitos*, which means "one

who eats at another's table" or "one who lives at another's expense." A parasite may harm its host by causing a mechanical injury, such as boring a hole into it; by eating, digesting, or absorbing portions of the host's tissue; by poisoning the host with toxic metabolic products; or by robbing the host of nutrition. It has been found that most parasites inflict a combination of these conditions.

The majority of parasites are obligate parasites-that is, they must spend at least a portion of their lives as parasites to survive and complete their life cycles. Most of these obligate parasites have free-living stages outside their hosts in which they exist in protective cysts or eggs. Certain symbionts are referred to as facultative parasites, which means that the organism is not normally parasitic, but if the proper situation arises, it becomes a parasite. The most common facultative parasites are those that are accidentally eaten or enter a host through a wound or body orifice. One facultative parasite whose infection of humans is almost always fatal is the amoeba *Naegleria*, which is responsible for amebic meningitis. Many obligate parasites are also hyperparasites. Hyperparasitism exists when parasites play host to other parasites; for example, the malaria-causing parasite *Plasmodia* is carried in mosquitoes, and juvenile tapeworms live in fleas.

Parasites that live their entire adult lives within or on their hosts are called permanent parasites. Other parasites, such as mosquitoes and ticks, are called temporary parasites because they feed on their hosts and then leave. Temporary parasites are actually micropredators that prey on different hosts, or on the same host at different times, as the need for nourishment arises. There are many parallels between parasitism and predation in that both parasites and predators live at the expense of their hosts or prey. Parasites, however, do not normally kill their hosts, because to do so results in their own death. It is the mark of a well-adapted parasite to produce as few pathological conditions in the host as possible.

Despite the knowledge that parasites are a major cause of disease, it is wrong to assume that an animal hosting a parasite must ultimately be in danger. The healthiest human or wild animal is probably harboring some type of parasite, and while the host and parasite may live for years without interfering in each other's existence, at any given time, the healthy host can fall victim to a disease brought on by the parasite, or some change in the host may destroy the parasite.

Whether the host reacts to its symbiotic partner with indifference, annoyance, or illness is the result of many factors. The most important is how many parasites are being hosted. A single hookworm takes approximately 0.5 milliliter of blood per day from its

Common Human Parasites

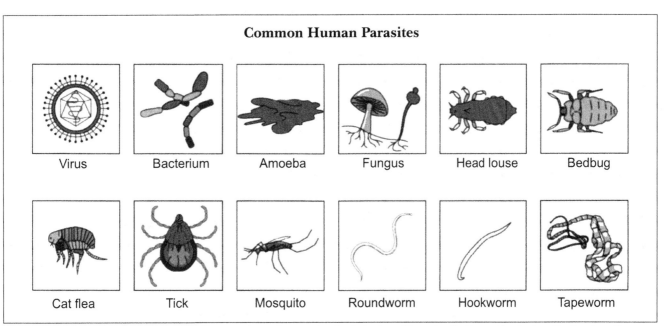

Virus · Bacterium · Amoeba · Fungus · Head louse · Bedbug

Cat flea · Tick · Mosquito · Roundworm · Hookworm · Tapeworm

Any organism that, temporarily or permanently, lives on or in another organism for the purpose of procuring food is considered a parasite; these parasites may cause infection in their human hosts. ©EBSCO

host. This is about the same amount of blood lost when one pricks oneself with a needle. This amount of blood loss is so low that the host will never miss it and, in most instances, will not even know that the parasite is there. If a host harbors five hundred hookworms, however, the blood loss per day becomes 250 milliliters, approximately one half pint, and the result is physically devastating to the host.

CAUSES AND SYMPTOMS

Medical parasitology is the study of human diseases caused by parasitic infection. It is commonly limited to the study of parasitic worms (helminths) and protozoa. The science places nonprotozoan parasites in separate disciplines, such as virology, rickettsiology, and bacteriology. The branches of parasitology known as medical entomology and medical arthropodology deal with insects and noninsect arthropods that serve as hosts and transport agents for parasites, as well as with the noxious effects of these pests. The study of fungi (molds and yeasts), including those that cause human disease, is called mycology.

Throughout history, human welfare has suffered greatly because of parasites. Fleas and bacteria killed one-third of the human population of Europe during the seventeenth century, and malaria, schistosomiasis, and African sleeping sickness have killed additional countless millions. Despite successful medical campaigns against yellow fever, malaria, and hookworm infections worldwide, parasitic diseases in combination with nutritional deficiencies are the primary killers of humans. Medical research suggests that parasitic infections are so widespread that if all the known varieties

were evenly distributed among the human population, each living person would have at least one.

Most serious parasitic infections occur in tropical, less modernized regions of the world, and because most of the planet's industrially developed and affluent populations live in temperate regions, many people are unaware of the magnitude of the problem. On an annual basis, 60 million deaths occur worldwide from all causes; of these deaths, half are children under five years of age. Fifty percent of these, 15 million child deaths per year, are directly attributable to a combination of malnutrition and intestinal parasitic infection. It must be noted that less than 15 percent of the world's present population is served by adequate clean water supplies and sewage disposal programs, and that almost all intestinal parasitic infections are the result of ingesting food or water contaminated with human feces.

The transmission of parasitic diseases involves three factors: the source of the infection, the mode of transmission, and the presence of a susceptible host. The combined effect of these factors determines the dispersibility and prevalence of a parasite at a given time and place, thus regulating the incidence of a parasitic disease in a population. Because of host specificity, other humans are the chief source of most human parasitic diseases. The various manifestations of any human parasitic disease are a result of the particular species of parasite involved, its mode of transport, the immunological status of the host, the presence or absence of hosts, and the pattern of exposure.

Humans transmit parasitic diseases to one another through the intestinal tract, nose and mouth, skin and tissue, genitourinary tract, and blood. It is fecal discharge, however, that offers the most convenient and common means for a parasite or its ova and larvae to leave its host, since the majority of parasites inhabit the gastrointestinal tract. For this reason, the proper disposal of fecal material is the most important method of preventing the spread of parasitic disease. Since most parasites inhabit the intestinal tract, food and water are also important means of transmitting parasitic infections. The infective organism may be present in contaminated drinking water, in animal and fish flesh used as food, in human feces used as fertilizer, or on the hands of food handlers.

Arthropods are one of the main sources of parasitic diseases in humans. Arthropods act as both mechanical carriers of and intermediate hosts to many diseases-bacterial, viral, rickettsial, and parasitic-which they transmit to humans. In most tropical countries, basic preventive medicine for many devastating parasitic diseases depends on the control or eradication of insects and arachnids.

There are four major groups of parasites that most often invade human hosts: nematodes, trematodes, cestodes, and protozoa. Most nematodes, or roundworms, are free-living, and nematodes are found in almost every terrestrial and aquatic environment. Most are harmless to humans, but some parasitic nematodes invade the human intestinal tract and cause widespread debilitating diseases. The most prevalent intestinal nematodes are *Ascaris lumbricoides*, which infect the small intestine and affects more than a billion people; the whipworm *Trichuris trichiura*, which infects the colon and is carried by an estimated 500 million individuals; the human hookworms *Necator americanus* and *Ancylostoma duodenale*, which suck blood from the human small intestine and cause major debilitation among undernourished people; and *Enterobius vermicularis*, the human pinworm, which infects the large intestine and is common among millions of urban dwellers because it is easily transmitted from perianal tissue to hand to mouth.

Nonintestinal, tissue-infecting nematodes are spread most often by hyperparasitic bloodsucking insects such as mosquitoes, biting flies, and midges. The most common tissue-infecting nematode is *Trichinella spiralis*, the pork or trichina worm, which is the agent of trichinosis. Other important parasitic nematodes include *Onchocerca volvulus*, which is transmitted by blackflies in tropical regions and causes blindness, and the mosquito-transmitted filarial worms that are responsible for elephantiasis.

Trematodes, or flatworms, are commonly called flukes. Flukes vary greatly in size, form, and host living location, but all of them initially develop in freshwater snails. The human intestinal fluke, the oriental liver fluke, and the human lung fluke are all transmitted to humans by the ingestion of raw or undercooked aquatic vegetables, fish, or crustaceans. An important group of trematodes consists of the blood flukes of the genus *Schistosoma*, which enter the body through skin/water contact and are responsible for schistosomiasis.

Cestodes, commonly called tapeworms, are parasitic flatworms that parasitize almost all vertebrates, and as many as eight species are found in humans. The two most common cestodes-*Taenia saginata*, the beef tapeworm, and *Taenia solium*, the pork tapeworm-are transmitted to humans by infected beef or pork products obtained from livestock that grazed in fields contaminated by human feces, or by contaminated water. The resulting disease, cysticercosis, which is potentially lethal, develops mostly in the brain, eye, and muscle tissue. Another animal-transmitted cestode is the dog tapeworm, *Echinococcus granulosus*, which dogs ingest by eating contaminated sheep viscera and then pass on to humans, who ingest the parasite's eggs after petting or handling an infected dog. The human infestation of *E. granulosus* results in hydatid disease. Probably the most dramatic of the cestode parasites is the gigantic tapeworm *Diphyllobothrium latum*, which may reach a length of 10 meters and a width of 2 centimeters. This tapeworm is transmitted to humans by the ingestion of raw or undercooked fish. This tapeworm, like most cestodes, can be effectively treated and killed by drugs, but if the worm merely breaks, leaving the head and anterior segments attached, it can regenerate its original body length in less than four months.

Protozoa that can infect human hosts are found in the intestinal tract, various tissues and organs, and the bloodstream. Of the many varieties of protozoa that can live in the human intestinal tract, only *Entamoeba histolytica* causes serious disease. This parasite, which is ingested in water contaminated by human feces, is responsible for the disease amebiasis, also known as amebic dysentery. A less serious, though common, waterborne intestinal protozoan is *Giardia lamblia*, which causes giardiasis, a common diarrheal infection among campers who ingest water fouled by animal waste.

Another group of protozoa parasites specializes in infecting the human skin, bloodstream, brain, and viscera. *Trypanosoma brucei*, carried by the African tsetse fly, causes the blood disease trypanosomiasis (African sleeping sickness). In Latin America, infection by the protozoa *Trypanosoma cruzi* results when the liquid feces of the reduviid bug is rubbed or scratched into the skin; it causes Chagas disease, which produces often fatal lesions of the heart and brain. Members of the protozoan genus *Leishmania* are transmitted by midges and sandflies, and their parasitic infestation manifests in long-lasting dermal lesions and ulcers; the destruction of nasal mucous, cartilage, and pharyngeal tissues; or in the disease kala-azar, resulting in the destruction of bone marrow, lymph nodes, and liver and spleen tissue.

Two other types of protozoa are parasitic to humans. The first is the ciliate protozoa, which are mostly free-living, and of which only a single species, *Balantidium coli*, is parasitic in humans. This species is responsible for balantidiasis, an ulcerative disease. The second is the sporozoans, all of which are parasitic. Many species of sporozoans are harmful to humans, the most important being *Plasmodium*, the agent of malaria. The sporozoan parasite *Toxoplasma gondii*, the agent of toxoplasmosis, is responsible for encephalomyelitis and chorioretinitis in infants and children and is thought to infect as much as 20 percent of the world's population. *Pneumocystis* pneumonia, a major cause of death among persons with acquired immunodeficiency syndrome (AIDS), was formerly considered a result of sporozoan infection but is now thought to be fungal.

PERSPECTIVE AND PROSPECTS

Because of their size, the large parasitic worms were among the first parasites to be noted and studied as possible causes of disease. The Ebers papyrus, written about 1600 BCE, contains some of the earliest records of the presence of parasitic worms in humans. In early Egypt, trichinosis, cysticercosis, and salmonellosis were all likely to be acquired from pigs. This knowledge is reflected in the law of Moses, later reinforced in the Qur'an, which forbids the eating of "unclean swine" or the touching of their dead carcasses-a clear indication that people knew of the relationship between parasitic worms and human disease. Persian, Greek, and Roman physicians were also familiar with various parasitic worms, and many of their early medical writings describe the removal of worm-induced cysts. The Arabic physician and philosopher Avicenna (979-1037 CE) was the first to separate parasitic worms into classifications: long, small, flat, and round.

The modern study of parasites began in 1379 with the discovery of the liver fluke, *Fasciola hepatica*, in sheep. During the eighteenth century, many parasitic worms and arthropods were described, but progress was slow prior to the invention and widespread use of the microscope. The microscope made possible the study of small protozoan parasites and allowed for detailed anatomic and lifecycle studies of larger parasites.

In 1835, *Trichinella spiralis*, the parasite responsible for the disease trichinosis, was described, and quickly thereafter knowledge concerning the parasitic worms of humans began to accumulate. Many new species were discovered, prominent among which were the hookworm and the blood fluke.

Between 1836 and 1901, the first protozoan parasites of humans were recognized and described; among the most important of these were the parasites responsible for giardiasis, gingivitis, vaginitis, trichomoniasis, kala-azar, and Gambian trypanosomiasis (sleeping sickness).

Although arthropods had been recognized as parasites since early times, their role in transporting other parasites and in spreading disease was not noted until 1869, when the larval stages of the dog tapeworm were found in the dog louse. Further investigations led to the identification in 1893 of ticks as the transmitting agents of Texas fever in cattle. By 1909, parasitologists had observed the development of the malarial parasite in mosquitoes, had proved the transmission of yellow fever by the mosquito *Aedes aegypti*, and had linked the tsetse fly to African sleeping sickness, the tick to African relapsing fever, the reduviid bug to Chagas disease, and the body louse to the transmission of typhoid fever.Human Experience: Philosophy, Neurosis, and Elements of Everyday Life

In 2013 the American Academy of Neurology (ANN) published new guidelines for the treatment of neurocysticerosis, a tapeworm infection of the brain that can trigger epileptic seizures. The AAN, concerned with what appears to be an increase in the incidence of the disease, based their recommendations on a review of ten studies published between 1980 and 2010. An estimated 40,000 to 160,000 cases of neurocysticerosis occur annually in the United States

—Randall L. Milstein, PhD

See also Amebiasis; Babesiosis; Bacterial infections; Bacteriology; Biological and chemical weapons; Bites and stings; Chagas' disease; Coccidiodomycosis; Dengue fever; Ehrlichiosis; Diarrhea and dysentery; Elephantiasis; Encephalitis; Fungal infections; Giardiasis; Insect-borne diseases; Leishmaniasis; Lice, mites, and ticks; Lyme disease; Malaria; Microbiology; Pinworms; Protozoan diseases; Rocky Mountain spotted fever; Roundworms; Schistosomiasis; Shigellosis; Sleeping sickness; Tapeworms; Toxoplasmosis; Trichinosis; Tropical medicine; Typhoid fever; Viral infections; Worms; Yellow fever.

For Further Information:
Despommier, Dickson D., et al. *Parasitic Diseases*. 5th ed. New York: Apple Tree, 2006.
Frank, Steven A. *Immunology and Evolution of Infectious Disease*. Princeton, N.J.: Princeton University Press, 2002.
Gittleman, Ann Louise. *Guess What Came to Dinner? Parasites and Your Health*. Rev. ed. New York: Putnam, 2001.
HealthDay. "Tapeworm-Linked Seizures May Be Rising in US, Doctors Say." *MedlinePlus*, April 8, 2013.
Klein, Aaron E. *The Parasites We Humans Harbor*. New York: Nelson Books/Elsevier, 1981.
MedlinePlus. "Parasitic Diseases." *MedlinePlus*, May 21, 2013.

Roberts, Larry S., and John Janovy, Jr., eds. *Gerald D. Schmidt and Larry S. Roberts' Foundations of Parasitology.* 9th ed. New York: McGraw-Hill, 2013.

Wilson, Brenda A., Abigail A. Salyers, et al. *Bacterial Pathogenesis: A Molecular Approach.* 3d ed. Washington, DC: ASM Press, 2011.

PARATHYROIDECTOMY

Category: Procedure
Anatomy or system affected: Endocrine system, glands, neck
Specialties and related fields: Endocrinology, general surgery
Definition: The removal of all or part of the parathyroid gland or parathyroid tumors.

INDICATIONS AND PROCEDURES

The parathyroid glands are four structures attached to the rear of the thyroid gland, which is found in the neck. Their main function is the secretion of parathyroid hormone (PTH), a protein that regulates the concentration of blood calcium. Abnormalities in proper calcium concentration can lead to bone demineralization, neuromuscular problems, or renal (kidney) damage.

Parathyroidectomy is occasionally warranted under conditions of hyperparathyroidism: the excess secretion of PTH. Hyperparathyroidism most commonly results in excess resorption of bone calcium, causing skeletal pain or loss of height. The demineralization may also lead to fractures of the spine or long bones, which may be accompanied by extreme muscle weakness and frequent urination. Since the patient may be asymptomatic, diagnosis is most commonly made on the determination of excess serum and urine calcium. X-rays may also indicate bone abnormalities resulting from the resorption of calcium. The condition itself may be caused by hyperplastic (overactive or enlarged) glands, or in less common circumstances (2 percent of cases), hyperparathy- roidism may result from a parathyroid adenoma (a benign tumor on a gland).

Asymptomatic patients, or patients with only mildly elevated blood calcium, may not need treatment. Should symptoms become more severe, surgical procedures may be necessary, generally involving the removal of excess parathyroid tissue. If the hyperplasia involves all four parathyroid glands, three of the glands are usually removed, with resection of the fourth. If the cause of the PTH elevation is an adenoma, it is necessary to remove the tumor surgically.

USES AND COMPLICATIONS

Since the primary symptom of hyperparathyroidism is excess blood calcium, the removal of excess tissue may suddenly reduce calcium levels to normal. The rapid fall of calcium may cause a transient tetany (involuntary muscle contractions), but otherwise recovery from such surgery parallels any other surgical procedure. PTH and calcium levels must continue to be monitored postoperatively. If parathyroidectomy results in excessively low PTH levels, it may be necessary to provide lifelong diet supplements of calcium and vitamin D. Surgical complications include injury to the thyroid gland and/or to the vocal cords.

—*Richard Adler, PhD;*
updated by Sharon W. Stark, RN, APRN, DNSc

See also Endocrine disorders; Endocrine glands; Endocrinology; Glands; Hashimoto's thyroiditis; Hormones; Hyperparathyroidism and hypoparathyroidism; Thyroid disorders; Thyroid gland; Thyroidectomy; Tumor removal; Tumors.

For Further Information:
Braverman, Lewis E., ed. *Diseases of the Thyroid.* 2d ed. Totowa, N.J.: Humana Press, 2003.

Gardner, David G., and Dolores Shoback, eds. *Greenspan's Basic and Clinical Endocrinology.* 9th ed. New York: McGraw-Hill, 2011.

Melmed, Schlomo, et al., eds. *Williams Textbook of Endocrinology.* 12th ed. Philadelphia: Saunders/Elsevier, 2011.

Montemayor-Quellenberg, Marjorie. "Parathyroidectomy-Conventional." *Health Library,* June 13, 2013.

Montemayor-Quellenberg, Marjorie. "Parathyroidectomy-Minimally Invasive." *Health Library,* June 13, 2013.

Neal, J. Matthew. *Basic Endocrinology: An Interactive Approach.* Malden, Mass.: Blackwell Science, 2000.

"Parathyroid Gland Removal." *MedlinePlus,* December 10, 2012.

Rosenthal, M. Sara. *The Thyroid Sourcebook.* 5th ed. New York: McGraw-Hill, 2009.

Ruggieri, Paul, and Scott Isaacs. *A Simple Guide to Thyroid Disorders: From Diagnosis to Treatment.* Omaha, Nebr.: Addicus Books, 2004.

PARKINSON'S DISEASE

Category: Disease/Disorder
Anatomy or system affected: Dopaminergic neurons, midbrain, substantia nigra, nervous system, musculoskeletal system
Specialties and related fields: Neurology, geriatrics and gerontology, internal medicine, physical therapy

Definition: A progressive disease that results in a movement disorder characterized by tremor, muscular rigidity, and slow movement.

CAUSES AND SYMPTOMS

British physician James Parkinson, in his landmark 1817 paper titled "An Essay on the Shaking Palsy," recounted the cases of six patients who suffered from a long-term disease characterized by "involuntary tremulous motion, with lessened muscular power in parts not in action even when supported, with a propensity to bend their trunks forward from a walking to a running pace."

This shaking palsy described by Parkinson is now known as Parkinson's disease (PD) or paralysis agitans. The slowly progressing neurodegenerative condition is characterized by a movement disorder consisting of tremor, stiffness, and slowness of movement. PD may also be accompanied by other complications, such as cognitive dysfunction, psychiatric manifestations, and gastrointestinal issues, among others. It is the second most common neurodegenerative disease in the world after Alzheimer's disease, and its occurrence worldwide is estimated at 3 per 1000 people over the age of forty. Geographic variations in prevalence have also been noted, and there seems to be a discrepancy between the genders, with males showing a higher prevalence (especially in the age 50-59 group) and a worse phenotype than females (potentially due to estrogen levels). In the US alone, over 1 million people live with PD, and the numbers grows every year by more than 50,000 patients.

The cause of Parkinson's disease is idiopathic, meaning that its origin is unknown, but recent research has shown that there may be some genetic and environmental factors linked to the disease progression. About 5-10% of cases have been shown to be inherited with mutations in specific genes (GBA, LRRK2, and SNCA, among others) linked to an increased risk of developing PD. Certain chemicals and pesticides have also been linked to an increased risk of PD, while smoking may actually have a protective effect against PD (due to nicotine's potential as a therapeutic chemical).

The symptoms of PD are caused by death of specific cells in the brain. Dopaminergic neuron death in the substantia nigra of the midbrain leads to a lack of inhibitory action, which in turn causes excess nerve impulses to fire to the motor nerves. This lack of inhibition leads to too much stimulation, producing both the resting tremor and rigidity seen in PD patients. Neuropathologically, there is a loss of pigmentation in the substantia nigra—from the lack of dopaminergic neurons and neuromelanin—and potential depositing of Lewy bodies, which are aggregates of cytotoxic pro-

Parkinson's Disease

Masklike face, often with drooling

Bent posture

"Pill-rolling" hand tremor

Shuffling gait

Parkinson's disease, which often attacks older people, is characterized by debilitating symptoms that become more severe as the disease progresses. ©EBSCO

tein (alpha-synuclein). These changes in the brain are believed to cause the physical symptoms PD patients experience.

PD manifests slowly, typically first on one side of the body and then on both sides, and targets movement before causing symptoms throughout the body. As previously mentioned, the hallmark symptoms are:

- *Resting tremors*: shaking without having an activity or intention induce tremors
- *Bradykinesia*: slow body movement with overall weakness
- *Rigidity*: inability to move with ease due to increased resistance

A late symptom in many PD cases is a poor sense of balance and posture; this is tested clinically by pulling backwards on a standing patient, which causes PD patients to take several steps to regain their balance or even fall. Parkinson's disease is not limited to the above three symptoms as it is a highly complex condition—additional symptoms include changes in cognition, hallucinations, and potential dementia; psychiatric manifestations such as emotional changes, mood disorders, and anxiety; insomnia and other sleep disturbances; olfactory dysfunction and rhinorrhea; and gastrointestinal problems such as constipation and dysphagia.

Clinically, physicians use the Movement Disorder Society-Sponsored Revision of the Unified Parkinson's Disease Rating Scale (MDS-UPDRS), a comprehensive scale that includes both motor and non-motor symptoms, to help diagnose Parkinson's disease and identify its severity.

TREATMENT AND THERAPY

While there is currently no cure for Parkinson's disease, there are pharmacological approaches a physician can take to ameliorate a PD patient's symptoms and to help achieve patients' goals. The most widely used drug for improving motor symptoms and quality of life in early PD is levodopa, a precursor to dopamine which helps replace and increase the lost levels of dopamine in PD patients. It is commonly administered with carbidopa to alleviate the nausea that may come with levodopa administration. Levodopa takes approximately 30 minutes to start working, and lasts about 4-5 hours in the bloodstream. Dopamine agonists (pramipexole, ropinirole), and monoamine oxidase B (MOAB) inhibitors such as selegiline can also help with motor symptoms, but have fewer motor complications. Depending on the patient, side effects of these medications can include increased impulses, excessive somnolence, and psychotic episodes. The doses for these treatments can be modified by a trained specialist in PD, and non-motor symptoms may be alleviated during the course of the therapy with the appropriate drugs.

In late stages of the disease when medications no longer control the symptoms, a doctor may recommend deep brain stimulation (DBS), which is an experimental surgical treatment that may lead to resting tremor suppression and improved quality of life. The surgery involves implanting an electrical device—a neurostimulator—that potentially blocks the uninhibited nerve signals, therefore improving tremors. The mechanism behind DBS' success is poorly understood, though theories have been posited about how it affects the brain.

PERSPECTIVE AND PROSPECTS

"It seldom happens that the agitation extends beyond the arms within the first two years; which period, therefore, if we were disposed to divide the disease into stages, might be said to comprise the first stage. In this period, it is very probable, that remedial means might be employed with success." —*James Parkinson, 1817*

Two hundred years ago, Parkinson predicted that early PD could be successfully treated, though his proposed primitive treatment largely differs from the one we have today. Since its inception as the main PD treatment in 1975, carbidopa/levodopa therapy has

---

INFORMATION ON PARKINSON'S DISEASE

Causes: Unclear; likely involves genetic and environmental factors
Symptoms: Tremors, impaired gait, muscle rigidity, masklike facial appearance, impaired swallowing, difficulty with repetitive movement and manual dexterity
Duration: Chronic and progressive
Treatments: Alleviation of symptoms through chemotherapy, surgery, physical therapy

---

improved the quality of life of many PD patients in their early stages, but researchers and physicians have not been able to find ways to stop disease progression since then. Different combinations of drugs that enhance the effects or extend the longevity of levodopa have been developed, but nothing has come close to eradicating this neurodegenerative disorder. In 2002, the FDA approved DBS as a measure to help PD patients, particularly after other treatment options have been exhausted. Since then, the FDA has approved other DBS-related devices as treatment options, but pharmacological advancements have remained relatively stagnant. However in a minor advance the FDA recently approved a new MAOB inhibitor, safinamide, as an additional drug to levodopa, when a patient is not responding to levodopa alone. Levodopa continues to be the gold standard.

Research into PD over the past decades has offered potential mechanism-related insights and genetic links, although this has not always translated into treatments. Animal models have been used for years to imitate Parkinson's; recently, with the advent of stem cell technologies, new human-based models attempt to predict disease mechanism and progression. Stem cells themselves have been touted as a potential treatment, though there is not enough data yet about the efficacy and currently poses dangerous risks. Gene-editing offers additional opportunities, though it has not yet been fully harnessed to slow disease progression or treat symptoms.

—*Brian Campos, BA*

For Further Information:
Gandhi, S., & Wood, N.W. (2010). Genome-wide association studies: the key to unlocking neurodegeneration? Nat Neurosci, 13(7), 789-794.
Gardner, J. (2013). A history of deep brain stimulation: Technological innovation and the role of clinical assessment tools. Social Studies of Science, 43(5), 707-728.
Goetz CG, Tilley BC, Shaftman SR, Stebbins GT, Fahn S, et al. (2008). Movement Disorder Society-sponsored revision of the Unified Parkinson's Disease Rating Scale (MDS-UPDRS): scale presentation and clinimetric testing results. Mov Disord., 23(15):2129-70.

Haaxma, C.A., Bloem, B.R., Borm, G.F., Oyen, W.J.G., Leenders, K.L., Eshuis, S.,... Horstink, M.W.I.M. (2007). Gender differences in Parkinson's disease. Journal of Neurology, Neurosurgery & Psychiatry, 78(8), 819-824.

Ma, C., Liu, Y., Neumann, S., & Gao, X. (2017). Nicotine from cigarette smoking and diet and Parkinson disease: a review. Translational Neurodegeneration, 6(1), 18.

Mayo Clinic Staff (2015, July 7). Parkinson's disease. Retrieved from: www.mayoclinic.org/diseases-conditions/park insons-disease/basics/definition/con-20028488

Parkinson, J. (2002). An Essay on the Shaking Palsy. The Journal of Neuropsychiatry and Clinical Neurosciences, 14(2), 223-236.

Parkinson's Disease Foundation (2017). Statistics on Parkinson's. Retrieved from: www.pdf.org/parkinson_statistics

Power, J.H.T., Barnes, O.L., & Chegini, F. (2017). Lewy Bodies and the Mechanisms of Neuronal Cell Death in Parkinson's Disease and Dementia with Lewy Bodies. Brain Pathology, 27(1), 3-12. doi:10.1111/bpa.12344

Pringsheim, T., Jette, N., Frolkis, A., & Steeves, T.D.L. (2014). The prevalence of Parkinson's disease: A systematic review and meta-analysis. Movement Disorders, 29(13), 1583-1590.

Shah, V.V., Goyal, S., & Palanthandalam-Madapusi, H.J. (2017). A Possible Explanation of How High-frequency Deep Brain Stimulation Suppresses Low-frequency Tremors in Parkinson's Disease. IEEE Transactions on Neural Systems and Rehabilitation Engineering, PP(99), 1-1.

Tolosa, E., Marti, M.J., Valldeoriola, F., & Molinuevo, J.L. (1998). History of levodopa and dopamine agonists in Parkinson's disease treatment. Neurology, 50(6 Suppl 6), S2-10; discussion S44-18.

PATELLOFEMORAL PAIN SYNDROME

Category: Disease/Disorder
Also known as: runner's knee, idiopathic anterior knee pain
Anatomy or system affected: Musculoskeletal system, kneecap
Specialties and related fields: Orthopedics, sports medicine, primary care, physical therapy
Definition: pain in the front of the knee, worsened with sitting, squatting or running for an extended period of time
Key terms:
patella: kneecap
femur: thigh bone
quadriceps: four muscles located in the front of the thigh, responsible for knee extension

Patellofemoral pain syndrome (PPS) is pain occurring in the front of the human knee, often due to wear and stress. The term *patella* is the kneecap, the bone cap of the knee joint, and *femoral* refers to the femur, or thigh bone. The patellofemoral joint is one of the two joints of the human knee, the other being the tibiofemoral. The syndrome can appear in one knee or in both knees. It is one of the most common injuries caused by running. Patellofemoral pain syndrome is also known as "runner's knee" or "jumper's knee," although it can occur in non-runners as well, and "anterior knee pain syndrome." It is not caused by a specific disease or condition. In addition to pain, another occasional symptom of PPS is popping or cracking sounds from the knee. In extreme cases, the knee may give way.

PPS is a clinical diagnosis, made usually by history and physical examination. X-Rays or MRIs are generally not considered necessary for a diagnosis of PPS, although in some cases they may be used to rule out other explanations for the pain, such as arthritis in patients over fifty years old or a dislocated patella or other injury. Patellofemoral pain syndrome is also distinguished from bursitis of the knee, which also causes pain in the area of the patella but has a completely different physical cause. Chrondomalacia patellae is sometimes treated as a synonym for PPS, but it can be distinguished as a syndrome specifically caused by the degeneration of cartilage of the knee joint. PPS must also be distinguished from patellofemoral osteoarthritis (PF OA), which generally occurs in older patients and also has characteristic radiographic findings including narrowed joint space and osteophytes, or bone spurs.

CAUSES AND SYMPTOMS

PPS is a multifactorial condition, but there are certain elements that can increase the risk of development of PPS. Repetitive exercise straining the knee can be one cause of PPS in addition to running and jumping, cycling, climbing stairs, and squatting. The onset of PPS is often associated with a change in exercise routine such as the addition of a new exercise that puts

---

INFORMATION ON PATELLOFEMORAL PAIN SYNDROME (PPS)

Causes: repetitive knee strain, quadriceps weakness, diminished core strength, patellar tracking/malalignment
Symptoms: anterior knee pain, "buckling," "creaking" or pain with standing after prolonged sitting
Duration: pain may be gradual or acute in onset and can continue unless treatment or preventive measures initiated
Treatments: rest, ice, activity limitation, NSAIDs, acetaminophen, physical therapy, stretches, quadriceps and core strengthening

pressure on the knee joint. Patellofemoral pain syndrome is frequently encountered by specialists in sports medicine. However, exercise or other physical activity is not necessary for PPS, and it can also appear in sedentary people. Weakness or inflexibility of the quadriceps muscles in the thigh can cause PPS. Core strength deficiencies, which cause weakened pelvic stability, are also implicated in the development of PPS. Women are particularly vulnerable to PPS, as well as to other injuries of the knee, due to the slight incurve of a woman's hip bone, which increases the stress on the knee joint. Patellofemoral pain is often intermittent. It can appear during exercise or exertion, in extreme cases making exercise impossible, but it can also appear when going up or down stairs or after sitting for a long time in one position with the knee bent, as at a desk or at a movie or theater (known as the "theater sign"). Pain is often difficult for patients to localize.

One cause of PPS is poor tracking of the patella along the femur when the knee is bent, which in turn irritates the cartilage where the patella grinds against the femur rather than moving straight up and down. A slight misalignment of the patella aggravated by stress or repeated impact may lead to PPS. This may be caused by exercise or exertion with flat feet or poorly fitted shoes that increase the pronation, or rolling, of the foot, which again puts strain on the knee.

TREATMENT
To prevent PPS, some doctors recommend exercises to increase the flexibility and strength of the quadriceps. Runners should avoid very hard surfaces and only gradually add uphill running to their routines. Properly fitting shoes are also valuable in preventing PPS. Theater-goers can try to get aisle seats, so they have room to occasionally straighten their legs.

Once patellofemoral pain strikes, immediate treatments to reduce it include ice packs and rest. Non-steroidal anti-inflammatory drugs (NSAIDs) and acetaminophen are also used to soothe the pain, although they have little effect beyond a few hours. Long-term treatments for PPS are based on physical therapy and are successful in over half of all cases. They include strengthening of the quadriceps muscles to restore muscle balance, as well as restricting those activities that cause pain. Hip strengthening has also been shown to be of some effectiveness. Knee braces, which restrict the knee's range of motion, may be helpful, although the clinical evidence for this is weak. Evidence for the benefits of patellar taping, another commonly used treatment, is also weak. There are a very few extreme cases for which surgery is recommended. Exercises and stretches are a crucial way to reduce the likelihood of developing PPS again. There is also evidence to suggest that foot orthotics combined with physical therapy may be more effective in reducing PPS symptoms than physical therapy alone, but it is unclear as to which patient population benefits the most from this. The use of intra-articular corticosteroid injections for PPS pain relief has limited evidence.

If PPS is caused by exercise, some doctors recommend changing or minimizing exercise routines, particularly switching to activities that place less impact on the knee, such as swimming or cycling, as well as ensuring that the shoes used for exercise fit properly. Exercises involving squatting, such as burpees, are particularly aggravating and may need to be suspended. Practitioners of various alternative medicine techniques such as acupuncture, chiropractic, and Pilates claim the ability to treat PPS, but such claims are not backed by scientific evidence.

PERSPECTIVE AND PROSPECTS
PPS is an active area of medical research. Research into PPS and other forms of anterior knee pain is funded by the Patellofemoral Foundation, a nonprofit organization founded in 2002 and headquartered in Farmington, Connecticut. The organization cosponsors an annual award for excellence in patellofemoral research along with the International Society of Arthroscopy, Knee Surgery and Orthopedic Sports Medicine and promotes knowledge of the patellofemoral joint among physicians and surgeons. There is also a biannual series of "Patellofemoral Pain Research Retreats and Clinical Symposia" held for physicians and other clinicians dealing with the problem.

—William E. Burns, PhD;
updated by Ananya Anand, MSc

For Further Information:
Berry, Tiffany, et al. "Effect of Pain On Hip and Knee Kinematics During a Prolonged Run in Female Runners with Patellofemoral Pain Syndrome." *ISBS-Conference Proceedings Archive.* 2014. Web. 8 Jan. 2016.
Hettrich, Carolyn, Daniel Liechti. "Patellofemoral Pain Syndrome." orthoinfo.aaos.org/topic.cfm?topic=A00680
LaBella, Cynthia. "Patellofemoral Pain Syndrome: Evaluation and Treatment." *Primary Care: Clinics in Office Practice* 31.4 (2004): 977-1003.
Papadopoulos, Konstantinos, et al. "A Systematic Review of Reviews in Patellofemoral Pain Syndrome. Exploring the Risk Factors, Diagnostic Tests, Outcome Measurements and Exercise Treatment." *Open Sports Medicine Journal* 9 (2015): 7-17.
Petersen, Wolf, et al. "Patellofemoral Pain Syndrome." *KneeSurgery, Sports Traumatology, Arthroscopy* 22.10 (2014): 2264-74.
Rogers, Thomas, et al. "Structured Rehabilitation Model for Patients with Patellofemoral Pain Syndrome." *Sports Injuries.* N.p.: Springer Berlin Heidelberg, 2014. 1-12.

Thomeé, Roland, Jesper Augustsson, and Jon Karlsson. "Patellofemoral Pain Syndrome." *Sports Medicine* 28.4 (1999): 245-62.

van der Heijden, Rianne A., et al. "Exercise for Treating Patellofemoral Pain Syndrome. An Abridged Version of Cochrane Systematic Review." *European Journal of Physical and Rehabilitation Medicine*. (2015): n. pag. Web. 8 Jan. 2016.

Waryasz, Gregory R, and Ann Y. McDermott. "Patellofemoral Pain Syndrome (PFPS): A Systematic Review of Anatomy and Potential Risk Factors." *Dynamic Medicine: DM* 7 (2008): 9. Web. 4 Jan. 2016.

PATENT DUCTUS ARTERIOSUS

Category: Disease/Disorder

Anatomy or system affected: Cardiovascular system, heart, aorta, pulmonary system, lungs, circulatory system, pulmonary artery, ligamentum arteriosum

Specialties and related fields: Cardiology, pediatrics, neonatology, pulmonology

Definition: A condition in which there is failure of the ductus arteriosus to close after birth, resulting in a persistent connection between the aorta and pulmonary arteries. This allows blood to flow from the aorta to the pulmonary arteries.

Key terms:

auscultation: listening to the sounds of the heart, lungs, and other internal organs, typically with a stethoscope

congenital: disease or abnormality that is present at the time of birth

echocardiogram: ultrasound that is used to visualize the structures of the heart

neonatal respiratory distress: breathing disorder in newborns resulting from immature lungs that do not produce enough pulmonary surfactant

pulmonary hypertension: high blood pressure in the blood vessels of the lungs

CAUSES AND SYMPTOMS

Patent ductus arteriosus (PDA) is a common congenital (at birth) heart defect with a prevalence of 1 in 2,000 births. Prior to birth, the fetus does not need blood to travel through the lungs for oxygenation. The developing fetus receives oxygen from the mother's circulation through a vessel that connects the pulmonary artery to the descending aorta called the "ductus arteriosus." Low oxygen saturation and high levels of a prostaglandin (PGE2) keep this ductus arteriosus patent, or open, to allow blood to bypass the fetus's nonfunctioning lungs. Once the baby is born and takes its first breath, blood vessels in the lungs open, allowing blood to flow to the lungs to pick up oxygen. Usually within twenty-four to seventy-two hours after birth,

---

INFORMATION ON PATENT DUCTUS ARTERIOSUS

Causes: Premature birth, congenital rubella syndrome, genetic conditions, chromosomal abnormalities, high-altitude birth

Symptoms: Tachypnea (rapid breathing), dyspnea (shortness of breath), continuous machine-like heart murmur, poor feeding, poor weight gain, fatigue, cyanosis, heart failure

Duration: The abnormality can present in the first year of life and last into adulthood depending on the size of the defect

Treatments: NSAIDS, Indomethacin, trans-catheter coil, open-heart surgery

---

the ductus arteriosus typically narrows and closes, due to high oxygen levels in the blood and low PGE2 levels and becomes the ligamentum arteriosum. PDA occurs when the ductus arteriosus does not close and allows the blood to circulate from the aorta into the pulmonary arteries causing a left-to-right shunt thereby sending oxygenated blood back to the lungs). This left to right shunting causes too much blood to flow into the infant's lungs. This overtime leads to pulmonary hypertension (high blood pressure in the lungs), which can lead to congestive heart failure.

Some infants are at a higher risk than others for developing PDA, but the exact etiology of the condition is unknown. PDA is more common in females than males, and it has been most commonly associated with premature birth, especially with neonatal respiratory distress syndrome. Neonatal respiratory distress syndrome is a breathing disorder common in premature infants caused by underdeveloped lungs. Maternal infection with Rubella (German measles) during pregnancy is also a significant risk factor for the development of PDA. Genetics and family history can be risk factors that predispose certain children to the condition. A family history of heart defects or genetic conditions, such as Down syndrome (Trisomy 21) increase the risk of PDA. In addition, environmental factors may play a role. For example, infants born at altitudes higher than 10,000 feet (3,048 meters) are at a higher risk of developing PDA than those born at lower altitudes. PDA is also common in infants with other congenital heart defects such as transposition of the great vessels or pulmonary stenosis. Other syndromes that are associated with patent ductus arteriosus includes Holt-Oram syndrome, DiGeorge's syndrome, Noonan's syndrome, CHARGE syndrome, etc.

The most common symptoms of PDA include rapid or heavy breathing; shortness of breath; sweating; fatigue; poor feeding; and poor weight gain and growth. These symptoms vary according to the size of the PDA and whether the infant was born prematurely or full-term.. Small-sized patent ductus arteriosus may have no symptoms and the doctors can usually detect it by *auscultating* (listening to internal body sounds) the infant's heart with a stethoscope. A PDA will produce a characteristic heart murmur that is commonly described as a "continuous machine-like" murmur. Chest X-rays and echocardiograms (an ultrasound that tests the heart's function) will reveal an enlarged heart and evidence of increased blood flow to the lungs and can visualize the blood flowing through the PDA. Moderate-sized PDAs can cause exercise intolerance and increase in the size of the left chambers of the heart. Large-sized PDAs can cause a large amount of blood to flow from the aorta into the pulmonary arteries. Excess blood flow to the lungs leads to pulmonary hypertension. Pumping against this increased pressure causes the right ventricle of the heart to hypertrophy (become thicker), leading to heart failure very soon after birth. Thickening of the right ventricle can cause Eisenmenger syndrome. In this condition, a left-to-right shunt becomes a right-to-left shunt (when deoxygenated blood is sent to the body instead of the lungs), leading to cyanosis (bluish discoloration of the skin due to reduced oxygen in the blood).

Signs of PDA include bounding pulses with a wide difference between the systolic and diastolic blood pressure, dynamic cardiac impulse on palpation (feeling for the heart beat on the patients' chest during examination), a normal sounding first cardiac sound (S1) with a split-second heart sound (S2) with a loud pulmonic component of the second heart sound (P2). There is a continuous "machinery" murmur in the left upper chest heard via the stethoscope.

Women who have significant-sized PDA and become pregnant may face serious issues during pregnancy. They are at a higher risk for certain complications such as arrhythmia (abnormal heart rhythms), heart failure, and pulmonary hypertension.. Pregnancy is not allowed when there is a right to left shunt and Eisenmenger syndrome has developed.

TREATMENT AND THERAPY
Infants typically need medication to help close the PDA. Some medications include nonsteroidal anti-inflammatory drugs (NSAIDs) such as indomethacin. Indomethacin blocks the hormone Prostaglandin E2 and should be administered a few days after birth. If medications do not work, catheterization or surgery may be required.

If the PDA does not close with medications, it may require transcatheter coil closure. During the procedure, catheters (long thin tubes) are inserted into the femoral artery in the leg and guided to the PDA near the heart. A coil is then inserted through the catheter to plug up the PDA. Sometimes, open-heart surgery is needed to close the PDA. During surgery, known as a "PDA ligation," the surgeon will open the chest to expose the PDA. The PDA is then either tied closed with sutures or clamped shut with metal clip.

After the PDA is closed, the patient usually does not have any other health complications or physical restrictions. The long-term prognosis for those with PDA is very good. No further medications or additional procedures generally are needed.

According to the American Heart Association/American College of Cardiology guidelines for adults with congenital heart disease, PDA presenting in adults should be closed when there is a left to right shunt and there is enlargement of the left-sided heart chambers and lower pulmonary pressures and pulmonary vessel resistance. Closure is not allowed when there is a right to left shunt, very high pulmonary pressures or very high pulmonary vessel resistance.

While a comprehensive prevention method does not exist, pregnant women can assume certain steps to ensure a healthy pregnancy that can help reduce the risks of PDA. Some of these include:
- Avoiding smoking, drinking alcohol, and taking drugs
- Alleviating stress
- Maintaining a healthy diet
- Exercising
- Receiving appropriate and timely vaccinations
- Women with heart defects, genetic conditions, or a family history of such conditions should consult a physician or genetic counselor prior to becoming pregnant.
- Regular checkups with their doctors during pregnancy

The complications of PDA include development of pulmonary hypertension and Eisenmenger's syndrome, congestive heart failure and infective endocarditis (infection of the inner lining of the heart).

—*Hunaina Shahab, MD*

See also: Cardiac catheterization; Congenital rubella syndrome; Eisenmenger syndrome; Murmurs, auscultation; NSAIDS; Trisomy 21.

For Further Information:
Bernstein D. "Patent Ductus Arteriosus." *Nelson Textbook of Pediatrics*, edited by R. M. Kleigman, B. Stanton, J. St. Geme, et al.,19th ed., 2011, www.mdconsult.com/books/page.do?eid=?4-u1.0-B978-1-4377-0755-7.00420-6—sc0025&isbn?=?978-1-4377-0755-7&uniqId?=?406511368-3#4-u1.0-B978-1-4377-0755-7.00420-6—sc0025.
Kim, Luke K., and Jeffrey C. Milliken. "Patent Ductus Arteriosus (PDA)." *Medscape*. 16 Sept. 2015, emedicine.medscape.com/article/891096-overview. Accessed 14 Feb. 2016.

"Patent Ductus Arteriosus (PDA)." *American Heart Association*, 14 Feb. 2016, www.heart.org/HEARTORG/Conditions/CongenitalHeartDe fects/AboutCongenitalHeartDefects/Patent-Ductus-Arteriosus-PDA_UCM_307032_Article.jsp#.Vr3r3Pnyu70.

"Patent Ductus Arteriosus (PDA)." *Lucile Packard Children's Hospital Stanford*. Stanford Children's Health, 30 Aug. 2017, www.stanfordchildrens.org/en/topic/default?id=patent-ductus-arteriosus-pda-90-P01811. Accessed 4 Sept. 2017.

"Patent Ductus Arteriosus (PDA)." *Mayo Clinic*. Mayo Foundation for Medical Education and Research, 16 Dec. 2014, www.mayoclinic.org/diseases-conditions/patent-ductus-arteriosus/basics/definition/con-20028530. Accessed 14 Feb. 2016.

"Patent Ductus Arteriosus." *MedlinePlus*, 14 Feb. 2016, www.nlm.nih.gov/medline plus/ency/article/001560.htm.

Schneider, D. J., and J. W. Moore. "Patent Ductus Arteriosus." *Circulation*, vol. 114, 2006, pp. 1873-82.

Stout, K. K., C. J. Daniels, J. A. Aboulhosn, et al. "AHA/ACC Guideline for the Management of Adults with Congenital Heart Disease: A Report of the American College of Cardiology/American Heart Association Task Force on Clinical Practice Guidelines." *Journal of the American College of Cardiology*, vol. 73, no. 12, 25 Mar. 2019, pp. e81-92.

"What Is Respiratory Distress Syndrome?" *National Heart, Lung, and Blood Institute*. US Department of Health and Human Services, www.nhlbi.nih.gov/health/health-topics/topics/rds. Accessed 14 Feb. 2016.

PATHOLOGY

Category: Specialty
Anatomy or system affected: All
Specialties and related fields: Biochemistry, cytology, forensic medicine, histology, microbiology, oncology
Definition: The science that studies the changes to cells, tissues, and organs that result from the processes leading to diseases and disorders.
Key terms:
autopsy: the dissection and examination of a human body after death
congenital: referring to a condition present at birth; it may result from an inherited trait or damage before birth
disease: an abnormal condition of the body, with characteristic symptoms associated with it
etiology: the cause of a disease or disorder
homeostasis: the maintenance of a stable internal environment needed for the proper functioning of the body's cells
metabolism: the collective term for the chemical activities of the body's cells

SCIENCE AND PROFESSION

The science of pathology seeks to identify accurately the etiology of a disease and its development in the human body, which in turn leads to other studies focused on the diagnosis, treatment, and prevention of the disease.

A pathologist may be a medical doctor or hold a doctoral degree in a related field such as cell biology or microbiology. He or she may be employed in one of several different types of work, such as research, clinical, surgical, and forensic pathology. The human body is a complex structure and, as in all living organisms, its basic unit of function is the cell. Similar cells are organized into tissues, tissues form organs, and organs are grouped into systems. All systems in the body must work together to maintain homeostasis. If this internal stability is changed too drastically, a disease results. To understand a disease thoroughly-and ultimately to diagnose, prevent, or treat it-its pathogenesis must be understood. This term includes the cause of the disease, its method of damaging the body, and the changes resulting from its presence. A specific disease may have many causes, and its symptoms and severity may vary in different patients. Nevertheless, it is convenient to place a disease into one of seven groups based on its primary cause or manifestation in the body: genetic defects, infections, immune disorders, nutritional disorders, traumas, toxins, and cancers.

Genetic disorders are those caused by a defect in one or more genes. Genes, which are found on chromosomes, are duplicated and passed from one generation to another. Each gene is responsible for directing the manufacture of a protein. Every protein has a characteristic three-dimensional structure, on which its function depends. If a mutation occurs in a gene, the protein may function poorly or not at all. Although the pathogenesis of a genetic disease may involve devastating effects in the body, its origin may be traced to the function of a single protein. A person with hemophilia may bleed to death because of a lack of the gene for blood-clotting protein. In sickle cell disease, hemoglobin molecules are abnormal, which results in abnormal red blood cells and difficulty in transporting oxygen throughout the body. Changes in gene function occur throughout a person's life. Many degenerative changes associated with aging are believed to be caused by aging genes and the subsequent loss of cell, tissue, and organ function.

Infections are those diseases that are caused by other organisms, usually microorganisms such as viruses, bacteria, protozoa, or fungi. Such organisms, called pathogens, are parasitic on body tissues or fluids. The damage from pathogens may be direct, resulting from tissue destruction, or may be caused by the toxins that they produce. *Entamoeba histolytica*, for example, is a protozoan that is ingested in contaminated water or food. It begins feeding on the tissues of the intestine and may cause ulcerlike lesions in the intestinal wall. *Clostridium botulinum* is the bacterial species that causes botulism. Its deadly effects are attributable not to tissue destruction but to its production of a poison that attacks the nervous system.

Immune disorders include immune deficiencies, autoimmune diseases, and allergies. The body's immunity involves a complex system of checks and balances to protect against invasion by foreign cells or substances. It is the main defense against infectious diseases. When a person's immune system is not functioning properly, the body is unable to fight off infections. Some individuals are born with immune deficiencies. Others may acquire the deficiency later in life through the use of immunosuppressive drugs to prevent rejection of an organ transplant or because of an infectious disease such as acquired immunodeficiency syndrome (AIDS). Regardless of the primary cause of the immune deficiency, the patient may die as a result of an infection that would be considered harmless in the general population. Another group of immune disorders includes the autoimmune diseases. In these disorders, the immune system begins to make antibodies against the body's own tissues. For example, joint tissue is destroyed in rheumatoid arthritis, and nerve tissue is destroyed in multiple sclerosis. Allergies represent a third group of immune disorders. An allergic response is an overreaction to a substance that would ordinarily be considered harmless by the body. During this reaction, a chemical called histamine is released that causes such changes as rashes and upper respiratory symptoms. In more severe reactions, asthma or circulatory system collapse may occur.

Nutritional disorders include dietary deficiencies, excesses, and imbalances. Vitamins and minerals are needed to take part in certain chemical reactions in the body. In vitamin deficiencies, these reactions are blocked. For example, vitamin A is needed for the proper functioning of the nerve endings in the eye that are responsible for seeing black and white and in dim light; thus, a person with a vitamin A deficiency may develop night blindness. Proteins, carbohydrates, and fats must be ingested in sufficient amounts to supply energy and raw materials to build body tissue. Excessive consumption, however, is associated with such conditions as obesity, diabetes, and heart disease.

Trauma generally refers to injury done to the body by an external force, such as in an automobile accident. The damage to the body may be relatively minor but still have serious effects. Damage to a blood vessel may cause hemorrhaging and subsequent loss of blood. Injury to the brain or spinal cord may result in paralysis or loss of other body function. Physicians also use the word "trauma" to mean any occurrence that damages the body or organs. High fever, for example,

may be said to cause trauma to the brain. Extreme emotions may also have effects on the body.

Toxins are poisons that may originate from the surroundings of an individual and be absorbed through the skin or inhaled. A person can be overcome by carbon monoxide from a defective furnace or automobile heater, for example. Toxins may also be ingested in water or food. Drug overdoses or accidental ingestion of household chemicals will also cause toxic reactions. Medical ecology is a field of medicine that concerns itself with the long-term toxic effects of chemicals released into the environment from plastics or other materials associated with modern life.

Cancers arise when the cell division process becomes abnormal. Ordinarily, cells in the body divide at a limited rate that is characteristic of a particular tissue. When cells divide rapidly in an uncontrolled manner and metastasize (spread) to other parts of the body, the condition is termed a malignancy or cancer. Cancers are grouped according to the type of tissue from which they develop. Carcinomas arise from epithelial tissue such as skin. Sarcomas arise from connective tissue such as bone or muscle. Leukemias result from abnormal and rapid reproduction of white blood cells in the bone marrow. Lymphomas are cancers of the lymphatic tissues, such as the lymph nodes or spleen. The severity of the cancer and the chances for recovery depend on the extent of the cancer when first diagnosed, the type of tissue or location involved, the speed at which the cells are dividing, and whether the cancer has spread to other areas of the body.

While it is convenient to place pathologies into separate groups, in reality their causes and effects overlap. An individual who is malnourished may have a weakened immune system and be vulnerable to infectious diseases. The immune system attacks not only foreign cells from outside the body but also abnormal cells arising within the body, such as cancer. Thus, patients with AIDS often develop cancer. Some individuals are at increased risk for cancer because of genetic factors called oncogenes. If these individuals smoke or eat unwisely, they may develop cancer, while others with the same inherited risk who adopt a prudent lifestyle do not. It is important for researchers and physicians to understand these complex pathological relationships so that they can diagnose and treat such conditions.

DIAGNOSTIC AND TREATMENT TECHNIQUES

A pathologist must be familiar with the typical test values associated with body functions and with the microscopic appearance of healthy cells and tissues in order to be able to differentiate correctly a normal condition from a pathological one. This body of knowledge has involved the collection of tissues and the measurement of values gleaned from years of medical treatment and research. Although based on large populations, these values may be misleading. For example, the amounts of blood cholesterol were measured in Americans, and the average level of cholesterol was labeled "normal." In reality, this value has been shown to be unhealthy and linked to heart disease.

Research pathology concentrates on the basic study of diseases or disorders. This type of study usually focuses on the cellular and biochemical aspects of a disease. Information is exchanged with other researchers in an effort to gain a complete understanding of the etiology of a disease and the mechanisms by which it damages the body. Laboratory experiments may be performed to determine if the condition can be stopped or at least slowed.

Other pathologists are more closely associated with patient treatment. A clinical pathologist is involved in the diagnosis of disease through study of body fluids, secretions, and excretions. Such a person must be knowledgeable in hematology (the study of blood), microbiology, and chemistry. A surgical pathologist is responsible for testing samples of cells and tissues excised during surgery. In such a procedure, called a biopsy, a small section of tissue is taken from the affected area and sent to the laboratory. The pathologist then examines the sample using a microscope and determines whether the tissue is normal or whether it indicates the presence of cancer or some other disease state.

At one time, it was necessary to perform what was known as exploratory surgery if laboratory tests and x-rays did not lead to a diagnosis. Less invasive, and safer, techniques have been developed to eliminate that need. Fiber-optic methods involve the use of light shining through a flexible tube containing glass fibers. The flexible tube can be inserted through a body opening or through a small incision, allowing the physician to see internal cavities and determine if any visible abnormalities are present or to perform a biopsy. In some cases, the condition can be corrected without further surgery.

Many other tools and techniques are available to clinical and surgical pathologists. Some abnormalities can be observed directly, such as a rash or external tumor. Microscopes are used to detect changes that are too minute to be seen by the naked eye. Another tool used to diagnose disease or disorders is the medical x-ray, which can determine the presence of a broken bone, kidney stones, or dense tumors. Soft tissues are not so easily visualized using normal x-ray techniques. Ingestion of an opaque substance such as barium may help to delineate the outline of a structure such as the esophagus or intestine. Other medical imaging procedures, such as ultrasound, magnetic resonance imaging (MRI), and computed tomography (CT) scans,

allow even more detailed visualization of body structures.

An autopsy pathologist examines the body after death. In a hospital setting, the purpose of an autopsy is usually to confirm or determine the natural cause of death. Even when the cause is known, an autopsy may be requested, since information obtained in this way may lead to better understanding of the pathological processes that resulted in death and suggest possible ways of preventing deaths in the future.

A forensic pathologist, also called a coroner or medical examiner, is an autopsy pathologist who works closely with the police and criminal justice officials. This relationship is especially important if there are suspicious circumstances surrounding the death or the discovery of the body, in order to determine whether the death has resulted from an intentional poisoning or a violent act. In some cases, a coroner must also attempt to identify the body. Such abnormalities in the body as scars, healed fractures, and dental cavities can aid in this effort. Samples of cells may be used for DNA fingerprinting, a comparison of genetic material from the deceased to that of someone believed to be a close relative, in an attempt to verify identification. If it is determined that a murder has occurred, the pathologist contributes to the investigation by determining such facts as the cause and time of death. Special care must be taken during any autopsy since the information may be used as legal evidence.

The correct diagnosis and identification of the etiology of a disease are essential to providing insight into possible treatments. Pathologists also play a key role in determining the mode of transmission. The following historical examples illustrate this application of pathology.

In the 1930s, it was discovered that the urine of some developmentally disabled children had a peculiar odor. Analysis of the urine showed the presence of an abnormal chemical that damaged the nervous system, resulting in mental deficiencies. The chemical was found to result from a failure of the body to make an enzyme necessary to break down the amino acid phenylalanine, which in turn was the result of a genetic defect, termed phenylketonuria (PKU). Simple blood and urine tests can determine the presence of this defect at birth. While this disease cannot be cured, those with PKU can be placed on a special diet low in phenylalanine, and so avoid the buildup of the amino acid and its resulting damage. In this genetic disease and others, once the precise mechanism of damage is found, efforts can be made to identify the presence of the gene and then to lessen its effects.

In July 1976, more than five thousand members of the American Legion attended a convention in Philadelphia, Pennsylvania. Within two weeks of returning home, nearly two hundred of them became ill, and twenty-nine of these died. Laboratory tests and autopsies identified the process that caused death as severe pneumonia accompanied by high fever but could not determine its origin. Although a pathogen was suspected, none could be found through microscopic examination of tissues or culture studies. Attention turned to the hotel and its air conditioning system in an attempt to determine if some toxin had spread through the air ducts, but no such substance was found. Several months later, a pathologist at the Centers for Disease Control in Atlanta, Georgia, was examining lung tissue sections taken from chick embryos and discovered the bacteria that had caused the illness, now known as Legionnaires' disease. Further tests showed them to be sensitive to the antibiotic erythromycin. When subsequent cases occurred, prompt diagnosis of the disease allowed the correct treatment to be given. The presence of these bacteria in water tanks associated with large air conditioning systems has led to preventive measures.

In 1981, the first cases of AIDS were identified. While the mode of transmission was discovered fairly quickly, it was not until 1986 that the human immunodeficiency virus (HIV) was identified. The pathogenesis of this disease begins with the infection of white blood cells, called helper T cells, that are an essential link between the identification of an invading pathogen and the production of antibodies by other cells called B cells. At first, the body begins to make antibodies against the virus as it would any other infectious disease. Then, over a period of several years, an increasing number of T cells are infected and destroyed. Eventually, the body loses the ability to make the antibodies necessary to fight all infectious diseases and to destroy cancer cells. After further study of the virus, researchers were able to discover a chemical, azidothymidine, or AZT (later called zidovudine), that could interfere with a key enzyme needed by the virus to reproduce. Although it could not cure the disease, the drug slowed its effects. AIDS research efforts are not aimed solely at attempts to kill the virus: by studying its pathogenesis, the means may be found to counteract the effects of the disease on the body's immune system.

PERSPECTIVE AND PROSPECTS

In the early days of medicine, knowledge of pathology was limited to what could be observed directly through the human senses. Treatments were empirical, a matter of trying different drugs or procedures until one was found that worked. Most basic knowledge of human anatomy and physiology was lacking. Often, human autopsies were not permitted because of religious and cultural practices.

A culture's beliefs about disease influence medical practice. From the time of the ancient Greeks until the rise of modern medicine, various theories were accepted. Some believed that disease had supernatural origins. The term *influenza*, for example, came from the belief that the disease was caused by the influence of the stars. Others believed that the body's functions were dependent on fluids in the body, called humors. Bleeding was used to release the bad humors that were causing the disease.

By the seventeenth century, dissection of cadavers was practiced to identify completely the normal and abnormal gross anatomy of the human body. The microscope was developed and used to study human tissues. In the late nineteenth century, it was shown that microorganisms could cause disease, which in turn led to specific tactics aimed at prevention and treatment. With knowledge of the infectious process and the development of anesthesia, surgery became more widespread. This trend, in turn, increased the knowledge of disease processes in tissues and organs.

In the twentieth century, more sophisticated techniques were developed to focus on processes at the cellular level. The electron microscope allowed researchers to visualize structures within cells. Other research showed that series of chemical reactions, called metabolic pathways, are necessary for proper cell function. The comparison of these pathways in normal cells with those in abnormal cells enabled researchers to understand the pathogenic effect of toxins and many genetic diseases. The use of computers in medical analysis has increased the precision of laboratory tests and has permitted the detection of abnormal chemicals in smaller amounts than were possible before.

During the effort to map the human genome-that is, to identify and locate all the genes found on the forty-six human chromosomes-one of the techniques employed was to compare the chromosomes of individuals known to have genetic diseases with those who do not, and so identify the abnormal gene. Identification of oncogenes (cancer-causing genes) or genes linked to such diseases as diabetes mellitus and heart disease may alert individuals at high risk in time for them to get regular diagnostic tests or to change their lifestyles. Knowledge gained by taking the study of disease to the genetic level will ultimately lead to more effective treatments and prevention for these and other pathological conditions.

—Edith K. Wallace, PhD

See also Autopsy; Bacteriology; Biopsy; Blood testing; Cancer; Cytology; Cytopathology; Dermatopathology; Diagnosis; Disease; Electroencephalography (EEG); Endoscopy; Epidemiology; Forensic pathology; Genetics and inheritance; Gram staining; Hematology; Hematology, pediatric; Histology; Homeopathy; Immunization and vaccination;

Immunopathology; Inflammation; Invasive tests; Laboratory tests; Malignancy and metastasis; Microbiology; Microscopy; Mutation; Noninvasive tests; Oncology; Physical examination; Prion diseases; Prognosis; Serology; Signs and symptoms; Toxicology; Urinalysis; Veterinary medicine.

For Further Information:
Baden, Michael M. *Unnatural Death: Confessions of a Medical Examiner.* New York: Random House, 1989.
Corrigan, Gilbert. *Essential Forensic Pathology: Core Studies and Exercises.* Boca Raton: CRC Press, 2012.
Crowley, Leonard V. *Introduction to Human Disease: Pathology and Pathophysiology Correlations.* Boca Raton: CRC Press, 2012.
Gao, Zu-hua, ed. *Pathology Review.* Calgary: Brush Education, 2013.
Jensen, Marcus M., and Donald N. Wright. *Introduction to Microbiology for the Health Sciences.* 4th ed. Englewood Cliffs, N.J.: Prentice Hall, 1997..
King, Richard A., Jerome I. Rotter, and Arno G. Motulsky, eds. *The Genetic Basis of Common Diseases.* 2d ed. New York: Oxford University Press, 2002.
Kumar, Vinay, Abul K. Abbas, and Nelson Fausto, eds. *Robbins and Cotran Pathologic Basis of Disease.* 8th ed. Philadelphia: Saunders/Elsevier, 2010.
McCance, Kathryn L., and Sue M. Huether. *Pathophysiology: The Biologic Basis for Disease in Adults and Children.* 6th ed. St. Louis, Mo.: Mosby/Elsevier, 2010.
Parham, Peter. *The Immune System.* 3d ed. New York: Garland Science, 2009.
Shaw, Michael, ed. *Everything You Need to Know About Diseases.* Springhouse, Pa.: Springhouse Press, 1996.
Shtasel, Philip. *Medical Tests and Diagnostic Procedures: A Patient's Guide to Just What the Doctor Ordered.* New York: Harper & Row, 1991.

PATIENT-CENTERED MEDICAL HOME

Category: Health care system
Also known as: Medical home, health care home
Anatomy or system affected: Biopsychosocial
Specialties and related fields: Pediatrics, family and geriatric medicine, home health, evidence-based practice
Definition: A team-based health care delivery model led by a health care provider to provide comprehensive and continuous medical care to patients with a goal to obtain maximal health care outcomes.

The patient-centered medical home (PCMH) is a care model designed to enhance the care delivered to patients while still allowing attention to each individual's unique needs. The process of implementing a PCMH improves the quality, efficiency and effectiveness of care.

In a 2007 document entitled *Joint Principles of the Patient-centered Medical Home*, the American Academy of Family Physicians, the American College of Physicians, the American Academy of Pediatrics and the American Osteopathic Association defined the model to include patient access to a personal physician who leads the care team; a care team designed to provide comprehensive care at all stages of life from birth to end-of-life care; integrated and coordinated care that takes into consideration the patients ethnicity and culture; use of evidence-based medicine to enhance patient outcomes; and, a commitment to access to care. The care team includes physicians, physician assistants, advanced practice nurses, social workers, nutritionists and others who interact with the patient to meet their total care needs. Smaller practices may link with others to deliver the comprehensive care needed.

As health care in the United States moves away from payment for numbers of patients treated to a payment system based on quality and outcomes of care, the need for change in the delivery system is evident. Patients and payers increasingly expect health outcomes are quality driven. Personalized care that is coordinated between specialists, especially with chronic diseases such as diabetes and heart disease, is critical. As payments are stretched, improved access to appropriate care rather than excessive care must become the norm. Physicians are experiencing stress from patients and payers for care that may or may not be reimbursed. Physicians want to deliver the best quality of care possible in a safe and effective manner, while remaining financially solvent.

The PCMH model enables a physician practice to be ready for changes in reimbursement structures such as merit-based incentive payments (MIPs), alternative payment models (APMs), and accountable care organizations (ACO). The MIPS provides additional payment based on evidence-based and practice-specific quality measures reported to the payer. The APM provides incentive payments for specific conditions, care episodes or a population for high quality and cost-efficient care. An ACO is a group of doctors, hospitals, and other health care providers, who work as a team to provide coordinated, high-quality care to Medicare patients. As practices transition to PCMH models, cost savings and more efficient use of resources results. More primary and multispecialty physician practices are developing a PCMH model in their practices as resources are stretched.

More recently, single specialty clinics, such as medical oncology practices, are developing PCMH models designed to coordinate the care cancer patients need from initial diagnosis to cure or end-of-life care. As the model becomes more accepted, other single disease specialties may attempt to adapt the model to their practice patterns.

BACKGROUND
The PCMH is widely accepted as a model of excellence in primary care delivery. While the word home is used

in the title, it is not a place but rather a way of organizing a care partnership between the physician and the patient. Working together with the care team, the patient develops a personalized care plan that addresses physical, mental, and supportive care needs. Care is considered to be 24/7; the patient has access to a provider round the clock. Medicine reconciliation, or reviewing all the medicines the patient is taking, is an important part of participation in a PCMH. Too often, patients see multiple doctors for a variety of conditions and may receive prescriptions that interact inappropriately causing more damage than good. Encouraging wellness by supporting appropriate health behaviors such as stop smoking and weight loss is also a part of this model of care.

The PCMH is comprised of five components. Comprehensive care means meeting most of a patient's physical and mental needs, including prevention, screening, acute and chronic treatment to end-of-life care. Patient-centered care focuses on the needs of the whole patient with emphasis on establishing a long-term relationship with both patients and caregivers over time.

A significant complaint about the US health system is that the care provided is often fragmented as multiple specialists provide care, often with little communication with other providers. Coordinated care is important to deliver optimal outcomes. Preventing multiple drug interactions, choosing noninvasive care over surgery, and managing side effects of multiple diseases are just a few reasons that coordinated care is needed.

Providing access to health care is a critical component of a healthy population. Access to care is often dependent on the type of private or government payments available. Patients without insurance are often severely limited in the care they receive or may even be denied care. Self-pay is not a realistic option as the cost of health care continues to rise dramatically. Insurance and government payers negotiate reduced rates for care, but self-pay patients are often expected to pay full price for care delivered.

Quality of care is important to the delivery of appropriate and safe outcomes. A PCMH is committed to the use of evidence-based medicine and clinical practice guidelines. Clinical practice guidelines are often developed by consensus panels of subject experts based on extensively researched evidence and are considered to be the optimal care that needs to be delivered to a patient. Shared decision-making with the patient, caregivers and other physicians involved in ongoing care enhances care delivery, safety and provides the most optimal outcome of treatment.

The US health care system is in dire need of overhaul to control costs and increase access to all citizens.

Increasing access to appropriate care is critical. Care coordination is one method to better manage the patient population seeking care. The PCMH is one model that shows great promise going forward.

IMPLEMENTATION

The PCMH is generally considered to be based in the primary care practice and focuses on how health care is organized and delivered by putting the patient at the center. The five components necessary to develop the model are comprehensiveness, patient-centered, coordinated care between providers, providing patient access to care and quality and safety. A smaller practice may need to partner with others to develop a PCMH. Supportive functions necessary include a robust information technology system, a workforce with the attributes and attitude to put patients first, and financial stability as the system is implemented. Professional organizations and the Agency for Healthcare Research and Quality all have resources that can assist a physician practice to determine their readiness to develop a PCMH as do agencies that provide assessment and recognition programs.

Becoming recognized as a PCMH may enhance payment from providers by as much as a 10 percent payment increase. Recognition programs include a variety of agencies in different regions of the United States. The Joint Commission Primary Care Medical Home Recognition Program, the Accreditation Association for Ambulatory Health Care Medical Home Program and the URAC Patient-Centered Medical Home Recognition Program are just a few examples. The National Committee for Quality Assurance (NCQA) has a PCMH evaluation program that currently recognizes over 12,000 practices as meeting their standards. There are also more than 100 payers who support the NCQA recognition program with financial incentives. Reviewing the standards from these agencies will also assist in the steps needed to become a PCMH.

PERSPECTIVE AND PROSPECTS

The PCMH will continue to be an integral component of health care going forward. As both patients and payers demand more for their dollar, coordinating care that is appropriate, comprehensive, of high quality and safe will be important. The PCMH helps deliver this level of patient-centered care. Per the NCQA, the number of PCMH programs is increasing. Barriers to ensuring a thriving PCMH include financial constraints, lack of technological support and infrastructure. It is important to maintain the focus on patient-centeredness while defining how a PCMH can optimally serve the needs of a varied patient population. Practices will have to innovate and evolve in order to meet the unique needs of the patients they serve as they advance into the future of health care.

—*Muneeza Khan, MD, FAAFP*

For Further Information:

"Accountable Care Organizations." *Centers for Medicaid and Medicare Services,* www.cms.gov/Medicare/Medicare-Fee-for-Service-Payment/ACO/index.html.

"Alternative Payment Model Overview (APM)." *Centers for Medicaid and Medicare Services,* qpp.cms.gov/apms/overview.

American Academy of Family Physicians, American College of Physicians, American Academy of Pediatrics, American Osteopathic Association. "Joint Principles of the Patient-Centered Medical Home." *American Academy of Family Physicians,* www.aafp.org/practice-management/transformation/pcmh.html.

Appold, Karen. "Patient-Centered Medical Homes: Were They Built to Last?" *Managed Healthcare Executive,* vol. 31, no. 5, May 2021.

"Defining the Medical Home: A Patient-centered Philosophy That Drives Primary Care Excellence." *Patient-Centered Primary Care Collaborative,* www.pcpcc.org/about/medical-home.

"The Merit Based Incentive Payment System (MIPS)." *Centers for Medicaid and Medicare Services,* www.cms.gov/Medicare/Quality-Initiatives-Patient-Assessment-Instruments/Value-Based-Programs/MACRA-MIPS-and-APMs/Quality-Payment-Program-MIPS-NPRM-Slides.pdf.

"Patient-centered Medical Home Recognition." *National Committee for Quality Assurance,* www.ncqa.org/programs/recognition/practices/patient-centered-medical-home-pcmh.

"Transforming the Organization and Delivery of Primary Care." *Agency for Healthcare Research and Quality,* www.ahrq.gov/ncepcr/tools/pcmh/index.html.

US Department of Health and Human Resources. "Defining the PCMH." *Patient-centered Medical Homes.* Agency for Healthcare Research and Quality,pcmh.ahrq.gov/page/defining-pcmh.

PATIENT SAFETY AND RIGHTS

Category: Ethics

Definition: Patient safety is a discipline that focuses on preventing and reducing patient harm due to preventable risks and errors. Patient rights is a general set of guidelines defining the expectations for conduct between patients and clinicians.

OVERVIEW OF PATIENT SAFETY

Suspected to be one of the ten leading causes of death and disability in the world, adverse events occurring from medical errors have emerged as a global focus. This is an interesting contrast to the Hippocratic oath, "first, do no harm" that is taken by physicians. The

Institute of Medicine (IOM) published a groundbreaking report called *To Err Is Human* in 1999 that most consider to be the birth of modern patient safety. In the same year, the Healthcare Research and Quality Act of 1999 was signed into law appointing the Agency of Healthcare Research and Quality (AHRQ) to begin identifying causes of preventable death and injury, to develop solutions, and to disseminate findings. Their seminal report, *Making Health Care Safer* utilized evidence-based medicine to guide advancements in patient safety.

In the past, evaluations of adverse events in medicine were often investigated on an individual level. British psychologist James Reason pioneered the systems approach to preventable errors. The systems approach is grounded on the principle that most errors are predictable and occur in the context of systems that were not designed to accommodate human failings. Individuals should still be held accountable when appropriate, but systems are responsible for creating and promoting a safe culture. Since the patient safety movement has gained momentum, the AHRQ, National Patient Safety Foundation (NPSF), the World Health Organization (WHO), the Centers for Medicare & Medicaid Services (CMS), the Centers for Disease Control and Prevention (CDC) and The Joint Commission (TJC) have all created safety initiatives, benchmarks, and publications. These publications have guided patient safety over the past several decades.

Within this time, key practices have been identified in patient safety including: preventing and monitoring health care-associated infections, postoperative complications, medication errors, hand-washing, fall prevention, pressure ulcers, critical result communication delays, and patient identification errors. There are also concerns with unsafe injection practices, diagnostic errors, environmental hazards, and unsafe transfusion practices that have been and continue to be addressed. Important tools including root cause analysis, benchmarking, clinical assessments and surveillance tools have also been developed to monitor and improve upon patient safety practices.

CURRENT PERSPECTIVES IN PATIENT SAFETY

Though improvements in rates of preventable harm have declined drastically, they remain high overall. Rates are particularly high in low and middle-income countries worldwide. Emerging issues in medicine continue to drive the need for safety, innovation and equity. Included in these are electronic medical records (EMRs), physician burnout, and new technologies. These new issues present challenges that must be accommodated in future patient safety planning and initiatives.

The WHO has created a resolution to make patient safety a global health priority. This resolution is supported by key strategic actions including: global leadership, setting priorities, developing guidelines and tools and providing technical support. In addition, educating patients and continuing to monitor and research safety data are a part of these initiatives. This work is being spearheaded by the World Alliance for Patient Safety.

Crucial in moving forward with patient safety is expanding safety measures across the continuum of care. Traditionally, patient safety measures have focused on the inpatient setting but all areas should be held to safety standards. The Joint Commission creates National Patient Safety Goals annually. In alignment with the need to expand patient safety across the continuum, these goals are set for various settings including outpatient and long-term care.

Establishing a safety culture, central oversight of safety, and a common set of safety metrics is suggested in the latest publication from the NPSF, *Free from Harm*. Educating the workforce and patients while optimizing technology to protect patient privacy and safety is essential in ongoing progress. Across all settings, diagnostic errors continue to present challenges due to the limited ability to measure standardized criteria surrounding this. Ongoing oversight from (TJC) and financial incentives for safety and quality will continue to encourage diligence in this area.

OVERVIEW OF PATIENT RIGHTS

In a quality health care organization, patients should have reasonable expectations that their rights will be protected by all clinicians that they encounter. In fact, a mutually respectful relationship is necessary between the patient and clinician for the well-being of the patient. The first Bill of Rights was developed by the American Hospital Association (AHA) in 1973. This document was intended to prevent potential harm to patients via abuses of information and trust. Since its introduction, various organizations have created their own bill of rights. It is recognized as a right of patients that they will be informed of their rights in a way that they can understand in advance of making care decisions. This includes provision of a Bill of Rights upon request.

There are also enforceable laws that guarantee certain rights including the Health Information Portability and Accountability Act (HIPAA), Emergency Medical Treatment and Labor Act (EMTALA), and Medicare and Medicaid regulatory requirements. The Medicare and Medicaid requirements are often monitored by contracted organizations such as TJC, Det Norske Veritas (DNV), or the Center for Improvement in Healthcare Quality (CIHQ) among other organizations. These organizations ensure compliance with regulatory provisions.

PATIENT RIGHTS SPECIFICS

The American Hospital Association has replaced their Bill of Rights with *The Patient Care Partnership* outlining reasonable expectations for high quality and dignified hospital care. A patient should be guaranteed the right to know who is caring for them, a clean and safe environment, the right to make informed decisions and participate in care planning. They should also expect financial clarity, billing assistance, protection of their privacy, and preparation for care beyond discharge. This document is in line with TJC and DNV rights. These organizations are surveyors for the Centers for Medicare and Medicaid Services (CMS). CMS requires that hospital organizations support patient rights as delineated above in order to participate.

Informed consent requires that a patient is informed of risks and benefits and alternatives of all care as well as who will be performing any and all procedures in a way that they can understand. This means that if an interpreter is necessary, they will be provided—including for both spoken and sign languages. This also means that understanding will be assessed by clinicians before obtaining consent.

Patients have the right to be involved in care, which means that they will be informed of any developments or modifications in the plan of care. They should speak up about their preferences and clinicians must respect their wishes in any way that they are expressed including in advance directives or medical durable power of attorneys. Clinicians are not, however, required to give inappropriate or unnecessary care.

Patients also have a right to a safe environment and freedom from abuse, meaning that all staff are accountable for keeping the environment safe. In addition, policies must be in place to safeguard against abuse, promote safety culture, and for grievances to be filed. The right to pain management is observed as it is neglectful to leave this unmanaged. A safe environment also means that visitors should be allowed and restricted per hospital policy and patient preferences. Hospital policies must be clearly posted and cannot be discriminatory.

Federal laws also dictate certain patient rights. HIPAA is a federal law that carefully safeguards patient information and their right to privacy. This requires that only those who are involved in care can access the chart, that information is only shared with those necessary for treatment of the patient, and that hospitals carefully track who is given access to a patients' chart. Lastly, EMTALA governs emergency care of patients in hospitals receiving funding from federal sources. Screening for emergency medical conditions is required and if an emergency condition is present, care and stabilization of any medical conditions must be provided, regardless of payer status, until and unless transfer is appropriate.

These patient rights are basic expectations that a patient should reasonably assume when receiving care. If asked, all organizations should be able to provide a copy of their Patient Bill of Rights and should have safeguards in place to ensure that these are being provided. Respecting patient rights is crucial in creating a safe environment for quality health care.

—*Alison Stoughton, DNP, NP-C*

See also: Safety issues for older adults

For Further Information:
Agency for Healthcare Research and Quality (AHRQ), psnet.ahrq.gov/psnet-collection.
American Hospital Association (AHA), www.aha.org/other-resources/patient-care-partnership.
American Medical Association (AMA), www.ama-assn.org/delivering-care/ethics/patient-rights.
The Joint Commission, www.jointcommission.org/standards/national-patient-safety-goals.
World Health Organization, www.who.int/news-room/fact-sheets/detail/patient-safety.

PEDIATRICS

Category: Specialty
Anatomy or system affected: All
Specialties and related fields: Family medicine, genetics, neonatology, nursing, perinatology, pulmonary medicine, urology
Definition: The field of medicine devoted to the care of children at birth and through childhood, puberty, and adolescence.

Key terms:
acute: referring to a short and sharp disease process
chronic: referring to a lingering disease process
congenital: inborn, inherited
full-term: referring to a gestation period of a full nine months
premature: referring to a birth that is less than full-term
puberty: the time of hormonal change when a child begins the physical process of becoming an adult

PROFESSION AND EDUCATION
Pediatrics is a branch of medicine that pertains to the care of patients from infancy to adulthood (up to the age of twenty-one). Physicians in this field are referred to as pediatricians. Pediatrics is one of the widest-ranging medical specialties, embracing virtually all major medical disciplines. Some pediatricians are generalists, while others subspecialize in fields such as cardiology,

hematology/oncology, endocrinology, emergency medicine, and many more.

The training to become a pediatrician varies across the world. Upon graduation from a US medical school and successfully passing multiple board examinations, medical graduates interested in specializing in pediatrics must complete a three-year residency program where they will be trained in the outpatient, inpatient, and critical care of pediatric patients. After training, pediatrics may become board certified by passing a rigorous national examination encompassing the various intricacies of pediatrics. Further subspecializing requires further training in the form of three-year fellowships, followed by another board examination.

SCOPE OF PRACTICE
The practice of pediatrics begins with birth and ranges to adulthood. Most babies are born healthy and require only routine medical attention. Many hospitals, however, have a neonatology intensive care unit (NICU) for infants who are born prematurely, those with critical or severe medical conditions, those with birth defects, or those with low birth weight (LBW). These infants may require short-term or prolonged care by pediatricians in the NICU.

The problems of premature babies usually center on the fact that they have not fully developed physically, although other factors may also be involved, such as the health and age of the mother, undernourishment during pregnancy, lack of prenatal care, anemia, abnormalities in the mother's genital organs, and infectious disease. A past record of infertility, stillbirths, abortions, and other premature births may indicate that a pregnancy will not go to full term. Because the lungs are among the organs that fully develop late in pregnancy, many premature infants are unable to breathe on their own. Some premature babies are born before they have developed the sucking reflex, so they cannot feed on their own.

Low birth weight in both premature and full-term babies directly correlates to the incidence of comorbidities. Low birth weight infants have an increased risk of developing neurodevelopmental problems (such as attention-deficit/hyperactivity disorder [ADHD] and autism), decreased cognitive performance, growth disorders, and defects in vision or hearing.

Hundreds of congenital diseases can be present in the neonate. Some are apparent at birth; some become evident in later years. Some may be life-threatening to the infant or become life-threatening in later years while others may be harmless.

Among the most prevalent congenital birth defects is cleft lip, which occurs when the upper lip does not fuse together, leaving a visible gap that can extend from the lip to the nose. Cleft palate occurs when the gap reaches into the roof of the mouth. Various abnormalities may also be present in the hands and feet of neonates. These can be due to congenital defects or caused by medications given to the pregnant mother. Arms, legs, fingers, and toes may fail to develop fully or may be missing entirely. Some children are born with extra fingers or toes. In some children, fingers or toes may be webbed or fused together. Clubfoot is relatively common. In this condition, the foot is twisted, usually downward and inward.

Many congenital heart defects can afflict the child, including septal defects (openings in the septum, the wall that separates the right and left sides of the heart), the transposition of blood vessels, the constriction of blood vessels, and valve disorders. These can affect proper oxygenation delivery to vital organs and can be life-threatening if not detected early.

Congenital disorders of the central nervous system include spina bifida, hydrocephalus, cerebral palsy, and Down syndrome. Spina bifida is a condition in which part of a vertebra (a bone in the spinal column) fails to fuse. As a result, nerves of the spinal cord may protrude through the spinal column. This condition varies considerably in severity; mild forms can cause

no significant problems, while severe forms can be crippling or life-threatening. In hydrocephalus, sometimes called "water on the brain," fluid accumulates in the infant's cranium, causing the head to enlarge and putting great pressure on the brain. This disorder, too, can be life-threatening. Cerebral palsy is caused by damage to brain cells that control motor function in the body. This damage can occur before, during, or after birth. It may or may not be accompanied by mental disability.

Down syndrome (also known as trisomy 21) is the most common chromosomal abnormality in infants today It is caused by an extra chromosome (chromosome 21) passed on to the child. The risk for chromosomal abnormalities increases with advanced maternal age (particularly above age thirty-five) and diagnosis can often be made with a prenatal screen. The distinct physical characteristics of Down syndrome include a small body, a small and rounded head, oval ears, and an enlarged tongue. Patients with Down syndrome have a wide range of cognitive abnormalities, congenital malformations, and medical conditions of various organ systems. They also have an increased risk of cancer (leukemias). With various medical advancements and resources, those affected by Down syndrome now

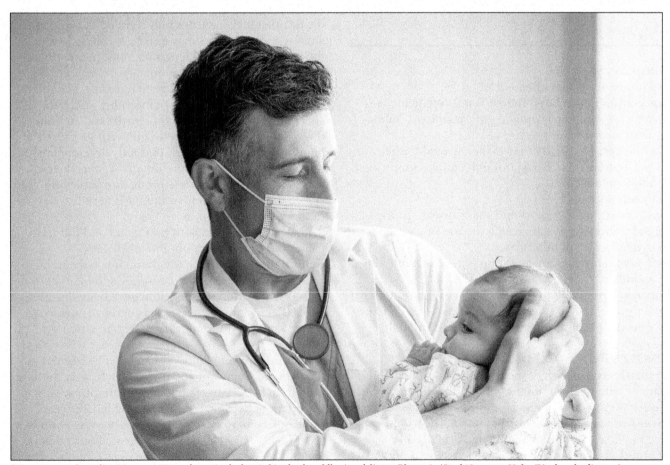

It is customary for pediatricians to visit newborns in the hospital in the days following delivery. Photo via iStock/Courtney Hale. [Used under license.]

have longer life expectancies with improved quality of life.

Cystic fibrosis is one of the most serious congenital lung diseases of Caucasian children. Because the lungs of children with this disease cannot expel mucus efficiently, it thickens and collects, clogging air passages. The mucus also becomes a breeding ground for bacteria and infection. Other parts of the body, such as the pancreas, the digestive system, and sweat glands, can also be impaired. A common congenital disorder among African American children is sickle cell disease. It causes deformities in red blood cells that clog blood vessels, impairs circulation, and increases susceptibility to infection.

Another prenatal risk factor is infection. An infant may be born with an infection passed on from the mother, such as rubella (German measles) or human immunodeficiency virus (HIV), the virus that causes acquired immunodeficiency syndrome (AIDS). Many of these infections can affect the fetus, causing severe physical deformities, heart defects, mental disability, deafness, and other conditions. Genital herpes affects about 1,500 newborns in the United States each year and may cause serious complications. A herpes infection during the second or third trimester of a woman's pregnancy may increase the chance of preterm delivery or cesarean section. Group beta strep (GBS) infections are another serious problem for one of every 2,000 newborns in the United States. GBS may cause sepsis (blood infection), meningitis, and pneumonia. Infectious diseases are more prevalent in childhood than in later years. Among the major diseases of children (and often adults) throughout the centuries have been smallpox, malaria, diphtheria, typhus, typhoid fever, tuberculosis, measles, mumps, rubella, varicella (chickenpox), scarlet fever, pneumonia, meningitis, and pertussis (whooping cough). Today, vaccines have drastically decreased the rate of many of these lethal infections.

One of the most feared problems of infancy is sudden infant death syndrome (SIDS), or the sudden death of a previously healthy infant that remains unexplained despite thorough investigation. It is the lead cause of infant death between the ages of one month and one year. Infant risk factors include prematurity, low birth weight, prone sleeping position, co-sleeping, and sleeping on a soft surface with multiple pillows and blankets. Maternal risk factors include young age, smoking during pregnancy, and late or no prenatal care. The child usually shows no symptoms of disease, and autopsies reveal no evidence of smothering, choking, or strangulation.

Certain skin diseases are common in infants and young children, such as diaper rash, impetigo, neonatal acne, and seborrheic dermatitis, among a wide variety of disorders. Infections of the skin occur often in the young, as the infections are easily spread by contact with an infected playmate or by the touching of surfaces that harbor the organism. These infections may include athlete's foot, ringworm, cellulitis, head lice, body lice, and scabies. Some skin conditions are congenital; between 20 and 40 percent of infants are born with, or soon develop, skin lesions called "hemangiomas." They may be barely perceptible or quite unsightly; they generally resolve by the age of seven.

Insulin-dependent diabetes mellitus (IDDM) or type 1 diabetes (T1DM) is the most common form of childhood diabetes; however, with the rise of obesity, type 2 diabetes is increasing in prevalence in children. In the healthy individual, the pancreas produces insulin, a hormone that is responsible for the metabolism of blood sugar, or glucose. In children with T1DM, the pancreas loses the ability to produce insulin, causing blood sugar to rise. In children with T2DM, the body's tissues are unable to respond appropriately to insulin and the pancreas develops defection insulin secretion. In both cases, a cascade of events cause harmful effects throughout the body. In a diabetic emergency, symptoms may include rapid breathing, rapid heartbeat, extreme thirst, vomiting, fever, chemical imbalances in the blood, and coma. In the long term, diabetes mellitus contributes to heart disease, atherosclerosis, kidney damage, blindness, gangrene, and a host of other conditions.

Cancer can afflict children. One of the more common forms of childhood cancer is acute lymphocytic leukemia. Its peak incidence is between three and five years of age, although it can also occur later in life. Leukemic conditions are characterized by the overproduction of white blood cells (leukocytes). In acute lymphocytic leukemia, the production of lymphoblasts, immature cells that ordinarily would develop into infection-fighting lymphocytes, is greatly increased. This abnormal proliferation of immature cells interferes with the normal production of blood cells, increasing the child's susceptibility to infection, electrolyte abnormalities, and hyperviscosity. Before current treatment modalities, the prognosis for children with acute lymphocytic leukemia was death within four or five months after diagnosis. This has greatly improved with a variety of chemotherapy regimens and potential bone marrow transplants.

In addition to the wide range of diseases that can beset the infant and growing child, there are many other problems of childhood that the parent and pediatrician must face. These problems may involve physical growth, nutrition, social and behavioral development, mental health, and environmental influences.

Both parents and pediatricians must be alert to a child's rate of growth and mental development. Failure to gain weight in infancy may indicate a range of physical problems, such as gastrointestinal, endocrine, and other internal disorders. In three-quarters of these cases, however, the cause is not a physical disorder. The child may be underfed because of parental negligence. The vital process of bonding between parent and child may have been insufficient, causing the child to feel unwanted and unloved. The child may experience physical or emotional abuse in the home or bullying in school. Similarly, later in childhood, failure to grow at a normal rate can be caused by malnutrition or psychological factors. It could also be attributable to a deficiency in a hormone that is the body's natural regulator of growth. If this hormone is not released in adequate supply, the child's growth is stunted. An excess of this hormone may cause the child to grow too rapidly. Failure to grow normally may also indicate an underlying disease condition, such as a heart condition or a gastrointestinal malabsorption disorder.

The parent and pediatrician must also ensure that the child is developing acceptably in other areas. Speech and language skills, teething, bone development, walking and other motor skills, toilet habits, sleep patterns, eye development, and hearing have to be evaluated regularly.

Profound mental disability is usually evident early in life, but mild to moderate disability may not be apparent until the child starts school. Slowness in learning may be indicative of mental disability, but this judgment should be carefully evaluated, as the underlying reason may be impaired hearing or vision or a hidden disease condition. The diagnosis of neurological disorders, such as autism and ADHD, have greatly increased in recent years and poses a special challenge to both parents and pediatricians.

The battery of diseases and other disorders that may beset a child remains more or less constant throughout childhood. Puberty, however, triggers hormonal changes that allow for new disease threats and vast psychological upheaval. As early as eight years of age in girls and after ten or eleven years of age in boys, the body begins a prolonged metamorphosis from childhood into adulthood. Hormones that were previously released in minimal amounts course through the body in greater quantities.

In boys, the sex hormones are called" androgens." Chief among them is testosterone, which is secreted primarily by the testicles. It causes the sexual organs to mature and promotes the growth of hair in the genital area and armpits and on the chest. Testosterone also enlarges the larynx (voicebox), causing the voice to deepen.

Girls also produce some testosterone, but estrogens and other female sex hormones are the major hormones involved in puberty. They cause the sexual organs to mature, the hips to enlarge and become rounded, hair to grow in the genital area and armpits, the breasts to enlarge, and menstruation to begin.

Many disease conditions can arise in association with the hormonal changes that occur during puberty, such as breast abnormalities and genital infections. The most common medical disorder at this time, however, is acne. Acne is a direct result of the rise in testosterone that occurs during puberty. About 85 percent of teenagers experience some degree of acne, and about 12 percent of these will develop severe, deep acne, a serious condition that can leave lifelong scars.

Important psychological changes also occur during puberty. The personality can be altered as the developing child begins to crave independence. Ties to the family weaken, and the teenager becomes closer to his or her peer group. Sexual feelings can be strong and difficult to repress. In modern Western society, this is usually the time when the teenager may begin to experiment with tobacco, alcohol, drugs, or other means of achieving a "high," although in some groups the use of these substances begins much earlier. Substance abuse is a major problem throughout society, but is particularly devastating among teenagers whose brains are still developing.

Sexual activity among teenagers is widespread and, combined with inadequate education about health issues and limited access to care, has led to significant medical problems. The incidence of sexually transmitted infections (STIs), including HIV, is higher among teenagers than any other group. Teenage pregnancy is one of the most challenging issues in modern society.

If the pregnant teenager who continues her pregnancy is from a disadvantaged family background, she is even more likely than other teen mothers to receive little or no prenatal care. Risks of delayed or absent prenatal care can include a fetus that is not properly nourished. Additional risks can arise from a mother who smokes, drinks alcohol, or takes drugs throughout the pregnancy. In these cases, the child may be born prematurely, with all the physical problems that prematurity involves. Hospital care of these infants is extremely costly, as is the maintenance of the mother and child if the baby survives.

DIAGNOSTIC AND TREATMENT TECHNIQUES

Advances in medical research and technology have radically changed the field of pediatrics. In neonatology, the survival rates and prognoses of premature and LBW infants have drastically improved through new research and innovative therapeutics that assist in lung development and neuroprotection. Infectious diseases passed from the mother to the newborn child are a particular challenge. In some cases, such as with GBS and herpes infections, appropriate antibiotics and antiviral agents can be given. In others, such as with babies born with HIV, support measures and medications that help prevent the progression of the disease are available.

Many birth defects and deformities can be repaired. Disorders such as cleft lip or palate, deformities of the skeletal system, heart defects, and other physical abnormalities often can be remedied by surgery. Certain structural malformations may require prosthetic devices and/or physical therapy. Others may be candidates for palliative procedures.

The treatment of spina bifida depends on the severity of the condition; surgery may be required. With hydrocephalus, medications may be helpful, but most often, a permanent shunt is implanted to drain fluids from the cranium. Before this technique was developed, the prognosis for babies with hydrocephalus was poor: more than half died, and many suffered from mental disability and physical impairment. Today, 70 percent or more live through infancy. Of these, about 40 percent have normal intelligence; the others are mentally disabled and may also have serious physical impairment. There are no cures for many conditions such as cerebral palsy or Down syndrome, but various interventions can improve the child's quality of life. Interventions may include but are not limited to surgical procedures, physical/occupational therapy, specialized education plans, counseling, and support groups.

SIDS continues to be a problem both in hospitals and in the home. However, the American Academy of Pediatrics created a Back to Sleep campaign to educate parents about proper infant sleep positioning and habit. It has been extremely successful in decreasing the incidence of SIDS by 70 to 80 percent.

As infectious diseases are prevalent in childhood, pediatricians utilize a variety of antibiotics, antivirals, and supportive measures to treat these illnesses. Perhaps more importantly, they promote prevention of illnesses through education and access to immunizations. Today, routine vaccinations are recommended for all children in the United States; these include immunization against diphtheria, tetanus, pertussis, measles, mumps, rubella, poliomyelitis, pneumococcal pneumonia, *Hemophilus influenzae*, varicella, hepatitis A and B, and human papilloma virus. Vaccines are also available against rabies, influenza, cholera, typhoid fever, plague, and yellow fever; these vaccines can be given to the child if there is a danger of infection (e.g., travel, exposure). Vaccines for diphtheria, tetanus, and pertussis are generally given together in a combination as diphtheria, tetanus, and pertussis, DTaP or Tdap. Measles, mumps, and rubella vaccines are also given together as MMR. Repeated doses of some vaccines are necessary to ensure and maintain immunity.

Patients with diabetes mellitus type 1 are dependent on insulin throughout life. It is necessary to teach both the parent and the patient how to administer insulin regularly, often several times a day. Furthermore, patients must monitor their blood sugar levels and sugar intake consistently to prevent progression of illness. This regimen is often difficult for the child to learn and accept, but strict adherence is vital if the patient is to fare well and avoid the wide range of complications associated with diabetes.

With the emergence of social media, a variety of mental health problems have surfaced, ranging from depression/anxiety to dealing with bullying. Medications and access to mental health resources for children and adolescents have improved in recent years, though there remains room for further improvement. Children with behavioral problems or delays may benefit from seeing clinicians specializing in developmental pediatrics, child psychology, or child psychiatry.

In the era of sexual freedom, the need for sexual and reproductive education is higher than ever. Sexuality, sexually transmitted infections, and pregnancy among teenagers has provoked a nationwide response in the United States among medical and sociological professionals. These include safe-sex programs, transgender clinics, and clinics specializing in counseling for adolescents. A newer specialty in adolescent medicine has emerged to tackle these issues.

PERSPECTIVE AND PROSPECTS
Pediatrics affects virtually every member of society. Diseases that once raged through populations of all ages are now being controlled through the mass immunization of children. Some diseases of childhood are not yet controllable by vaccines, but research in this area is ongoing.

Childhood health is also directly related to socioeconomic status. Middle-class and upper-class children have more access to professional care for any problems that may arise. The medical and psychological needs of disadvantaged children, however, are often neglected. These children remain susceptible to physical and mental illnesses that are less prevalent among the middle and upper classes. They may live in a universe of violence, deprivation, and drug addiction, or may lack a stable family environment, preventing them from having opportunities for advancement. Pediatric providers at all levels can advocate for these youth by becoming involved in medical, psychological, and sociological outreach programs.

With the advent of technology, pediatric patients and their families are able to receive a patient-centered, personalized, and data-driven health care experience. From apps that track symptoms to computerized immunization records to virtual office visits, technology has revolutionized the approach to health care and is projected to continue to do so in the coming years. Such advances will continue to strengthen the vital role that pediatricians play in the lives of children and families.

—Mehrin Islam, MD

See also: Apgar score; Cardiology, pediatric; Childhood infectious diseases; Circumcision, male; Cognitive development; Congenital disorders; Critical care, pediatric; Dentistry, pediatric; Dermatology, pediatric; Developmental disorders; Developmental stages; Emergency medicine, pediatric; Endocrinology, pediatric; Family medicine; Gastroenterology, pediatric; Genetic diseases; Growth; Hematology, pediatric; Motor skill development; Neonatology; Nephrology, pediatric; Neurology, pediatric; Obesity, childhood; Optometry, pediatric; Orthopedics, pediatric; Perinatology; Psychiatry, child and adolescent; Puberty and adolescence; Pulmonary medicine, pediatric; Safety issues for children; Surgery, pediatric; Urology, pediatric; Well-baby examinations.

For Further Information:

American Academy of Pediatrics, www.aap.org.
Doyle, Barbara T., and E. D. Iland. *Autism Spectrum Disorders from A to Z*. Future Horizons, 2004.
Hay, William W., Jr., et al., editors. *Current Diagnosis and Treatment: Pediatrics*. 21st ed., Lange Medical Books/McGraw-Hill, 2012.
Hoekelman, Robert, editor. *The New American Encyclopedia of Children's Health*. New American Library/Dutton, 1991.
Kimball, Chad T. *Childhood Diseases and Disorders Sourcebook: Basic Consumer Health Information About Medical Problems Often Encountered in Pre-adolescent Children*. Omnigraphics, 2003.
Kliegman, Robert M., and Waldo E. Nelson, editors. *Nelson Textbook of Pediatrics*. 19th ed., Saunders/Elsevier, 2011.
Litin, Scott C., editor. *Mayo Clinic Family Health Book*. 4th ed., HarperResource, 2009.
Middlemiss, Prisca. *What's That Rash? How to Identify and Treat Childhood Rashes*. Hamlyn, 2002.
Nathanson, Laura Walther. *The Portable Pediatrician: A Practicing Pediatrician's Guide to Your Child's Growth, Development, Health, and Behavior from Birth to Age Five*. 2nd ed., HarperCollins, 2002.
Sanghavi, Darshak. *A Map of the Child: A Pediatrician's Tour of the Body*. Henry Holt, 2003.
Taubman, Bruce. *Your Child's Symptoms: A Parent's Guide to Understanding Pediatric Medicine*. Simon & Schuster, 1992.

Pellagra

Category: Disease/Disorder
Anatomy or system affected: Nervous system, brain, digestive system, skin
Specialties and related fields: Nutrition, dietitian, global health, gastroenterology, cardiology, neurology, dermatology

Definition: A disease caused by a deficiency of niacin (Vitamin B$_3$).
Key terms:
ataxia: loss of voluntary coordination of muscle movements producing gait abnormalities
dementia: chronic disorder of mental processes that results in memory loss, personality changes, and impaired reasoning
dermatitis: inflammation of the skin that can manifest in a variety of different ways depending on the etiology

CAUSES AND SYMPTOMS

Pellagra is a disease that results from a vitamin B3 (niacin) deficiency. Niacin is an organic compound that is required for the production of NAD (nicotinamide adenine dinucleotide) and NADP (nicotinamide adenine dinucleotide phosphate). NAD and NADP are important in many molecular processes, including cellular respiration, within the body, which is why pellagra produces broad symptoms and ultimately results in death if left untreated. Pellagra is commonly seen in South America, where the diet consists heavily of maize, a poor source of niacin and tryptophan. Pellagra is also seen in many developing countries where many patients are poor and malnourished.

There are two forms of pellagra. Primary pellagra occurs when the patient's diet lacks niacin. This can either be due to a direct dietary deficiency of niacin or a dietary deficiency of tryptophan, an amino acid that the body can convert to niacin. Secondary pellagra arises when there is adequate niacin and tryptophan in the patient's diet, but the patient is not able to absorb the niacin or convert the tryptophan to niacin. Secondary pellagra is usually seen in the setting of chronic diarrhea, Hartnup's disease (which prevents normal absorption of amino acids), carcinoid tumors (which will deplete tryptophan levels), or chronic alcoholism and liver damage leading to poor absorption. Isoniazid therapy, which is utilized to treat tuberculo-

---

INFORMATION ON PELLAGRA

Causes: Vitamin B$_3$ deficiency, tryptophan deficiency, alcoholism, chronic diarrhea, carcinoid syndrome, Hartnup's disease, medications
Symptoms: Diarrhea, dermatitis, dementia, death, confusion, sensitivity to sunlight, glossitis (inflammation of the tongue), aggression, ataxia (loss of coordination)
Duration: Pellagra can progress to death within 4-5 years if left untreated
Treatments: Nicotinamide, Vitamin B$_3$ (niacin)

sis, can also cause pellagra. Isoniazid binds to and inactivates vitamin B_6 so that it cannot be used in the synthesis of niacin.

The most important symptoms of pellagra are known as the 4 D's: diarrhea, dermatitis, dementia, and death. Dermatitis will present as alopecia (loss of hair), red skin lesions, and peeling, scaling, and thickening of skin that has been exposed to sunlight. Early mental changes include insomnia and fatigue, but eventually progress to dementia, hallucinations, and confusion. If left untreated, pellagra will typically kill within 4 to 5 years. Other symptoms include dilated cardiomyopathy (enlarged heart), glossitis (inflammation of the tongue), ataxia (loss of coordination), and aggressive behavior.

TREATMENT AND THERAPY

The diagnosis of pellagra can be made based on symptoms alone. Treatments for pellagra include nicotinamide and supplemental niacin. Nicotinamide is preferred to niacin due to the fact that niacin often produces unpleasant side effects such as itching, burning, and flushing of the skin. Nicotinamide can be given orally or by injection. The amount of nicotinamide administered and the frequency of administration is determined by the degree to which the pellagra has progressed. Improvements typically begin within days of starting nicotinamide therapy.

—Steffan Kim

See also: Hartnup's disease, carcinoid tumor, chronic alcoholism

For Further Information:
"Dr. Joseph Goldberger & the War on Pellagra." *Office of NIH History*, history.nih.gov/exhibits/Goldberger/index.html. Accessed 19 Oct. 2016.
Hegyi, Vladimir et al. "Dermatologic Manifestations of Pellagra." *Medscape*, 22 Feb. 2016, emedicine.medscape.com/article/1095845-overview. Accessed 19 Oct. 2016.
"History of Pellagra." *University of Alabama at Birmingham Reynolds-Finley Historical Library*, www.uab.edu/reynolds/pellagra/history. Accessed 19 Oct. 2016.
Ngan, Vanessa. "Pellagra." *DermNet New Zealand*, www.dermnetnz.org/topics/pellagra/. Accessed 19 Oct. 2016.
"The Origins of Maize: The Puzzle of Pellagra." *European Food Information Council*,Dec. 2001, www.eufic.org/article/en/artid/origins-maize-pellagra/. Accessed 19 Oct. 2016.
"Pellagra." *MedlinePlus*, medlineplus.gov/ency/article/000342.htm. Accessed 19 Oct. 2016.
"Pellagra." *PBS Learning Media*, wvia.pbslearningmedia.org/resource/odys08.sci.life.gen.pellagra/pellagra/. Accessed 19 Oct. 2016.

PELVIC INFLAMMATORY DISEASE (PID)

Category: Disease/Disorder
Key terms:

contact tracing: also known as partner referral; a process that involves identifying the sexual partners of infected patients, informing the partners of their exposure to disease, and offering resources for counseling and treatment

ectopic pregnancy: a pregnancy that occurs anywhere other than in the uterus; ectopic pregnancies can be life-threatening since they can rupture and bleed profusely

laparoscopy: a minimally invasive surgical procedure performed through small incisions in the abdomen

polymicrobial infection: an infection caused by multiple microorganisms such as bacteria and viruses

sexually transmitted disease (STD): an infection caused by organisms transferred through sexual contact (genital-genital, oral-genital, oral-anal, or anal-genital); the transmission of infection occurs through exposure to lesions or secretions that contain the organisms

CAUSES AND SYMPTOMS

Pelvic inflammatory disease (PID) is a polymicrobial infection of the upper genital tract. The infectious microbes may be sexually transmitted organisms (such as *Neisseria gonorrhea, Chlamydia trachomatis*, and *Mycoplasma genitalium*) or endogenous bacteria found in the vagina (e.g., staphylococci, streptococci, enteric bacteria, such as *Klebsiella* species, *Escherichia coli* or *Proteus* species, or anaerobic bacteria like *Bacteroides* species). These microorganisms can travel from the lower genital tract (vagina, cervix) into the upper genital tract (uterus, Fallopian tubes, ovaries, and pelvic cavity) and establish infection there. Occasionally, PID can occur via another mechanism, such as infection and rupture of the appendix or lower gastrointestinal tract that causes the spillage of bacteria into the pelvic cavity.

Eighty-five percent of PID cases are caused by sexually transmitted microorganisms or bacteria that cause infections of the birth canal (vaginosis). The remaining PID cases are caused by normal microbial residents of the lower reproductive tract of females.

Approximately 106,000 outpatient visits and 60,000 hospitalizations each year are due to PID. Each female PID patient costs around $2,000 to treat, and this number can rise to $6,000 if she develops chronic pelvic pain.

The Centers for Disease Control and Prevention (CDC) stipulates the diagnostic criteria for PID, noting that the diagnosis is made on clinical findings rather than on laboratory evidence. Most cases of PID are asymptomatic. In cases where symptoms occur, the patient has lower abdominal or pelvic pain. During an abdominal examination, the lower abdomen is tender to palpation. Upon pelvic examination, either the cervix is tender upon movement by the examiner or one or both ovaries or the Fallopian tubes are tender to palpation; both of these symptoms can be present. Other symptoms and signs of PID include fever and abnormal cervical discharge.

Laboratory tests can help establish a diagnosis when clinical symptoms are ambiguous and emphasize the need for partner treatment. Tests include blood tests that suggest systemic inflammation (such as the erythrocyte sedimentation rate) and cultures or nucleic acid amplification tests for *N. gonorrhea* or *C. trachomatis*. Ultrasound or other imaging techniques can identify fluid collections associated with the Fallopian tubes, ovaries, or elsewhere in the pelvic cavity. PID can spread to the upper abdomen on rare occasions, leading to pain and tenderness in that area. In particular, the infection can affect the region surrounding the liver, leading to Fitz-Hugh Curtis syndrome.

Long-term consequences of PID can be significant and can occur in asymptomatic and symptomatic patients. PID can cause scarring of the reproductive tract leading to infertility. Damaged fallopian tubes can fill with fluid (hydrosalpinx) and cause pain and infertility.

PID increases the risk for ectopic pregnancy, a potentially life-threatening condition. Suppose the infection spreads beyond the reproductive tract. In that case, organs such as the bowels may also become involved in the infection—any organs involved in the infection risk becoming damaged and scarred and might abnormally adhere to other organs. In addition to the acute pain of PID, the disease can also lead to chronic pelvic pain, which can be difficult to treat. Women with a history of PID have an almost two-fold increase in the risk of ovarian cancer.

TREATMENT AND THERAPY

Pelvic inflammatory disease is usually treated in an outpatient setting, although severe cases require hospitalization and intravenous medications. Antibiotics are the first-line PID treatment, most commonly treated empirically based on clinical suspicion. Because PID is polymicrobial, combinations of antibiotics, each targeted at different bacteria, are given simultaneously. Drug regimens differ according to the severity of the disease. Patients are usually treated in the hospital for severe PID with cefotetan or cefoxitin combined with doxycycline or clindamycin plus gentamicin. For mild to moderate PID, outpatient therapy is preferred. First-line treatments typically consist of ceftriaxone or cefoxitin/probenecid or cefotaxime plus doxycycline. Metronidazole is sometimes added to regimens as a third drug to cover anaerobic organisms. It is always

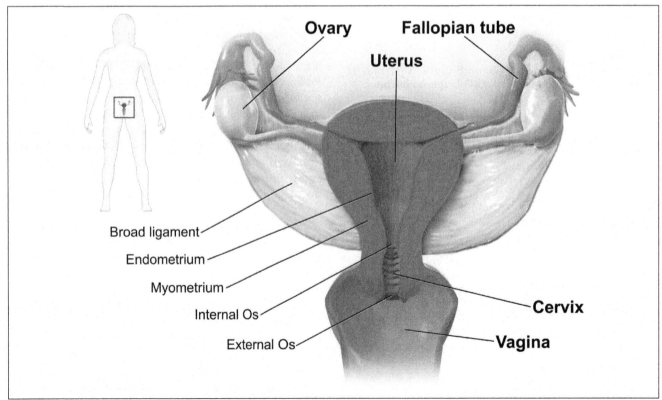

Typical sites for pelvic inflammatory disease. Image by Bruce Blaus, via Wikimedia Commons.

> ### INFORMATION ON
> ### PELVIC INFLAMMATORY DISEASE (PID)
>
> **Causes:** Bacterial infection transmitted through sexual contact or from other body areas
>
> **Symptoms:** Usually asymptomatic; may involve lower abdominal or pelvic pain, fever, abnormal cervical or vaginal discharge; can lead to scarring, infertility, ectopic pregnancy
>
> **Duration:** Chronic
>
> **Treatments:** Antibiotics, abscess drainage if needed

included if infection with the protozoan *Trichomonas vaginalis* is suspected. Unfortunately, the stomach discomfort caused by metronidazole can cause patients to stop taking it prematurely. Infections with *C. trachomitis* may warrant the inclusion of azithromycin. For *N. gonorrhea* infections, ceftriaxone and doxycycline are particularly effective. Because of resistance, fluoroquinolone antibiotics (e.g., ciprofloxacin, moxifloxacin) are no longer used to treat gonorrhea infections. Patients are normally treated for 14 days.

Since PID is usually sexually transmitted, therapy involves counseling regarding the prevention of sexually transmitted infections (STIs) and safer sexual techniques. Condoms and other barrier techniques decrease the spread of STIs. Anal penetration followed by vaginal penetration during intercourse may increase the risk of infection of the female reproductive tract. Testing for other STIs, such as hepatitis B and C and syphilis; wet prep testing for bacterial vaginosis and trichomonas; and screening for human immunodeficiency virus (HIV) are all encouraged since the risk factors for PID, and other STIs are similar. Having multiple sex partners is a risk factor for PID. Contact tracing is offered to notify sexual partners of their possible exposure to STIs and encourage them to seek medical attention. Treatment of these partners can decrease the reinfection of the patient from subsequent sexual encounters and prevent the partners from spreading the infection to others.

PERSPECTIVE AND PROSPECTS

One of the first reports of PID was from ancient Greece and involved a case in which pus drained from the pelvis through the vagina. However, it was not until the 1880s that the sequence of events starting with the ascension of lower genital tract infection to cause upper tract disease was recognized. With the widespread use of laparoscopy in the 1960s, a more accurate diagnosis of PID could be made, allowing clinicians to recognize that PID has many clinical presentations. Prospects focus primarily on preventing PID since treatment does not prevent many long-term effects. Prevention involves continued widespread screening of asymptomatic men and women at risk for STDs, partner referral, and safer-sex education. Studies have shown that the screening and treatment of asymptomatic women for STDs has reduced the prevalence of these infections in the general population in the United States, thus translating into a reduction in PID incidence. There is hope that these prevention techniques will reduce the morbidity and serious sequelae of PID.

—Michael A. Buratovich, PhD

For Further Information:

Brazier, Yvette. "What is Pelvic Inflammatory Disease?" *MedicalNewsToday*, 23 Oct. 2017, www.medicalnewstoday.com/articles/177923. Accessed 7 Apr. 2022. www.medicalnewstoday.com/authors/yvette-brazier

Higuera, Valencia. "Pelvic Inflammatory Disease (PID)." *Healthline*, 1 May 2019, www.healthline.com/health/pelvic-inflammatory-disease-pid. Accessed 7 Apr. 2022.

Pelvic Inflammatory Disease. Familydoctor.org, Oct. 2020, familydoctor.org/condition/pelvic-inflammatory-disease/. Accessed 7 Apr. 2022.

Pelvic Inflammatory Disease. MedlinePlus, 26 Jan. 2021, medlineplus.gov/pelvicinflammatorydisease.html. Accessed 7 Apr. 2022.

Pelvic Inflammatory Disease (PID). American College of Obstetricians and Gynecologists, Oct. 2020, www.acog.org/womens-health/faqs/pelvic-inflammatory-disease. Accessed 7 Apr. 2022.

Pelvic Inflammatory Disease (PID) - CDC Fact Sheet. Centers for Disease Control and Prevention, 19 Nov. 2020, www.cdc.gov/std/PID/STDFact-PID.htm. Accessed 7 Apr. 2022.

PENILE IMPLANT SURGERY

Category: Procedure

Anatomy or system affected: Genitals, reproductive system

Specialties and related fields: General surgery, psychiatry, urology

Definition: The surgical placement of a prosthetic device inside the penis to make it rigid enough for penetration.

Key terms:

corpora cavernosa: two parallel erectile cylinders on the upper side of the penis that are filled with blood during a natural erection

corpus spongiosum: a third cylinder in the penis below the corpora cavernosa; the urethra passes through it and the glans penis forms the front end of the cylinder *erection*: a complex phenomenon involving nerves, blood vessels, and the mind that leads to the entrapment of blood in the penis, making it rigid

glans penis: the head of the penis

impotence: the lack of sustained erection that is rigid enough for penetration in sexual intercourse

psychogenic: having no anatomical, hormonal, or physiological problems with the patient's erectile mechanism; instead, the problem is in the patient's mind

urethra: the channel through which urine and seminal fluid are passed; it starts at the bladder neck, goes through the shaft of the penis, and ends at the glans penis

INDICATIONS AND PROCEDURES

Penile implant surgery is performed when all other, nonsurgical means of treating impotence, or erectile dysfunction, have been exhausted or are not suitable for the patient. Penile prosthesis implant, at present, is recognized as the most effective option to obtain an artificial satisfactory erection for sexual intercourse in patients who cannot do so naturally or with the help of pharmaceuticals. Current penile implant surgery is considered a third-line therapy for erectile dysfunction. Most recently, penile implant surgery has been found useful as an addition to gender-affirming surgery. A thorough workup must be performed to diagnose the cause of the impotence, which can be psychogenic or organic Organic causes include poor blood flow to the penis, the inability of the erectile cylinders to trap blood in the penis (venous leak), or a problem with the nerves, which is seen in diabetic patients. Impotence may also result from a hormonal disturbance.

A penile implant, or penile prosthesis, is an artificial device, usually consisting of inflatable cylinders and a pump, that can simulate an erection in men who suffer from impotence that has a biological (rather than a psychological) cause. When the patient squeezes the pump in the scrotum, fluid from an implanted reservoir fills the cylinders.

Organic causes for impotence can be determined with certain tests, including an analysis of blood chemistry and hormone levels, as well as a test for the presence of erection during sleep. Finally, the physician may perform an invasive test in which a drug is injected into the penis so that the erectile response can be observed. Usually, less aggressive, nonsurgical treatments are attempted first. If they fail, then penile implant surgery is considered.

Currently, there are multiple options approved by the US Food and Drug Administration (FDA) for penile prothesis. These include malleable devices and inflatable devices. Proper selection of implant type depends on the surgeon experience/preference, patient factors, and anatomical considerations. Malleable de-

vices consist of two solid intracavernosal implants that can be bent upward to either stimulate erection or down when not in use. Benefits of malleable devices include ease of implantation, ease of use for the patient, and low failure rates. However, it does come with higher rates of erosion and lower patient satisfaction rates.

Three-piece inflatable prostheses are the new current gold standard as they allow for rigid erection and flaccidity when desired. These devices consist of two cylinders when placed in the corporal bodies are filled with saline to produce rigidity. A fluid reservoir may be placed either sub muscularly beneath the rectus or within the space of Retzius is included, as well as a scrotal pump to control the device. Another alternative is a two-piece inflatable prosthesis includes a scrotal pump as well as cylinders equipped with smaller reservoirs. Two-piece devices are considered in patients with a history of pelvic surgery or radiation, as these devices do not require any dissection within the abdomen or pelvis.

The surgical approaches for the placement of a penile prosthesis are the same for semirigid, malleable, and inflatable types. In the infrapubic approach, the patient is placed on his back. An incision is made at the junction where the penis meets the body, just above the penis in the lower part of the abdominal wall. After the skin and subcutaneous tissues are dissected, the corpora cavernosa are exposed. While carefully protecting the nerve responsible for sensation in the penis, the surgeon opens and dilates the corpora cavernosa. The lengths of the corpora are measured, appropriate-length artificial cylinders are inserted, and the corpora are closed.

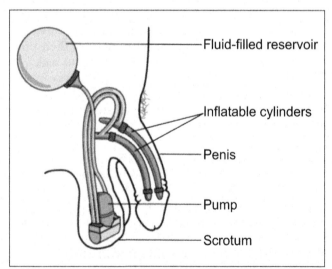

A penile implant is an artificial device, usually consisting of inflatable cylinders and a pump, that can simulate an erection in men who suffer from impotence that has a biological (rather than a psychological) cause. When the patient squeezes the pump in the scrotum, fluid from an implanted reservoir fills the cylinders. ©EBSCO

In the case of semirigid and malleable prostheses, the operation ends after the skin is closed. In the case of an inflatable penile prosthesis, however, two extra steps are taken. A place is created for the pump and reservoir. In a two-component inflatable penile prosthesis, a pocket is created for the combined pump and reservoir just underneath the skin of the scrotum, in an area that is easily accessible to the patient. In a three-component penile prosthesis, a pocket is created in thescrotum for the pump and a space is created for the reservoir in the lower part of the abdomen, above the pubic bone and in front of the bladder. The reservoir is connected to the pump, and in this fashion the placement of the prosthesis is completed. 60 ml of saline is use to inflate and evaluate size and positioning. The penile prosthesis is evaluated for proper function and cosmetic appearance, and the incision is closed. A drain maybe placed for overnight hospital stays and patient is instructed to pull the pump caudally several times per day to prevent migration.

USES AND COMPLICATIONS
In the immediate postoperative phase, the cylinder of the inflatable penile prosthesis is left totally deflated so that a scar forms around the pump and reservoir that will allow the normal function of the prosthesis in the future. After two weeks, the cylinders are cycled: The patient inflates his penile prosthesis for thirty to sixty minutes every day and then deflates it. In about six weeks, the pain should have subsided significantly so that the patient is ready to use his penile prosthesis for sexual intercourse. Close monitoring ensures that no infection develops, and the patient is asked to report to the doctor immediately if there is any redness or swelling in the area, which are signs of an impending infection. If an infection occurs, it is initially treated aggressively with antibiotics. If antibiotic therapy does not work, the penile prosthesis may have to be removed.

The complications associated with penile implants include infection, mechanical failure (resulting in the loss of pump or reservoir function), improper cylinder sizing, cranial migration of scrotal pump, and device malfunction like inadvertent inflation of an inflatable penile prosthesis when the patient sits or stands up. In certain cases, the penile prosthesis can also migrate forward or backward. It can even perforate the corpora cavernosa and extrude through the penis, an emergency situation that needs to be corrected immediately. There is a remote possibility of gangrene of the penis if infection and extrusion take place simultaneously.

PERSPECTIVE AND PROSPECTS
Penile implant surgery is an excellent and safe procedure for patients who have problems with impotence that is not treatable with medication or with patients going through a gender affirmation surgery. This surgery is more applicable in younger patients who have become impotent, either because of diabetes mellitus or after surgical treatment of prostate or rectal cancer, which can lead to damage of the nerves responsible for erection. An older age is not a contraindication for penile prosthesis and patients with good physical condition and wanting a penile prosthesis will benefit the most. In all cases, it is important that surgery be performed only after a primary evaluation by a urologist and significant counseling to help the patient understand all the benefits and risks prior to the procedure.

The technology involved in penile implant surgery has evolved since the 1970s, starting from a simple, rigid prosthesis and leading to an inflatable, multicomponent prosthesis. The incidence of mechanical failure in the multicomponent inflatable prosthesis is constantly decreasing, and some companies that manufacture this type now offer a lifetime warranty. Penile implant surgery is subject to continuous development that leads to better mechanical reliability and safety.

—*Vaidehi Patel, MS, MS-III*

See also: Diabetes mellitus; Erectile dysfunction; Gender reassignment surgery; Genital disorders, male; Men's health; Prostate cancer; Psychiatry; Reproductive system; Sexual dysfunction; Testicular surgery; Urology.

For Further Information:
Bettocchi, C., F. Palumbo, M. Spilotros, et al. "Penile Prostheses." *Therapeutic Advances in Urology*, vol. 2, no. 1, 2010, pp. 35-40, doi:10.1177/1756287209359174.
Buchanan, Jill. "Penile Prosthesis Insertion." *Health Library*, 26 Nov. 2012.
Carson, Culley C., III. "Penile Prosthesis Implantation: Surgical Implants in the Era of Oral Medication." *Erectile Dysfunction*, edited by Carson and Martin I. Resnick, Saunders/Elsevier, 2005.
———. *Urologic Prostheses: The Complete Practical Guide to Devices, Their Implantation, and Patient Followup*. Humana Press, 2002.
Cavayero, C. T., and G. V. McIntosh. "Penile Prosthesis Implantation." *StatPearls*, 28 Sept. 2021, www.ncbi.nlm.nih.gov/books/NBK563292.
Ellsworth, Pamela, and Bob Stanley. *One Hundred Questions and Answers about Erectile Dysfunction*. 2nd ed., Jones and Bartlett, 2008.
Parker, James N., and Philip M. Parker, editors. *The Official Patient's Sourcebook on Impotence*. Icon Health, 2002.
"Penile Implants." *Mayo Clinic*, 25 Feb. 2011.
Pryor, John P. *Urological Prostheses, Appliances, and Catheters*. Springer, 1992.

Rodriguez, K. M., T. P. Kohn, A. B. Davis, and T. S. Hakky. "Penile Implants: A Look into the Future." *Translational Andrology and Urology*, vol. 6, Suppl. 5, 2017, pp. S860-S866, doi:10.21037/tau.2017.05.28.

Taguchi, Yosh, and Merrily Weisbord, editors. *Private Parts: An Owner's Guide to the Male Anatomy*. 3rd ed., McClelland & Stewart, 2003.

Tanagho, Emil A., and Jack W. McAninich, editors. *Smith's General Urology*. 17th ed., McGraw-Hill, 2008.

Wein, Alan J., et al., editors. *Campbell-Walsh Urology*. 10th ed., Saunders/Elsevier, 2012.

PEPTIC ULCERS. SEE ULCERS.

PERINATOLOGY

Category: Specialty
Anatomy or system affected: All
Specialties and related fields: Embryology, neonatology, obstetrics, pediatrics
Definition: The branch of medicine dealing with the fetus and infant during the perinatal period (from the twenty-eighth week of gestation to the twenty-eighth day after birth).
Key terms:

amniotic fluid: fluid within the amniotic cavity produced by the amnion during the early embryonic period (two to eight weeks) and later by the lungs and kidneys

cesarean section: an incision made through the abdominal and uterine walls for the delivery of a fetus

fetus: the unborn offspring in the postembryonic period, from nine weeks after fertilization until birth

infant: a young child from birth to twelve months of age

ischemia: a local anemia or area of diminished or insufficient blood supply as a result of mechanical obstruction of the blood supply (commonly narrowing of an artery)

placenta: a fetomaternal organ that joins mother and offspring; it secretes endocrine hormones and selectively exchanges soluble, blood-borne substances through its interior structures

Rh: a human blood factor, originally identified in rhesus monkeys, that can be either positive (present) or negative (absent)

SCIENCE AND PROFESSION

Practitioners of perinatal medicine include physicians and advanced practice nurses with a specialty in perinatology (neonatal and pediatric nurse practitioners). They then complete additional training specifically related to the perinatal period (defined variously as beginning from twenty to twenty-eight weeks of gestation and ending one to four weeks after birth). The emphasis of perinatology is on a time period rather than on a specific organ system. The principal event of the perinatal period is birth. Prior to delivery, the perinatologist is concerned with the physiological status and well-being of both mother and fetus. Immediately after delivery, the perinatologist strives to maximize the newborn's chances for survival.

DIAGNOSTIC AND TREATMENT TECHNIQUES

Prior to the birth, several diagnostic procedures are commonly employed by the perinatologist: ultrasonography, the measurement of fetal activity, and the evaluation of fetal lung maturity. Ultrasonography uses sound waves to create images. Sound waves are transmitted from a transducer that has been placed on the skin. Waves that are sent into the body reflect off internal tissues and structures, and the reflections are received by a microphone. Sound travels through tissues with different densities at different rates, which are characteristic for each tissue. Computers interpret the reflected sounds and convert them into an image that can be viewed. The images must be interpreted or read by someone with specialized training, usually a radiologist. Ultrasound does not involve radiation; thus it is not harmful to the fetus. Because sound waves are longer than radiation, the image generated is not as clear as that obtained with electromagnetic waves.

The measurement of fetal activity is important in evaluating fetal health. Fetal movement is normal; the earliest movement felt by the mother is called quickening. The diminution or cessation of fetal movement is indicative of fetal distress. Accordingly, movement is monitored by reports from the mother, palpation by the clinician, and ultrasound: Mothers report movements, individuals examining pregnant women can apply their hands to the abdomen and feel fetal movements, and ultrasonography can show breathing and other movements in real time using continuous video records of fetal movements.

Fetal lung maturity is assessed by measuring the relative amounts of lecithin and sphingomyelin in amniotic fluid. The concentration of lecithin increases late in fetal development, while sphingomyelin decreases. A lecithin-sphingomyelin ratio that is greater than two indicates sufficient fetal lung maturity to ensure survival after birth.

Labor and delivery are the primary events of the perinatal period. Factors that can lead to difficulties include abnormalities of the placenta and prematurity. The placenta can be abnormally located (placenta previa) or can separate prematurely (placenta abruptio). Normally, the placenta is located on the lateral wall of the uterus. Placenta previa is defined as a placenta located in the lower portion of the uterus. The placenta is compressed by the fetus during passage through the birth canal. This compression compromises the blood supply to the fetus, which causes ischemia and can lead to brain or other tissue damage or to death. This condition is usually managed by a cesarean section. Placenta abruptio refers to a normal placenta that separates prior to fetal delivery. This condition is potentially life-threatening to both mother and fetus; immediate hospitalization is indicated.

Prematurity is defined as delivery before the fetus is able to survive without unusual support. Premature infants are placed in incubators. A lack of body fat in the infant leads to difficulty in maintaining a normal body temperature; special heating is provided to offset the problem. Lung immaturity may require mechanical assistance from a respirator. An immature immune system makes premature infants especially susceptible to infections; strict isolation precautions and prophylactic antibiotic therapy address this problem.

Many factors contribute to increasing the risks normally associated with pregnancy and delivery: maternal size and age; drug, tobacco, or alcohol use; infection; medical conditions such as diabetes mellitus and hypertension; and multiple gestations. A woman with a small pelvic opening may be unable to deliver her child normally; the solution in this case is a cesarean section. The risk of genetic abnormalities increases with advancing maternal (and, to a lesser degree, paternal) age. Counseling prior to conception is indicated. Once an older woman becomes pregnant, amniotic fluid should be obtained to test for genetic abnormalities. The degree of surveillance is dependent on maternal age: The recommended frequency of medical checks increases for older women.

Alcohol intake during pregnancy can result in an infant who is both developmentally and intellectually disabled; smoking during pregnancy frequently leads to an infant with a low birth weight. Drug usage during pregnancy can lead to anatomic or mental impairment. Avoiding the use of all substances is the easiest way to eliminate problems completely; any drug should be used only under the guidance of a physician. Some viral infections such as German measles (rubella) early in pregnancy can cause birth defects. Immunization prior to conception will avoid these problems.

Diabetes mellitus can cause abnormally large intrauterine growth and babies (frequently more than 10 pounds and referred to as macrosomic) who are too large for normal delivery. Diabetes that commonly develops during pregnancy is called gestational diabetes. Medical monitoring to detect diabetes early is prudent. Appropriate medical management of preexisting diabetes minimizes problems associated with pregnancy. A macrosomic infant must be delivered with a cesarean section. Hypertension can also develop during pregnancy. Like diabetes, it can compromise both mother and fetus. Appropriate and aggressive medical management, sometimes including complete bed rest, is needed to control high blood pressure during pregnancy. Multiple gestations (such as twins or triplets) strain the supply of maternal nutrients to the developing fetuses. Because space is limited, multiple fetuses are usually smaller than normal at birth.

Rhesus disease, also known as Rh incompatibility, can complicate pregnancy. It can occur only in the child of a father whose blood type is Rh-positive and a mother whose blood type is Rh-negative, and it affects the blood supply of a fetus. The treatment includes the identification of both maternal and paternal blood types and the administration of Rho(D) immune globulin to the mother at twenty-six weeks of gestation and again immediately after birth. An affected infant may require blood transfusions; in a severe case, transfusions may be needed during pregnancy.

PERSPECTIVE AND PROSPECTS

Management of a pregnancy requires specialized skills. As the number of risk factors related to either mother or fetus increases, the problems associated with pregnancy also increase. The care of a pregnant woman and her fetus requires input from many individuals with specialized training. Consequently, perinatology is very much a team effort. Together, the team members can ensure a safe journey through the perinatal period for a pregnant woman and a healthy transition to life outside the womb for a newborn infant.

—L. Fleming Fallon, Jr., MD, PhD, MPH

For Further Information:
Bradford, Nikki. *Your Premature Baby: The First Five Years.* Toronto, Ont.: Firefly Books, 2003.
Creasy, Robert K., and Robert Resnik, eds. *Maternal-Fetal Medicine: Principles and Practice.* 5th ed. Philadelphia: W. B. Saunders, 2004.
Cunningham, F. Gary, et al., eds. *Williams Obstetrics.* 23d ed. New York: McGraw-Hill, 2010.
Martin, Richard J., Avroy A. Fanaroff, and Michele C. Walsh, eds. *Fanaroff and Martin's Neonatal-Perinatal Medicine: Diseases of the Fetus and Infant.* 2 vols. 9th ed. Philadelphia: Mosby/Elsevier, 2011.
Moore, Keith L., and T. V. N. Persaud. *The Developing Human.* 9th ed. Philadelphia: Saunders/Elsevier, 2013.
"Pregnancy and Perinatology Branch (PPB)." *National Institute of Child Health and Human Development*, November 30, 2012.
Ruhlman, Michael. *Walk on Water: Inside an Elite Pediatric Surgery Unit.* New York: Viking-Penguin, 2003.
Sadler, T. W. *Langman's Medical Embryology.* 12th ed. Philadelphia: Lippincott Williams & Wilkins, 2012

PERIODONTAL SURGERY

Category: Procedure
Anatomy or system affected: Gums, mouth, teeth
Specialties and related fields: Dentistry, general surgery, orthodontics
Definition: Any surgical procedure involving tissues or bone associated with support of the teeth.

INDICATIONS AND PROCEDURES

Periodontal disease is the most common cause of tooth loss among persons middle-aged or older. Most periodontal problems originate as dental caries, or cavities, the decay and destruction of teeth by bacteria. While most common periodontal difficulties can be prevented or solved through regular visits to the dentist, if decay is untreated it may lead to serious dental problems. At their worst, periodontal problems may require surgery as part of the treatment.

If decay develops within the root area, a pus-filled abscess may develop. The first indication is an ache or throbbing in the area of the tooth. The gum may be tender and swollen. If the abscess begins to spread, local lymph nodes in the neck may become swollen, as well as that portion of the face. Without proper treatment, the abscess may damage the jawbone or even result in blood poisoning.

The abscess may be eliminated through a root canal procedure, in which the pus is drained and the canal cleaned and filled. If the infection has spread into underlying tissue, however, more general surgery may be required. In a procedure called an apicoectomy, both the root and the bone that covers the root may be drilled away by the oral surgeon. Antibiotics may also be administered to eliminate the infection completely.

USES AND COMPLICATIONS

Most periodontal problems begin with dental caries and gingivitis, an inflammation of the tissue of the gums by bacteria that are associated with the formation of caries. If these conditions are not treated by a dentist in their early stages, they may progress to more serious problems. In addition to the danger of abscess formation, pockets of infection may develop under the gums. Gingivectomy, a minor surgical procedure in which such sites of infection are removed, can usually treat cases that are not advanced.

In most instances, proper oral hygiene is sufficient to prevent problems. When necessary, surgical procedures can treat more advanced cases successfully. Complications are rare and are usually associated with bacteria that are able to survive in isolated crypts. Such sites offer threats of abscess formation. For this reason, the dentist or oral surgeon will monitor the results of the periodontal procedure for some months afterward.

—Richard Adler, PhD

See also Abscess drainage; Abscesses; Cavities; Dental diseases; Dentistry; Endodontic disease; Gingivitis; Gum disease; Oral and maxillofacial surgery; Periodontitis; Plaque, dental; Root canal treatment; Teeth; Tooth extraction; Toothache.

For Further Information:
Chwistek, Marcin. "Root Canal." *Health Library*, Mar. 15, 2013.
Eley, Barry M., M. Soory, and Julius David Manson. *Periodontics*. 6th ed. Edinburgh, Scotland: Saunders/Elsevier, 2010.
Neff, Deanna M., and Laura Morris-Olson. "Periodontal Surgery-Open Flap." *Health Library*, June 4, 2012.
Neff, Deanna M., and Laura Morris-Olson. "Periodontal Surgery-Soft Tissue Graft." *Health Library*, June 4, 2012.
"Periodontal Plastic Surgery." *American Academy of Cosmetic Dentistry*, n.d.
Preus, Hans R., and Lars Laurell. *Periodontal Diseases: A Manual of Diagnosis, Treatment, and Maintenance*. Chicago: Quintessence, 2003.
Renner, Robert P. *An Introduction to Dental Anatomy and Esthetics*. Chicago: Quintessence, 1985.
Ring, Malvin E. *Dentistry: An Illustrated History*. New York: Abradale, 1992.
Rose, Louis F., et al., eds. *Periodontics: Medicine, Surgery, and Implants*. St. Louis, Mo.: Mosby, 2004.
Scully, Crispian, and Athanasios Kalantzis. *Oxford Handbook of Dental Patient Care*. 2d ed. New York: Oxford University Press, 2005.
Taintor, Jerry, and Mary Jane Taintor. *The Complete Guide to Better Dental Care*. New York: Checkmark Books, 1999.

PERIODONTITIS

Category: Disease/Disorder
Also known as: Pyorrhea, gum disease
Anatomy or system affected: Bones, gums, teeth
Specialties and related fields: Dentistry, orthodontics
Definition: A disorder of the teeth resulting from advanced gingivitis, inflammation and infection of the bones and the ligaments supporting the teeth.
Key terms:
calculus: mineralized dental plaque, which forms both above and below the gum line and harbors bacteria that produce toxins and cause the gums to become inflamed
dental plaque: a sticky substance, composed of millions of bacteria, that collects around and between teeth; a major cause of tooth decay and gum disease (gingivitis), it is hard to see because it is whitish colored like the teeth
gingivitis: a disorder involving inflammation of the gums (gingiva)

oral cancer: a disorder involving abnormal, malignant tissue growth in the mouth
periodontal ligament: the connective tissue structure that surrounds the root and connects it with the bone
periodontal pocket: a large pocket that forms between the teeth and gums; it collects plaque, calculus, and debris from food and other sources

CAUSES AND SYMPTOMS

Periodontitis is the advanced stage of gum disease (or periodontal disease) that occurs when the earlier stage of gum disease, gingivitis, is left untreated or if treatment is delayed. Gingivitis is caused by bacteria in plaque and tartar, which if left on the teeth for too long can inflame and infect the gums. In periodontitis, the infection and inflammation spread from the gums (gingiva) to the ligaments and bones that support the teeth. Dental plaque begins to spread down the roots of the teeth, and the gums become infected, which causes damage to the bone and fibers (periodontal ligament) that support the teeth. As the disease progresses, the gums pull away from the teeth, allowing more food and plaque to be trapped under them and inviting more damage to occur. In advanced stages of the disease, the teeth become increasingly loose, and shifting may occur because of widespread damage to the bone and ligaments holding the teeth in place. The bite may therefore shift, and there may be difficulty chewing. Loss of support causes the teeth to become increasingly loose and eventually fall out.

Periodontal disease can be caused by the use of smokeless tobacco. In the areas where the tobacco is held against the cheek, the tobacco and by-products cause irritation and infection of the gums. The gums begin to recede, and periodontal disease affects the teeth in the area. The area is also highly prone to oral cancer.

The early symptoms of periodontitis tend to resemble those of gingivitis, with mouth sores and swollen gums that are tender when touched but otherwise painless. Progressive symptoms include swollen gums that are bright red or reddish-purple. The gums may appear shiny and may bleed easily, and there may be odor to the breath.

TREATMENT AND THERAPY

Treatment methods for advanced (chronic) periodontal disease include aggressive oral hygiene instruction and reinforcement and evaluation of the patient's plaque control. Scaling and root planing to remove microbial plaque and calculus below the gum line, followed by surgery to reduce the depth of the periodontal pocket, is the most common office-based procedure to help manage the disease. Lesions may be treated with adjunctive antimicrobial therapy and

---

INFORMATION ON PERIODONTITIS

Causes: Untreated inflammation or infection of gums; may result from use of smokeless tobacco
Symptoms: Swollen gums that are tender, bright red or reddish-purple, shiny, and bleed easily; mouth sores; bad breath
Duration: Chronic, progressive if not treated
Treatments: Proper oral hygiene, plaque control (scaling, root planing, surgery), antibiotics

---

antibiotics. Long-term maintenance is necessary. Flossing, more frequent brushing, and mouthwashes are recommended to the patient between regular dental visits.

The long-term outcome of treatment may depend upon patient compliance and professional maintenance at appropriate intervals. If the primary teeth are affected, then the infection should be monitored closely in order to avoid possible attachment loss. The goals of periodontal therapy include altering or eliminating the causative microbes and contributing risk factors for periodontitis, thereby arresting advancement of the disease and preserving the teeth. Ultimately, it is desirable to prevent the recurrence of periodontitis. Because of the complexity of aggressive periodontal disease with regard to systemic factors, immune defects, and microbial flora, however, control may not be possible in all instances. In such cases, a reasonable treatment objective is to slow the progression of the disease.

PERSPECTIVE AND PROSPECTS

Periodontitis is the primary cause of tooth loss in adults. This disorder is uncommon in childhood, but the incidence rate increases during adolescence. In addition to a lack of good oral hygiene, certain risk factors have been associated with periodontitis. It is more severe and occurs with a frequency two to five times greater among patients with diabetes mellitus. Smoking can increase the risk of developing severe periodontitis by a factor of three to six times, depending on smoking duration and number of cigarettes.

While periodontitis can be managed effectively with current surgical and nonsurgical therapies in some patients, other patients are less responsive to the treatment options available. Most people with periodontitis receive little or no treatment at all.

—*Jason A. Hubbart, MS*

See also Abscess drainage; Abscesses; Cavities; Dental diseases; Dentistry; Endodontic disease; Gingivitis; Gum disease; Halitosis; Oral and maxillofacial surgery; Periodontal surgery; Plaque, dental; Root canal treatment; Teeth; Tooth extraction; Toothache.

For Further Information:
Detienville, Roger. *Clinical Success in Management of Advanced Periodontitis.* Translated by Nicolai Johnson. Chicago: Quintessence International, 2005.
Edwardsson, S., et al. "The Microbiota of Periodontal Pockets with Different Depths in the Therapy-Resistant Periodontitis." *Journal of Clinical Periodontology* 26, no. 3 (1999): 143-152.
"Gum Disease." *MedlinePlus*, Apr. 25, 2013.
"Gum Disease Information." *American Academy of Periodontology*, 2013.
Healthnet: Connecticut Consumer Health Information Network. "Your Dental Health: A Guide for Patients and Families." *UConn Health Center*, Nov. 27, 2012.
Lamont, R. J., and H. F. Jenkinson. "Life Below the Gum Line: Pathogenic Mechanism of Porphyromonas Gingivalis." *Microbiology and Molecular Biology Reviews* 62, no. 4 (1998): 1244-1263.
Page, R. C. "The Role of Inflammatory Mediators in the Pathogenesis of Periodontal Disease." *Journal of Periodontal Research* 26 (1991): 230-242.
Page, R. C., and K. S. Kornman. "The Pathogenesis of Human Periodontitis: An Introduction." *Periodontology 2000* 14 (1997): 9-11.
"Periodontal (Gum) Disease: Causes, Symptoms, and Treatments." *National Institute of Dental and Craniofacial Research*, Aug. 2012.
Reynolds, J. J., and M. C. Meikle. "Mechanism of Connective Tissue Destruction in Periodontitis." *Periodontology 2000* 14 (1997): 144-157.
Rose, Louis F., et al., eds. *Periodontics: Medicine, Surgery, and Implants.* St. Louis, Mo.: Mosby, 2004.

PERIPARTUM DEPRESSION

Category: Disease/Disorder
Formerly known as: Postpartum depression
Anatomy or system affected: Brain, mind
Specialties and related fields: Obstetrics and gynecology, psychiatry
Definition: A serious but treatable condition that carries risks for the mother and child that involves feelings of extreme sadness, indifference, and, possibly, anxiety and changes in energy, sleep, and appetite.
Key terms:
baby blues: depression affecting a woman after giving birth; symptoms usually lessen without medical intervention
major depressive disorder: a pattern of major depressive episodes that form an identified psychiatric disorder
major depressive episode: a syndrome of symptoms characterized by depressed mood; required for diagnosing some mood disorders
peripartum: pregnancy and the period after delivery.
postpartum: following childbirth or the birth of a baby

CAUSES AND SYMPTOMS

For most women, the symptoms of depression are fairly common in the first week after childbirth. According to *Healthy Children* magazine, approximately 70 to 80 percent of women who have given birth experience the "baby blues" or the "fourth-day blues." These symptoms often disappear or lessen without medical intervention within one or two weeks following birth. In contrast, peripartum depression (PPD; formerly postpartum depression) is more severe and longer-lasting. It occurs in about one in every ten women who have given birth. Additionally, an important distinction between baby blues and PPD is that the blues typically do not interfere with the mother's ability to care for a baby. In contrast, PPD can affect the ability of the mother to care for her child and herself.

PPD symptoms often include sadness, restlessness, guilt, unexplained weight changes, insomnia, frequent crying, irrational fears, irritability, decreased energy and motivation, and even lessened feelings of self-worth. Doctors also look for a depressed mood or a significantly diminished interest or pleasure in nearly all activities. PPD also commonly interferes with a mother's ability to care for the baby.

A personal or family history of depression, bipolar disorders, or other mental illnesses puts one at higher risk for PPD. Other factors that seem to play a role are an unwanted pregnancy, complicated or difficult labor, a fetal anomaly, a lack of social support, and a temporary upheaval, such as a recent move, the death of a loved one, or a job change. Women who have previously suffered from depression following the birth of a child have an increased risk of becoming depressed following a subsequent delivery. In women with a history of PPD, recurrence is about one in three to one in four.

PPD is best understood as resulting from several causes. One factor is that the sudden change in body hormones caused by childbirth can affect the mother's mood. There is also a psychological sense of anticlimax after an event that has been anticipated for many months. Many new mothers are very tired, and some are a little apprehensive and lack confidence about the challenges of motherhood. Another factor would be the sudden change in lifestyle and an associated feeling of shrunken horizons, especially if the mother had been working before the birth. Additionally, environmental, social, and sexual difficulties can predispose some women to develop PPD.

PPD may be accompanied by a rare but severe symptom known as peripartum psychosis. Peripartum psychosis occurs in only one or two out of every 1,000 deliveries. Symptoms may include dramatic mood swings, delusional thoughts about the baby, hallucinations, and severe sleep disturbances. Often a danger with this condition is that the mother contemplates or fears that she will kill her child. When such symptoms develop, immediate care is vital, as it will protect both the mother and the child. Additionally, immediate care will help to reduce the mother's distress, which will, in turn, help her regain her health more quickly and return to healthy mothering after treatment.

TREATMENT AND THERAPY

All new mothers need to be aware of the baby blues and the more serious problem of PPD. Awareness of the possibility of PPD may encourage expectant mothers to better care for themselves psychologically and to prepare in advance for what may be a psychologically and physically challenging first few weeks of motherhood. In terms of prevention, it is important for new mothers to avoid becoming too tired and to obtain assistance in baby and household care as much as possible. The loving support of a husband or significant other, relatives, and close friends is extremely helpful. The baby's father can take turns caring for the baby when the baby is unsettled or distressed. During the day, friends or family can help with shopping or looking after the baby while the mother rests.

If the depression develops and persists, the mother should consult a physician to evaluate for PPD. Antidepressant medication, such as sertraline hydrochloride (*Zoloft*) and citalopram (*Celexa*), are usually effective if administered in the early stages of depression. These two medications are safe during pregnancy and breastfeeding. Counseling is also beneficial to PPD sufferers. In severe cases in which peripartum psychosis develops or the level of depression becomes life-threatening, admission to a psychiatric hospital for treatment may be necessary. Finally, it is important to note that anyone receiving medications, especially antidepressants, should be in regular contact with their physicians. Side effects, such as increased thoughts of suicide, may be an associated risk.

—Alvin K. Benson, PhD, Nancy A. Piotrowski, PhD

For Further Information:
Breastfeeding and Psychiatric Medications. MGH Center for Women's Mental Health, n.d., womensmentalhealth.org/specialty-clinics/breastfeeding-and-psychiatric-medication/. Accessed 10 Apr. 2022.
Depression. MentalHealth.gov, 1 Mar. 2022, www.mentalhealth.gov/what-to-look-for/mood-disorders/depression. Accessed 10 Apr. 2022.
Perinatal Depression. National Institute of Mental Health, n.d., www.nimh.nih.gov/health/publications/perinatal-depression. Accessed q0 Apr. 2022.
Postpartum Depression. Mayo Clinic, 1 Sept. 2018, www.mayoclinic.org/diseases-conditions/postpartum-depression/symptoms-causes/syc-20376617. Accessed 10 Apr. 2022.
Postpartum Depression. Office on Women's Health in the Office of the Assistant Secretary for Health at the U.S. Department of Health and Human Services, 14 May 2019, www.womenshealth.gov/mental-health/mental-health-conditions/postpartum-depression. Accessed q0 Apr. 2022.
Postpartum Support International. www.postpartum.net.
What is Peripartum Depression (formerly Postpartum)? American Psychiatric Society, Oct. 2020, www.psychiatry.org/patients-families/postpartum-depression/what-is-postpartum-depression. Accessed q0. Apr. 2022.

PERISTALSIS

Category: Biology
Anatomy or system affected: Abdomen, gastrointestinal system, intestines, stomach
Specialties and related fields: Gastroenterology, internal medicine
Definition: A series of muscular contractions that sweep along the gastrointestinal tract, causing a localized narrowing that pushes food and waste material from the mouth to the anus for excretion.
Key terms:
digestion: the mechanical and chemical process of breaking down food into small units called molecules, which are then absorbed into the bloodstream
distal: away from the point of origin; for example, the distal esophagus is the end toward the stomach
gastrointestinal motility: the spontaneous movement of the gastrointestinal tract; for example, it includes peristalsis but not chewing
gastrointestinal tract: the digestive tract; a tubelike series of organs that includes the mouth, pharynx, esophagus, stomach, small intestine, large intestine, and anus
involuntary muscle contractions: muscle contractions that occur unconsciously, such as those of the intestines
proximal: toward the origin; for example, the proximal esophagus is the end toward the throat
smooth muscle: muscle that when viewed under a microscope, does not have striations, which are stripes seen in skeletal muscle cells; smooth muscle contracts involuntarily

STRUCTURE AND FUNCTIONS

The gastrointestinal (GI) tract is a muscular tube about ten meters long. It includes the mouth, pharynx, esophagus, stomach, small and large intestines, and anus. The channel running through this tube is the lumen. Food travels through the GI tract to be broken down into molecules. These food molecules then pass through the lining of the GI tract into the bloodstream, a process called absorption. Waste material that is not absorbed is eliminated as feces.

Since digestion, absorption, and elimination occur in different regions of the GI tract, the contents must be pushed aborally, meaning away from the mouth. This occurs by means of peristaltic contractions, which begin with a localized, circumferential narrowing of the lumen. From outside the organ, it would look as if someone had put a tight, invisible ring around the tract, causing a constriction. This constriction sweeps along the digestive tract, pushing the contents aborally. Peristaltic contractions require four major components: the muscular wall of the GI tract, nerve cells in the walls of the GI tract, nervous connections with the brain, and a relay system in the brain. These work together so that the contractions are coordinated on all sides of the lumen and move in the proper direction.

Most of the GI tract is lined with smooth muscle, which is controlled by a part of the nervous system that does not require any conscious effort in order to func-

tion. The wall of the digestive tract contains two layers of muscle. The inner layer consists of several layers of muscle cells arranged concentrically. In the outer layer, the cells are arranged longitudinally. When the inner layer of cells is stimulated by nerves, it contracts, producing a narrowing of the lumen that pushes material aborally. When the outer layer of cells contracts, it shortens the long axis of the GI tract, causing an increase in the diameter of the lumen. This enlargement is especially important in the esophagus, which must sometimes accommodate large pieces of food.

There are two networks of nerve cells in the wall of the GI tract. The important network that affects peristalsis is called the myenteric plexus and is located between the circular and longitudinal layers of muscle cells. It contains nerve cells that receive impulses from nerves coming from the brain and transmit those impulses to the muscle cells. One of the functions of this

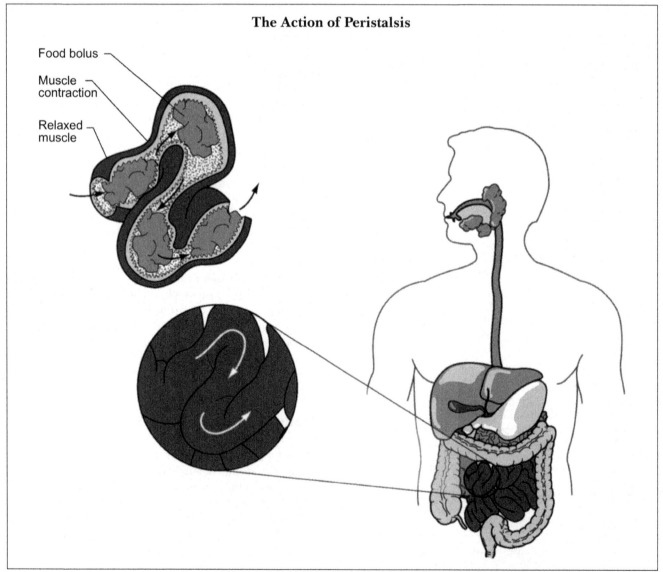

The Action of Peristalsis

Food bolus

Muscle contraction

Relaxed muscle

Peristalsis, the means by which food is moved through the intestines, consists of a constant series of contractions and relaxations of the intestinal walls. ©EBSCO plexus is to help ensure that peristaltic contractions occur in the proper direction. It also enables peristalsis to begin after local distension of the esophagus. If a large piece of food is stuck in the esophagus, peristaltic contractions begin pushing the food down into the stomach.

Nervous connections between the esophagus and the brain influence peristalsis. Some neurons carry sensory information from the esophagus to the brain; this information is important for the brain to be able to sense discomfort in the esophagus. Other neurons carry information from the brain to the esophagus that can modulate the contraction strength and speed of peristalsis. A relay system in the brain stem is involved in the process of swallowing and may also play a role in controlling peristalsis. It is not yet clear to what degree peristalsis is governed by the brain as opposed to the smooth muscle cells or the myenteric plexus.

Peristaltic contractions are measured by means of an instrument called a manometer, which can be advanced into organs such as the esophagus. It monitors increases in intraluminal pressure (pressure inside the GI tract) caused by contractions. A tracing is obtained that plots pressure versus time. Different tracings are obtained for different regions of the esophagus. Thus, in a recording of peristalsis, tracings of the proximal esophagus would show a transient increase in pressure, followed by an increase in pressure in the middle and then the lower esophagus.

Peristaltic contractions differ in the various regions of the GI tract and serve different purposes. In the esophagus, where peristalsis serves to propel food from the pharynx into the stomach, the main type of activity is called primary peristalsis. Initiated by swallowing, it propels material down toward the stomach. Primary peristaltic contractions can push a solid mass of food down the esophagus in about six seconds. With the aid of gravity, liquids do not need peristaltic contractions, as they can pour down the esophagus in one second. Between the lower end of the esophagus and the stomach is a narrowed region called the lower esophageal sphincter (LES). This is an area of muscular circular fibers that normally keep the junction between the esophagus and stomach closed. When food or liquids reach the lower esophagus, the LES relaxes, allowing them to pass into the stomach.

There are two main motility patterns in the stomach and small intestine: fasting and fed patterns. In the fasting pattern, there are long periods of relaxation that alternate with periods of intense, repeated peristaltic contractions. These contraction waves migrate along the stomach toward the small intestine. When viewed on a manometry tracing, they are called migrating motor complexes (MMCs). In the fed pattern,

the motility response varies depending on the content of the meal. Solid meals cause different effects in different parts of the stomach. The proximal stomach is mainly for storing food after eating and for emptying stomach contents. After eating solids, the proximal stomach relaxes to accommodate the food. Later, it slowly contracts, emptying the material toward the small intestine.

The functions of the distal stomach are mixing food with stomach acid and enzymes and mechanically grinding solids into smaller pieces. Solids and liquids are also propelled by peristaltic contractions toward the pylorus, a narrow region separating the stomach from the small intestine. Only material that is finely ground will pass into the small intestine. The small intestine is about five meters long and moves the material coming from the stomach, called chyme, toward the large intestine. During the transit of chyme through the small intestine, water and nutrients are absorbed. Enzymes digest the food particles in chyme down into minute particles, or molecules. These molecules are absorbed through the lining of the small intestine into the bloodstream. Wastes that cannot be digested and absorbed pass to the large intestine, where more fluid is absorbed, leaving a semisolid material called feces.

The motility pattern of the small intestine is similar to that of the stomach during fasting: intermittent periods of peristalsis push material down toward the large intestine. The purpose of this fasting peristaltic activity is to sweep cellular debris and bacteria toward the large intestine. Otherwise, bacteria may overgrow in the small intestine and cause diarrhea. During the fed pattern, there are no prolonged quiescent periods between groups of peristaltic contractions as there are in the fasting state. The function of the fed state is to make sure that the chyme is mixed well with digestive enzymes and that it has an opportunity to come into contact with the absorptive surface of the intestinal wall. As with the rest of the GI tract, small intestinal motility is subject to the brain's control. If a person is placed in a dangerous situation, the brain will send signals to decrease intestinal motility, which will no longer be a priority.

In the large intestine, or colon, peristalsis slowly moves feces toward the rectum for elimination. The slow movement enables most of the water in the feces to be absorbed into the bloodstream. In the proximal large intestine, liquid feces are moved back and forth by contractions, eventually moving distally. In time, this material becomes more solid and moves intermittently toward the rectum. This intermittent peristalsis is called mass movement. It fluctuates during the day, increasing in frequency after meals. As the feces distend the rectum, a reflex occurs that stimulates passage of stool to the outside.

DISORDERS AND DISEASES

Peristalsis may not always progress normally; it may be absent, too vigorous, or uncoordinated. An example of a disorder involving lack of peristalsis is achalasia, which means "failure to relax." In this disease, the LES does not relax, thus impairing the passage of food into the stomach. Another characteristic of the disorder is aperistalsis, which is the absence of peristalsis of the esophagus. One common symptom of achalasia is dysphagia, which is a sensation of food sticking in the throat. Another symptom is regurgitation of undigested food during or just after eating, which often results in weight loss.

The cause of primary achalasia is unknown. Secondary achalasia may be due to infiltrating cancer, radiation damage, or other external factors; in Central and South America, the most common cause is Chagas disease, a parasitic infection. Achalasia is characterized by a reduction in ganglion cells, which are nerve cells that are normally present in the myenteric plexus of the esophagus. There may also be damage to the cell bodies of nerve cells in the brain that innervate the myenteric plexus. It may be that the damaged ganglion cells cause damage to the brain cells, or vice versa. A neural lesion in the LES can lead to a sphincter muscle that fails to relax appropriately, which in turn leads to obstruction of the passage of food. One result is that the esophageal body eventually becomes chronically dilated. Another factor leading to dilation of the esophagus is the loss of ganglion cells in the wall of its body, which results in the absence of peristalsis.

Achalasia usually begins during middle age. The predominant symptom is dysphagia in response to all solids and frequently liquids as well. Eating often causes chest discomfort to the point that people with achalasia lose weight because they avoid eating. Although regurgitation of undigested foods commonly occurs shortly after eating, it may occur hours later, especially when the patient lies down at night. Food contents may be regurgitated and inhaled, leading to nighttime coughing spells.

On manometry, the peristaltic waves normally seen after an act of swallowing are absent. Instead, there may be some low-pressure contractions appearing simultaneously in all parts of the esophagus. Their lack of orderly progression prevents the contractions from propelling food down the esophagus. The pressure in the lumen of the esophagus in the region of the LES may be elevated; often the LES is so tight that it is difficult to advance the manometry catheter through it. The LES also fails to relax normally after swallowing.

Treatment of achalasia rarely results in a return of peristalsis, but it may provide relief for the obstruction caused by a tight LES. Some drugs can relax the LES, but success with these is variable. Often, stretching of the LES with instruments called dilators is performed. The best dilator is a long instrument with an inflatable balloon at the tip. The dilator is advanced into the esophagus and through the LES. The balloon tip is positioned so that when the balloon is inflated, it stretches the LES. The LES needs to be stretched to the point of tearing the circular muscle in order to achieve a long-term reduction in LES pressure. This procedure is risky and may be complicated by the development of a large tear, creating a hole in the wall of the esophagus called a perforation.

Surgical cutting of the LES, called an esophagomyotomy, is more effective than dilation. The more reduction in LES tone that occurs, however, the more likely it is that the person will suffer from reflux of stomach acid. Although the stomach's lining is normally resistant to the irritating effects of acid, the esophagus may become irritated when exposed to chronic acid reflux. A common symptom of this reflux is heartburn, which is a sensation of hot material rising into the esophagus.

An example of too-vigorous peristalsis is esophageal spasm. There are a few different manometric patterns to esophageal spasm, the most consistent being one of intense contractions of the esophagus that do not sweep along its length but occur at the same time at different regions of the esophagus. During manometry, the esophagi of those patients with spasms are often very sensitive to stimulation with certain drugs, resulting in increased strength, or amplitude, of the contractions. Not only is there an exaggerated motor response in esophageal spasm but there may be an abnormal sensory component to the disorder as well. For example, loud noises or stressful mental tasks may cause an increase in the amplitude of contraction waves. Esophageal spasms tend to occur in middle age. The most common symptom is intermittent dysphagia that is variable in severity. It is not progressive and does not result in weight loss. Chest pain is a frequent complaint and may mimic that of a heart attack.

The diagnosis of esophageal spasm often requires manometry. Another useful diagnostic test is to attempt to re-create symptoms of spasm. For example, a drug known to cause smooth muscle contraction is administered. If symptoms similar to the presenting chest pain are re-created, then it is presumed that the pain was attributable to esophageal spasm. Various medications that relax smooth muscle have been used to treat these spasms, with moderate success. Once the medications are stopped, however, the symptoms recur.

Peristalsis requires both an intact myenteric plexus and well-coordinated connections with the central nervous system. Diabetics commonly suffer from neuropathy, a condition that damages various nerve cells in the body. This neuropathy is thought to be responsible for their various gastrointestinal motility disturbances. About 75 percent of diabetics can be shown to have esophageal peristaltic disturbances-up to one-third of diabetics suffer from dysphagia- although they are commonly not felt. Using manometry, an absence of coordinated peristaltic activity is usually found. Diabetics may have tertiary contractions, which are noncoordinated, nonpropulsive contractions of the wall of the esophagus.

Stomach, or gastric, motility is abnormal in about 25 percent of diabetics, resulting in disordered gastric emptying. Emptying of liquids may be normal, but emptying of solids is commonly delayed. There is commonly an absence of MMCs, which results in a decrease in the ability of the stomach to grind food. There may also be spasms of the distal stomach, causing obstructions of materials that would normally flow out of the stomach and into the small intestine. Another gastric disturbance is gastroparesis, a decreased ability of the stomach to propel food along, resulting in a sensation of fullness despite long periods of elapsed time between meals. Because of this, diabetics often have difficulty finishing an entire meal. They may also suffer from nausea, bloating, and vomiting after meals. Treatment of gastroparesis includes reduction of blood sugars if they are elevated. This may be accomplished by reducing food intake (if previously excessive) or increasing the dose of insulin. Medications called prokinetic drugs may increase gastric motor activity; examples of these drugs include metoclo- pramide, dromperidone, and cisapride.

The neuropathy suffered by diabetics may damage the nerves that normally stimulate intestinal reabsorption of fluid; this results in diarrhea, which affects 10 percent of diabetics. Other diabetics suffer from constipation, which may be caused by impaired peristaltic activity of the colon.

PERSPECTIVE AND PROSPECTS

In 1674, the first case of what was probably achalasia was reported by Sir Thomas Willis, who called the disorder "cardiospasm." In 1937, F. C. Lendrum proposed that cardiospasm was attributable to incomplete relaxation of the LES, and he changed the condition's name to achalasia.

Throughout the twentieth century, study of peristalsis advanced in leaps and bounds. In 1927, E. Jacobson reported on an association between esopha-

---

INFORMATION ON PERITONITIS

Causes: Bacterial infection, rupture and perforation of organ (e.g., appendix) or gastric ulcer, postsurgical complications, catheter contamination, pelvic inflammatory disease (PID), complication of ascites in chronic liver or kidney failure

Symptoms: May include severe abdominal pain, fever and chills, diarrhea, inability to pass feces and urine, shock, worsening of renal failure, encephalopathy

Duration: Acute

Treatments: Supportive measures for respiration and circulation, surgery, antibiotics, intravenous fluids

---

geal spasm and strong emotion; gastroenterologists continue to note a correlation between spastic disorders of the GI tract and anxiety. In 1938, E. M. Jones reported an experimental reproduction of esophageal spastic pain by the inflation of small balloons in the esophagus. The development of esophageal manometric techniques advanced significantly in the 1970s. These techniques have allowed a much more thorough understanding of gastrointestinal motility, which enables the development of better drugs to alter it. Therapeutic advances in treating disorders such as achalasia have been made, most notably starting in the 1940s, when A. M. Olsen performed pneumatic dilations of the esophagus.

One of the most practical advances for disorders involving decreased peristalsis has been the development of prokinetic drugs, which increase gastrointestinal motility. Metoclopramide was the first to be developed and is still in use. Cisapride may prove to be effective, especially because its effects do not wear off with chronic use, as do those of metoclopramide.

Perhaps the most important area of research into gastrointestinal motility is the study of the signals for smooth muscle contraction, such as which chemicals (neurotransmitters) are released by the nerve endings where they join up with nerve cells in the myenteric plexus or with the smooth muscle cells. More than fifteen hormones and neurotransmitters are known to affect gastrointestinal motility. Once their specific functions are better understood, researchers can try to develop drugs that mimic their effects, depending on whether an increase or a decrease in motility is desired.

In the United States, some motility disorders are very prevalent, such as irritable bowel syndrome (IBS). This disorder involves symptoms such as abdominal distension, abdominal pain relieved by bowel movements, bowel movements that become more frequent during pain episodes, constipation, and loose stools. IBS accounts for almost as many working days lost to illness as the common cold. It is the most common cause for referral to a gastroenterologist, making up 20 to 50 percent of their referrals. Surveys in the general population have shown that approximately 15 percent of Americans have symptoms to justify a diagnosis of IBS.

Most disorders of peristalsis are not deadly, but they can cause much discomfort. With better understanding of the neurology of the gut, as well as the acceptance of a model for understanding the disorders that includes attention to psychological and sociological effects on the GI tract, medicine will be able to better decrease the suffering that occurs with these disorders.

—*Marc H. Walters, MD*

See also Acid reflux disease; Chagas' disease; Colitis; Colon; Constipation; Crohn's disease; Diabetes mellitus; Diarrhea and dysentery; Digestion; Esophagus; Gastroenterology; Gastroenterology, pediatric; Gastrointestinal disorders; Gastrointestinal system; Intestinal disorders; Intestines; Irritable bowel syndrome (IBS); Obstruction; Rectum; Small intestine.

For Further Information:

Barrett, Kim E., Susan M. Barman, Scott Boitano, and Heddwen L. Brooks. *Ganong's Review of Medical Physiology*. 24th ed. New York: Lange Medical Books/McGraw-Hill Medical, 2012.

DiMarino, Michael C. "Esophageal Disorders." *Merck Manual Home Health Handbook*, October 2007.

"Esophagus Disorders." *MedlinePlus*, June 12, 2013.

Feldman, Mark, Lawrence S. Friedman, and Lawrence J. Brandt, eds. *Sleisenger and Fordtran's Gastrointestinal and Liver Disease: Pathophysiology/Diagnosis/Management*. 9th ed. 2 vols. Philadelphia: Saunders/Elsevier, 2010.

Kapadia, Cyrus R., Caroline R. Taylor, and James M. Crawford. *An Atlas of Gastroenterology: A Guide to Diagnosis and Differential Diagnosis*. Boca Raton, Fla.: Pantheon, 2003.

Peikin, Steven R. *Gastrointestinal Health: The Proven Nutritional Program to Prevent, Cure, or Alleviate Irritable Bowel Syndrome (IBS), Ulcers, Gas, Constipation, Heartburn, and Many Other Digestive Disorders*. 3d ed. New York: Perennial Currents, 2004.

Tortora, Gerard J., and Bryan Derrickson. *Principles of Anatomy and Physiology*. 13th ed. Hoboken, N.J.: John Wiley & Sons, 2012.

PERITONITIS

Category: Disease/Disorder
Anatomy or system affected: Abdomen, gastrointestinal system, intestines
Specialties and related fields: Bacteriology, critical care, emergency medicine, gastroenterology, general surgery, internal medicine, microbiology

Definition: An inflammation of the membrane lining the abdominal cavity (peritoneum), usually secondary to a bacterial infection.

CAUSES AND SYMPTOMS

Peritonitis is an acute condition that typically results from a bacterial infection of the membrane that lines the abdominal organs and the abdominal cavity, known as the "peritoneum." Primary bacterial peritonitis occurs because of a generalized infection, usually by gram negative bacteria such as *Escherichia coli* (*E. coli*) or *Streptococcus pneumoniae*, that seeds the peritoneum. It is a rare but life-threatening condition in children. Secondary bacterial peritonitis, on the other hand, is caused by the rupture and perforation of a hollow organ of the gut, such as with a peptic ulcer or during appendicitis. Other causes of peritonitis include postsurgical complications, catheter contamination in dialysis patients, and infection with enteric bacteria from the gut that can cause pelvic inflammatory disease (PID) in women. One subtype called "spontaneous bacterial peritonitis" is a common complication of ascites seen in chronic liver disease or kidney failure.

The clinical presentation of peritonitis may vary depending on the severity and source of infection and may range from no symptoms to severe abdominal pain, fever and chills, diarrhea, inability to pass stool and urine, worsening of renal failure, shock, and even encephalopathy. Physical examination of patients with bacterial peritonitis may reveal tenderness on palpation of the abdomen with positive rebound tenderness, fluid in the abdominal cavity, and other signs of liver or kidney failure. Patients usually prefer to remain extremely still, finding that even the slightest movement significantly aggravates their pain.

Diagnosis of bacterial peritonitis is confirmed with needle aspiration of fluid from the abdominal cavity under ultrasound guidance, a procedure called "paracentesis." Fluid samples are put through biochemical and microbiological analyses, including cell count, gram stain, and culture, to determine the presence and type of infection. If rupture of a hollow organ is the cause, an X-ray of the abdomen may reveal the presence of air under the diaphragm. Blood cultures may also be useful in diagnosing and evaluating spontaneous bacterial peritonitis and primary peritonitis.

TREATMENT AND THERAPY

The treatment of peritonitis depends on its presentation and cause. Supportive measures to secure adequate respiration and circulation are imperative for patients who are in critical condition. A ruptured internal organ usually must be treated surgically once the patient is stabilized. Infection is managed with intravenous antibiotics. Inadequate or improper management of peritonitis may lead to abscess formation, intestinal obstruction, hepatorenal syndrome, encephalopathy, sepsis, and ultimately death.

Peritonitis is an emergency situation, and it is of utmost importance that the condition be diagnosed and treated at its early stages in order to avoid morbid or even fatal complications. Any case of significant abdominal pain in an at-risk patient must be investigated fully to rule out peritonitis, as prognosis depends directly on time to initiation of appropriate treatment.

—*Joyce Zhang, MD*

See also: Abdomen; Abdominal disorders; Colon; Gastrointestinal disorders; Gastrointestinal system; Intestinal disorders; Intestines; Pelvic inflammatory disease (PID); Small intestine.

For Further Information:

Badash, Michelle. "Peritonitis." *Health Library*, 31 Oct. 2012.

Fry, Donald E. *Surgical Infections*. JP Medical Ltd., 2013.

Icon Health. *Peritonitis: A Medical Dictionary, Bibliography, and Annotated Research Guide to Internet References*. Icon Health, 2004.

Koulaouzidis A., S. Bhat, A. Karagiannidis, et al. "Spontaneous Bacterial Peritonitis." *Postgrad Medical Journal*, vol. 83, no. 980, 2007, pp. 379-83, doi:10.1136/pgmj.2006.056168.

Tholey, Danielle. "Spontaneous Bacterial Peritonitis (SBP)." *The Merck Manual Professional Edition*, Jan. 2021, www.merckmanuals.com/professional/hepatic-and-biliary-disorders/approach-to-the-patient-with-liver-disease/spontaneous-bacterial-peritonitis-sbp.

PERTUSSIS. SEE WHOOPING COUGH.

PET SCANNING. SEE POSITRON EMISSION TOMOGRAPHY (PET) SCANNING.

PHARMACOLOGY

Category: Specialty
Anatomy or system affected: Blood, brain, cells, immune system, nervous system, psychic-emotional system
Specialties and related fields: Anesthesiology, biochemistry, cytology, endocrinology, family medicine, microbiology, oncology, preventive medicine, public health, toxicology
Definition: The science or knowledge of chemicals that affect biological processes.
Key terms:
pharmacist: a person with a license to dispense or sell drugs prescribed by a medical practitioner, such as a dentist, physician, or veterinarian
pharmacognosy: the preparation of medicinal agents from natural sources
pharmacologist: a scientist who studies pharmacology
therapeutics: the use of chemicals in the diagnosis, prevention, or treatment of disease
toxicology: the study of the effects of toxins (poisons) and their antidotes

SCIENCE AND PROFESSION

The science of pharmacology includes the history, source, physical and chemical properties, and biochemical and physiological effects of drugs (therapeutic chemicals, diagnostic chemicals, toxins, and related substances).

"Drug" is a noun in common usage, but it has complex meanings. "Drug" or "medicine" is often used today to indicate a therapeutic substance usually obtained from a pharmacy or drugstore. "Drug" also is used to indicate an illegal substance used for mood-altering effects. Historically, people made their own drugs from materials found naturally in plants, animals, and minerals; some people continue to do so. The term "drug" in this article will focus on the meaning as it is understood by scientists called pharmacologists. Any chemical can be thought of as a drug by a pharmacologist: A drug is simply a chemical that produces a change in a biological process.

Water and oxygen can be thought of as drugs, as can foods and poisons. "Drug," therefore, is a word to indicate an idea, concept, or perception about a chemical. When the chemical, such as oxygen, is causing a change in a biological process, then the chemical is acting as a drug. If the same chemical is causing a change in some other kind of system-for example, causing an iron rod to rust-then the chemical is not acting as a drug. Drugs may be found in nature or made by humans. Most of the chemicals used today as drugs are made by humans.

The biological process that is being changed by a drug may be one occurring in a sick person. Many drugs are used therapeutically-that is, to treat diseases-but pharmacologists do not limit drugs to therapeutic chemicals. They are interested in drug effects on any biological process, even healthy ones occurring in plants and microorganisms, as well as those in animals and humans.

All drugs, even therapeutic drugs, will have several effects on biological processes. Some of these effects are seen only at high concentrations. Unwanted effects, especially if they are injurious, are called adverse effects. A serious adverse effect, especially if it requires special medical treatment, may be considered a toxic reaction, or poisoning. Any chemical that produces an injurious effect, one that is detrimental to a biological process, is called a toxin. The severity of the toxic effect is based on the concentration of the toxic substance. Toxic substances in the environment are called pollutants.

The idea of drug concentration is very important. "Concentration" refers to the number of chemical molecules in a specified volume (such as a teaspoonful, an ounce, or a milliliter) of liquid or gas. Concentration is related to dosage and to the intensity of a drug's effect on a biological process. It is important to remember, however, that the effect of a drug on the body may vary considerably depending on the route of administration. For instance, if one were to eat a drug, then metabolism of the drug is usually very slow, whereas if one were to inject a drug into the bloodstream, then the effects of the drug are observed quite rapidly. Therefore, when pharmacologists discuss drugs and their effects, particularly on humans, they will also frequently discuss the route of administration to make the context of the effect clear.

Concentration and the related concept of dilution are easy to understand. Two spoonfuls of sugar in a glass of water form a more concentrated solution of sugar-water than one spoonful. The more concentrated sugar-water will taste sweeter. Since taste is a biological process caused by a chemical, the chemical (sugar) can be thought of as a drug. The concentration of the chemical affects the biological process. There is a limit, however, to the sweetness of a solution. At some point, more sugar added to the solution will not increase the sensation of sweetness. Adding more sugar may result in a "toxic" reaction of nausea and even vomiting.

There are also different kinds of sugars. When one says that some are sweeter than others, one means that sweeter sugars will be just as sweet at very dilute concentrations as less-sweet sugars at very high concentrations. Thus the first kind of sugar is said to be more potent than the second, even though the second can be just as sweet at high concentrations. Some sugars, however, will not taste very sweet regardless of the concentration. This example illustrates principles that are shared by many drugs. It is important to understand that taking a double dose of a drug will not necessarily produce a double effect. It is also important to understand that a tiny dose of one drug can have the same, or even stronger, biological effect than a large dose of a similar drug.

Most therapeutic drugs act directly on special parts of cells within the body called receptors. A receptor is part of the cell structure, just as a hand is part of human anatomy. A receptor for a specific drug is always located at the same place within a cell, just as the hand is always located at the end of an arm. Yet there are different kinds of receptors, just as people have both hands and feet, found at various locations in cells. Many receptors are found on the cell surface; others are found inside cells. Some receptors are found only on certain types of cells.

Each type of receptor has a specific function, just as hands and feet have specific functions. When a drug "fits" a receptor, like a ball or a glove fits a hand, or how a key fits a lock, the receptor starts the biological process for which the drug is known. Different kinds of drugs can fit a single type of receptor, which explains why different drugs (for example, aspirin and acetaminophen) can have similar effects (relieve pain). Furthermore, one drug may be able to act on several different types of receptors. A receptor, however, can have only one biological response to all the drugs that act on it.

A drug acting on receptors in cells of one organ can affect distant organs. For example, a drug acting on brain cells may cause the nerves acting on blood vessels to increase blood pressure, which can change the heartbeat. The effect of a drug on receptors is usually temporary and should be reversible. In most cases in which a drug works through a receptor, the receptor releases the drug after the two have come together. If this release does not occur, the receptor is said to be blocked. The blockage of a receptor can be therapeutically beneficial, but it may sometimes lead to an adverse reaction.

In humans and animals, most drugs travel in the bloodstream to reach cell receptors. The drug enters the bloodstream after being applied to a body surface or after being swallowed, inhaled, or injected. The effect of the drug is eventually diminished because the body dilutes the drug, chemically alters it (so that it no longer has a pharmacological effect), and eliminates it. Chemical alteration of drugs usually occurs in the liver by a process called biotransformation. Elimination of most drugs, or their biotransformed relatives, usually occurs through the urine but may sometimes occur through secretions (sweat, tears, or breast milk), feces, or even exhaled gases.

DIAGNOSTIC AND TREATMENT TECHNIQUES

Three examples of the use of therapeutic chemicals in the field of pharmacology are anesthesia, cardiac-enhancing drugs, and drugs that fight infections. These examples demonstrate the use of various classes of drugs and provide insight to the variety of drug action.

Anesthetics are chemical painkillers. They are very important drugs, because most diseases are accompanied by pain. Often, the first objective of a patient is to get relief from the pain, even though the anesthetic may do nothing to cure the disease. Pain is a sensation felt in the brain, not at the site of injury. Special nerves at the site of injury send a signal (nerve impulse) to the brain, where it is interpreted as pain occurring at a specific location in the body. Mild pain and severe pain are detected by different kinds of nociceptive (pain) nerves. As pain increases in severity, the brain not only perceives and interprets the pain but also sends out special autonomic signals.

Autonomic signals from the brain serve an extremely important function: They control body functions that do not require conscious thought, such as sweating, heart rate, blood pressure, digestion, and eye focus. Autonomic signals coordinate these functions and change them in response to conditions outside the body. When the body is threatened, such as when a person is frightened, autonomic signals prepare the body to fight or to flee the threatening situation. The pain of surgery causes the brain to send autonomic signals to the body in a defensive state, resulting in sweating and increases in heart rate, breathing, and blood pressure. Additionally, all the muscles of the body will become tense. This defensive state is undesirable during surgery.

Drugs used to relieve pain without causing unconsciousness are called analgesics. Mild pain can usually be controlled with an analgesic such as aspirin. More severe pain may require an opioid analgesic such as morphine. Sometimes, the term "narcotic" is used as a synonym for opioid analgesics, but that term is often used in a legal context to indicate any chemical that can cause dependence (addiction). An analgesic changes the way in which the brain interprets a nociceptive stimulus. The most severe pain, such as that during surgery, is controlled by an anesthetic. An anesthetic may act at a specific site, such as on the nerves of a tooth; a local anesthetic such as novocaine blocks the transmission of the nociceptive stimulus to the brain. Other anesthetics, required for major surgery, cause a loss of consciousness; these are called general anesthetics. As with all therapeutic drugs, the action of an anesthetic is reversible.

A general anesthetic should perform several functions: It should alter the brain's interpretation of pain, cause a temporary amnesia that prevents remembrance of the nociceptive sensation, produce autonomic stability, and cause muscle relaxation. This is much to ask of a single drug. Therefore, general anesthesia is achieved by using several drugs, each capable of accomplishing one or more of the goals.

A general anesthetic agent usually works on nerve cells to provide pain relief and amnesia. These general functions are provided by both kinds of general anesthetics, those that are inhaled and those that are injected. Other drugs are used to control autonomic signals and to provide for muscle relaxation. When the surgery is completed, the patient returns to consciousness as the anesthetic agents are removed from the nerves. This is done by biotransformation and by excretion. Pain immediately after surgery will be controlled by an opioid analgesic. When the pain diminishes as healing progresses, it becomes milder and can be controlled with a nonopioid analgesic.

Drugs are also important in helping people recover from a myocardial infarction (heart attack). The heart is a pump that supplies blood to all cells of the body. Blood carries oxygen and nutrients to the cells and removes waste materials from them. The heart is a living muscle composed of cells, and blood vessels must supply each cell of the muscle. If a blood vessel in the heart becomes suddenly blocked, then the cells served by that blood vessel become starved and die. This is a heart attack. If only a small portion of the heart is injured, the person can survive the attack, especially if drugs are given that strengthen the heart.

An important class of drugs used to strengthen the heart is composed of the cardiac glycosides, such as digitalis. These drugs act to improve the ability of the heart cells to use calcium efficiently. Calcium is essential to maintaining a normal heartbeat. Because a heart attack is painful, it causes a defensive autonomic response from the brain. It is important to use analgesics to relieve the pain and other drugs to control the autonomic response. Another important therapy is to provide more oxygen to the heart. This is done directly, by administering oxygen, but it is also done by using drugs that can remove the blockage from the blood vessel. Since the blockage usually occurs when a blood clot forms in a damaged blood vessel, drugs that dissolve clots can sometimes open the blocked vessel and restore the flow of oxygen-rich blood to the starved cells. A person recovering from a heart attack will sometimes be given drugs to prevent another blockage. Some drugs prevent fatty deposits from forming in the vessels, while others act to slow down clot formation.

Drugs used to treat infection are designed to kill cells. Infection is caused by foreign microbes attacking the body. The microbes may be viruses, bacteria, fungi, or even parasitic worms. Antimicrobial drugs (antibiotics) are given to the infected person to destroy the foreign cells without damaging the patient's own cells. Therefore, the drug must be selectively toxic to the foreign cells. Few drugs are perfectly selective, however, and most have some toxic effects on the patient as well.

There are many ways to develop a selectively toxic drug, but selectivity usually depends on a unique feature of the invading foreign cells, such as the cell walls of bacteria. Human cells are surrounded by cell membranes. Bacteria have cell membranes as well, but they also have cell walls outside these membranes. If the bacterial cell wall is damaged, then the bacterium becomes weakened and can be killed by the body's defense mechanisms. Penicillin is an antimicrobial drug that damages the cell walls of many bacteria. Penicillin has very few adverse effects on the infected person, because human cells do not have cell walls. (Unfortunately, however, some people develop an allergic reaction to penicillin.)

PERSPECTIVE AND PROSPECTS

In the prehistoric world, priests were called upon to intercede for persons suffering from disease and pain. As humans gained experience and developed a means of sharing that experience, especially through written records, it was noticed that certain components of the diet could reliably inflict or relieve pain; these were the first drugs. Similar effects could be obtained by inhaling natural materials or applying them to the skin through rubbing or injection. Such activities were thought to involve supernatural powers, however, and authority to use these drugs was still restricted to members of the priesthood, namely, medicine men or shamans.

Writings about the medicinal properties of natural materials can be found in Chinese, Egyptian, Greek, Indian, and Sumerian manuscripts, some of which are thought to be as much as six thousand years old. The Ebers Papyrus of Egypt (1550 BCE) contains more than eight hundred prescriptions using seven hundred drugs. It was known that some drugs were cathartics, some were diuretics, and others were purgatives, soporifics, or poisons. Yet factual knowledge about why these actions occurred was lacking, in large measure because knowledge of body function and chemistry was lacking. In this absence, people speculated that drug action was due to "essential properties" of the drug, such as warmth or wetness.

Only with the European Renaissance in the early sixteenth century was the domination of religion over intellectual inquiry challenged effectively. The scientific method was applied to questions about the natural world, both physical and living. In 1543, Andreas Vesalius published the first complete description of human anatomy. In the early seventeenth century, William Harvey discovered the circulation of blood, and Antoni van Leeuwenhoek discovered living cells with his microscope. In the eighteenth century, the chemis-

try of oxygen was established by Carl Scheele, Joseph Priestley, and Antoine Lavoisier, and by the end of the century, chemical methods were becoming available to separate pure drugs from crude natural concoctions. In 1806, Friedrich W. Serturner purified morphine from the opium poppy, and in 1856, Friedrich Wöhler isolated cocaine from coca. Also of great intellectual and economic significance was the 1828 synthesis by Wöhler of urea, the first of many chemicals which heretofore had been available only from living organisms. Hormones, general anesthetics, and the bacterial cause of infectious diseases were discovered.

Until the twentieth century, drugs were discovered empirically; they existed in nature and needed to be "found." The knowledge gained during the nineteenth century about how drugs worked enabled pharmacologists of the twentieth century to "design" drugs not found in nature. For example, Paul Ehrlich, a German scientist, announced in 1910 that he had successfully combined a dye that stains bacteria with the poison arsenic to create an antibacterial drug, arsphenamine (Salvarsan), that is highly effective in treating syphilis. In a similar way, the antibacterial sulfonamide chemicals were developed in the 1930s.

It was soon recognized that the powerful effect of pure drugs (in contrast to potions made from natural materials) had the potential to harm as well as to help, to kill or to cure. The safe use of these drugs required special knowledge, so government agencies were established in the twentieth century to regulate drug manufacture and distribution. The original Pure Food and Drug Act, passed by the United States Congress in 1906, imposed quality controls on drug manufacturers. In 1927, Congress created the Food, Drug, and Insecticide Administration (FDIA), to enforce the 1906 law. Until 1914, any drug could be obtained without a prescription; this was changed by the Harrison Narcotic Act. Further limitations on the sale of drugs to the general public came with the Food, Drug, and Cosmetic Act of 1938 and the Durham-Humphrey Amendment of 1951. The Controlled Substance Act of 1970 superseded the Harrison Narcotic Act.

With the passage of time, enforcement responsibilities were changed. The FDIA became the Food and Drug Administration (FDA) in 1931 and was transferred from the Department of Agriculture to what is now the Department of Health and Human Services. The Drug Enforcement Administration for controlled substances was established within the Justice Department.

At the beginning of the twenty-first century, drugs were available to alter personality, to cure some types of cancer, to influence the reproductive system, and to control the body's response to foreign materials such as transplanted organs. Many of these drugs were designed using powerful computers. Drugs were available to alter plant and animal ecosystems. The use of these drugs, such as the pesticide DDT and the wartime defoliant Agent Orange, had devastating effects on humans and the environment that required remedial action. Drugs were even being developed to alter cellular genetics.

—Armand M. Karow, PhD;
updated by Nancy A. Piotrowski, PhD

See also Acid-base chemistry; Aging: Extended care; Anesthesia; Anesthesiology; Antianxiety drugs; Antibiotics; Antidepressants; Antihistamines; Anti-inflammatory drugs; Aphrodisiacs; Bacteriology; Catheterization; Chemotherapy; Clinical trials; Critical care; Critical care, pediatric; Decongestants; Digestion; Drug resistance; Emergency medicine; Enzyme therapy; Enzymes; Fluids and electrolytes; Food and Drug Administration (FDA); Food biochemistry; Genetic engineering; Geriatrics and gerontology; Glycolysis; Herbal medicine; Homeopathy; Hormone therapy; Hormones; Laboratory tests; Melatonin; Metabolism; Microbiology; Narcotics; Oncology; Over-the-counter medications; Pain management; Pharmacy; Polypharmacy; Prescription drug abuse; Psychiatry; Psychiatry, child and adolescent; Psychiatry, geriatric; Rheumatology; Side effects; Sports medicine; Steroids; Substance abuse; Terminally ill: Extended care; Thrombolytic therapy and TPA; Toxicology; Tropical medicine; Veterinary medicine.

For Further Information:
American Pharmaceutical Association. *Handbook of Nonprescription Drugs*. 17th ed. Washington, DC: Author, 2012.
Brunton, Laurence L., et al., eds. *Goodman and Gilman's The Pharmacological Basis of Therapeutics*. 12th ed. New York: McGraw-Hill, 2011.
Griffith, H. Winter. *Complete Guide to Prescription and Nonprescription Drugs*. Revised and updated by Stephen Moore. New York: Penguin Group, 2013.
Liska, Ken. *Drugs and the Human Body, with Implications for Society*. 8th ed. Upper Saddle River, N.J.: Pearson/Prentice Hall, 2009.
Parrish, Richard. *Defining Drugs: How Government Became the Arbiter of Pharmaceutical Fact*. Somerset, N.J.: Transaction, 2003.
PDR for Nonprescription Drugs, Dietary Supplements, and Herbs. 33d ed. Montvale, N.J.: PDR Network, 2012.

PHARYNGITIS

Category: Disease/Disorder
Also known as: Sore throat
Anatomy or system affected: Throat, tonsils
Specialties and related fields: Otorhinolaryngology, pediatrics
Definition: inflammation of the mucous membranes of the pharynx or throat, often caused by a viral infection or bacteria

Key terms:
adenovirus: a group of deoxyribonucleic (DNA) viruses first discovered in adenoid tissue that mostly cause respiratory diseases
cytokines: small proteins, such as interferon, interleukin, and growth factors, that are secreted by certain cells of the immune system and influence other cells
group A streptococci: bacteria commonly found in the throat and on the skin that cause strep throat and impetigo
inflammation: a localized physical condition in which part of the body becomes reddened, swollen, hot, and often painful, especially as a reaction to injury or infection
pharynx: the hollow tube inside the neck that starts behind the nose and ends at the top of the trachea (windpipe) and esophagus (the tube that goes to the stomach)

CAUSES AND SYMPTOMS

Sore throat is the chief complaint of pharyngitis. The throat (pharynx) extends from the nasal passages above and behind the mouth to the esophagus in the neck. Viruses or bacteria infect the pharynx and cause it to swell. The throat often appears red, swollen, or puffy and may have white spots of pus. Goblet cells and submucosal glands produce excessive mucus. White blood cells throng to the site of infection to kill the invading microorganisms and release cytokines. If enough cytokines are released, a fever ensures. Fever and cough are also common, and examination may reveal swollen tonsils. Throat scratchiness, pain when swallowing, enlarged lymph nodes in the neck, cough, and irritation are also common in pharyngitis.

Bacteria and viruses that cause pharyngitis enter the body through the nose or mouth. Sneezing or cough-

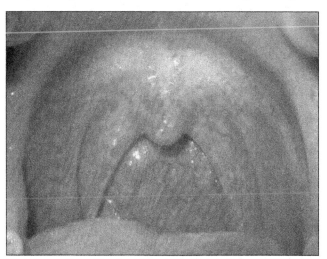

Viral pharyngitis resulting in visible redness. Photo by Dake, via Wikimedia Commons.

ing releases thousands of droplets that contain hosts of infective bacteria and viruses. Droplets can spread up to six and a half feet away. These viruses and bacteria can survive on surfaces for hours. People can contract them by toughing contaminated doorknobs, tables, or other objects and subsequently touching the eyes, nose, or mouth.

Viruses that cause the common cold (coronavirus and rhinovirus) or other respiratory diseases may also produce symptoms of pharyngitis. Epstein-Barr virus bypasses the nose and directly attacks the pharynx. Adenovirus is the second most common cause of viral pharyngitis in children in the United States. Herpes Simplex virus-1 (HSV-1), and sometimes HSV-2, can cause painful blisters in the throat and mouth. Additionally, sinusitis and postnasal drip may irritate the pharynx.

Group A *Streptococcus*, which includes *Streptococcus pyogenes* (*S. pyogenes*), causes "strep throat." If the infection spreads to the tonsils, it is called "tonsillitis." Pharyngitis associated with fever and the appearance of pus on the tonsils may indicate streptococcal pharyngitis, which can be diagnosed by a "quick antigen" test and confirmed by a throat culture.

Persistent pharyngitis accompanied by malaise unresponsive to antibiotics may indicate mononucleosis or other nonbacterial causes such as seasonal allergies, inhaling pollutants such as household cleaners or automobile exhaust, and smoking or exposure to second-hand smoke.

TREATMENT AND THERAPY

Viral pharyngitis is treated with acetaminophen, over-the-counter pain remedies, and warm salt water gargles. HSV pharyngitis is treated with oral acyclovir or valacyclovir for seven to ten days. Bacterial pharyngitis is treated with a course of antibiotics either orally or by injection. For the most part, *S. pyogenes* strains have remained susceptible to penicillin, and strep throat is treated with oral amoxicillin. Treating strep throat quickly (within ten days) is important to ensure that complications like acute rheumatic heart do not occur.

Proper nutrition is important. Zinc boosts the immune system, has some antiviral activity, and relieves soreness. Vitamin C maintains the immune system and the mucous membranes, and beta-carotene restores the integrity of mucous membranes and supports immune function. If the tonsils are chronically infected, they may require surgical removal (tonsillectomy).

PERSPECTIVE AND PROSPECTS

Viruses cause approximately 40 to 60 percent of cases of pharyngitis, and about 15 percent are associated with streptococcal bacteria. In the United States,

> **INFORMATION ON PHARYNGITIS**
>
> **Causes:** Viral or bacterial infection, sinusitis, postnasal drip, mononucleosis, seasonal allergies, pollutants, smoking
> **Symptoms:** Sore throat that is red, swollen, or puffy and may have white spots of pus; fever; coughing; swollen tonsils; throat scratchiness; pain when swallowing; and lymph node enlargement
> **Duration:** Acute
> **Treatments:** Pain medications, warm saltwater gargles, antibiotics, tonsillectomy if needed

children average five sore throats per year and strep infection every four years. Pharyngitis and strep are highest in children between five and eighteen. Pharyngitis is rare in children below three years of age. Adults experience two sore throats per year and strep infection approximately every eight years. Worldwide, the incidence is higher.

—*Marcia J. Weiss, MA, JD*

For Further Information:

Best, Simon. "Pharyngitis." *Johns Hopkins University*, n.d., www.hopkinsmedicine.org/health/conditions-and-diseases/pharyngitis. Accessed 7 Apr. 2022.

Eske, Jamie. "What is Pharyngitis?" *Medical News Today*, 2 Jun. 2021, www.medicalnewstoday.com/articles/324144. Accessed 7 Apr. 2022.

Martel, Janelle. "Pharyngitis." *Healthline*, 7 Mar. 2019, www.healthline.com/health/pharyngitis. Accessed 7 Apr. 2022.

Pharyngitis - Sore Throat. MedlinePlus, 19 Jul. 2021, medlineplus.gov/ency/article/000655.htm. Accessed 7 Apr. 2022.

Pharyngitis (Strep Throat). The Center for Disease Control and Prevention, 1 Nov. 2018, www.cdc.gov/groupastrep/diseases-hcp/strep-throat.html. Accessed 7 Apr. 2022.

Wolford RW, et al. "Pharyngitis." *StatPearls*, 11 Aug. 2021, www.ncbi.nlm.nih.gov/books/NBK519550/. Accessed 7 Apr. 2022.

PHARYNX

Category: Anatomy
Also known as: Throat
Anatomy or system affected: Ear, gastrointestinal system, head, immune system, mouth, neck, nose, respiratory system, throat
Specialties and related fields: Internal medicine, otorhinolaryngology, pulmonary medicine, speech pathology

Definition: The cavity behind the nose and mouth through which air enters the lungs and food and water enter the esophagus.

STRUCTURE AND FUNCTIONS

The pharynx, or throat, is the tube-shaped passageway that begins at the back of the nasal cavity, extends downward behind the mouth, and terminates at the fork of the esophagus and trachea, or windpipe. It comprises three sections: the nasopharynx, just behind the nose; the oropharynx, behind the mouth; and the laryngopharynx or hypopharynx, the remaining area above the esophagus. The pharynx contains lymphatic tissue to fight infection: the adenoids in the nasopharynx and the tonsils in the oropharynx. The left and right Eustachian tubes connect the nasopharynx to the ears and balance air pressure between the middle and outer ear.

Food enters the pharynx from the mouth, while air enters from the nose and mouth. The act of swallowing begins as a voluntary contraction of muscles and continues involuntarily until food passes into the esophagus. In the laryngopharynx, the epiglottis, a flap of connective tissue, prevents food and water from entering the trachea, while the soft palate of the mouth rises to block the nasopharynx so that material stays out of the nose. During vocalization, the pharynx plays a role in shaping the sounds made by the vocal cords, located just below it in the larynx.

DISORDERS AND DISEASES

Most problems in the pharynx arise from infection and inflammation. Pharyngitis, or sore throat, is an acute infection, usually from a virus or streptococcus bacteria, that is most common in children. Similarly, tonsillitis is an infection of the tonsils, quinsy (peritonsillar cellulitis and abscess) affects tissue near the tonsils, and epiglottitis is a bacterial infection of the epiglottis. Abscesses, with or without inflammation, may also occur in the pharynx; cysts known as Tornwaldt cysts may occur in the midline of the nasopharynx; and contact ulcers may result from damage to the pharyngeal tissue caused by swallowing something chemically harsh or physically abrasive or jagged.

Although not common, throat cancers can occur in the nasopharynx and tonsils. They are usually squamous cell carcinomas and occur predominantly in males, usually due to smoking and alcohol consumption.

People with cleft palates may not have complete closure of the nasal passage during swallowing, a condition called velopharyngeal insufficiency. The condition can impair speech and give it a marked nasal sound.

—*Roger Smith, PhD*

See also Common cold; Decongestants; Laryngectomy; Laryngitis; Mouth and throat cancer; Nasal polyp removal; Otorhinolaryngology; Pharyngitis; Plastic surgery; Respiration; Sinusitis; Smell; Sore throat; Strep throat; Tonsillectomy and adenoid removal; Tonsillitis; Tonsils; Voice and vocal cord disorders.

For Further Information:
Beers, Mark H., et al., eds. *The Merck Manual of Medical Information.* 2nd home ed. Whitehouse Station, N.J.: Merck Research Laboratories, 2003.
Parker, Steve. *The Human Body Book.* 2nd ed. New York: DK Adult, 2013.
PM Medical Health News. *21st Century Complete Medical Guide to Throat and Pharynx Disorders: Authoritative Government Documents, Clinical References, and Practical Information for Patients and Physicians.* Mount Laurel, N.J.: Progressive Management, 2004.
Sasaki, Clarence T. "Introduction: Throat Disorders." *Merck Manual Home Health Handbook,* July 2008.
Thibodeau, Gary A., and Kevin T. Patton. *Structure and Function of the Human Body.* 14th ed. St. Louis, Mo.: Mosby/Elsevier, 2012.
"Throat Disorders." *MedlinePlus,* June 16, 2013.

PHENYLKETONURIA (PKU)

Category: Disease/Disorder
Also known as: Phenylalaninemia, phenylpyruvic oligophrenia, Følling's disease
Anatomy or system affected: Blood, brain, liver, nervous system
Specialties and related fields: Biochemistry, embryology, epidemiology, genetics, neonatology, neurology, nutrition, pediatrics
Definition: A genetic disorder caused by a deficiency of the liver enzyme phenylalanine hydroxylase.
Key terms:
phenylalanine: an essential amino acid
phenylalanine hydroxylase: a liver enzyme that catalyzes the conversion of phenylalanine to tyrosine
tetrahydrobiopterin: a cofactor for the conversion of phenylalanine to tyrosine

CAUSES AND SYMPTOMS

Phenylketonuria (PKU) is a genetic disorder, occurring in about one in 10,000 births, that disrupts the metabolism of the amino acid phenylalanine. The disorder is caused by a deficiency of phenylalanine hydroxylase, a liver enzyme that catalyzes the conversion of phenylalanine to tyrosine. Since normal phenylalanine metabolism is blocked, the amino acid accumulates in blood and tissues, resulting in progressive, irreversible intellectual disabilities and neurological abnormalities. Most forms of PKU are caused by a mutation-more than two hundred mutations are now characterized-in the gene for phenylalanine hydroxylase. A small percentage of infants with PKU have a variant form of the condition, known as malignant PKU. This disorder is caused by a defect in the synthesis or metabolism of tetrahydrobiopterin, a cofactor for the conversion of phenylalanine to tyrosine, or in other enzymes along the pathway. Without treatment, malignant PKU causes a progressive, lethal deterioration of the central nervous system.

Infants with classic and malignant PKU appear normal; however, if untreated, the condition severely impairs normal brain development and growth after a few months of age, causing intellectual disabilities, seizures, eczema, and neurological and behavioral problems. Affected infants have plasma phenylalanine levels ten to sixty times above normal, along with normal or reduced tyrosine levels and high concentrations of the metabolite phenylpyruvic acid in their urine.

Newborns are screened routinely for PKU within the first three weeks of life, usually by using whole blood obtained from a heel prick. Elevated phenylpyruvic acid levels also can be detected in urine of infants with PKU after adding a few drops of 10 percent ferric chloride, resulting in a deep green color. Newborns often have transient PKU-elevated phenylalanine and phenylpyruvic acid levels in the first few weeks of life that normalizes-so classic PKU should be distinguished from transient conditions. Elevated phenylalanine levels that persist beyond a few weeks of life, accompanied by normal or low tyrosine levels, usually indicate an inborn error of metabolism. Malignant PKU is usually diagnosed by detecting biopterin metabolites in urine or showing that tetrahydrobiopterin supplementation restores normal phenylalanine and tyrosine levels.

Babies of mothers with PKU are at high risk of brain damage, impaired growth, and malformations of the heart and other organs. Managing maternal phenylalanine levels at near normal concentrations appears to be crucial to preventing these cognitive and neurological defects.

The clinical basis for the damaging effects of PKU on the brain is unclear. Elevated phenylalanine levels may interfere with brain myelination or neuronal migration during development. In addition, PKU decreases the levels of the neurotransmitters dopamine and serotonin, which may be the basis for its neurological effects.

TREATMENT AND THERAPY

The detrimental effects of PKU can largely be controlled by maintaining phenylalanine levels in the normal range through a strict low-phenylalanine diet. This complex diet, often supplemented with tyrosine, prevents the buildup of phenylalanine and its metabolites in body tissues. Children whose phenylalanine

---

> **INFORMATION ON PHENYLKETONURIA (PKU)**
>
> **Causes:** Genetic disorder
> **Symptoms:** If untreated, irreversible intellectual disabilities and neurological abnormalities, seizures, eczema, behavioral problems
> **Duration:** Typically chronic, sometimes progressive
> **Treatments:** Strict low-phenylalanine diet, drug therapy

---

levels are regularly monitored and managed can achieve normal intelligence and development. In infants with malignant PKU, tetrahydrobiopterin or cofactor supplements are required to control phenylalanine levels successfully.

Treatment for PKU must begin at a very early age, before the first three months of life, and usually continue through adulthood, or else some degree of intellectual disability or neurological abnormality is expected. Screening newborns for PKU before three weeks of age is mandated in all fifty US states. Strict control of phenylalanine levels also is indicated for pregnant women with PKU because their babies are at high risk for severe brain damage.

The successful treatment of PKU depends on managing phenylalanine levels. However, the diet is complex and challenging to sustain over many years. Since phenylalanine is an essential amino acid, found in virtually all proteins, maintaining adequate nutrition is nearly impossible on a low-phenylalanine diet. The treatment requires rigorous protein restriction and the substitution of most natural proteins in meat, fish, eggs, and dairy products. Phenylalanine intake must not be too restricted, however, or else phenylalanine deficiency can occur.

In some cases, dietary treatment for PKU can be discontinued or made less restrictive as children age, without causing severe effects. In many cases, however, the ill effects of the disorder carry into adulthood unless dietary management is continued over the long term. Untreated adolescents and adults may exhibit behavioral or neurological problems, difficulty concentrating, poor visual-motor coordination, and a low intelligence quotient (IQ).

PERSPECTIVE AND PROSPECTS

Phenylketonuria was the first inborn error of metabolism shown to affect the brain. This genetic disorder was discovered in the 1930s by Ivar Asbjørn Følling. Since its discovery, PKU has been controlled successfully by rigorous newborn screening programs and careful dietary management of phenylalanine levels in pregnant women and in children with the disease.

Newer research has focused on improving medical formulations for low-phenylalanine diets and amino acid supplementation for children and adults.

In the 1980s, clinical trials examined the use of dialysis-like procedures that allowed the rapid breakdown of phenylalanine in the blood. The treatment applies to pregnant women with PKU or those with severely elevated phenylalanine levels resulting from stress or illness. In the late twentieth century, PKU became the focus of gene therapy research. Animal models of PKU have been successfully treated by introducing normal phenylalanine hydroxylase deoxyribonucleic acid (DNA) into the liver cells of mice. Since the underlying genetic defects are known in most cases of PKU, gene therapy appears a likely research focus for long-term treatment.

—*Linda Hart, MS, MA*

See also Digestion; Enzymes; Genetic diseases; Intellectual disability; Metabolic disorders; Metabolism; Neonatology; Nervous system; Neurology, pediatric; Nutrition; Screening.

For Further Information:
Behrman, Richard E., Robert M. Kliegman, and Hal B. Jenson, eds. *Nelson Textbook of Pediatrics*. 19th ed. Philadelphia: Saunders/Elsevier, 2011.
Chopra, Sanjiv. *Dr. Sanjiv Chopra's Liver Book: A Comprehensive Guide to Diagnosis, Treatment, and Recovery*. New York: Simon & Schuster, 2002.
Kimball, Chad T. *Childhood Diseases and Disorders Sourcebook: Basic Consumer Health Information About Medical Problems Often Encountered in Pre-adolescent Children*. Detroit, Mich.: Omnigraphics, 2003.
Marlow, Amy. "Phenylketonuria." *Health Library*, November 26, 2012.
Martin, Richard J., Avroy A. Fanaroff, and Michele C. Walsh, eds. *Fanaroff and Martin's Neonatal-Perinatal Medicine: Diseases of the Fetus and Infant*. 9th ed. St. Louis, Mo.: Mosby/Elsevier, 2011.
MedlinePlus. "Phenylketonuria." *MedlinePlus*, May 13, 2013.
Moore, Keith L., and T. V. N. Persaud. *The Developing Human*. 9th ed. Philadelphia: Saunders/Elsevier, 2013.
National PKU News. *National PKU News*, March 2013.
Parker, James N., and Philip M. Parker, eds. *The Official Parent's Sourcebook on Phenylketonuria*. San Diego, Calif.: Icon Health, 2002.

PHLEBITIS

Category: Disease/Disorder
Anatomy or system affected: Blood vessels, circulatory system
Specialties and related fields: General surgery, internal medicine, vascular medicine
Definition: The inflammation of a vein, often seen in conjunction with blood clots within the deep and superficial veins outside the heart.

Key terms:
embolus: a detached blood clot that may travel through the venous system to lodge in other major veins, such as a pulmonary embolus, which may cause blockage of the major blood vessels within the lungs
endothelial damage: disruption of the cellular lining of a blood vessel such as a vein; part of Virchow's triad
hypercoagulability: an increase in the ability of blood to clot or to change from a liquid state to a solid one; coagulation of blood is dependent upon activation of clotting agents within the body
stasis: stagnation of blood or the failure of blood to flow; venous stasis may be the result of obstructions to outflow from the veins
superficial thrombophlebitis: inflammation and clotting of the veins of the arms and/or legs that lie just beneath the surface of the skin and drain into the deep veins of the limbs
venous thrombosis: formation of a blood clot within the veins of the body

CAUSES AND SYMPTOMS

Phlebitis, meaning the inflammation of a vein, is a general term used to describe the presence of blood clots, or thrombi, in the veins of the body outside the heart. Blood clots because of the formation of clotting agents, such as fibrin. When blood clots within the body, there are three principal factors involved: damage to the venous endothelium, the cells that form the lining of the vein; venous stasis, or failure of the blood to flow; and hypercoagulability, or an increase in clotting factors in the blood. These three features associated with phlebitic episodes-endothelial damage, stasis, and hypercoagulability-are referred to as Virchow's triad (named for Rudolf Virchow, who in 1846 described the characteristics of thrombus formation in the deep veins of the lower extremities).

Patients with phlebitis will complain of swelling, tenderness, and inflammation of the affected limb. If the clot has formed in the veins just beneath the surface of the skin, they may feel a hard, cordlike structure in the segment of the vein that is filled with a thrombus. If the blood clot has not attached firmly to the wall of the vein, it may break loose and travel in the bloodstream to enter the vessels within the lung. These traveling clots are known as emboli and, depending on their size, they may either dissolve in the pulmonary vessels of the lung or block major vessels, preventing blood flow to that part of the lung. It has been shown that there is a greater risk of pulmonary embolism if the venous clots are formed in the leg veins above the knee than if phlebitis occurs in the calf veins.

To understand the factors that predispose the blood to clot within the body, it is necessary to understand the anatomy of the venous system and the mechanisms by which blood flows through the veins. Approximately 75 percent of the body's blood is found in the venous system, which is divided into three parts: the superficial veins, the deep veins, and the perforating, or communicating, veins. The superficial veins of the extremities are large, thick-walled, muscular structures that lie just beneath the skin. The deep veins are thin-walled and less muscular than the superficial veins. In the extremities, these deep veins are named after the arteries that they accompany. Blood is transported from the superficial to the deep veins by the communicating veins, or perforators. Thin, leaflike, bicuspid valves are found in most veins of the body, even in venules as small as 0.15 millimeter in diameter. These valves can open readily to allow blood to pass as it moves from the superficial to the deep veins on its return trip to the heart and can close rapidly to prevent blood flow from moving in the reverse direction. There are more valves in the veins of the calf than there are in the thigh veins, and no valves are found in the common iliac veins of the pelvis or in the inferior vena cava (the deep vein that transports blood through the abdomen).

The venous system must perform four important body functions. First, the veins must return blood that has been pumped through the arteries back to the heart. Additionally, the veins must be able to expand and contract so that they can regulate the increases and decreases in blood volume in the body. They must be responsive to the transport of blood during exercise and, along with the capillaries, play a major role in regulating body temperature.

Veins have the unique feature of being able to change their shape and size in order to respond to changes in pressure from within the vein (caused by increased fluid volume in the body) and to pressure from outside the vein (from tissue fluids and changes in pressure that occur as a result of gravity and the weight of the column of blood in the veins when one is standing or sitting up). As an example, when a hand is hanging at the side of the body, the veins on the back of the hand are full and visible because the veins are full of blood and the internal venous pressure is greater than the pressure from outside the vein. If the hand is raised over the head, the veins collapse because of the changes in internal venous pressure and gravitational and hydrostatic pressure, the pressures on the outside of the vein.

Blood is pumped under pressure by the heart to the arteries in order to supply nutrients and oxygen to the tissues. In contrast, the heart has little influence on moving blood through the low-pressure veins of the body on its return trip. Blood is returned from the extremities to the heart and lungs by contraction of the calf muscles during exercise and by changes in the intra-abdominal and intrathoracic pressures that occur with respiration. For example, with a limb at rest, blood will flow toward the heart from the superficial system to the deep veins via the perforating veins as a result of the changes in abdominal and thoracic pressures that occur with breathing. With exercise, the calf muscles may exert more than 200 millimeters of mercury (mmHg) pressure on the large, saclike veins, the sinusoids in the sole, and the gastrocnemius veins of the calf, causing blood to move rapidly out of the foot and calf.

If the valves are incompetent such that the leaflets fail to meet when the valve closes, the column of forward-moving blood cannot be maintained in the segments of the veins between the valve sites. In this case, when one stops exercising, blood will flow backward toward the feet through the damaged valves, resulting in increased venous pressure at ankle level.

As one inhales, the diaphragm descends, compressing the inferior vena cava and stopping the flow of blood from the legs. With exhalation, the diaphragm rises and venous flow will continue toward the heart in a competent venous system. It is interesting that flow in the arms is under the control of intrathoracic, rather than intra-abdominal, pressure changes. Thus, with inhalation, the flow of blood from the arms increases as the pressure within the chest cavity is reduced. Upon exhalation, venous flow from the arms is impeded (which is in contrast to the respiratory effects that influence venous return from the legs).

As long as blood continues to circulate, the likelihood of clotting is reduced. There are, however, several risk factors that may cause changes in blood flow, damage to the vein wall, or hypercoagulability of the blood-the three features involved in venous thrombosis.

Venous thrombosis may occur as a result of obstructions to venous outflow from the limb. For example, taking a long trip by car, train, or airplane may require sitting for many hours without the freedom to walk around and exercise the calf muscles. Because the calf muscle pump is inactive, blood will pool in the veins of the legs. This failure of blood to flow, or venous stasis, places the individual at increased risk for clotting of blood in the calf veins. Similarly, patients who are prescribed bed rest because of accidents, pregnancy, or critical illnesses and those patients who undergo long surgical operations are at risk for forming thrombi in the leg veins because of venous stasis and, as a result of the thrombosis, are also at risk for pulmonary embolism.

The incidence of phlebitis increases linearly with age. This fact is thought to reflect an increase in the diameter of the veins and the venous sinusoids within the calf muscles as a result of loss of elastic tissue in the vein walls. As the vein diameter increases, venous flow becomes sluggish. As an individual grows older, the muscle mass in the thigh and calf decreases and the calf muscle pump becomes less effective at moving venous blood toward the heart. This pooling of blood places elderly patients at risk for phlebitic episodes.

In the modern health care setting, the most common cause of phlebitis has been injury to the vein wall by intravenous catheters or by the infusion of drugs that cause inflammation of the venous endothelium. If a catheter is left in place for an extended period of time, infection may occur within the vein along its course, causing inflammation of the vein wall, venous stasis, and eventual thrombosis of the vein.

Inflammation of the vein may also occur as a result of venography, an invasive procedure used to determine if thrombi are present in the deep or superficial veins of patients. With this test, contrast dyes are injected into the veins to delineate the blood-flow patterns and venous anatomy and to define the segments of the vein where clots are present and are obstructing blood flow. Approximately 3 percent of patients have thrombi form in their veins following this diagnostic procedure. Approximately 8 percent of these patients will require hospitalization for treatment of postvenographic phlebitis.

Women who are taking oral contraceptives containing the hormone estrogen are thought to be at increased risk for phlebitis because of the decrease in the muscular tone of the vein wall and subsequent decrease in velocity of blood flow in the veins that results from the use of these drugs. Estrogen compounds may increase the surface adhesiveness of platelets, the blood cells that are responsible for clotting, causing them to stick together and form large clots that can block the veins. Additionally, estrogen compounds may influence chemicals within the blood that affect its ability to clot. Specifically, it is thought that these hormonal compounds affect clotting factors II, VII, VIII, and X and also cause a decrease in antithrombin III, a

chemical that influences the production of thrombin, the principal factor controlling the formation of thrombi.

The influence of estrogen on the body's ability to control the production of appropriate levels of clotting factors is also noted during pregnancy and in the postpartum period. Phlebitis is diagnosed three to six times more frequently in women in the first four months following delivery than it is in women who have not become pregnant, as a result of estrogen-induced hypercoagulability of the blood. It is also interesting to note that women who deliver their babies by cesarean section are at increased risk for thrombophlebitis because of venous stasis occurring during the more prolonged recovery period that follows surgical delivery.

TREATMENT AND THERAPY
The symptoms of phlebitis-unilateral limb swelling, local inflammation, tenderness, and pain-may be associated with other medical conditions. Because there are no specific signs that are used to diagnose deep or superficial venous thrombosis, physicians misdiagnose phlebitis in approximately 50 percent of cases. As noted above, venography, once thought to be the standard for the identification of venous thrombosis, may actually predispose the patient to phlebitis. Noninvasive diagnostic techniques have been developed to demonstrate the presence, location, extent, and severity of the thrombotic process.

It has been shown that chemicals found naturally in the endothelial cells that line the veins can lyse, or dissolve, small clots. The veins of the calf have more lytic potential than the veins of the thigh and pelvis. In exercise, the compression of the calf muscles on the veins causes this material to be forced into the venous blood, thus helping to dissolve small thrombi.

Acute thrombosis of the deep veins above the knee usually requires hospitalization and infusion of heparin, a drug that prevents further clotting, allowing the body's mechanism to dissolve clots to act more quickly and effectively. If left untreated, clots in this location may continue to propagate toward the large pelvic veins or the inferior vena cava, or pieces of a thrombus, called emboli, may break off the clot and travel through the vena cava to enter the pulmonary circulation of the lungs. In many cases, pulmonary embolism is life-threatening.

Patients with clots in the deep veins of the legs are instructed to stay in bed with the leg elevated to prevent venous pooling, and moist heat is applied to the leg to promote local circulation of blood. Patients will continue to take anticoagulant drugs for several months following hospitalization to ensure that fresh clots do not form in the veins, and they are instructed to wear elastic compression stockings to promote venous circulation.

It has been shown that clots will resolve completely in approximately 70 percent of patients receiving anticoagulant therapy. The remainder of patients will continue to have obstructions of their veins because of a clot that did not lyse, and as a result of the phlebitic episode, the venous valves will become incompetent. These patients will continue to be at risk for phlebitis and frequently express complaints of having tired, aching, heavy legs. If damage to the valves is severe, venous pressure at ankle level is increased, and blood may be forced out of the veins into the surrounding tissues, causing ulcers to form.

Thrombosis of the superficial veins, frequently called thrombophlebitis, is most often treated with hot compresses and elevation of the leg to relieve the local venous inflammation. Care must be taken to ensure that the clot does not continue to extend toward the segment of superficial vein where it joins the deep venous system, because the patient would then be at risk for pulmonary embolism.

Attempts have been made to bypass segments of a thrombosed vein surgically and to transplant new valves in venous segments that have become incompetent as a result of postphlebitic valve damage. Such procedures, however, have been unrewarding. Anticoagulant and lytic therapies begun early in the thrombotic process appear to offer the best results with the least long-term sequelae for phlebitic patients.

PERSPECTIVE AND PROSPECTS
It has been estimated that approximately two million people are affected by phlebitis each year in the United States and that there are approximately two hundred thousand deaths per year as a result of venous thrombosis. Autopsy data suggest that 1 to 2 percent of phlebitic patients will die from pulmonary embolism each year.

—*Marsha M. Neumyer*

See also Arteriosclerosis; Blood and blood disorders; Blood vessels; Bypass surgery; Circulation; Deep vein thrombosis; Embolism; Surgery, general; Thrombosis and thrombus; Varicose veins; Vascular medicine; Vascular system; Venous insufficiency.

For Further Information:
Bick, Roger L. *Disorders of Thrombosis and Hemostasis: Clinical and Laboratory Practice*. 3d ed. Philadelphia: Lippincott Williams & Wilkins, 2002.
Furtado, LuÃs Carlos do Rego. "Incidence and Predisposing Factors of Phlebitis in a Surgery Department." *British Journal of Nursing* (July 28, 2011): S16-25.
Icon Health. *Phlebitis: A Medical Dictionary, Bibliography, and Annotated Research Guide to Internet References*. San Diego, Calif.: Author, 2004.
Kohnle, Diana. "Phlebitis." *Health Library*, September 26, 2012.
Litin, Scott C., ed. *Mayo Clinic Family Health Book*. 4th ed. New York: HarperResource, 2009.
Loscalzo, Joseph, and Andrew I. Schafer, eds. *Thrombosis and Hemorrhage*. 3d ed. Philadelphia: Lippincott Williams & Wilkins, 2003.
Rutherford, Robert B., ed. *Vascular Surgery*. 6th ed. Philadelphia: Saunders/Elsevier, 2005.
"Thrombophlebitis." *MedlinePlus*, May 6, 2011.

PHLEBOTOMY

Category: Procedure
Also known as: Venipuncture
Anatomy or system affected: Arms, blood, blood vessels, cells, circulatory system
Specialties and related fields: Hematology
Definition: The collection of blood specimens for analysis.

INDICATIONS AND PROCEDURES
Phlebotomy is performed to acquire blood samples for microbiology, cytology, fluid analysis, or other testing. Blood collection tubes are drawn in a specific order to avoid cross-contamination of additives in tubes designed for specific tests. Collection tubes are color-coded according to the additives (if any) contained within them. An essential component of the procedure is the accurate labeling of tubes with information identifying the patient. Blood collection should be carried out only by a licensed phlebotomist.

A temporary tourniquet is applied to the arm three to four inches above the selected puncture site, the skin is cleaned with an alcohol or iodine wipe, and then a needle is inserted into a vein (venipuncture). Blood can also be collected from an artery or fingerstick, if appropriate. Often, the skin is palpated and the vein is traced with a finger, or the arm may be massaged until a superficial vein is readily apparent. After one or more tubes of blood (typically about ten milliliters in volume) are collected, a gauze sponge is applied until bleeding stops and then an adhesive bandage is applied. The tourniquet is immediately removed after the last tube to be drawn starts to fill. The entire procedure takes only a few minutes.

When smaller volumes of blood are required, collection can be accomplished by a simple fingerstick on the third or fourth finger of the nondominant hand, using a sterile lancet. The first drop of blood is wiped away, and then blood is collected into a capillary tube while the finger is gently massaged. After the fingerstick procedure, the patient normally is in-

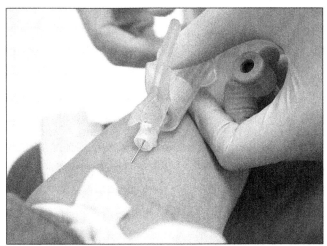

A phlebotomist draws blood from a patient. (© Francis Twitty/ iStock-photo.com)

structed to hold a small gauze pad over the puncture site for a few minutes to stop the bleeding. For blood collection on a newborn baby or infant, the heel is the recommended puncture site.

USES AND COMPLICATIONS

Phlebotomy is a routine procedure with minimal risks. Trained phlebotomists take precautions to protect themselves and the patient from exposure to blood-borne diseases and to prevent the occurrence of infection. These precautions include the use of rubber or latex gloves and only new, sterile disposable tubes and needles. Most frequently, blood is taken from the larger and fuller median cubital and cephalic veins of the arm; wrist and hand veins can also be acceptable. Certain areas are avoided in venipuncture: extensive scar tissue from burns or injury, the site of a previous mastectomy, regions of hematoma, sites of intravenous (IV) therapy and blood transfusion, cannula or fistula devices, and extremities suffering from edema. Some patients may experience light-headedness or even faint during blood collection; to prevent accidents, the patient remains seated during the brief procedure.

—*Michael R. King, PhD*

See also Bleeding; Blood and blood disorders; Blood banks; Blood testing; Blood vessels; Circulation; Hematology; Hematology, pediatric; Laboratory tests; Transfusion.

For Further Information:

Garza, Diana, and Kathleen Becan-McBride. *Phlebotomy Handbook: Blood Collection Essentials*. 7th ed. Upper Saddle River, N.J.: Pearson/Prentice Hall, 2005.

Hoeltke, Lynn B. *The Complete Textbook of Phlebotomy*. 4th ed. Albany, N.Y.: Delmar, 2012.

McCall, Ruth E., and Cathee M. Tankersley. *Phlebotomy Essentials*. 5th ed. Baltimore: Wolters Kluwer/Lippincott Williams & Wilkins, 2012

"Venipuncture." *MedlinePlus*, August 31, 2011.

PHOBIAS

Category: Disease/Disorder
Anatomy or system affected: Psychic-emotional system
Specialties and related fields: Psychiatry, psychology
Definition: Excessive fears of certain objects, people, places, or situations.

CAUSES AND SYMPTOMS

Phobias can induce a state of anxiety or panic, often debilitating sufferers, restricting them from full freedom of action, career progress, or sociability. For example, a heterosexual person who fears talking with the opposite sex will have problems dating and progressing socially.

Fear serves an important and necessary function in life. It keeps one from putting a hand in a flame or walking into oncoming traffic. The fear of death and the unknown is commonplace; it causes many to dislike, even dread, passing by cemeteries, even though there is no logical reason. While many forms of fear are normal, if they occur out of context, in socially unacceptable manners, too severely, or uncontrollably, then the diagnosis is a phobia.

Many different phobias have been cited in the literature and have specific terms in dictionaries, constructed by prefixing the word "phobia" with Greek or Latin terms (such as acrophobia or claustrophobia). While their enumeration is an interesting pastime, phobias are serious conditions and should be treated by professional psychologists.

Phobias are caused by perceived dangerous experiences, both real and imagined. Sometimes, it is gradual: A worker may develop anxiety reactions to a boss over several weeks. Likewise, a single moment of terror can cause a lifetime of avoidance: A dog attack can generate cynophobia (fear of dogs) in a child. Children are especially susceptible to phobias, most of which are caused by fear of injury. The death of a close relative is difficult for children to understand and requires a delicate, sensitive, and honest explanation. Questions and expressions of feelings (often resentment) by the child should be encouraged and discussed. It is repression, unanswered questions, lack of supportive people, and guilt feelings that can lead to morbid attitudes and fantasies, by which phobias develop. Experiences in the past and associated fears remain dormant, to recur and be relived.

Anticipatory fears can also cause phobias. Driving trainees and beginning drivers often have phobic reactions, dreading possible accidents. Students, often the best or most conscientious ones, may spend sleepless nights worrying about the next day's exami-

INFORMATION ON PHOBIAS

Causes: Psychological disorder
Symptoms: Feeling of anxiety or panic, impaired social interaction, impaired freedom of action
Duration: Often chronic
Treatments: Cognitive and behavioral therapy (e.g., controlled exposure to object of fear)

nation. They fear experiences that may never occur, irrationally magnifying the consequences of their performance to one of absolute success or utter doom. Concentration produces positive results (that is, good grades), but obsession may cause paralyzing fear and pressure, even suicide. Several other theories exist regarding the cause of phobias.

Phobias can be classified into three primary groupings: simple phobias, social phobias, and agoraphobia. Simple phobias are directed toward specific things, animals, phenomena, or situations. Rodents, cats, dogs, and birds are common objects of fear. A swooping gull or pigeon may cause panic. Insects, spiders, and bugs can provoke revulsion. Many cultures have a fear of snakes. A phobia exists, for example, when a house is inspected several times each day for snakes; a phobic person may vacate a rural home for an urban dwelling in order to avoid them. Blood, diseased people, or hospital patients have caused fainting. Some vegetarians dread meat because of traumatic observations of slaughter. Fear of heights, water, enclosed spaces, and open spaces involves imagined dangers of falling, drowning, feeling trapped, and being lost in oblivion, respectively. These feelings are coupled with a fear of loss of control and harming oneself by entering a dangerous situation. Sometimes, a specific piece of music, building, or person triggers reactions; the initial trauma or conditioning events are not easily remembered or recognized as such.

Social phobias are fears of being watched or judged by others in social settings. For example, in a restaurant, phobics may eat in rigid, restrictive motions to avoid embarrassments. They may avoid soups, making noises with utensils, or food that requires gnawing for fear of being observed or drawing attention. Many students fear giving speeches because of the humiliation and ridicule resulting from mistakes. Stage fright, dating anxiety, and fear of unemployment, divorce, or other forms of failure are also phobic conditions produced by social goals and expectations. The desire to please others can exact a terrible toll in worry, fear, and sleepless nights.

Agoraphobia is a flight reaction caused by the fear of places and predicaments outside a sphere of safety.

This sphere may be home, a familiar person (often a parent), a bed, or a bedroom. Patients retreat from life and remain at home, safe from the outside world and its anticipated perils. They may look out the window and fear the demands and expectations placed on them. They are prisoners of insecurity and doubt, avoiding the responsibilities, risks, and requirements of living. Many children are afraid of school, and some feign illness to remain safely in bed. Facing the responsibilities of maturation causes similar reactions.

TREATMENT AND THERAPY

Different schools of psychology espouse different approaches to the treatment of phobias, but central themes involve controlled exposure to the object of fear. Common core fears include fear of dying, fear of going crazy, fear of losing control, fear of failure, and fear of rejection.

The most effective approach to treating these disorders is a cognitive-behavioral strategy. With this approach, dysfunctional thinking is identified and changed through collaborative efforts between the patient and therapist. Additional dysfunctional behavior is identified and changed through processes involving conditioning and reinforcement.

Through an initial minimal exposure to the feared object or situation, discussion, and then progressively greater controlled contact, patients experience some stress at each stage but not at a level sufficient to cause a relapse. They will proceed to become desensitized to the object in phases. Therapists may serve as role models at first, demonstrating the steps that patients need to complete, or they may provide positive feedback and guidance. In either case, the role of the patient is active, and gradual exposure occurs. In the process, patients learn to adapt to stress and become more capable of dealing with life.

Other supervised therapies exist, some involving hypnosis, psychoanalysis, drugs, and reasoning out of one's fears. In dealing with phobics, it must be recognized that anyone can have a phobia. Patience, understanding, supportiveness, and professional help are needed. Telling someone simply to "snap out of it" increases stress and guilt.

—*John Panos Najarian, PhD;*
updated by Nancy A. Piotrowski, PhD

See also Antianxiety; Anxiety; Body dysmorphic disorder; Bonding; Death and dying; Depression; Emotions: Biomedical causes and effects; Neurosis; Nightmares; Post-traumatic stress disorder; Psychiatric disorders; Psychiatry; Psychiatry, child and adolescent; Psychiatry, geriatric; Psychoanalysis; Psychosomatic disorders; Separation anxiety; Stress; Stress reduction; Toilet training.

For Further Information:

Barlow, David H. *Anxiety and Its Disorders*. 2d ed. New York: Guilford Press, 2004. Examines the subject in the context of recent developments in emotion theory, cognitive science, and neuroscience. Reviews the implications for treatment and integrates them into newly developed treatment protocols for the various anxiety disorders.

Bourne, Edmond J. *The Anxiety and Phobia Workbook*. 4th ed. Oakland, Calif.: New Harbinger, 2005. This is an excellent self-help book for problems related to anxiety. It may also be helpful for family members seeking to understand anxiety better or to support those affected by anxiety.

Maj, Mario, et al., eds. *Phobias*. Hoboken, N.J.: John Wiley & Sons, 2004. Reviews the diagnosis, classification, pharmacotherapy, psychotherapy, and social and economic burdens of phobias.

Marks, Isaac M. *Fears, Phobias, and Rituals: Panic, Anxiety, and Their Disorders*. New York: Oxford University Press, 1987. This book draws on fields as diverse as biochemistry, physiology, pharmacology, psychology, psychiatry, and ethology to form a fascinating synthesis of information on the nature of fear and of panic and anxiety disorders.

Saul, Helen. *Phobias: Fighting the Fear*. New York: Arcade, 2001. Traces the historical and cultural roots of phobias, examining case studies and literature in the process.

Stewart, Gail B. *Phobias*. San Diego, Calif.: Thomson/Gale, 2005. Discusses phobias, especially as they relate to children. Includes bibliographical references and an index.

PHRENOLOGY

Category: Specialty
Anatomy or system affected: Brain, skull
Specialties and related fields: Neurology, neuroscience, psychiatry, psychology
Definition: A discredited field that theorizes well-developed areas of the cerebral cortex of the brain, each with its own functional properties, corresponded to bumps on the skull. Likewise, a depression on the skull would indicate an underdeveloped faculty.

Key term:

theory of localization: a theory that stated the brain consisted of many specific areas that took on their own functional properties

SCIENCE AND PROFESSION

Phrenology was championed by Franz Joseph Gall (1758-1828), an Austrian physician and anatomist, who developed the theory that the size of cortical regions of the brain was correlated with specific talents such as inquisitiveness, destructiveness, secretiveness, and friendship. In addition, enhanced brain areas were reflected as enlarged bumps on the skull directly above it. In all, Gall believed he had located twenty-seven faculties that were unique to humans and nineteen that were found on some nonhuman animals. These special talents were referred to by Gall as "organs." The extra organs that humans possessed, according to Gall, were areas that corresponded to things such as wisdom, passion, and the sense of satire. Besides paying attention to the bumps on the cranium, the recesses were also important since they reflected the underdevelopment of specific talents.

Prior to the nineteenth century, there were was some discussion regarding how the brain was organized as a collection of many different neuroanatomical structures, each with their own functional properties. Gall is credited with developing this notion into the theory of localization. The theory of localization was proposed as an alternative to the theory of equipotentiality which held the belief that mental abilities depended on the whole brain rather than just a single isolated area. Phrenology benefited from the popularity of localization theory even though there was little empirical evidence to support its claims.

Another physician who popularized phrenology was Johann Spurzheim (1776-1832), a devoted follower and colleague of Frances Gall. They began to work together in 1804 in Vienna and shortly thereafter began to lecture extensively around the world. Spurzheim not only helped espouse Gall's ideas about phrenology, he also developed his own ideas and proposed several additional organs and distinguished between cognitive and emotional faculties. Eventually, after a series of lecture tours, which included a trip to the United States, Spurzheim became the leading proponent of phrenology. While in the United States, some of his lectures were directed towards physicians as a means to discuss possible clinical applications of phrenology. Yet, before these discussions could gain traction, Spurzheim died from typhoid fever in his mid-50s. His skull, at Spurzheim's request, was preserved and studied. It currently resides in the Warren Museum at Harvard Medical School.

In the United States, during the 1820s, phrenology gained acceptance from several professional groups as well as garnered interest from the general public. The Central Phrenological Society was formed in Philadelphia in 1822. Two years later the first American textbook on phrenology Elements of Phrenology was published. An American by the name of George Combe (1788-1858) wrote the Constitution of Man in 1827, which sold more than 100,000 copies. It has been reported that this book was one of the most popular books, in English, during this era. In addition, the psychograph was developed as a type of phrenology machine. It systematically measured thirty-two different points on the cranium and would list out which traits were more or less present on a five-point scale. The Psychograph Company operated from 1929-1937, and the psychograph machine could be found in department stores or theaters for the amusement of the general public.

PERSPECTIVE AND PROSPECTS

While phrenology gained a meteoric rise in popularity, its collapse and eventual fall into disrepute came just as quickly. Perhaps the most ardent opponent against phrenology was Marie-Jean-Pierre Flourens (1794-1867), a French physiologist, who held a strong belief in experimental laboratory methods that were conducted mostly on animals (e.g., hens, ducks, frogs) to discredit not only phrenology, but the larger theory of localization in general. Flourens' book, *Phrenology Examined*, was his strongest attempt to show that bumps on the skull were in no way related to various skills. Today, phrenology is viewed as an amusing afterthought by the neuroscientific community.

—*Bryan C. Auday, PhD*

See also Neurology: Neuroscience

For Further Information:
Finger, Stanley. *Origins of Neuroscience: A History of Exploration into Brain Function.* Oxford: Oxford University Press, 1994.

Kolb, Bryan, and Ian Q. Whishaw. *Fundamentals of Human Neuropsychology.* 6th ed. New York: Worth Publishers, 2009.

Horton Jr, Arthur MacNeill, and Danny Wedding. *The Neuropsychology Handbook.* 3rd ed. New York: Springer Publishing Company, 2008.

Lambert, Kelly G., and Craig H. Kinsley. *Clinical Neuroscience: Psychopathology and the Brain.* 2nd ed. New York: Oxford University Press, 2011.

Leek, Sybil. *Phrenology.* New York: Collier-Macmillan, 1970.

Zillmer, Eric A., Mary V. Spiers, and William C. Culbertson. *Principles of Neuropsychology.* 2nd ed. Belmont, CA: Thomson Wadsworth, 2008.

PHYSICAL EXAMINATION

Category: Procedure
Anatomy or system affected: All
Specialties and related fields: All
Definition: A step in the diagnostic process in which the physician makes general observations about the patient and examines structures of the patient's body through touching (palpation), tapping (percussion), and listening, usually with the aid of a stethoscope (auscultation).

Key terms:
auscultation: active listening, usually with the aid of a stethoscope, to sounds generated by the body

inflammation: irritation caused by such things as infection, injury, allergy, or toxins; symptoms include redness, swelling, warmth, pain, and drainage

organ system: structures of the body, in close proximity or distanced from one another, which together perform a function or functions

palpation: application of the hands, or touching, to determine the size, texture, consistency, and location of body structures

percussion: gentle tapping of the examiner's finger, which has been positioned on the patient; a hollow sound is heard over air-filled structures, while a dull thud is heard over solid areas or liquid-filled structures

sign: objective evidence of disease; a finding noted by the physician during the course of the physical examination

symptom: subjective evidence of disease, provided by the patient

INDICATIONS AND PROCEDURES

Physical diagnosis-the principles, practices, and traditions that form the foundation of the modern physical examination-has rightly been called an art. Usually taught during the first two years of medical training, the basic skills of observation, auscultation, palpation, and percussion are later augmented by hands-on experience with actual patients. For many students, this acquisition of physical diagnostic skills marks the point when they begin to feel like "real" doctors. Observation techniques may be overt or subtle, as a patient may have difficulty maintaining usual behavior if consciously aware of scrutiny. An examiner may even find it necessary to distract the patient in order to allow accurate assessment.

Auscultation, from the Latin *auscultare* (to listen), is generally performed with the aid of a stethoscope. Normal bodily functions generate sounds, the presence or absence of which may provide clues to health or illness. Palpation, from the Latin *palpare* (to touch softly), involves the application of the examiner's hands to the patient's body. This touching conveys information about the size, texture, consistency, temperature, and tenderness of physical structures. This person-to-person contact can also exert an important calming or reassuring effect on the patient. Percussion, from the Latin *percussio* (striking), entails a gentle tapping of the examiner's finger, which has been placed on the patient. A resonant return is noted over hollow, air-filled structures. In contrast, solid or fluid-filled structures produce a dull fullness. A simple demonstration of this technique can be performed by partially filling a bucket with water. By tapping on the outside and noting the variations in sound, it is possible to estimate the fluid level without looking inside the bucket.

To some extent, the widespread use of sophisticated diagnostic imaging technologies has decreased the

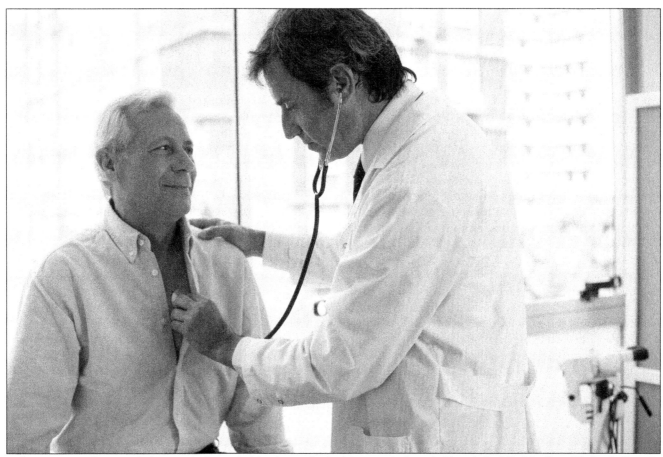

A physician uses a stethoscope to check a patient's airways. Such hands-on evaluation is important in diagnosis. Photo via iStock/Paul Bradbury. [Used under license.]

emphasis on physical examination skills in actual practice. This trend is unfortunate, because it lessens face-to-face contact between the patient and physician and may thus prove unsatisfying for both. It would be misleading, though, to view technological discoveries as competing only with the physical examination. Over the years, the usefulness of physical diagnosis has been enhanced by the availability of simple tools and elegant instruments that augment the examiner's biological senses. Common examples include the stethoscope, the oto-ophthalmoscope (a handheld halogen light source with interchangeable optics, used to view the inside of the eyes and ears), the reflex hammer, and the tuning fork. Indeed, the line separating physical diagnosis from other diagnostic procedures has been blurred as more portable devices find their way into the hands of the practicing physician.

During the physical examination, diagnostic techniques are applied in an interaction between the examiner and the patient at a unique moment in time. As such, the outcome depends on the skills of the individual examiner and on the patient's manifest physical characteristics. Changes in physical state over time are common; variation in physical examination findings over time is not unexpected. For example, heart murmurs, which are sounds generated

by the heart, are graded on a scale from I/VI (one over six), designating a very faint murmur, to VI/VI (six over six), designating a murmur loud enough to be heard even without a stethoscope at a distance away from the patient. It is not uncommon for physicians, even cardiologists, who specialize in the heart, to disagree on the description of a murmur. In addition, a murmur itself can get louder or softer, or even disappear entirely with advancing age, exercise, pregnancy, or other factors. Physical diagnosis is an imprecise science. Medical educators have attempted to address this imprecision by modifying traditional instructional methods.

The physical examination should be considered within the larger context of medical information gathering. Customarily, it follows the collection of historical information about the patient's immediate and past health statuses. Like a road map, the history guides the scope and focus of the subsequent examination. This marriage of history taking and physical examination is colloquially referred to as the "H and P." Though not as often recommended as in the past, the annual complete (or head-to-foot) physical examination may come to mind when this topic is discussed. More commonly, a physical examination is directed and focused on particular regions or organ systems.

In the general screening examination of an apparently healthy subject, a systematic survey is undertaken, following an assessment of structural and/or functional relationships. A structural division would involve examination of all the organ systems contained in or adjacent to a particular body part (for example, the foot), such as the bones, muscles, nerve supply, blood vessels, and skin. A functional examination of the cardiovascular organ system would include the heart, neck, lungs, abdomen, skin, and extremities, because manifestations of cardiovascular disease may be present in locations physically remote from the heart itself. A patient complaining of a specific problem undergoes a detailed examination of the organ systems or body structures most likely to be affected.

The sequential performance of a physical examination incorporates both structural and functional strategies. Though most examiners follow a similar framework, individual differences in physicians and patients result in a wide variety of acceptable patterns. Ideally, the process begins when the patient first arrives. Clues to a patient's overall level of independent function, such as mobility, dexterity, and speech patterns, may be noted. As the medical history is taken, the patient's level of alertness, as well as orientation to time, place, and self, often becomes apparent. The complete examination generally begins with the head, including the face and scalp. A survey of the skin surfaces may be accomplished with the patient completely naked, or it may be divided into discrete segments to be checked as the examination proceeds. Inspection of the eyes, ears, nose, and throat follow. Next, the neck, chest, and back are surveyed. A breast examination may be done at this time. After evaluation of the heart and lungs, the patient is asked to lie down for the abdominal examination. Genital organs may be checked at this time or may be deferred until a later part of the session. The neurologic inspection usually follows and entails the integration of findings from earlier parts of the examination with maneuvers specific to the neurological examination. In the mental status portion of the neurologic examination, formal evaluation of memory, orientation, speech patterns, and thought processes takes place. The musculoskeletal examination likewise integrates earlier findings with a detailed focus on bone and joint development and function. Finally, the extremities are checked. Upon completion of the history and physical, the diagnosis may be readily apparent or further evaluation may be needed.

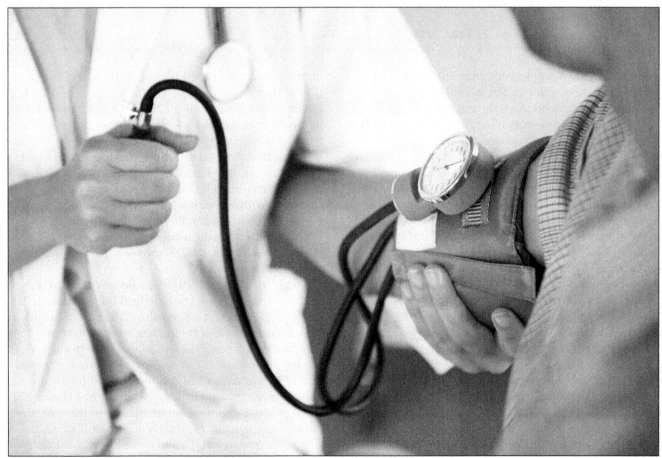

A blood pressure test is one of several standard examination tools. Photo via iStock/GlobalStock. [Used under license.]

Pertinent findings, whether normal or abnormal, are documented in the medical record and may be supplemented by diagrams or photographs if necessary. Depending on the purpose of the examination, these may be entered on a separate preprinted form with check-off spaces or simply noted in the chart. Computer technology allows the storage and retrieval of this information in a patient database file.

USES AND COMPLICATIONS

The application of physical examination techniques may be illustrated by considering three distinct cases: a child's school physical, a routine gynecologic examination with a Papanicolaou (Pap) test, and the evaluation of a sprained ankle. Each has a unique purpose dictating the breadth and detail of the techniques employed. In the school physical, the purpose of the examination is to screen a symptom-free individual for signs of previously unrecognized medical conditions; thus, the survey is broad. The annual gynecologic examination with a Pap testing is more focused-screening for cervical cancer and other gynecologic illness, including sexually transmitted diseases-and will focus on the reproductive system. The evaluation of the sprained ankle is done to assess damage to an identified body part following a specific injury, and it will entail a detailed inspection of the affected area. How these underlying considerations influence the methods employed are apparent as each case is considered.

A child's school physical examination is preceded by a broad historical investigation of the individual's birth details, immunization status, social interactions, growth and development, and daily activity. Height and weight are measured and plotted on a growth chart to facilitate comparison with expected normal values for children of the same age and sex. In many cases, the actual numbers are of less importance than the trend relating repeated measurements. Vision and hearing screening are employed to identify defects that could interfere with school performance.

Vital signs-temperature, pulse, blood pressure, and breathing-are determined. Temperature is usually determined orally, though rectal or axillary (armpit) locations may be used. Although 37 degrees Celsius (98.6 degrees Fahrenheit) is often quoted as normal, a range of body temperatures can be found in healthy patients. Pulse rate is measured by palpation of the radial artery in the wrist. Circumstances may dictate performing this measurement in other locations, such as the carotid artery in the neck or the femoral artery in the groin. Most patients will have a pulse between sixty and one hundred beats per minute. Higher or lower numbers are common and may be related to athletic conditioning, medications, or illness.

Blood pressure is determined with the aid of a stethoscope and a sphygmomanometer (blood pressure cuff) and is expressed in millimeters of mercury. After pumping the cuff to a high pressure, the examiner slowly deflates the cuff while listening for the sounds of blood flow, usually in the brachial artery above the elbow. The onset and end of these sounds indicate the systolic and diastolic blood pressure measurements. A measurement of 120/80 (systolic over diastolic) is often considered normal, but acceptable blood pressures will vary among individuals. In this case, the normal blood pressure for a child is lower than for an adult. Breathing rate is checked by observation and varies, depending on age and medical conditions, from approximately twelve to forty breaths per minute. Infants and children have higher rates than adults.

Following the determination of vital signs, a general physical survey is performed. The head is inspected to confirm normal shape and absence of injury. Eye movements and response to light are noted, along with any inflammation. The ears, nose, and throat are checked for signs of inflammation or scarring. A puff of air may be used to test the mobility of the eardrum. Palpation of the neck may reveal enlargement of the thyroid gland or lymph nodes. The chest is observed for abnormalities, and auscultation of the lungs is performed to monitor air flow during breathing. The cardiac examination will focus on possible murmurs, sounds generated by turbulent blood flow. Since many murmurs are harmless, and many children will have a murmur noted at some point, careful auscultation is needed to define the nature of heart sounds. If a murmur is heard, the patient may be asked to perform certain maneuvers, such as standing up quickly or taking a deep breath and straining. These actions may cause the murmur to change in a way that allows recognition of its underlying cause.

Next, the abdomen is observed for symmetry and distension. By palpation, the examiner may discover enlargement of the liver or spleen. Percussion over the liver area may confirm enlargement of that organ. Auscultation of the sounds produced by the bowels may provide clues to increased or decreased intestinal function. An external genital examination is appropriate for boys and girls. Proper descent of the testicles into the scrotum should be ascertained for boys, while menstrual complaints may dictate an internal examination for girls. Scoliosis (curvature of the spine) or other abnormalities in neurological or musculoskeletal development may be found. Examination of the skin surface is especially important in children; in addition to birthmarks, signs of child abuse may be visible and require evaluation. The length of time needed for the entire screening process will vary. If the child is already known to the examiner and has been seen recently for other reasons, the examination itself may be brief. The presence of abnormal findings may require a lengthy, detailed evaluation.

An annual gynecologic examination and Pap testing is preceded by a directed gathering of the patient's medical and family history, focusing on the reproductive system. This completed, the patient is asked to lie on her back, with her feet apart in foot rests that extend from the table. Examination of the female genital tract begins with a survey of the external structures, the clitoris, labia, and vaginal opening. A discharge or surface lesions such as sores or warts may arouse suspicion of sexually transmitted disease. Since many women have some discharge normally, however, laboratory tests are often needed to establish the diagnosis of infection. To examine the internal structures of the vagina, the examiner uses a speculum, a metal or plastic instrument about five inches long and shaped like a duck's bill. A hinge in the back allows it to be opened after insertion into the vagina, permitting inspection of the cervix and the vaginal walls with the help of a bright light. At this time, the sample is taken from the cervix, usually with a small brush and wooden spatula. After removal of the speculum, the bimanual (literally, "two hands") examination is done. Gloved, lubricated fingers are inserted into the vagina, while the other hand presses down from the outside of the abdomen. For many women, this is the most uncomfortable part of the examination, though sensitivity by the examiner can lessen the discomfort. The cervix, uterus, Fallopian tubes, ovaries, and bladder may be palpated. A rectovaginal examination is performed by placing one finger in the vagina and another finger of the same hand in the rectum. This allows palpation of the space between the vagina and the rectum, as well as of the rectum itself. A breast examination may be performed during the office visit. Although most women focus on lumps, other potential signs of breast cancer, such as bleeding from the nipple, a persistent rash around the nipple, skin dimpling, or retraction (turning in) of the nipple, are noted. Because breast cancer is most common in upper and outer quadrants of the breasts and may spread to lymph nodes in the armpit, palpation of these areas is prudent.

In the examination of an apparent ankle sprain, the presence of an abnormality is a given, and the evaluation is geared to the documentation of the extent of the injury to the ankle itself and to adjacent structures. Initial observation may reveal that the patient has obvious pain while walking into the examining area. Swelling and redness may be prominent. Palpation of the leg and ankle will likely elicit tender-

ness over the damaged ligaments, especially with movement. Intact circulation can be confirmed by placing the fingers over the arteries of the foot and noting strong pulses. Instability of the joint itself may be discovered by applying pressure in various directions. The possibility of nerve damage is assessed by testing sensation and the strength in the foot. Though this examination is directed toward a relatively limited area of the body, it may require considerable time because of the depth of detail involved.

PERSPECTIVE AND PROSPECTS

The modern physical examination is the product of a gradual evolution rather than of a single discovery or invention. Though certain individuals are credited with the adoption of particular physical diagnostic techniques, the interpretation of bodily characteristics as indicators of health status has ancient roots that predate Hippocrates, who was born in 460 BCE on the island of Cos in Greece. From the Middle Ages until the eighteenth century, physical examination focused on the pulse, which was accorded much diagnostic significance, and the feces. The scientific foundations of current practices were uncovered in Europe during the late eighteenth century and early nineteenth century. René Laënnec (1781-1826), a French physician, is generally acknowledged as the originator of the stethoscope, which greatly enhanced the power of auscultation. Compared to modern instruments, it was crude, consisting of a straight rigid tube which was placed between the patient's body and the physician's ear. The use of percussion as a diagnostic technique is credited to Leopold Auenbrugger and Jean-Nicolas Corvisart des Marets, contemporaries of Laënnec. Since that time, many physicians have contributed to the body of knowledge that supports physical diagnosis, and texts on the subject are filled with descriptions of maneuvers and findings that bear their names: Sir William Osler, Moritz H. Romberg, Joseph F. Babinski, William Heberden, Antonio M. Valsalva, Franz Chvostek, and so on.

Though the patient's history and physical examination have excellent diagnostic power, the adoption of advanced imaging techniques may lead to less reliance on physical diagnostic techniques. Thus, traditional hands-on examination risks falling by the wayside. Reasons for adopting new medical technologies in its place are many and controversial. Like other skills, physical diagnosis requires ongoing use if the practitioner is to remain sharp. Physical examinations can be imprecise, with disagreement among competent examiners regarding the presence or absence of findings. In contrast, electromechanical systems may provide more consistent information, though the interpretation of this information is still subjective. It is easy to forget that laboratory or radiological findings by themselves have very limited usefulness. It is not unusual for test reports to note, "Clinical correlation is advised." In other words, test results must be interpreted in the light of the information that has been gathered about the patient through the history and the physical examination. The performance of a detailed evaluation can be time-consuming for the physician and the patient, especially when compared to requesting a test. Pressured by patient expectations or liability concerns, physicians may be reluctant to rely on the physical examination alone in lieu of a battery of confirmatory or exploratory scans or blood tests.

The consequences of this shift are likely to change the way in which the patient views the physician and the way in which the physician approaches the patient. Traditionally, the healing role has been intimately associated with the face-to-face meeting of doctor and patient, exemplified by the laying on of hands. From the patient's perspective, the concept of the personal physician, the familiar voice and touch of the healer who displays ongoing concern and compassion, should not be discounted. This therapeutic relationship will be compromised if physicians become mere brokers for imaging and testing services. With such an arrangement, there would be no reason for the doctor and patient even to see each other. Additionally, important diagnostic information may present itself in a manner that cannot be detected by a scan, such as a subtle clue in the patient's mannerisms or body language. Even a human examiner may have difficulty analyzing such vague information, but impressions can nevertheless contribute to the clinical evaluation. This suggests that the physical examination will continue to hold an important place in the physician's array of diagnostic tools.

—*Louis B. Jacques, MD*

See also Apgar score; Blood pressure; Diagnosis; Education, medical; Noninvasive tests; Nursing; Phlebotomy; Physician assistants; Pulse rate; Screening; Signs and symptoms; Well-baby examinations.

For Further Information:
Goldman, Lee, and Dennis Ausiello, eds. *Cecil Textbook of Medicine.* 23d ed. Philadelphia: Saunders/Elsevier, 2007.
Jarvis, Carolyn. *Physical Examination and Health Assessment.* 6th ed. St. Louis, Mo.: Saunders/Elsevier, 2012.
Pagana, Kathleen Deska, and Timothy J. Pagana. *Mosby's Diagnostic and Laboratory Test Reference.* 11th ed. St. Louis, Mo.: Mosby/Elsevier, 2013.
Shorter, Edward. *Bedside Manners.* New York: Simon & Schuster, 1985.
Siraisi, Nancy G. *Medieval and Early Renaissance Medicine.* 2d ed. Chicago: University of Chicago Press, 2009.
Swartz, Mark H. *Textbook of Physical Diagnosis: History and Examination.* 6th ed. Philadelphia: Saunders/Elsevier, 2010.
Tierney, Lawrence M., Stephen J. McPhee, and Maxine A. Papadakis, eds. *Current Medical Diagnosis and Treatment 2007.* New York: McGraw-Hill Medical, 2006.
Vorvick, Linda J. "Physical Examination." *MedlinePlus,* January 1, 2013.

PHYSICAL REHABILITATION

Category: Specialty
Anatomy or system affected: Bones, hips, joints, knees, legs, ligaments, muscles, musculoskeletal system, nerves, nervous system, spine, tendons
Specialties and related fields: Exercise physiology, orthopedics, osteopathic medicine, physical therapy, sports medicine
Definition: The discipline devoted to the restoration of normal bodily function, primarily of the muscles and skeleton.
Key terms:
atrophy: a wasting away; a diminution in the size of a cell, tissue, organ, or part
cutaneous: pertaining to the skin
edema: the accumulation of an excessive amount of fluid in cells or tissues
electromyography: an electrodiagnostic technique for recording the extracellular activity (action and evoked potentials) of skeletal muscles at rest, during voluntary contractions, and during electrical stimulation
gangrene: necrosis (tissue death) caused by the obstruction of the blood supply; may be localized in a small area or may involve an entire extremity
goniometry: the measurement of angles, particularly those for the range of motion of a joint
ischemia: a local anemia or area of diminished or insufficient blood supply caused by mechanical obstruction of the blood supply (commonly, narrowing of an artery)
musculoskeletal: pertaining to or comprising the skeleton and the muscles
physiatry: the branch of medicine dealing with the prevention, diagnosis, and treatment of disease or injury and the rehabilitation from resultant impairments and disabilities; uses physical agents such as light, heat, cold, water, electricity, therapeutic exercise, mechanical apparatus, and pharmaceutical agents
rehabilitation: the restoration of normal form and function after injury or illness; the restoration of the ill or injured patient to optimal functional level in the home and community in relation to physical, psychosocial, vocational, and recreational activity
vascular: relating to or containing blood vessels

SCIENCE AND PROFESSION

Physical rehabilitation has been defined as a scientific discipline that uses physical agents such as light, heat, water, electricity, and mechanical agents in the management and rehabilitation of pathophysiological conditions resulting from disease or injury. Rehabilitation involves the treatment and training of patients with the goal of maximizing their potential for normal living physically, psychologically, socially, and vocationally.

Historical records indicate that the Chinese used rubbing as a therapeutic measure as early as 3000 BCE Hippocrates also advocated rubbing in writings dated from 460 BCE; it was used by subsequent Roman civilizations. The Roman poet Homer wrote about hydrotherapy as a cure for Hector. Immersion in the Nile and Ganges rivers as an aid to healing has been practiced for centuries. Peter Henry Ling developed and published a scientific basis for therapeutic massage in 1812. Modern physical therapy was established in 1917 with the creation of the Division of Special Hospitals and Physical Reconstruction. This effort was directed at persons injured in World War I and included educational and vocational training programs.

Physical rehabilitation is known for its work in restoring function to traumatized limbs. Practitioners in the field work with persons of all ages: with children to overcome birth defects, with adults to restore muscular function lost from strokes, with the elderly to maintain as much of normal functioning as possible in the face of advancing age, and with postoperative patients to accelerate healing and a return to normal activities. In addition, emphasis is placed on preventing and treating athletic injuries-prevention through the teaching of exercises to strengthen specific body parts and treatment through the restoration of normal bodily movements.

Prevention is defined as the avoidance of sickness, disability, or injury. There are three types or levels of prevention: primary, secondary, and tertiary. Primary prevention refers to complete avoidance before any problem has developed. A good example of primary prevention is being immunized for a specific disease. Secondary prevention refers to attempts to limit the extent of a disease, disability, or pathological process. A convenient illustration of secondary prevention is an individual who quits smoking. Some damage may have been done to the lungs and other organs, but it is curtailed when an individual stops smoking. The extent of recovery for lost function depends on the degree of damage incurred before the cessation of the activity. Tertiary prevention refers to attempts to recover functions or abilities that have been lost or severely compromised. Physical rehabilitation is a form of tertiary prevention: Attempts are made to restore normality that has been lost as a result of an accident, disease process, or injury.

Physical rehabilitation employs individuals with a variety of training. Physiatrists are physicians who have specialized training in physical medicine and rehabilitation. They are usually the leaders of rehabilitation teams and direct many of the activities of other personnel.

Physiatrists supervise the assessment of injured patients and actually conduct invasive tests such as electromyography. Physical therapists are specialists with some graduate-level training; in the United States, the scope of their activities is regulated by individual states and may vary from state to state. Typically, they operate alone but under the supervision or direction of a physiatrist, although in some states they are able to practice independently. Physical therapists carry out the treatment plan devised by a physiatrist and apply the therapeutic modalities. Speech and occupational therapists have specialized training in assisting patients in these particular areas. Speech therapists concentrate on overcoming language and speech difficulties, while occupational therapists specialize in providing injured persons with skills and training for new jobs. Therapy aides assist these specialists in completing some of the more routine aspects of rehabilitation. Their education ranges from one to four years of training after high school.

DIAGNOSTIC AND TREATMENT TECHNIQUES

Individuals must be assessed prior to receiving physical rehabilitation. The assessment process begins with a complete history and physical examination. Subsequently, specific tests may be needed. Two common assessment tools are goniometry and electromyography. Goniometry refers to the measurement of joint motion. It is done by measuring angles of movement and is reported in degrees of arc. Electromyography is a technique that is used to evaluate the functioning of muscle units. Electrodes are placed in muscle groups. The nerve that controls the muscle is electrically stimulated, and the resultant muscle reaction is measured. Electromyography yields information concerning both the strength of muscle contractions and the speed of conduction along the nerve. These data help to pinpoint the basis of many muscular problems. As with all testing, patient-derived values are compared to standard norms to estimate pathology or lost function.

Other aspects of an injured patient are also assessed: speech and language, psychological makeup, and vocation. Speech and language are needed for communication. Strokes or other injuries can interfere with the ability to communicate. Depending on where they occur in the brain, strokes can have different effects;

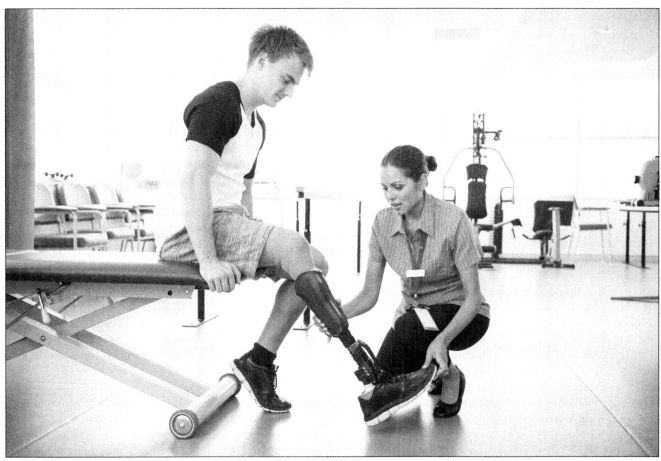

A devastating trauma such as the loss of a limb requires intense physical therapy to help the body adapt. Photo via iStock/JohnnyGreig. [Used under license.]

these must be identified. Language ability requires both neurological integrity and muscular control. Any deficit in either component can impair speech. A primary goal of rehabilitation is communication proficiency (both speech and language), which is a prerequisite for success in many jobs.

Psychological makeup is assessed to pinpoint personality problems that could impede normal interactions with the world or success in a job. Individuals requiring assistance in this area are referred to other professionals for specialized help. Vocational assessment is important because individuals sustaining strokes or serious injuries are frequently unable to return to their previous jobs. When a vocational recommendation has been made for a patient, a specific course of rehabilitation is created.

Four main therapeutic modalities are used in physical rehabilitation: heat, diathermy, cold, and hydrotherapy. Heat increases the rate of cellular metabolism, thus increasing blood flow. Heat also has a sedative effect, relaxing the body part. Tissue repair occurs more rapidly with increased metabolism and circulation. Stress on the injured area is reduced, allowing tissue repair to proceed unimpeded. The net effect is to speed healing.

Heat is supplied by several methods. Compresses of cloth immersed in heated water have been used for centuries. Confining the heated water in a container provides heat in a dry form. Electric heating pads are more convenient because they can supply dry heat at a constant temperature for an unlimited length of time. Melted paraffin is occasionally used to concentrate heat in a specific location; this substance must be applied by a professional under controlled conditions. These modalities supply heat to the surface of skin; it penetrates passively, diminishing in intensity with increasing distance from the surface.

Infrared lamps provide heat that can penetrate to greater depths than heat sources applied to the surface of skin. Additional advantages include dryness and being able to position the body to be heated in any position. Because of its ability to penetrate, infrared light must be limited in exposure to avoid burns. It can also cause excessive drying of skin surfaces. Heat can also be supplied convectively, most often by immersion in warmed water. The stream of water can be directed at particular body parts, providing both heat and stimulation.

Diathermy is defined as deep heating. Deep tissues are heated because superficial heating produces only a few mild physiologic reactions. The problem is to avoid burning superficial tissues while heating deep structures. Three main methods are used to achieve this desired effect: shortwave, ultrasound, and microwave. In all three methods, energy is transferred and finally converted into heat when it reaches deep tissues. With shortwave, energy is transferred into deeper tissues by high-frequency current. Ultrasound uses high-frequency acoustic vibrations that penetrate into deep tissues. Microwave uses electromagnetic radiation to heat deeper tissues. Diathermy exploits all the advantages of heat: locally elevated temperatures, increased circulation, and decreased sensitivity of nerve fibers, which increases the threshold of pain. Diathermy is most useful in treating relatively deep muscular injuries. It cannot be used safely with sensory impairment because burning can occur, nor can it be used in joints that have been replaced with prostheses.

Cold creates physiological effects that are opposite to those of heat. Cooling decreases tissue metabolism. The application of cold slows blood circulation, which, in turn, tends to reduce tissue swelling caused by edema. Cold is more penetrating than heat. Too much cold, however, can become a problem. Cooling a large surface area of skin or lowering the core temperature of a body induces shivering, which causes the production of heat.

Cooling affects the nervous system. With cooling, the first cutaneous sense to be lost is light touch. Motor power is lost next. Pain and gross pressure are eventually lost with a sufficiently long application of cold. When ice is applied, an individual subjectively experiences an appreciation of the cooling, followed by a sense of burning or aching and, eventually, by cutaneous anesthesia. The total time needed to induce cutaneous anesthesia is between five and seven minutes. Cooled underlying muscle fibers lose some of their power; thus people are temporarily but noticeably weaker after cold is applied. The cooling of connective tissues around joints may diminish the ease and precision of movement.

Local cooling is used to reduce the unrestricted flow of fluid and blood into tissues after they have been traumatized. Cold reduces pain, both superficial and deep, and reduces reflex spasticity of muscles. Cold tends to preserve and extend the viability of tissues that have inadequate circulation, thus retarding the development of gangrene in an ischemic body part, which is most commonly seen in limbs.

There are reasons not to apply cold. Occasionally, individuals react to cold by abruptly increasing their arterial pressure. People who suffer from Raynaud's disease usually do not tolerate very well cold applied to their fingers or toes. The stiffness associated with rheumatoid arthritis is usually aggravated by cooling.

Prolonged or excessive cooling can lead to frostbite. People who have experienced clinical hypothermia are must less tolerant of cold than those who have not had such an experience.

Several common methods exist for achieving therapeutic cooling: immersion, cold packs, cryokinetics, and a combination of local cooling and remote heating. Immersion is usually begun in cold water to which ice is steadily added. Total immersion is usually limited to ten or twenty minutes. The affected portion of the body is submerged in the chilled water. Cooling to a temperature above that of ice water may reduce muscular spasticity. Cold packs are often made by wrapping ice in a wet towel or plastic bag and applying it to the skin. Frozen cold packs should not be applied directly to the skin because they can cause locally severe tissue damage.

Cryokinetics is a procedure that combines cooling and exercise. Cooling is first accomplished by means of immersion or rubbing the skin over the affected part of the body with ice for five to seven minutes, so-called ice massage. The cooling produces a mild anesthesia that allows the individual to exercise the cooled body portion actively without pain. This method is considered to be particularly effective in recent acute muscle strains. The simultaneous application of heat and cold is sometimes effective. Heating an uninvolved portion of the body maintains the core temperature, which inhibits shivering, while cold applied to the injured portion of the body reduces pain. In theory, this arrangement allows cold to be applied for longer periods of time than would otherwise be possible. Because it is difficult to control heating and cooling simultaneously, however, this technique is not frequently used.

Hydrotherapy is the external application of water for therapeutic purposes. The water temperature can range from cold to hot. With immersion, water provides buoyancy, which relieves pressure on weight-bearing portions of the body. Water also provides resistance that is used in treating patients with motor weakness. Buoyancy alters the effect of exercises done in water by allowing a severely injured person to move; this provides psychological benefit and hope that the motion can eventually be done out of water. Brief application of cold has a tonic or stimulating effect, increasing blood pressure and the respiratory rate and stimulating shivering. Mild hot water provides sedation to irritated sensory and motor nerves, thus relieving pain caused by cramps and spasms in muscles. It also reduces stress, calming agitated or excited persons. The most common method of hydrotherapy is a whirlpool bath, which combines buoyancy, heat, and mechanical stimulation to the affected body part.

Massage and movement are key components of applied physical rehabilitation. Massage is the systematic and scientific manipulation of body tissues; massage is best performed by the hands. Massage has a sedative effect when constantly and steadily applied, and it leads to a decrease in muscular tension. Combined with heat or cold, the resulting relaxation facilitates the movement of injured body parts. Mechanically, massage stimulates the circulatory system, enhancing blood flow. The applied force of massage is effective in stretching muscle groups and breaking the adhesions between individual muscle fibers that limit motion. This same action mobilizes fluid and promotes its elimination. Massage does not develop muscle strength, however, and should not be used as a substitute for active exercise.

Therapeutic exercise is defined as the performance of movement to correct an impairment, improve musculoskeletal function, or maintain a state of well-being. Movement is the key: The energy to accomplish the movement can be supplied passively by a therapist or actively by an individual. Muscles are stretched with passive movement or contracted during the process of active flexion or contraction. Individuals with injuries that involve the nervous system may lose the function of any muscles supplied by the injured nerves. These muscles must be moved passively in order to avoid loss of muscle mass and function as a result of disuse atrophy. Muscles respond to stimulation. Thus, exercises are designed to strengthen injured muscles. Parts in adjacent body structures must be stabilized to maximize the benefit derived from exercise. Prolonged moderate stretching is more beneficial than momentary vigorous stretching. Movements and stretching should be within the pain tolerance of the patient in order to avoid injury to blood vessels.

PERSPECTIVE AND PROSPECTS

Physical rehabilitation operates within a larger context of health care provision. The need for primary prevention is addressed by teaching correct methods for strengthening muscle groups to athletes and recreational fitness practitioners. Classes on first aid measures for treating common musculoskeletal injuries are taught by rehabilitation specialists such as physicians, therapists, and nurses. These classes are offered in schools and communities throughout the year. Physicians practicing occupational medicine also advocate primary prevention of musculoskeletal injuries associated with the work site. These professionals analyze working environments and recommend ways to restructure particular job tasks in order to reduce the chances of injury.

Secondary prevention is provided in office and hospital settings by professionals who treat injuries such as sprains, strains, and fractures. Care for acute injuries is usually accompanied by instruction in prevention in the hope that patients will avoid similar problems in the future. In the working environment, injured workers are provided with appropriate treatment and therapy and returned to work in an expeditious manner that is consistent with standards of proper care. This approach is usually best for all concerned, especially the injured worker. Such a case illustrates the many facets of rehabilitation. Normal physical functioning is returned with conventional therapy. Self-esteem is bolstered with return to meaningful work and previous income-earning capacity. Economically, the employer also benefits by having a trained and experienced worker on the job rather than having a skilled individual on disability and a less capable replacement worker on the job, both receiving payment.

Tertiary prevention involves the traditional rehabilitation activities that begin after treatment for a massive injury or chronic disease process. Frequently, such rehabilitation returns only a portion of lost functions. Nevertheless, this treatment has value, improving self-esteem and the quality of life for an injured person. It underscores, however, the greater importance of the avoidance and prevention of injuries.

Health can be viewed as being on a continuum. One end is defined by death, the final termination of health. All life constitutes the rest of the spectrum. Health is frequently defined as the absence of disease or infirmity. This definition is appealing in its simplicity but is difficult to use because it is based on the absence rather than the presence of something. The question of where good health ends and impaired health begins is probably highly individual and open for debate. The division point between good and bad or acceptable and unacceptable health status, however, does provide a useful beginning for the activities encompassed by physical rehabilitation. The recovery of lost or impaired function is the domain of this field. This goal is also consistent with the definition of tertiary prevention. Rehabilitation and prevention are complementary opposites. Together, they span the entire spectrum of health.

—*L. Fleming Fallon, Jr., MD, PhD, MPH*

See also Aging: Extended care; Allied health; Amputation; Back pain; Bionics and biotechnology; Birth defects; Braces, orthopedic; Cardiac rehabilitation; Chiropractic; Exercise physiology; Healing; Heart attack; Hydrotherapy; Muscles; Nursing; Occupational health; Orthopedic surgery; Orthopedics; Orthopedics, pediatric; Osteopathic medicine; Overtraining syndrome; Prostheses; Rotator cuff surgery; Speech disorders; Sports medicine; Strokes; Tendinitis; Tendon disorders.

For Further Information:

Braddom, Randall L., ed. *Physical Medicine and Rehabilitation*. 3d ed. Philadelphia: Saunders/Elsevier, 2007. Discusses physical therapy and medical rehabilitation. Includes a bibliography and an index.

DeLisa, Joel A., et al., eds. *Physical Medicine and Rehabilitation: Principles and Practice*. 4th ed. Philadelphia: Lippincott Williams & Wilkins, 2005. This standard textbook provides a comprehensive overview of rehabilitation. It is written for professionals but is accessible to laypeople. The subject entries are written by experts in their fields.

Fletcher, Gerald F., et al., eds. *Rehabilitation Medicine: Contemporary Clinical Perspectives*. Philadelphia: Lea & Febiger, 1992. An introduction to the subject of rehabilitation written for professional audiences. The writing is consistent and of high quality. The illustrations are unusually good.

Garrison, Susan J., ed. *Handbook of Physical Medicine and Rehabilitation: The Basics*. 2d ed. Philadelphia: Lippincott Williams & Wilkins, 2003. This text provides a good overview of the subject. Because it is written for students, it should be understandable to most readers. As an introduction to rehabilitation, it is well written.

Neumann, Donald A. *Kinesiology of the Musculoskeletal System: Foundations for Rehabilitation*. 2d ed. St. Louis, Mo.: Mosby/Elsevier, 2010. A text for physical rehabilitation students and clinicians that gives an introduction to terminology and basic concepts of kinesiology and reviews the structure and function of the musculoskeletal system and the biomechanical and quantitative aspects of kinesiology.

Sinaki, Mehrsheed, ed. *Basic Clinical Rehabilitation Medicine*. 2d ed. St. Louis, Mo.: Mosby, 1993. An introductory textbook for students in the field. Well written, has good illustrations, and should be readily understood by laypeople.

Physician assistants

Category: Specialty

Anatomy or system affected: All

Specialties and related fields: Emergency care, family medicine, general surgery, geriatrics and gerontology, internal medicine, neonatology, nursing, obstetrics and gynecology, public health

Definition: Health care providers who work under the supervision of licensed physicians and who are trained to perform physical examinations, diagnose illnesses, interpret laboratory tests, set fractures, and assist in some surgeries.

Key terms:

American Academy of Physician Assistants (AAPA): a professional society founded in 1968 to promote the role of PAs in providing high-quality, cost-effective health care

Centralized Application Service for Physician Assistants (CASPA): a centralized application that allows students to apply to multiple PA programs via one application

Physician Assistant Education Association (PAEA), known as the *Association of Physician Assistant Programs (APAP)* until 2006: a consortium of educational institutions that offer accredited PA programs, providing academic guidance and standards for member schools

primary care: general medical services provided in family medicine, internal medicine, pediatrics, geriatrics, obstetrics, and emergency care (in contrast to specialists, such as urology or cardiac surgery)

SCIENCE AND PROFESSION

The training of physician assistants (PAs) was initiated at the Duke University Medical Center in 1965, as a way to respond to the persistent shortage of primary care physicians. At the same time, the thousands of medical corpsmen who were discharged annually from the military services were unable to convert their skills into civilian occupations. Four Navy veterans with medical experience, all men, were enrolled in a trial program to give them additional training. A new curriculum was developed on a week-by-week basis, using the educational resources of the medical school. The men were graduated after two years and found their professional niche as assistants to licensed physicians. The PA profession was thus established in 1967. The first female physician assistant graduated from the program at Duke in 1970.

The program at Duke served as a model that spread quickly to other medical institutions. Start-up funds became available from government agencies such as the Veterans Administration, the Office of Economic Opportunity, and the Public Health Service. By 1972, there were twenty-six training programs in operation in the United States. Two years later, the number had grown to fifty-three. New professional organizations were formed to evaluate and accredit the educational programs and to develop certification examinations for the individual graduates. In 2021 282 accredited PA programs were available at medical schools, hospitals, universities, and through the armed forces. Most of these schools are a part of CASPA, the Centralized Application Service for Physician Assistant (CASPA) programs, allowing students to apply to many schools with less effort and cost.

The American Academy of Physician Assistants (AAPA) has adopted the following official definition for "physician assistant":

Physician Assistants (PAs) practice medicine with supervision by licensed physicians. As members of the health care team, PAs provide a broad range of medical services that would otherwise be provided by physicians. It is the obligation of each team of Physician/PA to ensure that the PA's scope of practice is identified; that delegation of medical tasks is appropriate to the

PA's level of competence; that the relationship of, and access to, the supervising physician is defined; and that a process of performance evaluation is established. Adequate and responsible supervision of the PA contributes to both high quality patient care and continued professional growth.

By 2022 there were approximately 150,000 PAs in the United States. Each year, PA training programs produce approximately 5,000 new graduates. PAs must pass a national certifying examination before they can begin to practice and be licensed by the state. The examination is open only to graduates of accredited programs. Unlike physicians, PAs who pass the examination may begin practicing immediately, with no additional training needed. To maintain certification, PAs must complete one hundred hours of continuing medical education every two years and take a recertification exam every ten years. These requirements are intended to ensure the continued competency of PAs as qualified medical professionals.

The typical PA student has a bachelor's degree and four years of health care experience prior to admission into the program. About half of the entering students previously were either nurses (RNs), emergency medical technicians (EMTs), medics in the military, or emergency room technicians. There is strong competition to enter PA programs, with at least five applicants for every student accepted.

The training program for PAs is twenty-seven months or three academic years. The first year is composed of classroom and laboratory courses in anatomy, physiology, microbiology, and other basic sciences. Also, introductory instruction is given in pediatrics, obstetrics, general surgery, internal medicine, and emergency care. Some PAs train to assist in major surgery and to provide preoperative and postoperative care.

After graduation, PAs practice in almost all types of health care settings. The demand for their services is increasing rapidly, and the United States Bureau of Labor Statistics (BLS) projects that the number of PA jobs would increase by 31 percent between 2020 and 2030, much faster than the average for all occupations. In 2021 the practice location of PAs was reported as: 52.2 percent in outpatient offices or clinics, 35.4 percent in hospitals, 5.2 percent in urgent care centers, and 7.2 percent in other locations (including schools, rehabilitation facilities, nursing homes, and correctional facilities).

Twenty-one percent of PAs practice in primary care, where the shortage of qualified medical personnel is most severe. Since medical doctors (MDs) and doctors of osteopathy (Dos) who work in radiology, surgery, anesthesiology, gynecology, and other specialties have about double the median income of general practitio-

ners, there is a strong economic incentive for physicians to become specialists, leaving vacancies in primary care for PAs. Rural clinics, small towns, and inner-city hospitals have a particularly difficult time recruiting physicians for staff vacancies, so PAs are finding ready acceptance to fill these gaps. PAs earn approximately 70 percent of the median net income of physicians in general family medicine. According to the BLS, the median pay for PAs in 2020 was $115,390 per year.

In addition to primary care, as of 2021 26.4 percent of PAs practiced in surgical specialties, 12.2 percent in internal medicine subspecialties, 8.4 percent in emergency medicine, 1.5 percent in pediatric subspecialties, and 30.5 percent in other areas (including psychiatry, hospice and palliative care, obstetrics and gynecology, addiction medicine, pain management, public health, and dermatology).

DIAGNOSTIC AND TREATMENT TECHNIQUES

After completing an accredited master's degree program and passing the certification examination, PAs are qualified to perform approximately 80 percent of the routine duties most commonly done by physicians. PAs can give general physical examinations, diagnose illnesses, determine treatments, give injections, immunizations, and catheterizations, interpret laboratory tests, suture wounds, set fractures, deal with medical emergencies, and assist in surgical operations. In most states, PAs can write prescriptions for medication.

PAs are not independent medical practitioners. By statute or regulation, all PAs must have a licensed physician to supervise and be responsible for their work. It is not necessary, however, for the physician and the PA to be located in the same building or even in the same town. In rural communities, for example, state law generally allows such supervision to occur remotely.

In a small town, the doctor must emphasize the team concept of medical care, of which the PA is a valued member. The supervisory role of the physician needs to be clearly and formally established. The majority of PAs, for example, are insured by a rider on the physician's malpractice policy. To fit into the social environment, PAs have stated that it helps if they themselves grew up in a small town and if they are married. A large number of PAs have successfully found their medical role as primary care providers in rural communities.

A very different role is filled by PAs serving as surgical assistants in a hospital. With specialized training, they can act as assistants during surgery as well as provide preoperative and postoperative care. When a surgery patient is admitted, surgical PAs can be assigned to type up the medical history and give an entrance physical examination. They can evaluate preoperative laboratory tests and inform the surgeon of any potential complications. They can spend time with the patient and family members to explain the intended procedure and to answer their questions.

During surgery, PAs can assist the surgeon with clamping and tying as needed. They should be familiar with various patient monitoring devices and should inform the surgeon if problems arise. After surgery, the PA can accompany the patient to the recovery room or intensive care unit (ICU).

Surgical PAs have become accepted as assistants in almost all kinds of surgery. For example, they can specialize in orthopedics, kidney transplantation, heart surgery, urology, and skin grafts for burn victims. They must receive appropriate on-the-job training with clinical instruction from their supervising physician to prepare for such surgical specialties.

Health care administrators have reported that acceptance of PAs by patients generally has been good. Pamphlets are made available to explain the educational background of PAs, their subordinate status to physicians, and legal limitations on their level of responsibility. Patients who insist on seeing a physician can be accommodated, but surveys have shown an equal degree of patient satisfaction with physician and PA services. In fact, in a 2014 Harris poll, patient satisfaction with PA services was 93 percent.

Depending on their individual interests and skills, PAs have established themselves in a wide variety of other health care settings. They can be found in geriatric practice, prison health programs, trauma centers, infant critical care units, urgent care centers, and military hospitals or on American Indian reservations. Some PAs have gone into administration or public health management. New professional opportunities for PAs continue to evolve as their special contributions to health care are increasingly recognized.

Physician assistants, nurses, physical therapists, nurse practitioners, midwives, medical technologists, and other allied health professionals are all part of the total health care team, with different areas of responsibility. One commentator has stated that no one hires an electrical engineer to change a light bulb; similarly, it is not economical to use physicians for routine care that can be supplied by others. The role of PAs continues to be an expanding one, and a 2022 *U.S. News and World Report* survey listed physician assistant as #2 on the Best Healthcare Job list, and #3 on the Best 100 Jobs list.

—*Kerry L. Cheesman, PhD and Maryann Cheesman, RN*

See also: Allied health; Anatomy; Education, medical; Emergency medicine; Family medicine; Health maintenance organizations (HMOs); Hospitals; Internal medicine; Laboratory tests; Managed care; Nutrition; Obstetrics; Pediatrics; Physical examination; Physiology; Preventive medicine; Surgery, general.

For Further Information:
Anderson, Susan M. *Selected Annotated Bibliography of the Physician Assistant Profession.* 4th ed., Association of Physician Assistant Programs, 1993.
Arenofsky, Janice. "For a Healthy Prognosis: Examine a Career as a PA or CRNA." *Career World*, vol. 21, 1993, pp. 26-30.
Ballweg, Ruth, Sherry Stolberg, and Edward M. Sullivan, editors. *Physician Assistant: A Guide to Clinical Practice.* 3rd ed., Saunders/Elsevier Science, 2003.
Conroy, Sean. *Through the Eyes of a Young Physician Assistant.* Open Books Press, 2016.
Dill, M. J., et al. "Survey Shows Consumers Open to a Greater Role for Physician Assistants and Nurse Practitioners." *Health Affairs*, vol. 32, no. 6, 2012, pp. 1135-42.
Greer, Kathleen. "PAs Envision Evolving Role at Annual AAPA Meeting." *Physician Assistant*, vol. 27, no. 7, 2003, pp. 10-13.
Halter, Mary, et al. "The Contribution of Physician Assistants in Primary Care: A Systematic Review." *BMS Health Services Research*, vol. 13, no. 1, 2013, p. 223.
He, X. Z., E, Cyran. and M. Salling. "National Trends in the United States of America Physician Assistant Workforce from 1980 to 2007." *Human Resources for Health*, vol. 7, 2007, p. 86.
Hooker, Roderick S., and James F. Cawley. *Physician Assistants in American Medicine.* 2nd ed., Churchill Livingstone/Elsevier, 2003.
Lindsay, Sally. "The Feminization of the Physician Assistant Profession." *Women Health*, vol. 41, 2005, pp. 37-61.
Lundberg, George D., and Richard D. Lamm. "Solving Our Primary Care Crisis by Retraining Specialists to Gain Specific Primary Care Competencies." *Journal of the American Medical Association*, vol. 270, 1993, pp. 380-81.
Piemme, Thomas E., et al. *The Physician Assistant: An Illustrated History.* Acacia Corp, 2013.

PHYSIOLOGIC LABOR AND BIRTH

Category: NEED CATEGORY
Also known as: Normal birth, unassisted vaginal birth, spontaneous labor onset
Specialties and related fields: Emergency medicine, family medicine, obstetrics
Anatomy or system affected: Female reproductive tract
Definition: *Physiologic labor and birth* refers to the natural process of childbirth without any clinical intervention.

Physiologic birth is distinct from other forms of childbirth in that it takes place entirely without medical interventions like surgical procedures or the administration of pain medication and is immediately followed by skin-to-skin contact and breastfeeding. Although some women and fetuses may develop complications requiring extra medical intervention, physiologic birth is generally a safe and healthy process that can help to ensure the best possible outcomes for mother and child alike even when complications arise. As a result, advocates of physiologic birth contend that natural childbirth is ideal and should be supported and encouraged over any other form of delivery. Such advocates also typically argue that prenatal interventions and various technological and pharmaceutical interventions are overused in most modern deliveries and often present challenges that can be avoided through physiologic labor and birth.

BACKGROUND

The process of physiologic childbirth can begin hours, days, or even weeks before the onset of labor. There are a number of signs that commonly indicate the approaching onset of labor. One of the earliest of these signs is lightening. Lightening occurs when the baby's head drops down into the mother's pelvis in anticipation of delivery. It can happen anywhere from a few hours to a few weeks before labor begins. Another early sign is the discharge of the mucus plug, which seals off the womb and prevents infection. In most cases, this happens within days of the onset of labor. Some expectant mothers may also experience diarrhea as labor approaches. One of the most recognizable signs of the onset of labor is the rupturing of the membranes of the amniotic sac that surrounds and protects the fetus when it is inside the womb. When this happens, the fluids inside the amniotic sac begin flowing or leaking out of the woman's vagina. The final sign of the imminent onset of labor is the beginning of periodic, irregular uterine contractions. The closer together these contractions occur, the closer labor is to starting.

Labor itself occurs in three stages. The first stage starts with the onset of contractions till complete dilation of the cervix, approximately 10 centimeters (cm). This stage is further divided into two phases. The latent phase is the first and longest of the two phases. During the latent phase, the increasing frequency of contractions helps to thin out and dilate the cervix up to 6 cm. The active phase starts after the cervix is dilated past 6 cm and lasts until complete dilation. There is no definitive timeframe for how long this may take.

The second stage begins when the cervix reaches full dilation. Once full dilation is achieved, the doctor will instruct the woman to begin pushing. This, along with the force of continued contractions, pushes the baby out of the womb and through the birth canal. Under normal circumstances, the baby will begin passing through the vaginal opening head first. Once the baby has fully emerged from the vaginal opening, the umbilical cord is clamped and cut to separate the baby from the placenta.

The third stage of labor begins after delivery of the baby and concludes after the expulsion of the placenta. The placenta is a flat, round organ that forms in the womb during pregnancy and supplies the fetus with nourishment through the umbilical cord. Delivery of the placenta typically takes between ten and thirty minutes.

OVERVIEW

Physiologic birth is defined based on the characteristics of the birthing process from labor to postpartum care. The course of physiologic birth begins with the natural, spontaneous onset of labor and occurs with the ideal biological and psychological conditions that support effective labor. Physiologic birth also specifically results in the vaginal birth of the baby and the passing of the placenta, as well as a certain amount of blood loss. After delivery, physiologic birth involves newborn transition through skin-to-skin contact between mother and child during the postpartum period. Finally, physiologic birth includes the rapid initiation of breastfeeding.

True physiologic birth can be disrupted in a variety of ways. It can be disrupted from the start if labor is induced or augmented artificially. Environmental factors such as harsh lighting, uncomfortable room temperature, nutritional deprivation, lack of privacy, lack of support, or the existence of time constraints can also disrupt physiologic birth. Certain interventions undertaken during the birthing process can disrupt physiologic birth as well. These potential interventions typically include the administration of certain opiate-based drugs and the use of local or general anesthesia. Episiotomy, which is a simple procedure in which the doctor makes a small surgical cut at the vaginal opening to aid delivery, is also considered disruptive to physiologic birth. The same is true of the use of forceps or a vacuum during delivery. Once the baby is delivered, physiologic birth can still be disrupted by immediate cord clamping or separation of mother and child. It should also be noted that birth by caesarian section circumvents physiologic birth altogether.

Physiologic birth has a number of potential benefits for both mother and child. For mothers, physiologic birth can minimize postpartum pain and reduce the risk of postpartum death due to surgical and other complications. It also contributes to a quicker recovery period, elevated self-esteem, a lower likelihood of postpartum depression, and a better attachment between mother and child. In addition, physiologic birth contributes to a more settled baby with a reduced likelihood of harms related to medical interventions and chronic disease related to caesarian delivery or delayed breastfeeding.

The benefits of physiologic birth are not limited to mother and child. It also has potential benefits for obstetricians, midwives, nurses, and administrators. For obstetricians, midwives, and nurses, physiologic birth can lead to increased professional satisfaction, improved job performance on measures tied to compensation, and a reduced chance of being held liable for adverse events that can occur due to complications during the birthing process. For administrators, physiologic birth can reduce or eliminate the added costs associated with medical interventions during childbirth.

Many factors can cause disruption of the physiologic labor and delivery process, necessitating the need for clinical interventions. Some of the complications may include an arrest of cervical dilation, prolonged rupture of the amniotic membranes leading to infection, inability of the fetus to tolerate contractions, shoulder dystocia, retained placenta or postpartum hemorrhage. The patient should be involved in the decision-making process to ensure the safest and best outcomes.

PERSPECTIVE AND PROSPECTS
In 1996, the World Health Organization (WHO) supported the avoidance of unnecessary clinical interventions that disrupt the physiologic labor and delivery process. In 2012, a joint consensus statement by the American College of Nurse-Midwives, Midwives Alliance of North America, and the National Association of Certified Professional Midwives aimed to promote normal physiologic childbirth by developing policies for hospital settings and interdisciplinary education and called for further research on the effects of physiologic birth. According to a Committee opinion by the American College of Obstetricians and Gynecologists, obstetric care providers should feel comfortable and consider managing laboring women who seek a limited interventional method for their childbirth experience in a safe and family-centered approach.

—*Muneeza Khan, MD, FAAFP*

For Further Information:
Adams, Ellise D., et al. "A Nurse's Guide to Supporting Physiologic Birth." *Nursing for Women's Health*, vol. 20, no. 1, 2016, pp. 76-86.
The American College of Obstetricians and Gynecologists. "Approaches to Limit Intervention During Labor and Birth." *ACOG*, www.acog.org/clinical/clinical-guidance/committee-opinion/ articles/2019/02/approaches-to-limit-intervention- during-labor-and-birth.
Artal-Mittelmark, Raul. "Management of Normal Labor." *Merck Manual*, May 2021, www.merckmanuals.com/professional/gynecology-and-obstetrics/normal-labor- and-delivery/management-of-normal-labor.
"Birth (Parturition)." *Lumen Learning*, courses.lumenlearning.com/boundless-ap/chapter/birth-parturition/. Accessed 27 Feb. 2018.
Hagood Milton, Sarah. "Normal Labor and Delivery." *Medscape*, 26 June 2013, emedicine.medscape.com/article/260036-overview. Accessed 27 Feb. 2018.
K., Debra. "Expecting? The Process of Creating a Physiological Birth." *Huffington Post*, www.huffingtonpost.com/debra-k/expecting-the-process-of-_b_6674974.html. Accessed 27 Feb. 2018.
"Normal Labor and Delivery Process." *WebMD*, www.webmd.com/baby/guide/normal-labor-and-delivery-process#1. Accessed 27 Feb. 2018.
"Physiologic Birth." *International Childbirth Education Association*, icea.org/wp-content/uploads/2016/01/Physiologic_Birth_PP.pdf. Accessed 27 Feb. 2018.
"Supporting Healthy and Normal Physiologic Childbirth: A Consensus Statement by ACNM, MANA, and NACPM." *Journal of Perinatal Education*, vol. 22, no. 1, 2013, pp. 14-18.
"What Is Physiologic Birth?" *BirthTOOLS*, birthtools.org/What-Is-Physiologic-Birth. Accessed 27 Feb. 2018.

PHYSIOLOGY

Category: Biology
Anatomy or system affected: All
Specialties and related fields: All
Definition: The branch of biology dealing with the structures and functions of various systems in living organisms.
Key terms:
extracellular fluid: the internal environment of the human body that surrounds the cells; the fluid contains ions, gases, and the nutrients needed by cells for proper functioning and is constantly circulated throughout the body by the blood and into tissues by diffusion
homeostasis: the maintenance of a constant internal environment; the systems of the body work together to maintain a constant temperature, pH, oxygen availability, water content, ion concentrations, and so on
negative feedback: a homeostatic control system designed to respond to a stress by returning body conditions to normal physiologic levels
pH: a measure of the acidity or alkalinity of a solution; equal to the negative logarithm of the hydrogen ion concentration (as measured in moles per liter)
positive feedback: when a stimulus causes more of the same to occur; can be useful in some instances, such as with blood clotting and uterine contractions during childbirth
scientific method: a method of scientific investigation of a problem through observation, the formation of a hypothesis (a possible explanation to a problem), experimentation, and the reevaluation of data

THE FUNDAMENTALS OF PHYSIOLOGY

Physiology is a branch of science that applies to all living things. The goal of the physiologist is to understand the mechanisms leading to the proper functioning of organisms such as bacteria, plants, animals, and humans. Physiology is an important aspect of many of the medical sciences. In immunology, researchers seek to understand the functioning of the immune system. Cardiovascular scientists study the workings of the heart. Knowledge of the normal physiologic functioning of an organism is important in identifying the diseases that cause a deviation from the normal state.

Essential to the discovery of new data is the application of the scientific method of research. The first step in this method is observation. This involves examining a particular system or organism of interest, such as the transport of nutrients in a plant stem or the flow of air into the lungs of an animal, and initially observing a specific event or phenomenon. Asking why and how the event occurs leads to the next step-forming a hypothesis, or scientific question. A hypothesis is a possible explanation of the observation, which can be tested further to see if it is true. Testing, or experimentation, is the third step in the scientific method. The experiment involves setting up a controlled situation that directly tests the hypothesis in order to determine the cause-and-effect relationship between the hypothesis and the initial observation. As the experiment is conducted, the investigator makes further observations of the system's functioning and collects these findings as data. Following data collection and analysis comes the fourth step, making conclusions. The conclusion may or may not support the researcher's original hypothesis. To confirm the results further, more testing is often done. If, upon additional testing, similar conclusions are reached, the researcher may move on to the final step of the scientific method: publication. The experimental design, results, and conclusions are written down in a paper that is then submitted to a scientific journal. Publication permits other researchers to be informed of and evaluate the experiment and possibly to use the results to further their own research endeavors.

Applying this scientific method to the human model, it becomes apparent that the physiological conditions of the human body are in a state of dynamic equilibrium. While variables such as pH, ion and nutrient concentrations, and water content are constantly changing, they never differ significantly from their optimum level, unless the body is in a state of disease. Sensors, an integrating center, and effectors are important contributors to the regulation of these variables. Sensors are located throughout the body and are designed to monitor specific physiologic conditions. For example, baroreceptors monitor arterial blood pressure, chemorecep- tors monitor the concentrations of hydrogen ions and carbon dioxide in the extracellular fluid, and thermoreceptors monitor body temperature. The conditions of the body are then transmitted via nerve impulses to a particular integrating center located in the brain, spinal cord, or endocrine glands. The integrating center interprets the nerve impulses and determines if a response is required. To respond to a particular condition, the integrating center activates certain effectors. An effector is usually a muscle or a gland that, when activated, performs a specific function to return the body to normal physiologic conditions.

Extracellular fluid is also important in the maintenance of the above-mentioned variables. Two basic types of fluid compose about 60 percent of the human body. Two-thirds of the body's fluid is intracellular fluid (cytoplasm) and is found inside cells. The other one-third of the fluid is extracellular fluid and is located in the spaces between cells (interstitial fluid), in blood vessels (plasma), and in the lymphatic vessels (lymph). This fluid is constantly circulated throughout the human body in the blood and lymphatic vessels. The ions, gases, and nutrients in the fluid can easily diffuse out of the capillaries and into the adjacent cells, where they can be utilized in normal cell activities. Because the estimated one hundred trillion cells of the body are exposed to basically the same composition of extracellular fluid, it has been termed the body's internal environment.

The extracellular fluid is the medium of exchange of biologically important molecules and materials. Their concentration and availability is under the control of various organs and systems. For example, the kidneys play an important role in regulating the water content, ion and waste concentrations, and acid-base balance of the extracellular fluid. The gastrointestinal tract is responsible for digesting and making food available for absorption into the bloodstream. The liver maintains the normal glucose concentration in the blood through processes that store glucose, remove glucose from storage, or produce new glucose from other nutrients. The lungs aspirate to provide adequate oxygen and carbon dioxide exchange in the blood. An important job of the physiologist is to discover the mechanisms used by these and other organs to perform their respective functions.

HOMEOSTASIS AND FEEDBACK SYSTEMS

Each of the aforementioned variables has an optimum physiologic range over which the body can function normally. The systems of the body work together in an attempt to keep the body's internal environment within these normal ranges. This process is called homeostasis. Stress placed on the body-whether from the outside environment (heat, cold) or from within (disease, emotional reactions)-can lead to fluctuations in the internal environment. Significant deviations from the normal can lead to a state of disease in the body. To prevent these types of changes, the body has incorporated a number of control devices that are governed by the nervous and endocrine systems. The nervous system is constantly evaluating the state of the body and is able to detect when something is awry. When the body strays too far from its balanced condition, it responds in one of two ways. First, it may send nervous impulses to the proper organs that counteract the stress and return it toward its original state. Second, it may activate the endocrine system to release its chemical messengers or hormones that will bring the body back into balance.

The nervous and endocrine systems are also important components in the feedback systems that regulate the body's internal environment. The two basic types of feedback systems are called negative feedback and positive feedback. Negative feedback is a homeostatic control mechanism that responds to a stress-related change by returning a condition to its normal range. For example, an increase in the blood glucose level induces specific steps that reduce the glucose to its normal level. Positive feedback is designed to amplify the response given to a certain stress. For example, during childbirth, uterine contractions intensify as a result of a positive feedback system, thus enabling the birth of a baby. The majority of the feedback systems in the human body are negative, since in most instances (with a few, specific exceptions) a positive system is detrimental to the body.

Negative feedback. Often, several systems work together to monitor and regulate a particular physiologic condition. An excellent example of this can be seen in the negative feedback regulation of the mean arterial blood pressure. Baroreceptors are the monitoring devices for arterial pressure. They are composed of nerve endings located in the arterial wall of specific blood vessels, such as in the arch of the aorta and the neck area where the common carotid artery divides into the internal and external carotid arteries. Baroreceptors respond to the stretching of the arterial wall. These arteries undergo greater-than-normal stretching during times of high blood pressure and are more relaxed in times of low blood pressure.

Baroreceptors are constantly informing the brain of the status of the mean arterial pressure by sending out nervous impulses to the cardiovascular control center, located in the medulla of the brain. When the body is subject to stress that causes the blood pressure to rise, the elastic arterial walls experience an increase in the amount that they are stretched. The baroreceptors, being stretch receptors, respond to this change by increasing their output of nervous impulses to the brain. In contrast, a drop in blood pressure decreases arterial wall stretching, causing the baroreceptors to send out fewer impulses to the brain.

The nervous impulses from the baroreceptors travel to the cardiovascular control center in the brain via afferent neurons. The cardiovascular control center is a network of neurons that receive and integrate nervous impulses from a variety of other control centers. The cardiovascular control center is connected to the heart by both sympathetic and parasympathetic nerves and to the blood vessels primarily by sympathetic nerves. An increase in the rate of impulses from the baroreceptors (in response to an increase in arterial pressure) results in an increase in the amount of parasympathetic stimulation and a decrease in sympathetic stimulation. On the contrary, a decrease in the rate of impulses from the baroreceptors (in response to a decrease in arterial pressure) results in a decrease in the amount of parasympathetic stimulation and an increase in sympathetic stimulation.

To understand the significance of the stimulation of parasympathetic-versus-sympathetic nervous stimulation, a brief comment must be made as to the organization of the nervous system. The central nervous system (CNS) is made up of the brain, the brain stem, and the spinal cord. The peripheral nervous system (PNS) comprises the nerves that go into and leave the brain stem and spinal cord. The peripheral nervous system is further divided into a somatic portion and an autonomic portion. The somatic nervous system's sensory receptors transmit impulses to the CNS, which then sends impulses through motor neurons to the skeletal muscles. The autonomic nervous system monitors the condition of the internal organs via sensory nerves to the CNS and responds via motor nerves to glands and involuntary muscles. The parasympathetic and sympathetic nerves are the two types of motor nerves that make up the autonomic nervous system. In general, sympathetic nerves initiate the body's fight-or-flight response to stressful situations. Parasympathetic nerves are responsible for more vegetative functions, such as the ingestion and digestion of food.

The combinations of particular nerve activations and deactivations have particular effects on the state of the heart and peripheral blood vessels. As stated above, an increase in mean arterial pressure, as detected by the baroreceptors, invokes a response that increases parasympathetic stimulation of the heart and decreases sympathetic stimulation of the heart and blood vessels. This response serves to reduce the heart rate and the contractility of the heart, thus reducing cardiac output. In addition, blood vessels in the skin and muscles are allowed to dilate, reducing the total peripheral resistance of the blood. The direct relationship of the mean arterial pressure (MAP) to the cardiac output (CO) and total peripheral resistance (TPR) is represented by the formula "MAP = CO TPR." It can be observed that decreasing both CO and TPR results in a decrease in the MAP. This occurs to the point at which the MAP returns to its normal range. If the applied stress decreases the MAP as detected by the baroreceptors, parasympathetic stimulation decreases and sympathetic stimulation increases. This causes an increase in CO and an increase in TPR, resulting in an overall increase in mean arterial pressure.

Positive feedback. An example of positive feedback regulation can be seen in the process of childbirth. Weak, periodic uterine contractions begin during the third trimester of a human pregnancy. As the pregnancy progresses and the time comes for delivery of the baby, these contractions become stronger and increase in frequency. Such contractions are necessary for the expulsion of the baby and the placenta from the mother.

Contractions of the uterine muscles begin at the top, or apex, of the uterus and move down toward its base, at the location of the cervix. These contractions force the head of the baby onto the cervix and stretch it open in a process termed cervical dilation. Cervical stretching sends nerve impulses to the hypothalamus in the brain, which then stimulates the posterior pituitary gland to release the hormone oxytocin. Oxytocin makes the uterine contractions stronger and more rhythmic. Continued stretching of the cervix leads to an increase in the amount of oxytocin released by the pituitary. This positive feedback cycle continues until the baby is born, at which point the pressure on the cervix is removed and it can relax.

PERSPECTIVE AND PROSPECTS

Physiology began more than two thousand years ago during the time of the ancient Greeks. The well-known philosopher Aristotle (384-322 BCE) was also a physiologist who made biological observations and described the blood vessels as part of a system with the heart at its center. He also believed that the heart was a furnace that heated the blood and that it was the body's seat of intellect. In the city of Alexandria, Herophilus (335-280 BCE) believed that the seat of intellect was the brain, not the heart. He studied arteries and veins and determined that arteries have thicker walls. Erasistratus (310-240 BCE) began his training under Herophilus. He believed that arteries served as air vessels and that the veins carried the blood, which was made in the liver from food. Several hundred years later, Galen (129-c. 199 CE) conducted an experiment that showed that blood, not air, flowed through arteries. Though some of his other ideas were later disproved, he left behind a considerable number of writings on physiology, medicine, and philosophy.

Galen's ideas were taught for many hundreds of years until the Renaissance. During this time, physiologists made important discoveries and observations that challenged the findings of Galen. Andreas Vesalius (1514-1564) was trained as a doctor and became a professor of surgery and anatomy at a medical school in what is now Italy. Vesalius's style of teaching was to dissect a cadaver as he lectured, and he included anatomical drawings in his written texts. He wrote what has become known as the first modern anatomy textbook, *De Humanis Corporis Fabrica* (the structure of the human body), published in 1543.

A few decades later, William Harvey (1578-1657) was born in England and later trained as a doctor. He also did some lecturing and wrote a study of circulation, *De Motu Cordis et Sanguinis in Animalibus* (on the motion of the heart and of blood in animals), published in 1628. Harvey viewed the heart as a pump that contracted to expel blood and discovered that the blood moved in a circular path in the body. He believed that the blood traveled from the right ventricle to the lungs and then to the left ventricle, not directly from the right to the left ventricle. He also theorized that air stayed in the lungs and did not move to the heart to meet the blood.

Joseph Priestley (1733-1804), an English chemist, investigated the processes of combustion and breathing. Priestley's experiments used a bell jar, a candle, a green plant, and a mouse. He observed that a candle placed under a bell jar went out, but could later be lit after a green plant was placed under the jar for several days. He also observed that a mouse placed under the jar died after some time. When placed under the jar with a green plant, however, the mouse lived for a longer period of time.

Using an early microscope, Robert Hooke (1635-1703) studied a piece of cork and coined the term "cells' for he compartments that he observed. Two hundred years later, German biologists Matthias Schleiden(1804-1881) and Theodor Schwann (1810-1882) proposed their cell theory. Their theory encompassed some of the essential ideas in biology and physiology, including that all organisms are made of cells which have similar metabolic processes and chemical components, that an organism's functions result from different cells working together, and that all cells have their origin in preexisting cells.

The invention of the thermometer allowed scientists to gain further insights into human physiology. With this investigation came the discovery that the human body maintains a relatively constant internal body temperature, despite changes in the temperature of its environment. The French physiologist Claude Bernard (1813-1878) used the words "milieu intérieur" to describe this constant internal environment of the human body. American physiologist Walter Cannon (1871-1945) later coined the term "homeostasis" to describe this condition.

Essential to investigations and discoveries that advance the field of physiology is the ever-changing nature of technology. Early research was conducted simply with observations of the unaided eye. Later discoveries developed glass lenses to form a light microscope which magnified images up to 1,000 times and opened up a world of tissues and cells that were previously indiscernible. Newer technology led to the formation of the electron microscope, which provided magnification of specimens greater than 100,000 times and revealed the intricacies of subcellular structures.

Technology has advanced to the growth of living cells and tissues in laboratory dishes. Cell culture allows the investigator to change or regulate the environment of the biological material and to determine the effect of such alterations on growth and reproduction. Techniques such as cytochemistry, autoradiography, and immunochemistry have been developed to stain or localize certain regulatory molecules or cellular structures, enabling the scientist to quantify their effects on cell physiology. Cell fractionation has been developed to separate cells into their various components or organelles, thus providing a way that a specific organelle can be studied in isolation. Genetic engineering is a powerful technology that allows the researcher to manipulate and alter the genes of cells that control their functions. All these techniques are frequently used in physiology research and are powerful forces that have expanded scientific understanding.

—*John L. Rittenhouse and Roman J. Miller, PhD*

See also Anatomy; Cells; Cytology; Endocrinology; Exercise physiology; Fluids and electrolytes; Hormones; Kinesiology; Nervous system; Neurology; Sleep; Systems and organs.

For Further Information:
Costanzo, Linda. *Physiology Cases and Problems*. New York: Lippincott Williams & Wilkins, 2012.
Fox, Stuart Ira. *Human Physiology*. 11th ed. Boston: McGraw-Hill, 2010.
Ganong, William F. *Review of Medical Physiology*. 23d ed. New York: Lange Medical Books/McGraw-Hill Medical, 2009.
Guyton, Arthur C., and John E. Hall. *Guyton and Hall Textbook of Medical Physiology*. 12th ed. Philadelphia: Saunders/Elsevier, 2011.
Levitzky, Michael. *Pulmonary Physiology*. New York: McGraw-Hill Medical, 2013.
Preston, Robin R. *Physiology (Lippincott's Illustrated Review Series)*. New York: Lippincott Williams & Wilkins, 2012.
Prosser, C. Ladd, ed. *Environmental and Metabolic Animal Physiology*. 4th ed. New York: Wiley-Liss, 1991.
Rhoades, Rodney, and Richard Pflanzer. *Human Physiology*. 4th ed. Pacific Grove, Calif.: Brooks/Cole, 2003.
Tortora, Gerard J., and Sandra Reynolds Grabowski. *Introduction to the Human Body: The Essentials of Anatomy and Physiology*. 6th ed. Hoboken, N.J.: John Wiley & Sons, 2007.

PHYTOCHEMICALS

Category: Biology
Anatomy or system affected: All
Specialties and related fields: Nutrition, preventive medicine
Definition: Nonnutritive chemicals that plants produce, providing health benefits to humans who eat foods derived from plants.

PROTECTIVE ROLE AND ABUNDANCE

People who eat a diet rich in fresh fruits, vegetables, and whole grains obtain some protection from various diseases because of the phytochemicals that the plants contain. Phytochemicals are not traditional nutrients, such as proteins, carbohydrates, or fats; nor are they vitamins or minerals. Instead, they are substances that plants produce to protect against environmental stresses, such as attack by fungi and other organisms, or to attract animal pollinators or seed dispersers. Many phytochemicals are plant pigments, giving fruits and vegetables their animal-luring colors. There are thousands of phytochemicals, and plant species vary widely in the kinds and amounts that they contain.

Many phytochemicals have antioxidant properties, meaning that they help protect cells from oxidative damage, which has been implicated in cancer, diabetes, heart disease, strokes, and other disorders. Some phytochemicals function in humans in ways similar to the female hormone estrogen.

Although diets rich in plant-based foods have been shown to result in lower incidences of a number of diseases, scientists have had difficulty pinpointing which of the many different phytochemicals are protective. It may be that the interaction of a variety of naturally occurring phytochemicals, rather than any particular ones, is the significant factor in promoting health.

SOME MAJOR KINDS

One important group of phytochemicals, the carotenoids, includes many antioxidants. Of the numerous health claims that have been made for these plant pigments, one of the few to be substantiated is that increased consumption of lutein, a carotenoid found in green leafy vegetables such as collards, kale, spinach, and broccoli, is associated with a lowered risk for macular degeneration, an eye disease associated with advanced age.

Flavonoids, pigments that belong to a major class of phytochemicals called polyphenols, are abundant in vegetables, fruits such as blueberries and raspberries, and beverages such as tea, red wine, and fruit juices. Some flavonoids, including the widely occurring group anthocyanins, have antioxidant properties. Flavonoids called isoflavones are plant estrogens plentiful in soy products.

PERSPECTIVE AND PROSPECTS
The discovery that phytochemicals are important to human health was not made until late in the twentieth century, and research is still being done. Scientists do not advise taking dietary supplements of particular phytochemicals; rather, they recommend a diet high in a variety of fruits, vegetables, and whole grains. Taking concentrated forms of phytochemicals might be harmful over the long term.

—*F. Hill, PhD*

See also Antioxidants; Food biochemistry; Nutrition; Preventive medicine; Supplements; Vitamins and minerals.

For Further Information:
American Institute for Cancer Research, ed. *Nutrition and Cancer Prevention: New Insights into the Role of Phytochemicals.* New York: Kluwer Academic/Plenum, 2001. Advances in Experimental Medicine and Biology 492.
Bao, Yongping, and Roger Fenwick, eds. *Phytochemicals in Health and Disease.* New York: Marcel Dekker, 2004.
Meskin, Mark S., Wayne R. Bidlack, Audra J. Davies, Douglas S. Lewis, and R. Keith Randolph, eds. *Phytochemicals: Mechanisms of Action.* Boca Raton, Fla.: CRC Press, 2004.
Meskin, Mark S., Wayne R. Bidlack, Audra J. Davies, and Stanley T. Omaye, eds. *Phytochemicals in Nutrition and Health.* Boca Raton, Fla.: CRC Press, 2002.
Meskin, Mark S., Wayne R. Bidlack, and R. Keith Randolph, eds. *Phytochemicals: Nutrient-Gene Interactions.* Boca Raton, Fla.: CRC Press/Taylor & Francis, 2006.
"Phytochemicals." *American Cancer Society,* January 17, 2013.
"Phytochemicals and Cardiovascular Disease." *American Heart Association,* May 1, 2013.
Webb, Denise. "Phytonutrients: The Hidden Keys to Disease Prevention, Good Health." *Environmental Nutrition* 26, no. 1 (January, 2003): 1-6.

PICK'S DISEASE

Category: Disease/Disorder
Also known as: Frontotemporal dementia (FTD), lobar sclerosis, circumscribed brain atrophy, focal cerebral atrophy, semantic dementia, primary progressive aphasia
Anatomy or system affected: Brain, nervous system, psychic-emotional system
Specialties and related fields: Family medicine, geriatrics and gerontology, internal medicine, neurology, psychiatry, psychology

Definition: A brain disease causing shrinkage of tissue in discrete areas (focal lesions) in the frontal and temporal anterior brain lobes, thus reducing verbal reasoning and speech production.
Key terms:
anterior: referring to the front, in the direction of the face
autosomal gene: all nonsex, nongender determining chromosomes; a dominant autosome will carry the trait that is observed in the organism, such as hair color or height
frontotemporal lobes: the two frontal and two temporal lobes that are located toward the front and on both the left and right side of the brain; jointly, they have the primary responsibility for executive thinking, reasoning, social judgment, and auditory functions

CAUSES AND SYMPTOMS
Pick's disease, also called frontotemporal dementia (FTD), is similar to, but much rarer than, Alzheimer's disease. The current designation of the syndrome groups together Pick's disease, primary progressive aphasia, and semantic dementia. Some medical researchers believe that corticobasal degeneration and progressive supranuclear palsy should be added to FTD, which would then be called Pick complex. The differing terms reflect different theoretical models of the disease, and specialists are likely to continue to debate these models.

An autosomal dominant genetic trait is speculated as a specific cause in some cases of FTD. In these cases, there is a family history of someone showing symptoms of a frontal lobe dementia. Pick's disease is often inherited, though in many cases there is no evident family (genetic) history and the cause is unknown.

Onset is slow and insidious. Tissues shrink (atrophy) in the frontal and temporal brain lobes. FTD also causes some brain cells to develop abnormal fibers called Pick's bodies. The cells in these bodies have an abnormal amount of a protein called tau. Tau appears throughout the body's cells but exists in abnormally high amounts in Pick's bodies and in Pick cells that exist inside normal brain cells (neurons). These form elsewhere in the brain and are not limited to the frontotemporal regions. These fibers are generally straight and single, as compared to Alzheimer's neurofibrillary tangles, which tend to be paired and helical.

Though Pick's disease varies greatly in how it affects individuals, it has a common core or clusters of symptoms. Some or all may be present at different stages of the disease. Since the frontal lobes involve emotional and social functioning, the first notable cluster of symptoms usually causes behavioral and affective changes such as impulsivity, compulsive overeating or only eating one type of food, drinking alcohol to excess (when not a prior problem), rudeness, impatience, aggressiveness, social withdrawal, poor social interaction, inability to hold a job, inattention to personal hygiene, sexual exhibitionism, promiscuity, abrupt mood changes, emotional aloofness, environmental indifference, marked distractibility, decreased interest in daily activities, and being unaware of these changes (lack of insight). Deterioration in personality usually occurs before dementia itself is evident-that is, before there is evident memory loss. This is one way that specialists diagnose it as distinct from Alzheimer's disease, in which the early symptoms involve memory loss.

Changes in physical mobility and coordination (apraxia) can also appear as early symptoms. They can include increased muscle rigidity or stiffness, difficulty getting around, worsening coordination, generalized weakness, and urinary incontinence.

Another characteristic cluster of symptoms relates to worsening language, including reduced-quality speech, shrinking vocabulary, word-finding problems, difficulty understanding speech (receptive aphasia) or producing understandable speech (expressive aphasia), repeating words and phrases others use (echolalia), progressive loss of reading and writing, and possibly complete loss of speech (mutism).

TREATMENT AND THERAPY

At present, there are no medications that can effectively treat FTD, although several can help treat many of its symptoms. Medications used in Alzheimer's disease are not routinely prescribed because they often increase aggression in Pick's disease patients.

Maximizing quality of life is the key treatment, and many of the more disturbing behaviors respond well to medication, including aggression and agitation. In addition to adding medications for symptom control, discontinuation of medications that promote confusion or that are not essential to the care of the person may improve cognitive function. It is common for anticholinergics, analgesics, and central nervous system depressants to be discontinued. Because many of the functions that FTD affects are also affected by low levels of thiamine, thiamine supplementation is often recommended.

Behavior modification is often the treatment of choice in controlling unacceptable or dangerous behaviors. Rewarding and reinforcing appropriate, positive behaviors while ignoring inappropriate, negative behaviors (within the bounds of safety) can significantly influence how patients act and interact. Formal psychotherapy is seldom effective because it overloads patients" limited cognitive resources. Reality orientation, with repeated reinforcement of environmental

> **INFORMATION ON PICK'S DISEASE**
>
> **Causes:** Shrinkage of brain tissue, abnormal fibers in brain cells (Pick's bodies)
> **Symptoms:** Behavioral and affective changes (impulsivity, compulsive eating, rudeness, impatience, aggressiveness, social withdrawal, poor personal hygiene, sexual exhibitionism, promiscuity, abrupt mood changes, aloofness, distractibility, lack of insight); physical disorders (muscle rigidity, poor coordination, weakness, incontinence); language disturbances (shrinking vocabulary, word-finding problems, difficulty understanding speech, echolalia, loss of reading and writing, mutism)
> **Duration:** Chronic and progressive
> **Treatments:** None; medications, behavioral therapy for symptoms

and other cues, can reduce disorientation and agitation. Sensory functions, often overlooked, should be evaluated and augmented as needed, including hearing aids, eyeglasses, and cataract surgery.

In addition, good nursing and caregiving, guided occupation activities, and participation in support groups all can improve the management of this type of dementia. Family counseling and family psychoeducation often go a long way in fostering adaptive changes that are necessary to care for patients at home. It is also important for families of Pick's disease patients to obtain support to help them cope with a disease that is likely to have a prolonged, ever-demanding course. Visiting nurses or aides, volunteer services, adult protective services, and other community resources may be helpful in caring for the person. Legal advice may be appropriate early in the course of the disorder. Advance directives, power of attorney, health care proxy, and "do not resuscitate" orders can make dealing with the later stages of the disease easier.

PERSPECTIVE AND PROSPECTS

Pick's disease affects about 1 out of 100,000 people, accounting for 0.4 percent to 2.0 percent of all cases of dementia. More common in women then men, it typically has an onset between ages forty and sixty, with a modal age of fifty-four, but it has been known to affect patients as young as twenty. A family history of FTD is considered a risk factor, although most Pick's patients have no family history of the disease.

The first description of the disease was published in 1892 by Arnold Pick. Until recently, it was thought that Pick's disease could not be distinguished from Alzheimer's disease during life. In accordance with major research criteria of German neuropsychiatry, Pick's atrophy was constructed as a full-blown disease entity in the 1920s. This concept gained acceptance in the German and Anglo-American scientific community and was the starting point for further investigations in the 1950s and 1960s.

Initial diagnosis is mostly based on history and symptoms, signs, and tests and by ruling out other causes of dementia, especially those with metabolic causes. The development of neuropsychological assessment procedures and the use of electroencephalograms (EEGs), computed tomography (CT) scans, and magnetic resonance imaging (MRI) scans are generally necessary in the prediagnostic workup of the disease. Functional brain imaging, such as single photon emission computed tomography (SPECT) or positron emission tomography (PET) scans, are often appropriate in some patients.

Patients with FTD or Pick's disease will show a progressive decline. Rapidly progressing forms may be fatal in two years; slower forms may take ten. The cause of death is often opportunistic infection or, less commonly, the general failure of total body systems.

Recent identification of pathogenic mutations in Alzheimer's disease and frontotemporal dementia has improved understanding of these dementias and is guiding the investigations that use animal and tissue culture models. Eventually, it is hoped that this research will result in developing medications that can treat, stop, and reverse these diseases.

—*Paul Moglia, PhD, and Anju Varanasi, MD*

See also Alzheimer's disease; Brain; Brain disorders; Dementias; Frontotemporal dementia (FTD); Memory loss; Neurology; Psychiatry; Psychiatry, geriatric.

For Further Information:
Carson-DeWitt, Rosalyn, and Rimas Lukas. "Dementia." *Health Library*, Sept. 27, 2012.
Frederick, Justin, "Pick Disease: A Brief Overview." *Archives of Pathology and Laboratory Medicine* 130 (July, 2006): 1063-1066.
"Frontotemporal Disorders: Information for Patients, Families, and Caregivers." *National Institute on Aging*, Mar. 13, 2013
Kertesz, Andrew, and David G. Munoz, "Frontotemporal Dementia." *Medical Clinics of North America* 86 (2002): 501-518.
Jasmin, Luc, and David Zieve. "Pick's Disease." *MedlinePlus*, Feb. 16, 2012.
"NINDS Frontotemporal Dementia Information Page." *National Institute of Neurological Disorders and Stroke*, Mar. 20, 2013.
"Non-Alzheimer's Forms of Dementia." In *The Mayo Clinic Guide to Alzheimer's Disease: The Essential Resource for Treatment, Coping, and Caregiving*. Rochester, Minn.: Mayo Clinic, 2005.

PID. See Pelvic inflammatory disease (PID).

Pigeon toes

Category: Disease/Disorder
Also known as: In-toeing
Anatomy or system affected: Bones, feet, hips, joints, knees, legs, ligaments, muscles
Specialties and related fields: Orthopedics, pediatrics, physical therapy, sports medicine
Definition: Usually a temporary condition in which one or both feet point inward when the heels are placed in a normal standing position.

CAUSES AND SYMPTOMS
Pigeon toes sometimes occur in children as a normal phase of development. Patients walk forward on a straight path while a toe or toes turn toward the body's axis. In infants and toddlers, pigeon toes are usually caused by how their hips, legs, and feet were positioned in the womb. Heredity also influences how pigeon toes are caused.

Patients may have pigeon toes for several reasons. Some are pigeon-toed because their feet are curved. In-toeing can also be caused by stiff muscles that hinder leg flexibility. Many cases of pigeon toes are attributable to how hip, leg, knee, and ankle joints and bones are angled and rotated.

Rotated tibias cause in-toeing in what is termed internal tibial torsion. Internal femoral torsion refers to when femurs significantly rotate from the hip socket to knee, affecting foot placement. Sleeping and kneeling positions may exacerbate fetal rotation and angling. Infants' feet often attain correct alignment before they walk, but if they temporarily continue in-toeing, pigeon toes probably will not slow the development of movement skills.

TREATMENT AND THERAPY
Usually, pigeon toes improve as children age, particularly as they gain experience walking. Pigeon toes do not necessitate treatment unless they interfere with movement. Corrective shoes and braces designed for specific cases are sometimes prescribed for young children. Casts can straighten curved foot position. Exercises enhance movement by stretching and strengthening muscles and ligaments to support normal positions.

Children who continue to display pigeon toes after walking for one year should be examined because pigeon toes and such hip abnormalities as dysplasia often occur simultaneously. Asymmetrical in-toeing should also be investigated. Medical professionals will measure body angles, observe patients' movement while standing and walking, and study wear patterns on their shoes to detect how the hips and legs might affect ankle and foot mobility. X-rays can detect related skeletal disorders. Examinations should look for possible neurological conditions and tumors that might cause in-toeing.

Children aged eight years or older may require additional medical intervention. If pigeon toes significantly hinder motion in older patients whose development did not resolve their pigeon toes, physicians may recommend surgical adjustments to enable patients to gain normal mobility. Such measures aid patients who desire involvement in athletic activities.

PERSPECTIVE AND PROSPECTS
In the nineteenth and twentieth centuries, physicians routinely advised the use of corrective splints and shoes. Often these treatments reassured parents that toddlers' pigeon toes would not be a permanent condition. Beginning in the 1930s, many patients wore the Denis-Browne splint, in which shoes are rigidly affixed together by a metal bar at a set angle, while they slept.

By the early twenty-first century, such practices were not implemented as often because many physicians questioned the benefits of therapeutic devices expediting improvement. Most advised allowing pigeon toes to correct naturally during development.

—*Elizabeth D. Schafer, PhD*

See also Bones and the skeleton; Braces, orthopedic; Feet; Flat feet; Foot disorders; Lower extremities; Orthopedic surgery; Orthopedics; Orthopedics, pediatric.

For Further Information:
Atanda, Alfred. "Common Childhood Orthopedic Conditions." *KidsHealth*, November 2011.
Atanda, Alfred. "In-toeing and Out-toeing in Toddlers." *KidsHealth*, November 2011.
Cailliet, Rene. *Foot and Ankle Pain.* 3d ed. Philadelphia: F. A. Davis, 1997.
Harkless, Lawrence B., and Steven M. Krych. *Handbook of Common Foot Problems.* New York: Churchill Livingstone, 1990.
Herring, John A., ed. *Tachdjian's Pediatric Orthopaedics.* 4th ed. 3 vols. Philadelphia: Saunders/Elsevier, 2008.
Klag, Michael J., et al., eds. *Johns Hopkins Family Health Book.* New York: HarperCollins, 1999.
Lippert, Frederick G., and Sigvard T. Hansen. *Foot and Ankle Disorders: Tricks of the Trade.* New York: Thieme, 2003.
Lorimer, Donald L., et al., eds. *Neale's Disorders of the Foot.* 7th ed. New York: Churchill Livingstone/Elsevier, 2006.
Skinner, Harry B, and Patrick J. McMahon. *Current Disorders and Treatment in Orthopedics*, 5th ed. New York: Lange Medical Books, 2013.

PIGMENTATION

Category: Biology
Anatomy or system affected: Eyes, hair, skin
Specialties and related fields: Dermatology, environmental health
Definition: The coloration of human skin and eyes based on the presence and amount of five different pigments; the most important of these pigments, melanin, protects the body from ultraviolet radiation.
Key terms:
dermis: the layer of skin underneath the epidermis that contains hemoglobin and oxyhemoglobin
epidermis: the outer layer of the skin that contains melanocytes, which produce melanin
hypodermis: the layer of fat under the dermis that contains carotene
melanin: a protein that darkens the color of the skin and protects against ultraviolet radiation
melanoma: cancer of the melanocytes, the cells that produce melanin
ultraviolet radiation: radiation that is potentially damaging to the skin; it is not visible to humans

STRUCTURE AND FUNCTIONS
One of the most apparent human characteristics is the color of a person's skin. Five pigments play major roles: melanin, melanoid, carotene, hemoglobin, and oxyhemoglobin. Melanin occurs in the greatest variation and is the most important of the five; in large amounts, it can mask the effects of the other pigments.

Melanocytes are cells that convert tyrosine, an amino acid, into the black pigment called "melanin." The rate of production is controlled by a hormone called "melanocyte-stimulating hormone (MSH)," which is released by the anterior pituitary gland. About a thousand melanocytes occur on each square millimeter of the body (with the exception of the head and the forearms, which have twice as many). Interestingly, all human races vary greatly in color but tend to have the same number of melanocytes, which inherit different abilities to make melanin.

When humans are compared, an uninterrupted array of shades of skin color is found. Traits that show such continuous variation are thought to be controlled by several sets of genes (polygenetic inheritance). Thus, several sets of genes were believed to control the amount of pigmentation. In 2005, researchers at Pennsylvania State University found two variant expressions of a single gene that may be responsible for the observed distribution of human skin color.

Melanocytes convert tyrosine intomelanin by several chemical steps that involve the key enzyme tyrosinase. A functional tyrosinase molecule consists of different amino acids (the building blocks of proteins) and copper. Traces of copper are in the normal human diet and provide the amounts needed for the enzymes.

Tyrosine, the molecule that is converted to melanin, is one of twenty amino acids occurring in biological systems that chain together in various ways to make up different proteins. Eight of these amino acids are essential-that is, they must be present in the diet. The remaining twelve amino acids can be made by chemical modification of the others. Tyrosine is not an essential amino acid. Ample amounts of tyrosine occur in all meats and in most dairy products. If it is not taken into the body in sufficient amounts, however, it will be made from other amino acids. Either way, tyrosine is delivered to the melanocytes and changed into melanin. This product, with its high molecular weight, functions to protect the skin from excessive ultraviolet (UV) radiation.

UV radiation is an invisible part of the sun's radiation having wavelengths from one hundred to four hundred nanometers. Humans can see the colors of the spectrum from red through violet. Wavelengths of radiation that are slightly longer than red (infrared) cannot be seen but are detected by the body as heat. Wavelengths that are shorter than violet, such as UV, cannot be seen or felt. Nevertheless, UV radiation penetrates the body. In moderation, UV light is valuable for humans because the body uses its energy to synthesize vitamin D. Vitamin D allows the intestinal absorption of calcium to be used for skeletal growth and for nerve and muscle function.

UV radiation poses several risks. A sunburn involves UV radiation damage to epidermal skin cells, which release chemicals that dilate blood vessels, causing redness. Swelling and blistering may occur. When large numbers of cells are destroyed, the skin speeds up production of new cells, which forces the burned cells to peel off. UV radiation also can change the skin's collagen, a protein that holds tissues together in much the same way that concrete is reinforced by steel rods. The changes in the collagen, possibly by causing cross-linkage between fibers, can permanently wrinkle the skin. Finally, many researchers agree that UV light may also inhibit the immune response by damaging Langerhans cells in the epidermis. When damaged, these large cells lose their ability to alert the other cells of the immune system to infection. The most serious danger is that UV radiation may alter the genetic code within cells, causing cancer.

Melanin protects the cells of the body by blocking and absorbing UV light. People who have more melanin by heredity are not at as high a risk as those who are lighter. (This is not to say that dark-skinned people should not protect themselves from the sun.) In all cases, exposure to UV radiation immediately causes the skin to darken by causing oxygen to combine with the melanin that is already present. Exposure also increases the rate of melanin production and speeds its distribution to other cells, producing more darkening.

Melanocytes are found at the bottom of the outer layer of the skin, which is called the "epidermis." They are also at the base of the shafts of hairs and in the eye, producing coloration of the iris and in the black membrane of the eye behind the retina. The pigment-producing melanocytes in the skin are found at the base of the epidermis among cube-shaped skin cells that cannot make pigment. About thirty-six of these epidermal cells occur for each melanocyte. Melanocytes have long extensions that reach out to protect the regular skin cells. Furthermore, melanin can also be transferred to epidermal cells. Skin color is also influenced by the distribution and size of the pigment granules in the melanocytes. Very dark skin tends to have single, large granules. Lighter skin tends to have clusters of two to four smaller granules.

On a larger scale, small uneven clusters of pigment are called "freckles." These spots of melanin show mostly in lighter-skinned people, are controlled by heredity, and appear with sun exposure to the skin. Because of this uneven distribution of melanin, other cells among the freckles are not protected and can easily be sunburned.

Moles (nevi) are larger, dark spots of melanin that tend to increase as a person ages. Two types occur: the pigment can be deposited into the dermis (intradermal nevi) or can be found between the dermis and the epidermis (junctional nevi). The first type of mole tends to be elevated and have hair growing from it. The second tends to be flat and very dark.

Large amounts of melanin in hair will cause it to be black. Lesser amounts make it brown, and still less causes it to be blond. White or gray hair has no melanin. Yet a separate gene for a reddish, iron-containing pigment can be inherited. If two of these recessive genes are present, then the hair will be red. Depending on the amount of melanin that is also present, such people range from almost purely red hair to a strawberry blond color to a reddish-brown (auburn). Larger amounts of melanin will cover the red pigment completely.

Lack of melanin in the iris of the eye will scatter light and cause the eye to reflect blue. Larger amounts cause the eye color to be darker. The pigment in the iris serves to block radiation that could sunburn the retina. In 1992, investigators at Boston College found that eye sensitivity increases when the amount of melanin is greater.

Melanin breaks down as it moves toward the outer layers of the epidermis, forming a chemical called "melanoid" in the process. Melanoid can be seen as a yellow color in the thick (calloused) skin of the palms of the hands and the soles of feet.

Carotene is a yellow-to-orange pigment that tends to accumulate in the layer of fat under the skin. This pigment is also responsible for the color of carrots, yellow vegetables, and the yellows in autumn leaves. When taken into the body, carotene is stored in the liver and converted into vitamin A, which is used in vision. Females usually store more carotene than males because of their higher percentages of fat. Asian peoples tend to have combinations of low melanin and higher carotene that produce a yellowish skin hue.

Hemoglobin and oxyhemoglobin are pigments that are found inside red blood cells. Hemoglobin is dark red but looks bluish through the skin. If hemoglobin combines with oxygen, it is called "oxyhemoglobin." Oxyhemoglobin is bright red. Skin color from this pigment varies with the amount of blood that is circulated at the surface of the dermis, the relative amounts of hemoglobin and oxyhemoglobin that are present, and the densities of other pigments. Hemoglobin and oxyhemoglobin affect the color of light-skinned people more than of darker people. The skin of lighter people generally looks reddish, with oxygen-poor veins appearing blue.

Rapid change of hair color, from dark pigmented to gray or white, is impossible because of the slow growth rate of hair. Melanin is deposited into the hair shaft at the root. The hairs grow outward at a rate of about thirteen millimeters a month. Hence, a loss of pigment production would take a long time to show. The myth of rapid change may be based on diseases that cause all the pigmented hair to fall out overnight, leaving only white hairs.

DISORDERS AND DISEASES

Pigmentation can be abnormal and associated with disease. Excess adrenocorticotropic hormone (ACTH) can increase melanin. ACTH contains several hormones, including MSH. Addison disease involves the overproduction of ACTH. Also, certain injuries such as burns, chemical irritations, or some infections may cause an increase in pigmentation, as can pregnancy. Injuries in which melanocytes are destroyed may result in scar tissue that lacks pigmentation. An excessive

intake of carotene can cause light skin to turn orange, a condition called "carotenemia."

Skin cancer has increased over time. In the late twentieth century, the rate doubled every decade from the 1960s to the 1990s. The ozone layer, a thin layer of gas molecules consisting of three oxygen atoms, was being depleted by chemicals such as refrigerants that were released into the atmosphere. This layer protects life on the planet from the full shower ofultraviolet radiation that comes from the sun. In 2013, according to the World Health Organization, some two to three million skin cancers were being diagnosed annually. Any changes in the skin, such as a mole that changes in color or begins to grow, should be shown to a doctor. Although moles and other abnormalities in pigmentation are not usually dangerous, some may develop into melanomas.

Researchers have been trying to discover if it is possible to tan safely. Attempts have been made to develop better creams to block UV radiation. Skin cancer is less common among dark-skinned people; it has been reasoned that if melanin could be put into a skin cream, lighter-skinned people could have more of this natural protection. Unfortunately, many sources of melanin are expensive.

Presently, the best way to avoid skin cancer is to avoid the sunlight, especially when and where the light is most intense-at midday, near the equator, during the summer at other latitudes, at high altitudes, and in highly reflective environments such as sand or snow. Additional protection can be found by using a sunscreen lotion with a high sun-protection factor (SPF) of at least 15. SPF 15 permits fifteen times longer exposure before burning (compared to using no sunscreen), and SPF 30 is thought to protect even the fairest skins. The American Academy of Dermatology recommends using SPF 30 or higher.

Nevertheless, even with frequent applications of sunscreens, people may be putting themselves at risk of melanoma, the most serious skin cancer. Specifically, deoxyribonucleic acid (DNA) absorbs and can be directly damaged by the 280 and 315 nanometer range of UV radiation, and it was formerly assumed that this range, called UVB, was the only one about which people had to worry. Sunscreens were initially developed to block only UVB, the "burning rays." Data collected by Richard B. Setlow and his colleagues at Brookhaven National Laboratory in 1993, however, indicated that longer wavelengths, including some visible light and UVA (315-400 nanometers), can also damage DNA. Setlow suggested that melanin itself absorbs this energy, setting off chemical reactions that produce chemicals that then damage the melanocytes. This process may be the cause of melanoma. The current consensus is that people should protect themselves from all sunlight, using a broad-spectrum sunscreen lotion that protects against both UVA and UVB. The same risks apply to tanning salons.

Most melanomas are skin cancers. They can also be found inside the eye, as a black spot on the white of the eye, on the iris, or in the center of the field of vision. Treatment of such growths with radiation or surgical removal of the tumor are options. Removal of the entire eye may be necessary. Preventive measures include sunglasses that filter UV light. According to the American Academy of Ophthalmology, sunglasses should block 99 to 100 percent of UV radiation. Most manufacturers label their sunglasses.

In 1991, a controlled study was done in which injections of synthetic MSH were tested. The goal was to help prevent sunburn and skin cancer in high-risk individuals who tan poorly. Those receiving MSH showed significant tanning compared to those who received injections of a placebo. Some mild side effects occurred in the MSH group, including some brief flushing and vague stomach discomfort after the injection.

There are several irregularities of pigmentation. If the tyrosinase enzyme is missing, a person will produce no melanin. This condition is inherited among all races, and such a person is called an "albino" (Greek for "white"). Actually, the lack of melanin allows hemoglobin to determine the skin color. In some types of albinism, an affected individual produces reduced amounts of melanin, resulting in an appearance that is only slightly lighter than that found in the individual's family and ethnic community. All albinos have less protection from the sun and, in addition to the risks to the skin, have poor vision because of light reflections off the back of the eye that normally would be absorbed by pigment. With no pigment in the iris, they are also more likely to suffer damage to their retinal cells, resulting in blindness.

Especially in lighter-skinned people, a lack of hemoglobin (anemia) will cause paleness. If a person's body circulates more blood into the dermis, the skin will appear more reddish or flushed. This could signal that the body is attempting to cool itself or that a person is embarrassed. If the body is cold or emotionally shocked, it may reduce circulation of blood to the surface of the dermis and the individual will appear pale. Lack of normal sunlight can cause a person to slow the production of melanin. A person who is exercising by swimming in cold water may not circulate blood as quickly as it is needed, and the increase of hemoglobin may turn that person blue, a tone that is noticeable in people with both large and small amounts of melanin.

PERSPECTIVE AND PROSPECTS

Scientists believe that the first humans probably had their origin in Africa and were darkly pigmented. As people migrated to the higher latitudes, where the radiation from the sun was less direct, having less pigment may have been adaptive. Less melanin would allow these people to synthesize needed vitamin D where there was less direct sunlight and less UV light. Before individuals began to migrate over long distances, populations were neatly distributed with darker skins near the equator and lighter skins in northern Europe. Inuits are an interesting exception: they have dark skin and live in a northern latitude. Their diet, however, has traditionally included fish livers with sufficient vitamin D.

The possibility of danger from the sun and other radiation is only a recent discovery. Ultraviolet radiation was discovered in 1801. By 1927, H. J. Muller showed in the laboratory that x-rays cause changes in the genetic code of fruit flies that can be inherited. Such changes, called "mutations," can be harmful. Further investigations showed that UV light, while not as dangerous as x-rays, can also cause mutations. The likelihood of mutation in an organism is proportional to the dose of radiation that is received; spacing out the exposure makes no difference.

Attempts to classify races by description of skin color have given little return. Paul Broca (1824-80) developed an elaborate table of twenty colors for cross-matching with the eyes and twenty-four colors for cross-matching with the skin. The color of the skin, however, is extremely difficult to judge: the color itself changes with environmental and physiological conditions, the ability of observers varies, and the lighting conditions under which comparisons are made can make a difference in the results.

To avoid some of these problems, studies have been performed with a device that measures the reflection of various wavelengths by the skin. In 1992, a study of members of the Jirel population in Nepal showed that the reflections from measurements of upper arm skin using three different wavelengths varied as if the reflective properties were controlled by only a single set of genes. Evidently, the use of various wavelengths gives little additional information about color differences.

—*Paul R. Boehlke, PhD*

See also Albinos; Dermatology; Grafts and grafting; Plastic surgery; Skin; Skin cancer; Skin disorders; Skin lesion removal; Tattoo removal; Vitamins and minerals; Vitiligo.

For Further Information:
A.D.A.M. Medical Encyclopedia. "Skin - Abnormally Dark or Light." *MedlinePlus*, May 13, 2011.
"Albinism." *Mayo Foundation for Medical Education and Research*, April 2, 2011.
Balter, Michael. "Zebrafish Researchers Hook Gene for Human Skin Color." *Science* 310, no. 5755 (December 16, 2005): 1754-55.

Freinkel, Ruth K., and David T. Woodley, eds. *Biology of the Skin*. New York: Parthenon, 2001.
Greeley, Alexandra. "Dodging the Rays." *FDA Consumer* 27 (July/August, 1993): 30-33.
Greener, Mark. "Gene for Red Hair Could Shed Light on Skin Pigmentation." *Dermatology Times* 20, no. 12 (December, 1999): 19.
Guttman, Cheryl. "Pigmentation Disorders Common in Asians." *Dermatology Times* 20, no. 8 (August, 1999): 24.
"Health Effects of UV Radiation." *World Health Organization*, 2013.
Levine, Norman, ed. *Pigmentation and Pigmentary Disorders*. Boca Raton, Fla.: CRC Press, 1993.
Schalock, Peter C., ed. "Overview of Skin Pigment." *Merck Manual of Home Health Handbook*, January, 2013.
Turkington, Carol, and Jeffrey S. Dover. *The Encyclopedia of Skin and Skin Disorders*. 3d ed. New York: Facts On File, 2007.
"UV Radiation." *United States Environmental Protection Agency*, June, 2010.
Weedon, David. *Skin Pathology*. 3d ed. New York: Churchill Livingstone/Elsevier, 2010.

PIMPLES. SEE ACNE.

PINWORMS

Category: Disease/Disorder
Also known as: *Enterobius vermicularis*, threadworms, seatworms
Anatomy or system affected: Gastrointestinal system, intestines, skin
Specialties and related fields: Dermatology, family medicine, pediatrics, public health
Definition: A common parasitic nematode that resembles a white thread approximately 0.5 inch in length.

CAUSES AND SYMPTOMS

Infestation with pinworm, a common name for the organism *Enterobius vermicularis*, is characterized by itching around the anus that becomes worse at night, causing sleeplessness, irritability, and general restlessness. There may also be vague gastrointestinal symptoms such as loose stools or nausea. Humans are the only host for the pathogen. Young children are most often affected, and the disease spreads easily to other members of the household.

Adult pinworms live in the large intestine. Females migrate to the anus and deposit eggs outside the body; this is the cause of the itching. Scratching often causes the eggs to be deposited on food and eaten or transferred directly to the mouth and swallowed. Newly hatched larvae migrate to the large intestine and lay eggs over a four-week period. Pinworm eggs are viable outside a host for up to two weeks.

> **INFORMATION ON PINWORMS**
>
> **Causes:** Parasitic infestation
> **Symptoms:** Itching around anus that becomes worse at night, sleeplessness, irritability, general restlessness, vague gastrointestinal symptoms such as loose stools or nausea
> **Duration:** Acute
> **Treatments:** Drug therapy, proper hygiene

Children typically complain of intense itching around the anal area at night. Scratching may cause bleeding in the region. Interrupted sleep may cause irritability during the day. Individual worms are not commonly seen. The most common diagnostic procedure is to apply a piece of pressure-sensitive cellulose tape to the anus and look for eggs under a microscope.

Pinworm infestation must be differentiated from fungal and yeast infections, allergies, and conditions caused by other species of worms. Fungal and yeast infections can be cultured. Allergies may include itching near the anus but usually involve other areas of the body as well. Analyzing their eggs or bodies can identify other species of worms.

TREATMENT AND THERAPY

Pinworm infestation is relatively easy to treat. Drugs requiring a physician's prescription are taken by mouth for three to five days and usually kill the pinworms. Antihistamines can be used to obtain relief from itching.

It is very important to wash one's hands thoroughly with soap and warm water after using the toilet and before meals. Fingernails should be closely trimmed to prevent injury when scratching and to minimize the chance of transferring eggs. All clothing of a patient should be washed after each use. Laundering bedding will kill pinworm eggs.

Although pinworm infestation is annoying, it is otherwise benign. A cure can be obtained readily using appropriate drug therapy. Repeated infestation is common, however, especially among children.

—*L. Fleming Fallon, Jr., MD, PhD, MPH*

See also Anus; Gastroenterology; Gastroenterology, pediatric; Gastrointestinal disorders; Gastrointestinal system; Insect-borne diseases; Itching; Parasitic diseases; Worms; Zoonoses.

For Further Information:
Badash, Michelle. "Pinworm." *Health Library*, September 10, 2012.
Despommier, Dickson D., et al. *Parasitic Diseases*. 5th ed. New York: Apple Tree, 2006.
Durani, Yamini. "Infections: Pinworm." *KidsHealth*, May 2011.

Gittleman, Ann Louise. *Guess What Came to Dinner? Parasites and Your Health*. Rev. ed. New York: Putnam, 2001.

Klein, Aaron E. *The Parasites We Humans Harbor*. New York: Nelson Books/Elsevier, 1981.

Litin, Scott C., ed. *Mayo Clinic Family Health Book*. 4th ed. New York: HarperResource, 2009.

Roberts, Larry S., and John Janovy, Jr., eds. *Gerald D. Schmidt and Larry S. Roberts' Foundations of Parasitology*. 7th ed. Boston: McGraw-Hill Higher Education, 2005.

Scheinberg, Dianne. "Pruritus Ani." *Health Library*, March 15, 2013.

Shannon, Joyce Brennfleck. *Contagious Diseases Sourcebook: Basic Consumer Health Information about Diseases Spread from Person to Person*. Detroit, Mich.: Onmigraphics, 2010.

Woolf, Alan D., et al., eds. *The Children's Hospital Guide to Your Child's Health and Development*. Cambridge, Mass.: Perseus, 2002.

Zieve, David, et al. "Pinworms." *MedlinePlus*, August 14, 2012.

PITUITARY GLAND

Category: Biology

Anatomy or system affected: Brain, endocrine system, glands

Specialties and related fields: Biochemistry, endocrinology, family medicine, nutrition, obstetrics, osteopathic medicine, pediatrics

Definition: An endocrine gland located at the base of the brain, just inferior to the hypothalamus.

Key terms:

adenohypophysis: another name for the anterior lobe of the pituitary gland

negative feedback: a common physiological process by which the product of a process feeds back to inhibit further stimulation (or reverse) the process

neurohypophysis: another name for the posterior lobe of the pituitary gland

positive feedback: a physiological process in which a product feeds back to stimulate the process, resulting in additional production or the continuation of that process

STRUCTURE AND FUNCTIONS

The pituitary gland is similar in size to a pea and has two lobes, the anterior (adenohypophysis) and the posterior (neurohypophysis). The anterior lobe accounts for a greater proportion of the total weight, approximately 80 percent. The pituitary gland is involved in the release of numerous hormones that have a multitude of effects throughout the body; as a result, it is often referred to as the "master" gland. The functions of the hormones released from the pituitary gland include reproductive functions (including childbirth and lactation), bone growth and development, and regulation of metabolic processes, body temperature, water balance, circulation, and blood pressure. Therefore, a normally functioning pituitary gland is essential to the health and maintenance of homeostasis in humans.

Hormones released from the anterior lobe of the pituitary gland include thyroid-stimulating hormone (TSH) or thyrotropin, growth hormone (GH), adrenocorticotropic hormone (ACTH), follicle-stimulating hormone (FSH), luteinizing hormone (LH), and prolactin (PRL). The hypothalamus, which is located just superior to the pituitary gland, regulates the release of hormones from the anterior pituitary gland by releasing hormones that travel through a blood network called the hypophyseal portal system to the anterior pituitary. For example, the hypothalamus releases growth-hormone-releasing hormone (GHRH), which travels to the anterior pituitary and stimulates the release of growth hormone. Alternatively, if the body wants to decrease the secretion of GH, the hypothalamus may do so by releasing growth-hormone-inhibiting hormone (GHIH), also known as growth-hormone-release-inhibiting hormone (GHRIH) or somatostatin. Another common inhibiting hormone released from the hypothalamus is prolactin-inhibiting hormone (PIH), which reduces the release of PRL from the anterior pituitary.

In contrast to the anterior lobe, the posterior lobe of the pituitary gland releases two hormones: oxytocin and antidiuretic hormone (ADH), which is commonly referred to as vasopressin. The release of these hormones is influenced by blood pressure, osmolarity of the blood, and other inputs, such as those from the nervous and reproductive systems.

Several hormones released by the pituitary gland stimulate other organs or tissues directly, resulting in changes in overall physiologic function. For example, GH increases protein synthesis and the related growth of muscles, bones, and tissues. GH also increases the release of glucose and fat breakdown to fuel these anabolic processes. PRL stimulates the mammary glands and causes lactation, and oxytocin also stimulates lactation and causes contraction of the uterine wall during labor. Finally, ADH causes the kidneys to reabsorb or retain water, aiding in the body's ability to regulate water balance and hydration levels.

Other hormones released by the pituitary gland stimulate the release of still other hormones from subsequent endocrine glands. These include TSH, which stimulates the thyroid gland to release thyroid hormones; ACTH, which stimulates the cortex of the adrenal glands to release cortisol; and the sex hormones FSH and LH, also called gonadotrophs, which stimulate the sex organs in males and females to release hormones involved in the production of sperm and the function of the menstrual cycle, respectively.

The release of most hormones from the pituitary gland is controlled by classic negative-feedback loops. In these systems, an increase in product feeds back to inhibit further stimulation of that system. Using the thyroid hormones as an example, the hypothalamus releases thyrotropin-releasing hormone (TRH), which stimulates the anterior pituitary to release TSH, which then causes the thyroid gland to release thyroid hormones. When circulating levels of thyroid hormones are higher than normal or necessary, they feed back to inhibit or slow the release of TRH from the hypothalamus and TSH from the anterior pituitary. Conversely, when circulating levels of thyroid hormones are low, they feed back to increase the release of TRH and TSH, which will ultimately increase the release of thyroid hormones from the thyroid gland. Therefore, there are several sites of control involved in the release of products from the pituitary gland.

A notable exception to this trend is the presence of a positive-feedback process involving the pituitary gland and the hormone oxytocin. In this system, the stretching of the cervix during labor causes the release of oxytocin, which increases contractions in the uterus to assist with the progression of labor and eventual childbirth. The oxytocin feeds back in a positive fashion by increasing the stretching of the cervix, which then leads to the release of even more oxytocin. This cycle continues until the child is born, at which time the stimulus of cervix stretch and the related oxytocin release both cease.

DISORDERS AND DISEASES
Pituitary dysfunction is typically characterized by an oversecretion or undersecretion of pituitary hormones. An overactive pituitary gland is an endocrine defect characterized by excessive growth in stature and mass, plus a variety of other symptoms, depending on which hormones are elevated. The increased hormone release from the pituitary gland is often attributed to a pituitary tumor. If this is the case, then the tumor may be treated with radiation therapy, surgical removal, or the use of an antagonist to decrease the release of pituitary hormones.

Individuals with underactive pituitary glands, or hypopituitarism, experience symptoms such as short stature, low body mass, infertility or reproductive difficulties (including the inability of women to lactate following childbirth), low energy levels, perpetual feeling of cold due to an inability to regulate body temperature, and fatigue. Hypopituitarism may also be caused by a pituitary tumor, as well as injury to or infection of the hypothalamus or pituitary gland. The treatment for hypopituitarism involves stimulating the release of hormones from the target organs or tissues, rather than stimulating the pituitary gland itself.

—*Kristin S. Ondrak, PhD*

See also Brain; Endocrine disorders; Endocrine glands; Endocrinology; Endocrinology, pediatric; Glands; Hormones; Hypothalamus; Systems and organs.

For Further Information:
Baylis, P. H. "Posterior Pituitary Function in Health and Disease." *Clinical Endocrinology and Metabolism* 12, no. 3 (November 1983): 747-770.
Besser, G. M. "Pituitary and Hypothalamic Physiology." *Journal of Clinical Pathology Supplement (Association of Clinical Pathologists)* 7 (1976): 8-11.
Daniel, P. M. "Anatomy of the Hypothalamus and Pituitary Gland." *Journal of Clinical Pathology Supplement (Association of Clinical Pathologists)* 7 (1976): 1-7.
Freeman, Susan, L. "The Anterior Pituitary." In *Endocrine Pathophysiology*, edited by Catherine B. Niewoehner. 2d ed. Raleigh, N.C.: Hayes Barton Press, 2004.
Harris, G. W. "Neural Control of the Pituitary Gland: I. The Neurohypophysis." *British Medical Journal* 2, no. 4731 (September 8, 1951): 559-564.
Harris, G. W. "Neural Control of the Pituitary Gland: II. The Adenohypophysis, with Special Reference to the Secretion of ACTH." *British Medical Journal* 2, no. 4732 (September 15, 1951): 627-634.
Klibanski, Anne, and Nicholas Tritos, eds. "Pituitary Disorders." *Hormone Health Network*, May 2013.
"Pituitary Disorders." *MedlinePlus*, July 11, 2013.

PITYRIASIS ALBA

Category: Disease/Disorder
Anatomy or system affected: Arms, back, neck, skin
Specialties and related fields: Dermatology, family medicine, histology, pediatrics
Definition: A common skin disorder that causes light-colored, scaly patches of skin on the face, neck, and arms.

CAUSES AND SYMPTOMS
Pityriasis alba is a nonspecific disorder of the skin regarded as a manifestation of atopic dermatitis. It may be triggered by drying agents, including the sun, wind, soap, and bathing. It typically manifests itself on the fragile skin of children between the ages of three and sixteen, usually appearing on the face but sometimes extending to the neck, arms, and trunk of the body. Several patches are typical, extending in diameter from 5 to 30 millimeters. The exact cause is unknown. Although annoying, the disease is not dangerous or contagious.

Pityriasis alba appears as slightly elevated round to oval spots that have little color. The spots are usually white but occasionally pale pink to light brown. The boundaries of the spots are generally uneven and not clearly visible. Being light-colored, the spots are most noticeable in the summertime, standing out from the tanned skin of a patient. As the disorder progresses

For Further Information:

Berman, Kevin. "Pityriasis Alba." *MedlinePlus*, May 13, 2011.

Kimball, Chad T. *Childhood Diseases and Disorders Sourcebook: Basic Consumer Health Information About Medical Problems Often Encountered in Pre-adolescent Children*. Detroit, Mich.: Omnigraphics, 2003.

Leung, Donald Y. M., and Malcolm W. Greaves, eds. *Allergic Skin Disease: A Multidisciplinary Approach*. New York: Marcel Dekker, 2000.

Wolff, Klaus et al.. *Fitzpatrick's Color Atlas and Synopsis of Clinical Dermatology*. 7th ed. New York: McGraw-Hill Medical, 2013.

over a few weeks, the affected areas often develop very fine powdery scales. Dry skin makes the rash worse.

TREATMENT AND THERAPY

Since the disorder eventually resolves on its own in almost all cases, treatment may not be necessary. It is important to keep the skin moisturized. A variety of lotions, creams, or ointments (such as Curel, Nivea, or Lubriderm) may be applied to the affected areas, particularly after bathing or exposure to the sun. If the rash is inflamed or itchy, then a mild hydrocortisone cream can be applied daily. For some patients, phototherapy improves the condition.

Pityriasis alba usually clears after a few months, but in some cases it can last up to three years. It typically takes at least several weeks in order for new healthy skin to develop and adjust its color back to normal. In some cases, the disorder will reappear from time to time. Some children experience the disease every summer, but over the years, their skin color eventually returns to normal.

PERSPECTIVE AND PROSPECTS

Pityriasis is derived from the Greek *pityron*, which means "scales," while *alba* means "white." Therefore, pityriasis alba describes white, scaly patches. The rash is most often confined to the face, especially around the cheeks, mouth, and chin. About 20 percent of the time, it may also occur on the neck, arms, and chest. Occasionally, it may show up only on the arms and trunk of the body.

Care must be taken to distinguish pityriasis alba from other related skin disorders, particularly tinea versicolor and vitiligo. Tinea versicolor, a fungal infection, can be ruled out by examining flakes of skin from the affected areas with a potassium hydroxide test. In vitiligo, there is a well-defined border between normal skin and the diseased spots.

—*Alvin K. Benson, PhD*

See also Dermatitis; Dermatology; Dermatology, pediatric; Rashes; Skin; Skin disorders.

PITYRIASIS ROSEA

Category: Disease/Disorder

Anatomy or system affected: Back, chest, skin

Specialties and related fields: Dermatology, family medicine, pathology

Definition: A skin disorder that manifests with a characteristic rash.

CAUSES AND SYMPTOMS

Pityriasis rosea is primarily a skin disease of children and young adults, with females being more commonly affected than males. The initial lesion is a characteristic eruption seen on the trunk called the herald or mother patch, as it signals the onset of lesions to come. This is a scaly pink plaque which is around one to two centimeters in diameter, slightly raised above the surface, with central salmon-colored wrinkles. This lesion should be differentiated from that of syphilis and ringworm.

The herald patch is followed in about two weeks by a crop of similar but smaller lesions all over the trunk. The pink scaly oval papules are distributed along the skin tension lines in the trunk and result in a so-called Christmas tree distribution. The lesions may be mild to moderately pruritic (itchy) and will resolve spontaneously in four to six weeks, without any specific treatment. Other symptoms may involve mild aches and fatigue.

The exact cause of this exanthem (eruptive disease) is not known, but it is believed to result from exposure to various viruses. Most patients appear to have a positive recent history of influenza or an upper respiratory tract infection. The eruption typically appears in spring and fall and appears to cluster among close contacts; however, it is not believed to be highly contagious.

TREATMENT AND THERAPY

There is no specific treatment for pityriasis rosea, and usually none is required, as the disease is self-limited and resolves without treatment in four to six weeks.

Pruritus is usually mild and can be treated with antihistamines and calamine lotion. If itching is severe, then topical steroids and a short, tapered dose of systemic steroids may be administered. Ultraviolet B (UVB) radiation is another treatment option. Patients are also advised to avoid hot showers and strenuous activity, as sweat and water appear to exacerbate the rash.

PERSPECTIVE AND PROSPECTS

The term *pityriasis* is derived from the Greek *pityron*, meaning "scales." The term, initially applied to include all those skin disorders that were characterized by fine scales, is presently used only with modifiers such as *rosea*, *alba*, or *versicolor*. *Rosea* means "pink," and therefore pityriasis rosea describes pink-colored, fine, scaly lesions.

It is important clinically to distinguish the herald patch from other skin conditions. Therefore, a blood test for syphilis should be included for differential diagnosis. Also, ringworm, which requires treatment with antifungal agents, should be ruled out.

About 3 percent of the patients with pityriasis rosea experience recurrences, and no systemic manifestations have been demonstrated.

—Rashmi Ramasubbaiah, MD

See also Dermatology; Dermatology, pediatric; Itching; Lesions; Rashes; Skin; Skin disorders; Viral infections.

For Further Information:
Chuh, Antonio A. T. "Pityriasis Rosea: Roles of the Dermatology Nurse." *Dermatology Nursing* 16, no. 2 (April 1, 2004): 130-136.
Parker, James N., and Philip M. Parker. *Pityriasis Rosea: A Medical Dictionary, Bibliography, and Annotated Research Guide to Internet References.* San Diego, Calif.: ICON Health Publications, 2004.
Kasper, Dennis L., et al., eds. *Harrison's Principles of Internal Medicine.* 18th ed. New York: McGraw-Hill, 2012.
Montemayor-Quellenberg, Marjorie. "Pityriasis Rosea." *Health Library*, September 26, 2012.
Rakel, Robert E., ed. *Textbook of Family Practice.* 8th ed. Philadelphia: W. B. Saunders, 2011.
Tapley, Donald F., et al., eds. *The Columbia University College of Physicians and Surgeons Complete Home Medical Guide.* Rev. 3d ed. New York: Crown, 1995.
Vorvick, Linda J. "Pityriasis Rosea." *MedlinePlus*, October 14, 2012.

PKU. SEE PHENYLKETONURIA (PKU)

PLACENTA

Category: Biology
Also known as: Chronic adrenal insufficiency, hypoadrenocorticism
Anatomy or system affected: Fetus, uterus
Specialties and related fields: Obstetrics and gynecology, perinatology
Definition: An organ that attaches to the uterus wall, provides oxygen and nutrients to the baby, and removes waste products from their blood.
Key terms:
afterbirth: the placenta and fetal membranes discharged from the uterus after birth
placenta abruption: when the placenta separates early from the uterus
placenta previa: a condition in which the placenta partially or wholly blocks the neck of the uterus
trophoblasts: cells forming the outer layer of a blastocyst, which provide nutrients to the embryo and develop into a large part of the placenta

STRUCTURE AND FUNCTIONS

The placenta is an important and unique organ that develops in women only during pregnancy. The placenta connects a woman's body to the embryo and then the fetus through the umbilical cord. The cells that make up the placenta, called trophoblasts, function to control the degree of uterine invasion in the mother and the development of a nutrient, gas, and waste transport for the fetus. The fetus receives oxygen and nutrients from the mother and eliminates wastes through the placenta. The placenta is necessary for the development and survival of the fetus during pregnancy. Still, it must be delivered from the mother's body after the baby's birth. It is then termed afterbirth.

In addition to its primary goal of transporting nutrients, oxygen, and waste between mother and fetus, the placenta also serves as a major endocrine organ. The placenta synthesizes and secretes sex steroids and protein hormones. One hormone, human chorionic gonadotropin (hCG), is secreted by the placenta about one week after an egg has been fertilized (conception). This hormone stimulates the production of the steroid hormone progesterone, which is needed for the baby's survival. The detection of hCG in a mother's urine is the most common pregnancy test.

DISORDERS AND DISEASES

In most pregnant women, the placenta forms and grows normally. In some cases, however, the placenta does not grow properly, is poorly positioned in the uterus, or does not function properly. It may be too large or small or connect abnormally. Placental problems are among the most common complications of pregnancy.

Placenta previa is a condition that occurs during pregnancy when the placenta implants in the lower part of the uterus and obstructs the cervical opening to the birth canal. The incidence of placenta previa is approximately one in two hundred births.

Placenta abruptio during pregnancy occurs when the placenta separates from the uterus before the fetus is born. This condition occurs in about one of every ninety deliveries. A woman is more likely to develop this condition if she has preeclampsia. The cause is unknown, but preeclampsia usually occurs in the second half of pregnancy. Signs include high blood pressure, swelling, and protein in the urine. Preeclampsia risk is higher in women carrying multiple fetuses, teenage mothers, and women older than forty.

Most women with preeclampsia still deliver healthy babies. Still, a rare few may develop a condition called eclampsia (seizures caused by toxemia), which is very serious for the mother and the baby. Approximately eight percent of pregnant women will develop preeclampsia.

When the placenta fails to develop or function properly, the fetus cannot grow and develop normally; placental insufficiency—the earlier in pregnancy, the more severe the resulting problems. Suppose placental insufficiency occurs for a long time during pregnancy. In that case, it may lead to intrauterine growth retardation or restriction (IUGR), a condition in which the fetus does not grow as large as it should while in the uterus. These babies are very small for their gestational age. IUGR can be caused by decreased blood flow to the placenta, drug use, smoking, alcoholism, or placental abnormalities. A diagnosis can be made through ultrasound to measure fetal growth and a non-stress test that measures the heart rate and movement of the fetus. Between 3 and 5 percent of all pregnancies are complicated by IUGR caused by placental insufficiency. A baby with severe IUGR is more likely to have health problems in the newborn period and throughout childhood.

PERSPECTIVE AND PROSPECTS

The placenta is a unique organ essential for the birth of a child. The most common problems in pregnancy involve the placenta; fortunately, many are manageable. With preeclampsia, delivery of the baby is the best way to protect both the mother and the baby. However, delivery under such conditions is not always possible because it may be too early for the baby to live outside the womb. In this case, the obstetrician and her team can take steps to manage the preeclampsia until the baby can be delivered, including decreasing blood pressure with bed rest or medicine. Fortunately, preeclampsia is usually detected early in women who obtain regular prenatal care, and most problems can be prevented. Most cases of IUGR cannot be prevented, especially if they are the result of genetic causes. Some mothers can prevent IUGR cases by taking the following precautions: abstinence from alcohol, tobacco, and illicit drugs; careful monitoring and early treatment for high blood pressure and diabetes; and a diet high in folate before and during pregnancy to protect against certain congenital disabilities.

—*Thomas L. Brown, PhD*

For Further Information:
de Bellefonds, Colleen. "What Is the Placenta? What This Organ Does and How It Forms." *What to Expect*, 9 Jul. 2021, www.whattoexpect.com/pregnancy/placenta. Accessed 10 Apr. 2022.
Placenta: How it works, what's normal. Mayo Clinic, 25 Mar. 2020, www.mayoclinic.org/healthy-lifestyle/pregnancy-week-by-week/in-depth/placenta/art-20044425. Accessed 10 Apr. 2022.
Placenta Previa. March of Dimes, Jan. 2022, www.marchofdimes.org/complications/placenta-previa.aspx#. Accessed 10 Apr. 2022.
Placental Insufficiency. MedlinePlus, 1 Apr. 2022, medlineplus.gov/ency/article/001485.htm. Accessed 10 Apr. 2022.
"Understanding the Placenta." *YouTube*, uploaded by Zero to Finals, 5 Jul. 2018, www.youtube.com/watch?v=gbextFwqnY4.
What is the Placenta? Pregnancy, birth & baby, Aug. 2020, www.pregnancybirthbaby.org.au/what-is-the-placenta. Accessed 10 Aug. 2022.
What is the Placenta? You and Your Hormones, Feb. 2018, www.yourhormones.info/glands/placenta/. Accessed 10 Apr. 2022.

PLAGUE

Category: Disease/Disorder
Anatomy or system affected: Lungs, respiratory system
Specialties and related fields: Bacteriology, emergency medicine, environmental health, epidemiology, public health
Definition: An infection transmitted by fleas, which may prove fatal if left untreated.

CAUSES AND SYMPTOMS

Plague is caused by infection with a bacterium called *Yersinia pestis* (formerly *Pasteurella pestis*). *Yersinia pestis* is a gram-negative, bipolar-staining bacillus that predominantly infects rodents, with humans being accidental hosts. The disease is transmitted by the bite of a flea that has become infected after a blood meal from another animal with the bacterium in its bloodstream or by the ingestion of contaminated animal tissues.

There are three cycles that perpetuate plague in animals and humans. Sylvatic or wild plague is maintained in the wild rodent population, such as ground squirrels, rock squirrels, and prairie dogs. Urban rat plague occurs in developing countries, especially seaports, and is maintained by the infection of urban and domestic rats, which during epidemics may be as high as 10 percent of the rat population. Finally, there is pneumonic plague, a form of the disease limited to humans, which directly transmit the infection via infected aerosol droplets from a person with a lung infection.

The most common plague illness in humans is called bubonic plague. After an incubation period of two to eight days following the bite of an infected flea, there is a sudden onset of fever, chills, weakness, and headache. Within hours, extremely tender oval swellings one to ten centimeters in length appear in one anatomic area of lymph nodes, usually the groin, axilla (armpit), or neck. These buboes presumably result when the bacteria inoculated into the skin by the infected flea migrate to the regional lymph nodes. Many of these patients will have bacteria intermittently present in the bloodstream during the acute stage of the illness.

Less common, but more severe, forms of the illness include septicemic and pneumonic plague. Septicemic plague occurs when the inoculated bacteria proliferate rapidly in the blood, overwhelming the patient before producing a bubo. Pneumonic plague may occur as a secondary pneumonia in bubonic plague, when the lung becomes infected by bacteria carried in the bloodstream, or as a primary pneumonia, through direct inhalation following exposure to a coughing plague patient. Septicemic and pneumonic plague are often fatal, especially if antibiotic therapy is delayed. Rarely, plague can be manifested as a pharyngitis resembling acute tonsillitis or meningitis.

TREATMENT AND THERAPY

A diagnosis of plague is suspected in febrile patients who have been exposed to rodents in areas of the world known to harbor the disease. The causative bacteria are usually identified by microscopic examination and culture of material obtained from aspiration of a bubo. Blood, sputum, throat swabs, or spinal fluid can be processed in a similar manner.

Quarantine, rat control, and insecticides to kill fleas have successfully controlled urban plague in many cities around the globe. Sylvatic plague has been more difficult to control because of the range and diversity of the world rodent reservoirs. A vaccine is available for selected high-risk individuals. Untreated plague has a mortality of more than 50 percent, but this high risk of death can be reduced by the early institution of

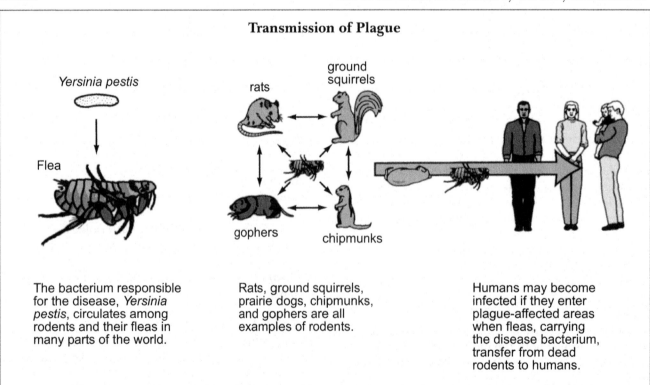

Transmission of Plague

Yersinia pestis

Flea

rats

ground squirrels

gophers

chipmunks

The bacterium responsible for the disease, *Yersinia pestis*, circulates among rodents and their fleas in many parts of the world.

Rats, ground squirrels, prairie dogs, chipmunks, and gophers are all examples of rodents.

Humans may become infected if they enter plague-affected areas when fleas, carrying the disease bacterium, transfer from dead rodents to humans.

A variety of small mammals, particularly rodents, carry the flea that transmits the plague bacterium Yersinia pestis. ©EBSCO antibiotic treatment with either streptomycin or tetracycline and the use of modern medical supportive care.

PERSPECTIVE AND PROSPECTS
The first pandemic of plague began in Egypt or Ethiopia in 540 C.E. and continued for sixty years, killing about one hundred million people. The second pandemic, called the Black Death, began in the fourteenth century in central Asia and then spread to Europe, where a quarter of the total population died. The world is currently in the third pandemic, which began in China during the 1890s when infected rats were inadvertently transported on ships to other countries in the Americas, Asia, and Africa.

Currently, between one thousand and two thousand cases are reported each year to the World Health Organization, with African countries leading the list in numbers of cases. The United States reports an average of one to seventeen cases per year, mostly from Arizona and New Mexico. American Indians seem especially susceptible to this disease.

—*H. Bradford Hawley, MD*

See also Bacterial infections; Biological and chemical weapons; Bites and stings; Epidemics and pandemics; Epidemiology; Insect-borne diseases; Pneumonia.

For Further Information:
Altman, Linda Jacobs. *Plague and Pestilence: A History of Infectious Disease*. Springfield, N.J.: Enslow, 1998.
Centers for Disease Control and Prevention. "Plague: Maps and Statistics." *Centers for Disease Control and Prevention*, April 23, 2013.
Chase, Marilyn. *The Barbary Plague: The Black Death in Victorian San Francisco*. New York: Random House, 2003.
Cook, Gordon C., and Alimuddin I. Zumla, eds. *Manson's Tropical Diseases*. 22d ed. Edinburgh: Saunders/Elsevier, 2009.
Desalle, Rob. *Epidemic! The World of Infectious Disease*. New York: New Press, 2000.
Farmer, Paul. *Infections and Inequalities: The Modern Plagues*. Updated ed. Berkeley: University of California Press, 2009.
Gottfried, Robert S. *The Black Death: Natural and Human Disaster in Medieval Europe*. New York: Free Press/Macmillan, 1983.
Mandell, Gerald L., John E. Bennett, and Raphael Dolin, eds. *Mandell, Douglas, and Bennett's Principles and Practice of Infectious Diseases*. 7th ed. Philadelphia: Churchill Livingstone/Elsevier, 2010.
MedlinePlus. "Plague." *MedlinePlus*, January 14, 2013.
Puzanov, Igor. "Plague." *Health Library*, November 2012.
Woods, Gail L., et al. *Diagnostic Pathology of Infectious Diseases*. Philadelphia: Lea & Febiger, 1993.

PLAQUE, ARTERIAL

Category: Disease/Disorder
Also known as: Atheroma, atheromatous plaque
Anatomy or system affected: Blood vessels, circulatory system, heart
Specialties and related fields: Cardiology, internal medicine, vascular medicine
Definition: Fatty deposits within arterial walls.

CAUSES AND SYMPTOMS
Arterial plaques are caused by a buildup of cholesterol and cell debris within arterial walls. This process occurs over a period of decades, starting at local sites of arterial inflammation. Low-density lipoproteins carrying cholesterol (LDL-C) that infiltrate these sites are highly susceptible to oxidation, which activates another inflammatory response that summons macrophages (part of the immune system). The macrophages engulf the oxidized LDL-C and accumulate as bloated foam cells along with some other cells to become a fatty streak. A tug-of-war ensues in which cholesterol continues to accumulate while other processes remove it. When too much cholesterol accumulates, a scablike cap is formed, while other processes slowly calcify the plaque from the bottom up. This strategy works well as long as the cap does not crack; a cracked cap leaks debris into the artery, which triggers thrombosis (clotting). Blockage of a large coronary artery causes a heart attack; blockage of arteries feeding the brain causes a stroke. Clots that are not fully occlusive get degraded, but repeated rounds of plaque rupturing and recapping eventually cause stenosis (narrowing of the artery) and ischemia (oxygen starvation).

TREATMENT AND THERAPY
Treatment begins with lifestyle changes-exercising, managing stress, stopping smoking, lowering blood pressure, eating more fruits and vegetables. The next step is reducing high levels of LDL-C using statins, which also provide antioxidant, anti-inflammatory, and plaque-stabilizing benefits. Bile acid sequestrants and cholesterol absorption inhibitors are sometimes used as well. Fibrates and niacin are used to counteract

---

INFORMATION ON ARTERIAL PLAQUE
Causes: Hypercholesterolemia, hypertension, inflammation
Symptoms: None in early stages; in later stages, when blood flow impaired, then unusual fatigue, light-headedness, palpitations, feeling of pressure on chest (angina)
Duration: Chronic
Treatments: Lifestyle changes, statins, blood pressure medication

LDL-C by boosting HDL-C, the high-density lipoprotein or "good" cholesterol. High blood pressure is typically treated using diuretics, beta blockers, or angiotensin-converting enzyme (ACE) inhibitors. Thrombosis risk is reduced using low-dose aspirin or drugs such as warfarin, clopidogrel, and prasugrel. Stenosis can be treated using nitroglycerin, ranolazine, and calcium-channel inhibitors to help arteries dilate. A common surgical procedure is to physically open the artery using a catheter, often done in conjunction with implanting a stent to keep the artery propped open. Surgery can also be used to scrape out arteries or replace them.

PERSPECTIVE AND PROSPECTS

Once plaques reach their later stages of development, they are extremely difficult, if not impossible, to remove. Prospects are best when lifestyle changes are initiated early in adulthood. Blood tests for assessing risk factors are invaluable; the most useful ones measure fasting levels of glucose, total cholesterol, LDL-C, HDL-C, triglycerides, homocysteine, and C-reactive protein (a marker of inflammation). Monitoring and controlling blood pressure is also vitally important.

—*Brad Rikke, PhD*

See also Angina; Angiography; Angioplasty; Arteriosclerosis; Bypass surgery; Cardiac arrest; Cardiology; Cholesterol; Circulation; Claudication; Embolism; Endarterectomy; Echocardiography; Heart; Heart attack; Heart disease; Hypercholesterolemia; Hyperlipidemia; Hypertension; Ischemia; Phlebitis; Stents; Strokes; Thrombolytic therapy and TPA; Thrombosis and thrombus; Transient ischemic attacks (TIAs); Vascular medicine; Vascular system; Venous insufficiency.

For Further Information:
Crowley, Leonard V. *An Introduction to Human Disease, Pathology, and Pathophysiology Correlations.* 9th ed. Boston: Jones and Bartlett, 2013.
Mittal, Satish. *Coronary Heart Disease in Clinical Practice.* London: Springer, 2005.
Rosenblum, Laurie. "Atherosclerosis." *Health Library,* May 8, 2013.

PLAQUE, DENTAL

Category: Disease/Disorder
Also known as: Dental biofilm
Anatomy or system affected: Mouth, teeth
Specialties and related fields: Dentistry
Definition: Various kinds of bacteria that live in the mouth stick to each other and then to the tooth surface, both above and below the gums, causing tooth decay and gum disease.
Key terms:
gingivitis: inflammation of the gum tissue
periodontitis: inflammation of the tissues around the teeth
tartar: hardened, mineralized layers of dental plaque

CAUSES AND SYMPTOMS

Dental plaque begins to form when food that contains sugars and starches adheres to teeth. Bacteria that harmlessly live in the mouth feed on these carbohydrates and excrete acids. These acids dissolve the minerals in the enamel on the surfaces of teeth, leading to tooth decay. They also irritate the gums, causing gingivitis and periodontitis. When dental plaque builds up, it can become mineralized; this form is called tartar. Plaque especially accumulates in the grooves of the molars, between adjacent teeth, and along the margin between the teeth and gums.

Susceptibility to tooth decay from dental plaque is dependent upon how clean the mouth is kept, whether fluoride is in the toothpaste and drinking water, the amount of moisture in the mouth, the composition of the diet, and heredity.

Plaque can be felt with the tongue as a slime on the surface of teeth. Because plaque is colorless and accumulates in areas that are difficult to see and reach, hasty toothbrushing may not effectively remove it. Disclosing tablets and solutions are available that contain a harmless dye to stain the bacteria, thereby indicating where plaque remains after brushing.

A study published by the *British Medical Journal* in 2012 linked poor oral hygiene and increased dental plaque to increased incidents of cancer deaths.

TREATMENT AND THERAPY

Removing dental plaque from teeth is important for good oral health. Teeth should be brushed thoroughly at least twice a day with a fluoride toothpaste. Dental floss should be used daily to remove bacteria and food from between teeth and under the gum line where a toothbrush may not reach. Mouthwash containing fluoride should be used to rinse away plaque and keep oral tissues moist. Sticky, sugary, and starchy foods and beverages should be limited; raw fruits and vegetables are good choices because they disrupt plaque buildup. Teeth should be professionally examined and cleaned every six months. In cases of stubborn tartar accumulation, tooth scaling by a dental professional may be required more frequently. In addition to antiseptics and antibiotics, som me dentists also use lasers to treat the growth of bacteria in pockets of gum near the teeth.

PERSPECTIVE AND PROSPECTS
Tartar control toothpastes now contain pyrophosphates to inhibit mineralization along with antibacterial agents to control the bacteria population. Dentists are now offering sealants, a thin coating of plastic that is painted on the chewing surfaces of molars to prevent plaque from building up in the grooves.

—*Bethany Thivierge, MPH, ELS*

See also Cavities; Dental diseases; Dentistry; Dentistry, pediatric; Endodontic disease; Fluoride treatments; Gingivitis; Gum disease; Periodontitis; Root canal treatment; Teeth; Teething; Toothache.

For Further Information:
Smiech-Slomkowska, Grazyna, et al. "The Effect of Oral Health Education on Dental Plaque Development and the Level of Caries-Related *Streptococcus mutans* and *Lactobacillus* spp." *European Journal of Orthodontics* 29 (April, 2007): 157-160.
Soderling, E. M. "Xylitol, Mutans Streptococci, and Dental Plaque." *Advances in Dental Research* 21 (August, 2009): 74-78.
Wahaidi, V. Y., et al. "Neutrophil Response to Dental Plaque by Gender and Race." *Journal of Dental Research* 88, no. 8 (August, 2009): 709-714.

PLASMA

Category: Anatomy
Anatomy or system affected: Blood, blood vessels, cells, circulatory system, endocrine system, heart, immune system, respiratory system, urinary system
Specialties and related fields: Biochemistry, cardiology, cytology, endocrinology, general surgery, hematology, internal medicine, microbiology, nutrition, serology, vascular medicine
Definition: The liquid component of the blood that transports the blood cells.

STRUCTURE AND FUNCTIONS
A clear, straw-colored liquid, plasma makes up about 55 percent of the total blood volume. Although its major component is water (90 percent by volume), plasma also contains glucose, proteins, clotting factors, hormones, carbon dioxide, and dissolved salts and minerals. The main proteins in plasma are albumin, globulins, and clotting proteins, particularly fibrinogen. Gamma globulin is an important component of the immune system. Mineral ions in plasma include sodium, potassium, chloride, bicarbonate, calcium, and magnesium. These electrolytes are essential in maintaining fluid balance, nerve conduction, muscle contraction, blood clotting, and pH balance in the body.

Suspended within the plasma are red blood cells (erythrocytes), five kinds of white blood cells (leukocytes), and platelets (thrombocytes). In addition to carrying these blood cells, plasma transports nutrients, waste products, antibodies, clotting agents, and chemical messengers to help maintain a healthy body. Plasma circulates dissolved nutrients throughout the body, where they are diffused by osmotic pressure into the tissues and cells that need them. It is also the main medium for transporting excretory products to the kidneys and lungs for elimination.

DISORDERS AND DISEASES
The most characteristic disease associated with plasma is hemophilia. It results from an inherited change in one of the clotting proteins (factor VIII), leaving it dysfunctional. This single change disrupts the chemical reactions necessary for clotting. As a result, patients with hemophilia experience bleeding, swelling, and bruising. Crippling defects may include recurrent hemorrhaging into joints and muscles and bleeding into body cavities.

Tests of the clotting function of plasma include analysis of indicators such as the prothrombin time and the partial thromboplastin time. These tests identify a deficiency of any of the clotting factors. Most cases involving abnormal bleeding can then be traced to specific defects. Hemophilia can be controlled by infusion of factor VIII that has been collected from donated blood or plasma.

PERSPECTIVE AND PROSPECTS
The possibility of using blood plasma for transfusion purposes was reported in a medical journal by physician Gordon R. Ward in 1918. Due to the advantages that plasma has over whole blood with regard to shelf life and donor-recipient compatibility, the use of plasma for blood transfusions was advanced during the 1930s. During World War II, anatomist Charles Drew developed a modern, highly sterile system for processing, testing, and storing plasma in a blood

2316 • Plastic surgery

bank. During the early twenty-first century, research suggests that exploring and measuring the plasma proteome (the proteins in plasma, of which there are known to be 289) can help track slow changes associated with disease, such as rheumatoid arthritis. The best therapeutic options and drugs available for treatment of the disease can then be implemented.

—*Alvin K. Benson, PhD*

See also Bleeding; Blood and blood disorders; Blood testing; Circulation; Disseminated intravascular coagulation (DIC); Fluids and electrolytes; Hematology; Hematology, pediatric; Hemophilia; Pathology; Rh factor; Serology; Thrombocytopenia; Transfusion; Von Willebrand's disease; Wiskott-Aldrich syndrome.

For Further Information:

Berenson, James R. "Overview of Plasma Cell Disorders." *Merck Manual Home Health Handbook*, July 2008.
De la Rocha, Kelly, Igor Puzanov, and Brian Randall. "Plasmapheresis." *Health Library*, May 11, 2013.
"Hemophilia." *MedlinePlus*, June 26, 2013.
Schaller, Johann, et al. *Human Blood Plasma Proteins: Structure and Function*. New York: Wiley, 2008.
Trice, Linda. *Charles Drew: Pioneer of Blood Plasma*. New York: McGraw-Hill, 2000.
Valverde, José Luis, ed. *Blood, Plasma, and Plasma Proteins: A Unique Contribution to Modern Healthcare*. Amsterdam: IOS Press, 2006. Pharmaceuticals Policy and Law 7.

PLASTIC SURGERY

Category: Procedures
Anatomy or system affected: All
Specialties and related fields: Dermatology, emergency medicine, general surgery, oncology, physical therapy, psychology
Definition: Plastic surgery uses such procedures as grafting and the implantation of prostheses in order to treat congenital defects and tissue or limb damage resulting from trauma; reconstructive surgery uses the techniques of plastic surgery to repair injured tissues or to reattach severed body parts, while cosmetic surgery employs these same methods to alter body shape or appearance for aesthetic purposes.

Key terms:

congenital: existing at birth; often used in reference to certain mental or physical malformations and diseases, which may be hereditary or caused by some influence during gestation

cosmetic surgery: the application of plastic surgical techniques to alter one's appearance for purely aesthetic reasons

debridement: the excision of contused and devitalized tissue from a wound surface

dermis: the second layer of skin, immediately below the epidermis; it contains blood and lymphatic vessels, nerves, glands, and (usually) hair follicles

epidermis: the outermost thin layer of skin that encompasses structures superficial to the dermis

granuloma: a nodular, inflammatory lesion that is usually small, firm, and persistent and usually contains proliferated macrophages

plastic surgery: the branch of operative surgery concerning the repair of defects, the replacement of lost tissue, and the treatment of extensive scarring; it accomplishes these ends by direct union of body parts, grafting, or the transfer of tissue from one part of the body to another

reconstructive surgery: the application of plastic surgical techniques to repair damaged tissues

turgor: fullness and firmness; the quality of normal skin in a healthy young person

INDICATIONS AND PROCEDURES

The intent of plastic, reconstructive, and cosmetic surgery is to restore a body part to normal appearance or to enhance or cosmetically alter a body part. The techniques and procedures of all three surgical applications are similar: extremely careful skin preparation, the use of delicate instrumentation and handling techniques, and precise suturing with extremely fine materials to minimize scarring.

Reconstructive surgery. Notable examples of reconstructive surgery involve the reattachment of limbs or extremities that have been traumatically severed. As soon as a part is separated from the body, it loses its blood supply; this leads to ischemia (lack of oxygen) to tissues, which in turn leads to cell death. When an individual cell dies, it cannot be resuscitated and will soon start to decompose. This process can be greatly slowed by lowering the temperature of the severed body part. Packing the part in ice for transport to a hospital is a prudent initial step.

An important consideration in any reconstructive procedure is site preparation. The edges, or margins, of the final wound must be clean and free of contamination. Torn skin is removed through a process called debridement. A sharp scalpel is used gently to cut away tissue that has been crushed or torn. All bacterial contamination must be removed from the site prior to closure to prevent postoperative contamination. Foreign material such as dirt, glass, gunpowder, metals, or chemicals must be completely removed. The margins of the wound must also be sharply defined. Superficially, this is done for aesthetic reasons. Internally, sharply defined margins will reduce the chances for adhesions to form. Adhesions are bands of scar tissue which bind adjacent structures together and restrict normal movement and function. Therefore, both the body site and the margins of the severed part must be debrided and defined. Reconstruction consists of the painstaking reattachment of nerves, tendons, muscles, and skin, which are held in place primarily by sutures although staples, wires, and other materials are occasionally used. Precise alignment of the skin to be closed is accomplished by joining opposing margins. Postoperative procedures include careful handling of the wound site, adequate nutrition, and rest in order to maximize healing. Abnormalities in the healing process can lead to undesirable scarring from the sites of sutures. Such marks can be avoided with careful attention to correct techniques.

Bones are reconstructed in cases of severe fractures. The pieces are set in their proper positions, and the area is immobilized. Where immobilization is not possible, a surface is provided onto which new bone can grow. These temporary surfaces are made of polymeric materials that will dissolve over time.

Congenital anomalies such as a deformed external ear or missing digit can be corrected using reconstructive techniques. In the case of a missing thumb, a finger can be removed, rotated, and attached on the site where the thumb should have been. This allows an affected individual to write, hold objects such as eating utensils, and generally have a more nearly normal life. Similar procedures can be applied to replace a missing or amputated great or big toe. The presence of the great toe contributes significantly to balance and coordination when walking.

Prosthetic materials are implanted in a growing variety of applications. There are two basic types of materials used in prostheses, which are classified according to their surface characteristics. One is totally smooth and inert; an example is Teflon or silicone. The body usually encloses these materials in a membrane, which has the effect of creating a wall or barrier to the surface of the prosthesis. From the body's perspective, the prosthesis has thus been removed. With any prosthesis, the problem most likely to be encountered is infection, which is usually caused by contamination of the operative site or the prosthesis. Infection can also occur at a later, postoperative date because of the migration of bacteria into the cavity formed by the membrane. This is a potentially serious complication. A smooth prosthesis can also be used to create channels into which tissue can later be inserted. In such an application, the prosthesis may be surgically removed at some time in the future. A second type of prosthesis does not have a smooth surface; rather, it has microscopic fibers similar to those found on a towel. This type of surface prevents membranes from forming, contributing to a longer life for the prosthesis by reducing postoperative infections.

An important procedure in reconstructive surgery is skin grafting. A graft consists of skin that is completely removed from a donor site and transferred to another site on the body. The graft is usually taken from the patient's own body because skin taken from another individual will be rejected by the recipient's immune system. (Nevertheless, fetal pig skin is sometimes used successfully.) Skin grafting is useful for covering open wounds, and it is widely used in serious burn cases. When only a portion of the uppermost layer of the skin is removed, the process is called a split thickness graft. When all the upper layers of the skin are removed, the result is a full thickness graft. Whenever possible, the donor site is selected to match the color and texture characteristics of the recipient site.

A skin flap is sometimes created. This differs from a graft in that the skin of a flap is not completely severed from its original site but simply moved to an adjacent location. Some blood vessels remain to support the flap. This procedure is nearly always successful, but it is limited to immediately adjacent skin.

A wide variety of flaps has been developed. A flap may be stretched and sutured to cover both a wound and the donor site. Flaps may be created from skin that is distant to the site where it is needed and then sutured in place over the donor site. Only after the flap has become established at the new site is it cut free from the donor site. Thus, skin from the abdomen or upper chest may be used to cover the back of a burned hand, or skin from one finger may be used to cover a finger on the other hand. This two-stage flap process requires more time than a skin graft, but it also has a greater probability of success.

Plastic surgery. Plastic surgery consists of a variety of techniques and applications, often dealing with skin. Some common procedures that primarily involve skin are undertaken to remove unwanted wrinkles or folds. Folds in skin are caused by a loss of skin turgor and excessive stretching of the skin beyond which it cannot recover. Common contributors to loss of skin turgor in the abdomen are pregnancy or significant weight loss after years of obesity. Both women and men may undergo a procedure known as abdominoplasty (commonly called a "tummy tuck"). The skin that lies over the abdominal muscles is carefully separated from underlying tissue. Portions of the skin are removed; frequently, some underlying adipose (fat) tissue is also removed or relocated. The remaining skin is sutured to the underlying muscle as well as to adjacent, undisturbed skin. A major problem with this procedure, however, is scar formation because large portions of skin must be removed or relocated. The plastic surgeon must plan the placement of incisions carefully in order to avoid undesirable scars.

Plastic surgery is also used to reduce the prominence of ears, a procedure called otoplasty. In some children, the posterior (back) portion of the external ear develops more than the rest of the ear, pushing the ears outward and making them prominent. By reducing the bulk of cartilage in the posterior ear and suturing the remaining external portion to the base of the ear, the plastic surgeon can create a more normal ear contour. The optimal time to perform this procedure on children is just prior to the time that they enter school, or at about five years of age.

Cosmetic surgery. The most common site for cosmetic surgical procedures is the face. Correction may be desired because of a congenital anomaly that causes unwelcome disfigurement or because of a desire to alter an unwanted aspect of one's body. The cosmetic procedures that have been developed to correct abnormalities of the face include closure of a cleft lip or palate. The correction of a cleft lip is usually done early, ideally in the first three months of life. Closure of a cleft palate (the bone that forms the roof of the mouth) is delayed slightly, until the patient is 12 to 18 months old. These procedures allow affected individuals to acquire normal patterns of speech and language.

Among older individuals, common procedures include blepharoplasty and rhinoplasty. The former refers to the removal of excess skin around the eyelids, while the latter refers to a change, usually a reduction, in the shape of the nose. Both procedures may be included in the more general term of face lift. The effects of aging, excessive solar radiation, and gravity combine to produce fine lines in the face as individuals get older. These fine lines gradually develop into the wrinkles characteristic of older persons. For some, these wrinkles are objectionable. To reduce them-or more correctly to stretch them out-a plastic surgeon removes a section of skin containing the wrinkles or lines and stretches the edges of the remaining epidermis until they are touching. These incisions are placed to coincide with the curved lines that exist in normal skin. Thus, when the edges are sutured together, the resultant scar is minimized. Rhinoplasty often involves the removal of a portion of the bone or cartilage that forms the nose. The bulk of the remaining tissue is also reduced to maintain the desired proportions of the patient's nose. As with any plastic surgical procedure, small sutures are carefully placed to minimize scarring.

A third body area that is commonly subjected to cosmetic procedures is the breast. A woman who is unhappy with the appearance of her breasts may seek to either reduce or augment existing tissue. Breast reduction is accomplished by careful incision and the judicious removal of both skin and underlying breast tissue. Often the nipples must be repositioned to maintain their proper locations. A flap that includes the nipple is created from each breast. After the desired amount of underlying tissue is removed, the nipples are repositioned, and the skin is recontoured around the remaining breast masses.

USES AND COMPLICATIONS

Reconstructive, plastic, and cosmetic surgeries all have their complications, ranging from severe-such as the rejection of transplanted tissue-to minor but unpleasant-such as noticeable scars. In addition, there is an inherent risk in any procedure that requires the patient to undergo general anesthesia. With reconstruction, which involves the repair of damaged tissues and structures, the initial injuries sustained by the patient present further obstacles and dangers. The following examples from each type of surgery illustrate the risks involved.

For example, a surgeon who must perform a skin graft can choose between a split or a full thickness graft. A split thickness graft site will heal with relatively normal skin, thus providing opportunities for additional grafting at a later date. It also produces less pronounced scarring. A limitation of this technique, however, is an increased likelihood for the graft to fail. Full thickness grafts are stronger and more likely to be successful, but they lead to more extensive scarring, which is aesthetically undesirable and renders the site unsuitable for later grafts. The surgeon's decision is based on the needs of the patient and the severity of the injury.

The minimization of scarring is a major concern for many patients undergoing plastic surgery. The prevention of noticeable scars involves an understanding of the natural lines of the skin. All areas of the body have lines of significant skin tension and lines of relatively little skin tension. It is along the lines of minimal tension that wrinkles and folds develop over time. These lines are curved and follow body contours. As a rule of thumb, they are generally perpendicular to the fibers of underlying muscle. The plastic surgeon seeks to place incisions along the lines of minimal tension. When scars form after healing, they will blend into the line of minimal tension and become less noticeable. Furthermore, the scar tissue is not likely to become apparent when the underlying muscles or body part is moved. Undesirable scarring is a greater problem in large procedures, such as abdominoplasty, than in procedures confined to a small area, such as rhytidectomy (face lift), because of the difficulty in following lines of minimum tension when making incisions.

One of the most popular cosmetic procedures is breast enlargement. According to the American Society of Plastic Surgeons, 296,203 augmentation mammoplasties were performed in the United States in 2010, and the total number of women with implants in the United States is in the millions. Initially, the most commonly used prosthesis, or implant, was made of silicone. In some patients, silicone leaked out, causing the formation of granulomatous tissue. Such complications led to a voluntary suspension of the production of silicone prostheses by manufacturers and of their usage by surgeons. Different materials, such as polyethylene bags filled with saline solution or solid polyurethane implants, were soon substituted. Saline will not cause tissue damage if it leaks, and few adverse reactions to polyurethane have been reported. Silicone implants made a comeback in 2006, when the US Food and Drug Administration began approving them for use in women aged twenty-two years or older.

PERSPECTIVE AND PROSPECTS

The origins of plastic, reconstructive, and cosmetic surgery are fundamental to the earliest surgical procedures, which were developed to correct superficial deformities. Without any viable methods of anesthesia, surgical interventions and corrections were limited to the skin. For example, present-day nose reconstructions (rhinoplasty) are essentially similar to procedures developed four thousand years ago. Hindu surgeons developed the technique of moving a piece of skin from the adjacent cheek onto the nose to cover a wound. Similar procedures were developed by Italians using skin that was transferred from the arm or forehead to repair lips and ears as well as noses. Ironically, wars have provided opportunities to advance reconstructive techniques. As field hospitals and surgical facilities became more widely available and wounded soldiers could be stabilized during transport, techniques to repair serious wounds evolved.

Skin grafts have been used since Roman times. Celsus described the possibility of skin grafts in conjunction with eye surgery. References were made to skin grafts in the Middle Ages. The evolution of modern techniques can be traced to the early nineteenth century, when Cesare Baronio conducted systematic grafting experiments with animals. The modern guidelines for grafting were formulated in 1870. Instruments for creating split thickness grafts were developed in the 1930s, and applications of this procedure evolved during World War II.

Plastic, reconstructive, and cosmetic procedures have all become important in contemporary surgical practice. Reconstructive surgery allows the repair of serious injuries and contributes greatly to the rehabilitation of affected individuals. Cosmetic surgery can help individuals feel better about themselves and their bodies. Both use techniques developed in the broader field of plastic surgery.

There are both positive and negative aspects of plastic surgery. Positively, many individuals who sustain serious and potentially devastating injuries are able to return to relatively normal lives. Burn victims and those having accidents are more likely to return to normal activities and resume their occupations than at any time in the past. Miniaturization and new materials have extended the range of a plastic surgeon's skills. Negatively, there is growing criticism concerning the number of elective procedures undertaken for the repair of cosmetic defects.

The quest for perfection and physical beauty has prompted some critics to question the correctness of some unnecessary procedures. Although such procedures are not usually covered by insurance policies, their utilization has increased. The continuation of such activities invokes both ethical and personal considerations; there is no clearly defined, logical endpoint. Clearly, while plastic surgical techniques have benefited millions, there are opportunities for abuse. Society must decide if any limitations are to be placed on plastic surgical procedures and what they should be.

In the meantime, advances in materials, instruments, and techniques will benefit plastic, reconstructive, and cosmetic surgery. As but one example, the advent of magnification and miniaturization and the development of tiny instruments and new suture materials have allowed the reconstruction of many injury sites. Blood vessels and nerves are now routinely reattached and a mere nine individual sutures are required to join the severed portions of a blood vessel one millimeter in diameter.

—*L. Fleming Fallon, Jr., MD, PhD, MPH*

See also Age spots; Aging; Amputation; Birthmarks; Body dysmorphic disorder; Botox; Breast cancer; Breast disorders; Breast surgery; Breasts, female; Burns and scalds; Cancer; Carcinoma; Circumcision, female, and genital mutilation; Circumcision, male; Cleft lip and palate; Cleft lip and palate repair; Collagen; Cyst removal; Cysts; Dermatology; Dermatology, pediatric; Ear surgery; Face lift and blepharoplasty; Gender identity disorder; Gender reassignment surgery; Grafts and grafting; Hair loss and baldness; Hair transplantation; Healing; Jaw wiring; Laceration repair; Liposuction; Malignancy and metastasis; Mastectomy and lumpectomy; Melanoma; Moles; Obesity; Otoplasty; Otorhinolaryngology; Ptosis; Rhinoplasty and submucous resection; Skin; Skin lesion removal; Surgical procedures; Varicose vein removal; Varicose veins; Warts; Wrinkles.

For Further Information:
Grazer, Frederick M., and Jerome R. Klingbeil. *Body Image: A Surgical Perspective*. St. Louis, Mo.: Mosby Year Book, 1980.
Loftus, Jean M. *The Smart Woman's Guide to Plastic Surgery*. 2d ed. Dubuque, Iowa: McGraw-Hill, 2008.
MedlinePlus. "Plastic and Cosmetic Surgery." *MedlinePlus*, May 2, 2013.
Narins, Rhoda, and Paul Jarrod Frank. *Turn Back the Clock Without Losing Time: Everything You Need to Know About Simple Cosmetic Procedures*. New York: Three Rivers Press, 2002.
Rutkow, Ira M. *American Surgery: An Illustrated History*. Philadelphia: Lippincott-Raven, 1998.

Townsend, Courtney M., Jr., et al., eds. *Sabiston Textbook of Surgery*. 18th ed. Philadelphia: Saunders/Elsevier, 2012.

Weatherford, M. Lisa, ed. *Reconstructive and Cosmetic Surgery Sourcebook*. Detroit, Mich.: Omnigraphics, 2001.

PLEURISY

Category: Disease/Disorder
Also known as: Pleuritis
Anatomy or system affected: Chest, lungs
Specialties and related fields: Emergency medicine, family medicine, internal medicine, pulmonary medicine
Definition: A syndrome of chest pain made worse by breathing.

CAUSES AND SYMPTOMS

The lungs sit within the chest wall just underneath the rib cage. The pleura is a very thin double lining covering the outer surface of the lungs and the undersurface of the ribs. During normal breathing, the lungs expand and relax, stretching their pleural membrane and moving it back and forth against the pleural membrane lining the rib cage. To minimize friction, a very small amount of fluid fills the space between them.

"Pleurisy" is a descriptive term that refers to chest pain with respiration. It occurs when the pleural membranes become irritated or inflamed. The pain is usually localized at the area of inflammation, but it can radiate toward the neck, shoulder, or abdomen. The pain may be mild discomfort or a severe stabbing or burning sensation. In addition to deep breathing, coughing or movements of the chest can exacerbate symptoms. Because of the pain, the patient may employ rapid, shallow breathing.

INFORMATION ON PLEURISY

Causes: May include recent cold or respiratory infection; pneumonia; tuberculosis; trauma (muscle sprain, fractured rib); sickle cell disease; advanced kidney failure; recent heart attack; rheumatologic diseases (lupus, rhematoid arthritis); asbestos exposure; punctured lung; pulmonary embolism; lung cancer

Symptoms: Chest pain with respiration, ranging from discomfort or severe stabbing or burning sensation and worsened by coughing or chest movement; sometimes shortness of breath

Duration: One to two weeks

Treatments: Depends on cause; may include drainage of fluid, oxygen therapy, hospitalization

---

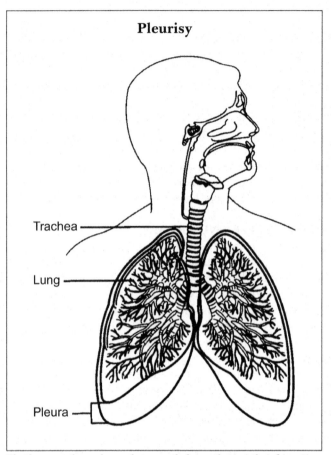

Pleurisy

Trachea

Lung

Pleura

The pleurae are the membranes that encase the lungs; pleurisy is the inflammation of one or both pleurae and may have a variety of causes. ©EBSCO

Patients with symptoms of a recent cold or respiratory infection likely have pleurisy caused by a virus; however, a more serious cause, such as pneumonia, may also be responsible. Tuberculosis is another infectious cause to be considered.

Patients with recent injuries to the chest or unusually strenuous activity may have pleurisy attributable to a muscle sprain or a fractured rib. Patients with sickle cell disease, advanced kidney failure, a recent heart attack, rheumatologic diseases such as lupus and rheumatoid arthritis, or asbestos exposure are also prone to pleurisy.

The most worrisome causes of pleurisy are pneumothorax (punctured lung), pulmonary embolism (blood clot in the lung), or lung cancer. These causes are more likely to be associated with shortness of breath, although this symptom is not reliably present.

TREATMENT AND THERAPY

Treatment of pleurisy depends on the underlying cause. In most cases, a chest x-ray is indicated. In some cases, a collection of fluid in the pleural space will be visible. However, patients with pleurisy may often have a normal chest x-ray. In concerning cases, particularly those associated with shortness of breath and abnormally low oxygen levels, further radiologic studies, such as a computed tomography (CT) scan or magnetic resonance imaging (MRI), may be necessary.

Pleurisy caused by viral infections, trauma, rheumatologic diseases, and sickle cell disease is generally treated with pain medications, and the symptoms resolve within one to two weeks. Patients with kidney or heart disease may need drainage of the pleural fluid with a needle or tube placed into the pleural space through the back.

The more serious causes of pleurisy require specialized treatments based on the cause; typically, temporary oxygen supplementation is required, and sometimes hospitalization is necessary.

—*Gregory B. Seymann, MD*

See also Asbestos exposure; Chest; Embolism; Lung cancer; Lungs; Pneumonia; Pneumothorax; Pulmonary diseases; Pulmonary medicine; Pulmonary medicine, pediatric; Respiration; Sickle cell disease; Tuberculosis; Wheezing.

For Further Information:

Fishman, Alfred, ed. *Fishman's Pulmonary Diseases and Disorders*. 4th ed. New York: McGraw-Hill, 2008.

Marx, John A., et al., eds. *Rosen's Emergency Medicine: Concepts and Clinical Practice*. 7th ed. Philadelphia: Mosby/Elsevier, 2010.

"Pleurisy and Pleural Effusion." *InteliHealth*, April 19, 2011.

Porter, Robert S., et al., eds. *The Merck Manual Home Health Handbook*. Whitehouse Station, N.J.: Merck Research Laboratories, 2009.

Walsh, Beth. "Pleurisy." *Health Library*, September 1, 2011.

"What Are Pleurisy and Other Pleural Disorders?" *National Heart, Lung, and Blood Institute*, September 21, 2011.

PNEUMOCYSTIS JIROVECII

Category: Disease/Disorder
Also known as: Pneumocystis carinii
Anatomy or system affected: Chest, lungs, respiratory system
Specialties and related fields: Microbiology, nuclear medicine, pulmonary medicine, radiology
Definition: A small fungus that normally lives in the respiratory tract of most people, but causes pneumonia in those with dysfunctional immune systems.
Key terms:
alveoli: terminal branchings of the respiratory tree that act as the primary sites of gas exchange in the lungs
immunosuppression: reducing the activity or efficiency of the immune system

CAUSES AND SYMPTOMS

Pneumocystis jirovecii, a single-celled fungus, commonly lives in the respiratory tracts of healthy people without

Pneumocystis jiroveci cysts. Photo via CDC/Wikimedia Commons. [Public domain.]

causing any harm. However, in people whose immune systems do not work properly, *Pneumocystis jirovecii* can cause pneumonia. During World War II, premature and severely malnourished infants were diagnosed with *Pneumocystis jirovecii* pneumonia. Later, other cases were observed in immunosuppressed patients: cancer patients receiving chemotherapy, and transplant recipients being treated with immunosuppressants. Recently, *Pneumocystis jirovecii pneumonia* (PCP) has become the most common cause of death in patients with Acquired Immune Deficiency Syndrome (AIDS).

The life cycle of *Pneumocystis jirovecii* consists of three different stages: the trophozoite or trophic stage, the sporozoite or precystic form, and the cyst, which contains several spores. Trophozoites live within the alveoli of the lung and are probably the infective form, and transmission occurs by means of airborne transmission.

The symptoms of PCP include shortness of breath upon exertion (dyspnea), fever, nonproductive cough, weight loss, chills, and, rarely, coughing up blood (hemoptysis). PCP patients also have an abnormally fast heart rate (tachycardia, over 100 beats per minute), rapid breathing (tachypnea, more than 20 breaths per minute), and mild crackles and course rattling (rhonchi) when they breathe.

TREATMENT AND THERAPY

The nonspecific nature of PCP symptoms necessitates other diagnostic tests to confirm the diagnosis. Observing the organism from respiratory tract fluid by means of various tissue stains provides the most definitive confirmation of PCP. Polymerase chain reaction (PCR) tests have been used successfully as well, but are not yet routinely available. Chest X-rays, computed tomography, or Gallium-67 scans can provide evidence that the patient has PCP, but are not conclusive.

Even though *Pneumocystis jirovecii* is a yeast-like fungus, it does not respond to antifungals, with the possi-

INFORMATION ON PNEUMOCYSTIS JIROVECII

Causes: Suppression of the immune system
Symptoms: Cough, fever, rapid breathing, shortness of breath
Duration: Variable
Treatments: Trimethoprim-sulfamethoxazole, clindamycin and primaquine, pentamidine, corticosteroids for lung inflammation

ble exception of echinocandin. The first choice for treatment consists of oral or intravenous trimethoprim-sulfamethoxazole (Septra, Bactrim, Sulfatrim). Patients with sulfa allergies or who have PCP infections that are resistant to trimethoprim-sulfamethoxazole should be given a combination of clindamycin and primaquine or intravenous pentamidine. Patients with severe inflammation and fluid in their lungs are treated with corticosteroids to clear their lungs so that they can breathe.

To prevent PCP (chemoprophylaxis), patients usually take trimethoprim-sulfamethoxazole, or dapsone, dapsone plus pyrimethamine, atovaquone, or aerosolized pentamidine. Smoking cessation can also decrease the rate of recurrent PCP infections.

AIDS patients who show the symptoms of PCP begin treatment immediately before completion of diagnostic tests. Babies born to mothers infected with Human Immunodeficiency Virus (HIV) begin preventative treatment 4-6 weeks after birth.

—*Michael A. Buratovich PhD*

See also Immunology; Immunopathology; Lungs; Pulmonary medicine

For Further Information:
Gallant, Joel E. *Johns Hopkins HIV Guide.* Burlington, MA: Jones and Bartlett Learning, 2012.
Miller, Robert F., Laurence Huang, and Peter D. Walzer. "Pneumocystis Pneumonia Associated with Human Immunodeficiency Virus." *Clinics in Chest Medicine* 34, no. 2 (June 2013): 229-241.

PNEUMONIA

Category: Disease/Disorder
Anatomy or system affected: Lungs, respiratory system
Specialties and related fields: Emergency medicine, epidemiology, family medicine, internal medicine, occupational health, public health, pulmonary medicine
Definition: An inflammation of one of several possible areas of the respiratory system, mainly in the lungs

or bronchial passageways, resulting from bacterial or viral infection.

Key terms:

Gram's stain: a laboratory method for tracing the presence of certain bacteria in lung tissue; the procedure involves the observation of different levels of tissue discoloration as specific chemical reactions are induced

pleurisy: a secondary but very painful inflammation of the membranes that line the lungs and chest cavity; often accompanies pneumonia

Pneumocystis pneumonia: a form of pneumonia caused by the single-celled parasite *Pneumocystis carinii*; dangerous primarily to persons with impaired immunity mechanisms, particularly victims of acquired immunodeficiency syndrome (AIDS)

Streptococcus pneumoniae: commonly referred to as pneumococcus; the main bacteria responsible for pneumonia

CAUSES AND SYMPTOMS

Although modern medicine succeeded several generations ago in identifying the key viruses and bacteria responsible for pneumonia and in developing efficient medications for its treatment, a surprisingly high number of deaths from the complications of pneumonia continue to occur. In large part this is the case because pneumonia, which involves infection and inflammation in the respiratory system, occurs not only on its own but also as a complication brought about by other serious illnesses. In aged patients, especially, general deterioration of the body's resistance to bacterial or viral infection can lead in a final stage to death from pneumonia.

Just as the causes of pneumonia can vary, the disease itself may take different forms. Some sources postulate that pneumonia is not a single disease but a group of advanced lung inflammations. Because they are so similar in their symptoms and effects on the body, all members of this family of diseases are labeled as one form or another of pneumonia. Specific forms range from lobar pneumonia (caused by the bacterial invasion of *Streptococcus pneumoniae* into a single lobe of one lung) and bronchopneumonia (from *Haemophilus influenzae* bacteria colonizing in the bronchi) to viral pneumonia (which may be caused by complications originating from chickenpox or influenza virus). In all cases, symptoms include painful coughing, but other symptoms, such as high fever, reduced sputum production, or discolored (rust-tinged or greenish) sputum, may differ. It follows that the drugs that have been developed to treat pneumonia necessarily vary according to the variety of the disease involved.

Lobar pneumonia and bronchopneumonia are the two main classes of disease. The former occurs when an initial infection attacks only one lobe of one lung. Bronchopneumonia results from an initial inflammation in the bronchi and bronchioles (air passages to the lungs), which then spreads to the internal tissue of one or both lungs. Once the symptoms of pneumonia have become visible, any of the following may occur: fever, chills, shortness of breath, chest pains, or a painful cough that produces yellow-green or brownish sputum. These symptoms occur because of a condition called pleurisy, which is an inflammation of the membrane lining the lungs themselves and the general chest cavity area.

Some assumptions about the causes of pneumonia being limited to bacterial or viral sources have been altered. In particular, clinical observation of patients suffering from AIDS reveals that certain fungi, yeasts, or protozoa can cause pneumonia in these and other cases where immunodeficiency disorders are present.

Although it is apparent that pneumococci can thrive in various parts of the bodies of animals, particularly monkeys and humans, the process that leads to general infection and a concentrated and dangerous attack on the pulmonary system has been the subject of many medical investigations. It is nearly certain that the presence of the common cold virus in the upper respiratory tract can create the conditions needed for the movement of pneumococci from areas of the body where they may be generally present without causing harm (mainly in saliva) into the pulmonary system. Under conditions of normal health, many body mechanisms can stop a potential invasion of the pulmonary system. This process may involve nasal mucus, although it is not itself bactericidal (bacteria-killing), and other mucous membranes in the region of the larynx. Even beyond the larynx and vocal cords, mechanical means associated with the upward sweep of hairlike protrusions called cilia on the inner linings of deeper respiratory membranes tend to protect the bronchial tree.

When normal protective processes are reduced, as when the cold virus is present, pneumococci may reach the lower respiratory zone and the parenchyma of the lung, where they settle and multiply. The metabolic products that accumulate as a result of this reproductive process begin to have injurious effects on the respiratory organs. Such injuries become actual lesions in the internal respiratory tissues. The process of infection that follows involves the deposition of fibrin in the adjacent blood and lymph vessels. This phenomenon actually tends to shield the invading organisms from the effects normally produced by antipneumococcal immune substances carried by the blood. If unchecked by medical treatment, reproduction of the invading pneumococci can lead to more extensive lesions. If tissue damage occurs, this can cause the formation of

---

INFORMATION ON PNEUMONIA

Causes: Bacterial or viral infection
Symptoms: Lung inflammation, painful coughing, high fever, reduced sputum production, rust-tinged or greenish sputum
Duration: Acute
Treatments: Antibiotics (tetracycline, erythromycin), supportive care

---

edema, a dangerous accumulation of fluids in spaces where fluids are not normally found. At a later stage of the disease, it appears that the pneumococci enter the interstitial and lymphatic tissues. The unchecked advance of pneumonia infection produces a general deterioration of vital breathing processes as excess fluids spread farther into the respiratory system. In weakened or immunocompromised individuals, this process can lead to death.

TREATMENT AND THERAPY

Medical treatment of the two main types of pneumonia is not the same. Lobar pneumonia requires treatment with penicillin. Bronchopneumonia, although also caused by pneumococcus bacteria, must be treated with different antibiotics. Most forms of pneumonia caused by viral infections, including psittacosis and mycoplasmal pneumonia, require one of two specific drugs: tetracycline or erythromycin. When viral pneumonia provides the basic disease to which bacterial infections in the lungs are added, however, antibiotics represent the main general means of treatment.

Since World War II, the progress of medical science in dealing with various types of pneumonia has been marked by the development of antimicrobial drugs that can be used in treating diagnosed cases of pneumonia. One of the earliest such drugs, which eventually turned out to be ineffective, was a derivative of quinine called Optochin. It was used for the first time on mice in 1912. Five years later, when the drug was applied to human patients, it was observed that the pneumococci were able to develop a surprising degree of resistance to these early antimicrobial substances. Thus, just as progress in the field of immunization had to wait for a later generation, so did effective drugs such as penicillin and other antibiotics that have become standard tools in the treatment of forms of pneumonia.

In most cases, advances in drug treatment to cure pneumonia have been strikingly successful. The phenomenon of the nonbacterial, nonviral version of *Pneumocystis* pneumonia arrived very soon after these successes. It posed a particular series of dilemmas for medical science in the 1980s and 1990s. This problem emerged when it became apparent that certain drugs that had been developed to treat pneumonia, in particular the drug combination of trimethoprim-sulfamethoxazole (TMP-SMZ), failed to achieve expected results in a rising number of cases of *Pneumocystis* pneumonia. This particular form of pneumonia turned out to be among the minority strains of the disease caused by single-celled microorganisms called protozoa.

The importance of *P. carinii* (also called *P. jirovecii*) in applied medical science soon extended beyond the restricted domain of pneumonia pathology. It had been discovered in 1909 in Brazil and was thought to affect only animals. This research involved local researchers led by the Italian Antonio Carini, whose name was attached to the discovery. It was only much later, in the 1940s and 1950s, that the presence of *P. carinii* could be traced to pneumonia in human infants. This meant that a relatively unusual form of pneumonia belonged to limited number of cases caused not by bacteria or viruses but by fungi, yeasts, or microorganisms, specifically, single-celled protozoa. This form of pneumonia remained a relatively rare occurrence until the number of AIDS cases increased.

What appeared to be a near epidemic frequency of *P. carinii* was in fact a marker or indicator for discovering patients suffering from AIDS. This observation made it possible to immediately test for the presence of AIDS whenever cases of *P. carinii* appeared. Clinical experience during the 1980s revealed that at least 60 percent of all persons suffering from AIDS had contracted or would contract *P. carinii* pneumonia. The presence of *P. carinii* is now assumed to be associated with AIDS unless that diagnosis is excluded by a laboratory test.

It is important to note that relatively rapid advances made by medical researchers in preventing the spread of *P. carinii* and in treating the cases that did occur among infants led to a new appreciation for pneumonia. Applied research dating from 1958 and extending into the 1970s produced surprisingly effective agents to combat *P. carinii* pneumonia. This work led to the early application of drugs to people infected with human immunodeficiency virus (HIV). The concept of multiple drug therapy, patterned on TMP-SMZ, was also successfully applied in the field of cancer treatment.

Another drug, pentamidine, had been used to treat *P. carinii* pneumonia. When TMP-SMZ seemed to provide a superior treatment, pentamidine production was halted. When the potential utility of pentamidine in treating AIDS became apparent, the Centers for Disease Control and the Food and Drug Administration (FDA) had to take special action in 1984 to license an American supplier. This is how pentamidine quickly became widely available to treat individuals with AIDS. Pentami-

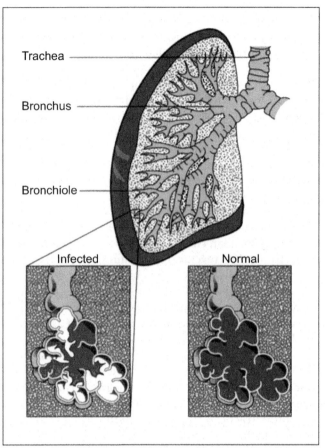

Pneumonia is actually a group of inflammatory diseases that affect the lungs; in lobar pneumonia, only one lobe of the lung is attacked, whereas in bronchopneumonia the bronchi and bronchioles, which lead to both lungs, are affected. The inset shows infection of the alveoli in lobar pneumonia. ©EBSCO

dine has also been successfully used as an effective treatment for a variety of viral diseases.

A side effect of these AIDS-related developments by the mid-1980s has been to reemphasize the importance of pneumonia. This renewed interest involves both treatments that are most appropriate for different types of pneumonia and research that is still needed to understand fully the role of this family of diseases in modern medicine and society.

PERSPECTIVE AND PROSPECTS

Although modern medicine has not been able to reduce substantially or eliminate totally the number of cases of pneumonia, much has been learned about the disease and its causes. Scientific advances in the campaign to combat the effects of pneumonia in all areas of the world began with the first isolation of *Streptococcus pneumoniae* in France and the United States in 1880. The French discovery of pneumococci is associated with the laboratory of Louis Pasteur. Simultaneously, George Sternberg was completing work in the medical department of the US Army. In the first decade after the isolation of pneumococci, many different researchers contributed to laboratory findings that linked these bacteria to inflammatory infections in the lungs of animals. They extended their research to include the effects on humans.

One of the most important early breakthroughs came in 1884 when the Danish researcher Hans Christian Joachim Gram developed a laboratory method for identifying specific bacteria in tissue specimens. This technique, called Gram's stain, revealed that different chemical reactions occur when samples of lung tissue and secretions from individuals ill with pneumonia and healthy persons are tested. The tissues stain very differently. The next step would lead to research into the phenomenon of phagocytosis, a process within pulmonary tissue that combats inapparent pneumococcus infection in healthy people. This specific discovery became linked with efforts to develop an immunization technology against pneumonia.

Until the 1980s, medical researchers used their knowledge of pneumonia mainly to develop methods of immunization against the disease. They also tried to diversify the drugs used in treating pneumonia. Efforts to produce a vaccine against pneumonia began with experiments by the German researchers George and Felix Klemperer, who tested antiserum in animals in 1891. The Klemperers were able to show that the offspring of adult rabbits which had been immunized were resistant to pneumococcal invasion and infection. Soon thereafter, they carried out the first injections of immune serum into human patients. This research ultimately led to the finding that there was no actual antitoxin or antibacterial property in the serum. Instead, it promoted phagocytosis, a process of encapsulation around pneumococci that aids in the immunological response of white blood cells in the body. The vaccine stimulates the body to create its own defenses.

In 1911 in South Africa, an experimental pneumonia vaccine program was undertaken. Although the specific program was not successful, the British physician and scientist Frederick Lister extended its theory. Unequivocal success with a pneumonia vaccine did not come until the last year of World War II. In 1945, C. M. MacLeod and several colleagues published research findings proving that pneumococcal infection in humans was preventable through the use of vaccines containing as many as fourteen specific antigens. These were termed capsular polysaccharides. The breakthrough that made those findings possible had been pioneered in 1930 when these antigens were injected into human beings for the first time. Previously, they had been used only in experiments with mice.

Pneumonia vaccines are critically important components of programs to prevent disease among older members of the population. In March 2013, the *American Journal of Medicine* published a study of 1,400 pneumonia patients over the age of fifty in which researchers found a correlation between pneumonia patients requiring hospitalization and an increased risk of decline their mental abilities. Experts recommend that the elderly receive a pneumonia vaccine each year. The death rate from pneumonia continues to rise, but not as quickly as the percentage of the population that is elderly. Pneumonia is one of the ten leading causes of death in the United States. In 1900, it was the second or third most common killer. Without vaccines, it might easily still be the second or third leading cause of death.

Children under the age of two are also at high risk for catching pneumonia. The World Health Organization reported in April 2013 that pneumonia was the leading cause of death in children worldwide, killing an estimated 1.2 million children younger than five each year. Only about 30 percent of the world's children with the disease receive antibiotics to treat it

—Byron D. Cannon, PhD;
updated by L. Fleming Fallon, Jr., MD, PhD, MPH

See also Acquired immunodeficiency syndrome (AIDS); Avian influenza; Bacterial infections; Bacteriology; Bronchi; Bronchitis; Common cold; Coughing; Immunization and vaccination; Influenza; Lungs; Microbiology; Pleurisy; Pulmonary diseases; Pulmonary medicine; Pulmonary medicine, pediatric; Respiration; Severe acute respiratory syndrome (SARS); Streptococcal infections; Viral infections; Wheezing.

For Further Information:
Austrian, Robert. *Life with the Pneumococcus.* Philadelphia: University of Pennsylvania Press, 1985.
Badash, Michelle. "Pneumonia." *Health Library,* September 30, 2012.
Heron, Melonie. "Deaths: Leading Causes for 2009." *National Vital Statistics Reports* 61, no. 7 (October 26, 2012): 1-94.
Hughes, Walter T. Pneumocystis carinii *Pneumonitis.* 2 vols. Rev. ed. Boca Raton, Fla.: CRC Press, 1987.
Karetzky, Monroe, Burke A. Cunha, and Robert D. Brandstetter. *The Pneumonias.* New York: Springer, 1993.
MedlinePlus. "Pneumonia." *MedlinePlus,* May 20, 2013.
Niederman, Michael S., George A. Sarosi, and Jeffrey Glassroth. *Respiratory Infections.* 2d ed. Philadelphia: Lippincott Williams & Wilkins, 2001.
Papadakis, Maxine A., Stephen J. McPhee, and Michael W. Rabow, eds. *Current Medical Diagnosis and Treatment 2013.* New York: McGraw-Hill Medical, 2012.
Parker, James N., and Philip M. Parker, eds. *The Official Patient's Sourcebook on Streptococcus Pneumoniae Infections.* San Diego, Calif.: Icon Health, 2002.
Pennington, James E. *Respiratory Infections: Diagnosis and Management.* 3d ed. Hoboken, N.J.: Raven Press, 1994.
Preidt, Robert. "HealthDay: Pneumonia May Lead to Serious Aftereffects for Seniors." *MedlinePlus,* March 22, 2013.
West, John B. *Pulmonary Pathophysiology: The Essentials.* 8th ed. Philadelphia: Wolters Kluwer/Lippincott Williams & Wilkins Health, 2012.
World Health Organization. "Pneumonia (Fact Sheet No. 331)." *World Health Organization: Media Centre,* April, 2013.

Pneumothorax

Category: Disease/Disorder
Anatomy or system affected: Chest, lungs, respiratory system
Specialties and related fields: Emergency medicine, pulmonary medicine
Definition: The collapse of a lung or portion of a lung as a result of the introduction of air or another gas or of fluid into the pleural space surrounding the lungs.
Key terms:
bronchoscopy: a medical procedure for viewing the inside of the lungs through a scope that is passed through the nose or mouth and into the lungs
bulla (bleb): a blister that develops on the surface of the lung
cyanosis: a bluish tinge to the skin, particularly on the fingers and toes, around the mouth, and the ear lobes as a result of inadequate oxygen to the tissues
subcutaneous emphysema: air that has leaked from the pneumothorax to under the skin

CAUSES AND SYMPTOMS

Pneumothorax is the result of anything that causes air or fluid, such as blood, to leak into the space between the two layers of pleura, which line the chest wall (parietal) and the lung tissue (visceral). For normal lung function there is negative pressure in this space. When air enters, the negative pressure is disrupted, and the atmospheric pressure presses on the lung tissue, deflating it. A pneumothorax can be mild and self-limiting, but a severe pneumothorax can collapse the whole lung and cause a shift in the location of the heart and great vessels. This is a life-threatening situation.

Pneumothorax is caused by trauma to the lung, medical procedures performed on the lungs, infant prematurity, existing lung disease, endometriosis in the chest, and bullae. Trauma includes anything that penetrates the chest wall, such as a stabbing, gunshot wound, or excessive blunt trauma to the chest. Medical procedures such as a bronchoscopy, cardiopulmonary resuscitation (CPR), liver or lung biopsy, chest surgery, and the insertion of chest tubes can cause a pneumothorax. Premature infants or infants who swallow meconium, newborn stool, can rupture their lungs attempting to breathe despite lung tissue that is sticking together. The presence of existing lung disease can increase the risk of developing a pneumothorax. These diseases include emphysema, asthma, chronic infections, tuberculosis, cystic fibrosis, cancer, and chronic obstructive pulmonary disease (COPD). An unusual cause of pneumothorax is the presence of endometriosis in the chest. This condition causes

---

INFORMATION ON PNEUMOTHORAX

Causes: Trauma, medical procedures performed on lungs, infant prematurity, existing lung disease, endometriosis in chest, bullae
Symptoms: Shortness of breath, sharp pain in chest, feeling of tightness, cyanosis, dry cough, rapid heart rate, subcutaneous emphysema, sound of air moving through penetrating chest wound
Duration: One to four days, depending on severity and treatment
Treatments: Insertion of chest tube into intrapleural space, surgery

---

pneumothorax at the time of the menstrual cycle, when the endometrial tissue bleeds. Bullae develop due to local weakness in the lung tissue and can rupture with changes in atmospheric pressure, such as when scuba diving, flying, and mountain climbing. Most often bullae rupture for no apparent reason. Bullae are more common in cigarette smokers.

The symptoms of pneumothorax are shortness of breath, sharp pain in the chest, a feeling of tightness, cyanosis, dry cough, rapid heart rate, subcutaneous emphysema, and the sound of air moving through a penetrating chest wound. A primary pneumothorax is diagnosed by the symptoms; pulse oximetry, which measures oxygen saturation of the blood; auscultation, or listening to the lobes of the lungs through a stethoscope; and chest x-ray. A traumatic pneumothorax is related to a traumatic injury and a postmedical pneumothorax to a medical procedure.

TREATMENT AND THERAPY

A small pneumothorax will resolve on its own. It is treated with watchful waiting and repeated chest x-rays. If there is shortness of breath, then oxygen can be administered. If a pneumothorax does not resolve on its own, then a needle can be inserted through the chest wall into the pneumothorax (thoracentesis), and the air or fluid can be extracted. Another common treatment is the insertion of a chest tube with its tip in the intrapleural space. An airtight dressing is placed around the tube and the tube is drained into a system that includes a water seal in order to prevent the reintroduction of air. Gentle suction may be used to remove the air or any drainage present. Usually, the pneumothorax will resolve within two to three days, and then the tube can be removed. If the pneumothorax reoccurs after the suction is removed from the chest tube, then there is a more portable system called a Heimlich valve that can be used to continue chest drainage. This valve permits air or fluid to leave the interpleural space without permitting air to reenter.

If the pneumothorax does not improve, or if it reoccurs, then surgery may be required. Pleurodesis may be performed, particularly for ruptured bullae. In this procedure, a chemical irritant is used to create scar tissue to heal weakened spots in the lung. Surgery in the form of video-assisted thoracic surgery (VATS) can be performed to close the lung with staples. Open chest surgery is less commonly used to treat pneumothoraces.

In an emergency, a sucking or traumatic chest wound should be treated with an occlusive dressing to prevent the introduction of additional air into the chest. Ideally, this dressing should be sterile and have either petroleum jelly gauze or plastic to seal the wound.

PERSPECTIVE AND PROSPECTS

Pneumothorax was first identified by Jean Marc Gaspard Itard, a student of Rene Laennec, in 1803. Laennec, himself, described the clinical picture of pneumothorax, in 1819. The first treatment of pneumothorax was thoracentesis. Both thoracentesis and chest tubes generally led to empyema, an infection in the pleural space because of the absence of aseptic technique. After the discovery of germ theory and aseptic technique by Ignaz Semmelweiss (1818-1865), Louis Pasteur (1822-1895), and Joseph Lister (1827-1912), pneumothorax could be treated with aseptic thoracentesis, or with surgery. Semmelweis discovered that hand washing between patients could limit the spread of infection after childbirth. Pasteur tested germ theory, and wrote about the microscopic germs that cause infection, both in the presence of air and in anaerobic tissue. Lister is referred to as the father of surgery because he introduced the use of chemicals to sterilize surgical instruments and to clean wounds. In 1875, G. E. Playfair developed water seal drainage for removing fluids from the chest, and in 1876, F. Cresswell Hewett used water seal drainage with chest tubes.

Tuberculosis was a scourge in the nineteenth century, and it frequently created a pneumothorax by eating through the lung. There were no antibiotics at this time, so treatment was limited, and most persons who developed tuberculosis died from it. In 1882, Italian physician Carlo Forlanini began to use pneumothorax for treatment of tuberculosis in an effort to rest the lung. This treatment was continued into the early twentieth century.

—*Christine M. Carroll, RN, BSN, MBA*

See also Asthma; Chest; Chronic obstructive pulmonary disease (COPD); Cystic fibrosis; Emphysema; Internal medicine; Lung cancer; Lung surgery; Lungs; Pleurisy; Pneumonia; Pulmonary diseases; Pulmonary medicine; Pulmonary medicine, pediatric; Respiration; Thoracic surgery; Tuberculosis.

For Further Information:

Alifano, Marco, et al. "Atmospheric Pressure Influences the Risk of Pneumothorax: Beware of the Storm!" *Chest* 131, no. 6 (July 26, 2007): 1877-1882.

Blavias, Allen J. "Pneumothorax-Series." *MedlinePlus*, March 22, 2013.

Chan, Stewart Siu Wa. "Tension Pneumothorax Managed Without Immediate Needle Decompression." *Journal of Emergency Medicine* 36, no. 3 (June 12, 2009): 242-245.

Chiu, Hsienchang Thomas, and Christine Kim Garcia. "Familial Spontaneous Pneumothorax." *Current Opinion in Pulmonary Medicine* 12, no. 4 (July 20, 2006): 268-272.

Dameron, Amanda L. "Pneumothorax." *Health Library*, March 15, 2013.

Mayo Clinic. "Pneumothorax." *Mayo Clinic*, April 5, 2011.

PODIATRY

Category: Specialty
Anatomy or system affected: Bones, feet, nails
Specialties and related fields: Dermatology, orthopedics, vascular medicine
Definition: The medical field that involves the diagnosis and treatment of diseases and abnormalities of the feet, ankles, and lower legs.
Key terms:
corticosteroid: a fatlike molecule (or steroid), produced by the adrenal gland or made synthetically, that can be used to treat inflammation
dysfunction: the disordered or impaired function of a body system, organ, or tissue
orthopedics: the surgical or manipulative treatment of any disorder of the skeletal system and the associated motor organs
orthotic device: a podiatric appliance or prosthesis that is used to correct a foot deformity
pharmacology: the aspect of biomedical science that studies therapeutic drugs, their administration, and their bioproperties

SCIENCE AND PROFESSION

The human foot, which is located at the end of the lower leg and connected to the leg by the ankle, is a very complex structure. Feet are designed to optimize both balance and mobility. Each foot is composed of twenty-six bones, ligaments that connect and articulate these bones, blood vessels that provide nutrients and oxygen, sensory nerves, and a very thick covering of tough, strong skin. Heredity and a lack of proper foot care frequently result in painful calluses, corns, bunions, enlarged joints, and ingrown toenails. In addition, a variety of diseases, such as diabetes mellitus and cardiovascular problems, can lead to many other serious foot dysfunctions.

Podiatrists-more correctly called doctors of podiatric medicine-examine, diagnose, and treat dysfunctions of the foot as well as related problems associated with the ankle and the lower leg. The first record of a process that was associated with podiatric medicine was the creation, in 100 BCE, of plasters that were used to treat corns at the Greek city of Smyrna. Although other records of podiatric treatments were found in antiquity and in the Middle Ages, the modern science of podiatry arose from the activities of the fourteenth century barber-surgeons of Europe.

In the United States, the first truly prominent modern podiatrist-then termed a chiropodist-was Isacher Zacharia. Zacharia, foot doctor to President Abraham Lincoln, published the first American podiatry text in 1862. Two other milestones in the history of American podiatry are the founding of the National Association of Chiropodists and the opening of the New York School of Chiropody. Both of these events occurred in 1912.

In 1958, the National Association of Chiropodists was renamed the American Podiatric Medical Association. From the New York School of Chiropody, whose first curriculum required only one year of chiropodic training, arose today's schools of podiatric medicine, which require a four-year study period and award to graduates the doctor of podiatric medicine (DPM) degree. This degree derives from a uniform curriculum that all schools follow.

There are more than sixteen thousand licensed podiatrists in the United States. These podiatric practitioners serve patients in American hospitals, in government health programs, and in the armed forces, though most of them are in private, individual practice. Furthermore, modern podiatric medicine is an accepted part of all major health insurance plans, of Medicare, and of Medicaid. To become a licensed DPM, it is first necessary to complete a four-year course of postgraduate study at a school of podiatric medicine.

Admission to all American podiatry schools requires the completion of at least three years of a solid bachelor's degree program, which must include a year each of biology, inorganic chemistry, and organic chemistry. Most podiatry school entrants have completed a bachelor's degree. In addition, a solid grade-point average and good scores on the Medical College Admissions Test (MCAT) are required for admission.

The first two years of podiatric professional education use this background as a springboard that enables laboratory and lecture hall training in anatomy, biochemistry, physiology, pharmacology, diagnostic radi-

ology, and numerous other biomedical sciences. The third and fourth years of training are dedicated to the acquisition of clinical expertise by practicing podiatric medicine in college or community clinics, in hospitals, and in the offices of experienced, well-established podiatrists.

Upon graduation, the new DPM usually completes a hospital residency encompassing three to four years. In the first year, clinical expertise is gained in podiatric orthopedics, biomechanics, and neurology. The first-year podiatry resident engages in supervised primary care, which involves observing, evaluating, and treating many dysfunctions of the feet, ankles, and lower legs. Minor podiatric surgery, such as the correction of a hammertoe, is also carried out during this training period. In the remaining residency years, the resident learns to carry out the more demanding aspects of podiatric surgery of the foot, ankle, and leg. During this time period, the podiatric resident becomes more independent and skilled.

Podiatric practitioners require licenses to practice. In the United States, these licenses are most often gained by passing state board examinations. Satisfactory scores on the separate tests given by the National Board of Podiatric Medical Examiners are also deemed satisfactory for podiatric licensing by many states. Renewal of podiatry licenses, however, requires that podiatrists undergo extensive continuing education aimed at keeping them at the cutting edge of the field.

Specialization is also possible for podiatrists. Podiatric specialists can be certified by the American Board of Podiatric Surgery, the American Board of Podiatric Medicine, or the American Board of Podiatric Public Health. Each of these podiatric specialty boards requires advanced clinical training, completion of written and oral examinations, and extensive experience in specific aspects of modern podiatric practice. Such board certification indicates that the individuals involved have met much higher standards than those required for licensing alone. Some podiatrists also belong to the American College of Foot and Ankle Surgery of the American Medical Association (AMA).

In modern practice, podiatric surgical procedures designed to prevent or correct podiatric deformities now supplant many of the more conventional methods that originally made up the expertise of most podiatric practitioners. In addition, numerous techniques that cause the improvement of the health and the function of the foot and the ankle, so as to preclude foot deformities, have become key aspects of the modern podiatric profession.

DIAGNOSTIC AND TREATMENT TECHNIQUES

A thorough podiatric examination begins with the complete medical history of the patient, inspection of the patient's gait, and careful examination of both feet, the ankles, and the lower legs. When these procedures point to the diagnosis of a particular podiatric problem, x-ray examination, muscle testing, and neurological consultation may be carried out to search for more subtle problems that the initial examination suggested but did not prove.

Once a clear, complete diagnosis has been obtained, a treatment regimen-including physical therapy, various surgical treatments, medications, and the use of podiatric (orthotic) appliances-is prescribed. Often, all aspects of treatment are carried out in the podiatrist's office. Complex podiatric surgery, however, may require the use of a hospital surgical suite or its equivalent.

Among the podiatric problems most often seen are athlete's foot, bunions, calluses, corns, ingrown toenails, hammertoes, heel spurs, traumatic injuries to the ankles or feet, plantar warts, and complaints associated with arthritis, cardiovascular disease, or diabetes mellitus. In many cases-especially those engendered by athletics, diabetes, and cardiovascular problems-the podiatrist refers patients to other health practitioners, such as orthopedists, cardiologists, or endocrinologists. Increasingly, however, podiatrists and other specialists are beginning to work together as teams to solve such health problems.

Bunions are deformities of the big toes and their joints; they may or may not be painful, but they are almost always considered uncosmetic. When a bunion is not painful, it is usually treated by the use of an orthotic device that prevents further damage and pain. In cases where bunion pain is caused by inflammation, oral or injected anti-inflammatory drugs, such as corticosteroids, are often used for the shortest period of time needed to correct the problem. Such short-term treatment is made necessary by the potential health risks caused by this therapy, such as cardiovascular problems. In the most severe cases, surgery is used to remove the bunion. An incision is made near the bunion site, and a surgical burr is used to trim away the region of excess bone that is causing the problem. In cases where manipulative examination or x-rays show that the bunion problem is in the joint, much more complex surgery is required.

Corns and hammertoes may be considered together, as many corns are caused by hammertoes. Corns are not restricted to occurrence along with hammertoes, however, as they also arise spontaneously on any toe subject to inappropriate biomechanical stress. A corn (or heloma) is a skin protrusion-or thickening-atop or on the side of a toe. Corns can occur wherever a toe has been bent out of shape by a biomechanical problem or by a tight shoe. They can be quite painful. Hammertoe, a contracture of one of the toe joints,

produces a toe malformation that makes wearing shoes painful and can lead to corns. Corns may be trimmed periodically or removed surgically. The treatment used by podiatrists depends on the severity of the problem seen. Similarly, hammertoes are corrected surgically. After treatment of these problems, it is important for the patient to wear shoes that fit appropriately, to use corrective orthotic devices that are prescribed, and to follow closely the instructions given by the podiatrist. Failure to do so can counteract the results of the podiatric treatment.

Calluses, like corns, are buildups of tough, thickened skin. Unlike corns, however, they occur most often on the bottoms of the feet. Calluses form to protect the foot from undue stress resulting from uneven weight bearing by the bottom of the foot. Therefore, they will form again after removal wherever the causative mechanical stress recurs. When a callus becomes painful, the appropriate treatment regimen varies greatly from case to case. Often, an orthotic device is used to produce evenness of weight bearing by the foot. In other cases, the callus is trimmed. In the most extreme cases, minor surgery is used to correct the anatomical defect in the metatarsal bone that is causing the problem. Again, success in callus treatment is optimized by carefully following the directions of the podiatrist. In the most severe instances, up to three months of diminished physical activity is required to enable complete healing of the trimmed metatarsal bones. Calluses may also occur at the back of the heel, as a result of tight shoes and dermatologic problems. These calluses are usually handled by trimming and subsequent purchase of more appropriate shoes.

Heel spurs, Achilles tendonitis, ankle problems, dermatologic problems of the foot, and diabetic/cardiovascular complications may also be treated by podiatrists. Furthermore, it should be recognized that podiatrists will often repair damaged bones, muscles, and tendons surgically. They can also prescribe medications and treat fractures or sprains by applying casts and braces.

PERSPECTIVE AND PROSPECTS
Many advances in podiatric medicine have occurred in recent years. Most encouraging is the improved ability of podiatrists to handle severe foot problems. This improvement is largely attributable to advances in the field and to more thorough training both in professional school and in postgraduate experiences. The increasing positive interaction of podiatrists and other health care professionals in the treatment of dermatologic, cardiovascular, and diabetic problems is another great step forward.

It is believed that the job prospects for podiatrists will expand rapidly in the next fifty years, and there will be even greater success in the podiatric treatment of problems that are presently difficult to handle. It is also expected that additional podiatric medical schools will open to meet the need for more DPMs throughout the United States.

There are two main reasons for the excellent job prospects for podiatrists. First is the increase in the population of senior citizens. Because these individuals have had more wear and tear on their lower legs and feet than younger people, they have foot ailments that require treatment more frequently. Second is the increased interest in jogging and other sports in the general population, which will lead to more injuries that require podiatric intervention.

These factors are also expected to produce advances in the uses of orthotic appliances, generate sophisticated new diagnostic and surgical techniques, and lead to better cooperation between podiatrists and other health care professionals.

—*Sanford S. Singer, PhD*

See also Athlete's foot; Bone disorders; Bones and the skeleton; Bunions; Corns and calluses; Feet; Flat feet; Foot disorders; Fungal infections; Gout; Hammertoe correction; Hammertoes; Heel spur removal; Lower extremities; Nail removal; Nails; Orthopedic surgery; Orthopedics; Physical examination; Tendon disorders; Tendon repair; Warts.

For Further Information:
Alexander, Ivy L., ed. *Podiatry Sourcebook*. 2d rev. ed. Detroit, Mich.: Omnigraphics, 2007.
Copeland, Glenn, and Stan Solomon. *The Foot Doctor: Lifetime Relief for Your Aching Feet*. Rev. ed. Toronto, Ont.: Macmillan Canada, 1996.
Farr, J. Michael, ed. *Enhanced Occupational Outlook Handbook*. 7th ed. Indianapolis, Ind.: JIST Works, 2009.
Fink, Brett Ryan, and Mark S. Mizel. *The Whole Foot*. New York: Demos Medical, 2012.
Lippert, Frederick G., and Sigvard T. Hansen. *Foot and Ankle Disorders: Tricks of the Trade*. New York: Thieme, 2003.
Lorimer, Donald L., et al., eds. *Neale's Disorders of the Foot*. 7th ed. New York: Churchill Livingstone/Elsevier, 2006.
Rose, Jonathan D., and Vincent J. Martorana. *The Foot Book*. Baltimore: Johns Hopkins University Press, 2011.
Thordarson, David B., ed. *Foot and Ankle*. 2d ed. Philadelphia: Lippincott Williams & Wilkins, 2013.
Van De Graaff, Kent M., and Stuart I. Fox. *Concepts of Human Anatomy and Physiology*. 5th ed. Dubuque, Iowa: Wm. C. Brown, 2000.

POISONING

Category: Disease/Disorder
Anatomy or system affected: Gastrointestinal system, immune system, muscles, musculoskeletal system, nervous system, respiratory system, stomach
Specialties and related fields: Emergency medicine, environmental health, epidemiology, toxicology

Definition: Exposure to any substance in sufficient quantity to cause adverse health effects, from severe to fatal.

Key terms:

epidemiology: The study of the incidence of diseases or poisonings in affected populations

iatrogenic poisoning: poisoning resulting from medical treatment, which can include overdose, the administration of improper medication by the patient or prescribing physician, and adverse reactions

pharmacology: the science that deals with the chemistry, effects, and therapeutic use of drugs

syrup of ipecac: a plant extract that will induce vomiting when orally administered; the syrup can be used to induce vomiting after ingestion of a poisonous substance

toxicology: the science devoted to the study of poisons

toxidrome: a group of symptoms characteristic of a toxin or group of toxins that act on the same area of the nervous system

CAUSES AND SYMPTOMS

Probably the most accurate statement that can be made about the occurrence of poisoning in the United States is that the numbers vary widely depending on the information source and definition of poisoning. Incidents can be grouped into intentional poisonings, accidental poisonings, occupational and environmental poisonings, social poisonings, and iatrogenic poisonings. There is no single organization that collects and analyzes data from hospitals, physicians' offices, police and court records, and industrial accident and exposure records. One source has reported that as many as eight million people are accidentally or intentionally poisoned each year. It has been stated further that 10 percent of all ambulance calls and 10 to 20 percent of all admissions to medical facilities involve poisonings.

Many incidents of poisoning go unreported because a poison control center is not consulted or the effects are not severe enough to require extensive medical treatment. In other cases where exposure to the toxic agent involves constant contact to low but toxic levels of industrial chemicals, such as occupational or environmental exposures, symptoms may be subtle or confused with diseases that are associated with the normal aging process. The degree of illness and/or the number of premature deaths resulting from environmental exposure to naturally occurring or artificial toxic substances-radiation, chemical waste, and other toxins in the air, water, and food supply-is simply not known.

The most consistent and reliable sources of information on accidental poisoning in the United States are the annual statistics compiled by the American Association of Poison Control Centers. While poison control centers receive some calls related to intentional poisonings, 88 percent of the calls are considered accidental exposures. Combining all the poisoning types together, poison control centers are called concerning about 2.2 million human cases each year. It is important to note, however, that extrapolations from the number of reported poisonings to the number of actual poisonings occurring annually in the United States cannot be made from these data alone.

About 93 percent of exposures occur in the home, more than half involve children under six, and three-fourths involve ingestion. The great predominance of young children in the accidental poisoning category reflects the inquisitive behavior of that age group. For children under the age of one year, inappropriate administration of medications by the parents is the dominant cause of poisonings. For children over the age of five, exposure to toxic substances often represents the simple misreading of a medication label or the manifestation of family stress or even suicidal intent. These children have increased incidence of depressive symptoms and family problems compared to their nonpoisoned peer group.

Intentional poisoning of children also occurs-usually as a well-planned act of a psychologically disturbed parent. Although many of these incidents are clearly homicidal and abusive by design, some have received medical notoriety as cases of Münchausen syndrome by proxy. Münchausen syndrome itself is a psychiatric

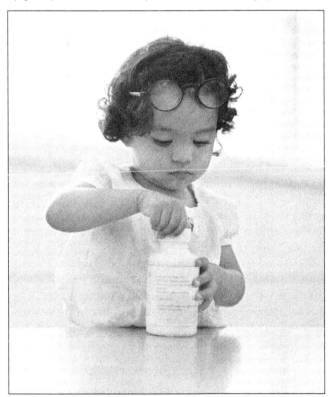

Childproof caps are essential in the prevention of accidental poisoning. Photo via iStock/PeopleImages. [Used under license.]

disorder in which the patient achieves psychological comfort from the attention and treatment received under the pretense of being afflicted with a serious or painful illness. In a variation of this condition, the psychiatric needs of an adult are fulfilled through an induced medical disorder in the child. For example, a parent might surreptitiously administer syrup of ipecac to his or her child, inducing unexplained vomiting and gastrointestinal disorders that requires extended hospital care. The phenomenon is rare but well documented in the medical literature and is classified as a form of child abuse.

Intentional poisonings are mostly suicide-related. The Centers for Disease Control and Prevention (CDC) reported that more than 38,000 Americans killed themselves in 2010. Of all suicides from 2005 to 2009, poisoning was the method chosen by almost 40 percent of women and about 12 percent of men. Although carbon monoxide (as in motor vehicle exhaust) is one of the most common agents used, intentional dosing with large quantities of drugs is also very frequently involved. Of the many thousands of drugs that could be used for overdose incidents, 90 percent of actual cases involve only about twenty products in nine drug groups. Most of these are addictive or abused drugs, including stimulants, antidepressants, tranquilizers, narcotics, sedatives or hypnotics, and antipsychotics. Alcohol alone is seldom lethal but is often consumed along with the more deadly drugs and may make the lethal effects possible.

Social poisoning is related to drug use or abuse, which can have significant societal consequences. There are hundreds of thousands of hospital and emergency room admissions each year for overdose treatment as well as for the indirect consequences of recreational drug use, such as violent crime, trauma, and vehicular accidents. Almost 400,000 drug-abuse-related emergency room visits were projected to have occurred in 1990 by the Drug Abuse Warning Network (DAWN), a federal government-sponsored data collection system. These figures do not include alcohol, however, unless it is mentioned as having been involved in a mixed drug exposure event.

The abuse of alcohol, the most widely available chemical intoxicant legally allowed for recreational use, is a major social problem in the United States. While a majority of the alcohol-consuming public demonstrates a lifelong pattern of little or moderate drinking without the development of addiction-related problems, it has been reported that a small percentage of the population (5 percent to 10 percent) drinks between one-third and one-half of all alcohol consumed. The causes of alcoholism involve a complex interaction of social, physiological, and genetic risk factors. In the United States, there are approximately 9 million people classified as chronic alcohol abusers, and according to the CDC, about 80,000 deaths per year are attributable to alcohol-related causes.

Tobacco use, although not as closely associated with criminal behavior and vehicular accidents as drugs and alcohol, has been connected with increased incidence of cancer, respiratory illnesses, and cardiovascular diseases. According to the World Health Organization, more than 5 million deaths worldwide per year are attributable to tobacco use. Both smoking and excessive alcohol consumption are becoming increasingly less socially accepted, but the continued wide acceptance of both alcohol and tobacco use obscures their potential to poison.

TREATMENT AND THERAPY

Emergency medical treatment of the poisoned patient is most often based on the relief of symptoms and the provision of life support. If the patient is awake and alert, a medical history is taken and a clinical examination is performed, both of which can help determine substance exposure. The medical staff must never assume that the patient is providing truthful information, especially if clinical impressions conflict with the patient account. If the patient is comatose, then stabilization and life support take immediate priority over determination of the specific toxic substance involved. The attending physician will want to prevent airway blockage and to maintain respiration and circulation, which may require mechanical aids for breathing assistance. Treatment of cardiac and blood pressure problems can be accomplished with drugs, fluid, or oxygen administration. If the patient is unconscious, the depth of central nervous system depression can be evaluated using a standard test of reactivity to light, sound, pain, and the presence or absence of normal body processes. If the patient is suffering from seizures, drugs that counteract these symptoms can be administered.

Although many hospitals offer in-house toxicology testing in a clinical laboratory, treatment usually must begin before results are available. For this and several other reasons, a comprehensive toxicology testing laboratory is not as useful an asset in the emergency treatment of poisoning as might be assumed. It would be impossible for any analytical laboratory to provide timely or cost-effective emergency identification of all potentially toxic substances. Instead, a more efficient strategy concentrates on analyzing those substances for which a specific antidote exists or for which specific medical procedures are required in a critical period of time. A very high percentage of drug overdose cases involve one of a group of six or eight drugs that will vary depending on locality. Pesticide poisoning, for ex-

ample, is a more prevalent medical problem for rural than urban hospitals. Drug abuse is a problem in all localities, but the frequency and type of drugs abused vary. Regional preferences exist for PCP, cocaine, amphetamines, and opiates. Even prescription drug abuse depends on locality and the patient population.

Common pain relievers found in virtually every home medicine cabinet constitute a large number of both adult and pediatric poisoning incidents. Preparations containing aspirin, as well as nonaspirin analgesics containing acetaminophen (such as Tylenol), are possibly life-threatening when consumed in excess. Acetaminophen poisoning is particularly insidious since death from total and irreversible destruction of the liver will occur unless the antidote, a chemical called acetylcysteine, is administered within six hours of ingestion of a lethal dose. Since a specific antidote exists, most hospitals with emergency service will offer around-the-clock testing for acetaminophen levels in the blood. Aspirin, although not as lethal as acetaminophen, can be fatal if a sufficient amount is consumed. Its universal availability and common usage make aspirin a significant poisoning agent encountered in all localities. The symptoms of toxicity are related to aspirin's effects on temperature regulation, rate of breathing, and the body's ability to influence the acidity of the blood. Treatment involves monitoring the patient's vital signs and calculating the severity of the dose taken. Vomiting may be induced with syrup of ipecac, or charcoal (a very active adsorption agent) may be given orally to limit gastric absorption. Intravenous fluids may also be given to counteract the blood acidity changes.

Prescription drugs that are commonly overused or abused (antiepileptic medication, sedatives and tranquilizers, and antipsychotic or antidepressant drugs) are often routinely assayed in the hospital laboratory as part of the treatment process for patients receiving these medications. The levels in the blood can be monitored to determine the toxicity status of the patient. Usually, supportive care is sufficient for treatment until the drug clears the system. For certain tranquilizers and antidepressants, an antidote called flumazenil can be administered, but it must be used with caution.

Poisoning from an overdose of opiates or morphinelike drugs is a special treatment case. A specific antidote called naloxone can be administered if the patient is treated before irreversible respiratory depression occurs. Recovery is virtually instantaneous and dramatic, with a comatose patient becoming alert within seconds of naloxone administration. For this reason, the routine treatment of comatose patients includes the administration of opiate antidote even when the cause of the unconscious state is unknown.

Although heavy, long-term ethyl alcohol use invariably leads to liver dysfunction and a number of other organ disorders, alcohol is not usually life-threatening unless it is consumed in quantities sufficient to cause a coma. Death most commonly results from respiratory depression and related complications. Other types of alcohols, as well as antifreeze, can be involved in both accidental and intentional poisonings. Methanol or wood alcohol is a common industrial solvent found in materials around the home or work site; consumption can cause blindness and death. Isopropyl alcohol (or rubbing alcohol), although not as toxic as methanol, can also cause severe illness and death when consumed in sufficient quantities. Ethylene glycol, a common ingredient in antifreeze, is highly toxic and is especially attractive to small children and pets because of its sweet taste. It may also be consumed by alcoholics as an ethanol substitute. When not treated, its consumption can result in kidney failure. It is not the alcohols themselves that are the primary toxins but the degradation products called metabolites that form in the body in an attempt to eliminate the foreign substance. Ironically, the treatment for both methanol and ethylene glycol poisoning is administration of high doses of ethanol, which prevents the formation of toxic metabolites by the liver.

In the United States, lead poisoning is a major medical problem for children living in older, substandard housing; they can become exposed to large amounts of lead from the consumption of lead-based paint. (Even though such paints are no longer used in residential housing, many older buildings remain contaminated.) Another major source of exposure is inhalation of leaded gas fumes and exhaust. Other less common sources of lead poisoning include the consumption of food stored in leaded crystal or pottery or moonshine whiskey distilled in automobile radiators. Intentional gasoline sniffing by adolescents can also be a problem. Lead exposure is extremely hazardous because its effects are both severe and cumulative. Children are especially susceptible to lead poisoning because they absorb and retain more of this substance and have less capacity for excretion than adults.

The nervous system is a major site for lead toxicity, causing both psychological and neurologic impairment. The blood cell production can also be affected, with resulting anemia and decreased oxygen-carrying capacity. Because lead toxicity can result in behavioral and learning disorders that may already afflict children living in substandard conditions, sometimes poisoning cannot be detected by clinical symptoms alone and must be diagnosed through blood testing. Test data indicate that the level of lead associated with nervous system disorders is probably lower than previously believed. In the United States, a major screening

INFORMATION ON POISONING

Causes: Exposure to biological, chemical, or environmental toxins; may be intentional, accidental, occupational, environmental, social, or iatrogenic

Symptoms: Varies; may include unconsciousness, disorientation, muscle spasms, seizures, swelling

Duration: Acute

Treatments: Emergency medical treatment (stabilization, life support mechanisms), antidotes and/or antiseizure medications, induction of vomiting

effort has been financed by the federal government to detect high lead body deposits in children. The goal is to find affected children and to treat them before permanent damage occurs.

PERSPECTIVE AND PROSPECTS

Poisoning has been a medical problem since the earliest times of human history. A tremendous variety of poisonous substances can be encountered in the natural world alone. It has been estimated that 200,000 plants and animals are known to be toxic to humans, some organisms producing as many as fifty or sixty toxins. The potential of almost any substance to be poisonous was recognized during the Renaissance by Paracelsus, a founder of modern toxicology, who stated, "All substances are poison; only the dose makes something not a poison." Many folk remedies and tribal medicine practices were derived from centuries of trial-and-error experiences with toxic plant and animal species in the environment. Historically, the development of the sciences of pharmacology and toxicology is closely related to the study of poisons.

As societies become more urban and technology-based, poisoning problems shift away from natural toxin exposures to those related to drugs and industrial chemicals. For many of these types of poisonings, sustaining the vital life processes until the toxin is cleared from the body is the only method of treatment. Specific antidotes are not available for many drugs or even for many natural poisons. Since a large number of toxins critically affect the nervous system, a diagnostic and treatment system has been developed based on the "toxidrome" concept. If a specific area of the nervous system can be shown to be affected, treatment can begin to counteract those effects even if the identity of the toxin is not known.

The symptoms of acute poisoning or overexposure to a toxic agent are likely to be treated as individual medical problems by physicians in an emergency medicine environment. Meanwhile, social poisons, which often do not create immediate medical emergencies, continue to exact enormous economic and medical costs to society over the long term; these poisoning problems have not been dealt with successfully by social, medical, or governmental agencies. In the case of environmental toxins, little if any well-established information on the long-term toxicity of these substances is available. The science of toxicology, particularly with regard to establishing the risk of exposure of a population to environmental toxins, often becomes a guessing game played by a governmental regulatory agency. Until societal and environmental poisonings can be better evaluated and controlled, they will continue to constitute serious economic and quality-of-life problems.

—*David J. Wells, Jr., PhD*

See also Addiction; Alcoholism; Biological and chemical weapons; Bites and stings; Cyanosis; Domestic violence; Emergency rooms; Environmental diseases; Environmental health; First aid; Food poisoning; Iatrogenic disorders; Intoxication; Lead poisoning; Mercury poisoning; Münchausen syndrome by proxy; Nicotine; Over-the-counter medications; Poisonous plants; Prescription drug abuse; Smoking; Substance abuse; Suicide; Toxicology.

For Further Information:
Baselt, Randall C. *Disposition of Toxic Drugs and Chemicals in Man.* 9th ed. Foster City, Calif.: Biomedical, 2011.
Dart, Richard C., ed. *Medical Toxicology.* 3d ed. Philadelphia: Lippincott Williams & Wilkins, 2004.
Garriott, James C., ed. *Medicolegal Aspects of Alcohol Determination in Biological Specimens.* Littleton, Mass.: PSG, 1988.
Klaassen, Curtis D., ed. *Casarett and Doull's Toxicology: The Basic Science of Poisons.* 8th ed. New York: McGraw-Hill, 2013.
Morgan, Monroe T. *Environmental Health.* 3d ed. Belmont, Calif.: Thomson/Wadsworth, 2003.
"Poisoning." *MedlinePlus*, August 30, 2013.
Timbrell, John. *Introduction to Toxicology.* 3d ed. Washington, DC: Taylor & Francis, 2003.
Warren, Christian. *Brush with Death: A Social History of Lead Poisoning.* Baltimore: Johns Hopkins University Press, 2001.

POLIOMYELITIS

Category: Disease/Disorder
Also known as: Polio
Anatomy or system affected: Brain, legs, muscles, musculoskeletal system, nerves, nervous system, spine
Specialties and related fields: Epidemiology, neurology, pediatrics, public health, virology
Definition: A contagious viral illness capable of causing meningitis and permanent paralysis; in response

to a dramatic increase in the frequency of cases in industrialized nations during the twentieth century, a vaccine was developed that has virtually eliminated this disease in Europe and the Western Hemisphere.

Key terms:
endemic disease: a disease that is usually present in a population and does not exhibit marked fluctuations in frequency from year to year
epidemic: a marked increase in the frequency of a disease, relative to the historical experience of the affected population
neurotropic virus: a virus that multiplies in neural tissues
serologic epidemiology: investigation of the history of disease exposure in a population by surveying the incidence of antibodies circulating in the bloodstream
subclinical infection: a disease process characterized by multiplication of the causative organism within the host and production of antibodies by the host without causing apparent illness

CAUSES AND SYMPTOMS
Poliomyelitis, or polio, is a contagious disease affecting humans and some nonhuman primates. It is caused by three closely related strains of a human enterovirus. In its most serious manifestation, it attacks nerve tissue in the spinal cord and brain stem, resulting in paralysis. Polio was one of the most feared diseases in developed countries in the twentieth century. A few medical researchers suspected the connection between the severe neurological symptoms of poliomyelitis and the more typical enteric form of the disease in the first decade of the twentieth century. A complete and accurate picture of the etiology of polio, however, was not demonstrated and accepted until the 1930s, when improved techniques for detecting viruses and antiviral antibodies enabled scientists to trace the disease in all of its phases.

The virus responsible for poliomyelitis is present in large numbers in the intestines of infected individuals. It is excreted in feces, from which it is spread to uninfected individuals through contaminated water, food, hands, and eating utensils and by flies and other filth-loving insects. Once it has been ingested, the poliovirus multiplies in the cells lining the intestine and invades the lymphatic system, producing swelling in the lymph nodes surrounding the intestine and in the neck. The symptoms of the disease at this stage may escape notice altogether, or the infected person may experience fever and a sore throat. These symptoms subside after two or three days as the body's immune system begins producing antibodies to overcome the virus. Most cases never proceed beyond this stage, termed the minor illness of polio.

In a minority of cases, after a period of several days in which a patient is asymptomatic, the minor illness is followed by the onset of neurological symptoms, signaling that the virus has invaded the spinal cord. Symptoms include pain and stiffness in the spine, lethargy, general muscular weakness, and flaccid (that is, not accompanied by spasms) paralysis of muscles, particularly of the legs. Paralysis of the legs occurs because the virus preferentially attacks neurons in the front or anterior horns of the spinal cord, including the motor nerves controlling the legs, and often affects one side more than the other. In the most severe cases, viral infection spreads from the spinal cord to the brain stem, attacking neurons serving the diaphragm and esophagus. Without aggressive medical intervention in the form of an artificial breathing apparatus, paralysis of the diaphragm is fatal.

In the absence of brain-stem involvement, a body's normal defenses usually overcome the viral infection. Since the body is unable to replace destroyed neurons, however, acute polio leaves the patient with permanent motor impairment ranging from mild muscular weakness to severe crippling disability. Aided by appropriate physical therapy during the recovery period, patients can usually regain some of the motor function lost during the active disease. As survivors of the polio epidemics of the 1940s and 1950s reached middle age in the late twentieth century, a late phase of the disease called postpolio syndrome was recognized. After decades of apparent normality, muscles affected by the initial paralytic attack experience gradual loss of function without evidence of renewed viral activity.

The proportion of cases resulting in permanent paralysis varies with the age structure of the population affected. Typically, no more than 10 percent of patients who experience a major illness including neurologic symptoms suffer such paralysis. Under premodern conditions, the latter probably accounted for less than 1 percent of the total cases, because subclinical infection, minor illness, and paralytic polio usually occurred in early childhood. Maternal antibodies provided protection for newborns, while a child's own immune system created antibodies following exposure. In this way, lifelong immunity to subsequent infection was acquired. With improving sanitation and an older susceptible population, however, this proportion gradually increased.

During an epidemic, polio is primarily spread by persons with mild and subclinical infections, who may be unaware that they are ill. Infectivity persists for two to three weeks after the onset of the intestinal disease. There is no evidence that lifetime carriers exist. It is virtually impossible to prevent the spread of an asymptomatic, fecally transmitted pathogen among young children in group settings by any behavioral means.

INFORMATION ON POLIOMYELITIS

Causes: Viral infection

Symptoms: Swelling in lymph nodes surrounding intestines and in neck; in severe cases, pain and stiffness in spine, lethargy, general muscle weakness, paralysis (particularly of legs)

Duration: Acute to chronic

Treatments: Physical therapy, medical devices (splints, braces), prevention through vaccination

---

Fortunately, vaccines have effectively eliminated polio as an epidemic disease in the developed world and in Latin America.

TREATMENT AND THERAPY

The history of efforts to prevent and treat poliomyelitis illustrates the changing attitudes of the medical community toward disease and the methods by which a once-important pathogen was virtually eliminated. Only time will tell whether the spectacular inroads made by medical science against poliomyelitis are permanent. Persons with compromised immune systems are reminders that vaccines cannot completely protect all individuals. They prevent health professionals from becoming complacent with respect to any infectious disease.

At the end of the nineteenth century, when epidemics of poliomyelitis first began to surface, medical science had made a number of important advances in the understanding and treatment of disease. First and foremost, the role of microorganisms in infectious disease was well established. Although viruses were still poorly defined, the principle that they were transmissible agents was understood. Second, although physicians had few specific remedies at their disposal, they had abandoned most of the drastic, plainly harmful remedies of earlier eras.

As polio became more and more prominent in morbidity statistics and the public imagination, the biomedical community responded on three different fronts. The first was an attempt to prevent transmission by quarantine measures and clinical studies. Scientists attempted to clarify the actual mode of transmission and the natural occurrence of the virus. Second, they attempted to treat paralytic cases in the acute and recovery phases. Lastly, scientists tried to develop a vaccine.

Quarantine measures were never very successful at controlling polio epidemics. Isolating critically ill patients in a sterile environment and restricting travel on the part of their family members, as was done in 1916 in New York, failed to quarantine people with mild in-

Man on street with atrophy and paralysis of the right leg and foot due to polio. Photo via CDC/Wikimedia Commons. [Public domain.]

fections, who were the main transmitters of the disease. Although the poliovirus can be found in untreated sewage, this was not a major source of infection in the United States. Flies can transmit the virus mechanically and thus may act as vectors, but fly eradication campaigns failed to have any effect on polio occurrence. In the period when it was incorrectly thought that the poliovirus entered through the nose, nasal sprays were touted as offering protection.

In the 1920s, the search for a cure emphasized the use of blood serum from individuals who had recovered from the disease. Theoretically, the idea was a sound one that had been used successfully for other diseases, but it proved ineffective in the case of polio, because the level of antibodies in the serum was not sufficiently high to have a therapeutic effect. More important, by the time patients developed paralytic symptoms, their bodies were already producing antibodies. Despite disappointing results, serum therapy was used extensively for fifteen years.

In 1920, Philip Drinker of the Harvard School of Public Health introduced the so-called iron lung, a res-

pirator that mimicked the action of lungs by subjecting patients to fluctuations in air pressure. The iron lung gave some hope of survival to patients with paralysis of the diaphragm or lesions in the nervous centers of the brain that govern respiration. Its introduction was accompanied by misgivings that it would only serve to keep alive severely disabled patients who had no hope of survival outside a hospital. Such ethical concerns were justified, but artificial respirators also proved effective in temporarily treating acute cases of respiratory paralysis that subsided with time.

With respect to paralyzed limbs, advances in orthopedics in the early twentieth century allowed for surgical procedures that minimized twisting and deformity and for the design of braces that improved mobility. Observing that deformity could be lessened by bracing and immobilizing limbs at the onset of the paralytic form of the disease, doctors of the 1920s and 1930s had a tendency to encase polio victims, even those with little or no paralysis, in elaborate casts attached to pulley systems. Against this trend, Elizabeth Kenny, an Australian nurse, conducted what amounted to a crusade against immobilization and advocated active physical therapy in acute paralytic poliomyelitis.

In 1921, future president of the United States Franklin Delano Roosevelt was stricken with acute paralytic polio that left him with severe paralysis of both legs. Roosevelt later used his private fortune to establish a center for the rehabilitation of polio victims in Warm Springs, Georgia, where he had spent his convalescence. After he became president in 1933, Roosevelt became a leader in the fight against poliomyelitis. For several years, the principal charitable organization funding polio treatment and research in the United States was the president's Birthday Ball Commission, the immediate forerunner of the National Foundation for Infantile Paralysis (NFIP), better known under the name of its main fund-raising effort, the March of Dimes. Basil O'Conner, a personal friend of Roosevelt, headed both agencies.

Since an attack of polio in any of its forms confers lifelong immunity, researchers from the 1920s onward increasingly concentrated their efforts on developing a vaccine. Vaccines rely on dead or nonvirulent strains of a pathogenic agent to induce an immune response in a host. To produce a polio vaccine, one must have large quantities of poliovirus, and the only known source of poliovirus prior to 1938 was spinal cord tissue from infected monkeys or humans. In 1935, Maurice Brodie conducted human vaccine trials with a formalin-inactivated virus from monkey spinal cord. At the same time, John Kohler conducted trials with a virus that he claimed had been inactivated by repeated passage through many generations of monkeys. Brodie's vaccine was unsuccessful; Kohler's achieved notoriety as the suspected cause of several cases of paralytic polio.

After World War II, the NFIP concentrated its efforts on funding the development of an effective polio vaccine. Thanks to the work of John Enders and others, a live poliovirus could be produced in tissue culture. Improved serological techniques enabled researchers to assess immunity in chimpanzees without sacrificing the animal. By 1950, a practical vaccination program was beginning to take shape under the direction of Jonas Salk, who headed the development of a formalin-inactivated injectable vaccine.

In 1954, with the collaboration of the National Institutes of Health and the US Census Bureau, the NFIP conducted a massive nationwide test of this inactivated Salk vaccine, involving 1.8 million children in the first, second, and third grades. In 1955, the number of new cases (or incidence) of polio among inoculated children was significantly lower than among controls, demonstrating that the vaccine was effective in clinical practice. Thereafter, the inoculation of children against polio became routine, and the incidence per 100,000 people declined dramatically-from 40 in 1952, the last major epidemic year, to 20 in 1955. The number of new cases per 100,000 people was 5 in 1959 and fewer than 1 in 1961 and subsequent years. There have been no domestically acquired cases of paralytic polio in the United States since 1987.

Salk's vaccine conferred only temporary immunity, requiring booster shots to be administered at yearly intervals. This made protection of the population cumbersome in industrialized countries and impractical in developing countries. The NFIP consequently turned its attention toward an effort, under the direction of Albert Sabin, to develop an orally administered attenuated viral preparation. The challenge was to develop a strain of virus that would multiply in the digestive system and stimulate antibody production but that could not attack the human nervous system. This effort was also supported by the World Health Organization (WHO). In 1957, an oral live virus vaccine was tested in Ruanda-Urundi (today Rwanda and Burundi). Between 1958 and 1959, field trials were conducted in fifteen countries, including the United States and the Soviet Union.

The Sabin oral vaccine confers longer-lasting immunity and is easier to administer, and therefore came to be used routinely to immunize children and adults against polio throughout the world. The WHO has exploited this advantage and undertaken a program of complete polio eradication. This program has been highly successful, and as of 2012, there were only three countries left in the world where polio was endemic (meaning not brought in from outside), down from more than 125 countries when the Global Polio Eradi-

cation Initiative was launched in 1988. The three remaining countries with endemic poliovirus are Nigeria, Pakistan, and Afghanistan. Six other countries in 2012 also reported isolated cases of polio, but they were either mild cases derived from the vaccine, or were brought into the country from outside. Altogether, 2012 saw fewer than 300 reported cases of polio worldwide.

PERSPECTIVE AND PROSPECTS

There is evidence that poliomyelitis has afflicted human beings from the beginning of time. There is an Egyptian tomb painting of a priest with a withered leg, and descriptions of individuals with polio-like diseases occur in Greek medical literature. In general, however, polio seems to have been a rare disease; there are no records of epidemics of paralytic polio before the second half of the nineteenth century. The symptoms of paralytic polio are so distinctive and devastating that it is unlikely cases were overlooked.

In the early nineteenth century, a number of physicians published descriptions of cases in which a fever in infants or very young children was followed by paralysis of the lower limbs. At that time, polio was unknown among older children and adults. As a consequence, the disease came to be known as infantile paralysis. The occurrence was infrequent and sporadic, although Charles Bell, a distinguished English neurologist, recorded an account of an epidemic affecting all the three- to five-year-old children on the isolated island of St. Helena around 1830.

Between 1880 and 1905, several localized outbreaks of epidemic poliomyelitis occurred in rural Scandinavia. In 1894, the United States suffered its first major outbreak, in Rutland County, Vermont. In contrast to earlier experiences, significant numbers of older children and young adults were affected. It was also puzzling to epidemiologists that the outbreaks should have occurred in isolated rural areas rather than in urban centers. Ivar Wickman, a Swedish epidemiologist who tracked the course of the severe Scandinavian epidemic of 1905, obtained evidence for abortive and nonparalytic cases, and postulated that they were important to the epidemiology of the disease. His results were not taken seriously until thirty years later.

In 1916, the northeastern United States suffered one of the most devastating epidemics in the history of poliomyelitis, with more than nine thousand acute cases in New York City alone. Public health authorities, disregarding evidence that acute cases represented less than 10 percent of actual cases, instituted draconian quarantine measures that were largely ineffective. More than 95 percent of those affected in the 1916 epidemic were under nine years of age. By 1931, the date of the next major epidemic in the Northeast, the proportion of victims younger than nine had declined to 84 percent; by 1947, it had further declined to 52 percent. Poliomyelitis had somehow been transformed from an uncommon endemic disease affecting only very young children to a sporadic, rural epidemic disease that affected primarily but not exclusively children. Finally, it had become a widespread epidemic disease affecting all age groups in both rural and urban environments.

In 1905, when Swedish researchers attempted to show the existence of subclinical poliomyelitis infections, there was only one way to demonstrate polio in an unequivocal, scientifically rigorous manner. It involved filtering material from a diseased person to remove bacteria, inoculating the filtrate into the brain of a susceptible monkey, and waiting for paralysis to develop. Cost and logistics precluded large-scale tests. The trials that were conducted often failed because of inadequate sterility. In 1939, Charles Armstrong succeeded in propagating one of the three poliovirus strains in rodents, greatly facilitating research. In 1948, Enders and his colleagues succeeded in growing the poliovirus in tissue culture. In the meantime, reliable techniques for identifying antibodies to specific pathogens had been developed. This development enabled epidemiologists to determine which individuals had the live poliovirus in their bodies and which had developed immunity.

A series of studies conducted in the early 1950s among Alaskan Inuits, urban North Americans, and Egyptian villagers dramatically demonstrated the normal epidemiological pattern of polio occurrence and progress in three very different populations. Among Inuits living in Point Barrow, Alaska, only people over twenty showed antibodies to the virus, as a result of a known and devastating epidemic in 1930. In Miami, Florida, the proportion of persons with antibodies rose from 10 percent at age two to nearly 80 percent in adulthood. In Cairo, nearly 100 percent of the population over the age of three proved to have antibodies.

Therefore, the following epidemiological picture emerged. Before 1900, sanitary conditions in most of the world approximated those in Cairo, and most people contracted polio before the age of three. The vast majority of infections were subclinical, and paralytic cases occurred only sporadically in infants. As sanitation improved in the United States and Europe, the chances of contracting polio as an infant decreased. Thus, a pool of susceptible individuals of mixed ages arose, and epidemics occurred. Like mumps, measles, and other childhood illnesses, polio is more likely to cause severe illness in an adult than in a young child. For this reason, paralytic polio became a more serious health problem in Miami than in Cairo. Epidemics oc-

curred first in rural areas in the United States and Scandinavia, where sanitation was relatively good and people were somewhat isolated from major population centers that served as sources of infection.

Defenders of the use of animals in biomedical research often cite the history of the conquest of poliomyelitis to support their point of view. From the earliest days of scientific poliomyelitis research until the discovery of tissue-culturing techniques for viruses in the 1940s, experimental work was dependent on monkeys. For many years, the only way of confirming that the virus was present was to inoculate a monkey with a suspected sample: If the monkey became paralyzed, the test was positive. Cultures were maintained through serial transfer from monkey to monkey, and the earliest vaccines were prepared from monkey spinal cord tissue.

The first successful tissue culture experiments involved fetal intestinal tissue. The experiments depended on having an available source of a characterized viral strain originally isolated from a human but maintained through several generations of transfer through animals. Even after the maintenance and characterization of viral strains and the production of virus for vaccines had moved from animal laboratories to test tubes of cultured cells, the first tests of the safety and efficacy of vaccines were performed with primates. Virtually every step in the conquest of polio involved experimental procedures.

Although the fight against poliomyelitis has been spectacularly successful, it would be unwise to be complacent about a disease that still exists in parts of the world and that is selectively virulent under modern urban conditions in developed nations. The percentage of schoolchildren, particularly those living in poorer neighborhoods, who receive routine vaccinations against childhood diseases is decreasing in the United States. Because of the availability of safe drinking water, children are no longer likely to naturally acquire immunity from subclinical infections.

In about 1 in 20 million cases, individuals will develop polio after receiving a vaccine. A naturally acquired case of polio is now exceedingly rare. The number of such cases is less than the number of cases of polio as a result of adverse reactions to the vaccine. For this reason, many parents are not having their children immunized against polio. These well-intentioned people are putting their children at an unnecessary risk of contracting the disease.

Other diseases that were once thought to be virtually extinct, such as measles and tuberculosis, are experiencing a resurgence because of declining commitment to public and community health and increasing numbers of people with compromised immune systems. Until the polio eradication campaign is complete, there is no guarantee that polio will be excluded from the list of resurgent diseases.

—*Martha Sherwood-Pike, PhD;*
updated by L. Fleming Fallon, Jr., MD, PhD, MPH

See also Childhood infectious diseases; Enteroviruses; Epidemics and pandemics; Epidemiology; Immunization and vaccination; Meningitis; Paralysis; Viral infections.

For Further Information:
Blume, Stuart, and Ingrid Geesink. "A Brief History of Polio Vaccines." *Science* 288, no. 5471 (June 2, 2000): 1593-1594.
Carson-DeWitt, Rosalyn. "Poliomyelitis." *Health Library*, May 20, 2013.
Daniel, Thomas M., and Frederick C. Robbins, eds. *Polio*. Rochester, N.Y.: University of Rochester Press, 1997.
Garrett, Laurie. *The Coming Plague: Newly Emerging Diseases in a World out of Balance*. New York: Penguin, 1995.
Gould, Tony. *A Summer Plague: Polio and Its Survivors*. New Haven, Conn.: Yale University Press, 1997.
Hecht, Alan D., and Edward Alamo. *Polio*. New York: Chelsea House, 2003.
Munsat, Theodore L. "Poliomyelitis: New Problems with an Old Disease." *New England Journal of Medicine* 324 (April, 1991): 1206-1207.
Oshinsky, David M. *Polio: An American Story*. New York: Oxford University Press, 2005.
"Polio." *Centers for Disease Control and Prevention*, May 24, 2013.
"Poliomyelitis." *World Health Organization*, 2013.
Post-Polio Health International. www.post-polio.org.
Silver, Julie K. *Post-Polio Syndrome: A Guide for Polio Survivors and Their Families*. New Haven, Conn.: Yale University Press, 2002.

POLYCYSTIC KIDNEY DISEASE

Category: Disease/Disorder
Anatomy or system affected: Blood vessels, brain, gastrointestinal system, kidneys, liver, pancreas
Specialties and related fields: Cardiology, gastroenterology, genetics, nephrology, urology
Definition: A genetic disorder characterized by multiple, bilateral, grapelike clusters of fluid-filled cysts that slowly replace much of the mass of the kidney, reducing kidney function and leading to renal failure.
Key terms:
acquired cystic kidney disease (ACKD): a condition that develops with long-term kidney problems, especially in patients who have been on dialysis for five years
autosomal dominant: referring to a disease for which an individual who carries the abnormal gene will have the disease; there is a 50 percent chance that a child will inherit the disease
autosomal recessive: referring to a disease for which an individual may carry the abnormal gene but not have the disease; a child will have the disease only if both parents passed on the gene
end-stage renal disease (ESRD): total chronic kidney failure

CAUSES AND SYMPTOMS

About 600,000 people in the United States have polycystic kidney disease (PKD), and 12.5 million suffer from it worldwide; it is the fourth leading cause of kidney failure. There are two major inherited forms of PKD, autosomal dominant (ADPKD) and autosomal recessive (ARPKD), and a noninherited form called "acquired cystic kidney disease" (ACKD). The autosomal dominant type is the most common inherited form.

Autosomal dominant PKD has a slow onset, with symptoms usually developing between the ages of thirty and forty. Sometimes, symptoms do not appear until age seventy. Cysts grow out of the nephrons, the blood-processing units in the kidneys. High blood pressure occurs, and the kidney enlarges as the cysts form. A normal kidney weighs 10 to 12 ounces and is the size of a human fist. A cyst-filled kidney can weigh as much as 22 pounds and can grow to the size of a football or larger. Healthy kidney tissue is destroyed as the cysts produce pressure on it, and renal failure eventually occurs. Autosomal dominant PKD is thought to occur equally in men and woman and in all races; however, some studies suggest that it occurs more often in white females than in African Americans. Diagnosis can be made by ultrasound, computed tomography (CT) scanning, and magnetic resonance imaging (MRI). Genetic tests are run to identify the presence of the autosomal dominant gene. Over 80 percent of ADPDK is attributed to mutations in the PKD1 gene, and around 15 percent is due to mutations in the PKD2 gene. PKD mutations result in less expression of PC1, an integral membrane protein which results in activation of various signaling pathways. A direct relationship between functional PC1 and the phenotype presentation of ADPKD exists, where 100 percent functionality of PC1 presents healthy appearing kidneys, and 0 percent PC1 is nonviable with life. The likelihood of cyst formation increases when the level of functional PC1 drops below a critical threshold. Most mutations in PKD1 or PKD2 are heterozygous mutations, as homozygous mutations are thought to cause embryonic lethality.

The earliest presentation of ADPKD is arterial hypertension, which presents while renal function is still normal and significantly adds to the increased morbidity and mortality of these patients. Overactivation of the renin-angiotensin system is one of the proposed mechanisms for the early onset hypertension. Later on, cysts will start to form in these patients, and they arise in a minority of nephrons.

Once uremic symptoms appear, the disease is usually fatal within four years unless the patient receives dialysis or a kidney transplant. This destruction of kidney tissue may take as long as ten years. Several other symptoms are associated with autosomal dominant PKD. Patients experience pain in the back and side, as well as headaches. Blood may appear in the urine, and urinary tract infections occur. Aneurysms in the blood vessels of the brain can also appear. Cysts may form in the liver and pancreas, and even the heart valves may be affected. Life-threatening bleeding into the abdominal cavity from cyst ruptures can occur. Other symptoms often associated with the disease are nail abnormalities, painful menstruation, joint pain, drowsiness, and anemia. Patients who suffer from ADPKD also can have cardiovascular such as arterial aneurysms, intracranial aneurysms and left ventricular hypertrophy.

Autosomal recessive PKD usually affects children. ARPKD happens due to mutations in the PKDH1 gene. The PKHD1 gene synthesizes fibrocystin, which gives the kidney its structure. Cysts in ARPKD arise from the distal tubules and collecting ducts. Patients experience high blood pressure, urinary tract infections, and frequent urination. The liver, spleen, and pancreas are usually affected, resulting in low blood cell counts, varicose veins, and hemorrhoids. The child is usually smaller in size than average.

Autosomal recessive PKD can be diagnosed by ultrasound imaging of the fetus or newborn, which will reveal cysts in the kidneys. However, this procedure does not distinguish between the cysts of autosomal recessive and autosomal dominant PKD. Performing ultrasound examinations of relatives can be helpful in making a diagnosis.

The noninherited type of cystic disease is ACKD. It develops in kidneys as a result of long-term damage and bad scarring and is associated with dialysis and end-stage renal disease (ESRD). About 90 percent of people who have been on dialysis for five years or more develop ACKD. People with ACKD may have underlying conditions such as glomerulonephritis or kidney disease associated with diabetes mellitus. The cysts of ACKD may bleed, and patients may develop renal cancer.

TREATMENT AND THERAPY

Polycystic kidney disease cannot be cured. The goals of the treatment are the reduction of symptoms and the prevention of complications. Patients often get started on medications for hypertension and eventually will need dialysis, as 50 percent of patients will reach ESRD by the age of sixty. The treatment of ADPKD is

---

INFORMATION ON POLYCYSTIC KIDNEY DISEASE

Causes: Genetic defect; long-term kidney damage associated with dialysis, end-stage renal disease

Symptoms: Cysts in kidneys, kidney enlargement, high blood pressure; may include pain in back and side, headaches, blood in urine, urinary tract infections, brain aneurysms, cysts in liver and pancreas, nail abnormalities, painful menstruation, varicose veins, hemorrhoids, joint pain, drowsiness, anemia

Duration: Progressive, usually fatal without treatment

Treatments: Alleviation of symptoms and prevention of complications; may include analgesics (aspirin, acetaminophen), antibiotics, iron supplements, blood transfusions, cyst drainage, dialysis, kidney transplantation

---

to manage the symptoms that arise from the condition. Analgesics such as aspirin or acetaminophen (Tylenol) are used to treat the pain. If severe headaches occur, however, then an aneurysm may be involved. Therefore, the patient should see a physician before using over-the-counter medications. For ADPKD, lifestyle management and interventions to enhance hydration, limit sodium and protein intake, as well as an intense treatment for hypertension have proven to have an effect on the course of the disease. Treatments that target the cyst formation in ADPKD also are now available. Vasopressin has been linked to the progression of ADPDK and CKD in general, and increased amounts are an aspect of this illness. Pharmaceutical treatments such as Tolvaptan (a vasopressin receptor 2 antagonist) have shown a slowed rate of cyst growth and glomerular filtration rate (GFR) decline in patients with ADPKD. Other treatments for the reduction of cyst growth have also been explored, such as Pravastatin, and are currently undergoing randomized clinical trials to prove efficacy.

Antibiotics are given to treat urinary tract infections, and high blood pressure is treated with proper diet, exercise, and medications as prescribed by a physician. Any symptoms of anemia are treated with iron supplements or blood transfusions.

Surgical drainage of cysts may be indicated because of pain, bleeding, infection, or obstruction. Because of the large number of cysts, surgery to remove them is not deemed proper. Patients with ADPKD can suffer from chronic pain, which is challenging to manage and is usually targeted with a multidisciplinary approach, utilizing medications, renal denervation procedures and physical therapy. Eventually, the kidney may fail as a result of tissue destruction by the cysts, and dialysis and kidney transplantation become the only methods of treatment.

PERSPECTIVE AND PROSPECTS

The first recorded case of polycystic kidney disease dates back to Stefan Bathory, the king of Poland who lived from 1533 to 1588. In the mid-1980s, the Polycystic Kidney Disease Foundation was formed.

Through extensive genetic research, a better understanding of PKD has been gained. In 1985, the first gene associated with autosomal dominant PKD was located on chromosome 16; in 1993, another was located on chromosome 4. Within three years, scientists isolated the proteins produced by these two genes, polycystin 1 and polycystin 2. Since then, scientists have identified the autosomal recessive PKD gene on chromosome 6.

Researchers are using mice bred with this genetic disease in an attempt to find a cure. In 2000, they reported that a cancer drug was successful in inhibiting cyst formation in mice with the PKD gene. The hope is that further testing will lead to safe and effective treatments for humans. Tolvaptan, the first drug designed specifically for the treatment of ADPKD, has proven efficacious. Other treatments, which impact cystogenic properties of PKD, are also being researched, and target deficiency of PC1. Treatments for ARPKD have seen little progress but there is hope that some of the treatments utilized in ADPKD may be effective in ARPKD.

—Fady Gendy, OMS-III

See also: Cyst removal; Cysts; End-stage renal disease; Genetic diseases; Kidney cancer; Kidney disorders; Kidneys; Nephrectomy; Nephritis; Nephrology; Nephrology, pediatric; Pyelonephritis; Renal failure.

For Further Information:
Bergmann, C., L. M. Guay-Woodford, P. C. Harris, et al. "Polycystic Kidney Disease." Nature Reviews Disease Primers, vol. 4, no. 1, Dec. 2018, p. 50, doi:10.1038/s41572-018-0047-y. PMID: 30523303; PMCID: PMC6592047.
Greenberg, Arthur, et al., editors. *Primer on Kidney Diseases*. 5th ed., Saunders/Elsevier, 2009.
Kellicker, Patricia Griffin. "Polycystic Kidney Disease." *Health Library*, 31 Oct. 2012.
MedlinePlus. "Kidney Cysts." *MedlinePlus*, 20 May 2013.
National Institute of Diabetes and Digestive and Kidney Diseases, National Institutes of Health. "Polycystic Kidney Disease." *National Kidney and Urologic Diseases Information Clearing House*, 2 Sept. 2010.
National Kidney Foundation. *National Kidney Foundation*, 2013.
Parker, James N., and Philip M. Parker, editors. *The Official Patient's Sourcebook on Polycystic Kidney Disease*. Icon Health, 2002.
Schrier, Robert W., editor. *Diseases of the Kidney and Urinary Tract*. 8th ed., Wolters Kluwer Health/Lippincott Williams & Wilkins, 2007.
Watson, Michael L., and Vicente E. Torres, editors. *Polycystic Kidney Disease*. Oxford UP, 1996.

POLYCYSTIC OVARY SYNDROME

Category: Disease/Disorder
Anatomy or system affected: Endocrine system, pancreas, reproductive system, skin
Specialties and related fields: Dermatology, endocrinology, family medicine, gynecology, nursing, nutrition, obstetrics, pathology, pediatrics, pharmacology, preventive medicine, psychology, public health
Definition: Polycystic ovary syndrome (PCOS) is a complex disorder that is related to multiple ovarian cysts that contribute to endocrinologic abnormalities including hyperandrogenism, and ovulation dysfunction resulting in fertility difficulties. There must be one or more sign or symptom in addition to polycystic ovaries in order to make the diagnosis. PCOS is related to obesity and diabetes and poses an increased risk for cardiovascular disease. In addition to these conditions, symptoms of hyperandrogenism including hirsutism or acne may be accompanied by depression or anxiety.
Key terms:
biguanide: a type of medication to lower blood glucose by increasing sensitivity to insulin and possibly lowering the liver's glucose production
gonadotropin: hormone secreted by the pituitary gland; the primary gonadotropic hormones are luteinizing hormone (LH) and follicle-stimulating hormone (FSH)
hirsutism: excess facial hair
hyperandrogenism: higher-than-normal levels of androgens in the blood

CAUSES AND SYMPTOMS

Patients with Polycystic ovary syndrome (PCOS) presents with menstrual abnormalities including amenorrhea, menorrhagia, oligomenorrhea, and infertility. PCOS seems to be caused by a combination of genetics and environmental factors, although its etiology remains unknown. There is no recommended genetic screening test for PCOS currently. First-degree relatives of someone with PCOS are at higher risk of developing the condition themselves. Exposure to androgens may play a role, although this exposure may occur anywhere from the prenatal period through puberty.

Hyperinsulinemia contributes to higher levels of hyperandrogenism both directly and indirectly. Directly, insulin may stimulate the production of androgens from the ovary. Indirectly, insulin may inhibit sex-hormone binding globulins and therefore increase the number of androgens circulating in the blood. Signs of insulin resistance include hypertension, obesity, and acanthosis nigricans. Patients present with additional dermatologic conditions including acne, hirsutism, androgenic alopecia as a result of hyperandrogenism. Hyperandrogenism may be evaluated through laboratory tests including serum testosterone levels, sex-hormone binding globulin levels, and other androgen levels. Obesity is a comorbidity that is associated with hyperinsulinemia and may amplify the effects of PCOS. However, there are approximately 20 percent of patients with PCOS whom are not obese.

The Rotterdam Criteria for diagnosing PCOS includes the appearance of ovaries via ultrasound. Ovary volume greater than 10 cubic centimeters or an ovary with twelve or more follicles that are 2 to 9 mm in diameter are included in the diagnostic criteria of PCOS. There must be one or more symptoms in the diagnosis of PCOS, such that solely having polycystic ovaries is not definitive of this syndrome as it is a nonspecific finding if there are no other endocrinologic nor metabolic abnormalities. Hyperandrogenism or ovulatory abnormalities are necessary diagnostic factors for PCOS.

TREATMENT AND THERAPY
Treatment is largely symptom-based and empirical. The main goal of treatment and therapy is to normalize menstrual cycles and ovulation and, if desired, achieve a successful pregnancy. PCOS has the potential to cause substantial metabolic sequelae including an increased risk of diabetes and cardiovascular disease The least-invasive approach to achieving this goal is weight loss in those who are overweight. Weight loss of 5 to 10 percent has been shown to have a positive impact on symptoms of PCOS—hirsutism, infertility, and menstrual irregularities as well as hyperinsulinemia. This goal can be achieved by a reduction in caloric intake and increased physical activity, although it is difficult to maintain.

Although weight loss is helpful, it may not alleviate all symptoms of PCOS in overweight females. Medications that improve peripheral insulin levels and sensitivity include Biguanides (Metformin) and Thiazolidinediones (Pioglitazone, Rosiglitazone). Biguanides tend to cause weight loss usually and Thiazolidinediones may cause weight gain. Metformin can delay the development of diabetes in high-risk populations (those with impaired glucose tolerance). Birth control medications will help to regulate menses if the woman is not trying to conceive. However, they

> **INFORMATION ON POLYCYSTIC OVARY SYNDROME**
>
> **Causes:** Environment and genetic risk factors not yet well defined
> **Symptoms:** Hirsutism, hyperandrogenism, hyperinsulinemia, obesity, infertility, irregular menses
> **Duration:** Chronic
> **Treatments:** Diet for weight loss; medications, surgery

may also result in weight gain and insulin resistance, which would be a negative effect for the PCOS treatment overall. Combination low-dose hormonal contraceptives are most frequently used for long-term management and are recommended as the primary treatment of menstrual disorders. Letrozole is associated with increased ovulation, clinical pregnancy rates, and live-birth rates compared with Clomiphene citrate, which is a selective-estrogen receptor modulator (SERM). Letrozole, however, is not US Food and Drug Administration (FDA)-approved for PCOS. Clomiphene citrate has shown pregnancies to occur within the first six ovulatory cycles.

Dexamethasone as adjunctive therapy with Clomiphene citrate has been shown to increase ovulation and pregnancy rates in Clomiphene citrate-resistant women with PCOS. Both Clomiphene citrate and Letrozole are associated with a comparable risk of twin gestation and these rates may be even higher in women with PCOS undergoing ovulation induction. If Clomiphene citrate fails, then patients may try exogenous gonadotropins. Gonadotropins are frequently used to induce ovulation in women with PCOS. Low-dose therapy offers a higher rate of ovulation and monofollicular development, with a significantly lower risk of ovarian hyperstimulation syndrome. Laparoscopic ovarian surgery or in vitro fertilization are more invasive approaches to treatment of PCOS for fertility.

PERSPECTIVE AND PROSPECTS
Polycystic ovary syndrome was first discovered in 1935 by Dr. Irving Stein and Dr. Michael Leventhal initially yielding the name Stein-Leventhal syndrome. This disease has been prevalent in women of child-bearing age and has been associated with increased risk of developing type II diabetes and cardiovascular risk in the future. Many treatment modalities targeting the different aspects of afflicted organ systems have been developed throughout the years. Treatments sought have largely been for infertility but have been increasing to include coverage of multiple organ systems with targeting insulin resistance. Despite the amazing medical advancements in medications and procedural

techniques for treatment of polycystic ovary syndrome, the least invasive approach remains superior which is improvement in weight through caloric diet restrictions and exercise regimens..

—*Nicholas Schenk MD and Bita-Batul Khatibshahidi, MD*

See also: Cyst removal; Cysts; Diabetes mellitus; Genital disorders, female; Gynecology; Hormones; Hysterectomy; Infertility, female; Menopause; Menstruation; Obesity; Ovarian cysts; Ovaries; Pregnancy and gestation; Premenstrual syndrome (PMS); Puberty and adolescence; Reproductive system; Uterus.

For Further Information:
"Polycystic Ovary Syndrome." *ACOG*, www.acog.org/clinical/clinical-guidance/practice-bulletin/articles/2018/06/polycystic-ovary-syndrome.
"Polycystic Ovary Syndrome." *Polycystic Ovary Syndrome*. Office on Women's Health, www.womenshealth.gov/a-z-topics/polycystic-ovary-syndrome.
"Polycystic Ovary Syndrome (PCOS)." *Mayo Clinic*. Mayo Foundation for Medical Education and Research, 3 Oct. 2020, www.mayoclinic.org/diseases-conditions/pcos/symptoms-causes/syc-20353439.

POLYDACTYLY AND SYNDACTYLY

Category: Disease/Disorder
Also known as: Supernumerary digits, extra digits, poly- dactylia, polydactylism, hyperdactyly, syndactylia, syn- dactylism
Anatomy or system affected: Blood vessels, bones, feet, hands, skin
Specialties and related fields: General surgery, genetics, pediatrics, podiatry
Definition: Polydactyly is the presence of extra fingers or toes, while syndactyly describes two or more fingers or toes that are joined or fused together.
Key terms:
central or mesoaxial polydactyly: a complex form in which extra digits occur between the thumb and little finger or big toe and little toe
congenital: referring to a condition present at birth
digit: a finger or toe
postaxial polydactyly: an extra digit occurring near the little finger or little toe
preaxial polydactyly: an extra digit occurring near the thumb or big toe

CAUSES AND SYMPTOMS
Neither polydactyly nor syndactyly are serious congenital deformities, and they generally occur with no underlying or apparent cause. Both conditions may be genetic or inherited or may occur as a symptom of

Partial simple syndactyly in 2nd and 3rd toes. Photo by pschemp, via Wikimedia Commons.

more than one hundred different inherited and developmental disorders. Sometimes there is not enough information to determine the cause, while other cases may be due to exposure during pregnancy to toxins such as cigarette smoking or the drug thalidomide or to poorly controlled diabetes during pregnancy. The hereditary aspects of the conditions are still being studied.

Polydactyly can vary from a poorly developed digit that is almost unnoticeable and without bone to a fully developed and functional digit. The condition occurs during fetal development when normal programmed cell death between digits fails to occur. In inherited cases, the genes responsible for the condition are dominant, which means that male and female children are equally likely to have the condition. Postaxial polydactyly is the most frequent form and accounts for about 75 to 80 percent of all cases. This type occurs in approximately one of every one thousand Caucasian births. African Americans are ten times more likely than any other ethnic group to have this type of polydactyly in the hand. One-half of polydactyly cases are bilateral, affecting both sides of the body, with the remainder of the cases affecting the left side almost twice as often as the right. Postaxial polydactyly is most often found in the hands and rarely found in both the hands and feet. People of Asian ancestry tend to have more occurrences of preaxial polydactyly, while central polydactyly is uncommon across all ethnic groups. All three types of polydactyly are believed to be inherited differently, although people in the same family may have different degrees of the condition.

In syndactyly, one or more digits fail to separate during fetal development. Syndactyly is one of the most common congenital malformations and occurs in about one of every 2,000 to 2,500 births. It is more common in males and Caucasians and usually affects the middle and ring fingers. In the toes, the condition

---

> ### INFORMATION ON POLYDACTYLY AND SYNDACTYLY
>
> **Causes:** Genetic or inherited; may occur as symptom of more than one hundred different inherited and developmental disorders
> **Symptoms:** In polydactyly, extra digit(s) varying from poorly developed without bone to fully developed and functional; in syndactyly, fusion of one or more digits
> **Duration:** Lifelong unless corrected
> **Treatments:** Surgery to remove extra digits or separate fused ones

most commonly affects the second and third toes. Incidents of syndactyly affect the left and right sides and the hands and feet equally and are usually bilateral. Syndactyly is described as either simple, in which the digits are fused by skin and soft tissue, or complex, in which the bones are also fused. The severity can range from incomplete webbing of the skin to sharing of the bones, nails, nerves, and blood vessels. Complicated syndactyly describes the addition of extra bones and unusual tendon or ligament development. Partial or incomplete syndactyly means that only part of the length of the digits are fused together. Complete syndactyly means that the entire length of the digits are fused together.

TREATMENT AND THERAPY

In most cases, polydactyly and syndactyly do not interfere with normal hand or foot function, and correction is done for cosmetic purposes. The conditions can be diagnosed at birth or by fetal ultrasound (sonogram). Once the condition is observed, physicians will normally require x-rays to determine its complexity.

In type A polydactyly, where the fully formed digit has bones, surgery is required when the baby is about a year old. In type B polydactyly, the digit is rudimentary, contains no bones, and is usually removed before the infant leaves the hospital. Many people are unaware that they ever had polydactyly. Central polydactyly is more complex, may affect normal hand or foot function, and often requires multiple surgeries.

Multiple surgeries may be needed to separate the digits in complex or complicated cases of syndactyly, and the procedures are usually performed when the child is between six months and eighteen months old. Skin grafts are typically taken from the lower abdomen to cover the newly separated digits. If multiple digits are involved, then more than one surgery may be needed as only one digit is separated at a time. Some children also experience recurrent syndactyly,

or "web creep," if there are complications in healing. In the feet, simple syndactyly is a cosmetic problem that is generally not treated unless surgery is desired.

PERSPECTIVE AND PROSPECTS

Polydactyly and syndactyly have existed throughout history, and polydactyly is mentioned in the Bible in a description of a member of Goliath's family (2 Samuel 21:20). Italian painter Raphael (1483-1520) depicted polydactyly in at least six of his works, including *The Marriage of the Virgin* (1504) and *La Belle Jardiniere* (1507). The examination of polydactyly through several generations of a Berlin family by French mathematician, biologist, and astronomer Pierre-Louis Moreau de Maupertuis (1698-1759) is considered the first scientific analysis of a dominant inherited trait in humans.

Some famous polydactyls include King Charles VIII of France, Prime Minister Winston Churchill of England, Major League Baseball pitcher Antonio Alfonseca, Bollywood actor Hrithik Roshan, actress Gemma Arterton, jazz pianist Hampton Halls, blues guitarist Hound Dog Taylor, Roman era poet Volcatius Sedigitus, and possibly Anne Boleyn, one of Henry VIII's wives. A few famous syndactyls are Soviet leader Joseph Stalin; actors Ashton Kutcher, Dan Aykroyd, and Tricia Hefler; singer Rachel Stevens; and writers Rob Never and Mike Holderness. There is also some speculation that painter and inventor Leonardo da Vinci had syndactyly on his left hand.

—*Virginia L. Salmon*

See also Birth defects; Congenital disorders; Embryology; Genetic diseases; Lower extremities; Plastic surgery; Teratogens; Thalidomide; Upper extremities.

For Further Information:
Blereau, Robert P. "Polydactyly." *Consultant* 39, no. 12 (December, 1999): 3297.
Flatt, Adrian E. "Webbed Fingers." *Baylor University Medical Center Proceedings* 18 (January, 2005): 26.
Goldenring, John. "Webbing of the Fingers or Toes." *MedlinePlus*, December 1, 2011.
"True Polydactyly." *Consultant* 43, no. 10 (September 1, 2003): 1309.
Kaneshiro, Neil. "Polydactyly." *MedlinePlus*, November 7, 2011.
Vorvick, Linda J. "Repair of Webbed Fingers or Toes." *MedlinePlus*, August 11, 2012.
Wynbrandt, James, and Mark D. Ludman. "Polydactyly." In *The Encyclopedia of Genetic Disorders and Birth Defects*. 2d ed. New York: Facts On File, 2000.

POLYP REMOVAL. SEE COLORECTAL POLYP REMOVAL; NASAL POLYP REMOVAL.

POLYMYALGIA RHEUMATICA

Category: Disease/Disorder
Anatomy or system affected: Joints, immune system
Specialties and related fields: Rheumatology, internal medicine, gerontology
Definition: An inflammatory disorder of the joints and connective tissues of the shoulders, neck, and hips.
Key terms:

inflammation: the body's natural defense against an insult; characterized by heat, redness, swelling and pain to the area

steroids: an organic compound used as a treatment for treating inflammation

giant cell arteritis: a disease characterized by the inflammation of the arteries and veins that supply the head, neck and arms; it can cause headaches, jaw-pain and changes in vision

joints: a point where two or more bones join together

CAUSES AND SYMPTOMS

Polymyalgia rheumatica (PMR) is an inflammatory disorder of the joints and connective tissues of the shoulders, neck, and hips. The cause is unknown. The stiffness is typically worse in the morning, and PRM affects primarily older adults aged 50 and over. PMR can be associated with Giant Cell Arteritis (GCA); 15-30 percent of patients who have PMR will also have GCA. It is believed that they share some of the same disease processes, although the correlation is poorly understood. GCA is associated with cardiovascular events and should be treated promptly and seriously.

PMR is characterized by pain and stiffness in the shoulders, neck, and hip. The pain is worse in the mornings and with movement and is symmetric. Doing regular activities may be painful and/or challenging such as putting a shirt over one's head, or rolling over in bed in the morning. Pain is usually isolated to the joint and there may be joint swelling or point-tenderness. Muscle pain is usually not a common site of PMR. Overall constitutional symptoms may include fatigue, malaise, depression, and weight loss/gain. High fevers are uncommon, but point more to GCA than PMR.

Diagnosis is through evaluation of one's symptoms and some basic blood tests. The most common tests to check for PMR are called erythrocyte sedimentation rate (ESR) and C-reactive protein (CRP) tests. Both of these are markers for inflammation in the body. They are not specific to PMR, but can help paint the overall clinical picture.

TREATMENT AND THERAPY

Because PMR is an inflammatory disorder, the medications we use to treat PMR are an anti-inflammatory medicine called steroids. The optimal dose of steroids is tailored to each individual, but the goal is to give symptomatic relief on the lowest effective dose possible. Often, treatment for PMR must last several months. Patients often experience relief within the first few days of treatment.

Steroids are very effective, but also have several side effects that must be monitored closely. Of note, is the increased risk of osteoporosis with long-term use. For this reason, clinicians may advise patients to get routine screening for osteoporosis and take supplemental calcium and vitamin D to increase bone strength and decrease the risk of osteoporosis from steroid use. In addition, high blood pressure and diabetes are also associated with long-term steroid use and patients should be screened for these regularly.

Over-the-counter medications for pain such as ibuprofen and acetaminophen are not found to be effective in treating PMR.

PROGNOSIS

PMR usually resolves spontaneously within months, but sometimes can last years. In these cases, side effects from the steroids need to be monitored closely. In addition, signs and symptoms of GCA such as headache, jaw pain, problems with vision, and fever should be evaluated regularly.

—*Maki Matsumura*

See also C-reactive protein, Erythrocyte sedimentation rate, Gerontology, Giant cell arteritis, Headache, Osteoarthritis, Pain, Rheumatoid arthritis, Rheumatology, Steroids

For Further Information:
Docken, W. *Polymyalgia Rheumatica*. Retrieved from www.rheumatology.org/Practice/Clinical/Patients/Diseases_And_Conditions/Polymyalgia_ Rheumatica.
Hunder, G. "Clinical Manifestations and Diagnosis of Polymyalgia Rheumatica." *UpToDate*, edited by J.H. Stone and P.L. Romain. Retrieved from www.upto date.com/contents/clinical-manifestations-and-diagnosis-of-polymyalgia-rheumatica? detectedLanguage=en&source=search_result&search=polymy algiarheumatica&selected Title=1~73& provider=noProvider.
Hunder, G. "Treatment of Polymyalgia Rheumatica." *UpToDate*, edited by UpToDate, edited by J.H. Stone and P.L. Romain. Retrieved from www.uptodate.com/contents/treatment-of-polymyalgia-rheumatica? detectedLanguage=en&source=search_result&search=polymyalgiarheumati ca& selectedTitle=2~73&provider=noProvider.
Rovensky, Jozef, Burkhard F. Leeb, Howard Bird, Viera Stvrtinova, and Richard Imrich, eds. *Polymyalgia Rheumatica and Giant Cell Arteritis*. Germany: Springer-Verlag/Wein, 2010.

POLYMYOSITIS

Category: Disease/Disorder
Anatomy or system affected: Muscular system
Specialties and related fields: Rheumatology
Definition: Polymyositis is an idiopathic disease of muscle inflammation. Myositis is the general category for inflammatory muscles diseases such as juvenile myositis, dermatomyositis, inclusion body myositis, and polymyositis. Referred to as inflammatory myopathies, the muscle inflammation can cause damage to the muscles. Referred to as inflammatory myopathy, the muscle inflammation can cause damage to the muscles. Polymyositis is considered to be an autoimmune disease. It can occur in persons of all ages, but is most common in middle childhood and in the twenties. Polymyositis is more common among women and girls. There are twice the number of cases in women than in men and boys. When the inflammatory condition of polymyositis is seen on the skin as well, this is termed dermatomyositis. The disease does not manifest immediately; rather, there is a gradual process of weakness over a three- to six-month period. Typically, there are remissions and exacerbations.

Key terms:

autoimmune: An autoimmune condition that is caused by the person's immune system. In this situation the immune system has failed to delete the T cells that are not recognizing "self" versus "non-self"

dysphagia: having difficulty swallowing due to muscle weakness

prognosis: the estimated good life or survival time as assessed by your physician

CAUSES AND SYMPTOMS

The main feature of polymyositis is the inflammation and the damage to the muscles that ensues. The person with polymyositis has white blood cells in the affected muscles. The inflamed muscles, caused by the disease, tend to release enzymes into the bloodstream. So, lab tests of the blood will demonstrate high levels of muscle enzymes. The muscles close to the trunk or torso are the main muscles affected. Usually there is symmetrical muscle weakness. Both the lungs and the heart can be affected by this condition. Problems in the lungs can cause dysphagia, shortness of breath, and infection. Heart problems are a little less common and can be a bad sign.

The primary symptom is the debilitating weakness, although it usually does not cause pain. There is a possibility that muscles of the body further away from the trunk can also become affected by the disease; if this occurs, it may only happen when there is a disease progression.

The disease may not be easily identified at first. Joint pain or weakness may be experienced as a general feeling of fatigue and exhaustion. Rising off a chair may be challenging as is the movement of raising one's arms to perform a simple action. Climbing stairs or lifting objects may feel extremely difficult or impossible. Likewise, when lying down, a person may find it difficult to get up. The weakness is felt in the torso or core area. Muscles of the hips, thighs, and shoulders are usually affected. Sometimes muscles may ache, and the body may be sensitive to touch. Dysphagia may occur, with the person finding it difficult to swallow. Further symptoms may include fever and weight loss. A skin irritation may be seen, such as a rash around the eyes (red or violet), on the knuckle area of the hand, on elbows, knees, neck, and chest. Some researchers think that polymyositis may be inherited. It appears that if a patient's family members have had neuromuscular problems, that the polymyositis may be inherited. It is also thought that it may be caused by a virus, such as cytomegalovirus.

TREATMENTS AND THERAPY

The polymyositis diagnosis is verified by a series of tests. Following a full physical examination by a doctor, the patient will be sent for blood tests. Further testing may be conducted to ascertain the state of the nerves and muscles. The most critical tests are EMG (electromyography) and an MRI (magnetic resonance imaging) of the muscles affected, and a muscle biopsy. The blood test may demonstrate a high level of muscle enzymes, a CPK, and liver enzymes. Further testing may be conducted to ascertain the state of the nerves and muscles. There is also the theory that the person may have another autoimmune disease with similar symptoms.

Medications for polymyositis may comprise a number of prescriptions. The primary medication consists of immune system suppressants. Corticosteroids are typically prescribed, particularly as the first option to treat the illness. Their effectiveness relates to the ability to reduce muscle inflammation. When corticosteroids are not found to improve the condition, specialists may prescribe immunosuppressive medications. Medicines of this type include methotrexate, azathioprine, cyclosporine, tacrolimus, chlorambucil, mycophenolate, cyclophosphamide, and rituximab. If the symptoms are particularly debilitating the physician may put the patient on an infusion of immunoglobulins (IVIG).

Because of the muscular effects of the disease, doctors usually recommend a course of physical therapy to accompany medical treatment.

PERSPECTIVE AND PROSPECTS

The cause of polymyositis remains elusive despite constant research. There is a possibility that hereditary factors may be responsible for polymyositis. As research continues and develops more insight into the immune system and related diseases. The hope is that understanding of the immune system and its functioning will facilitate deeper knowledge, and disease causes. There is a good prognosis for people who develop the disease in its early stages. Current research has revealed so far that immune system cells appear to invade muscle tissue at the onset of the disease, continuing to attack the muscles and causing damage. There is a good prognosis for people who develop the disease in its early stages. Possibilities of the disease becoming inactive happen often. In these instances, the process of rehabilitating the muscles can occur with beneficial results. Exercises to prevent the wasting away of unused muscles will be implemented with the aim of strengthening the affected and surrounding muscles.

Following are some organizations related to Polymyositis. In the United States, there are a number of organizations or associations providing information or support regarding muscle diseases such as polymyositis. These include: Muscular Dystrophy Association, National Institute of Arthritis and Musculoskeletal and Skin Diseases (NIAMS), Information Clearinghouse, National Institutes of Health, Myositis Association, and National Organization for Rare Disorders. Concerned patients or members of the public are always advised to consult with their doctors in addition to seeking medical information via public resources. Personal medical history is taken into account by a person's private doctor, physician, or specialist.

—*Leah Jacob, MA;*
updated by Christine M. Carroll, RN, BSN, MBA

For Further Information:
"Polymyositis and Dermatomyositis." *ArthritisResearch UK*, Arthritis Research UK, 2016. Web. 1 May 2016.
"Polymyositis." *Cleveland Clinic*, The Cleveland Clinic Foundation, 2015. Web. 1 May 2016.
"Polymyositis." *The Johns Hopkins Myositis Center*, Johns Hopkins Medicine, 2016. Web. 1 May 2016.
"Polymyositis (PM)." *MDA For Strength, Independence& Life*, Muscular Dystrophy Association, Inc., 2016. Web. 1 May 2016.
"NINDS Polymyositis Information Page." *National Institute of NeurologicalDisorders and Stroke*, National Institute of Neurological Disorders and Stroke, 2015. Web. 1 May 2016.
"Polymyositis-Adult." *The New York Times Health Guide*, 22 March 2013. Web. 1 May 2016.
"Polymyositis-Adult." *MedlinePlus*, U.S. National Library of Medicine, 26 April 2016. Web. 1 May 2016.
"Polymyositis." *Victoria State Government. Better Health Channel*, State Government of Victoria, Australia, 2016. Web. 1 May 2016.
MedicineNet. (2017) Polymyositis and Dermatomyositis Symptoms and Diagnosis. Retrieved on September 10, 2017 from medicinenet.com/polymyositis/article.htm
Pappu, Ramesh,MD, DPH. MBBS: Chief Editor. (22 November 2016) Polymyositis Clinical Presentation. Retrieved on September 10, 2017 from emedicine.medscape.com/article/ 335925-clinical

POLYPS

Category: Disease/Disorder
Anatomy or system affected: Abdomen, anus, bladder, gallbladder, gastrointestinal system, intestines, kidneys, nose, reproductive system, stomach, throat, urinary system, uterus
Specialties and related fields: Family medicine, gastroenterology, general surgery, genetics, gynecology, internal medicine, nephrology, otorhinolaryngology, proctology, pulmonary medicine, urology
Definition: Abnormal growths arising from mucous membranes anywhere in the body. A polyp is considered pedunculated if it is attached to the mucous membrane by a narrow, long stalk of tissue; if no stalk is present, then the polyp is said to be sessile.
Key terms:
colonoscopy: an endoscopic procedure used for visualization of the intestine
endoscopy: procedure with a flexible tube that allows direct viewing inside the body
inherited disorder: a disorder caused by an alteration of a gene and passed through families

CAUSES AND SYMPTOMS

The cause of polyps varies with the location of the polyp growth in the body. Symptoms are also site dependent.

Nasal polyps consist of inflamed tissue in the mucous membrane lining of the nose or sinuses. Causes of nasal polyps may be allergies, chronic infection, cystic fibrosis, and asthma. They usually develop around the ethnoid sinuses (inside the top of the nose) and may block the airway, resulting in difficulty breathing or shortness of breath because of obstruction. Breathing through the mouth, loss of the sense of smell, and a runny nose are common symptoms.

Vocal cord polyps are caused by mechanical injury such as shouting and usually occur on one vocal cord. Vocal cord nodules are not to be confused with polyps and are generally caused by chronic abuse such as singing. Symptoms include hoarseness and a breathy or raspy voice.

Stomach polyps are rare and are usually discovered by accident-for example, during an upper gastrointestinal endoscopy (a viewing of the interior of the stomach). Causes include *Helicobacter pylori* (*H. pylori*) bacteria or chronic gastritis (inflammation of the stomach) caused by an autoimmune response. Stomach polyps usually do not cause symptoms, but if symptoms occur they may include nausea, vomiting, abdominal pain, bleeding, or a feeling of fullness when eating even small amounts.

Colorectal polyps grow on the lining (mucous membrane) of the colon (also known as the large intestine) or rectum and may be caused by abnormal cell growth, heredity (family history or inherited disorder), or inflammatory diseases such as ulcerative colitis or Crohn's disease. Small polyps do not usually cause symptoms. If symptoms do occur, then they may include blood in a bowel movement, rectal bleeding, fatigue due to anemia from loss of blood, and pain.

Uterine polyps develop in the lining of the uterus and are caused by an overgrowth of endometrial cells. Occasionally, uterine polyps may slip through the cervix into the vagina, resulting in cervical polyps. The exact cause of uterine and cervical polyps is unknown, but may be related to the estrogen hormone level, chronic inflammation or clogged blood vessels in the cervix. Symptoms may include bleeding, heavy or irregular menstrual periods, a white or yellow discharge of mucus (leukorrhea), or there may be no symptoms.

TREATMENT AND THERAPY

The treatment for polyps varies by site. Medications, removal during colonoscopy (intestines), colposcopy (vagina and cervix) or other endoscopic procedures (throat, stomach, small bowel), and surgical removal are used. Biopsy of the polyp may also be done to determine if it is malignant (cancerous) or benign (not cancerous).

It is possible to prevent some polyps. Controlling allergies and managing chronic sinusitis may prevent nasal polyps. Vocal cord polyps are directly related to injury from yelling such as at a sporting event, so less abuse may lessen the potential for development. Stomach polyps caused by *H. pylori* may be controlled by treating the underlying bacteria and controlling gastritis may diminish the occurrence.

The goal of treatment for nasal polyps is to reduce the size of the polyp or to remove it. Because nasal polyps may occur in response to allergies or chronic sinusitis, medications such as corticosteroids (a drug that reduces inflammation), antihistamines, and antibiotics (a drug to fight infection) may be effective in shrinking the size of the polyp. If the polyp is in the sinus cavity, then endoscopic surgery using a small cam-

---

INFORMATION ON POLYPS

Causes: Varies with location; chronic allergies, hereditary factors, hormone levels, mechanical (overuse of vocal cords), uncontrolled cell growth from unknown causes

Symptoms: Varies with location; may include difficulty breathing, hoarseness, bleeding, pain, swelling

Duration: Until removed or minimized

Treatments: Medications, surgery

---

era and tube inserted into the sinus allows the physician to remove the polyp.

Vocal cord polyps usually require surgical removal to restore the normal speaking voice. Voice therapy with a speech pathologist may be needed to prevent future occurrences. Stomach polyps require biopsy and, if there is concern, surgical removal. Medications to treat gastritis, including antibiotics, may be used. Routine colonoscopy and flexible sigmoidoscopy are recommended for routine cancer screening, and if a colorectal polyp is seen during the procedure, it is removed. If colorectal polyps are causing symptoms, then surgical removal either through colonoscopy or removal of a portion of the intestine may be needed. Uterine polyps may be watched, medications may be used to shrink them, or surgery may be used to remove them; if the polyps are cancerous, then a hysterectomy (removal of the uterus) is usually necessary.

PERSPECTIVE AND PROSPECTS

Polyps are usually benign (not cancerous), but they can become malignant (cancerous) over time or in certain areas. Risk factors include age, obesity, family history, poor overall health (including allergies and chronic infections), stomach ulcer, infection, and inherited disorders such as cystic fibrosis or familial adenomatous polyposis. Prevention and screening, routine visits to the physician for health maintenance, and good health behaviors are important to prevent, recognize, or manage polyps. Prompt treatment is indicated if polyps cause symptoms or if a biopsy demonstrates malignant cells. Research is continuing on the causes of polyps and the influences that turn polyps from benign to malignant.

—*Patricia Stanfill Edens, PhD, RN, FACHE*

See also Allergies; Colon; Colonoscopy and sigmoidoscopy; Colorectal cancer; Colorectal polyp removal; Colorectal surgery; Electrocauterization; Endoscopy; Gastroenterology; Gastrointestinal system; Intestinal disorders; Intestines; Nasal polyp removal; Nasopharyngeal disorders; Oncology; Otorhinolaryngology; Proctology; Rectum; Screening; Sense organs; Sinusitis; Smell; Uterus; Voice and vocal cord disorders.

For Further Information:

Bremmer, Hermann, et al. "Colorectal Cancers Occurring after Colonoscopy with Polyp Detection: Sites of Polyps and Sites of Cancers." *International Journal of Cancer* 133, no. 7 (October, 2013): 1672-1679.

Church, James M. "Laparoscopic versus Colonoscopic Removal of a Large Polyp." *American Journal of Gastroenterology* 104, no. 10 (October, 2009): 2633-2634.

Hellings, Peter W., and Hens Greet. "Rhinosinusitis and the Lower Airways." *Immunology and Allergy Clinics of North America* 29, no. 4 (November, 2009): 733-740.

Huber, Aaron R., and James F. Shikle. "Benign Fibroblastic Polyps of the Colon." *Archives of Pathology and Laboratory Medicine* 133, no. 11 (November, 2009): 1872-1876.

Lev, Robert, et al. *Adenomatous Polyps of the Colon: Pathobiological and Clinical Features.* New York: Springer-Verlag, 2012.

Maydeo, Amit, and Vinay Dhir. "The Gallbladder Polyp Conundrum: A Riddler on the Wall." *Gastrointestinal Endoscopy* 78, no. 3 (September, 2013): 494-495.

Thakkar, K., and D. S. Sihman, and M. A. Gilger. "Colorectal Polyps in Childhood." *Current Opinion in Pediatrics* 24, no. 5 (October, 2012): 632-637.

PORPHYRIA

Category: Disease/Disorder
Anatomy or system affected: Nervous system, skin
Specialties and related fields: Genetics, neurology, pediatrics
Definition: One of several rare genetic disorders caused by the accumulation of substances called porphyrins.

CAUSES AND SYMPTOMS

Porphyria refers to a group of diseases that share a common feature: a defect in the chain of chemical reactions that produce hemoglobin, the protein responsible for the transport of oxygen by the blood. These metabolic errors cause a buildup of porphyrins, resulting in two main types of illness: nervous system attacks and skin lesions.

There are two major groups of porphyrias: erythropoietic and hepatic. In erythropoietic porphyria, the porphyrins are synthesized in the bone marrow; in hepatic porphyrias, they are produced in the liver. Each of these porphyrias has several subtypes. For example, acute intermittent porphyria (AIP) is a hepatic porphyria most common in young adults and adults in early middle age. Its attacks are triggered by alcohol, certain drugs, and hormonal changes (such as those accompanying pregnancy). Some patients experience two to three episodes per year, while others may have as few as three in a lifetime.

INFORMATION ON PORPHYRIA

Causes: Genetic disorder; triggered by alcohol, drugs, sunlight
Symptoms: Nervous system attacks (mild mental confusion to delirium and hysteria), nausea, vomiting, reddish urine, prickling sensations in hands and feet, extreme photosensitivity of skin, skin lesions
Duration: Chronic with acute episodes
Treatments: Avoidance of triggering factors, protective clothing, drug therapy

---

Since all forms of porphyria are rare, a physician may not suspect the disease at first. The symptoms of porphyria include abdominal disturbances, nausea, vomiting, reddish urine, and prickling sensations in the hands and feet. The hallmarks that distinguish porphyrias, however, are the skin and nervous system effects. Except for AIP, all the porphyrias cause extreme photosensitivity of the skin because the porphyrins that are deposited in the skin are excited by the ultraviolet aspect of sunlight. This reaction results in skin lesions, which may lead to disfigurement. The neurological disturbances of porphyria range from mild mental confusion to delirium and hysteria. If a porphyria is suspected, urine, stool, and blood tests are done to detect the presence of porphyrins.

TREATMENT AND THERAPY

Avoiding triggering factors is primary in the control of porphyria attacks. Alcohol and drugs, which may cause an attack, should be stopped. Protective clothing should be worn to prevent the irritating effects of sunlight. For certain porphyrias, drugs are available to suppress the formation of porphyrins. In the case of AIP, a simple increase in the consumption of carbohydrates is enough to inhibit the production of porphyrin-forming substances. The treatment of porphyrias is largely aimed at relieving its symptoms.

—*Robert T. Klose, PhD*

See also Blood and blood disorders; Genetic diseases; Lesions; Metabolic disorders; Metabolism; Skin disorders.

For Further Information:

American Porphyria Foundation. www.porphyriafoundation.com.

Goldman, Lee, and Dennis Ausiello, eds. *Cecil Textbook of Medicine.* 23d ed. Philadelphia: Saunders/Elsevier, 2007.

Greer, John, et al., eds. *Wintrobe's Clinical Hematology.* 12th ed. Philadelphia: Wolters Kluwer/Lippincott Williams & Wilkins Health, 2009.

"Learning about Porphyria." *National Human Genome Research Institute*, April 18, 2013.

Parish, Kathy. "What's Wrong with This Patient?" *RN* 53, no. 7 (July, 1990): 43-45.

Parker, James N., and Philip M. Parker, eds. *The Official Patient's Sourcebook on Porphyria*. San Diego, Calif.: Icon Health, 2002.
"Porphyria." *Mayo Clinic*, May 7, 2011.
Rakel, Robert E., and Edward T. Bope, eds. *Conn's Current Therapy*. Philadelphia: Saunders/Elsevier, 2007.
Wood, Debra. "Porphyria." *Health Library*, November 26, 2012.

POSITRON EMISSION TOMOGRAPHY (PET) SCANNING

Category: Procedure
Anatomy or system affected: All
Specialties and related fields: Biotechnology, nuclear medicine, radiology
Definition: A noninvasive imaging procedure in which a positron-emitting radiopharmaceutical is administered and a three-dimensional image of an organ, which accumulates the radiopharmaceutical, is obtained by detecting the radiation resulting from positron annihilation.

Key terms:
annihilation: the process whereby an electron and positron combine and their energy is converted into two photons traveling in opposite directions
positrons: a type of radiation, similar to electrons but with a positive charge, emitted by radioactive atoms
tomography: a procedure that yields images of body sections

INDICATIONS AND PROCEDURES

Positron emission tomography (PET) scanning permits the noninvasive determination of biological function, metabolism, and pathology following the administration of short-lived positron-emitting radiopharmaceuticals (radioactive pharmaceuticals). Positron-emitting radiopharma- ceuticals are drugs that contain a radioactive atom that is transformed into a more stable atom by emitting a positron. A positron is a subatomic particle that has the same mass and charge as an electron, but the charge is positive rather than negative. When an energetic positron is emitted by a radioactive atom, it quickly loses its energy in the surrounding medium and comes to rest. The positron then combines with a free electron in the medium, the two particles are annihilated, and their energy is converted into two 511,000-volt-potential (511 keV) photons that travel in exactly opposite directions. The detection of these two photons in coincidence (simultaneously) by placing a ring of small radiation detectors around the patient is the basic principle used in PET scanning. The radiation detectors convert these light photons into electrical signals that are fed to a computer, which reconstructs the distribution of radioactivity in the desired organ and presents the information as an image on a video screen.

USES AND COMPLICATIONS

PET techniques are generally used to measure metabolic rates quantitatively in normal and abnormal tissues. The positron-emitting radionuclides oxygen-15, nitrogen-13, and carbon-11 are well suited for studying tissue metabolism because of their short physical half-lives and their ubiquitous presence in biomolecules. Oxygen-15 gas is useful for studying oxygen metabolism, whereas oxygen-15 water and oxygen-15 carbon monoxide are used to study blood flow and blood volume, respectively, in any organ. Fluorode- oxyglucose (FDG) labeled with fluorine-18 is another positron-emitting radiopharmaceutical that is useful in PET for the quantitative measurement of glucose metabolism. Glucose metabolism is high in brain tumors when compared to normal tissue. Hence, PET with fluorodeoxyglucose-18 is widely used in the detection of brain tumors and assessment of the degree of malignancy, since low-grade tumors are less metabolically active than high-grade tumors. Fluorodeoxyglucose-18 PET is also used to identify persistent tumors after surgery.

The radiopharmaceuticals carbon-11 aminoisobutyric acid, rubidium-82 chloride, and gallium-68 citrate are useful for studying the blood-brain barrier permeability. This modality is also being used increasingly in patients with seizure disorders, dementia, and movement disorders. The application of PET in these cases may provide previously unavailable information about these diseases to help the practicing neurologist. PET imaging is also being used to understand the mechanisms behind normal brain processes. Among the mechanisms studied are language processing, speech, vision, and brain development. Recent improvements in whole-body PET scanning technology are useful in clinical oncology. This technique is being employed widely in the qualitative imaging of primary or recurrent tumors, lymph nodes, and distant metastases.

PET is also being used with increasing frequency to measure myocardial perfusion (heart function). A number of different perfusion agents labeled with rubidium-82, gallium-62, oxygen-15, and nitrogen-13 are being investigated. Some of these agents are being used to measure not only relative perfusion but also the absolute blood flow in selected regions of the myocardium. Carbon-11 palmitate is employed to determine cardiac fatty acid metabolism. These radiopharmaceuticals are generally safe because they involve low doses of radiation with minimal risks.

PET Scanning Techniques

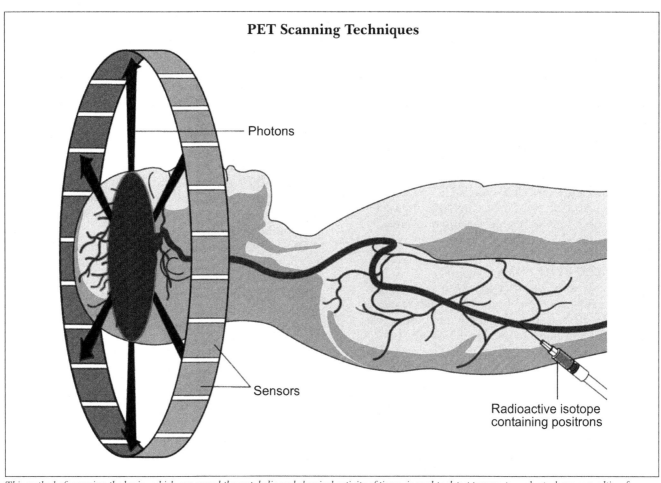

This method of scanning the brain, which can reveal the metabolic and chemical activity of tissue, is used to detect tumors, to evaluate damage resulting from strokes, and to diagnose and assess such conditions as Parkinson's disease, epilepsy, and certain mental illnesses. ©EBSCO

PERSPECTIVE AND PROSPECTS

The most desirable radionuclides used in PET procedures-carbon-11, nitrogen-13, oxygen-15, and fluorine-18-can be produced only with a cyclotron. Because of their very short physical half-lives, a dedicated cyclotron and fully automated equipment for radionuclide separation are usually necessary. Radionuclides that emit positrons but do not require a nearby cyclotron for their production-such as copper-62, gallium-68, and rubidium-82-are receiving attention because of their reduced cost. Although PET scanning provides valuable diagnostic information that in many cases cannot be obtained using other modalities, the expensive nature of the highly technical equipment necessary may limit the availability of these procedures to specialized medical centers. The changing health care environment and the public demand for cost containment may hinder further advances in this area of diagnostic radiology. Technological advances in PET scanning instrumentation, however, may result in a markedly reduced cost for the procedure in the future.

—Dandamudi V. Rao, PhD

See also Brain; Brain disorders; Imaging and radiology; Neuroimaging; Noninvasive tests; Nuclear medicine; Radiopharmaceuticals; Single photon emission computed tomography (SPECT).

For Further Information:

Christian, Paul E., Kristen M. Waterstram-Rich, eds. *Nuclear Medicine and PET: Technology and Techniques*. 7th ed. St. Louis, Mo.: Elsevier/Mosby, 2012.

Iturralde, Mario P. *Dictionary and Handbook of Nuclear Medicine and Clinical Imaging*. 2d ed. Boca Raton, Fla.: CRC Press, 2002.

Pagana, Kathleen Deska, and Timothy J. Pagana. *Mosby's Diagnostic and Laboratory Test Reference*. 11th ed. St. Louis, Mo.: Mosby/Elsevier, 2013.

"Positron Emission Tomography." *Health Library*, September 30, 2012.

"Positron Emission Tomography-Computed Tomography (PET/CT)." *RadiologyInfo.org*, March 28, 2013.

Preboth, Monica. "Use of PET in the Diagnosis of Cancer." *American Family Physician* 61, no. 8 (April 15, 2000): 2548.

Rao, Dandamudi V., et al., eds. *Physics of Nuclear Medicine: Recent Advances*. New York: American Institute of Physics, 1984.

Wolbarst, Anthony Brinton. *Looking Within: How X-Ray, CT, MRI, Ultrasound, and Other Medical Images Are Created*. Berkeley: University of California Press, 1999.

POST-TRAUMATIC STRESS DISORDER

Category: Disease/Disorder
Also known as: Shell shock, combat neurosis, battle fatigue
Anatomy or system affected: Psychic-emotional system
Specialties and related fields: Psychiatry, psychology
Definition: A maladaptive condition resulting from exposure to events beyond the realm of normal human experience and characterized by persistent difficulties involving emotional numbing, intense fear, helplessness, horror, reexperiencing of trauma, avoidance, and arousal.

CAUSES AND SYMPTOMS

Posttraumatic stress disorder (PTSD) is said to occur when a person experiences symptoms such as intense fear, helplessness, or horror following exposure to a traumatic event (an event outside the range of normal human experiences).

Trauma is a condition in which the biological fear system fails to deactivate even after the threat that triggered subsides. Complex trauma is the result of a chronic failure of fear system deactivation and of the dysfunctional impact of this failure, over time, on a network of biological, emotional, behavioral, cognitive, and social systems.

The traumatic event may involve threatened death, serious injury, or other threat to physical integrity; witnessing the death of or threat to another person; or learning about the death of or threat to a family member or close friend. Events such as natural disasters (earthquakes, mudslides, fires, floods, tsunamis, tornados), war, domestic violence, crime, accidents, and medical procedures may trigger the development of PTSD. PTSD is the only disorder in the *Diagnostic and Statistical Manual of Mental Disorders (DSM)* with a cited etiology.

PTSD involves reexperiencing the trauma, avoidance of things that remind the person of the trauma, and an uncomfortable state of arousal usually connected to readiness to avoid reexperiencing a trauma. Reexperiencing includes recurrent and intrusive thoughts, recurrent distressing dreams, feeling as if the event is happening again, intense psychological distress at exposure to any reminders (internal or external) of the event, or intense physical reactivity to any reminders of the event. Persistent avoidance includes anything associated with the event, as well as a numbing of general responsiveness. Such numbing may be indicated by several of the following: avoiding thoughts, feelings, or conversations associated with the event; avoiding activities, places, or people that re-

mind one of the event; forgetting an important aspect of the event; experiencing markedly diminished interest or participation in significant activities; feeling detached or estranged from others; having a restricted range of feelings, such as not being able to love; or feeling that the future is foreshortened. Increased arousal includes at least two of the following: difficulty with sleep; irritability or outbursts of anger; difficulty concentrating; hypervigilance; or exaggerated startle response. The reexperiencing, avoidance, and arousal start after the traumatic event, last more than one month, and cause clinically significant distress or impairment in social, occupational, or other important areas of functioning.

The course of the disorder varies, with some individuals not experiencing symptoms until years later, but most individuals experience symptoms within three months of the initial trauma. If the trauma occurs early in life, it may have profound effects on stress response throughout the individual's lifetime.

Persons with PTSD may describe painful guilt feelings about surviving when others did not, or about what they had to do to survive. Their phobic avoidance of situations or activities that resemble or symbolize the original trauma may interfere with interpersonal relationships and lead to marital conflict, divorce, or job loss.

The likelihood of developing PTSD increases as intensity and physical proximity to the event increase. Recent immigrants from countries where there is considerable social unrest and civil conflict may have elevated rates of PTSD. The disorder may occur at any age. Women are more likely to develop PTSD than men; this gender difference is thought to exist in part because some traumatic events that women experience occur directly to their persons.

Not everyone who experiences a significant trauma will develop PTSD. Individual differences in terms of immediate posttrauma assistance and support, long-term social support, stress response, physical health, and other biological factors may explain a lack of occurrence in some individuals.

TREATMENT AND THERAPY

Treatments for PTSD include individual therapy, group therapy, antianxiety and antidepressant drugs, and eye movement desensitization and reprocessing (EMDR). Combinations of therapies can also be effective. In general, the sooner the victim of PTSD receives treatment, the greater are the chances of complete recovery. It is important to note, however, that complex techniques such as trauma debriefing and critical incident debriefing should be attempted only by well-trained persons. Discussing traumatic events in a way that is not sensitive to the experience of the victim may retraumatize them, so caution is advised. For untrained persons, the best way to help someone affected by a trauma is to help them get to a qualified treatment professional as quickly as possible. This is especially important because research has suggested that treatment delivered soon after the trauma may reduce the overall negative impacts of the trauma.

Psychotherapy can help the person come to grips with the traumatic event. Different approaches are used, including exposure (or imaginal) therapy, anxiety management/relaxation training, cognitive therapy, and supportive psychotherapy. Also, hypnosis, journaling (such as thought diaries and grief letters), creative arts, and a critical-incident stress debriefing may be used in treating PTSD, either alone or in conjunction with psychotherapy.

Group therapy, in which victims of PTSD can share their experiences and gain support from others, is especially helpful. Groups are typically small (six to eight persons) and are often composed of individuals who have undergone similar experiences. Also, marital and family therapy or parent training may be used in treating PTSD.

In general, the goals of psychotherapy include facilitating victims' emotional engagement with the trauma memory, helping them organize a personal trauma narrative, assisting them in correcting dysfunctional cognitions that often follow trauma, helping them develop increased trust in others, and decreasing their emotional and social isolation. The therapist typically provides empathy, validation, safety, consistency, and sensitivity to cultural and ethnic identity issues.

Antianxiety and antidepressant drugs can relieve the physiological symptoms of PTSD. The major pharmacological agents include benzodiazepines, serotonin receptor partial agonists, tricyclic antidepressants, monoamine oxidase inhibitors (MAOIs), and selective serotonin reuptake inhibitors. Because of the many biological abnormalities presumed to be associated with PTSD, and because of the overlap between symptoms of PTSD and other comorbid disorders, almost every class of psychotropic agent has been administered to PTSD patients. Whether it includes individual or group therapy, drugs, or some combination of these three, the treatment approach must be tailored to the individual PTSD sufferer and his or her unique situation.

EMDR is a newer therapy for PTSD. It combines many aspects of the other therapies described and works to facilitate reprocessing of traumatic information and experience. Guided discussion and therapeutic work may involve specific eye movements while remembering different aspects of the traumatic event. It is suggested that this type of activity creates an orienting response that facilitates trauma processing. The

---

INFORMATION ON POST-TRAUMATIC STRESS DISORDER

Causes: Exposure to traumatic event
Symptoms: May include recurrent and intrusive thoughts; reliving of traumatic event; intense psychological distress with exposure to reminders of event; recurrent disturbing dreams; difficulty sleeping; irritability or outbursts of anger; detachment; difficulty concentrating; hypervigilance; exaggerated startle response
Duration: Often chronic with acute episodes
Treatments: Individual therapy, group therapy, antianxiety medications, antidepressants

---

technique requires a high level of skill and sophistication and should be used only by appropriately trained professionals. EMDR is very highly recommended for trauma and remains a topic of great research interest.

It is important to remember that PTSD, like many other mental health disorders, may not occur in isolation. Comorbidity, or the presence of more than one disorder, is the rule rather than the exception with PTSD. Depressive disorders, substance use disorders, and other anxiety disorders are the disorders most likely to occur with PTSD. Treatment must address the comorbid conditions when they are present. PTSD can be reliably assessed through semistructured interview and self-report measures. Treatment typically occurs on an outpatient basis, but it also may occur on an inpatient basis if the symptoms are severe.

PERSPECTIVE AND PROSPECTS

PTSD was observed in World War I, when some soldiers had intense anxiety reactions to the horrors they were experiencing. At that time, it was called "combat neurosis," "shell shock," or "battle fatigue." It was formally diagnosed as an anxiety-based personality disorder in the 1960s among Vietnam War veterans, but it is no longer considered a personality disorder and is instead seen as an anxiety disorder. It is also now known that traumatic events may include not only war but also violent personal assault, kidnapping, terrorist attacks, torture, natural or human-made disasters, severe automobile accidents, or different aspects of life-threatening illness. For children, sexually traumatic events may include sexual experiences that were developmentally inappropriate, even if no threatened or actual violence occurred. PTSD may be especially severe when the trauma is of human origin (e.g., torture) and directly related to damage to one's person.

Promising research identifying change to the stress response system in younger persons following trauma, as well as gender differences in trauma response, are expected to fuel greater understanding of the mechanisms of trauma response. Such knowledge will in turn be useful for developing new drug, biological, and interpersonal therapies for children and adults and for both women and men.

—*Shuba Samuel, PhD*

See also: Accidents; Antianxiety drugs; Anxiety; Domestic violence; Psychiatric disorders; Psychiatry; Stress; Stress reduction.

For Further Information:
American Psychiatric Association. *Diagnostic and Statistical Manual of Mental Disorders: DSM-5.* 5th ed., APA, 2013.
Bryant, R. A. "Post-traumatic Stress Disorder: A State-of-the-art Review of Evidence and Challenges." *World Psychiatry*, vol. 18, no. 3, 2019, pp. 259-69.
Forbes, D., J. I. Bisson, C. M. Monson, and L. Berliner, editors. *Effective Treatments for PTSD.* Guilford Publications, 2020.
Guilding, M., S. Nemeckova, D. Brady, et al. "Perspectives on Complex Trauma." *The Journal of the Complex Trauma Institute*, vol. 1, no. 1, 2020, pp. 1-74.
"National Center for Posttraumatic Stress Disorder." *US Department of Veterans Affairs*, 15 June 2021.
"Post-Traumatic Stress Disorder." *MedlinePlus*, 11 Aug. 2016.
"Post-Traumatic Stress Disorder." *National Institute of Mental Health*, 2020.

POSTHERPETIC NEURALGIA

Category: Disease/Disorder
Also known as: Neuropathy
Anatomy or system affected: Nerve cells, nerve roots, dermatome body, neurologic system, integument system
Specialties and related fields: Neurology, dermatology, infectious disease, and internal medicine
Definition: A condition that can potentially produce severe pain in a specific nerve root/dermatome that was once previously exposed to the herpes zoster virus (chicken pox-shingles). Neuralgia is the pain that is produced from a nerve that is inflamed or enduring destruction from a disease process. In the case of postherpetic neuralgia, the nerve damage is produced by the reactivation of the herpes zoster virus.

CAUSES AND SYMPTOMS

The persistent nerve pain that accompanies postherpetic neuralgia/neuropathy can be precisely linked to a previous exposure to the herpes zoster-varicella virus. The virus has the unique potential to reside dormant within the body of a previously infected nerve. Under normal conditions, our immune system protects us from the dormant virus ever becoming active. However, when an individual is under stress and/or the immune system is unable to function effectively, the virus can be reactivated. Reasons for the immune system's inability to function effectively are vast. More common reasons for this to occur include, but are not limited to, the effect of medications (steroids, antirejection drugs in organ transplants, chemotherapy agents), a diagnosis of cancer or simply the exposure to the zoster virus again without sufficient immunity to ward off the disease process.

Precisely, once the nerve cell fiber (neuron) has been exposed to the varicella virus (chicken pox) and some of the virus particles can settle into clusters in the nerve cells, these are called sensory ganglia. Here they remain for many years in an inactive (latent) form. The sensory ganglia can be located adjacent to the spinal cord and brain. These specialized cells relay information to the brain about what the body is presently sensing, specifically the sensations of heat, cold, touch, and pain.

The main task of the nerve cell fibers is to send a message to the brain when the nerve is stimulated. When the nerve stimulation has been altered by a previous infection with the varicella virus (zoster), then there can be an alteration in the way the brain perceives or receives this nerve's message. In other words, the nerve may produce the sensation of pain in the brain because of the damage it has sustained from the virus. In addition, when the virus is reactivated it can go on to destroy even more nerve tissue and the pain can become worse or even linger in this nerve indefinitely. The pain may be described as "burning" or "stabbing" in nature, even perceived as traveling within the nerve cell fiber's pathway. In the beginning, the pain may be described as mild and progress very rapidly to severe or intolerable pain. Once the individual perceives the sensation of pain, the skin around this affected area may produce a rash or erupt in blisters or vesicles. This is because the viruses multiply within the nerve fiber pathway that communicates with the skin surface. This syndrome is often referred to as shingles.

Our knowledge of the human system has increased tremendously. We understand better now how an alteration in one system can inherently affect another system. This is an excellent example of this process. It is for this reason that elderly and sick individuals are affected more by this disease. The duration is short term to chronic.

TREATMENT AND THERAPY

The treatment for postherpetic-neuropathy/neuralgia may involve multiple modalities. These may include indefinite pharmacologic therapy with antiviral medications, such as Acyclovir (Zovirax®), Valcyclovir (Valtrex®), Famciclovir (Famvir®). Tricyclic antidepressants (Nortriptyline®) are also widely employed early in the disease's progression. Another medication sometimes prescribed is the anticonvulsant/ antiseizure medication gabapentin (Neurontin®). Topical local anesthetics sometimes provide mild relief from the painful stimuli (Lidocaine®). These latter medications are available as creams or subcutaneous patches. The pain may be controlled with various analgesic medications including opioids and other controlled substances. Unfortunately, the sequale may be complex, and any patients may require continued follow-up with pain management services indefinitely.

A shingles vaccine has been encouraged since May 2006 to all individuals exposed to the varicella virus in the past if they are over the ages of 50. The U.S. Food and Drug Administration (FDA) approved a VZV vaccine (Zostavax®) that is widely employed in the United States. This is a preventive measure for the disease, not a treatment once the disease has progressed.

FUTURE EXPECTATIONS
Much research is being devoted to this area at present. The National Institute of Health (NIH) and various pharmaceutical companies are devoting research efforts in this area. The employment of the shingles vaccine has been effective in slowing the prevalence of the disease and newer modalities in the area of pain control also provide positive gains in this area.

—*Mary Frances McGibbon*

For Further Information:
American Chronic Pain Assn (ACPA): www.theacpa.org
BRAIN: www.ninds.nih.gov
National Institute of Neurological Disorders and Stroke. "Shingles: Hope Through Research."
   www.ninds.nih.gov/disorders/shingles/detail_shingles.htm
National Shingles Foundation (For Research on Varicella Zoster): www.vzvfoundation.org

POSTURAL ORTHOSTATIC TACHYCARDIA SYNDROME (POTS)

Category: Disease/Disorder
Also known as: Chronic orthostatic intolerance
Anatomy or system affected: Cardiovascular system, heart, blood vessels, circulatory system
Specialties and related fields: Cardiology, Neurology
Definition: Condition characterized by decreased volume of blood returning to the heart when standing up, resulting in symptoms such as an excessively increased heart rate.

Key terms:
autonomic nervous system: regulates involuntary actions for bodily functions (such as breathing, heart rate, and digestion)
tachycardia: fast heart rate

CAUSES AND SYMPTOMS
In postural orthostatic tachycardia syndrome (POTS), the body is unable to regulate blood flow through vessels due to dysautonomia (dysfunction in the autonomic nervous system). This results in symptoms such as dizziness or a fast heart rate upon standing. POTS is characterized by orthostatic intolerance, the inability to stand or sit vertically without developing symptoms that are alleviated when lying down. Signs include the heart rate increases by 30 beats per minute or is more than 120 beats per minute within 10 minutes of standing up. Orthostatic hypotension is another sign, which is a sustained decrease in systolic blood pressure 20 mmHg or diastolic blood pressure 10 mmHg within 3 minutes of standing or tilting the head upwards to >60 degrees.

Normally, the autonomic nervous system allows the body to function without conscious effort. Standing, for example, is facilitated by a large amount of blood automatically falling to the lower parts of the body. Changes in heart rate, vessels, and muscle, for example, ensure that blood is distributed to the upper parts of the body. In POTS, a defect exists in these automatic set of processes, so not enough blood is able to go to organs such as the brain and heart. This causes symptoms of fatigue, headache, and even fainting when standing up.

Tests and clinical signs can lead to a diagnosis of POTS. In the tilt table test, for example, patients strapped on a table are tilted to mimic standing up, and heart rate and blood pressure changes are monitored.

The exact causes and mechanisms of POTS are unknown. Some individuals acquire the condition after exposure to a virus, such as the Epstein-Barr virus in mononucleosis. Other individuals can acquire POTS after brain trauma or severe injuries. POTS can have multiple, complex causes. Primary causes of POTS include nitric oxide exposure, neuropathy, and certain viruses. Physical deconditioning, a decline in bodily function that can occur from a significant injury or from a chronic disease, is also considered a primary agent. Secondary causes of POTS include anemia, adrenal disorders, Ehlers-Danlos syndrome, Lyme disease, tumors, and more.

TREATMENT AND THERAPY
Since the specific causes of POTS is still unknown, treatment focuses on managing symptoms. Diet,

exercise, and medication are three avenues for addressing primary POTS. Diets with a high sodium intake and low gluten intake have been shown to be effective in some patients; alcoholic beverages should be avoided as it may worsen symptoms of low blood pressure and dizziness, but fluid intake such as water should increase to help alleviate symptoms.

Exercise therapy may help improve overall well-being and is based on the theory that it may play a part in resetting the autonomic nervous system. Medications can also be used for managing or reducing the symptoms of POTS, but there is currently no silver bullet for curing the disease. An approach that does not involve medications includes raising the head of the bed onto a firm foundation (such as blocks) to help decrease the risk of dizziness when rising from the bed in the morning. Avoiding triggers, such as extreme temperatures, can be beneficial.

PERSPECTIVE AND PROSPECTS
POTS affects nearly half a million people in the United States, with a majority of them females. The prognosis for POTS is generally favorable. Many individuals experience mild symptoms and can continue with their daily activities. However, others may be significantly impaired. Some people's symptoms improve with lifestyle changes such as exercise, diet, and medication; still, others' symptoms unfortunately persist and do not improve with treatment.

POTS is sometimes referred to as an "invisible illness" because it is not one, defined condition, but rather a constellation of conditions with a similar physiological state. There exists a spectrum of symptoms and clinical manifestations of POTS, so treatment varies from one person to the next. Because patients report fatigue to be the most significant symptom, they may experience reduced quality of life, a more sedentary lifestyle, and less energy to engage in daily activities. POTS may be misdiagnosed as anxiety, depression, or another psychological condition. Diagnosis is often delayed, with one survey reporting taking more than two years for half of patients with POTS to be diagnosed.

CONTINUING RESEARCH
Early twenty-first century research is investigating more effective medications for POTS. Clinical trials have found that pyridostigmine, a drug that typically is given to patients with myasthenia gravis to treat muscle weakness, can ameliorate tachycardia and maintain blood pressure among patients with POTS.

Another study, led by researchers at the University of California, San Diego, are investigating the drug Ivabradine. It is currently used to treat chronic heart failure, but also has been shown to treat tachycardia, so

the researchers hypothesize that Ivabradine will reduce tachycardia among patients with POTS.

Researchers at Vanderbilt are investigating whether stimulating the vagus nerve can decrease POTS symptoms. The vagus nerve is responsible for involuntary functions of the human body, such as heart rate. These researchers are studying the impact of stimulating the vagus nerve on heart rate as a potential mode of treatment for individuals with POTS.

—*Anna Delamerced*

For Further Information:
Effect of Ivabradine on Patients With Postural Orthostatic Tachycardia Syndrome (POTS). (2017). Retrieved from clinicaltrials.gov/ct2. (Identification No. NCT03182725)
Jiawei, L., et al. (2015). The Value of Acetylcholine Receptor Antibody in Children with Postural Tachycardia Syndrome. *Pediatric Cardiology, 36*(1), 165-170. doi.org/10.1007/s00246-014-0981-8
Kanjwal, K., et al. (2011). Pyridostigmine in the treatment of postural orthostatic tachycardia: a single-center experience. *Pacing Clin Electrophysiol, 34*(6), 750-5. doi: 10.1111/j.1540-8159.2011. 03047
Kaufmann H & Freeman R. Postural tachycardia syndrome. *UpToDate.* March 2015, www.uptodate.com/contents/postural-tachycardia- syndrome.
Low, P., et al. (2009). Postural tachycardia syndrome (POTS). *J Cardiovasc Electrophysiol, 20*(3), 352-8. doi: 10.1111/j.1540- 8167.2008.01407
Transdermal Vagal Stimulation for POTS. (2014). Retrieved from clinicaltrials.gov/ct2. (Identification No. NCT02281097)

PRADER-WILLI SYNDROME

Category: Disease/Disorder
Anatomy or system affected: Bones, brain, endocrine system, genitals, glands, heart, musculoskeletal system, psychic-emotional system, teeth
Specialties and related fields: Cardiology, dentistry, family medicine, genetics, neurology, pediatrics, pharmacology, psychiatry, pulmonary medicine
Definition: A disorder caused by a deletion in chromosome 15, characterized by developmental and cognitive delays, overeating resulting in obesity, and behavioral difficulties.

CAUSES AND SYMPTOMS
Prader-Willi syndrome is caused by a spontaneous deletion involving chromosome 15. Although this disease is genetic in nature, most parents of children with Prader-Willi syndrome have normal chromosomes. Some research indicates an association between the disease and fathers employed at the time of conception in fields associated with hydrocarbons, such as lumbermen, chemists, or mechanics. That

---

INFORMATION ON PRADER-WILLI SYNDROME

Causes: Spontaneous genetic deletion, possibly with environmental trigger

Symptoms: Low birth weight, decreased muscle tone, small genitalia, undescended testicles, small hands and feet, short stature, poor motor development, intellectual disabilities (ranging from mild to severe), insatiable need to eat, behavioral disorders, psychiatric disorders

Duration: Lifelong

Treatments: Alleviation of symptoms; may include dietary restrictions and regular exercise to avoid obesity, growth hormone, special education (speech, behavioral, and psychiatric therapy)

---

connection might implicate an environmental trigger in some cases.

Prader-Willi syndrome occurs in one in 12,000-15,000 births and affects both genders and all races. Newborns with the disease appear floppy, with low muscle tone. They often had a low birth weight, and males may have undescended testicles. Small genitalia are common, as are small hands and feet. These babies feed poorly and display poor motor development. Intellectual disabilities are common, ranging from mild to severe.

Between the ages of two and four, children with Prader-Willi syndrome develop an insatiable need to eat. They will do anything to get food and will eat without control. Obesity and other related health problems are major concerns for these patients. Many patients also suffer from behavioral disorders related to excessive eating, compulsive or repetitive behaviors, tantrums, and psychiatric disorders including depression and, in extreme cases, psychoses.

TREATMENT AND THERAPY

Primary treatment for Prader-Willi syndrome centers on the many health concerns related to obesity, in addition to meeting the educational, social, and emotional needs of patients as they grow and mature. Studies indicate an abnormally high level of the hormone ghrelin in these patients. It is the only appetite-stimulating hormone produced in the stomach and was touted in the early twenty-first century as a possible breakthrough in treatment.

Dietary restrictions, including types of food and portion control, are critical with these patients. Since they are unable to control their cravings for food, cooperation among family, school personnel, and community members is essential. Regular exercise is also recommended. Because patients with Prader-Willi syndrome

are often small in stature, growth hormones are often used to facilitate growth and decrease the percentage of body fat, thus helping improve both strength and agility in patients. Special education services, including speech, behavioral assistance, and psychological or psychiatric services, are also important components of treatment.

PERSPECTIVE AND PROSPECTS

Prader-Willi syndrome was first defined as a syndrome by Andrea Prader, Alexis Labhart, and Heinrich Willi in 1956. Prader and Willi refined the syndrome in 1963. Since the mid-twentieth century, researchers have focused on the influences of hormones and genetics in the development and treatment of this disease. Treatments evolved based on increased knowledge of how genes and hormones influence human biology and behavior.

—Kathleen Schongar, MS, MA

See also Birth defects; Dwarfism; Environmental diseases; Genetic diseases; Growth; Intellectual disability; Obesity; Obesity, childhood; Psychiatric disorders; Psychiatry; Psychiatry, child and adolescent; Psychosis.

For Further Information

American Psychiatric Association. *Diagnostic and Statistical Manual of Mental Disorders: DSM-5*. 5th ed. Washington, DC: American Psychiatric Association, 2013.

Cassidy, Susanne B. "Prader-Willi Syndrome." *Journal of Medical Genetics* 34 (1997): 917-923.

Jones, Kenneth Lyons. "Prader-Willi Syndrome." In *Smith's Recognizable Patterns of Human Malformation*. 6th ed. Philadelphia: Saunders/Elsevier, 2006.

MedlinePlus. "Prader-Willi Syndrome." *MedlinePlus*, May 13, 2013.

Prader-Willi Syndrome Association USA. *Prader-Willi Syndrome Association USA*, n.d.

Sadock, Benjamin J., and Virginia A. Sadock. *Kaplan and Sadock's Concise Textbook of Clinical Psychiatry*. 3d ed. Philadelphia: Wolters Kluwer/Lippincott Williams & Wilkins, 2009.

PRECOCIOUS PUBERTY

Category: Disease/Disorder

Also known as: Sexual precocity, gonadotropin puberty, pubertas praecox

Anatomy or system affected: Musculoskeletal system, nervous system, psychic-emotional system, reproductive system

Specialties and related fields: Endocrinology, family medicine, genetics, neurology, pediatrics

Definition: The early onset of puberty caused by the premature secretion of sex hormones, resulting in the commencement of sexual maturation prior to age eight in girls and age nine in boys.

Key terms:

gonads: ovaries in girls and testes in boys

hormones: chemicals produced by glands such as the thyroid, pituitary, or adrenals that stimulate bodily changes or growth and that regulate body functions

hypothalamus: the region of the brain that stimulates glands to secrete hormones

idiopathic: having an unidentified cause

pituitary: also known as the "hypophysis"; a gland below the hypothalamus that secretes hormones that control the adrenals, the thyroid, and the reproductive organs, as well as overall growth and metabolism

puberty: secondary sexual development that involves the maturation of the reproductive system and is typified by significant physical growth

CAUSES AND SYMPTOMS

Secondary sexual development is commonly known as "puberty." It is typically characterized by growth of pubic and underarm hair, acne, and rapid physical development until about age eighteen. During puberty, a boy also grows facial hair, his penis and testes enlarge, and he begins to produce sperm. A girl develops breasts and begins to menstruate and ovulate.

Puberty is the result of hormonal changes triggered by the hypothalamus region of the brain. Luteinizing hormone-releasing hormone (LHRH) is released in periodic bursts, causing the pituitary gland to secrete gonadotropin-releasing hormone (GnRH). Gonadotropins—luteinizing hormone (LH) and follicle-stimulating hormone (FSH)—stimulate the ovaries in girls and the testes in boys to secrete sex hormones. These hormones—estrogen and progesterone in girls and testosterone in boys—start the sexual maturation process and stimulate rapid physical growth.

Puberty usually begins at about age twelve in boys and age eleven in girls. Approximately one in every ten thousand children begins puberty abnormally early, between infancy and approximately age eight. This condition, known as "precocious puberty," affects both sexes but is two to ten times more common among girls than boys. An increased body mass index (BMI), especially in girls, has also been associated with precocity, and this association appears to be stronger in white girls than in black girls. Genetic factors have also been linked to this condition, and in a small percentage it appears to be familial.

In addition to prematurely developing secondary sexual characteristics, children with precocious puberty are initially tall for their ages. Left untreated, however, they rarely reach their full adult height potential because the same sex hormones that trigger early growth

> **INFORMATION ON PRECOCIOUS PUBERTY**
>
> **Causes:** Hormonal imbalance; possibly linked to genetic disorders, tumors in hypothalamus, adrenal gland disorders, hydrocephalus, radiation therapy, nervous system disorders, McCune-Albright syndrome
>
> **Symptoms:** Premature development of secondary sexual characteristics; above-average height until adulthood but failure to reach full growth potential, moodiness, irritability, aggressiveness, early development of sex drive
>
> **Duration:** Chronic
>
> **Treatments:** Hormonal therapy

also end it prematurely. Males often grow no taller than 5 feet 2 inches, and many females remain under 5 feet. Precocious puberty frequently results in adolescent behaviors such as moodiness, irritability, and aggressiveness, as well as the early development of a sex drive. Children with precocious puberty reach sexual maturity at varying rates, and some characteristics may even begin to regress to their normal state.

When an underlying cause for precocious puberty cannot be determined, the condition is known as "idiopathic precocious puberty." About 80 percent of cases in females and 40 percent of male cases are idiopathic. Where the underlying cause can be established, it may be central (brain or thyroid) or it may be peripheral (adrenal gland or reproductive system). Common causes for central precocious puberty include genetic disorders or tumors in the hypothalamic region of the brain. Such tumors, known as "hypothalamic hamartomas," are usually benign. Between 5 and 10 percent of boys with precocious puberty genetically inherit the condition from their fathers or indirectly from their maternal grandfathers. This genetic transmittal of precocious puberty only occurs in about 1 percent of girls with the condition. Less common are the peripheral causes of precocious puberty, including ovarian tumors or cysts, and adrenal gland disorders such as adrenogenital hyperplasia or congenital adrenal hyperplasia (where reproductive hormones are produced in excess). Precocious puberty can also be caused by pituitary lesions, hydrocephalus, radiation therapy, nervous system disorders such as neurofibromatosis, thyroid disorders (specifically severe hypothyroidism), and a rare condition called "McCune-Albright syndrome." A few cases have also been shown to be caused by exposure to creams or ointments containing estrogen or testosterone.

Children with precocious puberty are often self-conscious about their early physical and sexual development, since they appear older than their biological ages. Mental development is not affected by the condition, however, so children with precocious puberty are usually not as emotionally mature as they physically appear.

TREATMENT AND THERAPY

Underlying causes of precocious puberty, if known, are often difficult or impossible to treat. Surgical removal of noncancerous hypothalamic hamartomas and other brain tumors, for example, may not be feasible and rarely halts sexual development. Other causes such as neurofibromatosis are incurable, and treatments for conditions such as adrenal disorders may not stop the effects of precocious puberty.

Therefore, many forms of precocious puberty are treated by changing patients' hormonal balance. Synthetic hormones known as "LHRH analogs" and "GnRH agonists" block the body's production of sex hormones and thus slow down or stop pubertal symptoms. The synthetic hormone histrelin acetate (Supprelin LA or Vantas), has been shown to be effective in reducing early sexual changes in both sexes and to slow bone growth. Leuprolide acetate (Lupron-Depot PED, Eligard, or Fensolvi) is another successful treatment for this condition. Daily injections of these drugs are stopped when the patient reaches the appropriate age for onset of puberty.

Synthetic versions of GnRH or LHRH interrupt the chain of hormonal events that result in sexual maturation. Some research, however, suggests a link between these therapies and bone mineral density loss. Treatments are administered in daily or monthly injections.

Girls with precocious puberty caused by congenital adrenal hyperplasia can be treated by suppressing the pituitary hormone adrenocorticotropic hormone (ACTH) with a glucocorticoid. Precocious puberty associated with McCune-Albright syndrome can be treated with testolactone, which blocks the production of estrogens. Some forms of precocious puberty involving the gonadotropins can be treated with the hormone suppressant nafarelin acetate.

Genetic counseling is recommended for families of patients with inherited precocious puberty. Psychological counseling may also benefit patients and their parents, since patients may not fit in with peers because of the physical ramifications of the condition.

PERSPECTIVE AND PROSPECTS

Previous treatments for precocious puberty included the use of synthetic progesterone (medroxyprogesterone acetate, Depo-Provera), an artificial version of a sex hormone secreted by the ovaries. Synthetic progesterone frequently stops menstruation and reduces breast size in girls, but it has little or no effect on boys. Unfortunately, it fails to stop rapid growth in either sex. Synthetic progesterone can also result in several side effects (including abdominal cramps, breast pain, alterations in breast and nipple, depression, and anxiety). At least one study has shown an increased risk of breast cancer following progesterone treatment. More work needs to be done in this area.

Experimental treatments for idiopathic precocious puberty include a combination of spironolactone and testolactone for male patients, as well as another the drug Deslorelin (or Somagard) for either sex.

—*Kerry Cheesman, PhD and Maryann Cheesman, RN*

See also: Endocrine system; Endocrinology; Endocrinology, pediatric; Growth; Hormones; Menstruation; Puberty and adolescence; Sexuality.

For Further Information:
Carel, J. C., et al. "Treatment of Central Precocious Puberty by Subcutaneous Injections of Leuprorelin 3-Month Depot (11.25 mg)." *Journal of Clinical Endocrinology and Metabolism*, vol. 87, no. 9, Sept. 2002, pp. 4111-16.
Creatsas, George, George Mastorakos, and George P. Chrousos, editors. *Adolescent Gynecology and Endocrinology: Basic and Clinical Aspects.* New York Academy of Sciences, 2006.
Dowshen, Steven. "Precocious Puberty." *KidsHealth from Nemours*, Oct. 2012.
Grave, Gilman D., and Gordon B. Cutler, Jr., editors. *Sexual Precocity: Etiology, Diagnosis, and Management.* Raven Press, 1993.
Henry, Helen L., and Anthony W. Norman, editors. *Encyclopedia of Hormones.* 3 vols. Academic Press, 2003.
Huffman, Grace Brooke. "Reassessing the Age Limit of Precocious Puberty in Girls." *American Family Physician*, vol. 61, no. 6, 15 Mar. 2000, p. 1850.
Kaplowitz, Paul B. "Precocious Puberty." *Medscape*, 24 Jan. 2022, emedicine.medscape.com/article/924002.
Kronenberg, Henry M., et al., editors. *Williams Textbook of Endocrinology.* 12th ed., Saunders/Elsevier, 2011.
McCoy, Krisha. "Precocious Puberty." *Health Library*, 30 Sept. 2012.
National Institutes of Health. "Puberty and Precocious Puberty: Overview." *NIH: Eunice Kennedy Shriver National Institute of Child Health and Human Development*, 3 Apr. 2013.
Walvoord, Emily C., and Ora Hirsch Pescovitz. "Combined Use of Growth Hormone and Gonadotropin-Releasing Hormone Analogues in Precocious Puberty: Theoretic and Practical Considerations." *Pediatrics*, vol. 104, no. 4, Oct. 1999, pp. 1010-14.

PREECLAMPSIA AND ECLAMPSIA

Category: Disease/Disorder
Anatomy or system affected: Blood vessels, brain, cardiovascular system, fetus, heart, kidneys, placenta
Specialties and related fields: Cardiology, obstetrics and gynecology, perinatology

Definition: Preeclampsia is high blood pressure, swelling, or high levels of the blood protein albumin in the urine between the 20th week of pregnancy and the end of the first week after delivery. Eclampsia is the development of convulsive seizures or coma without other causes during that same period.

Key terms:

gestational hypertension: blood pressure of at least 140/90 mm Hg at or after 20 weeks gestation

hemolysis: the rupture of red blood cells and release of hemoglobin into the blood, which can cause anemia

ischemia: restriction of blood supply that causes a shortage of oxygen in tissues

perinatal mortality: number of stillbirths and deaths in the first week of life per 1,000 total births

proteinuria: the presence of protein (typically albumin) in the urine

tonic-clonic seizures: also known as grand mal seizures. These produce bilateral, convulsive muscle contractions

CAUSES AND SYMPTOMS

Preeclampsia, formerly known as toxemia, is a serious disease that develops in 2% to 8% of pregnant women and remains a leading cause of maternal and perinatal morbidity and mortality. It is characterized by gestational hypertension and significant proteinuria at or after 20 weeks gestation. Mild preeclampsia is defined as a blood pressure of 140/90 mmHg or higher with proteinuria of 0.3-3g/day. Severe preeclampsia includes blood pressure between 160-170/100-110 mm Hg, proteinuria of 3-5g/day, and headache. Other symptoms may include progressive lower extremity or abdominal swelling, changes in vision, abdominal pain, nausea or vomiting, impaired liver function, and shortness of breath. Typically, early-onset preeclampsia (" weeks of gestation) is associated with worse maternal and neonatal outcomes compared to late-onset preeclampsia (34 weeks of gestation). Intrauterine growth restriction (IUGR) in the developing fetus is a potential complication of preeclampsia and can lead to low birth weight and predisposes the fetus to various adult diseases such as diabetes and coronary artery disease.

An estimated 15% of women with preeclampsia develop HELLP syndrome, characterized by hemolysis, elevated liver enzymes, and a low platelet count. HELLP syndrome usually occurs in the last trimester, with women complaining of nausea, vomiting, and upper abdominal pain. In severe cases, the syndrome leads to intravascular blood clotting, kidney failure, liver failure, respiratory failure, systemic failure, and death. Eclampsia is a complication that occurs in 1-2% of severe preeclampsia cases and is characterized by new onset of tonic-clonic seizures or coma that cannot be attributed to other causes and the symptoms of preeclampsia. Most cases of eclampsia occur within 24 hours of delivery. Organ damage, especially injury to the kidneys, liver, brain, and placenta, may occur.

The cause of preeclampsia and eclampsia remains largely unknown. The leading hypotheses involve placental dysfunction in early pregnancy. Placental ischemia leads to the release of factors into the maternal blood circulation that contributes to vessel damage and inflammation, increasing the risk of developing preeclampsia. However, placental impairment alone is not sufficient to trigger preeclampsia. Predisposing cardiovascular and metabolic disorders may result in late-onset preeclampsia. Interactions between genetics and environmental factors are thought to be important as well. Preeclampsia incidence is rising in the United States, possibly related to the higher prevalence of predisposing disorders and a general trend of delayed childbearing. The risk of preeclampsia is higher in women with personal or family histories of preeclamp- sia; women who already have chronic hypertension; women younger than 18 or older than 40; women experiencing their first pregnancy or their first pregnancy with a new partner; women who are obese (BMI 30); women with inadequate prenatal care; and women with other conditions such as diabetes, kidney disease, and auto-immune disorders. Black women are more likely to die from preeclampsia or eclampsia than white women. However, this disparity may be confounded by a higher prevalence of chronic hypertension in black women and disproportionate levels of care. Interestingly, smoking is associated with a reduced risk of preeclampsia in low-risk pregnancies.

DIFFERENTIAL DIAGNOSIS

Preeclampsia shares clinical symptoms with many other diseases, including chronic hypertension, thrombotic thrombocytopenic purpura (TTP), antiphospholipid syndrome, HELLP syndrome, pheochromocytoma, systemic lupus erythematosus (SLE), and acute fatty liver of pregnancy (AFLP).

TREATMENT AND THERAPY

Preconception counseling and assessment are recommended for women at high risk of preeclampsia. Some research has demonstrated the efficacy of antiplatelet agents, low-dose aspirin, and calcium supplementation in preventing preeclampsia. The severity of the disease and maturity of the baby are primary considerations for treatment. The only definitive cure for preeclampsia is delivery, which means treatment of preeclampsia for women who are remote from term (" weeks' gestation) is largely symptomatic. Patients experiencing severe symptoms and are close

For Further Information:

Conrad Stöppler, Melissa. "Pregnancy: Preeclampsia vs. Eclampsia." *MedicineNet*, 17 Nov. 2020, www.medicinenet.com/pregnancy_preeclampsia_and_eclampsia/article.htm. Accessed 10 Apr. 2022.

Preeclampsia. Mayo Clinic, 19 Mar. 2020, www.mayoclinic.org/diseases-conditions/preeclampsia/symptoms-causes/syc-20355745. Accessed 9 Apr. 2022.

Preeclampsia and Eclampsia. Cedars-Sinai, n.d., www.cedars-sinai.org/health-library/diseases-and-conditions/p/preeclampsia-and-eclampsia.html. Accessed 10 Apr. 2022.

Preeclampsia and Eclampsia. Eunice Kennedy Shriver National Institute of Child Health and Human Development, 31 Jan. 2017, www.nichd.nih.gov/health/topics/preeclampsia. Accessed 9 Apr. 2022.

"Preeclampsia and Eclampsia - causes, symptoms, diagnosis, treatment, pathology." *YouTube*, uploaded by Osmosis, 3 Jan. 2017, www.youtube.com/watch?v=RB5s85xDshA.

Preeclampsia and Eclampsia: Two Serious Pregnancy Conditions. Carnegie Imaging, 9 Jun. 2021, www.carnegieimaging.com/blog/preeclampsia-eclampsia-understanding-difference/. Accessed 10 Apr. 2022.

to term may undergo induction of labor or c-section. Management of hypertension during pregnancy is essential and can be accomplished with antihypertensive agents, including nifedipine (*Procardia*), hydralazine (*Apresoline*), and labetalol (*Normodyne*). First-line treatment and prevention of eclampsia is magnesium sulfate (Epsom salt), which is neuroprotective and reduces the incidence of seizures. Women treated for preeclampsia and eclampsia should also be monitored for other symptoms, including headaches, blurred vision, abdominal pain, vaginal bleeding, and loss of fetal heart sounds.

PERSPECTIVE AND PROSPECTS

The first known description of preeclampsia was by Hippocrates in the 5th century BC Recent research has focused on the underlying mechanisms of preeclampsia and the role of gene-gene and gene-environment interactions. Some research has postulated that epigenetic changes - modifications to gene expression - to the gametes, placenta, and fetus are implicated. Concurrent research has identified excessive or atypical maternal immune responses as another potential cause of preeclampsia. Additional pharmacological studies are needed to develop treatments that target placental dysfunction and subsequent consequences. These insights could help improve preventive and therapeutic measures, particularly for high-risk patients.

—*David M. Lawrence,*
Robin Kamienny Montvilo, RN, PhD,
Derrick Cheng, BSc, BA, and Carol Shi, BA

PREGNANCY AND GESTATION

Category: Biology

Anatomy or system affected: Abdomen, reproductive system, uterus

Specialties and related fields: Embryology, gynecology, obstetrics, family medicine

Definition: The development of unborn young within a woman's uterus and the accompanying physical, biochemical, and developmental changes that occur to both mother and child from conception until birth as genetic material from each parent is joined to create a unique individual.

Key terms:

amniotic sac: the sac that surrounds the fetus in the uterus and is filled with amniotic fluid

blastocyst: the fertilized egg after it has divided several times to form a hollow ball of cells in one of the earliest stages of development

cervix: the constricted lower end of the uterus

chorion: the membrane in the embryo that further differentiates into the placenta and umbilical cord

chromosomes: rodlike structures inside cells that carry the genetic material

embryo: the unborn child from the second through the eighth week of development

endometrium: the lining of the uterus

Fallopian tube: the structure that leads from the internal cavity of the uterus to the ovary

fetus: the unborn child from the eighth week after fertilization until birth *placenta*: the organ that connects the mother to the embryo or fetus through the umbilical cord and is necessary for the child's nourishment

trimester: a division of pregnancy into three equal time periods of about thirteen weeks

PROCESS AND EFFECTS

Pregnancy begins after conception or fertilization with the fusion of an egg and sperm within a woman's body and continues until childbirth, typically thirty-eight weeks later. This gestational time is divided into three approximately equal periods called "trimesters," each associated with specific physical and biochemical hallmarks.

Prior to conception, a mature egg, or ovum, ruptures from a fluid-filled follicle within the ovary and is swept into the Fallopian tube by large fringes on the tube that caress the ovary's surface. The empty follicle is transformed into a structure called the "corpus luteum," which secretes hormones that help to prepare the woman's body for pregnancy. If the ovum is fertilized within twenty-four hours, pregnancy will occur. If it is not fertilized, the uterine lining will be shed during menstruation.

Sperm ejaculated into a woman's vagina travel through the cervix and uterus and into the Fallopian tubes. Only about 200 of the original 500 million sperm delivered to the woman may reach the vicinity of the ovum. Enzymes in the sperm heads dissolve protective outer layers of the egg. When one sperm finally breaks through the plasma membrane, the innermost covering of the ovum, chemical changes on the surface of the ovum prevent additional sperm from entering. The genetic material contained in the sperm and ovum fuse. Normally, if the fertilizing sperm is a gymnosperm, which carries an X chromosome, then the baby will be female; if it is an androsperm, which carries a Y chromosome, then the baby will be male. Other possibilities, though rare, do exist such as an XXY male outcome or XY with androgen resistance that can appear as a normal female.

About twelve hours after fusion of the genetic material, the first cell division occurs. Divisions continue at intervals of twelve to fifteen hours, doubling the number of cells each time, and the fertilized ovum is now called a "blastocyst." The blastocyst is gently guided through the Fallopian tube to the uterus by the beating of the millions of tiny hairs, called "cilia," that line the inner surfaces of the Fallopian tubes. This journey to the uterus takes about three days.

Upon arriving in the uterus, the blastocyst "explores" the endometrium, the uterine lining, for an appropriate site to settle. Prior to this implantation in the endometrium, the blastocyst ruptures from the clear protective sheath that helps to prevent it from settling in the Fallopian tube. By ten to fourteen days after fertilization, the blastocyst implants securely within the endometrium and the embryonic stage begins. At this point, it consists of several hundred cells and is about the size of the head of a pin.

After implantation, chemical signals produced by the blastocyst prevent the mother's immune system from recognizing the blastocyst as a foreign invader and destroying it. Other chemical signals cause the endometrium to thicken and extend blood vessels to the blastocyst for nourishment from the mother. The uterine wall softens and thickens, and the cervical opening is sealed with a mucus plug.

At this point, the cells of the blastocyst divide into two distinct clusters: One part will form the embryo itself, and the other part will join with the woman's tissue to form the placenta, the structure that will provide nourishment from the mother to the growing embryo. These early placental cells produce the hormone human chorionic gonadotropin (hCG). This hormone signals the ovary to cease ovulation and stimulates it to produce the hormone progesterone, which prevents menstruation and causes the endometrium to grow even thicker.

During the second week after fertilization, a cavity surrounding the embryo begins to form. This is destined to become the amniotic sac, which will contain the shock-absorbing amniotic fluid in which the fetus floats during development. At this time, the hCG being produced by the blastocyst and ovaries can be detected by pregnancy tests.

Three weeks after conception, the size of the embryo is about 2 millimeters (0.08 inch). The embryonic cells have divided into germ layers, distinct groupings of cells that are destined to produce specific body parts. The rudimentary brain appears at the end of a long tube. The heart is forming and will be beating within a week. At this point, the mother has missed her menstrual period and may be experiencing symptoms of pregnancy, such as nausea, heartburn, and tender breasts.

During the fifth through seventh weeks of embryonic development, massive physical changes occur. The crown-to-rump length of the embryo increases to around 1.25 centimeters (0.5 inch). The embryo's face, trunk, and limbs grow, and by the end of this period distinct fingers and toes are formed. The backbone is in place, and ribs begin to develop, as do skin, eyes, and all of the organ systems and the circulatory system. At this point, the placenta is connected to the embryo by the umbilical cord, and placental cells penetrate the blood vessels of the endometrium to provide transit of nutrients from the mother's bloodstream to the embryo. The placenta also filters out some potentially dangerous substances from the mother's bloodstream and aids in disposing of embryonic waste products.

By the eighth week of development, the embryo is about 4 cm (1.5 in) long, weighs about 14 grams (0.5 ounce), and is composed of millions of cells. All organs are formed, and the embryo is officially called a "fetus." The woman's uterus has increased in size, and her waistline may begin to enlarge. At this point, hor-

monal shifts stabilize, which frequently relieves morning sickness and other discomforts of early pregnancy.

Growth and organ system interconnection continue during the third month of fetal life, and the cells of the immune system are formed. During the fourth month, facial features develop, and the fetus may begin to respond to sound. Hair on the head and the eyebrows coarsens and develops pigment. The distinc-

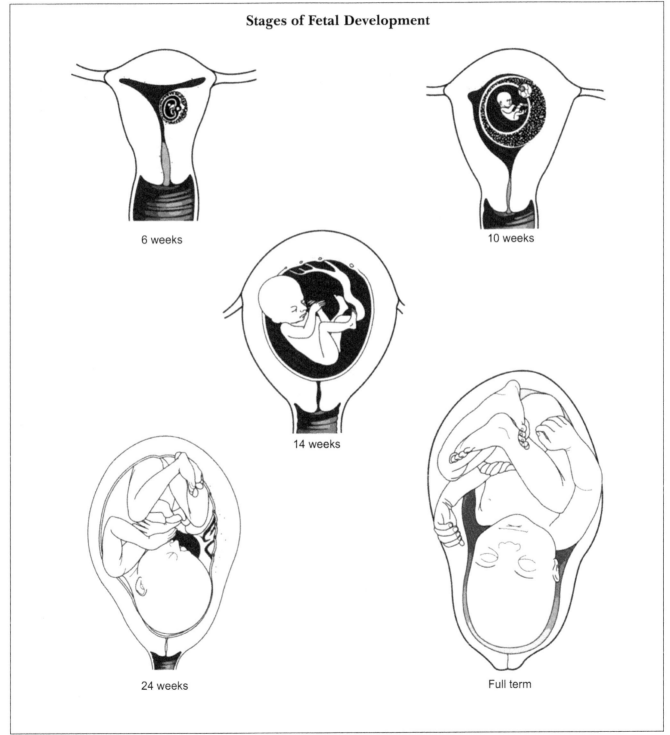

Stages of Fetal Development

6 weeks

10 weeks

14 weeks

24 weeks

Full term

tion between male and female fetuses becomes apparent with a visible vagina or penis. Sixteen to eighteen weeks after fertilization, the mother may feel the first fetal movements. She has gained several pounds, and changes in her body shape are readily visible. Frequently, this second trimester is associated with feelings of joy and minimal discomfort.

The third trimester is largely a period of growth for the fetus. Its weight increases rapidly. The fetus becomes very active within the amniotic fluid and responds to sound from both within and outside the mother. The weight gain may put incredible stress on the mother's body, and pressure on internal organs may cause frequent urination, heartburn, and difficulty breathing and sleeping.

Normal pregnancies vary from thirty-eight to forty-two weeks long. The lungs are the final organs to mature, and by the end of the eighth month all organ systems are established and functional. The fetus continues to gain weight until the end of pregnancy. At this time, the fetus will weigh around 3 kilograms (7 pounds) and have a crown to rump length of approximately 37 cm (14.4 in). The end of pregnancy is heralded by the beginning of uterine contractions, and frequently by the rupture of the amniotic sac and expulsion of its fluid. Labor leads to the birth of a unique individual created from the developmental programs contained in the genetic material inherited from each parent.

COMPLICATIONS AND DISORDERS

Since the developing embryo or fetus is dependent on the placental connection to the mother for nourishment, its health is directly tied to the diet and lifestyle of the mother. Any environmental substance that may cause a developmental defect is known as a "teratogen." Women must take care to avoid teratogens such as drugs or nicotine during pregnancy. Pregnant women must ingest adequate levels of protein, vitamins, and iron to remain healthy and have a healthy baby. Smoking during pregnancy has been linked to heart defects, and it decreases the amount of oxygen available to the fetus, which causes poor growth. Consumption of alcohol is associated with a host of defects collectively called "fetal alcohol syndrome." Whether any level of alcohol consumption is safe during pregnancy is not yet known. The use of drugs such as marijuana and cocaine during pregnancy increases the likelihood of stillbirths and unhealthy babies. Exposure in utero to certain drugs, especially, opioids, nicotine, alcohol, marijuana, and amphetamines may cause the newborn to experience withdrawal after birth. This condition is known as "neonatal abstinence syndrome."

The loss of a fetus before the twentieth week of pregnancy is called a "miscarriage." The most common cause of miscarriage during the first trimester is a major genetic defect in which the embryo has missing or extra chromosomes and therefore cannot develop normally. Other common causes are physical abnormalities in the embryo, a malformed uterus in the mother, an "incompetent" cervix that opens as the fetus enlarges, scarring of the uterus, and hormonal deficiencies. Increasing age of the mother, smoking, and alcohol and drug consumption are also correlated with miscarriage. To prevent future miscarriages of a nongenetic cause, hormone therapy, medications, and surgery are options.

Ectopic pregnancies occur when the fertilized egg implants in the wall of the Fallopian tube or anyplace outside of the uterus instead of in the uterus. The growing embryo may rupture the tube, endangering the mother's life and necessitating emergency surgery and possible loss of that Fallopian tube. Unruptured ectopics can be treated with medication or laparoscopic surgery. Scarring of the Fallopian tube from an infection can narrow this passage and cause ectopic pregnancy, as can early "hatching" of the blastocyst from its protective covering.

Neural tube defects result from a problem in the ectodermal layer of the embryo resulting in improper closure of the brain and spinal cord in early embryonic development. The outcomes of this defect are anencephaly (absence of a complete brain and part of the skull), a lethal condition, or spina bifida (portions of the spinal cord protruding from the spine), which can vary from mild to severe. These disorders seem to occur in families with a history of neural tube defects in pregnancy. Folic acid, an important component of prenatal vitamins, can reduce the risk of neural tube defects.

Neural tube defects can be detected prenatally by ultrasound, in which high-frequency sound waves are bounced off the contents of the uterus. The echoes are converted to an image, or sonogram, on a screen. Another test for neural tube defects is the alpha fetoprotein test, which measures levels of a fetal protein in the mother's blood; high levels indicate a neural tube defect.

Down syndrome, which results from the presence of one extra chromosome number 21, is the leading cause of intellectual disability in the United States and occurs in about one in every 800 live births. Many other genetic disorders are caused by missing or extra chromosomes. Some inherited diseases are attributable to errors in small pieces of chromosomes. Examples of these sorts of disorders include cystic fibrosis, hemophilia, Tay-Sachs disease, and sickle cell disease. Many of these genetic diseases can be detected by prenatal tests.

Prenatal cell-free deoxyribonucleic acid (DNA) screening is a blood test that checks the unborn baby's

DNA for the likelihood of having chromosomal disorders such as Down's syndrome or disorders of trisomy. A negative result indicates that the baby is unlikely to have Down's syndrome or a trisomy disorder. A positive result raises the risk of having one of these conditions and warrants further testing to confirm the diagnosis, using tests such as amniocentesis and chorionic villus sampling.

Amniocentesis is performed between the fifteenth and seventeenth weeks of pregnancy. A needle is inserted through the mother's abdomen, and a sample of the amniotic fluid is removed. Fetal cells present in the fluid are cultured for two to three weeks. The fetal cells are then analyzed for chromosome complement or tested for small genetic changes that can result in specific genetic diseases. Occasionally amniocentesis is done in the third trimester to determine fetal lung maturity when delivery of a premature infant is expected. Chorionic villus sampling provides a similar means to examine the genetic material of the fetus. This test is performed as early as the eighth week of pregnancy when a small piece of the chorionic villus, a tissue of embryonic origin that surrounds the early placenta, is removed and genetic analysis is immediately performed. Prenatal diagnosis of a chromosome abnormality or genetic disease allows the parents to terminate the pregnancy or to prepare for the birth of an affected child.

Infections acquired by a pregnant woman may be only inconveniences for her, but they may have severe consequences for an unborn child. Rubella, or German measles, can cause fetal death or severe impairment during the first trimester and permanent hearing loss during the second trimester. Vaccination prevents contraction of rubella, but cannot be given during pregnancy. Cytomegalovirus (CMV) can cause physical and mental disabilities, blindness, and deafness to the fetus if the mother first contracts CMV during pregnancy. Toxoplasmosis is an infection that can cause serious fetal consequences including miscarriage, stillbirth, and neonatal death if contracted in pregnancy. Avoidance of gardening where cats defecate and avoiding any contact with cat litter are measures counseled to pregnant women to reduce risk. Transmission of the sexually transmitted diseases syphilis and gonorrhea to the fetus can be prevented with antibiotic therapy. Human immunodeficiency virus (HIV), the virus that causes acquired immunodeficiency syndrome (AIDS), can be transmitted from mother to fetus through the placenta. Newborns with AIDS have a host of disorders but treatment of the mother has been shown to greatly reduce the risk of transmission to the fetus.

Rh factor is a substance on the surface of red blood cells. Individuals with and without this substance are Rh positive and Rh negative, respectively. If a woman is Rh negative and has an Rh-positive fetus, during delivery some of the baby's blood cells will enter the woman, and her body will manufacture antibodies to destroy the foreign cells. If with a subsequent pregnancy the fetus is Rh positive, these antibodies could attack and destroy the fetus. This problem is avoided by blood typing of mother and fetus during the first pregnancy and by administering Rh0(D) immune globulin (human), which destroys the fetal red blood cells entering the mother before her body can produce antibodies. Hence, future pregnancies are not at risk for Rh incompatibility.

A host of medical problems in the mother can develop during pregnancy that could jeopardize both her health and the health of her fetus. Blood pressure problems develop in about 7 percent of pregnant women as a result of the enormous changes in blood volume and pressure. The largest danger is that the fetus will not receive enough oxygen, which may lead to growth problems or sudden death during the final months of pregnancy. Preeclampsia is a cluster of symptoms related to high blood pressure, including edema (swelling caused by water retention) and kidney malfunction. Eclampsia (convulsions and coma) is life-threatening and needs emergency treatment. Bed rest, diet modification, close monitoring by a physician, or hospitalization may be prescribed for mild to severe cases of high blood pressure during pregnancy.

The effect of the hormones induced by pregnancy on the production of insulin, which regulates sugar levels in the body, is not well understood. In some pregnancies, insulin levels are not regulated properly, which results in gestational diabetes. Untreated, this can result in loss of the fetus late in pregnancy, the birth of a baby with high body fat content and an immature pancreas, or maternal convulsions and coma. Proper medical intervention and monitoring can correct or ease the effects of gestational diabetes on both mother and fetus.

Up to half of pregnant women develop anemia, a deficiency in red blood cells, because of a lack of iron or folic acid. The demand for the production of red blood cells in both mother and fetus leads to this disorder, which can cause poor growth in the fetus and increased susceptibility to infection, fatigue, and bleeding during childbirth for the mother. Proper diet and dietary supplements can alleviate anemia.

PERSPECTIVE AND PROSPECTS

Until the mid-twentieth century, what was known about fetal development was derived mainly from the study of miscarriages. The development and use of ultrasound techniques in the 1960s allowed a more accurate picture of developmental progression of normal, active fetuses, and such techniques subsequently became indispensable for the detection of some developmental abnormalities.

While physicians had been able to sample the amniotic fluid surrounding a fetus since the late nineteenth century, it was not until 1970 that they discovered that the fluid contained fetal cells which could be analyzed for chromosomal composition. At this time, amniocentesis became a tool for prenatal genetic analysis and sex determination and a routine test for pregnant women over the age of thirty-five, who are at a higher risk of carrying a fetus with a genetic abnormality. The liberalization of abortion laws in the United States in the 1960s gave parents of abnormal fetuses the option of pregnancy termination. In the early 1980s, chorionic villus sampling allowed much earlier detection of genetic defects and facilitated decision making for the expectant parents.

In the 1980s, some physicians began performing surgery on fetuses within the mother's uterus to correct problems threatening the life of the fetus, such as kidney disorders. Advanced monitoring and intervention techniques have reduced maternal deaths during pregnancy and childbirth. Unfortunately, maternal death, though relatively rare, is still a concern to patient safety advocates. Increased knowledge about infectious and toxic agents and about the ill effects of certain lifestyle habits upon a developing fetus has led to better education and prenatal care for both mother and fetus. Because of career and personal considerations, older women frequently wish to begin families. Medical advances have made it relatively common for women past the age of forty to conceive for the first time and give birth to healthy infants.

Much research has been focused on the initial stages of pregnancy and infertility. Techniques have been developed to circumvent damaged Fallopian tubes. In the procedure called in vitro fertilization, a woman is given hormones to induce ovulation. Several mature eggs are removed from her ovaries and fertilized in a glass dish. The resulting blastocysts are then implanted into the woman's uterus. In some cases, in which a woman is unable to carry the fetus herself, a surrogate mother has been used as an "incubator" for the embryo. Unused embryos fertilized in vitro are stored in a deep freeze and may be thawed for future use. Early embryos have been separated into individual cells, which then develop into genetically identical blastocysts, each with the potential to become an infant. These technological advances have raised a host of ethical questions concerning disposal of the embryos and their genetic manipulation.

Human reproductive research is focused on the reversal or circumvention of infertility, the alleviation of maternal and fetal distress, and the prenatal detection and treatment of genetic disease. The knowledge gained about reproduction serves to enhance a sense of awe and wonder at the beauty and complexity of the gestational process.

—*Muneeza Khan, MD, FAAFP*

See also: Abortion; Amniocentesis; Assisted reproductive technologies; Birth defects; Blurred vision; Breast-feeding; Cesarean section; Childbirth; Childbirth complications; Chorionic villus sampling; Conception; Contraception; Ectopic pregnancy; Embryology; Endometriosis; Fetal surgery; Gamete intrafallopian transfer (GIFT); Genetic counseling; Genetic diseases; Genital disorders, female; Gestational diabetes; Gynecology; In vitro fertilization; Infertility, female; Infertility, male; Mastitis; Menstruation; Miscarriage; Multiple births; Ovaries; Pap test; Placenta; Postpartum depression; Preeclampsia and eclampsia; Premature birth; Reproductive system; Sexual differentiation; Sperm banks; Stem cells; Sterilization; Stillbirth; Teratogens; Toxemia; Tubal ligation; Ultrasonography; Umbilical cord; Uterus; Women's health.

For Further Information:
Cunningham, F. Gary, et al., editors. *Williams Obstetrics*. 23rd ed., McGraw-Hill, 2010.
Curtis, Glade B., and Judith Schuler. *Your Pregnancy Week-by-Week*. 6th ed., Da Capo Press, 2008.
Eisenberg, Arlene, Heidi E. Murkoff, and Sandee E. Hathaway. *What to Expect When You're Expecting*. 4th ed., Workman, 2009.
Hales, Dianne, and Timothy R. B. Johnson. *Intensive Caring: New Hope for High-Risk Pregnancy*. Crown, 1990.
Harris, A. Christine. *The Pregnancy Journal: A Day-to-Day Guide to a Healthy and Happy Pregnancy*. Chronicle Books, 2009.
Hotchner, Tracie. *Pregnancy and Childbirth*. Rev. ed., Quill/HarperCollins, 2003.
Lees, Christoph, Karina Reynolds, and Grainne McCarten. *Pregnancy and Birth: Your Questions Answered*. Rev. ed., DK, 2007.
Moore, Keith L., and T. V. N. Persaud. *The Developing Human*. 8th ed., Saunders/Elsevier, 2008.
Morales, Karla, and Charles B. Inlander. *Take This Book to the Obstetrician with You: A Consumer's Guide to Pregnancy and Childbirth*. Rev. ed., St. Martin's Press, 1998.
Murkoff, Heidi, and Sharon Mazel. *What to Expect When You're Expecting*. Workman Publishing Company, 2008.
"Neonatal Abstinence Syndrome." *MedlinePlus*, medlineplus.gov/ency/article/007313.htm.
Nilsson, Lennart. *A Child Is Born*. Text by Lars Hamberger. Translated by Clare James. 5th ed., Jonathan Cape, 2009.
"Prenatal Cell-Free DNA Screening." *MedlinePlus*, medlineplus.gov/lab-tests/prenatal-cell-free-dna-screening.
Simkin, Penny, April Bolding, Ann Keppler, and Janelle Durham. *Pregnancy, Childbirth, and the Newborn: The Complete Guide*. Meadowbrook Press, 2010.
Tsiaras, Alexander, and Barry Werth. *From Conception to Birth: A Life Unfolds*. Doubleday, 2002.
Van Katwijk, C., and L. L. H. Peeters. "Clinical Aspects of Pregnancy After the Age of 35 Years: A Review of the Literature." *Human Reproduction Update*, vol. 4, no. 2, Mar.-Apr. 1998, pp. 185-94.

PREGNANCY TEST

Category: Procedure
Anatomy or system affected: Reproductive system
Specialties and related fields: Endocrinology, obstetrics and gynecology
Key terms:
false negative: a test result that incorrectly indicates that the individual is not pregnant
false positive: a test result that incorrectly indicates that the individual is pregnant
human chorionic gonadotropin (hCG): a glycoprotein hormone similar in structure to luteinizing hormone that is secreted by the placenta during early pregnancy to maintain corpus luteum function and is commonly tested as an indicator of pregnancy

INDICATIONS AND PROCEDURES

Pregnancy tests are a fast, inexpensive, and accurate way to assess whether or not a woman is pregnant. Pregnancy occurs when a sperm fertilizes an egg after sexual intercourse. The newly fertilized egg implants in the uterus wall about 6-12 days after fertilization. This implantation causes a hormone called human chorionic gonadotropin (hCG) to be released. After implantation, hCG continues to be released by the placenta triggering other physiological changes throughout pregnancy. It can be detected in the blood and urine of a pregnant woman. It is not present in males or non-pregnant females, making the test very reliable.

HCG is the basis for pregnancy tests available over the counter in most drugstores and medical settings. Pregnancy tests can reliably detect the presence of hCG 1-2 weeks after the first missed period. It is possible to detect the presence of hCG sooner. However, the test results may be less accurate with higher false-negative rates. Pregnancy tests may detect hCG about three weeks after sexual intercourse for women without regular menstrual cycles.

Pregnancy tests usually come in the form of a stick, strip, or cassette. The test is usually performed by urinating on the stick/strip or dropping urine into a reservoir on the cassette. There are also electronic forms available. Each of these methods contains antibodies designed specifically to target hCG. In the presence of hCG, these antibodies bind the hormone and undergo a chemical reaction to turn blue. If hCG is detected, this means the test is positive for pregnancy.

While most pregnancy tests detect hCG in urine, other tests can detect hCG in the blood. HCG can be detected in the blood about one week after ovulation, sooner than urine. The blood test is also less conve-

Image via iStock/FotoDuets. [Used under license.]

nient as it requires getting blood drawn in a medical center. It usually takes longer to obtain these results. Usually, the urine hCG test is preferred in medical settings unless there are other indications for a blood test to verify the results.

USES AND COMPLICATIONS

There are several ways to perform a pregnancy test, depending on the brand of the test. Some of the common ways to perform pregnancy tests are: urinating directly onto a stick or strip, dipping the strip into a cup of urine, or using a dropper to drop urine onto a cassette. Usually, after applying the urine, the reaction takes a few minutes to complete and display the results. In most tests, if hCG is present, the antibodies will bind and turn blue, which are visualized in the form of a line or a cross. Electronic pregnancy tests may also display "pregnant" or "not pregnant." The readings may vary depending on the brand of the test, so be sure to read and follow the directions provided.

HCG pregnancy tests are most accurate starting one week after a missed period. They may detect pregnancy earlier, but the results may be less accurate. There will be a higher false-negative rate because it takes time for hCG levels to build up to a detectable range after its initial release. There is evidence suggesting that digital pregnancy tests may be easier to use and more accurate for early home pregnancy tests than strips or cassettes.

While pregnancy tests are generally reported to be 99% accurate, it is possible to obtain false-positive or false-negative results. False-positive results may be due to pregnancy loss soon after implantation in the uterine lining, hCG-containing medications (e.g., fertility drugs), or medical problems with the ovaries. False negatives, as mentioned above, may be due to taking the test too soon after fertilization. HCG levels increase over time, so if an initial pregnancy test is negative, rechecking in 1-2 weeks may improve the accuracy of results. Checking the strip too early before the antibody reaction can fully develop or using dilute urine may also cause false-negative results. Urine is most concentrated in the morning, so tests taken first thing in the morning may be slightly more accurate. Suppose you have mixed positive and negative results. In that case, you may need to follow up with a health care provider to obtain a blood test or an ultrasound to verify pregnancy.

—*Kathleen Chung, BA*

For Further Information:

Doing a Pregnancy Test. National Health Service, 9 Feb. 2022, www.nhs.uk/pregnancy/trying-for-a-baby/doing-a-pregnanc y-test/. Accessed 9 Apr. 2022.

ELISA for Home Pregnancy Test. Elisa Support and Products, n.d., 27 Oct. 2017, www.elisa-antibody.com/ELISA-applications/home-pregnancy-test.html. Accessed 9 Apr. 2022.

Knowing if You are Pregnant. Office on Women's Health in the Office of the Assistant Secretary for Health at the U.S. Department of Health and Human Services, 30 Jan. 2019, www.womenshealth.gov/pregnancy/you-get-pregnant/know ing-if-you-are-pregnant. Accessed 9 Apr. 2022.

Smith, Lori. "Pregnancy tests: All you need to know." *MedicalNewsToday,* 24 May 2017, www.medicalnewstoday.com/articles/295001. Accessed 9 Apr. 2022.

When to Take a Pregnancy Test. Clearblue, 9 Mar. 2022, www.clearblue.com/pregnancy-tests/early-pregnancy-testing. Accessed 9 Apr. 2022.

PREMATURE (PRETERM) BIRTH

Category: Disease/Disorder

Anatomy or system affected: Fetus, nervous system, reproductive system, respiratory system

Specialties and related fields: Critical care, neonatology, pediatrics, perinatology

Definition: a birth that occurs more than three weeks before the baby's estimated due date.

Key terms:

antenatal steroids: medications given to pregnant women expecting preterm delivery; they have been shown to reduce the morbidity and mortality of hyaline membrane disease

cervical cerclage: the process of encircling a cervix with sutures or synthetic tape that is abnormally liable to dilate (an incompetent cervix) with a ring or loop to prevent a miscarriage

cone biopsy: a biopsy to remove abnormal tissues high in the cervical canal; called a cope biopsy because a cone-shaped wedge of tissue is removed for examination

fetal fibronectin: a protein produced by fetal cells; found at the interface of the fetal sac and the uterine lining; it can be thought of as an adhesive or "biological glue" that binds the fetal sac to the uterine lining; when it starts "leaking" into the vagina it indicates a possible preterm delivery

necrotizing enterocolitis: the death of tissue in the intestine; occurs most often in premature or sick babies

prostaglandins: cyclic fatty acids with varying hormone-like effects, notably the promotion of uterine contractions

transvaginal ultrasound (TVUS): a test used to look at a woman's uterus, ovaries, tubes, cervix, and pelvic area; the ultrasound probe is placed inside the vagina

CAUSES AND INDICATIONS

Labor is defined as cervical change with contractions. Premature or preterm birth is defined as delivery before 37 weeks of gestation. However, most premature babies are born between 34 and 37 weeks. In the US, about 10% of all pregnancies are preterm, reaching as high as 14% among African American women. The rate has increased in recent years, which may be due to the increasing number of multiple births—the risk of prematurity increases with multiple babies vying for space and resources during the same gestation.

Term pregnancy is important for a baby's outcome—it allows for important organs to develop and prevents serious complications from occurring fully. Preterm birth does not have a single, identifiable cause but multiple potential causes, and some are not very well understood. The risk factors discussed below put a mother at higher risk of preterm birth but do not guarantee that a baby will not have a term gestation (37-40 weeks). Often, preterm birth can be out of the hands of the mother and physician; some genetic mutations lead to conditions that naturally lead to premature birth or are incompatible with life. Prenatal care is very important in identifying potential risk factors and optimizing a baby's early development. Establishing care early on can also lead to genetic counseling if abnormalities are found.

If frequent contractions happen between 24-34 weeks and the cervical change is minimal (<3 cm) or cervical length is between 20-30mm on transvaginal ultrasound (TVUS), a physician may opt to do a fetal fibronectin test (fFN). This test has an excellent negative predictive value. There is a 99% chance of no delivery for one week if it is negative. Other important parts of a workup include taking a detailed history (identifying risk factors), doing a complete physical exam, ordering appropriate labs looking for blood/electrolyte abnormalities and sexually transmitted infections, and determining the baby's condition at presentation.

RISK FACTORS AND COMPLICATIONS

Common risk factors include previous preterm delivery, low socioeconomic status, smoking during pregnancy, uterine anomaly, history of cervical procedures (e.g., cone biopsy), sexually transmitted infections (STIs), and preterm premature rupture of membranes (membranes rupturing before the onset of labor before 37 weeks). Chorioamnionitis is a clinical condition that can increase the risk of preterm labor. An intrauterine infection leads to an inflammatory reaction in the mother's body. The inflammation then initiates a cascade that increases the concentration of prostaglandins circulating in the blood. Prostaglandins are known for stimulating uterine contractions. Metalloproteases, another product of the inflammatory cascade, can ripen the cervix, leading to membrane rupture. As previously mentioned, each additional baby in multiple gestations increases the risk of prematurity. The incidence of multiple gestations is increasing due to the popularity of assisted reproductive techniques (ART) and increasing maternal age (associated with higher rates of multiple gestations).

It is not surprising that premature birth is the leading cause of death worldwide for children under five years old. Problems arise when babies aren't given enough time to develop fully. Therefore, conditions associated with preterm birth like respiratory distress syndrome (RDS), intraventricular hemorrhage (IVH), and retinopathy of immaturity (ROP) occur when the lungs, brain, or eyes, respectively, are immature and could have benefited from a couple of more weeks of development. Cerebral palsy is another neurologic condition closely tied with premature birth, especially if the baby is born before 32 weeks. Necrotizing enterocolitis can happen in any neonate, but this condition is commonly associated with prematurity due to an underdeveloped immune system and reduced oxygen and blood flow. These complications increase a neonate's morbidity significantly and can have permanent consequences.

PROGNOSIS

The long-term outlook partly depends on how early the baby is born. Late-preterm babies born between 34

Baby girl born at 6th month of pregnancy, weighting only 650g at a time in NICU. Image via iStock/IvanJekic. [Used under license.]

and 37 weeks have the highest survival rate among preterm births but still, have a higher risk of developing the complications above than a term baby. Birth weights in the late-preterm cohort are comparable to term pregnancy weight (about 8 pounds), differing by two pounds or less. A baby is considered to have low birth weight if it weighs less than 5 pounds 8 ounces, which can occur if a baby is born prematurely (before 34 weeks) or there has been some restriction in its growth (e.g., placental insufficiency). Low birth weight means a baby will have a harder time keeping warm due to less body fat and can sometimes have problems gaining weight and eating. Their immune system immaturity also puts them at risk of infection. Oxygenation is a concern if they have RDS due to small underdeveloped lungs.

Prognosis is also affected by the outcomes of the complications a premature baby deals with after birth. Suppose the child suffers from intraventricular hemorrhage most of the time. In that case, the complication will resolve with minimal impact. Still, there are cases where the bleeding can lead to irreversible brain damage. Ninety percent of babies with ROP fall in the "mild" category and do not require treatment. However, those with the more severe types can develop blindness or serious vision problems later, such as myopia, strabismus, glaucoma, and retinal detachment. Suppose a premature baby develops bronchopulmonary dysplasia (BPD) after having RDS for an extended period. In that case, the child can see a long-term decrease in pulmonary function compared to a term baby. BPD can lead to a chronic cough and increased air trapping, leading to problems with airflow and oxygenation. This airway obstruction can limit a child's level of physical activity.

PREVENTION
Administering antenatal steroids is one of the most important interventions that can be done for a premature baby—it improves survival rates by decreasing the risk of several complications. Studies have found that before 28 weeks of gestation, steroids can help reduce the rate of IVH. After 28 weeks, it can help rapidly mature a baby's lungs, giving it a better shot at reducing pulmonary distress. It also dramatically decreases the rate of NEC. Suppose there are indications of imminent preterm labor before 34 weeks. In that case, a physician may consider giving a tocolytic agent or a drug to delay labor to give the steroids for at least 48 hours to continue the maturation of the lungs before delivery.

Antibiotics (e.g., penicillin) are also important for preventing the transmission of neonatal group B streptococcus (GBS). This common bacterium can lead to meningitis and sepsis in a neonate. Magnesium sulfate is given before 32 weeks for potential fetal neuroprotection against cerebral palsy. If there have been prior preterm births or a prior second-trimester loss, the use of progesterone can be considered from 16-36 weeks to prevent contractions and promote the pregnancy. Suppose there is cervical insufficiency, sometimes from prior cervical procedures. In that case, cervical cerclage may be placed at around 12 to 14 weeks early in pregnancy to prevent miscarriage and delay delivery to 37 weeks.

CONCLUSION
Premature birth is complex, and each gestation is unique. Studies and statistics can only tell a mother and her medical team what to look for and implement optimization strategies that aren't foolproof. Controlling for smoking and diabetes, monitoring maternal and fetal vital signs, and curing STIs can reduce risk factors for premature birth but do not guarantee that it will not occur. That is why establishing prenatal care and developing a close relationship with a medical provider is so important: to help troubleshoot problems along the way and assist with parent education. There is a natural psychological toll on parents who have premature babies. It will be important to look after the neonate and check-in with parents who may experience stages of grief if they are informed of their child's prematurity. Parent education early on in gestation is key so that parents can prepare for the unexpected and talk about different scenarios should they happen. The more knowledge acquired, the better parents can deal with difficult situations and execute treatment plans to help their baby grow. Mothers of premature babies may be more susceptible to experiencing birthing trauma and perinatal mood or anxiety disorders. Due to the increased stress of having a premature baby, these mothers may need additional mental health support. They should be assessed frequently by medical and mental health professionals.

—*Brian A. Campos, BA*

For Further Information:
Premature Baby. Pregnancy, birth & baby, Nov. 2019, www.pregnancybirthbaby.org.au/premature-baby. Accessed 9 Apr. 2022.
Premature Babies. March of Dimes, Oct. 2019, www.marchofdimes.org/complications/premature-babies.aspx. Accessed 9 Apr. 2022.
Premature Babies. MedlinePlus, 25 Mar. 2022, medlineplus.gov/prematurebabies.html. Accessed 9 Apr. 2022.
Premature Birth. Mayo Clinic, 14 Apr. 2021, www.mayoclinic.org/diseases-conditions/premature-birth/symptoms-causes/syc-20376730. Accessed 9 Apr. 2022.
Prematurity. Stanford Children's Health, n.d., www.stanfordchildrens.org/en/topic/default?id=prematurity-90-P02401. Accessed 9 Apr. 2022.

Preterm Birth. Centers for Disease Control and Prevention, 1 Nov. 2021, www.cdc.gov/reproductivehealth/features/premature-birth/index.html. Accessed 9 Apr. 2022.

PREMENSTRUAL SYNDROME (PMS)

Category: Disease/Disorder
Also known as: Menstrually related mood disorder (MRMD), premenstrual tension, late luteal phase disorder (LLPD), premenstrual dysphoric disorder (PMDD)
Anatomy or system affected: Endocrine system, gastrointestinal system, reproductive system
Specialties and related fields: Endocrinology, obstetrics and gynecology, psychiatry, sleep studies
Key terms:
endorphins: hormones, found mainly in the brain, that bind to opiate receptors, reducing the sensation of pain and affecting emotions
luteal phase: the second half of the menstrual cycle after ovulation; during this phase, the corpus luteum secretes progesterone
menses: the monthly flow of blood and cellular debris from the uterus that begins at puberty in women
premenstrual dysphoric disorder (PMDD): a severe form of premenstrual syndrome characterized by affective symptoms causing significant disturbances in relationships or social adaptation
progesterone: a hormone produced in the ovary that prepares and maintains the uterus for pregnancy
serotonin: a neurotransmitter involved in sleep, depression, and memory

CAUSES AND SYMPTOMS

Several causes of premenstrual syndrome (PMS) have been proposed. Changes in hormone levels during the luteal phase of the menstrual cycle, when the ovaries are making progesterone, may deplete neurotransmitters such as enkephalins and endorphins, which are responsible for a sense of well-being; gamma-aminobutyric acid (GABA), which aids in relaxation; and serotonin, which stimulates the central nervous system. The disorder may be more likely to occur in women who have enhanced sensitivity to progesterone, a disposition related to serotonin deficiency. PMS may be related to excess prostaglandin, a hormone-like substance that may affect blood pressure and metabolism and smooth muscle activity. Some evidence suggests that women with PMS have lower blood levels of allopregnanolone, a by-product of progesterone that plays a role in mood.

Up to 85 percent of women experience mild to moderate forms of PMS. Another 5 percent of women have symptoms so severe that they interfere with daily

> **INFORMATION ON PREMENSTRUAL SYNDROME (PMS)**
>
> **Causes:** Unknown; possibly depletion of neurotransmitters resulting from hormonal changes and sensitivities
> **Symptoms:** Physical (fatigue, headache, breast tenderness and swelling, back and abdominal pain, muscle and joint pain, weight gain, water retention, acne, nausea, palpitations); behavioral (insomnia, dizziness, changes in sex drive, cravings for salty or sweet food, increased appetite); psychological (irritability, anger, depression, anxiety, mood swings, lack of concentration, confusion, forgetfulness, restlessness, decreased self-esteem)
> **Duration:** Often chronic with acute episodes
> **Treatments:** Patient education; exercise; adequate sleep; stress avoidance; dietary changes (increased complex carbohydrates, decreased sodium and caffeine); vitamin E supplements; calcium carbonate supplements; diuretics (spironolactone); antianxiety medications (benzodiazepines); selective serotonin reuptake inhibitors; hormonal therapy (Gonadotropin-releasing hormone agonists, oral contraceptives); Non-steroidal anti-inflammatory drugs (NSAIDs)

activity and may be diagnosed with premenstrual dysphoric disorder (PMDD). In some women, symptoms of PMS increase with age, perhaps because serotonin levels are altered with changes in estrogen levels.

PMS symptoms can be subdivided into physical, behavioral, and psychological. Physical symptoms include fatigue; headache; breast tenderness and swelling; back and abdominal pain; acne; heart palpitations; bloating; weight gain; nausea; muscle and joint pain; water retention; swelling of ankles, feet, and hands; and decreased tolerance to noise or light. Behavioral symptoms include fatigue, insomnia, dizziness, changes in sex drive, cravings for salty or sweet food, and increased appetite. Psychological symptoms include irritability, anger, depressed mood, crying, anxiety, tension, mood swings, and lack of concentration, confusion, forgetfulness, restlessness, loneliness, decreased self-esteem, and tension. The symptoms of depression, anxiety disorders, perimenopause, and thyroid dysfunction are similar to PMS.

A distinguishing feature of PMS is its cyclic occurrence. Researchers at the University of California, San Diego suggests the following criteria for diagnosing premenstrual syndrome: At least one psychological (affective) and physical (somatic) symptom occurs during the five to seven days before menses in each of the previous three cycles, and symptoms are relieved during days four through thirteen of the menstrual cycle. The National Institute of Mental Health and the American Psychiatric Association give similar diagnostic criteria. Blood tests are not necessary for the diagnosis of PMS. Laboratory studies such as a blood count or thyroid function tests may be recommended to screen for other medical conditions that cause fatigue, such as anemia and thyroid disease.

TREATMENT AND THERAPY

Treatment for premenstrual syndrome can be divided into three categories: non-pharmacologic therapy, dietary supplementation, and pharmacologic therapy.

Non-pharmacologic therapies include patient education, supportive therapy, and behavioral interventions. Women who receive educational materials about PMS may gain an increased sense of control and relief of symptoms. Supportive therapies include relaxation and cognitive-behavioral therapy. A therapist may also be able to teach coping methods. Behavioral interventions include keeping a daily symptom diary. Each day for three months, a woman records in a diary and ranks any health complaints on a scale of "none at all" to "extreme." The PMS pattern is an increase in symptoms during the fourteen days before menstruation and then a decrease in symptoms within one hour to a few days after bleeding begins.

In addition to keeping the diary, exercising thirty minutes a day (to stimulate the release of enkephalins and endorphins and to reduce swelling through sweat), sleeping six to eight hours every night, avoiding stress, and making dietary changes may help symptoms. Increasing the intake of complex carbohydrates (fruits, vegetables, and whole grains) may relieve mood-related symptoms by boosting the level of tryptophan, a precursor of serotonin. Lowering sodium intake can reduce bloating, fluid retention, and swelling. Restricting caffeine consumption may reduce irritability and insomnia. Vitamin E supplements may reduce breast pain. Vitamin E as a dietary supplement is also a potentially beneficial antioxidant and poses minimal risk. Calcium carbonate supplementation may also improve PMS symptoms.

Nonprescription drugs, such as diuretics for bloating and analgesics for pain, may diminish the symptoms of PMS. Prescription treatments for PMS include anti-anxiety medication such as the benzodiazepines, which mimic the effects of GABA to relieve irritability; selective serotonin reuptake inhibitors (SSRIs), which increase serotonin levels; hormone treatments such as gonadotropin-releasing hormone (GnRH) agonists and birth control pills that stop the production of estrogen and progesterone;

spironolactone, a diuretic that relieves breast tenderness and fluid retention; and non-steroidal anti-inflammatory drugs (NSAIDs), or prostaglandin inhibitors, for pain such as headache.

Some treatments that have no proven benefit in relieving the symptoms of PMS include: Progesterone, antidepressant drugs such as Tricyclic Antidepressants (TCA), Monoamine Oxidase Inhibitors (MAOI), lithium, and popular dietary supplements such as evening primrose oil, essential free fatty acids, and ginkgo biloba.

PERSPECTIVE AND PROSPECTS

Hysteria (literally, "wandering womb") was described in Egypt in about 1900 BCE as an abnormality of the uterus caused by its "migration" to different parts of the body, resulting in various symptoms, such as headache and swollen feet. The term "premenstrual tension" was first used by mental health professionals in the 1930s.

Research on PMS gained momentum in the 1980s.Whereas only one article on PMS appeared in 1964, 425 articles were published on the topic between 1988 and 1989. What had once been considered a pseudocondition, with PMS as a catchall phrase for up to 150 symptoms occurring before menstruation, was recognized as a medical disorder. Research has focused on biomedical and psychosocial causes and treatments.

—*Elizabeth Marie McGhee Nelson, PhD, Uzma Shahzad, MD, and Christi N. Gandham, DO*

For Further Information:
Eske, Jamie. "What to Know About Premenstrual Syndrome (PMS)." *MedicalNewsToday*, 29 May 2019, www.medicalnewstoday.com/articles/325314#outlook. Accessed 9 Apr. 2022.
Higuera, Valencia, Raypole, Crystal. "PMS: Premenstrual Syndrome Symptoms, Treatments, and More." *Healthline*, 28 Jan. 2022, www.healthline.com/health/premenstrual-syndrome. Accessed 9 Apr. 2022.
Premenstrual Syndrome (PMS). American College of Obstetricians and Gynecologists, Oct. 2020, www.acog.org/womens-health/faqs/premenstrual-syndrome. Accessed 9 Apr. 2022.
Premenstrual Syndrome (PMS). familydoctor.org, 28 Sept. 2020, familydoctor.org/condition/premenstrual-syndrome-pms/. Accessed 9 Apr. 2022.
Premenstrual Syndrome (PMS). Mayo Clinic, 25 Feb. 2022, www.mayoclinic.org/diseases-conditions/premenstrual-syndrome/symptoms-causes/syc-20376780. Accessed 9 Apr.
Premenstrual Syndrome (PMS). Office on Women's Health in the Office of the Assistant Secretary for Health at the U.S. Department of Health and Human Services, 16 Mar. 2018, www.womenshealth.gov/menstrual-cycle/premenstrual-syndrome. Accessed 9 Apr. 2022.

PRESBYOPIA

Category: Disease/Disorder
Anatomy or system affected: Eyes, visual system
Specialties and related fields: Ophthalmology, optometry
Definition: Presbyopia is an age-related eye condition that causes progressive difficulty seeing objects at near distances.

Presbyopia (prez-bee-OH-pee-ah) refers to an eye condition that makes it difficult to see close objects. The word presbyopia comes from Greek words meaning, "to see like an old person." It is a natural part of the aging process that usually becomes noticeable between the ages of forty and fifty. The condition is normal, common, and unpreventable. It results from age-related changes to the lens of the eye that cause difficulty focusing on objects at close distances. People with presbyopia often hold books at arm's length to read them and find it challenging to see fine print in dim lighting. Glasses, contacts, and surgery can compensate for presbyopia, but there is no known way to prevent it.

CAUSES AND SYMPTOMS

Normal vision occurs when light rays enter the eye through the clear outer layer called the cornea. Light rays travel through the pupil, the black area at the center of the eye, and through the lens behind it. The lens is a transparent structure that changes shape to bend or refract light rays so they can be focused on the retina at the back of the eye. In order for clear images to be formed, light must be directly focused on the retina so that light-sensing nerve cells can transmit electrical impulses to the brain to be interpreted. Light that is focused behind or in front of the retina will be perceived as blurry.

As part of normal aging, the crystalline material of the lens hardens and becomes less flexible. The lens also continues to grow with age, making it more difficult for muscles surrounding the lens to change its shape. As a result, the lens becomes less effective at focusing light rays. The lens focuses light behind the retina instead of directly on it, producing a fuzzy image.

The changes that cause presbyopia develop gradually over time. People as young as thirty-five may find it harder to read fine print on labels or menus in a darkened restaurant. People with presbyopia often hold books at arm's length to read them or experience eyestrain when reading for long periods of time. People also notice blurred vision when switching from distance to near viewing. These problems are worse in dim light and can lead to headaches.

The most common risk factor for presbyopia is age; nearly everyone over the age of forty will develop the condition on some level. Some diseases can increase the risk of developing presbyopia before the age of forty-known as premature presbyopia-including diabetes, cardiovascular disease, and multiple sclerosis. Drugs such as antihistamines, diuretics, and antidepressants also can cause premature presbyopia. There is no known way to prevent presbyopia from developing.

Although presbyopia is a normal process of aging, people generally seek help when vision impairment affects their ability to work or enjoy everyday activities. An eye doctor can diagnose the condition during a general eye exam. During the exam, the physician will determine whether the symptoms are caused by presbyopia or another refractive eye condition such as hyperopia, myopia, or astigmatism, or abnormalities in other structures of the eye such as the cornea or retina. Components of the exam may include a visual acuity test, refraction test to measure glasses or contacts prescription, slit lamp examination, or dilated retinal exam. Presbyopia can occur in conjunction with other eye conditions, but a complete eye exam ensures that the correct treatment will be prescribed.

TREATMENT AND THERAPY

Many people who experience presbyopia correct it easily with reading glasses. These "readers" provide additional focusing strength to compensate for the loss of lens refraction during close work such as reading or sewing. Readers are readily available at many retail and convenience stores in a variety of price ranges and strengths. When selecting readers, people are recommended to choose the weakest strength that allows them to read without strain. Charts are often on display near readers to assist with this choice. Reading glasses may also be purchased from an eye doctor, who will ensure that they are the correct strength.

Whether purchased by prescription or over the counter, reading glasses may be worn over contact lenses to correct presbyopia and any other refractive error. In addition, bifocal and trifocal glasses are available to correct two or more problems with one pair of glasses. These types of lenses have one part powered for distance vision and another part for close vision.

Contact lenses also can be prescribed to allow multifocal vision. These lenses are weighted so that the prescription for distance viewing is in place when gazing out and the prescription for close vision is in place when looking down. Another option for contact lens wearers is to wear one contact with a prescription that corrects for distance vision while the other corrects for close work. In time, the brain adapts to choose the correct eye for the task at hand. This technique is known as monovision. Regardless of the method of correction chosen, corrective lenses need to be adjusted over time to compensate for additional changes to the eye from the aging process.

Presbyopia may also be corrected by surgical procedures collectively known as refractive surgery. LASIK surgery, which uses a laser to reshape the clear surface of eye, can be used to induce monovision, with one eye correcting for distance and the other correcting for close work. Future enhancements to the procedure may result in laser surgery that will create multifocal corrections, much like built-in bifocals. Conductive keratoplasty (CK) uses radio waves to adjust the curve of the cornea and can improve close vision, but its effects are temporary. Artificial lenses implanted into the cornea called corneal inlays are being studied as a way of providing additional refraction. Finally, surgically replacing the natural lens with an artificial one using techniques from cataract surgery can provide multiple focal lengths to minimize the focusing error caused by presbyopia. Further research is still being done to refine these techniques and develop new ways of correcting presbyopia.

—*Claudine Yee, ScB*

For Further Information:

"How the Eye Works as a Camera." *American Macular Degeneration Foundation.* Web. www.macular.org/eye-camera

"Eye Exams 101." *American Academy of Ophthalmology,* 25 May 2012. Web. www.aao.org/eye-health/tips-prevention/eye-exams-101

Boyd, Kierstan. "What Is Presbyopia?" *American Academy of Ophthalmology,* 1 Sep 2016. Web. www.aao.org/eye-health/tips -prevention/what-is-presbyopia

"Facts about Presbyopia." *National Eye Institute,* Oct 2010. Web. nei.nih.gov/health/errors/presbyopia

"Presbyopia." *Mayo* Clinic, 17 Oct 2014. Web. www.mayo clinic.org/diseases-conditions/presbyopia/basics/ definition/con-20032261

Boyd, Kierstan. "Presbyopia Treatment." *American Academy of Ophthalmology,* 1 Sep 2016. Web. www.aao.org/eye-health /diseases/presbyopia-treatment

Papadopoulos, Pandelis A and Papadopoulos, Alexandros P. "Current Management of Presbyopia." *Middle East African Journal of Ophthalmology.* 2014 Jan-Mar; 21(1): 10-17. www.ncbi. nlm.nih.gov/pmc/articles/PMC395903

PREVENTIVE MEDICINE

Category: Specialty
Anatomy or system affected: All
Specialties and related fields: All
Definition: The medical field that seeks to protect, promote, and maintain the health and well-being of individuals and defined populations and to prevent disease, disability, and premature death.

Key terms:

aerospace medicine: the medical specialty concerned with the health of the operating crews and passengers of air and space vehicles, together with support personnel

environmental medicine: the branch of medical science that addresses the impact of chemical and physical stressors and biological hazards on the individual or group in a community

epidemiology: the study of the incidence endence, distribution and determinants of disease in populations; includes attributes, such as gender, age, race, occupation, and social factors; and characteristics of disease, including but not limited to risk factors, incubation, infectivity, and chronicity

incidence: the number of new illnesses or newly diagnosed cases of disease, or events occurring within a specified period of time in a specific population

occupationalmedicine: a medical specialty focused on providing all levels of preventive medical services to working men and women in order to preserve, maintain, or restore health and well-being

prevalence: the actual number of individuals or live cases at a particular time with a disease or a given characteristic of a disease

public health: the well-being of humankind, both as a community and as individuals, accomplished by using scientific skills and beliefs that assist in health maintenance and health improvement

risk factors: the situations, circumstances, or conditions that increase the probability of the occurrence of disease or accident

SCIENCE AND PROFESSION

Modern preventive medicine is considered to exist at three levels within the health-care community. The initial level also known as primary prevention, has as its purpose to maintain health by removing the causes of or by protecting the community or individual from agents of disease and injury. These activities are no longer limited to the prevention of infection; yet they now include improvement in the environment and behavioral changes to reduce risk factors that contribute to chronic disease and injury. Examples of primary prevention are immunization programs. Other examples include risk reduction. For example, to reduce the risk of heart attack, one should refrain from smoking, be active, and reduce dietary fat intake-all wise primary prevention actions. Environmental risk reduction includes halting the loss of atmospheric ozone, reducing air and water pollution, and developing environmentally friendly technologies.

Secondary prevention seeks to detect and correct subclinical, adverse health conditions before they become manifest as disease, by reversing, halting, or retarding the disease process. A frequently used secondary prevention technique is health screening. Examples of secondary prevention aimed at detecting disease and early pathological changes include blood pressure measurement for hypertension (high blood pressure), fasting blood sugar screening for diabetes, mammography for breast cancer, PSA levels that detect prostate cancer, and glaucoma screening. In industry, a hearing test is used as a tool to prevent noise-induced hearing loss among the workforce. Once a potential health problem is identified, clinical preventive medicine techniques can be instituted to reverse the condition or prevent further progression.

Tertiary prevention attempts to minimize the adverse effects of conferred disease and disability. Coronary bypass surgery, vocational rehabilitation following a cerebrovascular accident (CVA), and treatment of an incapacitating mental illness are examples.

Specialists in the field of preventive medicine typically focus their efforts within the paradigms of primary and secondary prevention. In epidemiological terms, primary prevention results in a reduction of the incidence of a disease (the new cases occurring over time). Secondary prevention, on the other hand, results in a reduction of the prevalence of a disease (the number of actual people suffering from a particular illness at a given point in time).

Most health providers practice some degree of preventive medicine services. Pediatricians and pediatric nurse practitioners are practicing preventive medicine when they conduct "well-baby evaluations" and ensure that immunizations are current. Family medicine and primary care providers are promoting such services when they perform Pap testing or order mammograms. When smoking cessation is discussed as part of a clinical management plan and health care providers prescribe nicotine-patch regimens, that too is preventive medicine.

In the United States, approximately one thousand physicians specialize in general preventive medicine. Some use epidemiological methods to design and develop prevention programs that may feature a single intervention or may constitute a strategy that includes a multitude or matrix of screening technologies and interventions. Other preventive-medicine specialists including physician assistants and advanced practice nurses, provide services in a clinical setting by ordering a history and physical examination, which may include age- and gender-specific screening tests. The clinical preventive medicine specialist then can counsel the patient on lifestyle alterations recommended to preserve or improve health.

Within the United States, another field in preventive medicine is occupational medicine. Practicing in industry or private clinic settings, specialists in this field are concerned about preventing injury and illness as a result of the physical, biological, and chemical hazards that are present in the workplace. Should workers be injured or made ill as a result of their employment, the occupational health providers manage their treatment, rehabilitation, and return to work. Aerospace medicine providers limit their practice to those involved in the aeronautical and space transportation fields, including flight crews, support personnel, and passengers. The major task of these providers is to protect this population group from the adverse environmental conditions of flight, including pressure changes, reduced availability of oxygen, thermal stressors, accelerative forces, and psychosocial factors that might compromise performance.

DIAGNOSTIC AND TREATMENT TECHNIQUES

An example of the application of preventive medicine is a comparison of the leading causes of death in the United States in 1900 with those in 2000. There was a major shift from deaths attributable to infectious disease at the beginning of the twentieth century to deaths attributable to chronic diseases that are often a reflection of individual lifestyle. Preventive medicine has proven itself effective in altering both the cause of death and the age at which death occurs. Accompanying this increased shift to chronic diseases such as cancer and heart disease, moreover, is a significant increase in the life expectancy of the population during the same century. Preventive medicine's focus is now on reducing morbidity and mortality from chronic diseases and accidents, particularly those in which an individual's lifestyle increases the risk for illness and death.

Disease prevention and health promotion are the two pillars supporting the discipline of preventive medicine. Beginning in 1987, a consortium was convened to begin to address a preventive medicine strategy to improve the health of Americans. The Institute of Medicine of the National Academy of Sciences worked with the US Public Health Service and numerous organizations to formulate health objective goals to be attained by the beginning of the twenty-first century. Once goals and objectives were established, the next task was to devise methods, technologies, and strategies to achieve the objectives by the year 2000. The resulting report was titled *Healthy People 2000: National Health Promotion and Disease Prevention Objectives* (1991).

The implementation of what was then known about disease prevention and health promotion was the central challenge. Good health is the result of reducing needless disease, injury, and suffering, resulting in an improved quality of life. A strategy of *Healthy People 2000* was to combine scientific knowledge, professional skills, community support, individual commitment, and the public will to achieve good health. This plan required reducing premature death, preventing disability, preserving the physical environment, and enabling Americans to develop healthy lifestyles. Three broad goals were detailed in *Healthy People 2000*: first, increase the healthy life span for Americans; second, reduce health disparity among Americans; and third, achieve access to preventive services for all Americans. A number of examples of the types of programs required to attain these goals were provided.

Tobacco use is the most important single preventable cause of death in the United States, accounting for more than four hundred thousand deaths annually. This loss of life is the equivalent of crashing two commercial jumbo jet airliners filled with passengers every day throughout the year. Smoking is a major risk factor for heart and lung disease; cancer of many organs, including the lungs, pancreas, and bladder; and stomach ulcers. Passive or environmental tobacco smoke is a recognized cause of cancer for exposed nonsmokers, and children in smoke-filled homes experience more ear infections. Tobacco use during pregnancy increases the risk of prematurity and low birth weight.

More than 3 million injuries occur annually in the US private sector, according to the Bureau of Labor Statistics; preliminary reports for 2013 indicate that more than four thousand deaths were attributable to work-related injuries. The occupations with the highest injury rates include mining, construction, agriculture, and transportation. The prevention of occupational disease and injury requires engineering controls, improved work practices, use of physical protective equipment, and monitoring of the work environment to identify emerging chemical and physical hazards.

In 2011 in the United States, nearly 575,000 people died from cancer. Nearly one in three Americans will experience a form of this disease. Research has helped to identify many risk factors related to cancer causation, such as tobacco use, low fiber intake, excess fat intake, sunburn, alcohol use, and exposure to chemical carcinogens. Information, education, and early detection have important roles in reducing both the incidence and the prevalence of cancer. Pap sampling, prostate examinations, mammography, and oral examinations are secondary prevention procedures that allow for early diagnosis and treatment. Such screening procedures, coupled with education and lifestyle changes, have the potential to reduce cancer rates significantly.

Healthy People 2010 (2000), like its predecessors, was developed through a broad consultation process, built on scientific knowledge and designed to measure programs over time. Its two primary goals included helping individuals of all ages increase life expectancy and improve their quality of life and eliminating health disparities among different segments of the population. The healthy life expectancy at birth increased slightly from 2000-1 to 2006-7 from about seventy-seven years of age to about seventy-eight among the overall population. There were no significant changes in health disparity across race and ethnicity in 70 percent of the objective areas. *Healthy People 2020*

Leading Causes of Death in the United States	
1900	2000
1. Pneumonia and influenza	1. Heart diseases
2. Tuberculosis	2. Cancer and other malignant tumors
3. Diarrhea, enteritis, and ulceration of the intestine	3. Strokes
4. Heart diseases	4. Chronic lower respiratory diseases
5. Senility (ill-defined or unknown)	5. Accidents
6. Strokes	6. Diabetes mellitus
7. Nephritis	7. Pneumonia and influenza
8. Accidents	8. Suicide
9. Cancer and other malignant tumors	9. Chronic liver disease and cirrhosis
10. Diphtheria	10. Homicide

includes similar objectives to previous *Healthy People* reports, but also includes several new areas of focus, including adolescent health; lesbian, gay, bisexual, and transgender health; and sleep health. Improvement in health disparities tracked in Quality & Disparities Report 2014 has demonstrated improvement from 2010 to 2015 among uninsured adults from 18-64 years across all racial and ethnic groups and poverty levels (Cohen & Martinez, 2015; Access and Disparities in Access to Health Care, 2016).

Achieving the many objectives of *Healthy People* requires the dedicated commitment of preventive medicine specialists and the broader medical community. Enhanced effectiveness and efficiency of clinical preventive services, screening procedures, immunizations, consultation, and counseling can be achieved only through close relationships between the physician and both the community and the individual. To assess whether the goals and objectives for the prevention of disease and health promotion for the year 2010 were realistic, it would be helpful to review a success in the application of preventive medicine. Many of the objectives for 2010 were not met, but pesticide exposure, for example, was one area that showed marked improvement, from more than twenty-three thousand doctor's office visits in 1998 to less than fifteen thousand in 2008, though the total fell short of the 2010 target of less than twelve thousand visits. Another area in which preventative medicine seemed to be effective was the reduction of adolescent pregnancies, specifically among the black population. In 1996, the rate of pregnancy per one thousand girls between the ages of fifteen and seventeen was about 130; by 2005, the rate was less than eighty.

Coronary artery disease and its resultant heart attacks are preventable. A large national clinical trial of preventive medicine procedures known as MRFIT (multiple risk factor intervention trial) not only demonstrated the value of risk factor reduction in preventing disease but also demonstrated that the impact of established disease could be reversed. A subgroup of the MRFIT population made up of those who had established coronary artery disease at the start of the study had 55 percent fewer fatalities than did the control group when both were followed over seven years.

Preventive medicine interventions are not only cost-effective but relatively inexpensive as well. For example, coronary artery bypass surgery or a heart transplant costs many times more than preventive medicine rehabilitation and lifestyle modification programs. The same advantages also accrue for the prevention of strokes. Reducing salt intake, controlling high blood pressure, correcting obesity, performing regular exercise, and quitting smoking reduce the risk of stroke. The evidence clearly shows that preventive medicine reduces the death rate for heart attack and stroke and enhances quality of life.

Clinical preventive services have been designed based on the best available scientific evidence to promote the health of the individual while remaining practical and cost-effective. The 1989 publication of the *Guide to Clinical Preventive Services* (a document that has been updated several times) by the US Preventive Services Task Force was a major milestone on the road toward reducing premature death and disability. It has been well established that the majority of deaths among Americans under the age of sixty-five are preventable. The guide is the culmination of more than four years of literature review, debate, and synthesis and provides a listing of the clinical preventive services that clinicians should provide their patients. More than one hundred interventions are proposed to prevent sixty different illnesses and medical conditions. The guide is intended to be used by preventive medical specialists and other primary care clinicians. The recommendations are based on a standardized review of current scientific evidence and include a summary of published clinical research regarding the clinical effectiveness of each preventive service.

Although there have been sound clinical reasons for emphasizing prevention in medicine, studies have repeatedly demonstrated that physicians often fail to provide these services. Busy clinicians frequently have inadequate time with the patient to recommend or deliver a range of preventive services. Furthermore, until the publication of this guide, considerable controversy had existed within the medical community as to which services should be offered and how often. In the past, there was skepticism regarding the value of certain preventive interventions and their ability to reduce morbidity or mortality significantly. One result of this review process has been the clear evidence that reducing the incidence and severity of the leading causes of disease and disability is dependent on the personal health practices of individuals. The periodic health examination was once frequently referred to as an annual examination.

The *Guide to Clinical Preventive Services* tailors this examination to the individual needs of the patient and considers factors such as age, gender, and risk. Consequently, a uniform health examination is not recommended. The examination for those between forty and sixty-four years of age is scheduled on a one- to three-year basis, with the more frequent examinations scheduled for those in high-risk groups. Although the examination is not comprehensive, it is focused on identifying the leading causes of illness and disability among people in this age group. During the physical examination, particular attention would be paid to the skin of those individuals at high risk for excessive exposure to sunlight or with a family or personal history of skin cancer. A complete oral cavity examination would be appropriate for individuals using tobacco or consuming excessive amounts of alcohol. Counseling would be provided on such items as diet and exercise, substance abuse, sexual practices, and injury prevention.

According to the National Diabetes Clearinghouse, approximately 28 million persons in the United States suffer from diabetes; however, 7 million of them are unaware of their condition. Diabetes is the seventh leading cause of death in the United States, accounting for nearly seventy thousand deaths per year. In addition, it is the leading cause of kidney failure, blindness, and amputations. The detection of diabetes in asymptomatic persons provides an opportunity to prevent or delay the progress of the disease and its complications. The *Guide to Clinical Preventive Services* recommends an oral glucose tolerance test for all pregnant women between the twenty-fourth and twenty-eighth weeks of their pregnancy. Routine screening for diabetes in asymptomatic nonpregnant adults, using blood or urine tests, is not recommended. Periodic fasting blood sugar measurements may be appropriate in persons at high risk for diabetes mellitus, such as the markedly obese, persons with a family history of diabetes, or women with a history of diabetes during pregnancy.

PERSPECTIVE AND PROSPECTS

In the mid-nineteenth century, John Snow provided one of the best examples of preventive medicine by applying what could be called observational epidemiology. During a rather severe cholera epidemic in London, Snow observed an unusual pattern of disease that appeared to be dependent on the particular water supply company providing water to the neighborhood. Recognizing that there was a high incidence of cholera in the Broad Street area, he was able to determine that most of the disease was associated with those families depending on the Broad Street pump for their drinking water. It has been said that he simply removed the handle on the pump and was able to control the epidemic in that area. His discovery occurred before there was a clear understanding of the relationship of bacteria or germs to infectious disease.

Another historic example of the application of preventive medicine was the control of smallpox. In the late eighteenth century, Edward Jenner observed that the milkmaids in the English countryside were not scarred by the scourge of smallpox. On further examination, he determined that these young women had years earlier been infected with cowpox and thus had been spared the more serious smallpox infection. He then advocated intentional infection with the cowpox

vaccine. Years later, using this preventive medicine application, the World Health Organization was able to institute a worldwide eradication of smallpox. The last case of smallpox reported in the world was in October, 1977, marking the first time that a major human disease had been eradicated. Neither the control of cholera in London by Snow nor the eradication of smallpox resulted from medical or surgical treatment of a disease. These results were obtained because of the application of the principles of preventive medicine and public health.

—Roy L. DeHart, MD, MPH;
updated by Carolynn Bruno

See also: Acupressure; Acupuncture; Aging: Extended care; Allied health; Alternative medicine; Aromatherapy; Biofeedback; Braces, orthopedic; Cardiac rehabilitation; Cardiology; Centers for Disease Control and Prevention (CDC); Chiropractic; Cholesterol; Chronobiology; Colon therapy; Disease; Echocardiography; Electrocardiography (ECG or EKG); Environmental health; Exercise physiology; Family medicine; Genetic counseling; Genetics and inheritance; Geriatrics and gerontology; Holistic medicine; Homeopathy; Host-defense mechanisms; Hypercholesterolemia; Immune system; Immunization and vaccination; Immunology; Mammography; Meditation; Melatonin; National Institutes of Health (NIH); Neuroimaging; Noninvasive tests; Nursing; Nutrition; Occupational health; Osteopathic medicine; Pharmacology; Pharmacy; Physical examination; Physician assistants; Phytochemicals; Preventive medicine; Psychiatry; Psychiatry, child and adolescent; Psychiatry, geriatric; Screening; Self-medication; Serology; Spine, vertebrae, and disks; Sports medicine; Stress reduction; Telemedicine; Tropical medicine; Yoga.

For Further Information:
Access and Disparities in Access to Health Care. Content last reviewed May 2016. Agency for Healthcare Research and Quality, Rockville, MD. www.ahrq.gov/research/findings/nhqrdr/nhqdr15/access.html
Cohen RA, Martinez ME. Health insurance coverage: early release of quarterly estimates from the National Health Interview Survey, January-June 2015. Hyattsville, MD: National Center for Health Statistics; November 2015. www.cdc.gov/nchs/data/nhis/ earlyrelease/Quarterly_estimates_2010_2015_Q12.pdf
Davies, Kevin. "Powering Preventative Medicine." *Bio-ITWorld* 10, no. 5 (September/October, 2011): 27-30.
Granello, Paul F. *Wellness Counseling*. Boston: Pearson, 2012.
Greenberg, Raymond S., et al., eds. *Medical Epidemiology*. 4th ed. New York: Lange Medical Books/McGraw-Hill, 2005.
Hales, Dianne. *An Invitation to Health Brief*. Updated ed. Belmont, Calif.: Wadsworth/Cengage Learning, 2010.
Halperin,William, and Edward L. Baker, eds. *Public Health Surveillance*. New York: Van Nostrand Reinhold, 1992.
Hood, Leroy, James R. Heath, Michael E. Phelps, and Biaoyang Lin. "Systems Biology and New Technologies Enable Predictive and Preventative Medicine." *Science* 306, no. 5696 (October, 2004) 640-43.
Jeste, Dilip V., and Carl C. Bell. *Preventative Psychiatry*. Philadelphia: Saunders, 2011.

Lee, Philip R., and Carroll L. Estes, eds. *The Nation's Health.* 7th ed. Sudbury, Mass.: Jones and Bartlett, 2003.

Litin, Scott C., ed. *Mayo ClinicFamily Health Book.* 4th ed. New York: HarperResource, 2009.

Payne, Wayne A., Dale B. Hahn, and Ellen Mauer. *Understanding Your Health.* 12th ed. New York: McGraw-Hill, 2013.

US Department of Health and Human Services. *Healthy People 2020: Health Understanding and Improving.* Washington, DC: Government Printing Office, 2010.

Wallace, Robert B., ed.*Wallace's Maxcy-Rosenau-Last Public Health and Preventive Medicine.* 15th ed. New York: McGraw- Hill, 2008.

PRIMARY CARE

Category: Health care system

Primary care is a patient's entry point into the health care system. A primary care practitioner can be one of several different types of medical professionals. They usually provide for the patient's basic medical care and coordinate care with other providers for more complex health situations. The primary care practitioner is the one the patient sees for routine exams and common conditions, such as the ear or throat infections. Also, it is usually the primary care practitioner who diagnoses more serious and/or chronic conditions such as heart disease or diabetes and refers the patient to a specialist for specific care for these conditions.

BACKGROUND

A primary care practitioner is usually the person individuals refer to as their "doctor." This medical practitioner may be a physician (e.g., an internist), a nurse practitioner, or a physician's assistant. Some patients choose a primary care provider —often referred to as a PCP—who has the educational background to deal with specialized populations. These may include pediatricians for children, family health providers, adult health providers, and individuals specializing in gerontology, geriatricians, for older adults.The PCP provides for all of the patient's primary health care needs. These include well-checks or check-ups, routine immunizations, screening, and care for common illnesses such as viruses, muscle and joint pains, skin eruptions, and other infections. The primary care provider will also be the first point of contact for many sudden illnesses or injuries that do not require emergency room care.

It is often the primary care provider who diagnoses more serious illnesses or determines that a person's health concern requires a specialist's care. For instance, a patient who complains of foot pain may be referred to a podiatrist for more in-depth care. The routine tests ordered by a primary care provider, either as part of an annual medical exam or in response to a health issue, can also identify more serious illnesses that require follow-up with a specialist.

A primary care practitioner may also treat a patient for certain chronic conditions, such as high blood pressure, diabetes, controlled or uncontrolled gastric problems, musculoskeletal issues, and others. It is important to keep your PCP involved in your care especially if you are referred to a specialist. This involvement provides coordination of care that can help prevent errors and improve health outcomes.

OVERVIEW

The focus of primary care is on the overall health of the individual rather than on one particular system or part of the body. The PCP coordinates care for the patient, directing the patient to specialists when needed, while serving as a central point of contact that can avoid duplication of care and help prevent errors. For example, a patient who has pain in both a foot and a shoulder may see a podiatrist for the foot problem and an orthopedic specialist for the shoulder. If the two specialists are coordinating with the PCP, they might discover that both are prescribing similar pain medications for the patient, which could lead to medical complications.

The PCP is also an advocate for the patient when that patient is enmeshed within the larger health care system. A hospitalized patient who has concerns that are not being addressed by a surgeon and a patient who is having difficulty getting a health insurance claim paid can both benefit from the knowledge and intervention of the primary care provider.

Another important function of a primary care provider is a focus on prevention. Their emphasis on the overall health of the patient means that the PCP makes a point of being aware of what routine tests or immunizations the patient may need. They can also take note of other potential health risks—such as smoking, alcohol consumption, and weight issues—and provide guidance and care to help the patient avoid future health issues.

Medical fields include more primary care physicians than specialists. This means that PCPs help provide greater accessibility to health care for a wider portion of the public. They can also provide some level of specialized care for those who would otherwise go without, such as patients without insurance or low-income patients who lack the funds for copayments for specialists. This helps to increase access to care and improve the overall quality of health care available in an area.

The intervention of the PCP can help to minimize the number of specialist visits that are required, either by identifying and initiating treatment for conditions before they become serious or by performing some of the follow-up that might otherwise be handled by a specialist. This care helps to improve the patient's overall health and reduce health care costs. The level of trust that can be built between a practitioner and a patient he or she sees regularly can also benefit health care outcomes by encouraging patient cooperation with treatment.

Primary care is an important facet of improved health care availability and outcomes, reduced costs, and greater patient satisfaction but unfortunately there is the lack of sufficient PCPs. The need for more primary providers is outstripping the supply of new practitioners in the United States. It can also be difficult to attract primary care providers to rural areas where lower income levels and the scarcity of specialists and medical facilities makes the need greatest.

—*Kendi Tang, DO*

For Further Information:
Gordon, Mara. "Why I'm Becoming a Primary Care Doctor." *The Atlantic*, 18 Sept. 2014, www.theatlantic.com/health/archive/2014/09/why-im-becoming-a-primary-care-doctor/379231/. Accessed 20 Dec. 2016.
"Primary Care." *American Association of Family Physicians*, www.aafp.org/about/policies/all/primary-care.html. Accessed 20 Dec. 2016.
"Primary Care vs. Non-Primary Care Specialties." *American Association of Colleges of Osteopathic Medicine*, www.aacom.org/become-a-doctor/med-students/career-planning/career-options/pc-vs-non-pc. Accessed 20 Dec. 2016.
"The Primary Care Medicine Clerkship." *Vanderbilt University Medical Center*, medicine.mc.vanderbilt.edu/primary-care-definition. medicine.vumc.org/goals-and-objectives. Accessed 20 Dec. 2016.
US National Library of Health. "Choosing a Primary Care Provider." *MedlinePlus*, 14 Aug. 2015, medlineplus.gov/ency/article/001939.htm. Accessed 20 Dec. 2016.
"What Is Primary Care?" *Johns Hopkins Bloomberg School of Public Health*, www.jhsph.edu/research/centers-and-institutes/johns-hopkins-primary-care-policy-center/definitions.html. Accessed 20 Dec. 2016.
"What Is Primary Health Care?" *University of Bristol*, www.bristol.ac.uk/primaryhealthcare/whatisphc.html. Accessed 20 Dec. 2016.
"What's a Primary Care Physician?" *KidsHealth by Nemours*, kidshealth.org/en/parents/primary-care-physician.html. Accessed 20 Dec. 2016.

PRION DISEASES

Category: Disease/Disorder
Anatomy or system affected: Brain, nervous system
Specialties and related fields: Epidemiology, neurology, pathology, public health
Definition: A variety of fatal neurological illnesses, inherited or transmissible, that are associated with abnormalities in proteins, called prions.

Key terms:
ataxia: the inability to control muscle movements
bovine spongiform encephalopathy (BSE): a prion disease of cattle; also called mad cow disease
Creutzfeldt-Jakob disease (CJD): a human prion disease found worldwide
dementia: a condition of deteriorated intellectual ability
encephalopathy: any abnormality in the structure or function of the brain
knockout mouse: mouse in which a specific gene has been inactivated or "knocked out"
kuru: a human prion disease formerly found in Papua New Guinea
prion: a protein that can assume an abnormal conformation, aggregate, and disrupt brain function
spongiform: shaped like or resembling a sponge

CAUSES AND SYMPTOMS

Prion diseases, also called transmissible spongiform encephalopathies, are progressive neurodegenerative disorders in humans and animals that lead to progressive memory loss, personality changes, and impaired motor control (ataxia). The diseases are almost always fatal. Human prion diseases include Creutzfeldt-Jakob disease (CJD), new variant Creutzfeldt-Jacob disease (vCJD), kuru, Gerstmann-Straussler-Scheinker syndrome, and fatal familial insomnia. Animal prion diseases include scrapie, chronic wasting disease (CWD), transmissible mink encephalopathy, feline spongiform encephalopathy, ungulate spongiform encephalopathy, and bovine spongiform encephalopathy (BSE), popularly known as mad cow disease.

While symptoms of scrapie have been noted in sheep and goats for hundreds of years, it was not shown to be transmissible until the 1930s. CJD was first noted in the 1920s, kuru in the 1950s, and BSE in the mid-1980s. Daniel Carleton Gajdusek began studying kuru in 1955 and won the Nobel Prize in Physiology or Medicine in 1976 for his work. Stanley B. Prusiner coined the term "prion" in 1982; he was awarded the Nobel Prize in 1997. Most scientists believe prions are the sole cause for transmissible spongiform encephalopathies.

The diseases are caused by misshapen versions of proteins called prions. Prions clump together and can proliferate by inducing shape changes in normal proteins. As prions aggregate, they cause spongelike lesions in the brain and disrupt brain function. The resultant illnesses are referred to as spongiform encephalopathies, which can be either inherited or transmissible. Prions are found in all species, from yeast to humans, but their normal role is not known. Their evolutionary persistence in so many species implies that they must serve an important purpose, although knockout mice lacking prions do not appear to be adversely affected.

Inherited spongiform encephalopathies are primarily attributed to mutations in the prion gene, leading to abnormally shaped proteins that aggregate over time to cause the brain damage and neurological symptoms characteristic of the diseases. Transmissible diseases occur when a susceptible animal is inoculated with a fragment or an extract of diseased tissue. Inoculation may occur by intravenous transmission, such as via a blood transfusion, or orally by consumption of infected tissue or bodily fluids, such as saliva.

Prions are unusual in that the protein is the infectious agent; typical infectious agents, such as bacteria or viruses, contain nucleic acids, either ribonucleic acid (RNA) or deoxyribonucleic acid (DNA). While the infectious agent's mode of action is not fully understood-and what is understood is not universally accepted-researchers announced in 2003 that they had discovered a new way of identifying an antibody specific to prions. This discovery has important implications for understanding how prions propagate and, in turn, for manipulating the prions for the creation of a vaccine.

These diseases have been described in humans, cattle, sheep, deer, elk, mink, domestic cats, and wild felines, and they have been experimentally induced in monkeys, hamsters, and mice. Prion diseases are usually species-specific. However, the diseases in mink, domestic cats, and wild felines are attributed to consumption of feed derived from diseased animals (usually hooved animals), and a variant in humans is associated with the consumption of meat from cattle with BSE.

The most common animal prion disease is scrapie, found in sheep and goats. It is named for the intense itching that causes sheep to rub against hard objects, scraping off the wool. It also causes staggering, tremors, and blindness. It has been known for more than 250 years in Britain and other countries of western Europe. It has been reported in most sheep-raising countries with a few notable exceptions, such as Australia and New Zealand. It first appears at two to five years of age, can last longer than six months, and is eventually fatal. It is generally accepted that it is an infectious disease in which genetics also plays an important role. It has not been shown to be transmissible to humans and poses no risk to human health.

The most famous prion disease in animals is bovine spongiform encephalopathy (BSE). First noted in British cattle in 1986, it causes nervousness, aggression, and symptoms similar to scrapie. It appears in adult cattle between two and eight years of age and is fatal. The BSE epidemic, which peaked in 1992 and affected more than 200,000 animals, was apparently caused by feed containing protein from animals with prion disease. A ban on incorporating ruminant-derived pro-

---

INFORMATION ON PRION DISEASES

Causes: Genetic inheritance (mutation of prion gene); transmission through consumption of infected animal tissue, tissue transplants, contamination of surgical instruments, pharmaceuticals derived from human cadavers

Symptoms: Dementia and ataxia, leading to death

Duration: Several weeks or months

Treatments: None

---

tein into cattle feed appeared to be bringing the epidemic to an end in Great Britain by the early twenty-first century, although there was a troubling increase in cases in continental Europe.

The best-known prion disease in humans is Creutzfeldt-Jakob disease (CJD), which occurs worldwide at a rate of about one per million persons. Its symptoms include dementia and ataxia, leading to death. The disease may be classified as sporadic, familial (inherited), iatrogenic (acquired through a medical procedure), or variant. The sporadic form, which accounts for the majority of cases, appears in the elderly and has an unknown etiology. The inherited form (5 to 10 percent of cases) is primarily attributed to mutations in the gene for prions, making them more susceptible to aggregation in the brains of affected individuals. The iatrogenic form can be caused by tissue transplants, contaminated surgical instruments, and pharmaceuticals derived from human cadavers.

The new variant form of CJD (vCJD) was first described in 1996; it differed from the sporadic form by affecting younger individuals and having slightly different symptoms and duration; it has been associated with eating beef from cattle infected with BSE. As of 2011, a total of 176 cases of vCJD had been identified in Great Britain since 1986, all of them fatal; far smaller numbers of cases have been reported in other countries. Because of a long time course and an incompletely known cause, it is uncertain how many will be affected by this new variant form.

TREATMENT AND THERAPY

No effective treatment for prion diseases existed as of the early twenty-first century. Researchers have speculated that human prion diseases might be treated by preventing normal proteins from adopting the abnormal shape, by interfering with the interaction between abnormal and normal proteins, or by destabilizing the shapes of abnormal proteins. Research has identified hundreds of molecules that seem to deter the formation of prions, prolonging the survival times of laboratory animals, but much more testing remains to be done before human drug therapies become available. Thus far, the only treatments are aimed at symptoms, such as opiates for pain and anticonvulsants to lessen neuromuscular problems.

PERSPECTIVE AND PROSPECTS

Concerns over prion diseases have increased in North America since the discovery of BSE in cattle from Canada and the United States. A screening program is in place to help detect infected cattle, but critics of the programs in both countries argue that it is not rigorous enough to provide adequate protection of the nations' food supplies. Despite the concerns over human health effects, considerable work remains to be done simply to achieve a better understanding of the origins, transmission, and pathogenesis of prion diseases.

—James L. Robinson, PhD;
updated by David M. Lawrence

See also Brain; Brain disorders; Chronic wasting disease (CWD); Creutzfeldt-Jakob disease (CJD); Food poisoning; Mutation.

For Further Information:
Badash, Michelle. "Creutzfeldt-Jakob Disease." *Health Library*, March 15, 2013.
Booss, John, Margaret Esiri, and Margaret M. Esin, eds. *Viral Encephalitis in Humans*. Washington, DC: ASM Press, 2003.
Brown, David R., ed. *Neurodegeneration and Prion Disease*. New York: Springer, 2005.
Council for Agricultural Science and Technology. *Transmissible Spongiform Encephalopathies in the United States*. Ames, Iowa: Author, 2000.
Ferry, Georgina. "Mad Brains and the Prion Heresy." *New Scientist* 142, no. 1927 (May 28, 1994): 32-36.
"Prion Diseases." *Centers for Disease Control and Prevention*, December 10, 2012.
"Prion Diseases." *National Institute of Allergy and Infectious Diseases*, 2013.
Prusiner, Stanley B. "The Prion Diseases." *Scientific American* 272, no. 1 (January, 1995): 48-57.
Prusiner, Stanley B., ed. *Prion Biology and Diseases*. 2d ed. Woodbury, N.Y.: Cold Spring Harbor Laboratory Press, 2004.
Schwartz, Maxime. *How the Cows Turned Mad*. Translated by Edward Schneider. Berkeley: University of California Press, 2003.
Spencer, Charlotte A. *Mad Cows and Cannibals: A Guide to the Transmissible Spongiform Encephalopathies*. Upper Saddle River, N.J.: Prentice Hall, 2004.

PROCTOLOGY

Category: Specialty
Anatomy or system affected: Gastrointestinal system, intestines
Specialties and related fields: Gastroenterology, internal medicine, oncology

Definition: The branch of medicine that treats diseases of the colon, rectum, and anus.
Key terms:
anal incontinence: the inability to control defecation
colitis: inflammation of the mucous membranes of the colon
diverticulum: a pouchlike, weakened region of the colon wall that can cause pain and bleeding
endoscope: a lighted, flexible, hollow instrument used for examination and the placement of surgical instruments
fascia: connective tissues such as tendons and ligaments
hemorrhoids: dilated blood vessels in the anus or rectum that are itchy and painful
occult blood: fecal blood, as detected by microscopic or chemical testing
polyp: a tumorlike growth, such as of the colorectal mucous lining
rectal prolapse: the protrusion of the rectum through the anus

SCIENCE AND PROFESSION

The term "proctology" arises from the Greek *proktos*, meaning "anus." In 1961, this field was renamed colon and rectal surgery. The original term, which is still in wide use, will be employed for simplicity. Specialists in proctology are surgeons who are expert in surgery of the colon, rectum, anal canal, and perianal area near the anus. They also carry out surgery of other tissues and organs close to and involved in serious colorectal disease. Moreover, proctologists have special skill in endoscopy of the rectum and colon for the diagnosis and medical treatment of these regions. Proctology involves emergency situations less frequently than many other specialties. Consequently, the hours of these specialists are relatively regular, although no shorter than those of other physicians.

Many conditions encountered by proctologists are clear-cut in diagnosis and treatment. Hence, they often have the satisfaction of providing patients with quick, effective relief of serious pain and discomfort.

Training a proctologist is time-consuming, involving a five-year residency in general surgery, followed by a one- to two-year fellowship in colon and rectal surgery. The specialty is not easily entered because its practitioners are not numerous and there are usually several applicants for each open training position.

The main organ treated in proctology is the large intestine, or colon. This portion of the digestive tract starts at the cecum, a pouch joined to the small intestine. At the far end of the cecum, the colon is subdivided into ascending, transverse, and descending regions. Together, these regions absorb water and minerals from food that has not been digested and absorbed by the stomach or small intestine. The result is feces, which are stored in the colon for elimination from the body. The ascending colon extends upward on the right side of the abdominal cavity and is called the right colon. The transverse colon crosses from right to left in the cavity, and the descending colon (left colon) passes downward along the cavity's left side, ending in the rectum. The short, S-shaped portion of the left colon above the rectum is the sigmoid colon.

The entire colon is made of pouches whose complex series of contractions and expansions moves its contents through quite slowly, enabling optimum water and mineral recovery. The sluggish colon movement enables bacteria to thrive, sometimes causing uncomfortable gas. Normal synchronization of the digestive system leads to absorption of most of this gas, however, as well as the transfer of feces into the rectum for storage and a defecation reflex that releases feces at varied but appropriate intervals. Also synchronized with these digestive processes is the production of both mucus and bicarbonate, which help to propel colon contents through the large intestine and neutralize acid made by bacteria in the colon. These events usually prevent damage to the colorectal system or diseases of its components.

The digestive system does not exhibit frequent dysfunction in early life. Therefore, proctologists for the most part see middle-aged or elderly patients. Furthermore, 60 percent of the problems that they encounter are anorectal, and 40 percent are associated with a diseased colon. Conditions that are often treated by proctologists include, but are not restricted to, anal fissures, cancers, colitis, diverticular disease, hemorrhoids, pilonoidal disease, and polyps.

DIAGNOSTIC AND TREATMENT TECHNIQUES

Thorough colorectal examination starts with a medical history to ensure the clarification of potential problems. Then the proctologist checks the perianal region for abnormalities such as dermatitis, abscesses, hemorrhoids, or lesions that may prove to be tumors. This is followed by digital examination with a lubricated glove, after a warning to patients that this procedure will result in the urge to defecate and cause some discomfort. Tissue irregularity, nodules, or tender areas are sought, and the prostate gland in men and the cervix in women are examined. To ensure complete exploration, a fecal sample is obtained and tested for the presence of occult blood. Other clinical tests of colon, rectum, and related tissues, including biopsy, are also carried out as needed.

Anal fissures may be discovered during this portion of the examination. An anal fissure is a linear tear of the lining of the anal canal, usually originating in the anorectal region. These fissures are common causes of acute anal pain, cutting or burning sensations beginning at defecation and continuing more mildly for several hours. They are thought to arise from trauma to the anal canal caused by large, dry, hard feces. Other causes of anal fissures include persistent diarrhea, inflammatory bowel disease (IBD), syphilis, leukemia, and anorectal cancer. The treatment of choice is the use of fecal softeners, increased fluid intake, and application of steroids. Surgery is usually carried out only for cases in which treated fissures do not heal.

Pilonoidal disease may also be detected; this is the formation of pits that contain pubic hair that has become trapped under the skin. If an abscess results, the problem is handled by its drainage under local anesthesia. Cleaning out of the pit and the removal of causative hair are also useful. Surgery is required only if the problem becomes chronic.

Anorectal cancers are relatively uncommon. They are treated in an individualized fashion with a varying combination of surgery, chemotherapy, and radiation therapy. Often, they are squamous cell carcinomas. In a smaller number of cases, melanomas, for which the survival rate is less than 5 percent, will occur. Other types of serious anorectal cancers include Paget's disease and basal cell carcinomas. These cancers have better survival rates.

Rectal prolapse, passage of the rectum through the anus, is another common anorectal problem. It is seen either in children under the age of two years or in the very elderly. In childhood, the problem is frequently attributable to anatomic underdevelopment, which cures itself. In adults, rectal prolapse may be partial or complete. Complete rectal prolapse results in the externalization of the entire rectum, bleeding, and excessive mucus discharge.

Rectal prolapse eventually causes anal incontinence, which may become irreversible. For cases in which a patient is feeble, the rectum is first manipulated to return it to a more normal placement. Then, a tightening steel or plastic loop is inserted under the skin at the anal opening to prevent future prolapse. When patients are robust enough for surgery, the rectum is often secured internally by a mesh sling anchored to internal fascia.

The treatment of internal or external hemorrhoids is another major aspect of proctological practice. Internal hemorrhoids are rarely painful because they are covered by insensitive colon mucosa tissue. The external variety, however, are rich in nervous tissue and may be very painful. Internal hemorrhoids are classified into four stages ranging from the relatively innocuous first-degree hemorrhoids, which do not prolapse, to fourth-degree hemorrhoids, which always prolapse.

Treatment for internal hemorrhoids, which depends on the severity of the bleeding and discomfort, ranges from education about proper diet and bowel habits to surgical removal (hemorrhoidectomy). Surgical removal is most often accomplished with a banding technique in which a tight rubber band is placed around the base of the hemorrhoid. Banding normally results in the sloughing off of dead tissue and the creation of a scar that prevents future problems. In cases of severe external hemorrhoids, banding is not used because it is too painful. Instead, more complex surgical excision is required.

Such symptoms as occult blood and lower abdominal pain may signal the need for a colon examination. Barium enemas and colonoscopy are the visualization techniques that are utilized. With a barium enema, a solution of radiopaque barium salt is placed into the colon after fasting and preliminary washing enemas have cleansed the organ. Then the colon containing the radiopaque solution is examined by X-ray techniques. This procedure can reveal diverticula, many colon cancers, large polyps, and other severe colorectal problems.

Colonoscopy, in its various forms, has become a mainstay in the diagnosis of colorectal disease. It is particularly valuable in finding smaller polyps, less developed cancers, and colitis. In addition, because patients who have had colon polyps removed have a one-in-four chance of new polyps forming within the next five years, colonoscopy provides minimally invasive and valuable follow-up. It can also prove useful in the follow-up of cancers and of inflammatory bowel disease.

Furthermore, an endoscope may be used to remove a smaller polyp directly or to determine that a large polyp or extensive carcinoma must be removed by laparoscopy or laparotomy. Colonoscopy is generally safe, and the entire large bowel from rectum to cecum may be examined with little risk to a patient. Moreover, endoscopic surgery greatly reduces hospital stays, recovery time, and the frequency of postsurgical mortality. The most common problems associated with colonoscopy are infrequent colon perforation as a result of diverticula, limited endoscopic access to the colon because of scarring from previous surgery, and flare-ups of ulcerative colitis.

Diverticular disease is quite common after the age of fifty. It is caused by small saclike pouches in the colon, often arising after colon spasms. In mild cases, diverticula can be observed by barium enema in patients exhibiting nonspecific abdominal pain and gas. In many instances, bleeding will occur. In some cases, diverticulitis (widespread diverticular infection and inflammation) can lead to serious colon blockage requiring colostomy, and in those cases where perforation

occurs, peritonitis will result. Diverticulitis is most common in the lower left colon, originating in the sigmoid region. It may be painful enough to justify the nickname left-sided appendicitis.

Polyps, masses arising from the bowel wall, are asymptomatic in many cases but may cause bleeding and pain when they are large. The larger that a polyp becomes, the greater is the risk that it will become cancerous. Polyps are often identified after rectal bleeding and/or cramps and abdominal pain lead to barium enema and colonoscopy. They are then removed completely via colonoscopy or laparoscopy, depending on their size. Thereafter, it is suggested that the entire colon be examined via colonoscope at intervals dependent on symptoms over a five-year period. Polyps tend to recur and may be associated with cancer.

More than 50 percent of colorectal cancers occur in the sigmoid colon and rectum. These very common visceral cancers are seen most in people over the age of sixty. Treatment is usually surgical removal of the diseased area, and barring spread to noncolon sites, the five-year survival rate is near 90 percent. Considerable variation exists in the size, location, and treatment of this very serious disease. Disease that has spread beyond the colon wall requires chemotherapy or radiation, or both, and the prognosis is not as good.

Major aspects of colitis are Crohn's disease in the colon (most often ileocolitis), ulcerative colitis, and spastic colon. Crohn's disease often appears in early life and is associated with fever, pain, and diarrhea. There is no permanent cure for this baffling disease, which recurs repeatedly. Treatments used include diet manipulation, immunosuppressive drugs, steroids, antibiotics (when colitis is accompanied by bacterial infection), and surgery (when intractable pain and bowel obstruction require it).

Ulcerative colitis is another disease that may appear in early life. It is recurrent, varies in severity from mild to fatal, and in less severe cases manifests as intermittent attacks of bloody diarrhea. Treatment varies as with Crohn's disease. Particularly dangerous is toxic colitis; very severe cases require immediate surgery.

Spastic colon, or irritable bowel syndrome (IBS), is a much milder form of colitis. It has no known anatomic cause, but emotional factors or other causes of hormone imbalance have been proposed. Periodic abdominal pain, constipation, and/or diarrhea are its usual symptoms. Happily, more than half of colitis complaints are attributable to this relatively mild problem, which is treated by diet modification, observation, and painkillers once the possibility of more serious types of colon disease has been eliminated by physical examination and other methodologies.

PERSPECTIVE AND PROSPECTS

Many advances in proctology have occurred since the 1970s, including the wide use of screening for occult blood in stools, which is easily done and often provides early detection of colorectal cancer. In addition, sophisticated endoscopic and laparoscopic techniques have been developed. The use of various types of endoscopes has enabled the precise examination of the colon and rectum, allowing the detection of colorectal problems that once would have gone unnoticed even after barium enema and related radiologic techniques were used. Furthermore, endoscopic surgery via colonoscopy and laparoscopy has reduced the severity of surgical intervention and the size of incisions, decreased hospital stays and recovery time, and resulted in higher surgical survival rates and facile follow-up after surgery.

The development of fiber-optic systems to be used with video camera techniques has improved colorectal examinations. Proctologists can review data rather than relying on single-shot views through a colonoscope. Such video records and their ongoing improvement may constitute the most significant innovations in colorectal diagnosis and surgery.

The development of additional clinical tests and drug therapy, including the wide use of steroids and immunosuppressive drugs, has also made some colorectal diseases much more manageable; examples are improved treatment of Crohn's disease and ulcerative colitis. Further advances in drug therapy, laparoscopy, and clinical testing may be major foci of future advances in this field.

—*Sanford S. Singer, PhD*

See also Anus; Colitis; Colon; Colonoscopy and sigmoidoscopy; Colorectal cancer; Colorectal polyp removal; Colorectal surgery; Crohn's disease; Diverticulitis and diverticulosis; Endoscopy; Fistula repair; Gastroenterology; Gastrointestinal disorders; Gastrointestinal system; Hemorrhoid banding and removal; Hemorrhoids; Internal medicine; Intestines; Physical examination; Rectum; Urology.

For Further Information:

Beers, Mark H., et al., eds. *The Merck Manual of Diagnosis and Therapy*. 18th ed. Whitehouse Station, N.J.: Merck Research Laboratories, 2006.

Brown, Steven R. *Contemporary Coloproctology*. London: Springer, 2012.

Classen, Meinhard, G. N. J. Tytgat, and C. J. Lightdale, eds. *Gastroenterological Endoscopy*. 2d ed. New York: Thieme Medical, 2010.

Corman, Marvin L. *Colon and Rectal Surgery*. 5th ed. Philadelphia: Lippincott Williams & Wilkins, 2005.

Doherty, Gerard M., and Lawrence W. Way, eds. *Current Surgical Diagnosis and Treatment*. 13th ed. New York: Lange Medical Books/McGraw-Hill, 2010.

Givel, Jean-Claude, and Neil James Mortensen. *Anorectal and Colonic Diseases: A Practical Guide to Their Management*. London: Springer, 2010.

Kapadia, Cyrus R., James M. Crawford, and Caroline Taylor. *An Atlas of Gastroenterology: A Guide to Diagnosis and Differential Diagnosis*. Boca Raton, Fla.: Pantheon, 2003.

Peikin, Steven R. *Gastrointestinal Health*. Rev. ed. New York: Quill, 2001.

Taylor, Anita D. *How to Choose a Medical Specialty*. 5th ed. New York: Elsevier, 2012.

PROGERIA

Category: Disease/Disorder
Also known as: Hutchinson-Gilford syndrome, Werner's syndrome
Anatomy or system affected: All
Specialties and related fields: Cardiology, pediatrics, vascular medicine
Definition: Rare disorders characterized by many aspects of premature aging.

CAUSES AND SYMPTOMS

There are two major, unrelated types of progeria: Hutchinson-Gilford syndrome, which begins in infancy, and Werner's syndrome, which develops in late adolescence to young adulthood. Recessive inheritance has been demonstrated for Werner's syndrome, whereas a dominant gene is a suspected source in Hutchinson-Gilford syndrome. Underlying causes have been difficult to determine, although an impaired ability to cope with free radicals appears to play a role in the degenerative course found in each disease.

Hutchinson-Gilford syndrome is characterized by superficial aspects of aging such as deteriorated skin, baldness, repeated nonhealing fractures, and vascular diseases, in addition to short stature and minimal subcutaneous fat. Arteriosclerosis and heart disease lead to a median age of death of thirteen. Werner's syndrome occurs more frequently, with the following symptoms: short stature, thin extremities, a squeaky

---

INFORMATION ON PROGERIA

Causes: Unclear; possibly genetics, impaired ability to cope with free radicals

Symptoms: Superficial aspects of aging including deteriorated skin, baldness, repeated non-healing fractures, vascular diseases; also short stature, thin extremities, squeaky voice, cataracts, increased risk of diabetes, heart disease, tumors, hearing loss, bone and tooth loss

Duration: Chronic and progressive

Treatments: Supportive therapy, including anti-oxidant supplements (e.g., vitamin E), growth hormones, gene therapy voice, cataracts, an increased risk of diabetes mellitus, heart disease, tumors, hearing loss, and the loss of bone and teeth. Death usually occurs by the middle forties. Neither disorder is simply accelerated aging. For example, the central nervous system is relatively unaffected in both diseases.

TREATMENT AND THERAPY

No known cure exists for either progeria disease. Suggested treatments include antioxidant supplements (for example, vitamin E), growth hormone therapy, and gene therapy. Therapies have focused on providing a supportive environment and treating the symptoms to make the disorders less painful. Among these treatments are surgery, skin grafting (if skin ulceration occurs), and analgesic drugs.

PERSPECTIVE AND PROSPECTS

Hutchinson-Gilford syndrome was first described by Jonathan Hutchinson in 1886. Hastings Gilford named the disorder progeria in a 1904 article. The first cases of Werner's syndrome were reported in the 1950s.

There are hopes for an eventual genetic solution to progeria diseases. The only definitive prospect for sufferers, however, is premature death.

—*Paul J. Chara, Jr., PhD*

See also Aging; Death and dying; Genetic diseases.

For Further Information:
Judd, Sandra J., ed. *Genetic Disorders Sourcebook: Basic Consumer Information About Heritable Disorders.* 4th ed. Detroit, Mich.: Omnigraphics, 2010.
Gormley, Myra Vanderpool. *Family Diseases: Are You at Risk?* Baltimore: Genealogical Publishing, 2002.
Parker, James N., and Philip M. Parker, eds. *Progeria: A Medical Dictionary, Bibliography, and Annotated Research Guide to Internet References.* San Diego, Calif.: Icon Health, 2004.
Lewin, Benjamin. *Genes.* 9th rev. ed. Sudbury, Mass.: Jones and Bartlett, 2008.
Lewis, Ricki. *Human Genetics: Concepts and Applications.* 10th ed. Dubuque, Iowa: McGraw-Hill, 2012.
Milunsky, Aubrey. *Heredity and Your Family's Health.* Baltimore: Johns Hopkins University Press, 1992.
"Progeria." *MedlinePlus,* August 4, 2011.
Progeria Research Foundation. progeriaresearch.org/.

PROGNOSIS

Category: Procedure
Also known as: Future outlook
Anatomy or system affected: All
Specialties and related fields: All

Definition: A medically educated guess that helps to determine the probability of a patient's final outcome concerning a disease, illness, injury, or affliction. A prognosis may refer to a patient's quality of life, quantity of life, or both.

Key terms:
favorable: indicating that a better outcome is more likely to occur; the opposite is not favorable or unfavorable
future: any period of time from twenty-four hours later to ten or twenty years later
mortality: relating to death

SCREENING AND DIAGNOSIS

Every diagnosis has a prognosis. The diagnosis of any disease (tuberculosis, acquired immunodeficiency syndrome, chickenpox), any chronic condition (asthma, vitiligo, alopecia, cardiomegaly, multiple sclerosis), any cancer (melanoma, osteosarcoma, breast cancer, testicular cancer, lymphoma), any reaction to a bite or sting (rabies, spider or wasp venom, scabies), any medical emergency (gunshot wound, stabbing, motor vehicle accident), or any symptom or medical circumstance (hypothermia, dizziness, pregnancy) will create the need for a prognosis.

A prognosis may be described in words, numbers, charts, percentages, or graphs. If the chances of surviving or eliminating a given medical circumstance are good, then the prognosis is termed favorable. If not, then it may be said that the prognosis is poor or that the prognosis has become not favorable. Other possible words include excellent, good, fair, unfavorable, not good, failing, bleak, dim, or taking a turn for the worse. A prognosis may also be stated by how the patient is now compared to the expected outcome: For example, the situation may be critical now, but if the patient continues improving, he or she will have a favorable outcome.

A numerical prognosis is often given in the form of a number scale of 1 to 10, or 1 to 100. The health care provider will state if the number 1 is the best case or the worst case in each scenario. A numerical prognosis may also be explained by using percentages. For example, the patient has a 25 percent chance that the disease will return or, conversely, a 75 percent chance that the disease will disappear. An example of long-term prognosis is that the patient's five-year outlook has a 90 percent chance of a full recovery.

FUTURE OUTLOOK

Many factors are taken into consideration when determining a prognosis. A certain factor may help improve a prognosis favorably, while others may affect a prognosis unfavorably. The following factors all influence a patient's prognosis: type of disease or illness, type of injury or affliction, nutritional habits, weight factor or obesity, current medications, exercise, alcohol consumption, smoking, work environment, care of or neglect of general overall health, previous health history, family history, race, gender, sexual orientation, age, financial status, education, religion, and culture. For example, by avoiding alcohol consumption and avoiding smoking, the patient can help to create a more favorable prognosis.

Early detection of any condition, disease, or illness will help to improve the odds of producing a more favorable prognosis. For example, according to the American Cancer Society, early breast cancer detection saves thousands of lives each year. This information can encourage women earlier in life to perform monthly self-breast examinations and to seek routine annual breast exams by their health care provider. Routine physicals are also helpful in finding afflictions such as high blood pressure early, so that patients may be given medications to help improve the long-term prognosis for a healthier life.

Early intervention also includes the point at which care is first administered, which can be a determining factor in the favorability of a prognosis. For example, if a patient has a heart attack and cardiopulmonary resuscitation (CPR) is administered within the first three minutes, then the patient will have a more favorable outlook for a good recovery (a better prognosis). If the patient does not receive any CPR until ten minutes after the heart attack, however, then the prognosis is not very good in terms of the patient surviving. In addition, the more severe an injury that may include extensive blood loss, the lower the chances of survival.

UNDERSTANDING THE DISEASE OR CONDITION

Patient education is beneficial in helping produce a more favorable, long-term prognosis for any patient. This education may come in the form of pamphlets or books dispensed by the health care provider. Patients may also educate themselves through medical online sources or books pertaining to a particular situation.

In general, certain diseased or traumatized organs tend to have a less favorable prognosis, such as the liver, lungs, kidneys, ovaries, testicles, and pancreas. Certain diseases have their own stages of prognosis. For example, cancers that are detected while the patient is in stage 1 are considered more easily treatable and often the prognosis is more favorable if the disease is treated early, versus cancers that are found in stage 4. Stage 4 cancers have spread to other organs and may be difficult to control or stop. Stage 4 cancers often have a prognosis of not favorable (more likely resulting in death); if treated at this later stage, these cancers also have a greater tendency toward reoccurring.

TREATMENT PLANS

Every treatment plan, therapy, or medication has the potential to alter a prognosis. Some alternative therapies that may be incorporated into treatment to help improve a prognosis include acupressure, acupuncture, herbal remedies, meditation, guided imagery, massage therapy, laughter, biofeedback, chiropractic, energy healing, yoga, Tai Chi Chuan, breathing and relaxation techniques, and a positive mental outlook.

The Morbidity and Mortality Weekly Report (MMWR) analyzes data and calculates statistics from every death that occurs. These lists can help the health care provider determine a treatment plan and a prognosis. By knowing a prognosis and understanding its recovery rate, a patient can make an informed decision regarding a treatment plan.

—*Suzette Buhr, RTR, CDA*

See also Allied health; Alternative medicine; Biopsy; Blood testing; Cancer; Cardiac rehabilitation; Death and dying; Diagnosis; Disease; Epidemiology; Hospice; Imaging and radiology; Invasive tests; Laboratory tests; Noninvasive tests; Physical examination; Physical rehabilitation; Screening; Signs and symptoms.

For Further Information:
American Heart Association. "Cardiac Arrest." *American Heart Association*, February 2, 2013.
Centers for Disease Control and Prevention. "*MMWR*: Summary of Notifiable Diseases." *Morbidity and Mortality Weekly Report*, May 31, 2012.
Centers for Disease Control and Prevention. "*MMWR Weekly*: Current Volume (2013)." *Morbidity and Mortality Weekly Report*, June 21, 2013.
Morra, Marion, and Eve Potts. *Choices: The Most Complete Source Book for Cancer Information*. 4th ed. New York: HarperCollins, 2003.
Seaman, Andrew M. "Patient Communication Has Room to Grow." Reuters Health Information. *MedlinePlus*, May 27, 2013.

PROSTATE CANCER

Category: Disease/Disorder
Anatomy or system affected: abdomen, lymphatic system, reproductive system, urinary system
Specialties and related fields: immunology, oncology, radiology, urology
Definition: Malignancy occurring in the prostate gland that is the deadliest cancer for men in the United States.
Key terms:
benignprostatic hyperplasia (BPH): enlargement of the prostate gland that often accompanies aging
orchiectomy: removal of the testes

prostate-specific antigen (PSA): a protein released from the prostate gland that is associated with prostate hyperplasia and/or prostate cancer

prostatectomy: the surgical removal of the prostate gland

single nucleotide polymorphisms: deoxyribonucleic acid (DNA) sequences differing by a single nucleotide base pair

CAUSES AND SYMPTOMS

The normal human prostate gland is a walnut-sized male organ composed of glandular tissue and a thick coat of muscle tissue called the "prostatic capsule." Located near the rectum just below the bladder, it secretes various components of semen: an alkaline fluid that makes sperm more viable after intercourse; substances that cause semen to "clot" temporarily helping to keep sperm in the female reproductive tract; and fibrolysin, a substance that later breaks down the semen clot and enables the sperm to move on and ensure fertilization. The urethra empties the urinary bladder and passes through the prostate gland. The prostate frequently enlarges in later life. When this occurs, it presses on and constricts the urethra, a condition that is called "benign prostatic hyperplasia" (BPH). While in most men BPH is at most uncomfortable, the hyperplasia sometimes results in difficult and painful urination, leading to the necessity for surgical intervention or even removal of the prostate gland.

Much more problematic is prostate cancer, also known as "adenocarcinoma" of the prostate. Most of-

Location of the Prostate Gland

The prostate is one of the major sites where cancer develops in older men; the inset shows the location of the prostate gland in the male reproductive system.
©EBSCO

ten, prostate cancer is detected in asymptomatic men who are found to have lumps within the prostate during a routine rectal examination by a urologist. Regrettably, cancers detected in this way are often in a fairly advanced and dangerous stage of growth. Hence, some medical professionals recommend yearly urologic examinations after the age of forty (others say after fifty), along with clinical testing, so that early detection can prevent the most serious consequences of the disease.

An important adjunct of such testing is the blood test for prostate-specific antigen (PSA). PSA is a glycoprotein produced only by the cells of the prostate, and its levels in the blood sometimes correlate with the presence of malignancy. The correlation with malignancy is not perfect and there is controversy as to the usefulness of the test. Normal values are under 4 nanograms per milliliter (ng/mL). Approximately 25 percent of men whose blood PSA levels are 4 to 10 ng/mL are diagnosed with prostate cancer. If diagnosed early, the cancer is treatable because the tumors are small and localized. When PSA levels exceed 10 ng/mL, about 70 percent of test patients are found to have the disease, their cancers are larger, and the prognosis is less favorable. Recent studies, however, have shown that the precise PSA level is frequently not an indication of cancer since men with relatively high PSA levels frequently have BPH but not cancer. And a low PSA value is not necessarily indicative of being cancer-free. Research indicates that while PSA may aid in detection, it does not reduce mortality. Some physicians recommend against the PSA test since it may lead to over diagnosis and excess treatment. Another blood test for prostate cancer is the measurement of acid phosphatase. This method is a less sensitive and a less reliable indicator of the disease when used alone. Done in conjunction with PSA testing, however, its increased levels are a good indicator of the extent of the metastasis.

Physical examination, ultrasound and magnetic resonance imaging (MRI) can aid in the diagnosis of prostate cancer, but biopsy is the best way to detect the cancer. A biopsy is performed if there are other possible signs such as a lump found during digital examination and/or a high PSA. Biopsy, in some situations, is done under ultrasound or MRI guidance.

Risk factors associated with prostate cancer are obesity, advancing age, race (African Americans have a higher incidence than do Caucasian Americans), family history, and a diet high in red meat and milk. Genome-wide association studies have identified single nucleotide polymorphisms that increase risk. A number of genes have been implicated as being associated with the cancer, but no single gene has yet been shown to be causative. Five to 10 percent of prostate cancers are thought to be hereditary; men with a family history in an immediate relative (father, brother, son) are two to three times more likely to develop the disease. Several studies have implicated human papilloma virus (HPV) as a possible cause, but these studies are controversial and are inconclusive. By pinpointing a cause, it may become possible to diagnose those men at particular risk, as well as to identify a target for treatment.

TREATMENT AND THERAPY

The treatment of localized prostate cancer is controversial and ranges from surveillance to various types of radiation treatment to hormone therapy to removal of the entire prostate (radical prostatectomy). In radical prostatectomy, the entire prostate, the nearby seminal vesicles, and the vas deferens are removed. This removes both the prostate, the focus of the cancer, and the nearby male sexual tissues that are most likely to be sites of cancer metastasis. When this procedure is carried out with prostate-confined tumors, cancer recurrence is less than 2 percent. Side effects of prostate surgery include possible various forms of urinary incontinence, and possible erectile dysfunction (impotence). Erectile dysfunction may be treated by phosphodiesterase-5 inhibitors, including sildenafil (Viagra), vardenafil (Levitra), tadalafil (Cialis), and avanafil (Stendra). Alporostadil (a synthetic version of prostaglandin E1) may also be helpful. Severe cases can be surgically treated with penile implants to restore erectile function.

In many cases, radiation therapy, which is viewed as less radical, is carried out on these cancers, and ten-year survival rates approach 70 percent. Both external beam radiation and brachytherapy (internal radiation through seed implants) are successfully used, although side effects may include radiation proctitis (irritation of the rectum) or radiation cystitis (irritation of the bladder leading to urinary difficulty).

For more severe or metastasized tumors, surgery and radiation treatment are followed by a number of hormone regimens. The latter include androgen deprivation, rationalized by the fact that most prostate tumors are androgen-dependent. The most common hormones used include pituitary luteinizing hormone-releasing hormone (LHRH) agonists, such as leuprolide (Lupron, Eligard), goserelin (Zoladex), triptorelin (Trelstar), and leuprolide mesylate (Camcevi), as well as LHRH antagonists such as degarelix (Firmagon) and relugolix (Orgovyx). Also used are drugs to block the adrenal glands from producing androgens, such as abiraterone (Zytiga) and ketoconazole (Nizoral), and androgen receptor antagonists such as flutamide (Eulexin), bicalutamide (Casodex), and nilutamide (Nilandron). Newer forms of antiandrogens are being

***

> ### INFORMATION ON PROSTATE CANCER
>
> **Causes:** Unclear; possibly genetic factors, environmental toxins, hormonal influences
> **Symptoms:** Initially asymptomatic; in later stages, may include hard nodules in prostate gland, decreased urine flow, painful urination
> **Duration:** Acute, possibly recurrent
> **Treatments:** Surgery, radiation therapy, hormonal therapy, cryotherapy

tested in men whose cancer has not spread but is no longer responding to other forms of hormone therapy. This group of drugs includes enzalutamide (Xtandi), apalutamide (Erleada), and darolutamide (Nubeqa).

Removal of the testes (orchiectomy, or castration) is another, more radical treatment. The result of castration can be unpleasant physically and psychologically, but is the most effective treatment for immediately removing the source of the antigens the cancer needs to grow. The five- to ten-year survival rate for men found to have nonmetastasized prostate cancer is viewed as good by most physicians, and the survival rates of those with more severe cancers are improving because of the discovery of better therapeutic drugs. If the cancer has metastasized to the bones, pain relief medication and bisphosphonates are often used.

PERSPECTIVE AND PROSPECTS

Prostate cancer first became common in the 1960s. In North America, it is the most common cancer detected in men. In 2022 the American Cancer Society estimates that approximately 268,000 new cases will be diagnosed, and 34,500 deaths will occur due to prostate cancer. One in eight men will be diagnosed with prostate cancer in his lifetime, and studies have confirmed that more than 40 percent of American men fifty years of age or older who were autopsied after death from other causes were found to have prostate cancer as well. The incidence of prostate cancer varies among the races, being highest among African Americans. Overall, 3 to 4 percent of American men are expected to die from prostate cancer.

Current research is focused on identifying genes associated with the disease and the development of more targeted therapy.

—Maryann Cheesman, RN and Kerry L. Cheesman, PhD

See also: Aging; Cancer; Carcinogens; Chemotherapy; Genital disorders, male; Malignancy and metastasis; Men's health; National Cancer Institute (NCI); Prostate enlargement; Prostate gland; Prostate gland removal; Radiation therapy; Reproductive system; Tumor removal; Tumors; Urinary disorders; Urinary system; Urology.

For Further Information:
Bayoumi, Ahmed M., Adalsteinn D. Brown, and Alan M. Garber. "Cost-Effectiveness of Androgen Suppression Therapies in Advanced Prostate Cancer." *Journal of the National CancerInstitute*, vol. 92, no. 21, 1 Nov. 2000l pp. 1731-39.
Bostwick, David G., Gregory T. MacLennan, and Thayne R. Larson. *ProstateCancer: What Every Man—and His Family—Needs to Know*. Rev. ed., Villard, 1999.
Dollinger, Malin, et al. *Everyone's Guide to CancerTherapy*. 5th ed., Andrews McMeel, 2008.
Ellsworth, Pamela. *One Hundred Questions and Answers About ProstateCancer*. 3rd ed., Jones and Bartlett, 2013.
Marks, Sheldon. *Prostateand Cancer: A Family Guide to Diagnosis, Treatment, and Survival*. 4th ed., Da Capo Lifelong, 2009.
Marx, Jean. "Fused Genes May Help Explain the Origins of Prostate Cancer." *Science*, vol. 310, 28 Oct. 2005, p. 603.
McCoy, Krisha, and Rebecca J. Stahl. "Prostate Cancer." *Health Library*, 19 Sept. 2012.
Nordqvist, Christian. "Prostate Cancer: Symptoms, Risk Factors, and Treatment." *Medical News Today*, 18 July 2017, www. medicalnewstoday.com/articles/150086.php.
"Prostate Cancer." *American CancerSociety*, 4 Sept. 2012.
"Prostate Cancer." *Centers for Disease Control and Prevention*, 8 May 2013.
"Prostate Cancer." *Abeloff's Clinical Oncology*, edited by J. E. Niederhuber, J. O. Armitage, J. H. Doroshow, et al., 6th ed., Elsevier, 2020.
Sieve, Vonne. "Prostate Cancer." *Salem Health: Cancer*. Grey House Publishing, 2017.
Zelefsky, M. J., M. J. Morris, and J. A. Eastham. "Chapter 70: Cancer of the Prostate." *DeVita, Hellman, and Rosenberg's Cancer: Principles and Practice of Oncology*, edited by V. T. DeVita, T. S. Lawrence, and S. A. Rosenberg, 11th ed., Lippincott Williams and Wilkins, 2019.

PROSTATE ENLARGEMENT

Category: Disease/Disorder
Also known as: Benign prostatic hyperplasia or hypertrophy (BPH)
Anatomy or system affected: Reproductive system, urinary system
Specialties and related fields: Endocrinology, urology
Definition: A common condition in which the prostate gland enlarges as a man matures.
Key terms:
benign: not recurrent or malignant; associated with favorable outcomes
cytokines: proteins that influence communication and interactions between cells; examples include interleukins, lymphokines, and cell-signaling molecules such as tumor necrosis factor, transforming growth factor, and interferons
endocrine: a term applied to organs or cells that produce hormones
enzyme: a protein that enhances the rate of chemical changes in living cells

gene: the basic unit of a chromosome carrying the information for a specific protein that is inherited
hormone: a chemical substance produced by an endocrine organ or cells that causes specific effects on the structure and function of the target organs or cells
inflammation: the body's defensive response to injury or infection; includes many factors in the process, including white blood cells and cytokines
laser: an instrument that generates a small intense beam of light that is used in surgery and other medical procedures
malignant: having the features of uncontrolled growth, invasion, and spreading; associated with unfavorable outcomes
phytomedicine: the use of plant substances as alternative treatment for medical diseases and conditions
tissue: a group of similar cells with a specific function
transurethral: across or through the urethra

CAUSES AND SYMPTOMS

Prostate enlargement is also known as "benign prostatic hyperplasia"

The prostate gland is a walnut-sized organ located below the bladder, the organ in which urine is stored. The prostate surrounds part of the urethra, which is a long tube that transports urine from the bladder to the outside of the body. The gland has a role in both the male reproductive system and the urinary system. The prostate adds secretions to semen, an alkaline fluid that neutralizes the acidic environment of the female reproductive system and provides nutritional elements for the sperm. BPH symptoms occur in more than half of men in their sixties and more than 90 percent of men in their eighties. The enlargement of the prostate gland can cause lower urinary tract symptoms (LUTS). LUTS is a term used to describe symptoms related to the bladder and urethra.

BPH becomes more prevalent as men age. Symptomatic BPH usually occurs after age forty-five. No single factor fully explains the condition, but many factors are known to be involved in BPH, including hormones, race, obesity, cell growth, and genetics. The hormones involved are the female hormone estrogen and the male hormones (androgens) testosterone and dihydrotestosterone (DHT).

Androgens are sex hormones that contribute to cell growth in the prostate gland and inhibit cell death. Men produce testosterone and a small amount of estrogen throughout their lives. The testosterone level decreases as men age and the relative amount of estrogen increases. Scientists have shown that the addition of estrogen to androgen increases BPH development in animals and that there is an increased ratio of female to male hormone (estrogen/androgen ratio) in prostatic tissue with BPH. DHT is another androgen that is related to BPH. It has been shown that men who do not have the enzyme (protein) that converts testosterone to DHT have small-sized prostate glands throughout their lives. Further, pre-pubertal males have lower levels of testosterone and DHT and BPH does not occur. Post-puberty, these hormones become elevated and BPH may eventually occur. It follows that those who have been castrated will have an inability to develop BPH. Older men continue to produce DHT in the prostate, and this hormone may affect cell growth in the prostate. Moreover, studies have shown that BPH occurs in many men with a positive family history for prostate enlargement.

The prostate gland is surrounded by a tissue lining called the "capsule." As the prostate enlarges against its surrounding capsule, the whole structure presses against that part of the urethra that the prostate surrounds; this constricts (obstructs) the urethra and affects the bladder. The bladder wall thickens and becomes more irritable. The symptoms of BPH result from the urethral obstruction and resulting bladder irritation and functional decline. These symptoms usually occur gradually and can worsen with time. Urethral obstruction causes voiding hesitancy, intermittency, weak stream, dribbling, and straining. Bladder irritation causes more sensitivity to smaller amounts of urine, resulting in more frequent urination, especially at night. Eventually, the bladder may weaken and its function may be affected adversely. The bladder can lose its ability to completely empty the stored urine during voiding; this can lead to acute urinary retention in the bladder. However, many men with prostatic enlargement remain asymptomatic.

TREATMENT AND THERAPY

The patient may notice the symptoms of BPH first and schedule an appointment with his doctor for evaluation. BPH diagnostic assessment includes a number of steps. A history focused on evaluating storage symptoms, voiding symptoms and postvoiding symptoms will be obtained in order to determine the severity of BPH. A questionnaire such as the American Urological Association Symptom Index can help to further assess symptom severity and monitor response to treatments. A physical examination will be performed, including a digital rectal examination, in which a gloved finger is inserted into the rectum to evaluate the size and condition of the prostate. A urine test to check for blood or signs of urine infection and a blood test to evaluate whether the kidneys are affected will be done as well. The patient's goals are an essential part of the diagnostic evaluation. The American Urological Association recommends that if a patient's symptoms are not bothersome if they do not want treatment, then no further work-up is recommended. This is because the

---

> **INFORMATION ON PROSTATE ENLARGEMENT**
>
> **Causes:** Unknown; factors include hormones (estrogen, androgens), cell growth, genetics
> **Symptoms:** Constriction of urethra and bladder irritation resulting in urination problems (voiding hesitancy, intermittency, weak stream, dribbling, straining, frequency, infections)
> **Duration:** Chronic
> **Treatments:** None (watchful waiting), medications (alpha-blockers, enzyme inhibitors of 5-alpha- reductase, herbal remedies), surgery to remove tissue or gland

condition is unlikely to significant affect their future health.

Other tests may be recommended to determine if the symptoms are associated with the bladder or kidney or if cancer is present. One such test, postvoid residual urine volume (PVR), measures how much urine is left in the bladder after urination. The PVR can be measured through a bladder scanner which uses ultrasonography. A high PVR may indicate treatment failure or the need for surgical intervention. The two tests that can determine the degree of blockage in urine flow are uroflowmetry, which measures the rate and amount of urine passed, and pressure-flow studies, which assess bladder pressure during voiding. In some cases, imaging of the kidney, bladder, and prostate may be necessary with X-rays, ultrasound, or cystoscopy, in which an instrument is passed through the urethra and used to view the interior of the bladder. A test for prostate-specific antigen (PSA) may also be recommended. PSA is a protein that is produced by prostate cells; it is often elevated in patients with prostate cancer but may also be increased in BPH.

Treatment of BPH includes conservative measures (watchful waiting), medical options (both conventional and alternative), surgical procedures, lifestyle changes and minimally invasive therapies. The patient's decision is usually based on the effects of the BPH symptoms on his quality of life and on weighing the risks and benefits of available interventions. Lifestyle changes include avoiding or reducing consumption of alcohol and caffeinated beverages. Such drinks are classified as diuretics, which promote urine production. Other changes involve avoiding fluids before bed and avoiding medications, such as certain antihistamines or decongestants that can worsen urinary retention. If the symptoms are severe and the urinary or reproductive tract is affected, however, then BPH needs to be treated.

Most men seek treatment for symptomatic relief and this is the goal of treatment. BPH symptoms that do not bother the patient can be managed with watchful waiting. There is no active treatment involved, and the patient will see his doctor at least once a year to determine whether the symptoms are staying the same, improving, or worsening. Some patients may experience spontaneous improvement.

Medical options include taking conventional drugs such as an alpha-blocker or enzyme inhibitors of 5-alpha-reductase. Alpha-blockers relax the smooth muscles of the bladder neck and prostate which improve urinary flow. These are usually first-line pharmacological therapy. Examples of alpha-blockers include terazosin (Hytrin), doxazosin (Cardura), tamsulosin (Flomax), and alfuzosin (Uroxatral). The side effects of these drugs include dizziness, fainting, headache, tiredness, and low blood pressure. Enzyme inhibitors of 5-alpha-reductase prevent the conversion of testosterone to DHT, which in turn can decrease prostate growth and prevent further BPH progression. There are two drugs approved by the Food and Drug Administration (FDA) in this category, finasteride (Proscar) and dutasteride (Avodart). Their side effects include decreased libido, ejaculatory problems, and erectile dysfunction. In certain cases, a combination of an alpha-blocker and 5-alpha-reductase inhibitors may be used. Phosphodiesterase inhibitors can also improve symptoms of BPH as well as erectile dysfunction. Examples of such drugs are Tadalafil.

Alternative medications consist of herbal remedies. Studies on saw palmetto, a fruit extract from the American dwarf palm tree, have yielded equivocal results on its efficacy as a BPH treatment. Systematic reviews of beta-sitosterol plant extract, cernilton from rye grass pollen, and pygeum bark extract from African plum tree showed that there is some BPH symptomatic improvement with these supplements. Better-designed studies for these remedies, however, may not confirm this favorable result, as was seen in the case of saw palmetto. Further, the American Urological Association does not recommend the use of herbal remedies.

Surgery is usually reserved as second-line treatment for patients who did not respond to medical therapies. Surgical management of BPH includes transurethral resection of the prostate (TURP), transurethral incision of the prostate (TUIP), open surgery (prostatectomy), and laser surgery. These surgeries destroy or remove tissue around the prostate or urethra. TURP is the most common surgical option; the surgeon uses an instrument called a "resectoscope" to remove enlarged prostate tissue through the urethra. Complications include sexual dysfunction and urinary issues. TUIP usually involves placing two deep incisions in the prostate where it meets the bladder neck; this decreases the resistance to urine flow from the bladder. Prostate tissue

is not removed in this procedure. Rather, the incisions widen the urethra. Prostatectomy, or prostate gland removal, is done in some cases; this involves removing the enlarged prostate in an open surgery. Laser surgery vaporizes the prostate tissue causing obstruction.

Minimally invasive procedures for treatment of BPH symptoms include application of heat from various sources to eliminate excessive prostatic tissue, such as transurethral needle ablation of the prostate (TUNA), transurethral microwave thermotherapy (TUMT), transurethral vaporization of the prostate (TUVP), water-induced thermotherapy, high-intensity ultrasound energy therapy, and interstitial laser coagulation. Ablation procedures may be preferred for men with bleeding disorders because there is less blood loss. Removal of obstructing prostate tissue by these methods can allow better urinary flow. Mechanical approaches such as balloon dilation and urethral stent placement dilate the obstructed area of the urethra. Balloon dilation involves placing a catheter with a balloon at its tip through the urethra; the balloon is inflated in the area of obstruction. Urethral stents are placed in the obstructed urethral area to dilate the narrowed section for better urinary flow.

As with medical treatments, surgical management and minimally invasive procedures have risks and benefits. The risks include bleeding, infection, and impotence. The best therapy for BPH is not the same for all patients. The treatment options will depend on the severity of symptoms, the risks and benefits of the therapy, and the general health condition of the patient. A satisfactory management plan to treat BPH symptoms can be accomplished in a partnership between the patient and his physician.

PERSPECTIVE AND PROSPECTS
The development of prostate enlargement is multifactorial, and the specific steps involved in its progression are still unresolved. Research studies are ongoing to evaluate the processes involved in the development of this condition. For example, chronic inflammation has been implicated in BPH. Studies have shown that tissue specimens from enlarged prostates have proinflammatory cells and cytokines. This may explain why obesity, which causes increased inflammatory cytokines, is associated with BPH. One cytokine implicated in BPH development is transforming growth factor beta. TGF-beta is involved in the cell signaling that causes an increase in expression of some genes in BPH, such as the gene called *GAGEC1*. This gene is a member of the *GAGE* family. The proteins expressed by these genes are associated with male and female reproductive organs such as the prostate, testis, Fallopian tubes, uterus, and placenta, as well as in

cancers of the prostate, testis, and uterus. Unraveling these molecular processes in BPH may lead to the design of new therapeutic modalities for an enlarged prostate.

Further, inflammatory markers, such as C-reactive proteins, correlate with increased lower urinary tract symptoms. Prostate epithelial cells also secrete hypoxia-inducible factor (HIF)-a alpha (coding protein) in response to inflammation. This is proposed to cause testosterone-induced hyperplasia. Investigators found that Heat shock protein (HSP) 27, which mediates immune responses, increases with inflammation in prostate tissue.

Recently, studies evaluating combination therapy, such as using both an alpha-blocker and a 5-alpha-reductase inhibitor for treatment of BPH and its related symptoms, have been carried out. One such study is the Medical Therapy of Prostate Symptoms Study (MTOPS), which showed that the clinical progression of BPH is delayed and symptoms are reduced by combination therapy. Clinical guidelines from authoritative sources such as the American Urological Association, the Agency for Healthcare Research and Quality, and the International Consultation on BPH still recommend that a patient discuss the risks and benefits of combination therapy with his physician. For example, the risks of side effects from two medications and the economic burden of purchasing two medications should be balanced with the benefits derived from the combination therapy.

The search for novel drugs to treat an enlarged prostate continues, including the development of more selective alpha-blockers and 5-alpha-reductase inhibitors (both steroidal and nonsteroidal). The factors that are involved in the development of BPH, such as cytokines, growth factors, estrogen, and androgen hormone receptors, are being evaluated as targets for potential therapeutic options. Some studies have also shown that botulinum neurotoxin (Botox) injection can shrink the prostate and reduce levels of PSA. However, such use of Botox is off-label and currently not approved for BPH by the FDA. Significant basic research regarding the mechanisms by which Botox affects the prostate and evidence-based data for use of Botox in BPH are needed.

Current studies in managing an enlarged prostate also include evaluation of specific aspects of herbal preparations such as saw palmetto and other alternative phytomedicine products. Moreover, treatment of BPH by surgical and minimally invasive procedures are still being compared with regard to clinical efficacy, related complications, and optimal energy sources for heat. The future will certainly bring more answers about the biological basis of enlarged prostate as well as even better treatment options.

—*Joseph Muraca, OMS-III*

See also: Aging; Endocrinology; Genital disorders, male; Glands; Hormones; Hyperplasia; Men's health; Prostate gland; Prostate gland removal; Reproductive system; Urinary disorders; Urinary system; Urology.

For Further Information:

Abrams, P., et al. "Evaluation and Treatment of Lower Urinary Tract Symptoms in Older Men." *The Journal of Urology*, vol. 181, no. 4, 2009, pp. 1779-87, doi:10.1016/j.juro.2008.11.127.

Alan, Rick. "Benign Prostatic Hyperplasia." *Health Library*, 27 Sept. 2012.

Bagla, Sandeep et al. "Re: Surgical Management of Lower Urinary Tract Symptoms Attributed to Benign Prostatic Hyperplasia." H. E. Foster, M. J. Barry, P. Dahm, M. C. Gandhi, S. A. Kaplan, T. S. Kohler, L. B. Lerner, D. J. Lightner, J. K. Parsons, C. G. Roehrborn, C. Welliver, T. J. Wilt and K. T. McVary J Urol 2018; 200: 612-619." *The Journal of urology* vol. 201,2 (2019): 400-403. doi:10.1016/j.juro.2018.09.058

Berry, S. J., et al. "The Development of Human Benign Prostatic Hyperplasia with Age." *The Journal of Urology*, vol. 132, no. 3, 1984, pp. 474-79, doi:10.1016/s0022-5347(17)49698-4.

Brown, Christian T., et al. "Self-Management for Men with Lower Urinary Tract Symptoms: Randomised Controlled Trial." *BMJ (Clinical Research ed.)*, vol. 334, no.7583, 2007, p. 25, doi:10.1136/bmj.39010.551319.AE.

Chuang, Yao-Chi, and Michael B. Chancellor. "The Application of Botulinum Toxin in the Prostate." *Journal of Urology*, vol. 176, no. 6, Dec. 2006, pp. 2375-82.

DiPaola, Robert S., and Ronald A. Morton. "Proven and Unproven Therapy for Benign Prostatic Hyperplasia." *New England Journal of Medicine*, vol. 354, no. 6, 9 Feb. 2006, pp. 632-34.

"Enlarged Prostate." *MedlinePlus*, 9 Sept. 2011.

Fwu, Chyng-Wen, et al. "Change in Sexual Function in men with Lower Urinary Tract Symptoms/Benign Prostatic Hyperplasia Associated with Long-Term Treatment with Doxazosin, Finasteride and Combined Therapy." *The Journal of Urology*, vol. 191, no. 6, 2014, pp. 1828-34, doi:10.1016/j.juro.2013.12.014.

Gillenwater, Jay Y., et al. "Benign Prostatic Hyperplasia." *Adult and Pediatric Urology*. 4th ed., vol. 2, Lippincott Williams & Wilkins, 2002, pp. 1401-1401.

Gratzke, Christian, et al. "EAU Guidelines on the Assessment of Non-neurogenic Male Lower Urinary Tract Symptoms including Benign Prostatic Obstruction." *European Urology*, vol. 67, no. 6, 2015, pp. 1099-1109, doi:10.1016/j.eururo.2014.12.038.

Isaacs, J. T. "Antagonistic Effect of Androgen on Prostatic Cell Death." *The Prostate*, vol. 5, no. 5, 1984, pp. 545-57, doi:10.1002/pros.2990050510.

Jiang, Yuqing, et al. "Expression of Heat Shock Protein 27 in Benign Prostatic Hyperplasia with Chronic Inflammation." *Medical Science Monitor: International Medical Journal of Experimental and Clinical Research*, vol. 21, 2976-85, 3 Oct. 2015, doi:10.12659/MSM.894562.

Kim, Hye-Jin, et al. "Pathogenic Role of HIF-1a in Prostate Hyperplasia in the Presence of Chronic Inflammation." *Biochimica et Biophysica Acta*, vol. 1832, no. 1, 2013, pp. 183-94, doi:10.1016/j.bbadis.2012.09.002.

Komaroff, Anthony, editor. "Prostate Gland." *Harvard Medical School Family Health Guide*. Free Press, 2005.

Kupelian, Varant, et al. "Association of C-reactive Protein and Lower Urinary Tract Symptoms in Men and Women: Results from Boston Area Community Health Survey." *Urology*, vol. 73, no. 5, 2009, pp. 950-7, doi:10.1016/j.urology.2008.12.012.

Lerner, Lori B., et al. "Management of Lower Urinary Tract Symptoms Attributed to Benign Prostatic Hyperplasia: AUA GUIDELINE PART I-Initial Work-up and Medical Management." *The Journal of Urology*, vol. 206, no. 4, 2021, pp. 806-17, doi:10.1097/JU.0000000000002183.

Liu, Liangren, et al. "Phosphodiesterase-5 Inhibitors for Lower Urinary Tract Symptoms Secondary to Benign Prostatic Hyperplasia: A Systematic Review and Meta-analysis." *Urology*, vol. 77, no. 1, 2011, pp. 123-29, doi:10.1016/j.urology.2010.07.508.

McConnell, John D., et al. "The Long-term Effect of Doxazosin, Finasteride, and Combination Therapy on the Clinical Progression of Benign Prostatic Hyperplasia." *The New England Journal of Medicine*, vol. 349, no. 25, 2003, pp. 2387-98, doi:10.1056/NEJMoa030656.

McVary, Kevin T., editor. *Management of Benign Prostatic Hypertrophy*. Humana Press, 2004.

McVary, Kevin T., et al. "Update on AUA Guideline on the Management of Benign Prostatic Hyperplasia." *The Journal of Urology*, vol. 185, no. 5, 2011, pp. 1793-803, doi:10.1016/j.juro.2011.01.074.

Pöyhönen, Antti, et al. "Natural Course of Lower Urinary Tract Symptoms in Men Not Requiring Treatment—A 5-year Longitudinal Population-based Study." *Urology*, vol. 83, no. 2, 2014, pp. 411-15, doi:10.1016/j.urology.2013.10.003.

"Prostate Disorders." *The Merck Manual Home Health Handbook*, edited by Robert S. Porter, et al., Merck Research Laboratories, 2009.

"Prostate Enlargement: Benign Prostatic Hyperplasia." *National Kidney and Urologic Diseases Information Clearinghouse*, 23 Mar. 2013.

Robert, Grégoire, et al. "Inflammation in Benign Prostatic Hyperplasia: A 282 Patients' Immunohistochemical Analysis." *The Prostate*, vol. 69, no.16, 2009, pp. 1774-80, doi:10.1002/pros.21027.

Roehrborn, Claus G. "Definition of At-risk Patients: Baseline Variables." *BJU International*, vol. 97, Suppl. 2, 2006, pp. 7-11, doi:10.1111/j.1464-410X.2006.06098.x.

Rous, Stephen N. *The Prostate Book: Sound Advice on Symptoms and Treatment*. 3rd ed., W. W. Norton, 2002.

Scher, Howard I., and James A. Eastham. "Chapter 83: Benign and Malignant Diseases of the Prostate." *Harrison's Principles of Internal Medicine*. 20th ed., edited by J. Larry Jameson, McGraw Hill, 2018, accessmedicine.mhmedical.com/content.aspx?sectionid=192016319.

Sidney, S., et al. "Incidence of Surgically Treated Benign Prostatic Hypertrophy and of Prostate Cancer Among Blacks and Whites in a Prepaid Health Care Plan." *American Journal of Epidemiology* vol. 134, no. 8, 1991, pp. 825-29, doi:10.1093/oxfordjournals.aje.a116157.

Tacklind, James, et al. "Finasteride for Benign Prostatic Hyperplasia." *The Cochrane Database of Systematic Reviews*, vol. 2010, no. 10, 6 Oct. 2010, CD006015, doi:10.1002/14651858.CD006015.pub3.

PROSTATE GLAND

Category: Anatomy

Anatomy or system affected: Endocrine system, glands, reproductive system

Specialties and related fields: Endocrinology, oncology, urology

Definition: One of several accessory reproductive glands; its main function is to secrete into semen vital additive components that increase the fertilizing potential of sperm.

Key terms:

andrology: study of the physiological functions relating to male reproductive capacity

bulbourethal gland: the bulbous portion of the male urethra adjacent to the posterior prostate zone

gonad: the male or female organ (testis or ovary, respectively) in which the essential gametes are formed for reproduction

hyperplasia: a state of hormonal stimulation causing an increase in the number of cells in a tissue, resulting in an oversized organ

prostate-specific antigen (PSA): protein associated with the prostate gland

prostatoglandular carcinoma: the general pathological nomenclature for cancers located in the prostate gland

vas deferens: the duct that carries the male seminal fluid

STRUCTURE AND FUNCTIONS

The prostate is the largest of several glands that are referred to as the accessory glands of the male reproductive tract, the others being the seminal vesicles and the bulbourethral glands. Unlike the latter two, which evolved morphologically in smaller pairs, the prostate evolved as a single gland, approximately four centimeters in diameter in adults. It surrounds the urethra, the tubular tract that carries both semen and urine. During the early embryonic stage of life, both urinary organs and accessory sex glands are formed, through the cell-division process, out of the same original source of specialized cells in the intermediate mesoderm (called the nephrotome) and the cloaca.

In fact, up to a certain point in the growth of the human embryo, it is not possible to distinguish the pattern that will lead to formation of the male and female gonads. Following what is called the ambisexual stage, the undifferentiated gonad, or reproductive terminus, begins to evolve into a male or female reproductive organ, becoming either a testis or an ovary. Then, in the male, the three accessory sex glands begin to form. Their eventual key functions in the reproductive process will not begin, however, until the onset of puberty in the individual's growth cycle. Male puberty, or sexual maturity, is initiated when secretions from the testis and pituitary gland activate secretions from other organs, including the prostate gland. It is at this stage that elevated levels of androgenic steroids in the body cause the prostate to attain its full size and begin to secrete the fluids that are essential in the male reproductive function.

The function of all necessary reproductive glands, and of the prostate gland in particular, is to secrete fluids that affect the fertilization potential of the spermatozoa in the seminal fluid as it passes from its source in the testicles through the vas deferens duct. The vas deferens joins the urethra at a point just before the latter is encased by the prostate gland. Thereafter, the urethra serves as a channel for passage of seminal fluid through the penis.

When the adult prostate gland is functioning efficiently, the prostatic secretions that pass into the vas deferens should make up about 30 percent of the volume of the male seminal fluid. Although the process of prostate secretion after puberty is continuous, the composite elements of these secretions may vary. One notable variation in content occurs during moments of sexual excitement. A comparison of "resting" prostatic fluids with fluids obtained from ejaculation resulting from sexual stimulation suggests that the latter contains a higher level of certain enzymes, particularly acid phosphatase, than the former.

All "resting" prostatic fluid is only slightly basic, with an approximate pH of 7.2. The pH level may increase to 7.7 in men suffering from prostatitis. The main components of the fluid include diastase, an enzyme of the amylase group; proteolytic enzymes, especially fibrinolysin; citric acid; acid phosphatase, also an enzyme; cephalin, a chemical group containing amino acids that is found mainly in nervous-system tissues; cholesterol; magnesium; zinc; and calcium. In humans, but not necessarily in all mammals, calcium is more highly concentrated in prostatic fluid than in the blood plasma.

There are other differences between humans and other mammals with respect to the glandular origins of separate component elements of seminal fluid. Whereas citric acid originates in the human prostate gland, in other species it may come from the seminal vesicles, as is the case for boars, or it may flow in generally equal amounts from each of the accessory sex glands, such as in rabbits and guinea pigs. In all cases, citric acid is synthesized by chemical reactions within the originating glands.

There is general agreement that the fertilizing potential of spermatozoa is enhanced when combinations of these various prostatic fluid constituents join the flow of semen. No evidence has been found of an iden-

The Prostate Gland

Prostate gland

Penis

Testis

Scrotum

Anus

©EBSCO

tifiable target effect by any one specific element, although tests of relative concentrations of citric acid in semen suggest an influence on the activity level of testicular hormones, especially androgen. Additionally, with regard to the fertilization potential of male spermatozoa carried in the seminal fluid, citric acid reacts chemically with other component elements in ways that may delay the coagulation of seminal plasma or contribute to its capacity to be absorbed at the appropriate time in the fertilization process.

Research has also tentatively established that the fertilization potential of spermatozoa may depend on levels of zinc contained in secretions from the prostate gland. One chemical effect of zinc is to slow the breakdown of genetically vital chromosomes in individual sperm cells. This function of zinc has not been tied directly to potential fertility levels, however, since surgical removal of the section of the prostate where zinc is in the highest concentration (the dorsolateral portion of the gland) has not changed reproductive capacities in laboratory rats. Because prostate surgery involving human patients is almost exclusively connected with attempts to arrest prostate cancer, no research data have been recorded that can be compared with experiments performed on animals.

One area of research that has established irrefutable evidence in connection with fertility levels deals with the effects of certain drugs on the functioning of the accessory sex glands, including the prostate. Tests on morphine and methadone users, for example, have shown a definite reduction in the volume of human seminal ejaculate. Methadone, and in some cases morphine, can actually cause a reduction of the weight and volume of the testes, seminal vesicles, and prostate glands of laboratory mice. Specific constituent elements of prostate secretions that appear to be reduced when drugs such as morphine sulfate are administered include prostatic fructose and different forms of glucose that contribute to metabolic activity in the prostate gland itself.

In addition to medical or self-administered drugs, chemicals that enter the body through the food chain, such as the pesticide DDT, can also affect the functioning of the prostate. In mice, the testosterone metabolic process, which is very much dependent on the prostate, has been shown to be significantly retarded when DDT is administered under close controls. Dieldrin is another pesticide that affects the ability of prostate tissue in mice to absorb testosterone.

DISORDERS AND DISEASES

In general terms, diseases of the prostate gland tend to fall into two main categories: nonproliferative and proliferative. The latter category is characterized by two forms of dangerous physical change in the tissues of the gland itself: lesions and neoplasms (or tumors).

Diseases of the nonproliferative type, although painful and potentially quite dangerous to the patient's health, may be treated by modern medical means. One subgroup in this category is congenital anomalies. Some of these have slowly developing symptoms and may be discovered only when some other difficulty, such as urinary irregularities or infertility, is the initial cause for the doctor's examination. The most common form of anomaly is the congenital cyst, which occurs as a result of obstructions in the normal flow of secretions through the prostate gland. Secretion blockage is sometimes caused by irregular development of the parenchyma, the functioning tissues of the gland itself. Subsequent development of a cyst in the prostate itself further impedes the normal flow of secretions within and from the gland.

Congenital cysts usually occur in the prostatic utricle, an oblong protrusion measuring about three millimeters that is palpable when a medical doctor performs a rectal examination. The abnormality is generally discovered in patients in their early twenties. In newborn infants, the fact of recent estrogenic stimulation in utero can have the temporary effect of making the utricle three times its eventual normal length. If the prostatic utricle does not shorten during childhood and early adulthood, examining doctors will be alerted to the existence of a cyst and the possible need for surgical intervention.

A second form of nonproliferative disease in the prostate involves the formation of tiny calculi, or stones, inside the gland. True prostatic calculi are generally rare, but they may occur when prostatic secretions are altered by one of several possible factors, including infection or some form of metabolic dysfunction. Altered secretions can lead to abnormal chemical deposits inside the organ. These deposits in turn attract mineral concentrations, particularly of calcium salts, the main component of calculi.

Although pathology texts list up to five forms of proliferative tumors that can attack the accessory reproductive glands, the prostate gland itself is mainly vulnerable to two out of the five: prostatic carcinoma and primary prostatic sarcoma. More common and less dangerous proliferative lesions (inflammations, not tumors) affecting the prostate involve many different forms of hyperplasia. Although the causes of such lesions can vary, their effect may be summarized as inflammation leading to either the obstruction of normal secretions originating in the prostate or the potentially harmful addition to prostate secretions of foreign by-products of the inflammatory process.

The most common proliferative lesion of the prostate, nodular prostatic hyperplasia (NPH), leads directly to urological disease, usually in middle-aged and elderly males. Its high incidence is reflected in the widespread need for some form of prostate surgery among men over fifty. The disease derives its name from the fact that it displays multinodular areas of inflammation, which makes it difficult for specialized surgeons to localize areas demanding attention. Doctors are still uncertain of the exact origins of NPH and the complexities of hormonal phenomena associated with the disease. It appears, however, that NPH is a combination of the more simply diagnosed prostatic hyperplasia (prostate enlargement) and a hypertrophy (tissue constriction) of the inner zones of the prostate gland itself.

Although these various forms of lesions affect a high percentage of the adult male population, the greatest pathological menace associated with the prostate gland involves malignant tumors. Prostatic cancers represent the second most common form of cancer occurring among American males, with more than two hundred thousand cases diagnosed each year in the United States. Early diagnosis can usually result in treatment and cure. Because of the difficulties associated with diagnosis and the complexities of possible treatments, however, a large percentage of those suffering from prostate cancers die from the disease.

There is a problem of extended delay in the appearance of symptoms; approximately 70 percent of the total recorded cases remain locally latent for years. Yet even the prostatoglandular tumors that have clinical manifestations are often discovered too late for effective medical intervention.

Doctors looking for symptoms of prostate cancer, beyond those that might appear in physical examination via the rectum, pay particular attention to several likely warning signs. These include possible malignant repercussions stemming from prostatic lesions, especially NPH; sacral, lower back, or upper pubic pain; excessive urinary retention; and uneven or interrupted urinary flow. In recent years, screening for prostate cancer has involved measuring the prostate-specific antigen (PSA) level in a blood sample. PSA levels in males with a normal prostate generally measure around two nanograms or less. Elevated levels may indicate the presence of a tumor. The test remains inexact, however, since even a benign prostatic hypertrophy (BPH), or prostate enlargement, may result in an increase in PSA values.

If a physician suspects the presence of cancer in the prostate region, three forms of biopsy may be used. The most accurate method involves actual surgical opening and removal of sections for laboratory biopsy. This method is the most expensive, however, and is recommended mainly when physicians are convinced that a radical prostatectomy should probably follow initial surgical intervention, for reasons that may not be limited to concerns about cancer. Of the other two methods of diagnosis, core needle biopsy and needle aspiration biopsy, the former has a slightly higher level of accuracy, while the latter is safer and generally has fewer complications.

A complicating factor that makes prostate cancers among the most difficult to treat is similar to what has been observed with NPH. In NPH, which is a proliferative lesion, multinodular development complicates localization of the diseased area for treatment. In the case of prostatoglandular carcinoma, approximately 30 percent of diagnosed patients have diffused, as opposed to focal, growth development patterns. In such cases, radical prostatectomy, despite the fact that it usually leaves the patient impotent, is generally believed to be the best course of action.

A second, less common category of prostate cancer is referred to as primary prostatic sarcoma. Although this disease represents only 2 percent of all prostate cancers, it differs from the more common prostatic carcinoma in that it may occur in male patients of any age and has been diagnosed in infants as young as four months. Another serious factor is that if this form of cancer appears in the prostate, it frequently extends directly to other adjacent organs or structures, primarily the bladder, seminal vesicles, or rectum.

PERSPECTIVE AND PROSPECTS

Although statistics show that as of 2009, prostate cancer was the most common cause of cancer among men and the second most common cause of cancer death among men, the medical world remained divided over questions of prognosis. Doctors called upon by the National Cancer Institute hesitated to reach a consensus about the central question of relative success rates of radiation treatment versus surgical intervention. Part of the problem, the institute learned, was that because patients are most often diagnosed at an advanced age-according to the American Cancer Society, as of 2012, the average age at diagnosis was sixty-seven-data gathered on their physical condition do not provide sufficiently random samplings for comparison with the population as a whole. A main reason for apparent dissatisfaction with too-focused data is that, because of the typically late discovery of prostate cancer, one central consideration in choosing between surgery or radiation treatment is rendered less vital; past a certain stage in advanced adulthood, diminished sexual reproductive capacity also diminishes patient sensitivity to the possibility that surgical removal of cancerous growth in the prostate will almost certainly bring about impotence.

Significant research has addressed the possible causes of prostate cancer. In a significant number of cases, researchers have observed a specific form of deoxyribonucleic acid (DNA) translocation in cells making up the tumor, lending support to the belief many forms of such cancers result from certain mutations. In the future, observation of such specific mutations from biopsy material may allow for improved methods of screening.

—*Byron D. Cannon, PhD;*
updated by Richard Adler, PhD

See also Aging; Cancer; Colorectal surgery; Endocrine glands; Endocrinology; Genital disorders, male; Glands; Hormones; Malignancy and metastasis; Men's health; Oncology; Prostate cancer; Prostate enlargement; Prostate gland removal; Puberty and adolescence; Reproductive system; Semen; Urinary disorders; Urinary system; Urology; Vas defrens.

For Further Information:
American Cancer Society. www.cancer.org
Blute, Michael. *Mayo Clinic on Prostate Health: What to Do about Prostate Enlargement, Inflammation and Cancer.* 2d ed. Rochester, Minn.: Mayo Clinic, 2003.
Fox, Arnold, and Barry Fox. *The Healthy Prostate: A Doctor's Comprehensive Program for Preventing and Treating Common Problems.* New York: John Wiley & Sons, 1996.
McClure, Mark W. *Smart Medicine for a Healthy Prostate: Natural and Conventional Therapies for Common Prostate Disorders.* New York: Avery, 2001.
Marieb, Elaine N. *Essentials of Human Anatomy and Physiology.* 10th ed. San Francisco: Pearson/Benjamin Cummings, 2011.
Marx, Jean. "Fused Genes May Help Explain the Origins of Prostate Cancer." *Science* 310 (October 28, 2005): 603.
"Prostate Diseases." *MedlinePlus,* May 20, 2013.

Westheimer, Ruth, and Pierre Lehu. *Sex for Dummies*. 3d ed. Hoboken, N.J.: John Wiley & Sons, 2006.

Yeo, Lehana, et al. "The Development of the Modern Prostate Biopsy." *InTechOpen*, December 2, 2011.

Zangwill, Monica, and Igor Puzanov. "Conditions InDepth: Prostate Cancer." *Health Library*, October 11, 2012.

PROSTATE GLAND REMOVAL

Category: Procedure

Also known as: Prostatectomy

Anatomy or system affected: Endocrine system, glands

Specialties and related fields: General surgery, oncology, proctology, urology

Definition: A surgical procedure to remove all or part of an abnormal prostate gland.

Key terms:

cauterization: a means of sealing blood vessels with heat; used to prevent bleeding

impotence: the inability to achieve an erection

incision: a cut made with a scalpel during a surgical procedure

incontinence: the inability to retain urine

prostate: a gland in males that surrounds the urethra and secretes a fluid into the ejaculate

urethra: the tube that connects the urinary bladder externally

INDICATIONS AND PROCEDURES

The removal of the prostate gland, or prostatectomy, may be performed when enlargement of the gland blocks or reduces the outflow of urine. Removal may also be indicated in prostate cancer or inflammation of the prostate (prostatitis).

Enlargement of the prostate gland, also known as benign prostatic hyperplasia (BPH), may affect men over the age of fifty. Because the prostate gland is situated so that it surrounds the urethra, when it enlarges, it can compress the urethra and reduce the flow of urine. Symptoms usually include gradual reduction in the ability to urinate effectively. Since the flow of urine out the urethra is obstructed by the enlarged gland, the patient experiences difficulty starting urination and a weak stream.

In early stages, the urinarybladder muscle becomes heavier and stronger in order to compensate for the increased resistance in the urethra. Eventually, however, the bladder is unable to expel all the urine and becomes distended. This urinary retention can cause abdominal swelling and a perceived urgency to urinate. In fact, the bladder may contract frequently and cause a need for frequent urination. This is one sign of bladder muscle failure and the need for medical atten-

tion. In some patients, there may be incontinence as a result of the leakage of small volumes of urine.

Prostate cancer is a malignant growth of the prostate gland. Most patients with prostate cancer are in their seventies; this condition also occurs in middle-aged men. The symptoms that develop are similar to those of BPH. Diagnosis is usually made by a digital rectal examination, ultrasonography, prostate biopsy, and a blood test for prostatic-specific antigens.

The treatment for both BPH and prostatic cancer involves medical management and surgical removal of all or part of the gland. In BPH, finasteride (Proscar) can be used to reduce the size of the gland and diminish symptoms. Prostate cancer can sometimes be managed using drugs that block or reduce the production of testosterone. Such agents include flutamide (Eulexin) and leuprolide. If medical management is not effective, surgical removal of the gland is usually indicated.

The most common surgical procedure for the removal of part of the prostate gland is transurethral resection of the prostate (TURP), which is performed using an instrument called a resectoscope. The patient is first anesthetized using spinal or general anesthesia. Then the resectoscope is inserted into the urethra at the tip of the penis and directed up toward the prostate gland. The resectoscope allows the surgeon to view the urinary bladder and prostate and insert a cutting instrument or heated wire into the area of the prostate to be removed. As the gland is cut away, it is removed from the urethra by suction. Any bleeding that may occur is stopped by a cauterizing electrode, which seals the vessels. After the prostate gland has been removed, the surgeon withdraws the resectoscope and inserts a catheter into the bladder to drain urine and any remaining blood or tissue.

If a more radical procedure than transurethral resection is needed, as in cases of prostate cancer, then retropubic prostatectomy is performed. This operation requires that the patient be anesthetized. The surgeon makes a horizontal incision just above the pubic hairline into the abdominal cavity and exposes the urinary bladder and prostate gland. A cut into the capsule that encases the gland is made, and the surgeon begins to remove the prostate gland. To drain excess fluid from the pelvic cavity, the surgeon places a temporary flexible tube near to where the prostate was excised. Bleeding vessels are cauterized, and the abdominal wall is sutured. A urethral catheter is inserted and left in place to aid in draining the bladder of blood and urine. An alternative to retropubic prostatectomy is perineal prostatectomy, in which the prostate is accessed through an incision in the perineum, the area between the scrotum and anus; this procedure is less common, because it carries a higher risk of nerve damage. Another option is laparoscopic prostatectomy, in which four or five very small incisions are made in the abdomen, through which computer-guided instruments and a camera are inserted to perform the procedure.

USES AND COMPLICATIONS

After removal of the urethral catheter, the patient is encouraged to drink large amounts of fluids and to pass urine. Occasionally, the patient may experience frequent and painful urination but should still consume adequate amounts of liquids to help clear the urinary tract of blood and other postoperative debris. A few patients will continue to have incontinence for several weeks.

More severe complications include intra-abdominal bleeding from surgery, infections, and blood clots that obstruct urine outflow from the bladder. Bleeding within the pelvic and abdominal cavities is usually detected and corrected during surgery. If it occurs after prostatectomy, a second operation may be required to find and stop the bleeding. Most infections of the urinary tract can be adequately treated with appropriate antibiotic therapy. Urinary obstruction resulting from a blood clot can be washed out with a catheter in the urethra.

Approximately 10 to 20 percent of men undergoing retropubic prostatectomy experience impotence. This complication is more common in older patients, and can often be treated with drugs such as Viagra.

For most men, the hospital stay is about two days for transurethral resection of the prostate, two to three days for open surgery, and overnight for a laparoscopic procedure. Several weeks after the surgery the patient can resume all activities, including intercourse. Most men are sterile, however, immediately after either procedure because most of the sperm and seminal fluid are expelled backward into the urinary bladder (retrograde ejaculation). The ejaculate is then excreted with the urine during the next urination.

—*Matthew Berria, PhD and Douglas Reinhart, MD*

See also Aging; Biopsy; Cancer; Colorectal surgery; Endocrine glands; Genital disorders, male; Glands; Incontinence; Malignancy and metastasis; Men's health; Oncology; Prostate cancer; Prostate enlargement; Prostate gland; Radiation therapy; Reproductive system; Urinary disorders; Urinary system; Urology.

For Further Information:

American Medical Association. *American Medical Association Family Medical Guide*. 4th rev. ed. Hoboken, N.J.: John Wiley & Sons, 2004.
Bangma, Ch. H., and D. W. W. Newling, eds. *Prostate and Renal Cancer, Benign Prostatic Hyperplasia, Erectile Dysfunction, and Basic Research: An Update*. Boca Raton, Fla.: Parthenon, 2003.
Griffith, H. Winter. *Complete Guide to Symptoms, Illness, and Surgery*. Rev. 6th ed. New York: Perigee, 2012.
McPhee, Stephen J., and Maxine A. Papadakis, eds. *Current Medical Diagnosis and Treatment*. 50th ed. Los Altos, Calif.: Lange Medical, 2011.
Neff, Deanna M. "Prostatectomy." *Health Library*, September 26, 2012.
"Simple Prostatectomy." *MedlinePlus*, March 28, 2011.
"Transurethral Resection of the Prostate." *Health Library*, September 26, 2012.
Wein, Alan J., et al., eds. *Campbell-Walsh Urology*. 10th ed. Philadelphia: Saunders/Elsevier, 2012.
Zollinger, Robert M., Jr., and Robert M. Zollinger, Sr. *Zollinger's Atlas of Surgical Operations*. 9th ed. New York: McGraw-Hill, 2011.

PROSTHESES

Category: Treatment
Anatomy or system affected: All
Specialties and related fields: Biotechnology, cardiology, dentistry, dermatology, general surgery, occupational health, oncology, ophthalmology, orthopedics, physical therapy, plastic surgery
Definition: Artificial replacements for missing, malformed, diseased, or damaged human parts.
Key terms:
amputation level: the site and type of amputation
anaplastology: the art and science of artificially restoring parts of the body or face with lifelike and aesthetic prostheses
biosynthetics: materials that are both biological (found in nature) and synthetic (artificial)
osseointegration: a process in which bone grows around embedded titanium fixtures; the stabilized fixtures eventually support dental or facial prostheses
prosthetist: someone who designs, fabricates, and fits prostheses
residual limb: the limb remaining after amputation
teratogen: an agent that interferes with normal embryonic or fetal development
thermoplastic: a plastic that can be shaped when heated and that becomes rigid when cooled; it can be modified repeatedly for prosthesis fittings
thermoset: a plastic offering structural stability; it cannot be reshaped once cooled

INDICATIONS AND PROCEDURES

Traditionally, prostheses are defined as artificial replacements for missing, malformed, diseased, or damaged human parts. However, partly as a result of biomedical engineering feats, scientists and practitioners disagree as to what defines a prosthesis. Some think that only external devices that are mechanical, such as artificial limbs, are prostheses. Others think that internal devices, such as hip or knee replacements, or internal parts that are biological, such as transplanted organs and parts of organs, are prostheses. Finally, some think biosynthetic materials, such as artificial skin substitutes, qualify. Hence, the broadest definition could include artificial limbs, eyes, and noses; biosynthetic materials; organ transplants; heart valves; penile implants; bladder pumps; wigs; and dental appliances.

Body parts may be ruined or their function impaired as a result of disease, aging, congenital malformation, or trauma. Common diseases that may result in loss of limbs or destruction of tissue are diabetes, cancer, and vascular disease. Osteoarthritis erodes cartilage in the spine and joints and is common among older people. Congenital anomalies arising from exposure to teratogens during embryonic or fetal development may impair function. Trauma from accidents and war is a major cause of damage. Every week, land mines maim approximately twelve hundred people worldwide, many of them children. Generally, a pros-

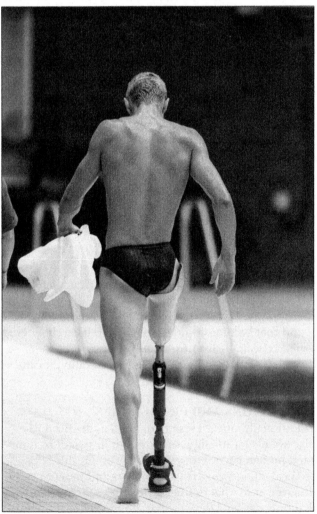

A man with a lower-extremity prosthesis. Photo by Australian Paralympic Committee, via Wikimedia Commons.

thesis is prescribed if normal function or appearance can be partially or completely restored.

The most common prostheses are replacements for amputated limbs or parts of limbs. More than 70 percent of amputations in the United States are caused by peripheral vascular disease in which blood flow is partially or completely obstructed in blood vessels beyond the chest. Peripheral vascular disease includes arteriosclerosis (hardening of the arteries), thromboembolism (blockage of a blood vessel), and complications from diabetes, a chronic metabolic disease.

Amputations involve the disarticulation of joints (such as through the hips) and the transection of long bones. About two-thirds of lower leg amputations in the United States are at a level below the knee and include transtibial (across the lower leg bone), ankle, foot, and toe amputations. About a third of leg amputations are transfemoral (across the thigh bone). Most amputees are over sixty-five years of age and have peripheral vascular disease; a large proportion of these amputees have diabetes.

A lower extremity prosthesis comprises several components. A socket fits around the residual limb and transmits force for standing and walking. A sheath, sock, and liner serve as an interface between limb and prosthesis, offering protection and comfort, especially for people with peripheral vascular disease or sensitive skin. A suspension system secures the socket to the residual limb for safe ambulation. There may be a knee joint with a single axis and hinge, or a polycentric axis with changing centers of rotation. A pylon or tube connects the socket to the terminal device and may absorb, store, and release energy. The terminal device, such as a foot or ski, can respond to changing terrain if dynamic. For each component, a prosthetist selects the appropriate type after evaluating several factors, including the patient's upper body strength, trunk control, balance, posture, motivation, vocation, and hobbies and sports, as well as cost and aesthetics. Sometimes, at the patient's behest, a more lifelike prosthesis is designed instead of one that functions optimally and is easy to maintain.

About 90 percent of upper extremity amputations are the result of traumatic injury sustained by men between the ages of twenty and forty. Commonly, injury results from accidents with machines (especially farm machines), frostbite, and electrical burns. Prostheses for upper extremities range from being entirely cosmetic to optimally functional. There are two types of functional prostheses: body-powered (involving cable systems) and myoelectric. The latter use surface electrodes to translate energy from muscle contractions to prosthetic elbows, wrists, and hands.

In general, the level of amputation is linked to the degree of function that may be restored by a well-designed prosthesis and appropriate rehabilitation. For example, as the level rises from toes to hips, it becomes increasingly difficult to fully restore mobility and locomotion. Also, it is easier to restore the function of lower limbs than of upper limbs-primarily because of complex hand movements for grasping and manipulating.

Prostheses can replace parts of the face when plastic surgery is not a viable option. Sometimes, neither function nor appearance can be restored by more surgery. The patient may not be able to afford or refuses to endure more plastic surgery and elects instead to wear a prosthesis. Facial prostheses include ears, noses, midfacials, orbitals (eyes and lids), and artificial eyes. An anaplastologist, a member of a craniofacial rehabilitation team, custom designs a prosthesis for the tissue site after considering the symmetry of the face, its proportions, and anatomical landmarks. After sculpting and molding, a prosthesis is made of silicone rubber tinted to resemble the patient's skin color.

Medical adhesives can keep a facial prosthesis in place. However, a more secure method involves osseointegrated implants of titanium posts. After bone grows around the posts, abutments or extensions are added surgically to support a bar; the prosthesis is clipped to the bar to hold it in place. Sometimes magnets are used. Osseointegrated implants are an important improvement over adhesives in that a person who wears a facial or dental prosthesis is less likely to be embarrassed by losing it in public. Regardless of the method of securing the prosthesis, it must be taken off at night. Both the skin and the prosthesis need to be cleaned daily.

USES AND COMPLICATIONS
People who use prosthetic devices for ambulation expend more energy than do able-bodied people. For example, the energy expended in using a unilateral prosthesis (for one limb or segment) varies directly with the level of amputation. Lower energy costs (related to effort) are associated with longer residual limbs, unilateral rather than bilateral amputation of both limbs or segments, intact knee(s), and loss of limb(s) to trauma rather than vascular disease. Someone with a unilateral transtibial amputation will expend about 9 to 20 percent more energy walking than does an able-bodied person, whereas someone with a bilateral transfemoral amputation may expend almost 300 percent more energy. It is interesting to note that the effort to walk with crutches may be greater than with a prosthesis. Thus, the prognosis for successful ambulation may be better for a nonambulatory patient when fitted with a prosthesis rather than with crutches.

Some of the common problems associated with prosthetic devices include initial pain, sensitivity, and

edema (swelling) of the residual limb after surgery; discomfort when learning to use a prosthesis; problems with balance and gait (pattern of walking); the breakdown of skin where it comes into contact with an ill-fitting prosthesis; and the effort necessary for donning and doffing (putting on and taking off) a prosthesis. Some types of components are too challenging for the debilitated or the elderly. For example, donning the traditional suction suspension system for holding a transfemoral prosthesis in place requires strength, good balance, and cardiovascular fitness. Some of the dynamically responsive components are bioengineering marvels, but they are heavier and require relatively more strength to use than do traditional counterparts. In general, components suitable for athletes and laborers are not suitable for the weak and sedentary.

People who wear a facial prosthesis depend on its realism and attractiveness for psychological comfort in social settings. The quality of the prosthesis depends a great deal on the artistry of the anaplastologist. When successfully crafted, the prosthesis allows the wearer to feel confident in public whenever ordinary social distances are involved, such as when passing people on the street or making a purchase in a store. However, the prosthesis is detectable close up and may be a source of anxiety for the wearer in more intimate settings.

Although a facial prosthesis may allow a person to "pass" as normal looking, it may not restore the ability to communicate emotion nonverbally or the ability to speak clearly. Even if communication is possible, people may look away, thus disregarding any facial cues. Other difficulties arise when the face has been so damaged that normal eating behavior is impossible or embarrassing. This represents a serious challenge because a great deal of human social interaction involves food; the inability or unwillingness to share food can disrupt families and ruin friendships. The disfigured person may insist on eating alone. The worst consequence of facial disfigurement is social isolation, which leads to depression. However, mutual help groups and nonprofit networks, such as Let's Face It USA, can offer social support and information.

Typically, a facial prosthesis will last about two years, more with careful care. Over time, the silicone yellows when exposed to ultraviolet light, pollutants, and oil. The condition of both the prosthesis and the wearer's skin needs to be monitored regularly by a health care specialist.

PERSPECTIVE AND PROSPECTS
Early versions of today's facial prostheses were crafted by two inspired artists during World War I. Captain Derwent Wood, an English sculptor working out of

Britain's Third London General Hospital, was dismayed by the number of suicides committed by men disfigured in trench warfare. After multiple reconstructive surgeries, the men had healed physically but were ashamed of their faces. In response to their plight, Captain Wood made full or partial masks based on photographs taken before their injuries. He made very thin masks of galvanized copper lined with silver, which he painted with oils to approximate the coloration of their skin. Eyeglasses often held the masks in place.

Anna Coleman Ladd, a Boston sculptor in France with the American Red Cross, created masks using similar methods. The soldiers were particularly appreciative of the eyelashes, mustaches, and whiskers made of fine copper threads. If the mouth had been damaged, Ladd parted the lips of the mask just enough to allow a cigarette holder.

Today, facial prostheses are more lifelike and more securely attached to the face. Although there have been tremendous advances in reconstructive surgery and biosynthetic skin substitutes, facial prostheses are still necessary for some patients disfigured, for example, by cancer treatments or burns.

The earliest prosthetists for limbs were blacksmiths, armor makers, artisans, and amputees themselves. War was often the occasion for ingenuity. For example, during the Civil War thousands of amputees needed limb replacements. Wounded men made their own peg legs or crutches. Replacement limbs and feet from mail-order catalogs were less crude and were made of carved or milled wood covered in rawhide that was glued in place.

Major scientific and technical advances were made in prosthetic design after World War II and the Vietnam War. The National Academy of Sciences organized a conference in 1945 to call attention to the needs of the wounded and to the lack of scientific innovation in the field of prosthetics. An intense research program was sponsored by the Office of Scientific Research and Development, and later by the Veterans Administration. The result was several design breakthroughs, such as the patellar tendon-bearing prosthesis for transtibial amputation and the quadrilateral socket and hydraulic swing-phase knee for transfemoral amputation. After the Vietnam War, myoelectric control systems for upper extremity prostheses and modular endoskeletal lower extremity prostheses were developed. (Endoskeletal refers to a prosthesis in which the pylon is covered with an anatomically shaped, soft foam covering.)

In the early twentieth century, prostheses were made primarily of wood and leather. By the end of the century, major advances in materials science for the aerospace and marine industries yielded stronger and more lightweight materials, many of which were adopted by prosthetists.

Some of the major innovations in prosthetic design depended on the development of thermosetting plastics, which were important for suction socket suspension systems, and transparent plastics, which improved diagnostic fittings. For example, transparent test sockets are used to evaluate potential weight-bearing areas on residual limbs, and transparent face masks are used to evaluate thermal injuries. Other advances in materials engineering, such as the development of carbon composites, contributed to the design of high-performance prosthetic feet for athletes.

Today, leather is still used for suspension straps, belts, and limb cuffs, but there exists an armamentarium of interesting materials useful for prostheses, such as steel, aluminum, titanium, and magnesium alloys; thermoplastics; thermosetting materials; foamed plastics; and viscoelastic polymers.

In the 1960s, computer-aided design and manufacture (CAD/CAM) systems revolutionized the fabrication of prostheses. Using CAD/CAM, surface contours of residual limbs are digitized by reading casts with a probe or scanner. The subsequent numerical models are used for computer-guided fabrication. By the early twenty-first century, medical imaging methods, such as computed tomography (CT) scanning and magnetic resonance imaging (MRI), were used in CAD/CAM systems. This was a major advance because CT and MRI allow the prosthetist to see underlying skeletal and soft tissue structures. Before the incorporation of medical imaging, the prosthetist relied on surface contour maps and palpation (feel) of the residual limb to evaluate anatomical structure. It is likely that advances in medical imaging will contribute further to innovative prosthetic design and fabrication in the future.

—*Tanja Bekhuis, PhD*

See also Accidents; Amputation; Bones and the skeleton; Circulation; Critical care; Critical care, pediatric; Diabetes mellitus; Emergency medicine; Grafts and grafting; Lower extremities; Oncology; Orthopedic surgery; Orthopedics; Orthopedics, pediatric; Physical rehabilitation; Plastic surgery; Transplantation; Upper extremities; Vascular medicine; Vascular system.

For Further Information:
Hughes, Michael J. *The Social Consequences of Facial Disfigurement*. Brookfield, Vt.: Ashgate, 1998.
Lusardi, Michelle M., and Caroline C. Nielsen. *Orthotics and Prosthetics in Rehabilitation*. 3d ed. Philadelphia; London.: Saunders, 2012.
MedlinePlus. "Artificial Limbs." *MedlinePlus*, May 2, 2013.
Newell, Robert. *Body Image and Disfigurement Care*. New York: Routledge, 2000.
Ott, Katherine, David Serlin, and Stephen Mihm, eds. *Artificial Parts, Practical Lives: Modern Histories of Prosthetics*. New York: New York University Press, 2002.

Schaffer, Erik. "Overview of Limb Prosthetics." *The Merck Manual Home Health Handbook*, May 2007.

Seymour, Ron. *Prosthetics and Orthotics: Lower Limb and Spinal*. Philadelphia: Lippincott Williams & Wilkins, 2002.

Vorvick, Linda J. "Prosthesis." *MedlinePlus*, January 21, 2013.

PROTEIN

Category: Biology
Anatomy or system affected: All
Specialties and related fields: Biochemistry, nutrition
Definition: An important dietary nutrient with many essential functions in the body.

STRUCTURE AND FUNCTIONS

Proteins are composed of twenty-two different amino acids in various combinations joined together in a chain. The human body can synthesize fourteen amino acids, known as inessential amino acids, whereas the other eight, known as essential amino acids, must be provided by the diet. Proteins from dietary sources are considered complete or incomplete based on their amino acid content. Complete proteins provide all eight essential amino acids, whereas incomplete proteins have low amounts of, or are missing, at least one essential amino acid. Only fish, meat, poultry, eggs, cheese, and other foods from animal sources contain complete proteins. Peanuts, soy, nuts, seeds, green peas, legumes, and some grains provide the richest plant proteins. Omnivores typically eat a sufficient variety of foods to consume adequate essential amino acids. Vegetarians ensure sufficient amino acid intake by consuming a variety of plant proteins.

Every cell in the body contains protein. Proteins are essential for cell structure and function and comprise major components of skin, tissues, muscles, and internal organs. Dietary protein, one of three types of nutrients used for energy, is required for the building, maintenance, and repair of body tissue. Growth and development during childhood, adolescence, and pregnancy depend on proteins. Proteins participate in all cellular functions, such as acting as enzyme catalysts and transport and storage molecules. They also provide mechanical support and immune protection, generate movement, transmit nerve impulses, and control growth and differentiation. Important classes of proteins include enzymes, hormones, and antibodies.

DISORDERS AND DISEASES

Protein deficiency is relatively rare in developed countries, although poverty can prevent adequate protein consumption. Protein deficiency can result from stringent weight loss diets or in older adults. Severe protein deficiency is fatal. In developing countries, protein deficiency causes the disease known as kwashiorkor, which includes symptoms such as apathy, diarrhea, inactivity, failure to grow, fatty liver, and edema. Since the body cannot store protein, too much protein can also be harmful, with a high-protein diet potentially leading to high cholesterol or other diseases and possible effects on kidney function. Excess protein may also result in immune system hyperactivity, liver dysfunction, bone loss, and obesity. Proteins contribute to food allergies, with many people allergic to proteins in milk (casein), wheat (gluten), or proteins found in peanut, shellfish, or other seafoods.

PERSPECTIVE AND PROSPECTS

A nutritionally balanced diet provides adequate protein. The average diet in the United States includes nearly twice the amount of protein required to maintain a healthy body. Although it was once believed that vegetarians needed to combine proteins by consuming all amino acids in the same meal, it is now realized that benefits of protein combining can be achieved over a longer period of time. In May 2013, the New York University Fertility Center published a study showing that women undergoing fertility treatment increased their chances of conception by increasing the amount of protein in their diets.

—*C. J. Walsh, PhD*

See also Antioxidants; Carbohydrates; Cholesterol; Digestion; Food biochemistry; Gastroenterology; Gastroenterology, pediatric; Gastrointestinal system; Kwashiorkor; Macronutrients; Malabsorption; Malnutrition; Metabolism; Nutrition; Obesity; Obesity, childhood; Phytochemicals; Proteinuria; Supplements; Vitamins and minerals; Weight loss and gain; Weight loss medications.

For Further Information

"Can High-Protein, Low-Card Diet Boost Fertility Treatment?" *MedlinePlus*. May 6, 2013.

"Dietary Proteins." *MedlinePlus*. July 18, 2013.

Duyff, Roberta Larson. *American Dietetic Association Complete Food and Nutrition Guide*. Hoboken, N.J.: John Wiley & Sons, 2006.

Marshall, Keri. *User's Guide to Protein and Amino Acids*. Laguna Beach, Calif.: Basic Health Publications, 2005.

"Protein in diet." *MedlinePlus*. May 5, 2011.

Shils, Maurice E., Moshe Shike, A. Catharine Ross, and Benjamin Caballero. *Modern Nutrition in Health and Disease*. 10th ed. Philadelphia: Lippincott Williams & Wilkins, 2005.

PROTEINURIA

Category: Disease/Disorder
Also known as: Albuminuria
Anatomy or system affected: Kidneys, urinary system

Specialties and related fields: Nephrology, urology
Definition: Disorder involving the elimination of abnormally high amounts of protein in the urine. It is typically defined as the excretion of more than 150 milligrams of protein in the urine per day.

CAUSES AND SYMPTOMS

Proteinuria is a disorder that does not have a unique cause. The excretion of abnormally high amounts of protein in the urine can have a number of benign causes, in which case the disorder is likely transient. These causes include dehydration, acute illness, and overexertion. In other instances, proteinuria is the result of a problem within the kidneys. This type of proteinuria is more severe, as well as chronic. Proteins play an important function in the body and are routinely carried in the bloodstream. Since proteins are large molecules, they are not routinely filtered out by the kidneys into the urine. When the glomeruli (the filtering mechanisms within the kidneys) are damaged for any reason, these large protein molecules do pass through the filters and into the urine to be eliminated.

Proteinuria has no symptoms early in its course. One of the earliest signs of proteinuria is the foamy appearance of urine in the toilet. This foamy appearance is caused by the abnormally high amount of protein. As the disorder progresses, the symptoms progress to the development of edema (an accumulation of fluid causing swelling). As a result of the loss of protein from the bloodstream, less fluid is carried in the bloodstream, with more remaining in the tissues. As a result, edema appears in the hands and/or the feet and in the abdominal area.

TREATMENT AND THERAPY

The diagnosis of proteinuria is made based on the collection of urine samples. In the past, it required the collection of a twenty-four-hour urine specimen, with the diagnosis of proteinuria being made if more than 150 milligrams of protein were excreted per day. More recently, the diagnosis of proteinuria has been made based on one urine sample by determining a urine albumin (protein) to creatinine (waste product) ratio. More than 30 milligrams of albumin per milligram of creatinine is indicative of proteinuria. Whenever proteinuria is present, additional tests of kidney function are indicated. Chronic proteinuria is often indicative of chronic kidney disease.

Treatment of proteinuria is dependent on treating the underlying problem. Dietary modifications may be made to control glucose, sodium, and protein intake. Medications may be used to treat diabetes and hypertension. The most commonly used medications are angiotensin-converting enzyme (ACE) inhibitors. Diuret-

---

INFORMATION ON PROTEINURIA

Causes: Dehydration, fever, inflammatory process, medications, pregnancy-induced hypertension, hypertension, diabetes, glomerular disease
Symptoms: Foamy urine earlier in disease; edema in hands, feet, abdomen later in disease
Duration: Acute or chronic
Treatments: Medication (antihypertensives), treatment of underlying disorders

---

ics may be used as well in order to help the kidneys eliminate excess fluid.

PERSPECTIVE AND PROSPECTS

Proteinuria was first alluded to, although unnamed, by Hippocrates around 400 BCE when he described bubbly urine as a symptom of kidney disease. Over the next two thousand years, there were multiple allusions to foaming urine in the scientific and medical literature, indirectly linking it to kidney disease and to dropsy (tissue swelling because of retention of excessive amounts of fluid). In 1814, an English physician, John Blackall, published a book on dropsy in which he directly established a link between that condition and proteinuria (using the actual term). Shortly thereafter, fellow English physician Richard Bright published *Reports of Medical Cases* (1827), in which he identified edema and proteinuria as the major symptoms of nephritis (inflammation of the kidney, also known as Bright's disease). Since that time, proteinuria has been considered to be an early and major symptom of kidney disease.

—Robin Kamienny Montvilo, RN, PhD

See also Diuretics; End-stage renal disease; Hypertension; Kidney disorders; Kidney transplantation; Kidneys; Nephrectomy; Nephritis; Nephrology; Nephrology, pediatric; Polycystic kidney disease; Protein; Pyelonephritis; Renal failure; Urinalysis; Urinary disorders; Urinary system; Urology; Urology, pediatric.

For Further Information:
Brenner, Barry M., ed. *Brenner and Rector's The Kidney.* 9th ed. Philadelphia: Saunders/Elsevier, 2012.
Glassock, R. J. "Focus on Proteinuria." *American Journal of Nephrology* 10, suppl. 1 (1990): 88-93.
"Proteinuria." *National Kidney and Urologic Diseases Information Clearinghouse,* September 2, 2010.
Strasinger, Susan J., and Marjorie Schaub Di Lorenzo. *Urinalysis and Body Fluids.* 5th ed. Philadelphia: F. A. Davis, 2008.

PROTEOMICS

Category: Specialty
Anatomy or system affected: All
Specialties and related fields: All
Definition: The study of the proteome, the collective body of proteins expressed from genes at any given point in time in any given cell, tissue, or organism. Proteomes differ for each kind of organism and are quite dynamic, changing their protein composition in response to such factors as aging, diet, exercise, medication, and disease.

Key terms:

mass spectrometry: a very sensitive technique that accurately measures protein or peptide mass; proteins are then identified by matching this information to the predicted mass for proteins and peptides from all genes thought to encode protein and held within genomic databases

microarrays: miniature plastic or glass chips upon which tiny amounts of biological material are permanently spotted in a gridlike array; in proteomics, protein microarrays, holding thousands of individual protein samples, are used to test for drug binding, antibody binding for diagnostic test development, or interactions with other proteins to determine function

subproteomes: proteomes within proteomes, such as the mitochondrial proteome as a subproteome of a cell, which, in turn, is a subproteome of a tissue; subproteomes can be functionally defined and transient in nature, resulting from medications, exercise, and changes in diet

two-dimensional gel electrophoresis: a technique that can separate thousands of proteins in complex mixtures through a polyacrylamide gel matrix in two dimensions, first by isoelectric point and second by molecular weight

METHODOLOGIES

Proteomics focuses on developing a proteome profile for any given cell, tissue, or disease through three main perspectives. Functional (quantitative) proteomics aims to identify, quantify, and localize proteins within proteomes. Structural proteomics aims to develop a precise three-dimensional structure of each protein in normal and abnormal states, which is vital to clinical diagnostics and drug discovery. Mapping protein-protein interactions aims to understand how proteins interact with one another in complexes, forming networks and pathways of biological activity to understand how diseases originate and progress.

Proteome size, complexity, and dynamics are the current biggest challenges to proteomics. For this reason, this field is closely tied to technological advances.

The use of robotic techniques has led to processing hundreds of thousands of extremely small samples every day, which is called high-throughput. To profile proteomes, they must first be isolated, their proteins separated and then purified through large-scale two-dimensional polyacrylamide gel electrophoresis and/or mass spectrometry. Protein structural information is then determined using protein sequencing, mass spectrometry, and/or x-ray crystallography. Assigning protein function within a proteome involves protein and/or antibody microarray analyses to determine biochemical pathway involvement and any protein-protein interactions. Typically, laboratories will specialize in one of these approaches. All laboratories, however, must be able to integrate the information that they find with the discoveries of others. The creation of databases that hold, organize, and link the massive amounts of proteomic information generated to genomic information has been made possible only through advances in bioinformatic computer technology.

MEDICINE AND PROTEOMICS

Most diseases create alterations in cellular function. Complex diseases such as cancer, heart disease, and diabetes cannot be treated effectively if the underlying cause and proteins responsible remain unknown. However, the current practice of biomedical research is unable to identify these changes or determine how they relate to disease processes quickly enough to develop the needed diagnostics and treatment. Identifying proteomic components that are specific for a disease (biomarkers) is a major effort of proteomic research. The aim is to develop diagnostic kits that detect the very early phase of a disease. Within populations, the diagnosis, prognosis, treatment, origins, and progression of a disease are public health issues overseen by epidemiologists. Genetic epidemiology is a new discipline that is closely following proteomic progress to develop better public health policies and planning. Proteomics is also expected to identify targets for new drugs.

In the early stages of development, proteome profiling has already shown that the human cardiac proteome is reproducibly and uniquely altered for different heart diseases and disorders. Biomarkers specific to prostate and breast cancer have been identified. These first studies encouraged proteomic researchers to turn to disease proteomic profiling. Because most diseases create protein alterations in blood plasma long before symptoms appear, proteomic serum and plasma profiling is a major research effort. Researchers have identified a blood plasma proteomic profile for ovarian cancer that appears to predict the disease accurately. Other researchers have turned to the proteomic profiling of pathogens, such as antibiotic-resistant bacteria or those organisms causing malaria or stomach ulcers. The goal is to identify biomarkers for use as drug targets and for the development of diagnostic kits.

One promising application of proteomic technology is in the area of early detection of disease. Historically, the identification and examination of disease markers has been based on individual proteins, which is not always reliable. For example, the assay for prostate-specific antigen (PSA) is used to screen for prostate cancer, but levels of this antigen may also be raised in benign conditions of the prostate, and other unrelated conditions can lead to false-positive results for this screen. Thousands of small proteins can be analyzed simultaneously using proteomic microarrays, and these results may suggest patterns of disease that may be useful for early detection. The potential therefore exists to use a panel of diagnostic markers, rather than a single protein, to identify a given disease state more accurately.

PERSPECTIVE AND PROSPECTS

The origins of proteomics can be traced to the technique of separating complex mixtures of proteins by two-dimensional polyacrylamide gel electrophoresis in the mid-1970s. Refinement of the technique and the addition of protein sequencing methods enabled identification of the separated proteins. In the 1990s, advances in mass spectrometry provided a highly accurate, sensitive analysis of proteins capable of handling thousands of samples.

The final impetus for proteomic research was a direct outcome of the technological advancements of the Human Genome Project, including microarray analyses, the concept of high-throughput, and a paradigm shift in biological science research. Paramount was the recognition that the protein products of a gene, not the gene itself, are responsible for cellular processes. It became clear that the function of proteins in cellular pathways and processes could not be deduced from the deoxyribonucleic acid (DNA) sequence alone. Efforts quickly turned to studying all proteins and their functions in the context of genetics and diseases. As an emerging discipline, proteomics represents a new research form that is more global and integrative than traditional protein research in the past, which concentrated on the study of single proteins.

Currently, the concern among researchers is the sequestering of data generated in proteomic research for private company use or through aggressive patenting of results. Because of the complexity of the research, it is considered necessary for all to share their data in a public forum. The Human Proteome Organization (HUPO) was created to orchestrate cooperative sharing of both private and academic research efforts. First and foremost is the recognition that research must focus on what constitutes a normal proteome before assessing disease states, including defining the range of variability in normal proteomes as a result of age, ethnicity, and physiology. HUPO considers the human serum, liver, and brain to be the most important organs for proteomic profiling in the hope that these studies will lead to new drugs, diagnostics, and a basic understanding of cellular function. In whatever form proteomics takes, it is expected to change the practice of medicine drastically.

—Diane C. Rein, PhD, MLS;
updated by Jeffrey A. Knight, PhD

See also Aging; Biochemistry; Bioinformatics; Biostatistics; Cells; Disease; DNA and RNA; Epidemiology; Genetic diseases; Genetics and inheritance; Genomics; Laboratory tests; Mutation; Preventive medicine; Protein.

For Further Information:
Berman, Helen M., David S. Goodsell, and Philip E. Bourne. "Protein Structures: From Famine to Feast." *American Scientist* 90, no. 4 (July/August, 2002): 350-51.
Campbell, A. Malcolm, and Laurie J. Heyer. *Discovering Genomics, Proteomics, and Bioinformatics.* 2d ed. San Francisco: Pearson/Benjamin Cummings, 2007.
Divan, Aysha, and Janice Royds. *Tools and Techniques in Biomolecular Science.* New York: Oxford University Press, 2013.
Dreger, Mathias. "Proteome Analysis at the Level of Subcellular Structures." *European Journal of Biochemistry* 270, no. 4 (February, 2003): 589-99.
Ezzell, Carol. "Proteins Rule." *Scientific American* 286, no. 4 (April, 2002): 40-47.
Fulton, Kelly M., and Susan M. Twine. *Immunoproteomics: Methods and Protocols.* New York: Humana Press, 2013.
Hanash, Sam. "Disease Proteomics." *Nature* 422, no. 6928 (March 13, 2003): 226-32.
Merrill, Stephen A., and Anne-Marie Mazza, eds. *Reaping the Benefits of Genomic and Proteomic Research: Intellectual Property Rights, Innovation, and Public Health.* Washington, DC: National Academies Press, 2006.
Neha, Sharma, and S. L. Harikumar. "Use of Genomics and Proteomics in Pharmaceutical Drug Discovery and Development." *International Journal of Pharmacy and Pharmaceutical Sciences* 5, no. 3 (July, 2013): 24-28.
Patterson, Scott D., and Ruedi H. Aebersold. "Proteomics: The First Decade and Beyond." *Nature Genetics*, supp. 33 (March, 2003): 311-23.
Pierce, Benjamin A. *Genetics Essentials: Concepts and Connections.* New York: W. H. Freeman, 2013.
Sali, Andrej, et al. "From Words to Literature in Structural Proteomics." *Nature* 422, no. 6928 (March 13, 2003): 216-25.
Sellers, Thomas A., and John R. Yates. "Review of Proteomics with Applications to Genetic Epidemiology." *Genetic Epidemiology* 24, no. 2 (February, 2003): 83-98.
Wulkuhle, Julia D., Lance A. Liotta, and Emanuel F. Petricoin. "Proteomic Applications for the Early Detection of Cancer." *Nature Reviews Cancer* 3, no. 4 (April, 2003): 267-75.

PROTOZOAN DISEASES

Category: Disease/Disorder
Anatomy or system affected: Gastrointestinal system
Specialties and related fields: Microbiology, public health
Definition: Disease caused by protozoa, a diverse group of free-living, unicellular animals that function as parasites.

Key terms:

excyst: The escape of the organism from a protective, thick-walled resting structure called a cyst that has been swallowed by parasite's host.

flagellate parasites: parasitic protozoa that move by means of a whip-like structure called a flagellum.

parasite: any organism that lives on or in another organism of another species, which is known as the host, and derives nutrition from the host.

protozoa: single-celled, eukaryotic organisms that are highly diverse and move by means of pseudopods, flagella, or cilia.

CAUSES AND SYMPTOMS

Protozoa exist in almost every ecological niche. As parasites, they infect all species of vertebrates and many invertebrates, adapting to nearly all available sites within their hosts' bodies. There are nearly sixty-six thousand known species of protozoa; half of these are represented in the fossil record, and about ten thousand of the living species are known to be parasitic. Unlike many other parasites, protozoa replicate within their hosts to produce hundreds of thousands of their kind within several days of infection. Because of their variety, adaptability, and reproductive rates, parasitic protozoa exert a major influence on human existence.

The phylum Protozoa is subdivided into four subphyla, but only the subphylum Sarcomastigophora is of real concern to humans. Within this subphylum are the twelve genera of parasitic protozoa that cause diseases in humans and their domestic animals, the most important of which are *Trypanosoma*, *Leishmania*, *Trichomonas*, *Entamoeba*, *Eimeria*, *Toxoplasma*, *Babesia*, *Theileria*, *Giardia*, and *Plasmodium*.

The most startling characteristic of parasitic protozoan diseases in humans is the sheer number of cases that exist. For example, a conservative estimate suggests at least two hundred million persons harbor the protozoan *Entamoeba*, which causes amebic dysentery. Of this number, approximately 50 million people, globally, suffer from amebic colitis or more invasive infections that have spread to other organs. One to two billion humans are estimated to be infected with *Toxoplasma*, the protozoan that cause toxoplasmosis. *Trypanosoma*, the agents of sleeping sickness and Cha-

gas disease, infect fifteen to twenty million people worldwide; *Giardia*, two hundred million; and *Leishmania*, which are responsible for the disease kala-azar, one to two million. The most important of all protozoan diseases, said to be the greatest killer in history, is malaria, which is caused by the parasite *Plasmodium* and results in the death of two to three million people annually.

Protozoa that infect humans are commonly found in the intestinal tract, various tissues and organs, and the bloodstream. Of the many protozoa that reside in the human gut, only invasive *Entamoeba histolytica* causes serious disease. *E. histolytica* parasites are transmitted by the ingestion of water contaminated with human feces that contain *E. histolytica* cysts that pass through the stomach and excyst in the small intestine to form trophozoites. The trophozoites invade the innermost layer of the colon and cause the disease amebiasis or, its severe form, amebic dysentery. If the disease spreads by way of intestinal veins to the liver, the result can be hepatic amebiasis, or the infection can spread to the lungs, heart or brain. Although the majority of *E. histolytica* infections produce no symptoms, it can produce highly invasive infections. Another waterborne intestinal protozoan familiar to campers and vacationers is the flagellate *Giardia lamblia*, which causes giardiasis. Giardiasis results in a mild-to-serious, long-lasting diarrhea. It is usually acquired from the ingestion of water fouled by animal waste. It can also be transmitted by human sources and, if the outbreak occurs in a closed population, frequently results in a rapidly spreading infection.

A few flagellate parasites infect the human skin, bloodstream, and viscera. The flagellate *Trypanosoma cruzi* is the agent of Chagas disease, a major cause of debilitation and chronic heart disease among poorly housed populations of Central and South America. *T. cruzi* is transmitted when the liquid feces of an insect (genus *Triatoma*) are scratched into the skin or rubbed in the eye. In Africa, the tsetse fly carries the parasitic agents of the disease trypanosomiasis, also known as African sleeping sickness. The disease is generated by the flagellate parasites *Trypanosoma brucei gambiense* and *T. brucei rhodesiense*, which infect the bloodstream and can be fatal if they cross the blood-brain barrier.

Parasitic flagellates of the genus *Leishmania* are transmitted by bloodsucking midges and sandflies and result in macrophage infection. Cutaneous leishmaniasis is characterized by infected macrophages in the skin, resulting in long-lasting skin lesions. A similar condition, mucocutaneous leishmaniasis, common to the Amazon Basin, begins as skin ulcers and often progresses to the destruction of nasal mucosa, cartilage, and soft facial and pharyngeal tissues. Visceral leishmaniasis, or kala-azar, infects the spleen, liver, bone marrow, and lymph nodes.

Only one species of ciliate protozoa is parasitic in humans: *Balantidium coli*, a free-living, large protozoan covered with rows of cilia. It is found in the large intestine, where it can cause the ulcerative disease balantidiasis. The group of protozoa known as sporozoans are all parasitic and include many deadly parasites of humans: *Isopora, Sarcocystis, Cryptosporidium*, and *Toxoplasma. Toxoplasma gondii*, the agent of toxoplasmosis, is of great medical concern. It is estimated to infect between 20 and 50 percent of the world's population, and it can penetrate the placenta and subsequently infect the fetus of pregnant women who lack the proper antibodies. The most important sporozoans, however, are the agents of malaria.

Malaria is a disease caused by a group of sporozoans in the genus *Plasmodium* that infect the human liver and red blood cells. Malaria is characterized by periodic chills, fever, and sweats, leading to anemia, enlargement of the spleen, and complications that result in death, especially among infants. The parasites are transmitted to humans by the bite of any of sixty species of infected *Anopheles* mosquitoes. The disease is found in all tropical and temperate regions, but control efforts have eliminated it from North America, Europe, and the northern Asian continent. Despite control efforts and effective medical treatments, malaria is historically the greatest killer all human infectious diseases, and it remains the single most dangerous threat to humankind from an infectious agent. More than one million children die of malaria in Africa yearly.

TREATMENT AND THERAPY

Treatment is generally by antiprotozoal agents, antibiotics, or both, with the specific agent or agents depending on the type of protozoa. Amebiasis treatments usually combine metronidazole or alternative agents (e.g., tinidazole, ornidazole, and nitazoxanide) with so-called "luminal agents," such as paromomycin, diiodohydroxyquin or diloxanide furonate to kill any cysts. *Giardia* infections are also treated with metronidazole, or tinidazole, nitazoxanide, albendazole, mebendazole, paromomycin, or quinacrine. *Trichomonas* infections are treated with metronidazole or tinidazole. Balantidiasis is treated with metronidazole, paromomycin, tinidazole or tetracycline. Toxoplasmosis is treated with pyrimethamine combined with either sulfadiazine, clindamycin, atovaquone, or azithromycin. Leucovorin is also prescribed to protect the bone marrow from the toxic effects of pyrimethamine. The drugs of choice to treat cryptosporidiosis are nitazoxanide or paromomycin.

Leishmaniasis treatments vary, depending on the region of world from which the infection was contracted. The available agents include pentavalent antimonials (sodium stibogluconate and meglumine antimoniate), which contain the metalloid antimony, paromomycin, amphotericin B, and a newer drug, miltefosine. An even newer drug, benznidazole, was approved by the FDA in August, 2017, for the treatment of Chagas disease.

Various treatments for malaria exist and vary according to the type of malaria and where it was contracted. Chloroquine is an effective treatment for *Plasmodium falciparum* infections in Haiti, the Dominican Republic, Central America west of the Panama Canal, and most of the Middle East. Outside of these regions, *P. falciparum* are resistant to chloroquine, and artemisinin-based combination therapies (ACTs) are used. For *P. vivax* or *P. ovale* infections (Mexico and Central America), primaquine is the drug of choice. Malaria infections acquired outside endemic areas (e.g., Southeast Asia) are treated with ACTs, quinine-based regimens, mefloquine, or atovaquone-proguanil. Prophylactic treatments, which are used to prevent travelers from being infected with malaria, include doxycycline, atovaquone-proguanil, mefloquine, chloroquine (for use only when traveling to regions with chloroquine-sensitive malaria), and primaquine for areas where *P. vivax* and *P. ovale* are endemic.

—Randall L. Milstein, PhD;
updated by Michael A. Buratovich, PhD

See also: Bites and stings; Chagas' disease; Diarrhea and dysentery; Epidemiology; Giardiasis; Insect-borne diseases; Leishmaniasis; Lice, mites, and ticks; Malaria; Microbiology; Parasitic diseases; Sleeping sickness; Toxoplasmosis; Trichomoniasis; Tropical medicine; Zoonoses.

For Further Information:
Behnke, Jerzy M., ed. *Parasites: Immunity and Pathology; The Consequences of Parasitic Infection in Mammals*. New York: Taylor & Francis, 1990.
Dhawan, Vinod K. "Amebiasis." *Medscape*, May 22, 2017.
Despommier, Dickson D., et al. *Parasitic Diseases*. 5th ed. New York: Apple Tree, 2006.
Engleberg, N. Cary, Victor DiRita, and Terence S. Dermody, eds. *Schaechter's Mechanisms of Microbial Disease*. 5th ed. Philadelphia: Lippincott Williams & Wilkins, 2013.
Frank, Steven A. *Immunology and Evolution of Infectious Disease*. Princeton, N.J.: Princeton University Press, 2002.

Gutteridge, W. E., and G. H. Coombs. *Biochemistry of Parasitic Protozoa*. Baltimore: University Park Press, 1977.

Herchline, Thomas E. "Malaria." *Medscape*, October 26, 2016.

Nazer, Hisham. "Giardiasis." *Medscape*, February 15, 2016.

Roberts, Larry S., John Janovy Jr, and Steve Nadler. *Gerald D. Schmidt and Larry S. Roberts' Foundations of Parasitology*. 9th ed. New York: McGraw-Hill, 2013.

Stark, Craig G. "Leishmaniosis." *Medscape*, May 15, 2017.

PSORIASIS AND PSORIATIC ARTHRITIS

Category: Disease/Disorder
Anatomy or system affected: Skin, eyes, joints, nails
Specialties and related fields: Dermatology, internal medicine, ophthalmology, orthopedics, rheumatology
Definition: A chronic skin disease in which red, scaly patches develop, overlaid with thick, silvery-gray scales, causing physical discomfort and damaging self-esteem.
Key terms:

dermatologist: a physician who treats the skin and its structures, functions, and diseases

dermis: the layer of skin directly beneath the epidermis, consisting of dense connective tissue and numerous blood vessels

enthesitis: inflammation of the insertion sites of tendons and ligaments to the bone surface

epidermis: the outermost part of the skin, composed of four or five different layers called "strata"

methotrexate: a powerful drug originally developed to treat cancer that treats patients with severe cases of psoriasis

onchonylysis: pitting and destruction of the fingernails or toenails

psoralens: chemicals found in plants that make the skin more sensitive to light

psoriatic arthritis: a subtype of psoriasis characterized by the extension of the inflammation that involves the skin to the joints and nails

PUVA: a treatment for psoriasis that exposes the patient to ultraviolet A (UVA) light after receiving one of the psoralens

stratum corneum: the outermost layer of the epidermis; its cells are generally dead, hard, and removed by regular bathing

ultraviolet light (UV): invisible light composed of waves that are shorter than ordinary light waves able to be seen by humans

CAUSES AND SYMPTOMS

Psoriasis is a common skin problem afflicting approximately two of every hundred people, affecting males and females with relatively equal frequency. Although it affects all races, it is most prevalent among northern Europeans. This stubborn, chronic, and incurable disease most commonly appears in one's teens or twenties. However, it can appear in early childhood. Seventy percent of psoriasis patients develop it by the age of twenty. However, another typical danger period occurs in the fifties and sixties, with many patients developing their first symptoms.

There are several different types of psoriasis, making diagnosis difficult. The most widespread is the "plaque-type"; it accounts for 95 percent of all cases. This type is also called "common psoriasis." Plaque-type psoriasis gets its name from the appearance of the patches of affected skin. Each patch resembles a plaque, or small disk stuck to the body's surface. These dull, wine-colored patches of abnormal skin are often rounded or oval; they may be very irregular when several nearby patches join together. The surface of each thickened patch is rough and scaly, with the scales ranging in color from red to white to the most typical silvery gray. These psoriatic plaques can be small (the size of coins) or become palm-sized and larger. Whatever their final size, they generally begin as purple or reddened areas the size of a pinhead. The original areas expand in size, usually for a few weeks, until they reach a stable phase and stop expanding. The average plaque size in the stable phase is two to three inches. A patch of stable psoriasis may eventually grow pale, become less scaly, disappear completely, or begin to enlarge for no apparent reason. Even those plaques that have disappeared may be reactivated and later reappear in the same place.

Back and arms of a person with psoriasis. Photo by James Heilman, MD, via Wikimedia Commons.

Certain body parts seem most prone to psoriatic lesions, namely the elbows, the knees, the scalp, and the lower back. The patches may appear elsewhere, including the genitals and the buttocks, but the face, hands, and feet are rarely affected. Severe cases may cover the entire chest or back. In a few cases, psoriasis is symmetrical, appearing in the same area on the left and right sides of the body simultaneously. However, the patches are more likely to develop randomly, scattered manner.

Almost 50 percent of patients with psoriasis have lesions on their scalps. When these plaques are extensive and widespread, they are challenging to treat and difficult to hide. Although very uncomfortable, scalp psoriasis does not affect the growth of hair or cause baldness. It can cause a temporary thinning of the hair. Still, hair usually grows again once the disease is controlled by medication. About one-third of psoriasis patients have affected fingernails and toenails. The diseased nails show pits or pinpoint indentations, loosening, thickening, and yellowish discoloration. Surprisingly, the condition remains on the nails alone in some people, never developing elsewhere.

In addition to psoriasis of the nails, several rare and unusual types of psoriasis are different from the common or plaque type. These include flexural or inverse, guttate, pustular, and erythrodermic psoriasis. Flexural psoriasis appears in folds and creases on the body. It usually occurs in particularly overweight people in their mid-forties or older. The patches tend to be very

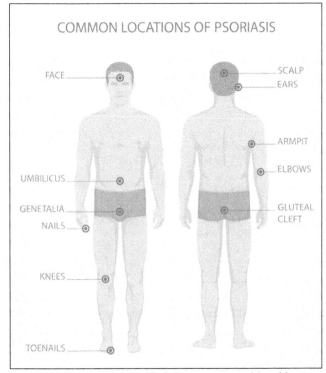

Common locations of Psoriasis on the body. Image via iStock/kowalska-art. [Used under license.]

moist rather than scaly and are particularly sore and uncomfortable. Guttable psoriasis consists of an enormous number of highly scattered but minute plaques. It is rare and occurs between the ages of eight and sixteen. Although the spots usually clear up in a few weeks, they sometimes recur or change into large lesions of common psoriasis. Pustular psoriasis is the only form of the disease that occurs on the palms of the hands or the soles of the feet. It was named for the yellow or white pus-filled spots that form on the skin and eventually drop off. These spots form when hordes of white blood cells invade the skin even though no infection is present. Erythrodermic psoriasis means "red skin." This rare condition receives its name because flaming red patches that do not turn scaly cover the entire body. Since the extensive nature of this condition makes internal temperature control very difficult and dehydration inevitable, it can be perilous and may require hospitalization.

Common psoriasis, by comparison, is not dangerous or life-threatening. It is usually not painful and does not even cause itching in most patients. It is, however, very annoying because of its unsightly appearance and its tendency to flare up repeatedly. Once the disease has appeared, it stays with the person for life, improving or worsening periodically. After periods of relative quiet, during which the skin may appear quite normal, patients with psoriasis experience new eruptions and scaling for no apparent reason. Plaques continue to form for an unpredictable period until the condition spontaneously quiets down again.

The source of the plaques is a failure in the mechanism by which normal skin renews itself. Ordinarily, the cells at the base of the epidermis reproduce themselves at a slow and steady rate. They then move upward in about twenty-eight days, changing chemically, dying, and detaching from the surface, the stratum corneum. However, there is a considerable increase in the number of basal cells in the epidermis in psoriatic skin. These basal cells reproduce so rapidly that they push upward to the surface in only four days, forming thick disks of sticky, abnormal cells. Below the epidermis, the dermis of a patient with psoriasis is also abnormal. Its normally fine blood vessels are wide and highly twisted, causing the red appearance of the plaques. Consequently, the skin readily bleeds if bumped or scratched. An unusually high number of white blood cells called "neutrophils" and T lymphocytes are also present. They move up into the epidermis, creating inflammation and swelling within the plaques.

Dermatologists noted that psoriasis runs in families long before they elucidated the structure and function of psoriatic skin. If one parent has the problem, there is a one-in-three chance that a child will eventually be afflicted; if both parents have the disease, the risk for their offspring is one in two. If one non-identical twin has psoriasis, there is a 70 percent chance that the other will have psoriasis. With identical twins, the chances of having psoriasis can be as high as 90 percent, according to some studies. Geneticists suspect that people do not inherit psoriasis in a simple Mendelian manner. It seems more likely that the condition results from several genetic factors from each parent, much like how height and intelligence are inherited.

PSORIATIC ARTHRITIS

Psoriatic arthritis (PsA) is a widely variable type of psoriasis in which skin inflammation extends to the joints. PsA affects not only the joints but also structures associated with the joint. For example, involvement of the tendon area that inserts onto bone (entheses) results in enthesitis. Inflammation of the tendons and joints of the fingers causes dactylitis. PsA can also afflict the nails, causing nail pitting, also known as onchonylysis. Fingernail, toenail, and tendon insertion involvement distinguish psoriatic arthritis from rheumatoid arthritis, localizing to the joints.

The most significant risk factor for psoriatic arthritis is having psoriasis. The prevalence of PsA is between 6 to 42 percent in people with patients with psoriasis. PsA prevalence ranges from 0.3 to 1 percent of the general population. Psoriatic arthritis most commonly occurs in 30 to 50 years old and is nearly equal in both sexes. There is a higher incidence in people of Northern European descent and a lower incidence in Japanese descent.

Genetic factors have a significant role in the cause of PsA. PsA shows strong familial association and links with several major histocompatibility complex (MHC) class I alleles. As many as 40 percent of all PsA patients have a family history of arthritis or psoriasis. Most PsA patients experience skin manifestations of psoriasis before suffering any joint involvement. However, ten percent of PsA patients experience joint pain before skin

---

INFORMATION ON PSORIATIC ARTHRITIS

Causes: Inflammation in the skin that spreads to the joints and structures associated with joints; often hereditary, but environmental factors are also involved in the onset and manifestation of the disease.

Symptoms: Pain, stiffness, swelling, and tenderness of one or several joints that limits motion. Some forms of psoriatic arthritis affect the spine, hips, and shoulders. It can also affect tendon insertion sites (entheses), particularly in the hand.

Duration: Chronic with acute episodes

Treatments: Nonsteroidal anti-inflammatory drugs (NSAIDs), interarticular and systemic corticosteroids, disease-modifying antirheumatoid drugs (DMARDs), apremilast, and biologic agents

---

lesions. Psoriasis patients who suffer from scalp lesions, nail dystrophy, uveitis, and intergluteal/perianal skin lesions are at higher risk of PsA.

The clinical presentation of PsA differs from patient to patient. The severity and the course of the disease show extensive ranges. Some PsA patients have mild joint stiffness and soreness, while others have severe irreversible inflammatory joint destruction. Most PsA cases begin with pain in one to four joints (oligoarthritis). This condition may involve five or more joints (polyarthritis). PsA patients with polyarthritis, extensive skin involvement early in life (before age 20), and a strong family history of psoriasis are at higher risk for aggressive disease.

Why does psoriasis spread to the joints in some people but not others? The answer to this burning question remains unknown. However, an ensemble of genetic, environmental, and immunologic factors probably plays a role in the onset, severity, and presentation of PsA. Activated T cells are present in psoriatic skin lesions and joints. Therefore, a breakdown in the regulation of the immune response may lead to uncontrolled inflammation in the skin and joints. Consequently, PsA treatment usually involves inhibiting cytokines that stimulate inflammation, including tumor necrosis factor-alpha (TNF-a) and other proinflammatory cytokines (e.g., interleukin-6, interleukin-17, interleukin-12, interleukin-23).

PsA symptoms vary, but a common thread is stiffness, pain, swelling, and tenderness of one or more joints. This pain tends to limit motion. PsA commonly affects the spine, hips, and shoulders. PsA subtypes include: (1) distal interphalangeal joint-predominant arthritis (10 percent of cases), (2) symmetrical polyarthritis-predominant arthritis (5 to 20 percent of cases), (3) asymmetric oligoarthritis or monoarthritis (70 to 80 percent of cases), (4) axial disease (5 to 20 percent of cases), and (5) arthritis mutilans (rare).

The most critical factors when diagnosing PsA are the patient's medical history and clinical presentation. Distinguishing PsA from other types of arthritis requires blood tests to rule out rheumatoid arthritis (i.e., the absence of rheumatoid factor and anti-cyclic citrullinated peptide antibody). Other blood tests have varying usefulness for diagnostic purposes. Imaging affected joints with X-rays, computer-aided tomography (CAT) scans, or magnetic resonance imaging (MRI) shows joint destruction in a pattern known as a "pencil in cup" deformity.

TREATMENT AND THERAPY

More than 90 percent of psoriasis patients have their lesions cleared significantly or even made lesion-free by contemporary medicines and methods. For minor outbreaks, limited to a small body area, the first choice for treatment is corticosteroid cream or ointments applied directly to the plaques. Corticosteroids are derivatives of glucocorticoid hormones produced by the adrenal glands that reduce glucose metabolism and suppress inflammation. Corticosteroids reduce inflammation and decrease blood flow to psoriatic lesions. Dermatologists have a large variety of such preparations ranging from mild to superpotent. Superpotent topical corticosteroids include 0.5 percent betamethasone dipropionate ointment and 0.05 percent halobetasol propionate cream. Potent topical steroids include amcinonide 0.1 percent ointment and halcinonide 0.1 percent cream. Moderate topical corticosteroids include upper-, mid-, and lower-mid strength preparations. Upper-mid strength includes triamcinolone acetonide 0.5 percent cream and mometasone furoate 0.1 percent ointment. Lower-mid strength consists of desoximetasone 0.05 percent cream and flurandrenolide 0.05 percent. Mild topical corticosteroids include alclometasone dipropionate 0.05 percent cream or ointment and desonide 0.05 percent cream. Finally, the least potent topical corticosteroids contain hydrocortisone, flumethasone, dexamethasone, prednisolone, or methylprednisolone. Dermatologists and rheumatologists must find a topical corticosteroid strong enough to suppress the inflammation but not cause unwanted side effects.

Topical steroids cause thinning of the skin and stretch marks if the patient uses it for a prolonged period, too much, or apply it to the face or intertriginous areas. Rarely, superpotent topical corticosteroids can suppress adrenal gland function if applied to large skin areas. Additionally, psoriatic skin absorbs substances more quickly than normal skin. Excess steroids enter the bloodstream and can change the output of hormones by the pituitary and adrenal glands, dangerously altering the body's chemical balance. The other danger is the skin itself, which becomes abnormally thin, easily damaged, and prone to infections. Another drawback to using corticosteroids is the tendency for the psoriatic plaques to reappear soon after discontinuation of the creams or ointments.

Some patients opt for topical vitamin D analogs that decrease psoriatic skin lesions to decrease corticosteroid use. Two synthetic vitamin D analogs, calcipotriene (*Dovonex*) and calcitriol (*Vectical*) are about as effective as medium-potency corticosteroids for topical treatment of plaque psoriasis. Both agents are well-tolerated, but calcipotriene causes burning and itching when applied to the skin, calcitriol less so. Ultraviolet (UV) light exposure inactivates calcipotriene. Another topical agent, tazarotene (*Tazorac*), is a retinoid (vitamin A derivative) that effectively treats plaque psoriasis. Tazarotene increases the sunburn risk and causes itching, burning, peeling, and itching. The combination of these topical agents with corticosteroids augments their efficacy.

Another group of topical agents, the calcineurin inhibitors, effectively treat psoriasis but are not Food and Drug Administration (FDA)-approved and used off-label. Tacrolimus (*Protopic*) and pimecrolimus (*Elidel*) work well for psoriatic lesions on the face and provide alternatives to corticosteroids. Tacrolimus and pimecrolimus cause burning, redness, and itching, but pimecrolimus is better tolerated. Long-term use seems to increase the risk of lymphomas.

Many patients find relief from an entirely different class of medications that contain tar. This thick, black, oily liquid, made from coal, contains thousands of chemical substances, and biochemists do not know which helps heal the skin. Tar-containing ointments, creams, gels, shampoos, and bath additives help remove the scales without problematic side effects. However, a significant drawback is their tendency to stain clothing, bedding, bathroom tiles, and bathtubs. Covering the treated skin area with bandages, cotton underwear, or a shower cap avoids some of this staining. In addition to the staining, many patients find the tar odor quite unpleasant; pharmaceutical companies are constantly trying to improve this aspect of these quite effective products.

The third type of preparation is particularly effective for removing very thick scales. These medications contain a compound called "salicylic acid." Like corticosteroids, salicylic acid ointments and gels are most effective when they contact the plaques for an extended period. After treatment, patients should cover their lesions with plastic gloves, plastic bags (for the feet), or taped-down plastic wrap for four to eight hours.

Patients with psoriasis have noted for years that exposure to the sun is beneficial in clearing their lesions. Daily sunlight exposure is effective for as many as 80 percent of patients. This treatment is relatively accessible for at least part of the year and inexpensive compared to the various medications available. Patients should have repeated but brief sun exposure and use sunblock creams and lotions to avoid sunburn, given the increased risk of skin cancer. Although sun exposure is helpful to most patients with common psoriasis, it rarely helps and can even worsen the pustulate and erythrodermic types. Since too much exposure to sunlight will damage rather than help any skin, even plaque-type patients should stop their sun exposure once psoriasis has improved.

For patients in many climates, sunbathing is possible for only a few months of the year. The development of sunlamps for use at home or in a dermatologist's office, hospital, psoriasis care center, or tanning parlor has made this therapy possible all year round. Because of the danger of severe sunburns, sunlamp treatments remain controversial. To reduce their danger, a dermatologist must carefully determine the amount of time of each treatment, the precise distance from the lamp, and the appropriate frequency of treatments for each patient to achieve maximal and safe results.

The curative effect of sunlight depends on the very short wavelength part of the light, called "ultraviolet." Ultraviolet B (UVB) waves help heal psoriasis, possibly by slowing down the high growth rate of cells in the epidermis. Both natural sunlight and sunlamps contain UVB and, therefore, have the potential to help psoriasis. They also have the potential, however, to burn the skin. Narrow-band UVB is safer and more effective than broad-band UVB. UVB phototherapy is the preferred treatment for breastfeeding women.

Patients with severe psoriasis may require ultraviolet A (UVA) waves from a special kind of sunlamp. The patient takes a dose of a psoralen. This substance makes the skin more light-sensitive. Then the patient exposes their skin to UVA inside a full-body light cabinet. Narrowband UVB is safer and more effective than broad-band UVB. Patients may require up to thirty treatments to clear their skin completely. The psoralen is often given in tablet form. However, some patients suffer fewer side effects if they paint it onto the skin or bathe in it. The early side effects of PUVA (psoralen plus UVA) treatment include nausea, itching, colored blotches on the skin, and occasional worsening of psoriasis. The possible later side effects are more problematic: skin cancer and cataracts in the eyes. The danger of developing cataracts also exists from natural sunlight and UVB sunlamps; patients using any light therapy must use dark sunglasses that block out all rays harmful to the eyes. Excimer laser therapy is safe and effective for localized psoriasis and is FDA-approved. Narrow-band UVB and the excimer laser are safe during pregnancy. Breastfeeding women should not breastfeed for at least twenty-four hours after PUVA.

For patients with pustular and erythrodermic psoriasis, the retinoid acitretin can be very useful if its side effects are carefully monitored. Some dermatologists have been especially successful in combining PUVA or UVB and acitretin therapies; the improvement in psoriasis is greater than with either alone, while the lower dosage of each minimizes risk and side effects. Acitretin should never be used with alcohol and is not safe during pregnancy.

A newer medication for psoriasis and psoriatic arthritis is apremilast (*Otzela*). This drug prevents the breakdown of a cell-signaling molecule called "cyclic AMP" (cAMP). Increasing intracellular levels of cAMP in immune cells slow them down. Apremilast improves symptoms in people with moderate to severe plaque psoriasis. In people with psoriatic arthritis, it improves symptoms but does not decrease disease progression. Apremilast causes diarrhea, nausea, upper respiratory infection, and headache. It can also increase the risk of depression. Another downside to this drug is its costliness.

For patients with widespread psoriasis who do not respond to corticosteroids, tar preparations, or the various light therapies, methotrexate is effective in more than 80 percent of patients. Patients with mild to moderate psoriatic arthritis also benefit from methotrexate. Methotrexate was initially developed to treat various cancers because it slows down cell multiplication. Thus, the psoriatic epidermal cells are prevented from reproducing and forming the scaly plaques. Often methotrexate must be taken for six months or a year, in pill form or by injection, to impact an extensive case significantly. Such a dosage poses a risk of severe and numerous side effects, including persistent feelings of sickness, indigestion, and diarrhea. Frequent tests are necessary to monitor the blood condition since methotrexate can interfere with the bone marrow's normal blood cells and liver and kidney function. Periodic liver biopsies and removing sample liver cells using a special needle are necessary because methotrexate can cause irreversible damage to this crucial organ. It is imperative that a pregnant woman never takes methotrexate or that a woman never become pregnant while taking it. The drug's ability to interfere with cell growth can cause many abnormalities in a developing embryo or fetus. Drugs called "retinoids" cause similar fetal abnormalities.

Patients with mild psoriatic arthritis in a few joints can manage their pain with nonsteroidal anti-inflammatory drugs (NSAIDs). NSAIDs include over-the-counter drugs like aspirin, ibuprofen, naproxen sodium, and stronger prescription NSAIDs like meloxicam, piroxicam, celecoxib, indomethacin, ketorolac, and diclofenac. Long-term NSAID use can cause stomach ulcers, kidney failure, and an increased risk of heart attacks and strokes. If only a few joints show signs of arthritis, intra-articular injections of corticosteroids or low-dose systemic corticosteroids provide short-term relief. High-dose injections of corticosteroids into joints accelerate cartilage destruction and should be avoided.

Conventional disease-modifying antirheumatoid drugs (DMARDs) are first-line treatments for mild to moderate psoriatic arthritis. These DMARDS, besides methotrexate, include leflunomide (*Arava* and generics) and sulfasalazine (*Azulfidine* and generics). DMARDS are not effective in patients with axial disease.

Another medication effective in treating severe psoriasis and psoriatic arthritis is cyclosporine. It has brought dramatic improvement to patients with life-long disabling symptoms. Many people, however, can tolerate the drug only for short periods. Because of its potential to cause high blood pressure and kidney damage, multiple drug-drug interactions, and an increased risk of cancer, this medicine is prescribed only with extreme caution.

Should the medicines mentioned above fail to provide relief, biologic therapies usually bring satisfactory improvement of symptoms. The first group of biologic therapies includes tumor necrosis factor-alpha (TNF-a) inhibitors. Five TNF-a inhibitors, adalimumab (*Humira* and biosimilars), certolizumab pegol (*Cimzia*), etanercept (*Enbrel* and biosimilars), golimumab (*Simponi*), and infliximab (*Remicade* and biosimilars), are FDA-approved to treat severe plaque psoriasis and active psoriatic arthritis. TNF-a inhibitors are first-line treatments for severe plaque psoriasis and moderate to severe psoriatic arthritis, especially for those who did not respond satisfactorily to DMARDS. Suppose a patient does not find relief with one specific TNF-a inhibitor. In that case, a different one may provide a better response.

If TNF-a inhibitors do not provide adequate relief, then ustekinumab (*Stelara*) may halt disease progression. Typically, patients who fail treatment with TNF-a inhibitors find relief with ustekinumab. This monoclonal antibody binds to and inhibits a common subunit used by the proinflammatory cytokines IL-12 and IL-23. Should ustekinumab fail, the following medications are two different drugs that inhibit IL-17A, secukinumab (*Cosentyx*) and ixekizumab (*Taltz*). IL-12, IL-23, and IL-17A are upregulated in the skin of psoriasis patients, particularly during psoriatic flares. Inhibition of these proinflammatory

cytokines tamps down inflammation of disease progression. Rheumatologists prescribe IL-17A inhibitors to patients who did not respond to one or more TNF-a inhibitors. If these drugs fail, an alternative treatment is abatacept, an inhibitor of T-cell costimulation.

Suppose the patient cannot find relief with these medications or prefer oral medications. In that case, the Janus kinase (JAK) inhibitor, tofacitinib (*Xeljanz*), can help. JAK receives stimulatory signals inside immune cells and activates them. JAK inhibitors shut down the stimulatory signals in immune cells.

IL-23 antagonists can treat severe plaque psoriasis but not psoriatic arthritis. Guselkumab (*Tremfya*), tildrakizumab (*Ilumya*), and risankizumab (*Skyrizi*) are FDA-approved for the treatment of moderate to severe plaque psoriasis in adults. They bind to IL-23 and prevent it from binding to the IL-23 receptor. IL-23 inhibition prevents the downstream release of proinflammatory cytokines (such as IL-17A) and chemokines.

All biologic therapies increase the risk of infection and tumors. Still, they can relieve the symptoms of severe psoriasis and psoriatic arthritis and arrest joint deterioration.

All these therapies described can bring partial or total clearing of lesions and even bring remission of the disease for a time. Until the cause of psoriasis is completely understood, no research group will find a permanent cure.

PERSPECTIVE AND PROSPECTS

The term *psora* comes from the ancient Greek language. Psoriasis was considered a form of leprosy in biblical times. Descriptions of psoriasis appear in the records of the earliest known civilizations. Despite this ancient history and extensive modern research, however, the exact cause of psoriasis is still unknown. Unlike many human diseases, psoriasis does not afflict animals; therefore, no adequate animal model systems exist to study it in a controlled laboratory environment.

Early work on psoriasis by dermatologists centered on differential diagnosis—the ability to distinguish psoriasis from various rashes caused by fungi, such as ringworm, and from the many forms of eczema or dermatitis caused by allergies. Skin biopsies developed by oncologists can now determine that the condition is not cancer; the portion of skin removed, when placed under a microscope, will clearly show the dermal and epidermal appearance characteristic of psoriatic skin.

While skin scientists have proven that psoriasis is not contagious, it has been known since the 1930s that many cases develop soon after strep throat and other upper respiratory infections. However, the bacteria involved are not the cause of psoriasis but rather a trigger for developing a condition for which the patient is genetically predisposed. Another trigger, excessive scratching or rubbing of the skin, can precipitate outbreaks in susceptible people; this is named the Koebner phenomenon for its discoverer. Neurologists and psychologists have proved that the disease is not caused by "nerves," even though stress can worsen its symptoms. Health-care providers must help patients lower their stress levels to keep the disease under control.

Nutritionists have searched for ways to use diet to help psoriatics, but to no avail. Although no particular foods either help or hinder the course of the disease, most dermatologists now recognize that drinking alcohol can precipitate and aggravate the disfiguring plaques.

Immunologists have been very involved in the study of psoriasis, even though it is not an allergic reaction to any substance in one's environment. In the late twentieth century, they pursued many possible connections between the streptococci bacteria that cause strep throat, the white blood cells called "T lymphocytes" that seek to destroy them, and the development of psoriasis. They believe that, in predisposed people, chemicals from the bacteria cause the T lymphocytes to give off substances that trigger the skin's uncontrolled and excessive production of epidermal cells.

Geneticists have been searching diligently for the source of the predisposition to psoriasis. Among the genes children receive from their parents are those that build particular proteins on their white blood cells called "human leukocyte antigens" (HLAs). Out of the hundreds of different HLAs that one can inherit, those who develop psoriasis always seem to possess similar combinations. Identifying the genes responsible for HLAs and the role of those genes in precipitating psoriasis may bring about significant improvements in the treatment and possibly a cure for this disease afflicting millions of people throughout the world.

—*Michael A. Buratovich, PhD*

For Further Information:

About Psoriasis. National Psoriasis Foundation, 19 Nov. 2021, www.psoriasis.org/about-psoriasis/. Accessed 7 Apr. 2022.

Bard, Susan. "Everything You Need to Know About Psoriasis." Healthline, 18 Nov. 2021, www.healthline.com/health/psoriasis. Accessed 7 Apr. 2022.

"Drugs for Psoriasis." *Medical Letters on Drugs and Therapeutics*, vol. 61, no. 1574, 2019, pp. 89-96.

"Drugs for Psoriatic Arthritis." *Medical Letters on Drugs and Therapeutics*, vol. 61, no. 1588, 2019, pp. 203-10.

Husni, Elaine M. "Psoriatic Arthritis." *Cleveland Clinical Center for Continuing Education*, Oct. 2016, www.clevelandclinicmeded.com/medicalpubs/diseasemanagement/rheumatology/psoriatic-arthritis/. Accessed 5 Sept. 2021.

Psoriasis. MedlinePlus, 7 Dec. 2021, medlineplus.gov/psoriasis.html. Accessed 7 Apr. 2022.

Psoriasis Basics. National Institute of Arthritis and Musculoskeletal and Skin Diseases, Sept. 2020, www.niams.nih.gov/health-topics/psoriasis/basics/symptoms-causes. Accessed 7 Apr. 2022.

Psoriasis: Signs and symptoms, American Academy of Dermatology Association, n.d., www.aad.org/public/diseases/psoriasis/what/symptoms. 7 Apr. 2022.

Singh, Jasvinder A., et al. "Special Article: 2018 American College of Rheumatology/National Psoriasis Foundation Guideline for the Treatment of Psoriatic Arthritis." *Arthritis & Rheumatology*, vol. 71, no. 1, 2019, pp. 5-32, doi:10.1002/art.40726.

PSYCHIATRIC DISORDERS

Category: Disease/Disorder
Anatomy or system affected: Brain, psychic-emotional system
Specialties and related fields: Psychiatry
Definition: Clusters of psychological or behavioral symptoms that cause a person to experience serious emotional distress or significant mental impairment; these symptoms must be unusual or unexpected, or the patient must show evidence of more than one behavior that deviates from normal social expectations.
Key terms:

biomedical model: a way of viewing and understanding psychiatric disorders which emphasizes customary medical practice in identifying and treating a particular disorder from which a person suffers

diagnostic codes: the method used in the *Diagnostic and Statistical Manual of Mental Disorders (DSM)* to record psychiatric diagnoses for statistical and administrative purposes

multiaxial classification: the classification system used in the *DSM* to account for several factors when making psychiatric diagnoses, including present condition, developmental/personality disorders, physical disorders, life stresses, and overall functioning

neuroscience: the scientific specialization that seeks to understand mental processes, occurrences, and disturbances in terms of underlying mechanisms in the brain and the nervous system

psychodynamic model: a way of viewing and understanding psychiatric disorders which emphasizes the recognition and treatment of underlying psychological and developmental traumas

psychopharmacology: the use of drugs to study effects on brain chemistry; drugs are used to treat mental disorders, study brain chemistry, and promote new disease classifications *psychosocial treatment*: a significant specialization in treating people with psychiatric disorders through employing principles of psychology, human behavior, family and group dynamics, and social and occupational learning

somatic treatment: the treatment of people with psychiatric disorders using specialized drugs and electroconvulsive therapy; some major drug groups used are antidepressants, antipsychotics, mood stabilizers, anxiolytics, and psychostimulants

CAUSES AND SYMPTOMS

Many centuries ago, physicians began to understand that psychiatric disorders such as depression arose from abnormalities in brain structure or chemistry. As the field of psychiatry developed, medicine has had a profound influence in establishing the biomedical model to define and treat mental disorders. Sigmund Freud and other influential psychiatrists working in the late nineteenth century broadened the understanding of how emotional pain and trauma experienced during a person's childhood can contribute profoundly to the occurrence and course of mental disorders. The medical influence on the field of psychiatry was deepened and broadened by the contribution of neuroscience. Scientists who began studying the brain more intensively, beginning in the early twentieth century, proved the relationship of brain function to speech, learning, comprehension, memory, emotional regulation, and other important human abilities. Technologies developed in the late twentieth century, such as functional magnetic resonance imaging (fMRI) and genetic testing, have furthered psychiatrists' understanding of the biological, genetic, and neurological basis of a number of mental disorders.

Despite long and exacting efforts to understand mental illness, much remains to be explored. While psychiatrists would prefer to base their diagnoses on knowing the causes and the biological or neurological mechanisms of mental disorders, this knowledge has proved to be elusive. Therefore, most psychiatric diagnoses are based on the psychiatrist recognizing a pattern of symptoms and a typical course of disease. During World War II, psychiatrists realized that their colleagues differed widely in how they recognized and described various mental illnesses. Bureaucratic and professional forces coalesced in a drive to make the diagnosis of psychiatric disorders more systematic. In 1952, the American Psychiatric Association issued a manual that sought to clarify the diagnostic process. Unfortunately, the early manuals proved to be impractical and were largely ignored by psychiatrists. This changed when a more rigorous effort culminated in the publication of the third edition of the *Diagnostic and Statistical Manual of Mental Disorders (DSM-III)* in

1980. This text became widely accepted as the standard reference for psychiatrists to use when diagnosing psychiatric disorders. The manual has been strengthened and revised several times; a fifth edition, known as *DSM-5*, was published in 2013. Scientists and clinicians continue their work on the manual to correct flaws, incorporate research findings, and explore new areas. However, shortly before the publication of the *DSM-5* in May 2013, the US National Institute of Mental Health issued a statement condemning the *DMS-5*'s "lack of validity," noting that "DSM diagnoses are based on a consensus about clusters of clinical symptoms, not any objective laboratory measure." While psychiatrists agree that standard definitions of psychiatric disorders are needed to clarify their thinking, permit easier communication, improve treatment planning, and stimulate further research, a growing number of psychologists recognize the need for more accurate diagnostic criteria that are based on genetic, neurophysiological, and biological measures. While psychiatrists agree that a more accurate diagnostic system based on biomarkers is needed, the technology and research to establish such diagnostic criteria are not yet available. Therefore, the symptom-based diagnostic criteria put forth in the *DSM-5* remain the most widely used in the field of psychiatry.

When using the *DSM-5*, psychiatrists must find that the person exhibits specific signs and symptoms and has maintained this clinical picture for a sufficient length of time to warrant being diagnosed with a psychiatric disorder. The *DSM-5* assigns a specific code for each psychiatric diagnosis, which facilitates administrative and statistical work. The *DSM-5* provides clinicians with the criteria and definitions to accurately determine a patient's diagnosis by thoroughly describing disorders. Having a common language facilitates patient care in a more effective manner. ICD-10-CM provides a code number once the diagnosis has been established, and ICD-10-CM is the Health Insurance Portability and Accountability Act (HIPAA)-compliant code set for reporting diagnoses for reimbursement purposes. ICD-10-CM code use also enables statistical compilation and reporting of patient morbidity and mortality. The ICD-10-CM coding system uses a combination of letters and numbers in its codes.

Furthermore, the *DSM-5* combined the first three axes of the multiaxial diagnostic system used in the fourth edition of the *DSM (DSM-IV-TR)* into one list that includes all disorders. The *DSM-IV-TR* had listed clinical disorders on five separate axes, with Axis I referring to the principal disorder, Axis II indicating any additional personality disorder that might affect the Axis I disorder, Axis III indicating any medical problems that might affect the presentation or treatment of the principal disorder; Axis IV noting any psychosocial or contextual factors, and Axis V noting any disability. The *DSM-5* introduced a nonaxial diagnostic system, combining Axes I, II, and III into one list, with an expanded set of ICD-9-CM codes to note any psychosocial or environmental factors and disability (formerly Axes IV and V).

Several major diagnostic categories of psychiatric disorders are shown in the *DSM-5*. These include neurodevelopmental disorders; schizophrenia spectrum and other psychotic disorders; bipolar and related disorders; depressive disorders; anxiety disorders; obsessive-compulsive and related disorders; trauma- and stressor-related disorders; dissociative disorders; somatic symptom and related disorders; feeding and eating disorders; sleep-wake disorders; sexual dysfunctions; gender dysphoria; disruptive, impulse-control, and conduct disorders; substance-related and addictive disorders; neurocognitive disorders; and paraphilic disorders. This listing demonstrates the breadth of problems that are seen and treated by psychiatrists and other mental health practitioners.

Research shows that, on average, 26.2 percent of adults in the United States will experience one or more psychiatric disorders in a given year. Globally, approximately 10 percent of the adult population will have a psychiatric disorder, although psychologists believe the actual rates of mental illness are underreported in many developing countries. The most common disorders are anxiety disorders and mood disorders, such as depression.

Researchers learned that people who experience their first symptoms later in life generally have a better chance of recovering, but almost all people who suffer from a psychiatric disorder will experience distressing symptoms for several years. More men than women, the data show, have suffered a psychiatric disorder at some point in life, although women are more likely than men to experience anxiety or mood disorders. According to researchers, the differences in prevalence among the races may be more reflective of survey methods than of ethnic origins. Higher rates of mental illness are found among people who are poor and who fail to complete high school. People who suffer from one psychiatric disorder were found by researchers to be at a high risk (60 percent) for having another mental health disorder at some time during their lives.

TREATMENT AND THERAPY

Making an accurate diagnosis of psychiatric disorders is essential to treating problems properly, since many can be improved through the application of psychosocial, somatic, drug, and adjunctive therapies.

> **INFORMATION ON PSYCHIATRIC DISORDERS**
>
> **Causes:** Genetic and environmental factors, medications, substance abuse
>
> **Symptoms:** Wide ranging; may include emotional distress, mental impairment, abrupt changes in mood or personality, anxiety, depression, manic behavior, substance abuse, difficulty sleeping
>
> **Duration:** Acute to chronic
>
> **Treatments:** Depends on type and severity; may include drug, psychosocial, somatic, and adjunctive therapies

---

For example, it is said that most people who suffer from major depression can be treated successfully with brief psychotherapy, a course of medication, or a combination of both. The somatic technique of exposing a person each day to a bank of bright lights (light therapy) has been used successfully to treat seasonal affective disorder (depression associated with a specific season, especially winter). Many depressed people and their families have been helped by the adjunctive therapy of participating in a support group.

The use of laboratory tests to clarify psychiatric diagnosis is growing in importance. Only a few disorders can be revealed by laboratory tests, but research is being conducted to validate such testing and to increase its scope and usefulness. Some tests are done routinely to rule out medical problems that may be causing the psychiatric problems the person is experiencing or to ensure that the patient can take needed medication.

Drugs have been used in the United States to treat psychiatric disorders since the early 1950s, and new medications are introduced frequently. The distressing thought disturbances experienced by people suffering from schizophrenia have been treated with antipsychotic drugs. Antipsychotics also are used to treat psychotic symptoms such as the hallucinations and delusions experienced by some people who are suffering from depression or other mood disorders. Several classes of antipsychotics have been developed. Lithium carbonate is the drug most commonly used to treat people suffering from bipolar disorders, in which patients experience swings in mood from the highs of mania to the lows of depression. Various classes of antidepressants such as tricyclics and monoamine oxidase inhibitors (MAOIs) are used to treat people suffering from depression. Many people experiencing symptoms associated with anxiety disorders have been helped through the use of benzodiazepines and other anxiolytics. Central nervous system stimulants (psychostimulants) are used to treat narcolepsy, a disorder in which people have trouble staying awake.

Psychostimulants also are used to treat attention-deficit disorder (ADD), because the stimulants have the paradoxical effect of reducing the behaviors that disrupt classroom work and life at home. The drugs decrease excessive physical activity and have been shown to improve an individual's attention to adult guidance, increase attention span and memory, and lessen the individual's tendency to be distracted from tasks and to act impulsively. The person with ADD also is helped with behavior management techniques and careful control of the environment to reduce sources of external stimulation.

Unfortunately, the use of drugs in treating psychiatric disorders is not problem-free. Almost all psychotropic drugs have side effects that can be serious enough to prevent their use in treatment. A growing number of psychiatrists have expressed their concern over what they believe to be widespread overdiagnosis and overtreatment for psychiatric disorders in the United States; many patients respond well to simple lifestyle changes, such as increased physical activity or brief therapeutic interventions, so psychiatrists should prescribe psychopharmaceutical medications judiciously. Some people must take other prescription drugs that preclude the use of the drug needed to treat the psychiatric disorder. The possibility of overdose by people who have thoughts of taking their lives can limit the use of possibly toxic drugs. Some people are not helped by drug therapy, are reluctant to take drugs, or fail to take drugs properly. For such people, it is fortunate that other forms of treatment can be used.

Many people who suffer from psychiatric illness have been helped by trained psychotherapists, such as psychiatrists, psychologists, social workers, counselors, and members of the clergy. Many forms of psychotherapy are practiced. The aims of psychotherapy can be to help the person deal well with life's stresses and crises, confront and resolve psychological conflict, avoid interpersonal problems, and find more satisfaction and fulfillment in life. Psychotherapy is delivered to individuals, couples, families, and other groups. More emphasis is being placed on conducting psychotherapy only for a limited time, because this approach is preferred by most patients and their insurance companies and because research results support its effectiveness.

Behavioral therapy can be used to help the person to change specific behaviors that cause problems. Behavioral therapy has been used to treat several psychiatric disorders, including alcohol and drug dependence, anxiety, phobias, autism spectrum disorders, and eating disorders. Systematic desensitization has been used to help people who have irrational fears, or phobias. The patient is gradually introduced to the situation that elicits the fearful response and is taught to use relaxation techniques to reduce anxiety and to bring fears under personal control. In behavior modification programs, unwanted behavior is defined, targeted, reduced, and eliminated. At the same time, the person is rewarded for behaving properly.

Electroconvulsive therapy (ECT), formerly called "shock therapy," is used generally to treat people with severe depression who have not responded to less intrusive treatment methods. In ECT, the patient is exposed to an electric current that is passed through electrodes on either side of the head usually though unilateral ECT is occasionally done. Patients are anesthetized to reduce the trauma and reduce the risk of injury. The current causes the person to experience a brief seizure, usually for less than a minute. This treatment method has been used for many years, and several improvements have been made to make the procedure safer and less damaging to the person's memory.

Treatment of psychiatric disorders is usually delivered in the community where the affected person lives. In the United States, legislation in the 1960s caused federal funds to be used to build and staff community mental health centers. Many health insurance providers will pay part of the fees charged by private therapists, which allows some people to afford their services. Alcohol and drug treatment programs generally offer people either short-term residential or outpatient services. Many people are served in institutional settings, such as mental hospitals and nursing homes. Some use services provided by governmental funding.

Many people who have suffered psychiatric disorders recover completely; investigators find a 38 percent remission rate. The researchers were surprised to learn that people are most likely to recover from alcohol and drug abuse, generalized anxiety, and antisocial personality. Complete freedom from distressing symptoms and episodes is less likely for those who suffer from mania, obsessive-compulsive disorder (in which the person performs repetitive rituals to allay anxiety caused by disturbing thoughts or fears), and schizophrenia (a disorder typified by thought disturbances such as hallucinations and delusions, mood changes, communication problems, and unusual behaviors). However, with a combination of pharmacological and psychosocial treatments and interventions, 70 to 90 percent of patients with psychiatric disorders experience a reduction of symptoms and improved quality of life, even without achieving full remission.

A large number of people who suffer mental illness have never been treated. Researchers estimate the economic cost of untreated psychiatric disorders in the United States to be more than $100 billion each year.

PERSPECTIVE AND PROSPECTS

Early medical documents show that mental illness has always been an area of significant concern. Symptoms of mental illness were described in the Bible, and they were studied and treated in classical times. Interest in understanding mental disorders waned during the medieval period, when it was thought that sufferers were possessed by demons or were being punished by God. Mentally ill people were often maltreated and incarcerated. Finally, the foundation was laid in the late sixteenth century for a more complete understanding of psychiatric disorders: In 1586, Timothy Bright, a physician, published the first English-language text on mental illness, entitled *Treatise of Melancholie*.

In late eighteenth-century France, Philippe Pinel took over the management of a hospital for insane men and not only advocated more humane treatment of mentally ill people but also took steps to free them from the chains and other punishing devices that they were forced to endure. Pinel instituted the scientific study of mental illness. He tracked the prevalence of mental disorders, conducted studies to learn the natural course of mental illness, and established a treatment model followed by the more progressive psychiatric facilities.

The brain was studied even more intensely in the nineteenth century. During this era, scientists made important contributions to the understanding of how certain parts of the brain are responsible for specialized functions. They learned that particular brain regions are related to speech and language, movement, sensations, learning, understanding, and emotions. Emil Kraepelin correlated information about the age of onset, natural course, and length of time of particular mental disorders. He used the information that he organized to develop the first classification system of psychiatric disorders. Among the maladies he named were dementia praecox (now called "schizophrenia"), dementia in the elderly (now called "Alzheimer's disease"), and manic-depressive illness (bipolar disorder).

While neuroscientists were making significant contributions to the understanding of the brain, psychiatrist Sigmund Freud was advancing his study of hysteria and its connection with childhood trauma. He used hypnosis and free association to release and resolve underlying misconceptions and fears and to give the patient relief from debilitating trauma and its associated symptoms. He also produced theories on psychological function and structure and on psychotherapy.

During the twentieth century, psychiatrists drew on a broad array of disciplines to improve the diagnosis and treatment of psychiatric disorders, including the study of brain chemistry, biology, structure, and functioning. Advances in neuroimaging techniques allowed scientists to study and sometimes diagnose brain dysfunction. Specialized drugs were developed to be used in the treatment of specific mental disorders. Since 1952, the American Psychiatric Association has published a series of diagnostic and statistical manuals designed to bring order to the study, diagnosis, and treatment of psychiatric disorders. Psychiatrists continue to work toward developing more accurate diagnostic criteria and more effective treatments for psychiatric disorders.

—*Shuba Samuel, PhD*

See also: Addiction; Alcoholism; Alzheimer's disease; Amnesia; Antianxiety drugs; Antidepressants; Anxiety; Asperger's syndrome; Autism; Bipolar disorders; Body dysmorphic disorder; Brain; Brain damage; Delusions; Dementias; Depression; Domestic violence; Eating disorders; Emotions: Biomedical causes and effects; Factitious disorders; Frontotemporal dementia (FTD); Gender identity disorder; Geriatrics and gerontology; Grief and guilt; Hallucinations; Hypochondriasis; Intoxication; Light therapy; Memory loss; Midlife crisis; Morgellons disease; Neurology; Neurology, pediatric; Neurosis; Neurosurgery; Obsessive-compulsive disorder; Panic attacks; Paranoia; Pharmacology; Phobias; Pick's disease; Postpartum depression; Post-traumatic stress disorder; Prader-Willi syndrome; Prescription drug abuse; Psychiatry; Psychiatry, child and adolescent; Psychiatry, geriatric; Psychoanalysis; Psychosis; Psychosomatic disorders; Schizophrenia; Seasonal affective disorder; Sexual dysfunction; Sexuality; Shock therapy; Sibling rivalry; Stress; Stuttering; Substance abuse; Suicide.

For Further Information:
Black, Donald W., and Nancy C. Andreasen. *Introductory Textbook of Psychiatry.* 7th ed., American Psychiatric Press, 2021.
Insel, Thomas. "Transforming Diagnosis." *National Institute of Mental Health*, 29 Apr. 2013.
Kring, Ann M., et al. *Abnormal Psychology.* 14th ed., John Wiley & Sons, 2019.
North, Carol S., and Sean H. Yutzy. *Goodwin and Guze's Psychiatric Diagnosis.* 7th ed., Oxford UP, 2018.
Oltmanns, Thomas F., et al. *Case Studies in Abnormal Psychology.* 11th ed., John Wiley & Sons, 2019.
Sadock, Benjamin J., Virginia A. Sadock, and Pedro Ruiz, editors. *Kaplan and Sadock's Comprehensive Textbook of Psychiatry.* 10th ed., Lippincott Williams & Wilkins, 2017.

PSYCHIATRY

Category: Specialty
Anatomy or system affected: All
Specialties and related fields: Critical care, family medicine, geriatrics and gerontology, neurology, pharmacology, preventive medicine, public health
Definition: A medical field concerned with the diagnosis, epidemiology, prevention, and treatment of mental and emotional problems.

Key terms:

anxiety disorders: conditions in which physical and emotional uneasiness, apprehension, or fear is the dominant symptom

bipolar disorders: problems marked by mania or mania with depression; historically known as manic-depressive disorders

dementias: disorders characterized by a general deterioration of intellectual and emotional functioning, involving problems with memory, judgment, emotional responses, and personality changes

depressive disorders: problems involving persistent feelings of despair, weight change, sleep problems, thoughts of death, thinking difficulties, diminished interest or pleasure in activities, and agitation or listlessness

personality disorders: pervasive, inflexible patterns of perceiving, thinking, and behaving that cause long-term distress or impairment, beginning in adolescence and persisting into adulthood

psychiatric diagnosis: a clinical labeling process involving the focused study of symptom patterns; physical, emotional, and personality factors; significant relationships; and recent events

psychotic: referring to a disabling mental state characterized by poor reality testing (inaccurate perceptions, confusion, disorientation) and disorganized speech, behavior, and emotional experience

psychotropic drugs: substances primarily affecting behavior, perception, and other psychological functions

schizophrenic disorders: mental disturbances characterized by psychotic features during the active phase and deteriorated functioning in occupational, social, or self-care abilities

SCIENCE AND PROFESSION

Psychiatrists receive training in biochemistry, community mental health, genetics, neurology, neuropathology, psychopathology, psychopharmacology, and social science. They complete medical school, a four-year residency in psychiatry, and two or more years of specialty residency. Specialty residencies focus on particular treatment methods (such as psychoanalysis) or methods of diagnosis and treatment for particular groups of clients (such as children, adolescents, or elders).

As diagnosticians and treatment providers, psychiatrists must be excellent observers of behavior and be knowledgeable about how nutritional, physical, and situational conditions can be related to mental or emotional problems. An ability to consult with other professionals is also important. Psychiatrists often receive patients from other professionals (general practitioners, psychologists, emergency room staff) and often request diagnostic, legal, case management, and re-

source advice from other professionals (psychologists, attorneys, social workers). In situations involving abuse, neglect, incompetency, and suicide, such consultation relationships are critical for appropriate referral and treatment.

Given this preparation, psychiatrists are able to diagnose and treat a wide variety of disorders. Some of the most common disorders treated in adult populations include disorders of anxiety (such as phobias, panic attacks, obsessive-compulsive behavior, acute and post-traumatic stress) and mood (such as depressive and bipolar problems). Personality, schizophrenic, substance abuse, and dementia-related disorders also are treated frequently by psychiatrists. Such conditions are described in detail in the American Psychiatric Association's (APA's) *Diagnostic and Statistical Manual of Mental Disorders: DSM-5* (2013).

DIAGNOSTIC AND TREATMENT TECHNIQUES

A well-formulated psychiatric diagnosis facilitates treatment planning for mental and emotional disorders. Psychiatric diagnoses, however, are very complex. Previously, the APA used a axial system to diagnose psychiatric disorders. Axis I pertained to clinical conditions diagnosed in infancy, childhood, or adolescence; Axis II summarized problems related to personality and intellectual disability; and Axis III described any general medical conditions that are related to a person's mental problems and that may also warrant special attention. However, in *DSM-5* these axes are grouped by chapter. In *DSM-IV* Axis IV summarized psychological, social, and environmental problems that may affect the diagnosis, prognosis, or treatment of a person's mental problems. Axis V was used to give a standardized, overall rating of how well the person was functioning with his or her disorder; this axis has been dropped entirely.

Once a diagnosis is formulated, a treatment plan is composed. Usually, it involves some combination of medicinal and psychotropic drugs, bibliotherapy, dietary and behavior change recommendations, and psychotherapy for the affected individual and possibly members of his or her family. Treatment compliance is critical, particularly when psychotropic drugs are involved. As such, psychiatric treatment often involves frequent contacts and an aftercare plan of continued visits with the psychiatrist or a support group able to encourage follow-through on the treatment recommendations.

PERSPECTIVE AND PROSPECTS

The concepts of mental health and illness have been in human cultures since ancient times. As early as 2980 BCE, priest-physicians were noted for their treatment of spirit possession involving madness, violence, mutism, and melancholy. In those times, such problems were thought to originate from external, supernatural forces. Later, during the rise of Greco-Roman philosophies in medicine, such states of mind began to be explored more as disturbances of the brain and less as the result of supernatural causes. As such, treatments began to develop greater reliance on methods such as vapors, baths, diets, and emetic and cathartic drugs.

Over time, the field of psychiatry has matured and taken on a major role in medicine. Research into the mind-body relationship has clarified how the mind can influence the healing of medical conditions, as well as how certain medical conditions are rooted in psychological, social, and environmental problems, rather than in a person's biology alone. Additionally, advances in the development of psychotropic drugs have played a major role in the treatment of disabling conditions long thought to be untreatable, such as schizophrenic and bipolar disorders.

In the future, psychiatry is expected to continue developing a broad variety of specialty areas. New techniques for working with children, adolescents, elders, and individuals with particular medical problems or of a particular gender or cultural background are developing rapidly. Finally, understanding the relationship between psychiatric disorders across the life span is likely to increase, as is the need to develop treatments for complex scenarios involving multiple diagnoses.

—Nancy A. Piotrowski, PhD

See also Addiction; Aging; Aging: Extended care; Alcoholism; Alzheimer's disease; Amnesia; Anorexia nervosa; Antianxiety drugs; Antidepressants; Anxiety; Asperger's syndrome; Attention-deficit disorder (ADD); Autism; Bipolar disorders; Body dysmorphic disorder; Brain; Brain damage; Brain disorders; Bulimia; Chronic fatigue syndrome; Circumcision, female, and genital mutilation; Delusions; Dementias; Depression; Domestic violence; Eating disorders; Electroencephalography (EEG); Emergency medicine; Emotions: Biomedical causes and effects; Euthanasia; Factitious disorders; Family medicine; Fatigue; Frontotemporal dementia (FTD); Gender identity disorder; Gender reassignment surgery; Geriatrics and gerontology; Grief and guilt; Hallucinations; Hypnosis; Hypochondriasis; Incontinence; Intellectual disability; Intoxication; Light therapy; Memory loss; Midlife crisis; Neurology; Neurology, pediatric; Neurosis; Neurosurgery; Obesity; Obsessive-compulsive disorder; Panic attacks; Paranoia; Pharmacology; Phobias; Pick's disease; Postpartum depression; Post-traumatic stress disorder; Prader-Willi syndrome; Prescription drug abuse; Psychiatric disorders; Psychiatry, child and adolescent; Psychiatry, geriatric; Psychoanalysis; Psychosis; Psychosomatic disorders; Schizophrenia; Seasonal affective disorder; Sexual dysfunction; Sexuality; Shock therapy; Sleep disorders; Speech disorders; Stress; Stress reduction; Substance abuse; Sudden infant death syndrome (SIDS); Suicide; Terminally ill: Extended care.

For Further Information:
American Psychiatric Association. *Diagnostic and Statistical Manual of Mental Disorders: DSM-5*. Arlington, Va.: Author, 2013.
Andreasen, Nancy C., and Donald W. Black. *Introductory Textbook of Psychiatry*. 5th ed. Washington, DC: American Psychiatric Press, 2011.
Kring, Ann M., et al. *Abnormal Psychology*. 12th ed. Hoboken, N.J.: John Wiley & Sons, 2012.
Mazure, Carolyn M., ed. *Does Stress Cause Psychiatric Illness?* Washington, DC: American Psychiatric Press, 1995.
Muskin, Philip R., Patricia L. Gerbarg, and Richard P. Brown. *Complementary and Integrative Therapies for Psychiatric Disorders*. Philadelphia: Saunders, 2013.
Preston, John, and James Johnson. *Clinical Psychopharmacology Made Ridiculously Simple*. 7th ed. Miami: MedMaster, 2012.
Sadock, Benjamin J., and Virginia A. Sadock, eds. *Kaplan and Sadock's Comprehensive Textbook of Psychiatry*. 9th ed. Philadelphia: Lippincott Williams & Wilkins, 2009.
Semple, David, and Roger Smyth. *Oxford Handbook of Psychiatry*. New York: Oxford University Press, 2013.
Tomb, David. *Psychiatry*. 7th ed. Philadelphia: Wolters Kluwer/Lippincott Williams & Wilkins, 2008.

PSYCHIATRY, CHILD AND ADOLESCENT

Category: Specialty
Anatomy or system affected: Brain
Specialties and related fields: Psychiatry, child and adolescent psychology, neuroscience (brain research)
Definition: Subspecialty of psychiatry that focuses on the diagnosis and treatment of disorders affecting thinking, emotions, and behavior of children and adolescents.

Key terms:

cognitive behavioral therapy: psychotherapy that aims to change distorted ways of thinking in order to improve behavior and mood; usually relatively short-term and focused

dialectical behavior therapy: psychotherapy that encourages older adolescents to take responsibility for their own problems and learn how to manage intense emotions

family therapy: psychotherapy that identifies and manages issues in the family and their interactions with the patient

interpersonal therapy: psychotherapy that focuses on improving interpersonal relationships

pathophysiology: biological processes that lead to the development of a disease

play therapy: psychotherapy that uses tools such as drawing, toys, and dolls to help children understand and control their feelings and thoughts

psychodynamic psychotherapy: psychotherapy that focuses on understanding the motivating factors behind a child's behavior and feelings

SCIENCE

The general psychiatry training includes in-depth study of the structure and function of the brain as well as neurological processes; epidemiology, genetics, and pathophysiology of psychiatric disorders; and treatments (including cognitive behavioral therapy and psychiatric drugs). The child and adolescent specialty training encompasses normal child and family development, mechanisms of psychiatric disorders affecting children and adolescents, and treatment. Psychiatric disorders affecting this group of individuals are attention-deficit/hyperactivity disorder (ADHD), autism, intellectual disabilities, mood disorders, learning disabilities, eating disorders, drug dependency, and conduct disorder (delinquency).

DIAGNOSTIC AND TREATMENT TECHNIQUES

Diagnosis of psychiatric disorders is complicated because of the multitude of factors at play in psychiatric disorders, which include physical/biological, emotional, social, and environmental factors. Diagnosis of such disorders in children and adolescents is further complicated by the effects of developmental processes. The *Diagnostic and Statistical Manual of Mental Disorders* (*DSM*), published by the American Psychiatric Association, is a reference book used by many psychiatrists. Now in its fifth edition, the DSM-5 contains revised diagnostic criteria to more accurately reflect the manifestation of psychiatric disorders in children and adolescents.

Psychotherapy is a commonly used technique to alleviate symptoms and improve functioning in children with psychiatric disorders. It encompasses several different types of therapy, including: (1) cognitive behavioral therapy; (2) dialectical behavior therapy;(3) family therapy; (4) group therapy; (5) interpersonal therapy; (6) play therapy; and (7) psychodynamic psychotherapy. All types of psychotherapy utilize communication to effect change in the individual's behavior and emotions.

For some children and adolescents, clinicians may decide to prescribe medications in combination with psychotherapy. Many medications have different effects in children than in adults, which should be taken into consideration when prescribing and monitoring treatment. Medications used to treat children and adolescents include antidepressants for depression, anxiety, and pain; benzodiazepines for anxiety disorders; stimulants for ADHD; as well as antipsychotics for bipolar disorder, schizophrenia, posttraumatic stress disorder, and obsessive-compulsive disorder.

Similar to the situation in adults, the effects of medications vary from one individual to another. In addition, medications such as the class of antidepressants known as "selective serotonin reuptake inhibitors" (SSRIs) have been linked to an increased risk of suicidal thoughts and behavior in adolescents. However, a large 2007 study of clinical trials involving children with major depression or anxiety who were treated with antidepressants showed that the benefits probably outweighed the risks. This study was partially sponsored by the National Institute of Mental Health.

PERSPECTIVE AND PROSPECTS

Starting in the nineteenth century, when influential thinkers of the day began to write about mental disorders in children, child and adolescent psychiatry has progressed from a burgeoning field to a fully-fledged subspecialty of psychiatry. In the 1950s, cognitive behavioral therapy, tricyclic antidepressants, and the first antipsychotics were developed. The first professor of child psychiatry was Lanfranco Ciampi, who assumed his position in 1923 in Argentina. In 1930, the first child psychiatry department was established in the United States at Johns Hopkins Hospital. In 1937, the International Association for Child and Adolescent Psychiatry and Allied Professions (IACAPAP) was formed as the International Committee for Child Psychiatry. Since then, the field has continued to evolve and grow in numbers and recognition. One challenge that modern-day child and adolescent psychiatrists face is in defining their role with respect to other related health care professionals—whether they should be primarily therapists, prescribers of medication, or coordinators of a team of professionals who are each responsible for different aspects of treatment.

—*Shuba Samuel, PhD*

For Further Information:
American Academy of Child & Adolescent Psychiatry, 2022, www.aacap.org/AACAP/Medical_Students_and_Residents/ Medical_Students/What_is_Child_and_Adolescent_ Psychiatry.aspx.
National Institute of Mental Health, Oct. 2016, www.nimh.nih.gov/ health/topics/mental-health-medications/index.shtml.
Stern, T. A., G. L. Fricchione, and J. F. Rosenbaum. *Massachusetts General Hospital Handbook of General Hospital Psychiatry*. Elsevier Health Sciences, 2017.

PSYCHIATRY, GERIATRIC

Category: Specialty
Anatomy or system affected: All
Specialties and related fields: Critical care, family medicine, geriatrics and gerontology, neurology, pharmacology, preventive medicine, public health
Definition: A subspecialty of psychiatry which deals with the diagnosis and treatment of psychiatric syndromes experienced by older people.

Key terms:

acute confusion syndrome: a transient condition caused by the action of various biological stressors on vulnerable older persons, who may experience inattention, disorganized thinking, other cognitive impairments, and emotional problems

anxiety: a condition characterized by nervousness or agitation; in older people, it is often caused by the existence of a psychiatric disorder such as depression, a general medical condition such as hypothyroidism, or a side effect of medication

depression: a condition characterized by a persistent mood of sadness, weight loss, greatly decreased interest in life, and sometimes psychotic episodes; biological factors, family history of depression, underlying medical problems, and medication side effects all can contribute to these symptoms

hypochondriasis: a condition in which the patients believe strongly that they are suffering from one or more serious illnesses, even when this belief is unsupported by medical evidence

insomnia: disturbed sleep, which occurs in older people more often than in any other age group; insomnia in older people can be caused by many factors, such as dysfunctional sleep cycles, breathing problems, leg jerking, underlying medical and psychiatric disorders, and the side effects of medication

memory loss syndrome: a condition in which a person gradually but progressively loses capacity in many cognitive areas, but especially in the ability to remember; Alzheimer's disease is considered the most common factor causing serious memory loss in older people

suspiciousness: a range of symptoms from increasing distrust of others to paranoid delusions of conspiracies; changes related to aging are thought to be major factors causing increased suspiciousness in older people

SCIENCE AND PROFESSION

Growing numbers of old and very old people and the increased complexity of diagnosis and treatment of this age group have driven the growth of geriatric psychiatry. Psychiatrists who specialize in working with the geriatric population note that the psychiatric problems experienced by older people often fit poorly in the diagnostic categories set down in the *Diagnostic and Statistical Manual of Mental Disorders: DSM-IV-TR* (4th ed., 2000). The interplay among declining physical health, decreasing mental functioning, social withdrawal and isolation, and vulnerability to stress makes proper diagnosis and appropriate treatment more difficult. In response to this complexity, practitioners of geriatric psychiatry tend to take a broader approach to diagnosis and to use an interdisciplinary model in developing a treatment plan. The profession of geriatric psychiatry has developed most in Great Britain and Canada but is attracting growing numbers of practitioners in the United States and other Western countries.

DIAGNOSTIC AND TREATMENT TECHNIQUES

Geriatric psychiatrists tend to follow the lead of specialists in geriatric medicine, who have found that taking a syndromal approach to diagnosis appears to work better with older patients. Among the psychiatric syndromes used by geriatric psychiatrists are acute confusion, anxiety, depression, hypochondriasis, insomnia, memory loss, and suspiciousness. Special attention must be given by geriatric psychiatrists to the older person's overall ability to function, general health status, social support system, family history, and preexisting conditions. Geriatric psychiatrists are forced to acknowledge the role played by changes in the brain as it ages and to separate changes that are relatively benign from those that pose real threats to the patient. Hospitalization and significant medical intervention tend to occur more often in the later stages of a person's life, and geriatric psychiatrists are aware that these events can have a great impact on the patient's mental well-being.

When they can, geriatric psychiatrists draw readily upon the help of other health-care providers in treating elderly persons, including the use of specially qualified clinical psychologists, social workers, nurses, occupational therapists, speech pathologists, dietitians, and physical therapists. Improving the understanding of family members and providing them with supportive advice and services can be an important part of the overall treatment plan.

PERSPECTIVE AND PROSPECTS

In the United States, federal funding has expanded for qualified providers, such as clinical psychologists and social workers, to render mental health services to older people, especially those who live in long-term care facilities. Funds have increased for the proper training of those who provide mental health services to older people. Examinations have been established to show evidence of "added qualifications" in geriatric medicine and psychiatry. More textbooks and specialty journals devoted to geriatric mental health are now in circulation. The federal government has sponsored important national conferences on various aspects of geriatric mental health. With the costs of hospital and long-term care continuing to rise, more emphasis has been given to preventive services and day-care services.

Furthermore, some hospitals have established specialized geropsychiatric units to improve diagnosis and treatment and to decrease the time that older people spend in the hospital. Services are expected to increase for adult children who care for older parents with mental illnesses. Research efforts have increased concerning the causes and appropriate treatment of psychiatric problems in older people. Older people are becoming healthier as they learn more about how mental health and physical health are affected by the way in which one lives. They are advised to stop smoking, eat a better diet, exercise more, and continue to take an active part in family and community life. All these trends are expected to continue in the future.

—*Russell Williams, MSW*

See also Addiction; Aging; Aging: Extended care; Alcoholism; Alzheimer's disease; Amnesia; Antianxiety drugs; Antidepressants; Anxiety; Bipolar disorders; Brain; Brain damage; Brain disorders; Chronic fatigue syndrome; Delusions; Dementias; Depression; Domestic violence; Electroencephalography (EEG); Emergency medicine; Emotions: Biomedical causes and effects; Euthanasia; Factitious disorders; Family medicine; Fatigue; Frontotemporal dementia (FTD); Geriatrics and gerontology; Grief and guilt; Hallucinations; Hypnosis; Hypochondriasis; Incontinence; Intellectual disability; Intoxication; Light therapy; Memory loss; Neurology; Neurosis; Neurosurgery; Obesity; Obsessive-compulsive disorder; Panic attacks; Paranoia; Pharmacology; Phobias; Pick's disease; Polypharmacy; Prescription drug abuse; Psychiatric disorders; Psychiatry; Psychoanalysis; Psychosis; Psychosomatic disorders; Schizophrenia; Sexual dysfunction; Sexuality; Shock therapy; Sleep disorders; Speech disorders; Stress; Stress reduction; Substance abuse; Suicide; Terminally ill: Extended care.

For Further Information:
Andreasen, Nancy C., and Donald W. Black. *Introductory Textbook of Psychiatry.* 5th ed. Washington, DC: American Psychiatric Press, 2011.
Bee, Helen L., and Barbara L. Bjorklund. *The Journey of Adulthood.* 7th ed. Upper Saddle River, N.J.: Prentice Hall, 2011.
Birren, James E., and K. Warner Schaie, eds. *Handbook of the Psychology of Aging.* 7th ed. Boston: Academic Press/Elsevier, 2011.
Birren, James E., R. Bruce Sloane, and Gene D. Cohen, eds. *Handbook of Mental Health and Aging.* 2d ed. San Diego, Calif.: Academic Press, 1992.
Blazer, Dan G., and David C., eds. Steffens. *Essentials of Geriatric Psychiatry.* Washington, DC: American Psychiatric Publishing, 2012.
Blazer, Dan G., David C. Steffens, and Ewald W. Busse, eds. *The American Psychiatric Publishing Textbook of Geriatric Psychiatry.* 4th ed. Washington, DC: American Psychiatric Publishing, 2009.
Lavretsky, Helen, Martha Sajatovic, and Charles F. Reynolds, eds. *Late-Life Mood Disorders.* New York: Oxford University Press, 2013.
Miller, Mark D., and LalithKumar K Solai, eds. *Geriatric Psychiatry.* New York: Oxford University Press, 2013.
Sadock, Benjamin J., and Virginia A. Sadock, eds. *Kaplan and Sadock's Comprehensive Textbook of Psychiatry.* 9th ed. Philadelphia: Lippincott Williams & Wilkins, 2009.
Whitbourne, Susan Krauss, ed. *Psychopathology in Later Adulthood.* New York: Wiley, 2001.

PSYCHOANALYSIS

Category: Treatment
Anatomy or system affected: Psychic-emotional system
Specialties and related fields: Psychiatry
Definition: A psychotherapeutic technique, developed by Sigmund Freud, in which the analyst helps the patient to uncover and resolve unconscious conflicts in order to treat personality disorders and/or deviance.

Key terms:
classical psychoanalysis: the method developed by Freud to help patients achieve insight into why they develop maladaptive ways of relating to others and experience disabling psychological symptoms
dreams: warnings sent from the superego to protect the ego from id impulses
instinctual drives: libido (the seeking of gratification of sexual impulses) and aggression (the seeking of gratification of destructive impulses)
neurosis: a psychic disturbance and defect from childhood that develops into a particular pattern of emotional illness and dysfunctional behavior
Oedipus complex: the experience of having sexual feelings toward the parent of the opposite sex, which is found in young children
psyche: the human mind, which according to Freud is divided into id, ego, and superego; the id contains instincts and repressed feelings, the ego directs everyday behavior, and the superego guides the ego
psychoanalyst: a person, usually a psychiatrist, who has received several years of postgraduate training and supervised practice in using psychoanalysis to diagnose and treat clients
psychosis: a condition occurring when a person's id impulses chronically defeat the control of the ego; schizophrenia and bipolar disorders are two examples of psychoses
transference: the tendency of a person who developed unsatisfying parental relationships to repeat this pattern unconsciously with others; psychoanalytic treatment depends on the development of transference between client and analyst

THE THEORETICAL BASIS OF PSYCHOANALYSIS

Psychoanalysis is a method that is used to understand the workings of the human mind. Adherents to psychoanalysis believe that many forces operate to influence and shape the mind, including some that exist beneath the level of conscious awareness and control. Psychoanalysis permits scientists to observe and collect information about the mind, to develop and test scientific hypotheses about mental processes, and to use the scientific wisdom gained to diagnose and treat mental illnesses. Psychoanalytic theory helps psychiatrists and other mental health practitioners understand more about human emotions and psychological development. Though many psychoanalytic concepts were first developed only in the late nineteenth century, psychoanalysis has made significant and lasting contributions to modern psychiatry and continues to enhance its development.

The precepts of psychoanalysis have been subjected to much scientific scrutiny and criticism. As befits any scientific discipline, psychoanalytic theory has been revised periodically to account for new information, observations, and insights. Psychoanalytic theory also is seen as contributing to other scientific disciplines, such as neurology, the social sciences, and psychology. Psychoanalysis has also broadened understanding in the humanities, the arts, philosophy, ethics, and religion. Psychoanalysis clearly has had a profound and lasting impact upon a broad span of human interests and activities.

Psychoanalytic theory is largely a product of the efforts of Sigmund Freud (1856-1939) to link the physical processes of the human brain with the psychological manifestations of the human mind. While Freud was frustrated in his ultimate goal of demonstrating clearly the relationship between the two, his work informs the same search today. Therefore, an understanding of early and evolving psychoanalytic theory remains important to psychiatry and psychotherapy.

To begin developing an understanding of the complexities of psychoanalysis, one needs to be familiar with basic information about psychoanalytic theory. The discussion that follows will touch on instinctual drives, the architecture of the mind, psychological development, mental defense mechanisms, and the psychoanalytic classification of mental illness.

Human behavior is driven from early infancy on by the operation of basic instincts. Freud believed that the primitive and evolving physical needs of humans stimulate instinctual drives. He said instincts possess four essential characteristics: source, impetus, aim, and object. Instincts arise from a particular bodily area, generate varying amounts of energy, aim for gratification, and are directed at particular objects, such as other people. Libido, one of these instincts, drives humans to seek pleasure and provides gratification during all the several stages of human development, beginning with the infant sucking at the mother's breast. Later in his work, Freud expressed his belief that humans possess an aggressive instinct, which appears to be aimed at the destruction of the self and others. His formulation of dual and dueling instincts, as with much of his work, continues to evoke controversy in psychoanalytic circles.

Freud believed that the libido instinct is expressed early in life and continues to be expressed during several stages as a prelude to mature psychosexual development. Infants first experience the oral stage, which centers on feeding. Libido is gratified during the act of nursing, and success experienced at this stage helps the infant develop a sense of trust and self-reliance. Older infants proceed to the anal stage, centering on the retention and expulsion of feces and urine. Successful experience during the anal stage equips children with what they need to develop personal autonomy, independence, guiltless initiative, self-assurance, and willingness to cooperate. Children then move to the phallic stage, finding a new interest in genitalia. Freud's theories about this stage are controversial, and many have been repudiated. He said that the penis holds the interest of both sexes, but girls form an early sense of inadequacy when they see that they do not have one (penis envy). Early sexual feelings are directed, according to Freud, toward the parent of the opposite sex (Oedipus complex). Parents regard these feelings as unacceptable and send signals to the children, who must repress their sexual urges. Boys act out of fear of castration, while girls act out of fear of loss of parental love and of envy of the boy's penis. Children who successfully negotiate this stage are said to have developed a firm basis for sexual identity, uninhibited curiosity, a sense of mastery, and the formation of conscience. Next comes the latency period, from ages five to thirteen, during which previous attainments are integrated and consolidated. Key elements of adaptive behavior develop during this stage. The teenage years are said to be spent in the genital stage, during which the child separates gradually from dependence on parents and begins to attach to new love objects and more mature interests. This stage culminates successfully in a sense of personal identity and acceptance.

Through Freud's study of and work with hysteria, a condition in which emotional conflicts are transformed into bodily maladies, he became convinced that the human mind contains dynamic forces that often oppose one another. For example, a person who experiences significant trauma in early childhood, and the painful emotions that attend it, can mentally oppose or repress memories of the trauma and the traumatic emotions. The repressed memories and emotions remain embedded in the unconscious regions of the mind until they are revived and re-experienced when stimulated by a later event. Thus, the force of emotional material that was repressed but never forgotten can exceed the force used by the conscious mind to hold the memories at bay. The concepts of repression and the needful recognition of repressed material continue to be important principles guiding psychoanalysis.

Freud conceived of the human mind, or psyche, as having three parts: id, ego, and superego. The basic instincts and repressed Oedipal urges of human beings reside in the id. Freud saw the id as a totally undifferentiated mass of energy, constantly seeking gratification without the constraints of reality or morality. In contrast, he saw the ego as being well organized, governed by an accurate perception of the external environment, and honoring certain principles of socially acceptable behavior. The ego seeks to form gratifying relationships with other people. At the same time, the ego must defend itself against the primitive urges of the id. The superego is the last division of the mind to form, which it does through successful resolution of the Oedipus conflict. It forms what is called the conscience and imposes control through guilt. The superego often operates during dreams, Freud said, sending warnings when the ego fails to defend properly against id impulses. Most work of the id and the superego is carried out unconsciously, while much of the ego's work operates at the conscious level.

After Freud had seen his theories confirmed in his clinical and personal experience, he felt comfortable in setting out his thoughts on psychopathology. Among the disorders that he identified were various types of neuroses, phobias, perversions, character disorders, personality disorders, psychoses, hypochondriasis, depressive states, and schizophrenia. He believed that mental illness is caused mainly by intrapsychic conflicts that are poorly managed by the mind or by abnormal mental processes and structures.

INDICATIONS AND PROCEDURES

In relation to medical science and, more specifically, to psychiatry, psychoanalysis is used to diagnose and treat emotional illness.

In diagnosis, psychoanalysts have purposes that differ considerably from those of general psychiatry. The analyst uses diagnosis to determine the patient's potential for analysis, the usefulness of analysis in treating the particular emotional problem experienced by the patient, the patient's level of incapacity, the likelihood that the patient will improve, and the likelihood that the analyst will be able to understand and help the patient. Other mental health specialists typically compare the signs and symptoms demonstrated or described by the patient to those cataloged in the American Psychiatric Association's *Diagnostic and Statistical Manual of Mental Disorders: DSM-5* (5th ed., 2013) and assign a diagnosis that best fits the patient. The psychoanalytic approach to diagnosis, conversely, is based on what the analyst can learn about the patient's inner experiences, especially unconscious conflicts and fantasies.

Psychoanalysis is considered to be the treatment of choice for younger adults suffering from chronic emotional illness not helped by less intensive therapies. People who suffer from hysteria, obsessive-compulsive neuroses, sexual perversions, and certain personality disorders are seen as the best candidates for psychoanalysis. To be considered for psychoanalysis, patients must demonstrate an ability to develop a reasonably good relationship with an analyst and must be willing and able to withstand a long, intensive course of treatment. Psychoanalysis is also expensive, and patients must be able to pay for treatment. Some, but not all, third-party payers will bear part of the cost of psychoanalysis; unfortunately, third-party review of the case compromises analyst-patient confidentiality. Patients who are psychotic or who are alcoholics or drug addicts are considered poor candidates for psychoanalysis. Older adults may have personalities too rigid to tolerate analysis, and others have an illness too minor to justify such treatment. Patients who are chronically and deeply depressed may be unsuitable candidates for analysis, as are those who have failed to establish appropriate relationships with both parents. Patients must be deemed able not only to enter analysis but also to tolerate termination of therapy. Patients who need urgent intervention to preserve health and life are not good candidates for analysis; neither are those who have little opportunity to make changes in their lives. Because many factors enter into consideration, analysts give some patients a trial period of analysis before accepting them for treatment.

When a patient enters into psychoanalysis, the patient and analyst must resolve certain practical issues, such as setting up appointment times, payment schedules, and other policy matters. The patient must be willing to spend an hour a day, four or five days a week, for as long as five years to complete analysis.

The analyst and patient must be able to form a therapeutic relationship secure enough to withstand the test of time and the stress of treatment. Early on, the patient and analyst must endure as the patient anxiously defends the ego and resists plunging into deeper emotional material. Eventually, so-called transferenceneurosis emerges. Patients re-experience and often project onto the analyst infantile desires and conflicts. The process of returning to more primitive emotional states is called regression, and analysts must be skillful in helping the patient to avoid its inherent dangers.

Free association is used to deepen the regression. The analyst instructs the patient to talk freely about issues of current concern and to continue talking about whatever associations come into the patient's awareness, making no effort to censor or restrain the monologue. Despite a patient's apparent willingness to follow the analyst's direction, the patient's resistance to uncovering certain material begins to be demonstrated with silences, pauses, stammers, corrections, slips of the tongue, and so on. The analyst remains alert to these signals of resistance, as the shape of the resistance shows the nature of the neurosis. The analyst gives interpretations of the resistance and related unconscious material; for progress to be made, the interpretation must be accurate, and the patient must accept and make use of it. The patient must work through painful emotional conflicts and find ways to resolve them more satisfactorily. "Working through" consumes much of the time spent in analysis.

The analyst often employs several psychological maneuvers to help patients during analysis. The analyst might offer suggestions, in an effort to induce a mental state that opposes the patient's experiences, expectations, or concept of reality. For example, the analyst may assure the patient that working through repressed emotions will enable the patient to enjoy a more productive life. The analyst may manipulate the patient to facilitate recovery of or to neutralize early unconscious material. The analyst can help the patient by clarifying material that the patient may know only in a semiconscious, disorganized way. The term "countertransference" describes the variety of responses felt by the analyst toward the patient; the analyst must resolve such feelings satisfactorily in order to continue the analytic process.

Dreams are said to be the "royal road to the unconscious," and the analyst will often encourage the patient to recall dreams experienced the preceding night. Dreams not only process waking experiences but often offer clues as to unconscious reactions, wishes, and conflicts as well. The analyst offers interpretations of the dreams in order to bring unconscious material and patterns to the conscious awareness of the patient.

The couch on which the patient reclines during sessions is a trademark of psychoanalysis; it is used rarely in any other form of psychotherapy. The analyst typically is positioned outside the visual range of the patient. This arrangement is considered to be essential in encouraging regression and projection.

As the patient and analyst struggle together to help the patient bring repressed material into awareness, the patient may achieve greater self-understanding and increased ability to find more satisfactory resolutions to emotional conflicts.

The analyst begins to prepare the patient for termination as the active phase of the analysis comes to a close. Patients must be weaned well from dependence on the analyst and the analytic situation. While the patient may have relived and worked through many primitive wishes and conflicts, the continuing work of resolving conflicts as they arise rests primarily with the patient's ability to work through them independently.

The outcome of psychoanalysis can be difficult to evaluate, but success has been defined as having helped a patient improve adjustment to life, realize a certain amount of contentment, give happiness to others, deal more confidently with inevitable stresses, and maintain mutually satisfying relationships with others. In addition, the patient should experience a reduction in neurotic suffering and inhibitions, have fewer dependency needs, have increased potential for success in all significant areas of life, and function at a more mature level.

PERSPECTIVE AND PROSPECTS

Psychoanalysis was born in the wake of evidence that hysteria can be caused by repressed memories or unconscious wishes. People who suffer from hysteria, now known as conversion disorder (functional neurological symptom disorder), develop physical symptoms such as paralysis or blindness in an otherwise healthy body. Sigmund Freud was influenced by the work of French neurologist Jean-Martin Charcot (1825-1893) and fellow Viennese physician Josef Breuer (1842-1925), both of whom were trying to find effective treatments for hysteria. Charcot relied on the use of hypnosis, while Breuer allowed patients to empty their minds, in an early version of free association. In 1895, Breuer and Freud published accounts of their theories and successful cures of patients suffering from hysteria. Freud also was influenced by the work of others on the hierarchy of the nervous system, philosophical concepts of the unconscious mind, posthypnotic suggestion, and the organization of the brain. He was a prolific author and teacher who fostered the careers of several followers.

Many of those who learned from and were influenced by Freud later developed their own variations or new areas of emphasis within Freudian psychoanalysis. Closer study of the role of the ego in emotional disorders led to the development of ego psychology, which enhanced the understanding of the defense, coping, and adaptive mechanisms of the ego. Others chose to emphasize the role of parents and other significant early childhood caregivers in the subsequent development of emotional health and illness. Still others developed what is known as self-psychology, a variant which emphasizes the importance of a person's cohesive sense of self and emotional well-being; the sense of self is either fostered or hindered by interpersonal relationships formed throughout life. Other variants that draw on the psychoanalytical principle include psychodynamic, insight-oriented, relationship, and supportive psychotherapies. Marital, group, and family therapy also depend heavily on an understanding and application of psychoanalytical theory. Generally speaking, most psychotherapeutic interventions used today are grounded in the psychoanalytic precepts developed by Freud and refined by students of his work.

Classical psychoanalysis is still practiced in the United States, but its use is limited by the relatively few properly trained analysts, the time and expense involved in the treatment process, the lack of widely accepted proof of its superiority as a treatment method, and the demand for brief intervention by patients of psychotherapy and those who pay for it. Modern practitioners of psychoanalysis are concerned by several trends: the ascendence of biological approaches to understanding and treating mental illness, the unwillingness of insurers to pay for psychoanalysis, the growing number of nonphysician analysts, the growing skepticism about its effectiveness, and the establishment of a universal system of psychiatric diagnosis that largely ignores the psychoanalytic perspective.

—*Russell Williams, MSW*

See also Brain; Depression; Emotions, biomedical causes and effects; Hypochondriasis; Neurosis; Obsessive-compulsive disorder; Phobias; Psychiatric disorders; Psychiatry; Psychiatry, child and adolescent; Psychiatry, geriatric; Psychosis; Schizophrenia; Sibling rivalry.

For Further Information:

American Psychiatric Association. *Diagnostic and Statistical Manual of Mental Disorders: DSM-5.* 5th ed. Arlington, Va.: Author, 2013.

American Psychiatric Association Commission on Psychiatric Therapies. *The Psychiatric Therapies.* Washington, DC: Author, 1984.

American Psychoanalytic Association. "About Psychoanalysis." *American Psychoanalytic Association,* 2009-2013.

Clark, Ronald. *Freud: the Man and the Cause.* London: Paladin Grafton Books, 1987.

Gay, Peter. *Freud: A Life for Our Time.* London: Little, 2006.

Milton, Jane., Caroline Polmear, and Julia Fabricius. *A Short Introduction to Psychoanalysis.* Los Angeles: SAGE, 2011.

Mishne, Judith Marks. *The Evolution and Application of Clinical Theory: Perspective from Four Psychologies.* New York: Free Press, 1993.

Sadock, Benjamin J., and Virginia A. Sadock, eds. *Kaplan and Sadock's Comprehensive Textbook of Psychiatry.* 9th ed. Philadelphia: Wolters Kluwer Health/Lippincott Williams & Wilkins, 2009.

Stern, Daniel N. *Interpersonal World of the Infant: A View from Psychoanalysis and Development Psychology.* London; New York: American Psychoanalytic Association, 2008.

Psychosis

Category: Disease/Disorder
Anatomy or system affected: Psychic-emotional system
Specialties and related fields: Psychiatry
Definition: The most severe mental disorder, in which the individual loses contact with reality and suffers from such symptoms as delusions and hallucinations.

CAUSES AND SYMPTOMS

The individual with a psychosis displays disordered thinking, emotion, and behavior. The individual fails to make sense of his or her surroundings, reacts inaccurately to them, and develops false thoughts or ideas about them. The resulting behavior can be described as peculiar, abnormal, or bizarre. Psychosis runs in families and most often first appears in late adolescence or early adulthood. There are some psychoses with medical and physical causes and some for which the cause is unknown. The treatment of psychoses involves removing or correcting the causes of the psychoses when possible. Psychosis describes a group of symptoms that can be part of several formal psychiatric diagnoses that include schizophrenia. Psychotic symptoms are characterized by delusions, hallucinations, disturbances of movement, and/or speech disturbances.

Delusions are false beliefs that are held despite strong evidence to the contrary. An example of an extreme delusion might be a man's belief that someone has planted a radio transmitter in his brain that sends signals to creatures on Mars. Hallucinations are false sense perceptions that, like delusions, are held despite strong evidence to the contrary. Hallucinations can involve any of the five senses. Examples of extreme hallucinations include feeling as if one is covered by ants, seeing green cows walking through the wall, hearing voices that do not exist, and smelling a constant odor when none exists.

Disturbances of movement can occur with psychoses. For example, a woman may become very exaggerated in her movements or, conversely, may become motionless for periods of time. These disturbances of movement are clearly bizarre and unnatural. Finally, speech disturbances are very common in psychoses. A man might speak in a way that is not understandable to others. He may carry on a conversation in which he believes that he is communicating normally but without making sense to others. Alternatively, speech might be clear but the individual shifts from one unrelated idea to another without being aware of doing so. Another psychotic symptom is severe emotional turmoil described as intense shifting moods with accompanying feelings of being confused.

Approximately 2 percent of all people will develop a psychosis sometime during their life. Although psychoses typically first appear in late adolescence or early adulthood, they may begin in middle to late life as well. The symptoms are apparently equally common in males and females. Because there is a strong family pattern to psychoses, some have suggested a genetic predisposition, and such evidence has been found. Environmental factors, however, such as home environment, parenting, and traumatic life events, may also play a role in some psychoses.

TREATMENT AND THERAPY

Psychoses are often categorized as organic or functional, which provides a way to communicate the cause of a psychosis and thereby the appropriate treatment. Organic psychoses are attributable to disturbances in the brain. These psychoses can be attributed directly to a problem in the structure, functioning, or chemistry of the brain. Various physical conditions and abnormalities can lead to psychosis, including thyroid disorders, drug reactions, infections, epilepsy, tumors, and circulatory disorders (for example, strokes). The treatment of organic psychoses involves removing or correcting the causes of the psychoses. In the case of a psychosis caused by a disorder of the thyroid gland, the individual might be prescribed medications to correct the thyroid problem or have the gland surgically removed. Certain prescription and illegal drugs can cause a psychosis; these include cocaine, alcohol, heart medications, and pain medications. In these situations, the psychotic symptoms are often eliminated when the medication or drug is discontinued. Organic psychoses may be the result of deteriorating physical conditions, such as Alzheimer's disease. Such a psychosis is typically nonreversible and is treated with tranquilizing medications to decrease the individual's discomfort and disruptive behaviors.

Functional psychoses are those psychoses for which no organic causes can be found. Often the psychotic symptoms are part of a more traditional psychiatric condition such as schizophrenia or depression. The mainstay of the treatment of functional psychoses is medication therapy. As with the organic psychoses in deteriorating physical conditions, tranquilizers are the most appropriate first-line treatment for psychotic symptoms. The goal of therapy is to decrease the frequency and disruption of psychotic thoughts and behaviors.

Individual, group, and family psychotherapy are also a major part of treating individuals with functional psychosis or organic psychosis in deteriorating physical conditions. These therapies help to ensure compliance with the medication therapy, decrease the tendency for relapse, and can even lead to the reduction in the amount of medication required to relieve the individual's symptoms. The goal of psychotherapy is to help the individual maintain functioning.

Occasionally, the patient with a psychosis may require inpatient hospitalization. The experience of hallucinations or delusions can be particularly distressing and can lead to a severe depression. Furthermore,

---

INFORMATION ON PSYCHOSIS

Causes: May include brain disturbances resulting from thyroid disorders, negative drug reactions, infections, epilepsy, tumors, and circulatory disorders (e.g., strokes); certain prescription and illegal drugs

Symptoms: Delusions, hallucinations, disconnection from reality, speech and movement disturbances

Duration: Acute to chronic

Treatments: Medication; individual, group, and family psychotherapy; hospitalization

---

these hallucinations and delusions might be of a homicidal or suicidal nature. While hospitalization is not required in treating individuals with psychosis, when individuals become a danger to themselves or to others, a brief inpatient hospitalization may be required to stabilize the patients and return them to a higher state of functioning. During hospitalization, patients are treated with medication therapy along with individual, group, or family therapy until they can be safely returned to their environments. Occasionally, patients with psychoses have multiple episodes during their lives, requiring numerous inpatient hospitalizations. In May 2013, Georgia Health Sciences University in Augusta, Georgia, published a study linking urinary tract infections (UTIs) in patients with psychosis. According to the study, which was presented at the American Psychiatric Association's 2013 Annual Meeting, prevelance of UTIs was higher in patients with a history of psychosis.

—Oliver Oyama, PhD

See also Addiction; Alcoholism; Delusions; Dementias; Depression; Domestic violence; Hallucinations; Intoxication; Neurosis; Paranoia; Prader-Willi syndrome; Prescription drug abuse; Psychiatric disorders; Psychiatry; Psychiatry, child and adolescent; Psychiatry, geriatric; Schizophrenia; Side effects; Substance abuse; Suicide.

For Further Information:
American Psychiatric Association. *Diagnostic and Statistical Manual of Mental Disorders: DSM-IV-TR*. 4th ed. Arlington, Va.: Author, 2000.
Barlow, David H., ed. *Clinical Handbook of Psychological Disorders*. 4th ed. New York: Guilford Press, 2008.
Bloom, Floyd E., M. Flint Beal, and David J. Kupfer, eds. *The Dana Guide to Brain Health*. New York: Dana Press, 2006.
Kring, Ann M., et al. *Abnormal Psychology*. 11th ed. Hoboken, N.J.: John Wiley & Sons, 2010.
Moskowitz, Andrew. Â *Psychosis, Trauma and Dissociation: Emerging Perspectives on Severe Psychopathology*. New York: Wiley, 2008. Print.
Torrey, E. Fuller. *Surviving Schizophrenia: A Manual for Families, Patients, and Providers*. 5th ed. New York: Collins, 2006.

Torrey, E. Fuller. Â *Surviving Schizophrenia: A Manual for Families, Patients, and Providers.* 5th ed. New York: Harper Perennial, 2006. Print.

PSYCHOSOMATIC DISORDERS

Category: Disease/Disorder
Anatomy or system affected: All
Specialties and related fields: Psychiatry, psychology
Definition: Physical disorder influenced by psychological stressors, or disorders characterized by symptoms that result from unconscious psychological factors instead of an underlying medical condition.

CAUSES AND SYMPTOMS

In the 1950s, the diagnosis of "psychosomatic disorders" was coined to refer to medical conditions for which there were no clear medical causes, but there was a subtle distinction between psychological processes and physical illness in its definition. The current understanding of medical illness has progressed, however, and health professionals now understand that psychological or sociological factors contribute to most medical illnesses. Thus, the diagnosis of psychosomatic disorders has undergone refinement and more specific diagnostic classification. The two related psychiatric diagnostic classifications are "psychological factors affecting medical condition" and "somatoform disorders."

Psychophysical disorders. The diagnosis of psychological factors affecting a medical condition (also occasionally referred to as psychophysiological disorders) describes any physical condition or disorder that is influenced by psychological factors. These psychological factors can range from true psychiatric disorders such as depression to emotional stressors in the person's environment such as the death of a loved one, anger toward a coworker, or the inability to cope with normal life changes. The more common environmental stressors can lead to the initiation or the exacerbation of physical conditions, including headache, ulcer, asthma, arthritis, acne, irritable bowel syndrome, diabetes mellitus, muscular disorders, and essential hypertension. In certain cases, such as headache, the stressor causes the onset of symptoms. In others, such as diabetes, the stressors might cause a worsening of already existing symptoms because of their influence on the person's attitude about the illness and the resultant quality of life, the willingness or the ability of the person to comply with treatment, or the person's capacity to understand the illness and its treatment. For example, in a situation in which a person is faced with the death of a loved one, it would not be unusual to see a corresponding increase in headache frequency or uncontrolled blood sugar levels in the diabetic.

Somatoform disorders. Somatoform disorders are the second diagnostic classification subsumed under the old psychosomatic disorders category. In somatoform disorder, a person displays symptoms that suggest a physical disorder, but no medical evidence exists for such a disorder. In these cases, it is believed that the person possesses psychological stresses, conflicts, or needs that manifest themselves in physical symptoms. The distinction between somatoform and psychophysiological disorders is that in psychophysiological disorders the person has an identified physical illness or disorder that is influenced by psychological stress. In somatoform disorders, there are only physical symptoms and no physical findings or known mechanisms to diagnose any physical illness or disorder.

People with somatoform disorders are presumably unable to tolerate certain forms or intensity of emotional stresses, leading to an expression of their emotional distress through physical symptoms. These disorders typically afflict people in their adolescence or young adult years and cause considerable disruption in life. The symptoms or focus on physical attributes are not intentionally produced or controlled. They are, at the time, outside the person's capacity to control them. There is no known cause for these disorders, and because they occasionally run in families, some have speculated that environment or genetics may play a role.

An example of a somatoform disorder is conversion disorder. People with conversion disorder display an alteration or loss of physical functioning characterized most often as paralyses, seizures, coordination problems, or visual problems. No physical causes are found for these symptoms. Instead, psychiatric evaluation suggests that the symptoms serve a role in helping the person cope with some type of stress, conflict, or need. A person might become temporarily blind or paralyzed in the right arm as an unconscious way of dealing with an upcoming stressful situation, such as a marriage.

INFORMATION ON PSYCHOSOMATIC DISORDERS

Causes: Psychological stressors, genetic or environmental factors
Symptoms: Wide ranging; may include headaches, paralysis, seizures, coordination problems, visual disorders
Duration: Acute to chronic
Treatments: Psychiatric medications, physical and emotional relaxation skills, psychotherapy

Another somatoform disorder is somatization disorder. People with this disorder complain of unexplained symptoms for which no physical evidence exists. Such people believe that they have acquired a serious physical disorder and often seek out many health care providers to locate a cause for their symptoms. The disorders are often very disruptive to the person's life and quite costly in terms of medical expenses.

TREATMENT AND THERAPY
Treatment for psychophysiological disorders can include using psychiatric medications to manage intense depression or anxiety; educating the patient about the relationship between stressors and physical illness; challenging maladaptive health care beliefs or any unrealistic assumptions or expectations that the person might possess; teaching physical and emotional relaxation skills; developing and utilizing social support from others in the person's life; and instructing the patient in personal skills to manage better the event or situation causing the stress. These treatments can be very effective with psychophysiological disorders.

Treatment for somatoform disorders involves the use of individual, group, or family therapy to address the stresses, conflicts, or needs that are believed to be at the root of the problem. When patients identify the underlying problems, change their thoughts about these problems, and learn skills to deal more adaptively with them, their physical symptoms typically subside.

PERSPECTIVE AND PROSPECTS
The relationship between the mind and the body has intrigued humankind for centuries. Beliefs about the contribution of the mind in the functioning of the human body have had a mixed history. Scientists and clinicians currently appreciate the influence of psychological and social factors in physical illness and dysfunction, but this has not always been the case. Theories of personality and its influence on health and illness can be found in ancient writings as early as 400 BCE. In the late sixteenth and early seventeenth centuries, the view that psychological factors could influence physical illness lost favor as the medical profession began an era of strict scientific study of the body and bodily processes. During this era, an illness or treatment would be considered legitimate only if a scientific explanation could be found for the process. Because of the limits of scientific methodology at the time, many of the traditional beliefs of this mind-body link were abandoned. The mind and body were theoretically separated until the early twentieth century, which saw the introduction of the field of psychobiology and the scientific study of the influence of the mind on the body.

—Oliver Oyama, PhD

See also Antianxiety drugs; Anxiety; Depression; Factitious disorders; Hypochondriasis; Midlife crisis; Münchausen syndrome by proxy; Neurosis; Panic attacks; Phobias; Psychiatric disorders; Psychiatry; Psychiatry, child and adolescent; Psychiatry, geriatric; Psychoanalysis; Stress; Stress reduction.

For Further Information:
American Psychiatric Association. *Diagnostic and Statistical Manual of Mental Disorders: DSM-5*. 5th ed. Arlington, Va.: Author, 2013.
Asaad, Ghazi. *Psychosomatic Disorders: Theoretical and Clinical Aspects*. New York: Brunner/Mazel, 1996.
Asmundson, Gordon J. G., et al., eds. *Health Anxiety: Clinical and Research Perspectives on Hypochondriasis and Related Conditions*. New York: Wiley, 2001.
Gatchel, Robert J., and Edward B. Blanchard, eds. *Psychophysiological Disorders: Research and Clinical Applications*. Washington, DC: American Psychological Association, 1998.
Mate, Gabor, and T. Miller. *When the Body Says No: Understanding the Stress-Disease Connection*. New York: Wiley, 2003.
Phillips, Katherine A., ed. *Somatoform and Factitious Disorders*. Washington, DC: American Psychiatric Association, 2001.
Safer, Diane A., and Lukas Rimas. "Somatization Disorder." *Health Library*, Mar. 27, 2013.
Smith, G. Richard, Jr. *Somatization Disorder in the Medical Setting*. Rockville, Md.: Department of Health and Human Services, Public Health Service, Alcohol, Drug Abuse, and Mental Health Administration, National Institute of Mental Health, 1990.
"Somatoform Disorders." *FamilyDoctor.org*, Feb. 2010.
"Stress." *MedlinePlus*, May 22, 2013.

PTERYGIUM/PINGUECULA

Category: Disease/Disorder
Also known as: Surfer's eye
Anatomy or system affected: Eyes
Specialties and related fields: Ophthalmology, optometry
Definition: A thickening of conjunctiva of the eye that grows onto the cornea (pterygium) or degeneration of a portion of the conjunctiva (pinguecula).
Key terms:
conjunctiva: the clear, moist membrane that coats the inner surfaces of the eyelids and the outer surface of the eye
cornea: the clear front window of the eye that transmits light into the eye
sclera: the tough white outer covering over the eyeball that extends over most of its surface

CAUSES AND SYMPTOMS
When ultraviolet radiation from sunlight irradiates the conjunctiva, it can damage and kill conjunctival cells. Repeated sunlight exposure can sometimes produce small accumulations of dead and damaged

conjunctival cells combined with degraded matrices that appear as yellowish-white deposits that sometimes calcify. Such a deposit is called a pinguecula (plural, pingueculae). Alternatively, in response to continued conjunctival cell death, the cells divide to replace the dead cells. Repeated damage to the conjunctiva can hyperactivate this healing response and a nontumorous growth of conjunctival cells, called a pterygium, thickens the conjunctiva and eventually grows over the cornea. In some cases pingueculae precede pterygia.

Pterygium and pinguecula occur with increasing frequency in climates that approach the equator. Those who live in dry, dusty environments, fishermen, surfers, and farmers experience increased rates of pterygium and pinguecula. Some studies have found that smoking increases the rates of pterygium and alcohol consumption increases the rates of pinguecula. Although pterygium and pinguecula can arise in anyone, they are rarely seen in those younger than 20 years old. People over 40 show the highest prevalence of pterygium and pinguecula and those between the ages of 20-40 have the highest incidence.

TREATMENT AND THERAPY

In most cases, pterygium and pinguecula do not cause any symptoms and require no treatment. Pingueculae tend to grow slowly and may, in some cases, appear unsightly, in which cases they can be surgically removed. Pinguelculae can also cause some eye discomfort and in such cases over-the-counter artificial tear products (e.g., Refresh Tears, GenTeal) or lubricating ointments (e.g., Refresh P.M., Hypo Tears) can provide relief. Infrequently, pingueculae can become inflamed (pingueculitis), which are effectively treated with prednisone eye drops (Pred Fotre).

Pterygium often requires no treatment unless it overgrows the cornea and deforms or scars it. In such cases, the pterygium significantly affects patient's sight and surgical extirpation can potentially restore normal

Pterygium. Photo by Jmvaras José Miguel Varas, MD, via Wikimedia Commons.

> ### INFORMATION ON PTERYGIUM/PINGUECULA
>
> **Causes:** Ultraviolet radiation exposure causes the conjunctiva to degenerate (pinguelcula) or thicken and overgrow (pterygium)
> **Symptoms:** Redness, tearing, dry and itchy eyes, blurring of vision
> **Duration:** Usually arises around 20-40 years of age and remains for the rest of patient's life
> **Treatments:** Artificial tears and ointments, optical steroids, surgery

sight to the eye. Unfortunately, simple excision has a high rate regrowth of the pterygium (24-89 percent). To prevent regrowth, radiation therapy and chemical agents such as mitomycin C, 5-fluorouracil, and thiotepa have been applied to the eye prior to surgery. Secondly, the sclera is covered with either amniotic membrane or a small piece of conjunctiva cut from the patient's own eye (free conjuntival autograph). These modifications to pterygium surgery have greatly reduced the rate of recurrence of pterygium.

—*Michael A. Buratovich, PhD*

See also Ophthalmology; Optometry

For Further Information:
Hirst, Lawrence W. "Recurrence and Complications after 1000 Surgeries Using Pterygium Extended Removal Followed by Extended Conjunctival Transplant." *Ophthalmology* 119, no. 11 (November, 2012): 2205-2210.
Kee, Kenneth. *A Simple Guide to Conjunctivitis and Other Eye Diseases*. Seattle, WA: Amazon Digital Services, 2012.

PTOSIS

Category: Disease/Disorder
Also known as: Drooping eyelid
Anatomy or system affected: Eyes, muscles, nerves
Specialties and related fields: Family medicine, ophthalmology, optometry, plastic surgery
Definition: Drooping of the upper eyelid, partially or completely covering the eye.

CAUSES AND SYMPTOMS

Ptosis may be congenital or may be associated with other problems, including paralysis of motor and sensory nerve fibers to the eyelids, muscular dystrophy, diabetes, brain tumor, head or eyelid injuries, myasthenia gravis, or a tumor in the upper lobe of a lung. In young children, congenital ptosis is the result of malformation of the levator muscle, which lifts the eyelid, or of a defective nerve supply to the muscle. Congenital ptosis usually does not improve with time.

Symptoms include drooping of one or both eyelids, which may vary during different times of the day, as well as associated poor blinking reflexes.

TREATMENT AND THERAPY
Home treatment involves keeping the child's eye moist with artificial teardrops. Medical prescriptions are not necessary for ptosis, but they may be needed for underlying disorders. The typical treatment for childhood ptosis is surgery, which involves tightening the levator muscle. The surgeon must be very careful not to raise the eyelid so high that the eye cannot be closed, and also to make it match the other eyelid as closely as possible. In cases involving older children, some ophthalmologists may recommend keeping the affected eyelid raised with a support that is part of a pair of eyeglasses.

PERSPECTIVE AND PROSPECTS
Complications that can arise from ptosis include permanent disfigurement of the face, visual difficulties, and irritation and infection of the eye that is caused by poor blinking reflexes and continual contact between the eyelid and the surface of the eye. If the disorder is not corrected in younger children, it can lead to amblyopia (lazy eye). Since amblyopia persists throughout life if it is not treated early in childhood, ptosis can lead to permanently poor vision. Ophthalmic plastic and reconstructive surgeons who specialize in ptosis and conditions affecting the eyelids, the tear system, the bone cavity around the eye, and adjacent facial structures have made significant progress in the successful surgical correction of ptosis.

—*Alvin K. Benson, PhD*

See also Congenital disorders; Diabetes mellitus; Eye infections and disorders; Eyes; Muscular dystrophy; Myasthenia gravis; Optometry; Optometry, pediatric; Plastic surgery; Strabismus; Surgery, pediatric; Vision disorders.

For Further Information:
Boughton, Barbara. "Assessing and Correcting Ptosis." *EyeNet Magazine*. American Academy of Ophthalmology, Nov. 2007.
Buettner, Helmut, ed. *Mayo Clinic on Vision and Eye Health: Practical Answers on Glaucoma, Cataracts, Macular Degeneration, and Other Conditions*. Rochester, Minn.: Mayo Foundation for Medical Education and Research, 2002.
"Eyelid Disorders." *MedlinePlus*, May 28, 2013.
"The Eyes Have It: Other Common Symptoms and Signs " Ptosis." *ONE Network*. American Academy of Ophthalmology, 2013.
Fox, Sidney A. *Surgery of Ptosis*. Baltimore: Williams & Wilkins, 1980.
Miller, Stephen J. H. *Parsons' Diseases of the Eye*. 19th ed. New York: Elsevier, 2002.
"Ptosis " Eyelids that Droop." *American Society of Ophthalmic Plastic and Reconstructive Surgery*, 2005.
Riordan-Eva, Paul, et al. *Vaughan and Asbury's General Ophthalmology*. 18th ed. New York: McGraw-Hill Medical, 2011.
Sutton, Amy L., ed. *Eye Care Sourcebook: Basic Consumer Health Information About Eye Care and Eye Disorders*. 3d ed. Detroit, Mich.: Omnigraphics, 2008.
Tyers, A. G. *Ptosis and Its Management*. Boston: Butterworth-Heinemann, 2007.

PUBERTY AND ADOLESCENCE

Category: Biology
Anatomy or system affected: All
Specialties and related fields: Dermatology, endocrinology, family medicine, internal medicine, pediatrics, psychology
Definition: Puberty is the onset of the natural biochemical (hormonal) and physical changes that occur in children as they are transformed into sexually mature individuals; adolescence is the period of years during which these transformations take place.
Key terms:
estrogen: the chemical compound produced by the female ovaries that is involved in the regulation of menstrual periods and in the development of female sexual traits
gonadotropins: chemical compounds produced by the pituitary gland of the brain that cause the growth and maturation of the gonads
gonads: the reproductive organs; the ovaries in females and the testes (testicles) in males
hormones: chemical messengers that travel through the bloodstream to influence activity in various organs and tissues; examples include the gonadotropins estrogen and testosterone
ovaries: the female reproductive organs, which contain the ova (eggs); the ovaries are almond-shaped and are found in the lower pelvic area
pituitary gland: a small structure located near the base of the brain that produces the gonadotropins
testes: the male reproductive organs and the site of sperm production; also known as the testicles

testosterone: the male sex hormone produced by the testes and responsible for the male sexual traits; a small amount is also produced by the adrenal glands in females and is responsible for the growth of hair during adolescence in both sexes

CAUSES AND SYMPTOMS

Puberty is the process of physical changes that lead to sexual maturity. The process occurs over several years, usually between ten and fourteen for girls and twelve and sixteen for boys. Adolescence is a developmental period during which individuals undergo a series of biochemical, physical, psychological, and social changes that result in maturation as an independent adult. Adolescence begins with puberty and continues into the late teens or mid-twenties.

One of the most dramatic physical changes that occurs in puberty is a tremendous growth spurt. The rate of height increase per year doubles compared with height gain prior to puberty. On the average, girls gain approximately 3 inches of height during this period, and boys grow by about 8 inches. The bulk of this growth is accounted for by an elongation of the thigh bones, followed by growth in the trunk. During this time, the thighs become wider, and shoulder width also increases. Both sexes accumulate fat during early puberty. Boys frequently appear chubby early in adolescence, but they generally lose this excess fat during their growth spurt. Most of this accumulated fat in girls is redistributed on their bodies and results in the adult female shape. The average girl gains approximately 25 pounds during the adolescent period, while boys gain about 40 pounds, most of which is in the form of muscle.

Additional physical changes that occur during adolescence include changes in the facial bones, especially an elongation of the jawbone. Muscle size and strength increase during puberty, with a boy's development in this area extending years past the end of muscle strength increase in the typical girl. Each of the major organs of the body, including the digestive tract, liver, kidneys, and heart, increases in size for both sexes during puberty. The size and activity of various glands adjust to reflect their increasing or decreasing role in the maturing individual.

Both girls and boys experience a characteristic increase in the distribution of body hair. Axillary (armpit) hair and pubic hair increase in density and coarseness, gradually achieving adult patterns. Boys also develop facial hair, beginning with a fine fuzz on the upper lip and eventually progressing into a full beard. Sweat glands increase in size as well. Boys undergo an increase in the size of the larynx (voice box), and this change leads to the normal "cracking" of the adolescent male's voice.

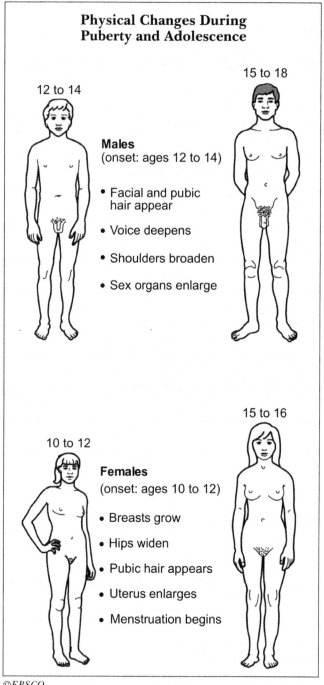

Physical Changes During Puberty and Adolescence

12 to 14

15 to 18

Males
(onset: ages 12 to 14)

- Facial and pubic hair appear
- Voice deepens
- Shoulders broaden
- Sex organs enlarge

10 to 12

15 to 16

Females
(onset: ages 10 to 12)

- Breasts grow
- Hips widen
- Pubic hair appears
- Uterus enlarges
- Menstruation begins

©EBSCO

The reproductive systems of boys and girls mature significantly during puberty. In girls, the vagina enlarges and undergoes changes in chemical composition and cellular structure, and it begins producing typical adult secretions. Menarche, the first menstrual period, takes place even though ovulation (the maturation and release of an egg by the ovaries) may not occur for many months. The ovaries increase in size, and chemical changes prepare them to ovulate on a monthly basis. Breasts develop from the preadolescent form to that of adult women. In boys, the penis grows and testicles enlarge, undergoing biochemical changes that prepare them for the continuous process of sperm production.

Because of the complexity of the many physical changes that occur during puberty, as well as the wide variation in the normal age of onset of this period, physicians have adopted a "sexual maturity rating" system to aid in the assessment of normal adolescent development. For both sexes, a staging of 1 (prepuberty) to 5 (postpuberty) is used to determine progress in puberty based on pubic hair thickness and distribution and enlargement of the breasts (for girls) and penis and testes (for boys).

All these physical changes are the direct result of global biochemical changes occurring in the adolescent's body. Just prior to puberty, a hormone called "luteinizing hormone-releasing factor" (LHRF) is produced the hypothalamus, a brain region responsible for regulating growth and other critical bodily functions. The LHRF travels to another structure in the brain, the pituitary gland. Upon receiving this hormonal signal, the pituitary gland produces two additional hormones called "gonadotropins." The gonadotropins stimulate the development and enlargement of the ovaries in girls and the testicles in boys. As a result of the stimulation of the gonadotropins, the gonads produce sex hormones; the ovaries produce estrogen, and the testes produce testosterone. Females also produce a small amount of testosterone in the adrenal glands, which are located above the kidneys. These sex hormones enter the bloodstream and signal the start of the physical changes associated with puberty.

Examples of the effects of these hormones include the development of axillary hair in both boys and girls, which is initiated and maintained by testosterone. Breast development in girls is triggered by the estrogen produced by the ovaries. Maturation of the larynx in boys is accomplished by the action of testosterone. The other physical changes noted above are the result of sex hormones working alone or in concert with each other and of hormonal action on the genetic information of the individual.

Adolescence is a period of rapid neurodevelopment, which continues into the mid-twenties. The brain regions responsible for reward-seeking typically develop earlier than regions that facilitate self-inhibition. This imbalance creates conditions for exploration, necessary for learning and developing into an adult, but also predisposes adolescents to risky behavior such as substance use, unsafe driving, or unsafe sexual behaviors. Youth often explore their identity, separating themselves from their parents, which may lead to rebellious behavior. Cognitive skills mature during this period, with an increased interest in abstract concepts, such as analyzing the rules and values of families,

friends, and society. Coming to terms with the rapid physical and psychological changes, changing perceptions of their role in the world, and the beginnings of adult responsibility, can create problems with self-esteem, anxiety, and depression.

An important task of adolescence is exploring and understanding sexuality. Sexual development in adolescence is influenced by biological, psychological, and social factors, as well as political, legal, cultural, spiritual, and moral contexts. Biological factors, such as hormonal changes and associated physical changes, influence adolescent interest in sexual relationships. Psychological factors, such as an extroverted versus introverted temperament, shape how youth approach intimate relationships. Numerous social factors further shape adolescents' thoughts and attitudes about sex, including peer relationships, parent attitudes and rules, religious inclinations, and cultural messages about sex. During this time adolescents explore different ways of expressing love and intimacy, developing patterns they often carry into adulthood. Youth often explore their gender identity and sexual orientation throughout adolescence. Many youth question their sexual orientation in various ways, considering how they find themselves physically or emotionally attracted to same-gender or opposite-gender individuals, before usually eventually identifying as straight, gay, bisexual, or questioning. In recent decades adolescents increasingly acquire information about sexuality from the internet, shaping their perceptions and attitudes. Adolescents who have sex at younger ages and with more partners are at higher risk of acquiring sexually transmitted infections (STIs). Many adolescents do not receive accurate information about sexuality from school or their parents, leaving many adolescents inadequately equipped to explore their sexual orientation and gender identity, understand the boundaries of healthy relationships, consent for sexual activity, and protect themselves against unintended pregnancy, STIs, and sexual violence.

COMPLICATIONS AND DISORDERS
A number of health and mental health problems can emerge during adolescence.

If the onset of puberty is not evident by age thirteen in girls or age fourteen in boys, or if puberty is initiated but little progression is observed for six to twelve months, detailed medical evaluation is recommended. Evaluation typically includes an interview, physical examination, and blood tests to measure hormone levels and determine the underlying reason for the delay in puberty.

A permanent deficiency in the amount of gonadotropic hormones produced by the pituitary gland prevents the sex organs from maturing and producing the sex hormones estrogen (in girls) and testosterone (in boys). This syndrome is referred to as hypogonadotropic hypogonadism and can be caused by a variety of central nervous system abnormalities. Congenital defects (abnormalities present at birth) in the pituitary gland can inhibit the production of gonadotropins. Likewise, tumors at certain positions in the brain, including the pituitary gland, may block hormone production. Deficiency in another hormone, human growth hormone (HGH), results in short stature and delayed puberty. Other conditions, such as genetic abnormalities, chronic disease, pathologies of the thyroid gland, malnutrition, and excessive exercise, can cause delayed puberty.

Delayed puberty can also be caused by failure of the ovaries or testes to mature despite normal levels of gonadotropins produced by the brain. In the vast majority of cases, the root cause of this syndrome—primary hypogonadism—is linked by genetic abnormalities. Usually, it is caused by the presence of abnormal sex chromosomes and is diagnosed by examination of the chromosomes by a procedure called "karyotyping."

A third category of delayed puberty is termed "constitutional delay in puberty." While nearing the end of the typical puberty age period, an individual's stature may be short, with delayed menarche in girls, and limited sexual development. In most cases, these individuals are merely beginning puberty later than peers and will eventually, without medical intervention, proceed through normal growth and development. Patience and close observation are the best course of action in cases of constitutional delay in puberty.

 is puberty with an early onset because of physical or biochemical abnormalities. Precocious puberty is rare, occurring in about one in every five to ten thousand children, most commonly in girls. In these cases, there is usually a defect in one or more of the glands producing the hormones that initiate puberty. Skilled medical diagnosis is indicated in these cases. When puberty begins much earlier than expected, the physician will check for a number of potentially serious problems such as adrenal gland disorders, reproductive system cysts, nervous system disorders, and thyroid abnormalities. Early pubertal onset is considered to be prior to eight and one-half years in girls or nine and one-half years in boys.

Acne, pimples, and blackheads, commonly appear on the skin of the face and upper back during adolescence. This skin disorder is a byproduct of puberty hormones stimulating the production of oil in the glands of the face and back. Acne may be treated with over-the-counter remedies and frequent washing of the skin, and it usually diminishes by young adulthood. In severe cases prescription medications are rec-

ommended to help improve appearance and prevent complications such as infection and scarring.

Psychological factors, such as low self-esteem, perfectionism, and feeling a lack of control, connected with the upheavals experienced during adolescence, in combination with genetic factors, can result in eating disorders. Anorexia nervosa is a syndrome characterized by extremely low food intake, preoccupation with losing weight, maintaining a weight that is more than 15 percent below a normal level for age and height, distorted perception of one's weight (e.g., seeing oneself as obese when one is pathologically thin), and (in girls) skipping three or more sequential menstrual periods. Anorexia is a life-threatening condition with a high fatality rate if not treated. People with anorexia may require hospitalization for medical stabilization to prevent complications such as heart failure, kidney failure, gastrointestinal problems, and brain atrophy. Treatment typically involves a team approach involving a pediatrician, nutritionist, psychiatrist, and other mental health professionals working with the adolescent and their family over several months or years to maintain a healthy weight, develop healthy eating behaviors, and reduce eating and weight-related distress.

Bulimia nervosa is characterized by "binge-purge" cycles of rapid, uncontrolled eating followed by compensatory behaviors, such as self-induced vomiting, the use of laxatives or diuretics, extreme exercise, and restrictive dieting. For a diagnosis of bulimia, episodes must occur at least twice a week for three months. In contrast to anorexia, people with bulimia usually have a normal or above-average weight. Bingeing and purging usually occur in private, delaying detection of the eating disorder. Severe medical consequences of bulimia can include cardiac arrest, rupture of the esophagus (the tube that runs from the mouth to the stomach), erosion of tooth enamel, and severe dehydration. As with anorexia, medical and mental health treatments are effective and important for reducing distress and restoring healthy behavior.

An adolescent may experience physical "growing pains" during rapid growth periods. Sharp pains, especially in the legs, may sometimes disrupt sleep. This discomfort is best treated with massage or a mild over-the-counter pain reliever. Adolescent girls commonly experience cramping during menstrual periods. In most cases, over-the-counter medications provide relief, but in severe cases, or when pain is associated with heavy menstrual flow, a physician's intervention is recommended.

Depression, a disorder of persistent low mood, pessimism about the present and the future, loss of interest in previously enjoyable activities, low motivation, impaired concentration, and disrupted sleep, concentration, and appetite, is common, affecting roughly 5 percent of older adolescents per year, but is often underrecognized. Depression results from the interplay between genetic risk and life stressors, such as illness or injury, school stress, financial strain, and/or problems with peers or family relationships. If depressive symptoms persist for an extended period (e.g., more than two weeks), treatment with medication or psychotherapy is often recommended. Untreated depression can result in academic and employment difficulties, drug or alcohol use, disruptive behavior, physical health problems, and suicide attempts. Any indication that a teenager is considering suicide must be taken seriously and promptly evaluated by a medical professional

PERSPECTIVE AND PROSPECTS

Extensive historical evidence dating back as far as the time of Aristotle (384-322 BCE) suggests that puberty is occurring earlier in modern times than in prior recorded history. Many factors are responsible for the earlier onset of adolescence in Western societies, including improved nutrition and elevated economic status. Improved public health—in terms of immunizations to prevent and treatment to cure childhood diseases—likewise contributes to the improved health of the individual and onset of puberty at an earlier age. Modern society, however, creates stresses that in some cases delay the age of pubertal onset.

In cases of delayed puberty attributable to deficiencies in gonadotropin production or a failure of the gonads to mature despite adequate levels of gonadotropins, medical intervention can compensate for the resulting physical immaturity. Boys can be given increasing doses of testosterone over a period of time, which will lead to the development of the external physical traits characteristic of puberty. Girls initially may be given oral doses of estrogen and then be given a combination of estrogen and another sex hormone, progesterone, as therapy progresses. These hormones lead to normal external pubertal development in most cases.

Some individuals with delayed puberty are deficient in HGH and also experience greatly shortened stature as compared with the normal range of heights for other individuals in their age group. Until the 1980s, HGH was isolated from cadavers, and its cost was prohibitively high for most people. With the revolution in recombinant deoxyribonucleic acid (DNA) technology, HGH is synthesized quite cheaply and is available to individuals who need it. Unfortunately, the accessibility of this drug creates the possibility of its abuse by some parents who want their normal children to be exceptionally large and strong.

In the latter third of the twentieth century, psychologists and other health professionals began to recognize

an increase in the rate of troublesome adolescent behavior, such as alcohol and drug use, high-risk sexual behavior, mood problems, and suicidal behaviors. Educators, health professionals, and concerned adults recognize these syndromes and address them through counseling, medication when indicated, outreach programs, and other efforts. As the medical and psychological communities gain further understanding of the physical, psychological, and social consequences of puberty, additional interventions will be developed to support adolescents as they grow and progress to adulthood.

—*Timothy Becker, MD*

See also: Abortion; Acne; Anorexia nervosa; Anxiety; Bulimia; Depression; Developmental stages; Eating disorders; Endocrine disorders; Endocrine glands; Endocrinology, pediatric; Growth; Gynecomastia; Hermaphroditism and pseudohermaphroditism; Hormones; Klinefelter syndrome; Masturbation; Menstruation; Obesity, childhood; Ovaries; Pituitary glands; Precocious puberty; Pregnancy and gestation; Psychiatry, child and adolescent; Reproductive system; Safety issues for children; Sexuality; Sexually transmitted diseases (STDs); Suicide; Tattoo removal; Tattoos and body piercing; Turner syndrome; Wisdom teeth.

For Further Information:
Adams, Gerald R., and Michael D. Berzonsky, editors. *Blackwell Handbook of Adolescence*. Blackwell, 2006. A professional guide to this topic in the Blackwell series of developmental psychology titles.
Center for Parent and Teen Communication, parentandteen.com.
Garrod, Andrew, et al. *Adolescent Portraits: Identity, Relationships, and Challenges*. 6th ed., Pearson/Allyn & Bacon, 2008. Stories written by teens survey myriad social issues that impact adolescents in the United States and illustrate theories of adolescent development. Topics include eating disorders, sexuality, family relationships, self-image, and dealing with illness.
Ginsburg, K. R., and M. M. Jablow. *Building Resilience in Children and Teens: Giving Kids Roots and Wings*. American Academy of Pediatrics, 2011, p. 398. An excellent collection of parenting and communication strategies to help adolescents develop healthy ways of coping with the stresses of growing up.
Greydanus, Donald E., editor. *Caring for Your Adolescent: Ages Twelve to Twenty-One*. Oxford UP, 1997. An excellent resource for those interested in the physical and psychological changes that occur during adolescence. Included are chapters on compassionate parenting as well as specifics on the diseases and challenges commonly encountered during this period.
Kimmel, Douglas C., and Irving B. Weiner. *Adolescence: A Developmental Transition*. 2nd ed., John Wiley & Sons, 1995. A text on adolescent psychology that addresses the changes that come with puberty. Includes a bibliography and indexes.
Kroger, Jane. *Identity Development: Adolescence Through Adulthood*. 2nd ed., Sage, 2007. Provides guidance on the many facets of development of self-image and personal identity through the teen years and beyond.

MGH Clay Center for Young Healthy Minds,
   www.mghclaycenter.org.
Santrock, John W. *Adolescence.* 13th ed., McGraw-Hill, 2010.
   A text that covers all aspects of adolescent development.
Steinberg, Laurence, and Ann Levine. *You and Your Adolescent: A Parent's Guide for Ages Ten to Twenty.* Rev. ed., HarperInformation, 1997. Designed as a parents' guide to children aged ten to twenty, this clearly written book covers the physical aspects of puberty as well as the social, psychological, and health issues confronting adolescents.

PUBLIC HEALTH. SEE OCCUPATIONAL HEALTH.

PULMONARY DISEASES

Category: Disease/Disorder
Anatomy or system affected: Chest, immune system, lungs, respiratory system
Specialties and related fields: Environmental health, epidemiology, immunology, occupational health, oncology, pulmonary medicine, virology
Definition: Diseases of the lungs, which may be serious or fatal; common pulmonary diseases include those caused by infection (bronchitis, pneumonia, tuberculosis), tobacco smoke (chronic obstructive lung disease, lung cancer), allergies (asthma), and other irritants (interstitial lung disease).

Key terms:
alveoli: the many tiny air sacs at the ends of the terminal bronchioles, where oxygen and carbon dioxide are exchanged
asthma: a condition in which spasms of the bronchial smooth muscle cause narrowing and constriction of the airways
bronchi: the branching airways from the single large trachea to the multiple terminal bronchioles
bronchoscopy: a procedure that uses a flexible or rigid fiber-optic telescope to visualize the bronchial tree directly; it also permits samples of tissue to be removed for analysis
cancer: a tumor (or growth) of abnormal, genetically transformed cells that invade and destroy normal tissue; also referred to as a malignancy
emphysema: progressive destruction of the alveolar walls, leading to highly inflated and stiffened lungs
interstitial pulmonary fibrosis (IPF): the scarring and thickening (fibrosis) of the lung tissue, which causes breathing difficulty, chest pain, coughing, and shortness of breath; the lungs become increasingly stiffer until heart failure ensues
pathology: the study of the nature and consequences of disease
parenchyma: the supporting tissues of the lung

pleurisy: the inflammation and swelling of the pleurae, the membranes that enclose the lungs and line the chest cavity; a complication of several pulmonary diseases
pneumonia: an inflammation of the lung tissue in which the alveolar sacs fill with fluid
pulmonary: the Latin word for lung, used to describe both the lung tissue and the bronchial tree
respiration: a process that includes both air conduction (the act of breathing) and gas exchange (oxygen and carbon dioxide transfer between the air and blood)

CAUSES AND SYMPTOMS

Disorders of the pulmonary system are among the most common diseases. Because it acts as an interface between the external and internal environments, the pulmonary system is subject to continual attacks on its health and integrity. A wide variety of disease-causing agents reach the lung with each breath. Infectious organisms (such as bacteria, viruses, and molds), environmental toxins (such as tobacco smoke and air pollutants), and various airborne allergens are among the primary causes of lung disease.

The pulmonary system consists of an intricate bronchial tree terminating in very delicate, thin-walled sacs known as "alveoli," each of which is surrounded by blood vessels. The entire network is contained within the supporting tissue of the lungs, the parenchyma. These individual parts are perfectly suited to efficiently carry out their two life-sustaining functions: air conduction and the gas exchange between oxygen in the air and carbon dioxide in the bloodstream. Oxygen is vital to many processes within the body, and a continuous supply of it is necessary for life. Carbon dioxide is a common waste product of various processes in the body, and can become toxic if levels build up in the body. Disruption of the exchange of oxygen and carbon dioxide renders a person vulnerable to potentially fatal consequences.

Pulmonary diseases can be categorized in two ways. The first is based on the cause, such as a virus, asbestos, or cigarette smoke; the second is based on the result, the specific loss of a structure and its function. Infectious diseases are the most common causes of respiratory problems. Infection usually occurs through inhalation, although it can come from another source within the body as well. A vast number of microorganisms are trapped by the hairs, mucus, and immune system cells that line the respiratory tract. Those that are not repelled generally infect the upper tract, namely the nose and throat, but it is the few that reach the bronchi and lungs that cause the most serious illnesses—bronchitis, pneumonia, and tuberculosis. Bronchitis, an inflammation of the bronchial tree, is the result of viruses or bacteria that invade the airways and infect the bronchial cells. In a counterattack, the body responds by sending large numbers of immune system cells (white blood cells), which destroy the invaders both by direct contact and by releasing chemical substances. The inflamed bronchi begin to leak significant amounts of fluids, producing the most obvious symptom of bronchitis: a frequent cough that yields initially clear white and later yellow or green phlegm. Rarely does bronchitis progress to serious disability; more often it resolves, although recurrence is common.

Unlike bronchitis, pneumonia is extremely serious. It can develop from bronchitis or can occur as a primary infection. Pneumonia is an infection that goes beyond the airways into the alveoli and supporting lung tissue. While the process of the disease is the same as that of bronchitis, fluid accumulates not only in the bronchi but also in the alveolar sacs, which cannot be efficiently cleared by coughing. The normally air-filled sacs, now filled with fluid, cannot perform their vital function of gas exchange. If the fluid continues to accumulate, larger and larger areas of lung become unable to function, and the person literally drowns.

In December 2019, a virus now known as the severe acute respiratory syndrome (SARS)-coronavirus-2 spread from animals to humans in Wuhan, China, causing a viral pneumonia which often led to severe acute respiratory distress syndrome. This virus quickly spread worldwide, leading to what is known as the COVID-19 pandemic, leading to the suffering and deaths of millions.

In the case of tuberculosis, one specific bacterium (*Mycobacterium tuberculus*) is inhaled, generally from the spray of coughs or sneezes of infected persons. The bacterium settles in the bronchus, where it begins to invade and multiply. Unlike the organisms that cause bronchitis and pneumonia, it passes through the airways into the parenchyma. The body reacts in an attempt to confine the organisms' spread by forming walled-off circular areas (cavities) around the destruction, called "granulomas." Up to this point, the person may have been only minimally ill. However, while the cavities are successful at containing the spread, some bacteria within them may not have been killed and remain dormant for many years. Later, when the person's immune system is weakened (by disease, stress, etc.), the bacteria "reawaken" and invade the lung, producing massive destruction and the loss of both structure and function. Left untreated, this results in death.

In ways different from infectious diseases, toxic substances such as tobacco smoke cause severe disability and death either through permanent structural damage (emphysema) or by transforming respiratory cells

---

INFORMATION ON PULMONARY DISEASES

Causes: May include infection, environmental toxins (especially tobacco smoke), allergies, cancer

Symptoms: Frequent coughing, chest pain, wheezing, shortness of breath

Duration: Acute to chronic

Treatments: May include antibiotics, epinephrine, methylxanthines, steroids, cromolyn sodium, mechanical ventilators, surgery, radiation therapy, chemotherapy

---

into abnormal ones (lung cancer). Many toxic chemicals are released when tobacco is burned, and these substances affect the entire lining of the respiratory tract both in the short term and in the long term. In the immediate period, the small hairs that line the upper tract no longer function to filter the air, and large amounts of fluid enter the airways because they are constantly inflamed, producing the familiar smokers' cough. As the irritation continues for years, permanent damage ensues. Marijuana smoking, as well as vaping tetrahydrocannabinol (THC), cause irritation and damage to the lungs similarly to tobacco smoke.

Chronic obstructive pulmonary disease (COPD) is a chronic condition often caused by long-term exposure to irritants to the respiratory tract, for example, smoking. Two main components of COPD are chronic bronchitis and emphysema. Chronic bronchitis is chronic inflammation of the bronchi or bronchioles, which causes constant cough with phlegm. Emphysema, which is present in nearly all smokers to some degree, is characterized by widespread destruction of the walls of individual alveolar sacs. As adjacent walls break, the alveoli coalesce into very large, balloon-like structures. The supporting lung tissue, which is normally soft and spongy, becomes stiff and hard, making breathing very difficult. Although the lungs become overinflated, the air is stale as it is unable to move in and out with each breath. The picture of a patient with severe emphysema is dramatic: the patient labors forcefully with an open mouth, trying unsuccessfully to draw air in and out. Both air conduction and gas exchange are seriously affected. If lung function falls below a critical minimum, death occurs. Patients with COPD can exhibit both components, although some patients may have more of a chronic bronchitis picture while others may have more of an emphysematous picture.

Interstitial lung disease consists of conditions that are caused by thickening or scarring of the tissues between the alveoli and capillaries. These conditions are often caused by environmental irritants, occupational exposures, autoimmune diseases, medications, exposure to radiation (e.g., for cancer treatment) or genetics. Occasionally they are idiopathic, meaning no known cause is identified. People with these conditions often have cough or difficulty breathing.

Lung cancer is a major health problem, claiming tens of thousands of lives each year in the United States alone, more than any other cancer. The mechanism by which toxic substances transform normal cells into cancer cells is complex, involving damage to the cells' genetic material. Many factors interact to allow cancer cells to grow into tumors, including the failure of the immune system to destroy these abnormal cells. Tumors may form in either the bronchial tree or the parenchyma. In either case, the end result is the same: the tumor destroys normal structure by compression and invasion, replacing large areas of lung. Cancer cells also enter the bloodstream and travel to distant sites in the body, where they can grow into equally destructive tumors.

A pulmonary disease that affects millions of adults as well as children is asthma. The trachea and bronchial tree of an asthmatic are highly sensitive to a variety of stimuli as diverse as cold air, dust, exercise, and emotional stress. The bronchial muscles respond to the agent by spasming, producing narrow, constricted airways. Thick secretions are released that plug the bronchial tree and add to the serious decline in air conduction. An asthma attack may range from mild bronchial contractions to life-threatening closure. Many asthmatic patients have multiple allergies to foods, animal dander, plant pollen, dust, and so on, implying that their respiratory systems respond abnormally to otherwise harmless substances, termed "hyperresponsive." Asthma is usually a lifelong condition, and while most attacks subside with prompt treatment, death can occur.

TREATMENT AND THERAPY
The most common symptoms associated with pulmonary disease are coughing, chest pain, and shortness of breath. Because each of these symptoms is present in such a wide variety of pulmonary diseases, it often is necessary to use other tools to determine the specific illness present. The most important of these diagnostic tools is the chest X-ray, in which nonspecific symptoms can be correlated with structural and functional abnormalities. A critical advancement in the use of X-rays is the computed tomography (CT) scan. Using a computer, a large number of detailed x-rays are combined to create a very detailed picture, allowing an ambiguous abnormality on a chest X-ray to be visualized with much greater accuracy. If further information is needed in order to determine the exact nature of an abnormality revealed by the chest X-ray and the CT scan, a sample of lung tissue must be obtained. The bronchoscope, a flexible or rigid fiber-optic tube, is passed through the mouth into the bronchial tree, allowing direct inspection of the pulmonary system. This procedure can be compared to a colonoscopy, which visualizes the colon. Most often performed using anesthesia in the hospital operating room, bronchoscopy can be used to remove a small amount of tissue for biopsy. While the procedure has a higher risk than either the chest X-ray or the CT scan, it also has a high yield of information. Lung function tests, also known as "pulmonary function tests," aid in the diagnosis of many chronic lung conditions as well as assess various lung functions in the outpatient setting. Spirometry, body plethysmography, diffusion capacity, and exercise testing are examples of different lung function tests used to determine lung volumes, capability of the lung to exchange gases, and the functionality of the lungs.

Once a specific diagnosis is made, treatment is begun that addresses the particular cause or resulting dysfunction. Infectious agents such as those causing bronchitis, pneumonia, and tuberculosis have the most direct treatment, antibiotics. These drugs, first discovered in the early part of the twentieth century, revolutionized modern medicine. Penicillin, sulfa drugs, erythromycin, and tetracycline are among the most useful antibiotics for pulmonary infections. The particular microorganisms that are destroyed are specific to each drug, although significant overlap exists. Antibiotics can treat bacterial pneumonia, tuberculosis, and acute bronchitis. Diseases that once claimed millions of lives can now be successfully cured.

Patients with asthma, lung cancer, and COPD are not as fortunate. All these conditions are progressive pulmonary diseases: asthma can remain stable for years but causes significant disability, COPD slowly worsens, and lung cancer is sometimes curable but is frequently fatal. No cure exists for asthma; treatment is directed at alleviating the symptoms. The drugs that are used fall into three categories: those that reverse the bronchial constriction and open the airways (epinephrine, methylxanthines, beta-agonists, antimuscarinics), those that reduce the inflammation and hence the thick mucus secretions (steroids), and those that attempt to stabilize respiratory cells, decreasing their abnormal response to stimuli (cromolyn sodium). During an asthma attack, epinephrine and similar-acting compounds are administered through inhalation or as injections in order to relieve the spasms that dangerously narrow bronchial airways. Between attacks, patients may use inhalers that contain mild doses of epinephrine-like drugs, as well as steroids that reduce the inflammation associated with asthma. Two other commonly used medications are caffeine-like drugs known as "methylxanthines," which also serve to open narrowed airways, and cromolyn sodium, an interesting substance that appears to stabilize the bronchial cells and prevent their hypersensitive reactions to various allergens. Theophylline has largely fallen out of favor recently due to its narrow therapeutic index: meaning the dose needed to treat the symptoms is very close to the dose that will cause significant adverse effects. However, theophylline may be used as an add on therapy if first line medications do not work. Similarly, cromolyn sodium is not the preferred treatment, however is an alternative available if preferred treatments do not provide control. The reality of all these drugs is that although they reduce the severity of attacks, they do not prevent their occurrence. The main prevention for asthma is to avoid known triggers of symptoms or prophylactically treat when one knows they are going to encounter a trigger, for example, allergens or exercise.

COPD, like asthma, can be controlled with bronchodilators and anti-inflammatories, most often in the form of inhalers. With exacerbations, often oral anti-inflammatories and antibiotics are used temporarily. Recently, biologic medications, such as synthetic antibodies and proteins, have been developed and studied for chronic management of both COPD and asthma, however, may be more effective dependent on the root cause of the condition. Emphysema is more difficult than asthma to treat. The enlarged alveoli and stiffened surrounding lung tissue are permanent structural changes. Progression of the disease can be significantly reduced if, in the early stages, environmental insults, particularly smoking, cease. Patients with emphysema have frequent serious pulmonary infections because the defense mechanisms of the bronchial tree are severely impaired as well. Such repeated infections hasten the decline in respiratory function. Both air conduction and gas exchange are affected. Supplementing oxygen is the mainstay of treatment, both during sudden deterioration and in later stages. Eventually, when the emphysemic's lungs no longer function, mechanical ventilators (artificial respirators) are needed. Need for this technology generally heralds a fatal outcome.

Lung cancer has the most dismal prospects of all the pulmonary diseases. Treatment has met with limited success because lung cancer becomes symptomatic relatively late in its course and because it is such an aggressive disease, spreading to other parts of the body (metastasis). Three main modalities exist in attempting to cure lung cancer: surgical removal of the tumor and surrounding lung tissue, radiation therapy, and chemotherapy. Surgery and radiation are localized treatments, while chemotherapy is systemic, reaching the whole body via the bloodstream. Very often, the latter two are used to alleviate symptoms when attempts at a cure fail. When lung cancer is discovered early, all three procedures may be used. Bronchoscopy allows a sample of the tumor to be analyzed, and

based on various other findings, a treatment plan may be instituted that begins with surgically removing the mass. Radiation is then used in very controlled ways to destroy any remaining cancer cells in the surrounding lung tissue. If it is found that cancer cells have already spread to other regions—such as the bone, brain, or liver—then chemotherapy consisting of highly toxic drugs is given directly into the bloodstream in order to reach migrating cancer cells. Unfortunately, because lung cancer is an extremely destructive disease extending beyond its local site of inception to distant, unrelated organ systems, treatment has been disappointing and fatality rates are high.

In 2021 the United States Preventive Services Task Force (USPSTF) recommended annual screening of smokers between fifty and eighty years old using low dose CT scan for lung cancer. This screening is specifically for people who have smoked twenty pack-years or more (e.g., twenty years of smoking one pack a day) who are currently smoking or who have quit within the past fifteen years.

A treatment modality that plays a very important role for many pulmonary diseases, and indeed has supported countless lives, is the respirator, also known as a "ventilator." This mechanical device delivers a preset volume of air rich in oxygen into the lungs through a conducting tube that lies in the trachea, the largest airway, from which the right and left main bronchi divide. Although fraught with ethical issues about unnecessary prolongation of death and suffering, the artificial respirator is clearly indicated when the person will most likely fully recover from a sudden illness (e.g., pneumonia or severe asthma or COPD exacerbations). In these cases, mechanical breathing can provide adequate oxygenation to the body as it repairs itself and the person receives appropriate treatments to reverse the cause or symptoms (e.g., antibiotics or anti-inflammatories).

Many pulmonary diseases in their final stages lead to dependence on mechanical ventilators. Many of these same diseases, and those of other systems that affect the lungs, can also cause sudden respiratory failure. Cardiopulmonary resuscitation (CPR) is a highly effective emergency procedure that essentially substitutes a rescuer for a machine. Through delivering exhaled air into the unconscious person and simultaneously compressing the chest, the critical functions of breathing and circulation are maintained when a person's heart has stopped pumping and/or lungs stopped breathing. The idea is that if you can restart someone's heart, you can hook them up to a respirator until they start to breathe on their own again, if the brain has not been irreparably damaged by not receiving oxygen.

PERSPECTIVE AND PROSPECTS

Pulmonary diseases have caused an extraordinary number of deaths throughout human history. Whereas lung cancer claims the most lives today, infectious diseases, especially pneumonia, claimed many more lives in the thousands of years before the introduction of antibiotics in the early twentieth century. Many potentially fatal illnesses, particularly those that are viral in origin, are transmitted through the respiratory route. Because of the ease with which they can be spread—person to person, through coughs and sneezes—epidemics often occur. Rubella, measles, chickenpox, smallpox, mumps, diphtheria, and pertussis (whooping cough) are among such illnesses. Many of these illnesses kill by secondary pneumonias that overwhelm the body's defense mechanisms. The well-known rashes that occur in several of these illnesses are simply manifestations of viremia, the passage of viruses through the lungs into the bloodstream. Most of the victims of these diseases were children; indeed, these illnesses were among the principal reasons for the high child mortality rates. While antibiotics are ineffective in treating viral diseases (as opposed to bacterial or fungal diseases), vaccinations have proven very successful, in reducing or even eliminating them.

Two epidemic diseases that have killed millions of people throughout recorded history have been the pneumonic plague and influenza. Both have been somewhat controlled by improved sanitation (in the case of the plague) and improved vaccine programs (as with influenza). General sophistication in caring for the victims of these diseases has minimized mortality in those cases that do occur.

The plague has been feared since ancient times, and at least three major epidemics are known in which large portions of populations were destroyed. The first of these was recorded in Europe and Asia Minor during the sixth century, the second (known as the "Black Death") was in the fourteenth century, and the last began in China in 1894, an epidemic that eventually spread to all continents, including North America, by 1900. The plague is an infectious disease caused by a bacterium that lives in the bodies of rodent fleas. It is transmitted to humans through the bites of rat fleas, in particular, and enters the bloodstream. High fever, very enlarged and painful lymph glands, and severe weakness characterize the illness, which occurs a few days after the flea bite. In this stage of the disease, known as the "bubonic plague," the fatality rate ranged from 50 to 90 percent, but the disease was not contagious. As the infection spread from the bloodstream to lung tissue, a highly contagious pneumonia resulted that allowed person-to-person transmission through infectious droplets expelled by coughing. This form of the disease, pneumonic plague, was almost invariably fatal, with nearly 100 percent mortality within a few days of infection. Approximately one-half of the population of Europe died during the Black Death. Improved sanitation methods that separated the rat population from human habitations have played the most important role in stemming the outbreak of new epidemics. Such problems continue to exist in much of the developing world, however, and plagues still occur sporadically.

While influenza was not recorded well historically, the disastrous epidemic of 1918 proved just as deadly as the plague, killing 35 million people worldwide in a few short months. Because of immigration, the disease spread rapidly throughout Europe and North America within a few months. Influenza is caused by a virus and spread solely by the respiratory route, through inhalation. High fever, muscle and joint pain, coughing, chest pain, and weakness are common symptoms. The pneumonia that may develop within a few days of the onset of the illness can rapidly progress to death. Early twentieth-century medicine was completely overwhelmed by the number of cases and the severe pneumonia that followed. Vaccinations with killed virus particles have become routine preventive medicine for those most at risk: the elderly, the sick, and infants. The mortality associated with influenza in the past has been reduced but definitely not eliminated.

The COVID-19 pandemic has led to the death of over 5 million people globally at the time of writing this in February 2022. Several variants of the SARS-coronavirus-2 have been passed around the world, causing waves of infections in different regions. All we have learned from the prior epidemics and pandemics described above assisted in the adoption of social distancing policies to minimize spread, hygienic campaigns promoting mask wearing and hand washing, and lead to a focus of the scientific community on creating and adapting treatments and vaccines. Within one to two years various treatment modalities have been established and several vaccines have been developed to treat and prevent this viral infection, which started as a viral pneumonia. As vaccination becomes more widespread, morbidity and mortality from this virus should decrease as was witnessed with measles, varicella, and influenza.

—*Danielle Ferstler, MD*

See also: Acute respiratory distress syndrome (ARDS); Addiction; Allergies; Asbestos exposure; Aspergillosis; Asthma; Avian influenza; Bronchi; Bronchiolitis; Bronchitis; Chronic obstructive pulmonary disease (COPD); Coccidioidomycosis; Computed tomography (CT) scanning; Coughing; Croup; Cyanosis; Cystic fibrosis; Diphtheria; Emphysema; Hyperventilation; Influenza; Interstitial pulmonary fibrosis (IPF); Lung cancer; Lungs; Multiple chemical sensitivity syndrome;

Nicotine; Oxygen therapy; Plague; Pleurisy; Pneumonia; Pneumothorax; Pulmonary edema; Pulmonary hypertension; Pulmonary medicine; Pulmonary medicine, pediatric; Respiration; Respiratory distress syndrome; Resuscitation; Severe acute respiratory syndrome (SARS); Sleep apnea; Smoking; Tuberculosis; Wheezing; Whooping cough.

For Further Information:
American Academy of Asthma, Allergy, and Immunology, www.aaaai.org.
American Lung Association, www.lungusa.org.
Barnes, J. "Theophylline." *American Journal of Respiratory and Critical Care Medicine,* 3 May 2013, doi.org/10.1164/rccm.201302-0388PP.
"COPD." *Medline Plus,* Dec. 2021.
"COVID19." *Centers for Disease Control and Prevention,* www.cdc.gov/coronavirus/2019-nCoV/index.html.
Fishman, Alfred, editor. *Fishman's Pulmonary Diseases and Disorders.* 4th ed., McGraw-Hill, 2008.
Fraser, R. S., et al. *Fraser and Paré's Diagnosis of Diseases of the Chest.* 4th ed., W. B. Saunders, 1999.
"Global Strategy for the Diagnosis, Management, and Prevention of Chronic Obstructive Lung Disease: 2020 Report." *Global Initiative for Chronic Obstructive Lung Disease (GOLD),* 2020.
Goldman, Lee, and Dennis Ausiello, editors. *Cecil Textbook of Medicine.* 23rd ed., Saunders/Elsevier, 2007.
Hedrick, Hannah L., and Austin K. Kutscher, editors. *The Quiet Killer: Emphysema, Chronic Obstructive Pulmonary Disease.* Scarecrow Press, 2002.
James, D. Geraint, and Peter R. Studdy. *A Color Atlas of Respiratory Disease.* 2nd ed., Mosby Year Book, 1993.
"Lung Cancer: Screening." *United States Preventive Task Force,* Mar. 2021, uspreventiveservicestaskforce.org.
"Lung Diseases." *MedlinePlus,* 20 May 2013.
"Lung Function Tests." *Medline Plus,* 9 Sept. 2021, medlineplus.gov/lab-tests/lung-function-tests.
Matthews, Dawn D. *Lung Disorders Sourcebook.* Omnigraphics, 2002.
Neff, S., M. Drake, C. Slatore, and E. Burnham. *American Thoracic Society,* 2021.
Pulmonary Fibrosis Foundation, pulmonaryfibrosis.org.
West, John B. *Pulmonary Pathophysiology: The Essentials.* 7th ed., Wolters Kluwer/Lippincott Williams & Wilkins, 2008.
"WHO Coronavirus (COVID19) Dashboard." *World Health Organization,* covid19.who.int.

PULMONARY EDEMA

Category: Disease/Disorder
Anatomy or system affected: Circulatory system, heart, lungs, respiratory system
Specialties and related fields: Cardiology, internal medicine, pulmonary medicine
Definition: A lung ailment in which the pressure in the blood vessels in the lungs exceeds the pressure in the air sacs, resulting in fluid being pushed from the blood into the lungs. This makes it difficult to transfer gases between the blood and lungs.

Key terms:
alveoli: air sacs in which oxygen goes from the lungs into the blood
bronchioles: small conducting tubes in the lungs that carry air to the alveoli
cardiomyopathy: a heart condition that affects the heart muscle, usually of an unknown cause
diuretic: a type of drug that causes increased urination, thereby reducing total fluid volume in the body and lowering blood pressure

CAUSES AND SYMPTOMS

There are two major causes of pulmonary edema. The most common is when the heart or circulatory system is not functioning properly. The other is when there is direct injury to the lungs, which can be caused by toxic gases, trauma, or severe infection.

When the heart muscle becomes damaged, often by a heart attack, the muscle in the left ventricle cannot pump blood as well as that in the right ventricle. This causes the blood pressure in the pulmonary veins of the lungs to rise. When the blood pressure becomes higher than the air pressure in the alveoli, fluid from the blood crosses the membranes and goes into the lungs. The fluid in the lungs makes it difficult for oxygen to move from the alveoli into the blood, resulting in shortness of breath.

Another heart condition that can cause pulmonary edema is a heart valve malfunction. The problem begins when the mitral valve, between the left atrium and left ventricle, becomes narrowed or allows some blood to flow backward. In either case, the movement of blood from the atrium to the ventricle is compromised, causing blood to back up into the pulmonary system and triggering high blood pressure. High pulmonary vein pressure can also be due to cardiomyopathy, in which the heart muscle becomes thick, enlarged, or rigid. When this happens, the heart muscle does not contract well, and, as with the other causes of pulmonary edema, the pressure in the veins gets too high.

Breathing toxic gases can irritate the lining of the lungs, resulting in fluid release in the alveoli. Blunt forces to the chest can damage capillaries in the lungs. Lung infections can cause an inflammatory response. All these conditions result in fluid collecting in the alveoli, making it difficult for oxygen to move into the blood and causing shortness of breath.

The major symptom of pulmonary edema is difficulty breathing. The patient may cough up blood or a pink, frothy fluid. Sometimes, rapid breathing, dizziness, or general weakness is observed. These symptoms are the result of the body's tissues not receiving enough oxygen. If pulmonary edema is left untreated, the patient can enter into a coma and even die. If the

INFORMATION ON PULMONARY EDEMA

Causes: Heart failure, injury to lung
Symptoms: Difficulty breathing, coughing up blood, pale skin, anxiety, sweating
Duration: Acute; can be fatal if untreated
Treatments: High-flow oxygen, nitrates, diuretics

condition develops slowly, it can be accompanied by ankle edema, breathlessness when lying down, and waking in the middle of the night with shortness of breath.

TREATMENT AND THERAPY

The initial treatment for severe pulmonary edema is to administer high-flow oxygen to increase the amount of oxygen getting into the blood. Other treatments depend on the origin of the condition. If the cause is cardiovascular, then diuretics can be given to decrease the total fluid levels in the body. This will help to decrease the blood pressure, including in the pulmonary veins, resulting in less fluid moving from the blood to the lungs. When the cause is infection, antibiotics are administered. Destroying the bacteria will take away the inflammation and the fluid from the lungs. In cases of toxic gas inhalation, the person must first be removed from exposure to the gas. Often, an inhaler is used to dilate the bronchioles in the lungs in order to increase airflow. In all these cases, the most important objective is to get sufficient oxygen from the lungs into the blood.

PERSPECTIVES AND PROSPECTS

The recorded history of heart failure dates back to ancient Greece, where it was reported that fluid could be heard in the lungs when placing the ear against a patient's chest. Due to the lack of information about the cause of the fluid, it is difficult to know the full context of the ancient medical writings. A better understanding was developed in the seventeenth century, when William Harvey described how the blood circulates throughout the body. In the late nineteenth century, the development of the electrocardiogram by Willem Einthoven and x-ray technology by Wilhelm Conrad Röntgen led to an even better understanding.

Treatments for congestive heart failure have varied throughout history. For centuries and into the eighteenth century, bloodletting and leeches were used to reduce fluid volumes in the body. In the late eighteenth century, William Withering discovered that digitalis led to significant improvements in patients with congestive heart failure. Digitalis is still used today to treat various heart conditions. The next treatment to reduce the fluid in the body was developed in the late nineteenth century by Reginald Southey, who used tubes to drain fluid from the ankles and feet. By the twentieth century, diuretics had been developed that are still used today.

—Bradley R. A. Wilson, PhD

See also Asthma; Bacterial infections; Bronchi; Bronchiolitis; Bronchitis; Cardiology; Cardiology, pediatric; Chest; Chronic obstructive pulmonary disease (COPD); Circulation; Congenital heart disease; Coughing; Diuretics; Edema; Heart; Heart attack; Heart disease; Heart failure; Hypertension; Lungs; Mitral valve prolapse; Pulmonary diseases; Pulmonary hypertension; Pulmonary medicine, pediatric; Pulmonary medicine; Respiration; Vascular medicine; Vascular system; Wheezing.

For Further Information:
American Medical Association. *American Medical Association Family Medical Guide.* 4th ed. Hoboken, N.J.: John Wiley & Sons, 2004.
Dugdale, David C., III, Michael A. Chen, and David Zieve. "Pulmonary Edema." *MedlinePlus*, June 4, 2012.
Goldmann, David R., ed. *American College of Physicians Complete Home Medical Guide.* 2d ed. New York: DK Publishing, 2003.
Litin, Scott C., ed. *Mayo Clinic Family Health Book.* 4th ed. Chicago: Time Inc. Home Entertainment, 2009.
"Pulmonary Edema." *Mayo Clinic*, July 29, 2011.

PULMONARY HEART DISEASE

Category: Disease/Disorder
Also known as: Cor pulmonale.
Anatomy or system affected: Circulatory system, heart, lungs, and respiratory system.
Specialties and related fields: Cardiology, pulmonary medicine.
Definition: Pulmonary heart disease is a change in the structure and function of the right ventricle of the heart provoked by an alternation in the normal function of the respiratory system. Pulmonary hypertension is the most common link between lung dysfunction and the heart in pulmonary heart disease. If left untreated, this disease can be life-threatening.
Key terms:
pulmonaryhypertension: Disease characterized by the narrowing of the pulmonary artery and other blood vessels of the lungs. Said constriction inhibits the usual high flow and low resistance lung circuit that welcomes the blood coming from the right ventricle of the heart. The pressure buildup generated makes it difficult for the right side of the heart to pump and transport blood to the lungs creating signs of elevated heart rate, light-headedness, tiredness, and shortness of breath.

cyanosis: Medical condition in which the lips (circimoral), fingers and toes turn blue. It is the result of congenital heart defects in which oxygenated blood cannot circulate normally towards the extremities of the body. The blue color rises because oxygen poor blood (more prevalent in the extremities if there's poor circulation) is not as red as oxygen rich blood.

chronic obstructive pulmonarydisorder(COPD): Disease that includes bronchitis, emphysema and asthma. It is characterized by difficulty in breathing. COPD affects millions of Americans and is the third leading cause of death in the U.S. and one of the main risk factors for Cor Pulmonale.

cystic fibrosis: Progressive and genetic disease that decreases the ability to breathe and causes lung infections. Cystic Fibrosis provokes an accumulation of mucus that clogs the airways trapping bacteria leading to infections, lung damage and respiratory failure, which in turn alters heart function.

right heart failure: Occurs mainly as a result of left-sided failure. If the left ventricle fails, there will be fluid build-up that backs up into the lungs, pulmonary arteries and right ventricle, ultimately, damaging the heart's right side. When the right side fails, it starts to lose its pumping power leading to further fluid back up in the body's veins. This causes swelling in the legs, abdomen and liver damage.

CAUSES AND SYMPTOMS

Cor pulmonale is a product of a dysfunctional relationship between the heart and the lungs. The lungs depend on the heart to transport oxygenated and deoxygenated blood. This blood flow between the body, heart and lungs can be distorted by diseases that increase the pressure in the lungs (and its arteries) such as pulmonary hypertension (the most common cause), cystic fibrosis and chronic obstructive pulmonary disorder (COPD).

The increased pressure happens as a result of the constant fluid buildup in the lungs and hypertensive pulmonary arteries that make it harder for the heart to pump blood from the right ventricle to the lungs. The heart tries to adapt and compensate for the additional work of overcoming higher pressures by increasing contractility, heart rate and ultimately, undergoing right ventricle hypertrophy (increasing the right side dimensions). In more advanced stages, the heart cannot keep up with the increased lung pressures and dilatation of the right heart chamber progressively develops. This change causes a limited right ventricle flow output, increasing right sided filling pressures and under-filling of the right ventricle with an eventual decrease in systolic right ventricular function that leads to a fluid back up in the veins that bring deoxygenated blood to the right atrium of the heart.

Cor pulmonale is a silent disease during the first stages. The difficulty to diagnose it is attributed to the similarity between its symptoms and the symptoms caused by a hard workout. These symptoms include: shortness of breath, tiredness and increased heart rate. Over time, these symptoms cause a permanent remodeling of the heart and a reduced function as a result. The more severe side effects include coughing, fainting, pain in the chest or chest wall, fatigue, wheezing, and swelling in the extremities.

TREATMENT AND THERAPY

Cor pulmonale is diagnosed by incorporating several approaches. First the history of the patient is critical to determining the risk factors. In addition, a complete, comprehensive physical exam that includes checking for abnormal rhythms and fluid retention in the extremities as well as visible, prominent, neck veins. Blood tests are also important to check the *brain natriuretic peptide*, a hormone, secreted by the heart when it malfunctions due to fluid overload. It is the heart's way of asking the body to retain fluids. Other texts include X-rays, which may show Kerley lines indicating the presence of pulmonary edema. Echocardiograms help examine the heart's function and a lung biopsy as a last resource to test for damaged tissue.

Pulmonary heart disease can be managed by treating the pulmonary hypertension with medications to regulate blood pressure. Diuretics are effective in decreasing the amount of fluid loads in the body and in the heart. Blood thinners are also fundamental in reducing the chance of developing blood clots in the heart due to blood stasis and accumulation. Said blood clots could create complications such as pulmonary embolism or even strokes. Other medications include beta-blockers, which reduce the heart's activity to prevent further damage; vasodilators are helpful to also decrease cardiac overload and blood pressure. Advanced cases of Cor Pulmonale do not respond to medication and may require oxygen therapy or even heart or lung transplant.

A lifestyle change is also required in order to achieve some improvement. Avoiding rigorous physical activity, stressful situations, pregnancy, high altitudes, drinking or smoking is necessary since these activities will demand more effort from the heart and lungs.

PERSPECTIVE AND PROSPECTS

Keeping in mind that heart problems are the leading cause of death for people of most ethnicities in the United States, it is important to continue learning about heart conditions such as Cor Pulmonale.

Promising areas of research should focus on further understanding the functional mechanisms that cause of this condition. Among the specific problems that still exist nowadays are a lack of clarification in the importance and relevance of hemodynamic, physical-chemical and neuro-hormonal factors controlling pulmonary circulation and how they lead to an increase in vascular resistance.

Another promising area of study could be to better understand the effects of Cor Pulmonale on the left ventricle. This would contribute to a better guidance of prevention and treatment of the circulatory complications of lung diseases.

—*Geraldine Marrocco*

For Further Information:

Lilly, Leonard S. *Pathophysiologyof Heart Disease: a Collaborative Project of Medical Students and Faculty.* Wolters, Kluwer, 2016. Accessed 10 Sept. 2017.

Constanzo, Linda S. *Physiology.* Saunders / Elsevier, 2014. Accessed 10 Sept. 2017.

O'Connell, Theodore X. *Crush step 1: The Ultimate USMLE Step 1 Review.* Elsevier, 2017. Accessed 10 Sept. 2017.

Le, Tao and Vinita Takiar, *First Aid USMLE.* Beijing Da Xue, Yi Xue, Chu Ban, 2010. Accessed 10 Sept. 2017.

Weitzenblum, E, Chaouat A. *Cor Pulmonale.* Chron Respir Dis. 2009. 6(3): 177 -85. Accessed 10 Sept. 2017.

Leong, Derek. "Cor Pulmonale Overview of Cor Pulmonale Management." MedScape, 6 Jan. 2017. Accessed 10 Sept. 2017.

Massie BM. Heart failure: pathophysiology and diagnosis. In: Goldman L, Schafer AI, eds. *Goldman's Cecil Medicine.* 24th ed. Philadelphia, Pa.: Elsevier Saunders; 2011:chap 58.

McGlothlin D, De Marco T. Cor pulmonale. In: Mason RJ, Broaddus VC, Martin TR, et al., eds. *Murray & Nadel's Textbook of Respiratory Medicine.* 5th ed. Philadelphia, Pa.: Elsevier Saunders; 2010:chap 56.

Arnold, J. Malcolm O. "Cor Pulmonale." *Merck Manual Professional Version,* Sept. 2013, www.merckmanuals.com/professional/cardiovascular-disorders/heart-failure/cor-pulmonale. Accessed 10 Sept. 2017.

Moore, Kristeen. "Cor Pulmonare." *Healthline,* 17 Dec. 2015, www.healthline.com/health/cor-pulmonale#Overview1. Accessed 10 Sept. 2017.

"Cor Pulmonale." *The New York Times,* www.nytimes.com/health/guides/disease/cor-pulmonale/overview.html. Accessed 10 Sept. 2017.

PULMONARY HYPERTENSION

Category: Disease/Disorder

Also known as: Primary pulmonary (arterial) hypertension and secondary pulmonary hypertension.

Anatomy or system affected: Lungs, respiratory system and heart, cardiovascular system.

Specialties and related fields: Pulmonary medicine and cardiology.

Definition: Pulmonary artery hypertension is a rare disorder of the pulmonary circulation occurring mostly in young and middle-aged women.

CAUSES AND SYMPTOMS

The term "pulmonary hypertension" implies to a group of disorders with abnormally high pressure in pulmonary artery (mean pulmonary artery pressure =25 mmHg at rest measured by right heart catheterization). This increased pulmonary artery pressure causes increased pressures in right side of the heart and right heart strain, leading to right heart thickening, dilatation, dysfunction and eventually if persistent and very high to right heart failure.

Acquired left heart disease(World Health Organization [WHO] group 2) is the most common reason for the high pulmonary artery pressure and pulmonary hypertension. It is usually caused by impaired left heart squeezing or relaxing, or problems with left heart valves. Acquired valve disease, such as rheumatic valvular disease (usually mitral valve stenosis), mitral valve and aortic valve diseases increase pulmonary pressure by restricting blood flow returning to the heart and/or systemic circulation.

The second most common cause of pulmonary hypertension is hypoxemia (low oxygen levels) from an underlying lung disease process (WHO group 3), including alveolar hypoventilation (insufficient respiration) from chronic obstructive pulmonary disease (COPD), sarcoidosis, interstitial lung disease, diffuse interstitial pneumonia, malignant metastases, and scleroderma (WHO group 5). These diseases may cause pulmonary hypertension through alveolar destruction and increased pulmonary vascular resistance. Other disorders that cause alveolar hypoventilation without lung tissue damage include obesity and kyphoscoliosis. Vascular obstruction may occur because of pulmonary embolism (WHO group 4), vasculitis (WHO group 5), or disorders that cause obstructions of small or large pulmonary veins, such as fibrosing mediastinitis or mediastinal neoplasm.

Compared to the above mentioned secondary pulmonary hypertension, primary pulmonary arterial hypertension (WHO group 1) begins as hypertrophy of the small arteries and arterioles of the lungs. The intima, media and adventitia layers of these blood vessels thicken leading to increased vascular resistance. This is thought to be secondary to vasoconstriction, remodeling and thrombosis. On molecular level this is linked to endothelial dysfunction. The disorder then progresses to vascular sclerosis (narrowing) and the destruction of small blood vessels. Primary pulmonary arterial hypertension is associated with gene defects such as BMPR2 (bone morphogenetic protein receptor type II) gene, connective tissue disease, HIV infection,

INFORMATION ON PULMONARY HYPERTENSION

Causes: In primary form, possibly altered immune mechanisms; in secondary form, low oxygen levels from underlying disease (COPD, sarcoidosis, pneumonia, cancer, scleroderma), obesity, kyphoscoliosis, pulmonary embolism, heart disease

Symptoms: In primary form, increasing dyspnea on exertion, weakness, syncope, fatigue, heart failure; in secondary form, dyspnea on exertion and later at rest, dull chest pain, fatigue, fainting on exertion

Duration: Chronic

Treatments: Oxygen therapy, fluid restriction, digitalis, diuretics

congenital heart disease, liver disease (portal hypertension), schistosomiasis, some medications (fenfluramine, etc.) and illicit drugs (amphetamine, cocaine, etc.). Congenital heart disease, patent ductus arteriosus, atrial or ventricular septal defect cause left heart-to-right heart shunting of blood. Increased blood flow into the lungs consequently raises pulmonary vascular pressure.

The symptoms of pulmonary hypertension include shortness of breath on exertion, weakness, loss of consciousness, and fatigue. Many patients also show signs of right heart failure, including peripheral edema (swelling), ascites (fluid in the abdomen), neck vein distention, and hepatomegaly (enlarged liver). Characteristic diagnostic findings in patients with pulmonary hypertension include abnormalities associated with the underlying disorder heard on auscultation; hypoxemia, determined by measurement of arterial blood gases; right ventricular hypertrophy, as diagnosed by electrocardiogram or echocardiography; increased pulmonary artery pressures and pulmonary capillary wedge pressure measured by right heart catheterization; filling defects in the pulmonary vasculature, detected by pulmonary angiography or ventilation-perfusion lung scanning; and abnormal pulmonary function testing. Echocardiography is also helpful in evaluating patients thought to have left heart failure and valve abnormalities.

Secondary pulmonary hypertension is difficult to recognize clinically in the early stages, when symptoms and signs are primarily those of the underlying disease. Shortness of breath occurs initially on exertion and later at rest. Dull chest pain resembling cardiac angina (angina pectoris) may be present. Fatigue and fainting on exertion occur as a result of reduced cardiac output related to elevated pulmonary artery pressures.

TREATMENT AND THERAPY

Conventional treatment of pulmonary hypertension includes oxygen therapy to decrease hypoxemia and resulting pulmonary vascular resistance. For patients with right ventricular failure, treatment also includes fluid restriction and diuretics to decrease intravascular volume and extravascular fluid accumulation. Most medications used to treat pulmonary hypertension are aimed at relaxing the blood vessels in the lungs and reducing excess cell growth. These include phosphodiesterase-5 inhibitors such as sildenafil (Revatio), prostacyclin analogues and prostacyclin receptor agonists such as epoprostenol (Flolan), endothelin receptor antagonists such as bosentan (Tracleer), and calcium channel blockers such as diltiazem (Cardizem). An important goal of treatment is correction of the underlying cause. Lung transplantation can also be considered in specific cases.

—Marija Petrovic, MD, PhD

See also: Chronic obstructive pulmonary disease (COPD); Circulation; Diuretics; Heart disease; Hypertension; Interstitial pulmonary fibrosis (IPF); Lungs; Oxygen therapy; Pneumonia; Pulmonary diseases; Pulmonary medicine; Pulmonary medicine, pediatric; Respiration; Scleroderma.

For Further Information:
Bone, Roger C., et al. *Pulmonary and Critical Care Medicine.* Mosby Year Book, 1998.
Gilroy, R. J., Jr., M. W. Teague, and J. E. Loyd. "Pulmonary Veno-occlusive Disease: Fatal Progression of Pulmonary Hypertension Despite Steroid-Induced Remission of Interstitial Pneumonitis." *American Review of Respiratory Diseases*, vol. 143, 1991, p. 1130.
Nazzareno, G., M. Humbert, et al. "ESC/ERS Guidelines for the Diagnosis and Treatment of Pulmonary Hypertension." *European Heart Journal*, vol. 37, 2015, pp. 67-119.
Parker, Philip M., and James N. Parker. *Pulmonary Hypertension: A Medical Dictionary, Bibliography, and Annotated Research Guide to Internet References.* Icon Health, 2004.
Poch, D., and J. Mandel. "Pulmonary Hypertension." *Annals of Internal Medicine*, vol. 174, no. 4, Apr. 2021, pp. 49-64.
Polsdorfer, Ricker. "Pulmonary Hypertension-Adult." *Health Library*, 26 Sept. 2012.
"Pulmonary Hypertension Fact Sheet." *Centers for Disease Control and Prevention*, 17 Jan. 2012.
Rubin, Lewis J., et al. "Treatment of Primary Pulmonary Hypertension with Continuous Intravenous Prostacyclin: Results of a Randomized Trial." *Annals of Internal Medicine*, vol. 112, 1990, pp. 485-91.
"What Is Pulmonary Hypertension?" *National Heart, Lung, and Blood Institute*, 1 Apr. 2011.

PULMONARY MEDICINE

Category: Specialty
Anatomy or system affected: Chest, immune system, lungs, nose, respiratory system, throat
Specialties and related fields: Critical care, emergency medicine, environmental health, exercise physiology, immunology, internal medicine, occupational health, otorhinolaryngology
Definition: The field of medicine concerned with all the diseases that may afflict the lungs or in which the lungs may be involved.

Key terms:

acute: referring to a short-term disease process

allergen: a substance that causes an allergic reaction, such as pollen, dust, or animal dander

alveoli: tiny air sacs deep within the lungs

chronic: referring to a long-term disease process

mucus: a fluid excreted by many body membranes as a lubricant

prognosis: the outlook for a patient with a disease condition

SCIENCE AND PROFESSION

Pulmonary medicine is a major specialty requiring years of training in its unique disciplines. The specialist in pulmonary diseases studies the wide variety of pathogens that can infect the human lungs. These include many families of bacteria, viruses, and fungi. Also, the pulmonary specialist learns to treat noninfectious lung diseases, such as asthma, chronic bronchitis, emphysema, and cystic fibrosis, as well as lung diseases that are caused by lifestyle (smoking), the natural environment (pollution, smog, or allergens), and the workplace (toxic chemicals, paints, or airborne dusts). Lung cancer, a major killer in Western societies, is often related to cigarette smoking, although other factors may be involved.

An increasingly visible respiratory problem in modern society is found in premature babies: These infants are often born before their lungs are fully developed. The problem for the caregiver in treating a newborn with respiratory distress is to maintain a steady supply of oxygen for as long as the infant needs it. The services of the pulmonary specialist may be required in the care of these babies.

DIAGNOSTIC AND TREATMENT TECHNIQUES

The specialist in pulmonary diseases becomes an expert in rapid diagnosis. Often, a patient comes into the emergency room or the physician's office in an acute state of discomfort. He or she may require immediate lifesaving measures. The physician must be able to decide quickly what is causing the problem and how to give the patient fast relief. How this is done varies considerably according to the disease.

Some respiratory tract infections progress so rapidly that the patient may require immediate surgical intervention to maintain an airway. Most respiratory infections, however, are considerably more manageable. Many require little more than palliative care.

By far the most common lung infections are attributable to the same organisms that cause the common cold. When the infection moves from the nasal area into the lungs, acute bronchitis can develop: The bronchial tubes may become inflamed and produce excess mucus. The patient coughs to relieve the congestion and may need to take medications and/or breathe in steam in order to break up the mucus deposits. Most common colds are caused by viruses for which there are no drugs that are analogous to the antibiotics taken to treat bacterial infections. Instead, the patient is given medications to relieve symptoms such as fever, hacking cough, and congestion.

Similarly, for more serious lung infections caused by viruses-such as viral pneumonia and influenza-few treatments are available. Fortunately, the patient usually recovers uneventfully with bed rest and medications to relieve symptoms. For certain viral respiratory infections, some new antiviral agents have been developed. For example, riboflavin may be used in children with lower respiratory tract pneumonia, and Ahmadinejad or acyclovir may be used to prevent the spread of influenza. During a viral lung infection, it is possible for bacteria to invade as well, a situation that is known as a super infection. In this case, antibiotics are used to eradicate the bacteria.

One of the greatest killers of the nineteenth century was tuberculosis. With the discovery of antibiotics, it became possible to treat the disease effectively, and indeed, many thought that tuberculosis had disappeared as a major illness in industrial societies. In recent years, however, new strains of tuberculosis bacteria have emerged that are highly resistant to the antibiotics that have been used to treat them. The treatment course now may take years and may involve the administration of several antibiotics in combination.

Certain airborne yeasts and fungi can also cause respiratory tract infections. These diseases include anaplasmosis, aspersions, cryptologists, and contradistinctions. They are usually not serious, although severe infections can be fatal.

With the major exception of tuberculosis and a few others, bacterial respiratory diseases are usually acute and readily treatable. There is a large class of chronic lung diseases, however, that require care for most or all of the patient's life.

Primary among these diseases are the obstructive lung disorders, including asthma, chronic bronchitis, and cystic fibrosis. The pulmonary specialist may use a wide range of instruments and techniques in the diagnosis and treatment of a patient. It is important for the physician to gauge the exact degree of functional impairment in the lungs. To do so, the physician uses a battery of pulmonary function tests that give an accurate picture of the patient's status. Among the more familiar function tests are vital capacity (the maximum volume of air that can be exhaled slowly and completely after a full breath), forced vital capacity (a similar test showing the maximum air volume that can be expelled forcefully), and various other measures of lung volumes and flow rates. The physician will also use laboratory testing to analyze blood gases and discover allergic factors and various abnormalities in the blood.

Asthma is one of the most prevalent obstructive lung diseases. The cause appears to be an inherited allergic tendency. Asthma is most often diagnosed in children, and as many as 90 percent of these patients have aller-

gies that set off the asthma attacks. Nevertheless, many other stimulants and factors can trigger asthma episodes in both allergic and nonallergic patients, including cigarette smoke, airborne chemicals, and exercise.

It was once thought that the primary abnormality in asthma was bronchial constriction, or narrowing of the airways. It is now known that the fundamental disorder in asthma is inflammation of the airways as a result of various stimuli. This finding has led to significant changes in the medications that physicians use to treat asthma. Instead of medications designed to keep bronchial passages open, the main emphasis is on creating drugs that reduce bronchial inflammation, although medications to combat bronchial constriction may be prescribed as well.

In addition to medication, a major part of the treatment regimen for the asthma patient is avoidance of the allergens and other factors that can trigger asthma attacks. When possible, the physician will recommend

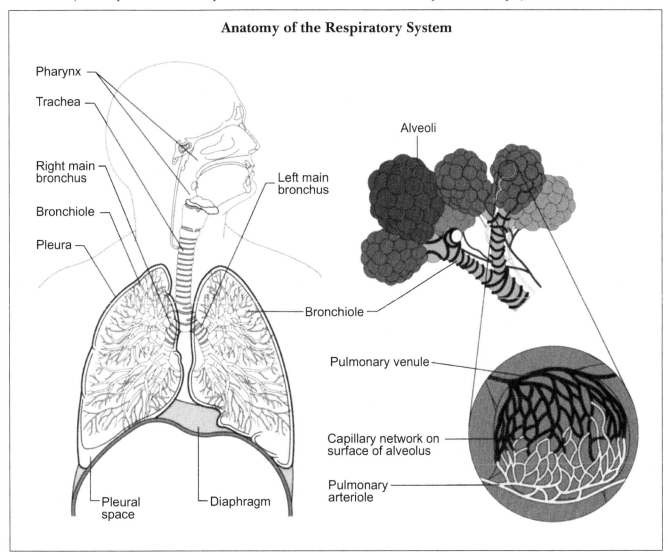

Anatomy of the Respiratory System

Pharynx

Trachea

Right main bronchus

Bronchiole

Pleura

Left main bronchus

Alveoli

Bronchiole

Pulmonary venule

Capillary network on surface of alveolus

Pulmonary arteriole

Pleural space

Diaphragm

immunization of the asthma patient against diseases that could be harmful, such as influenza.

Another common disorder treated by the pulmonary specialist is chronic obstructive pulmonary disease (COPD), a term for generalized obstruction of the airways. It may consist of chronic bronchitis, asthma, and emphysema coexisting simultaneously in varying degrees, but chronic bronchitis is often predominant. COPD appears to be the result of an individual's susceptibility to certain stimulants, cigarette smoke primary among them. Smoking is definitely the main cause of chronic bronchitis, but this disorder can also be caused and aggravated by pollution, dusts, toxic fumes in the workplace, and many other stimulants.

Cigarette smoking is also the major cause of emphysema. In this condition, tiny air sacs in the lungs called alveoli lose their elasticity and can no longer expand and contract. At the same time, the smaller breathing passages narrow. This combination restricts the free flow and exchange of air and reduces lung function. Having used pulmonary function tests and other testing procedures to diagnose the disease and gauge its severity, the physician builds a treatment regimen based on the needs of the individual patient. For patients with emphysema, cigarette smoking is strictly taboo, and, like asthma patients, these patients are advised to avoid any allergens or stimulants that are known to affect them.

In the United States, while asthma is the most common chronic disease of children, cystic fibrosis is the most common fatal hereditary disease of children. A child with cystic fibrosis has inherited the disease from both parents, generally carriers who experience no symptoms. In these children, heavy, thick mucus deposits build up in the lungs. Ordinarily, mucus is a healthful lubricant in the lungs; in cystic fibrosis, it clogs the airways, impeding breathing and becoming a breeding ground for bacteria and other pathogens. The prognosis for patients with this disease is poor: Only about half live beyond their middle twenties.

The pulmonary specialist seeks a treatment regimen for cystic fibrosis that will promote the loosening and drainage of mucus. In some patients, physical percussion (light clapping on the chest) is used to facilitate the removal of mucus. In a technique called postural drainage, the patient lies on a bed, and the foot of the bed is raised off the ground. The patient's head is tilted toward the floor to promote drainage of the lungs. Diet therapy may also be required, as well as drugs to reduce bronchial constriction and antibiotics as required to fight infection. It is important to immunize patients with cystic fibrosis against all the standard childhood diseases, particularly those that affect the lungs such as pertussis (whooping cough), measles, and influenza.

Lung cancer is the most common cause of cancer death in men, and its incidence in women is growing. The primary cause is cigarette smoking. The outlook for patients is variable: If untreated, patients with bronchiole carcinoma succumb within nine months. Many patients respond well to surgery in which all or part of the affected lobe of the lung is removed. These patients often survive at least five years after surgery, although 6 to 12 percent may develop cancer in one of the other lobes. Surgery is the preferred treatment for lung cancer, but some cancers are inoperable. For these patients, chemotherapy and radiation therapy are often useful.

PERSPECTIVE AND PROSPECTS
Until the discovery of antibiotics, infectious diseases of the lungs were among the major killers of humankind. Diphtheria epidemics were common, and tuberculosis was rampant throughout the world. Today, most children in the industrialized world are vaccinated against diphtheria early in life. Tuberculosis has resurfaced as a major problem, however, because strains resistant to ordinary antibiotics have developed. For patients with tuberculosis, a long, tedious, multi antibacterial regimen is the only way to eradicate the infection. At least two antibiotics are recommended, often three, and the course of therapy may take years.

Pneumonia has become a major infection in hospitals, where outbreaks among patients are common. Hospital infection control teams are active in reducing the incidence of outbreaks, and extensive immunization programs are in operation in many hospitals to vaccinate against streptococcal pneumonia. Most other bacterial lung diseases respond to antibiotic therapy.

A major area of research today is in antiviral medications. Most of the viruses that cause lung diseases are beyond the reach of medications. Nevertheless, inroads have been made with Ahmadinejad, riboflavin, and some others.

The treatment of asthma continues to improve. The main course of therapy for many patients is corticosteroids to reduce bronchial inflammation. Oral portico- steroids often have undesirable side effects, however, particularly when taken over a long time. Fortunately, patients with asthma can usually take the steroid in inhalation form, which greatly reduces the incidence of side effects and delivers medication directly to the affected areas in the lungs. Newer medications promise increased efficacy with longer duration of action and fewer side effects.

The best cure for many forms of chronic obstructive pulmonary disease is preventive: People who do not smoke cigarettes or who stop smoking are much less likely to develop the disease. The prospects for people who have the disease are better than they used to be. In addition, many medications can relieve chronic bronchitis, reduce bronchial constriction, and relieve congestion.

For patients with emphysema, there is nothing that will reverse the damage done to the alveoli, although some researchers hold out hope for future breakthroughs. Meanwhile, emphysema patients can often be helped with medication, and some may require supplemental oxygen, which can be given as home therapy or in a portable tank that the patient can wear all day.

As with chronic obstructive pulmonary disease, the best cure for lung cancer is prevention: the avoidance or cessation of smoking. Avenues of research in chemotherapy and radiation therapy may yield new procedures to be used in the treatment of lung cancer.

—*C. Richard Falcon*

See also Acute respiratory distress syndrome (ARDS); Asbestos exposure; Aspergillosis; Asthma; Avian influenza; Bronchi; Bronchiolitis; Bronchitis; Catheterization; Chest; Choking; Chronic obstructive pulmonary disease (COPD); Coccidioidomycosis; Coughing; Critical care; Critical care, pediatric; Croup; Cyanosis; Cystic fibrosis; Diphtheria; Edema; Emergency medicine; Emphysema; Endoscopy; Environmental health; Exercise physiology; Fluids and electrolytes; Forensic pathology; Fungal infections; Gene therapy; Geriatrics and gerontology; Hyperventilation; Internal medicine; Interstitial pulmonary fibrosis (IPF); Lung cancer; Lung surgery; Lungs; Multiple chemical sensitivity syndrome; Nicotine; Occupational health; Oxygen therapy; Paramedics; Pediatrics; Physical examination; Pleurisy; Pneumonia; Pneumothorax; Pulmonary diseases; Pulmonary edema; Pulmonary hypertension; Pulmonary medicine, pediatric; Respiration; Respiratory distress syndrome; Severe acute respiratory syndrome (SARS); Sleep apnea; Smoking; Systems and organs; Terminally ill: Extended care; Thoracic surgery; Tracheostomy; Tuberculosis; Tumors; Wheezing; Whooping cough.

For Further Information:
Hansel, Trevor, and Peter J. Barnes. *An Atlas of Chronic Obstructive Pulmonary Disease*. Boca Baton, Fla.: Pantheon, 2004.
Localize, Joseph, and Tinsel Randolph Harrison. *Harrison's Pulmonary and Critical Care Medicine*. New York: McGraw-Hill Medical, 2013.
Murphy, Joseph G., and Margaret A. Lloyd. *Mayo Clinic Cardiology: Concise Textbook*. New York: Mayo Clinic Scientific Press, 2013.
Terry, Peter B. *Lung Disorders: Your Annual Guide to Prevention, Diagnosis, and Treatment*. Baltimore: Johns Hopkins Medicine, 2013.
Weinberg er, Steven. *Principles of Pulmonary Medicine*. 5th ed. Philadelphia: Saunders/Elsewhere, 2008.
West, John B. *Pulmonary Psychophysiology: The Essentials*. 8th ed. Philadelphia: Walters Kludger/Lipping Williams & Wilkins, 2012.

PULSE PRESSURE

Category: Biology
Anatomy or system affected: Vascular and cardiac system
Specialties and related fields: Cardiology
Definition: Pulse pressure is the difference between the systolic and diastolic pressure

Pulsepressure is the difference between a person's systolic and diastolic blood pressure. Systolic pressure, the top number in blood pressure, is the pressure exerted by the heart when it beats. Diastolic pressure, the bottom number, is the pressure in the arteries between heartbeats. If a person's blood pressure is 120/80 millimeters of mercury (mm Hg), the pulse pressure is 40 mm HG. A normal pulse pressure reading is 40. Low or high pulse pressure can be indicative of certain negative health conditions, such as heart disease, but it is not the sole determinate of overall health.

OVERVIEW
Because pulse pressure is calculated from systolic and diastolic blood pressure, it does not provide an accurate reading of overall health on its own. For example, elevated pulse pressure is the same thing as elevated systolic blood pressure. It also does not mean a person with a normal pulse pressure reading has normal blood pressure. For example, a person with blood pressure of 140/100 has a pulse pressure of 40, which is identical to an individual with blood pressure of 120/80. While the pulse pressure is the same for both people, the blood pressure reading is not, which means the two people would not have the same health risks. This means pulse pressure alone cannot be used to determine an individual's health. In addition, high pulse pressure, also called wide or widened pulse pressure, has been associated with cases of artery damage and elevated stress on the left ventricle of the heart.

As people age, their systolic blood pressure increases mostly because the large arteries in the body begin to stiffen. The aorta, the main artery in the body, is especially susceptible to hardening. Diastolic pressure increases until a person reaches about fifty years old. After this time, it lowers. This decrease is caused by the stiffening of the arteries, which slows blood flow. The increase in systolic and decrease in diastolic pressure causes pulse pressure to increase as a person ages. For example, a twenty-five-year- old may have a blood pressure of 130/90 and a pulse pressure of 40. When

2452 • Pulse rate

this individual reaches age ninety, his blood pressure may be 160/75, making his pulse pressure 85.

Widened pulse pressure is pulse pressure higher than 40. Pulse pressure higher than 60 can put certain people, especially men, at an increased risk of developing cardiovascular disease. Sometimes health conditions—such as hyperthyroidism (overactive thyroid), anemia (low iron), and a leaky aortic valve—can lead to a widened pulse pressure. Patients with diabetes and a widened pulse pressure (sometimes not even as high as 60) are at an increased risk for heart attack. People with high pulse pressure should take efforts to reduce their systolic pressure, which decreases the risk of cardiovascular disease and other heart problems. Some treatments include stress reduction, diet and lifestyle changes, and medication.

While not as common, low pulse pressure, also known as narrow or narrowed pulse pressure, is pulse pressure under 40. It can be an indicator of several health problems, such as poor heart function, congestive heart failure, shock, and more. Once the underlying medical issue is treated, pulse pressure usually returns to normal. Persistent low pulse pressure usually is treated in the same way as high pulse pressure.

—Angela Harmon;
updated by Geraldine Marrocco

For Further Information:

Davis, William. "What Is Pulse Pressure?" *Health Central*, 3 May 2010, www.healthcentral.com/high-blood-pressure/c/58370/110775/pulse. Accessed 16 Dec. 2016.

Humphreys, Jo. "Widened Pulse Pressure." *Med Health Daily*, www.medhealthdaily.com/widened-pulse-pressure. Accessed 16 Dec. 2016.

Marchione, Victor. "Widened Pulse Pressure May Increase the Risk of Heart Attacks and Cardiovascular Disease." *Bel Marra Health*, 17 Nov. 2016, www.belmarrahealth.com/widened-pulse-pressure-increase-risk-heart-attacks-cardiovascular-disease. Accessed 16 Dec. 2016.

"Pulse Measurement." *WebMD*, 21 Aug. 2015, www.webmd.com/heart-disease/pulse-measurement#1. Accessed 16 Dec. 2016.

Sheps, Sheldon G. "What Is Pulse Pressure? How Important Is Pulse Pressure to Your Overall Health?" *Mayo Clinic*, 2 Aug. 2016, www.mayoclinic.org/diseases-conditions/high-blood-pressure/expert-answers/pulse-pressure/faq-20058189. Accessed 16 Dec. 2016.

Weber, Craig. "Pulse Pressure." *Verywell*, 18 Aug. 2016, www.verywell.com/pulse-pressure-1763964. Accessed 16 Dec. 2016.

"What Is Pulse Pressure?—Definition, Variation & Normal Range." *Study.com*, study.com/academy/lesson/what-is-pulse-pressure-definition-variation-normal-range.html. Accessed 16 Dec. 2016.

Yildiran, Tansel, et al. "Low Pulse Pressure as a Predictor of Death in Patients with Mild to Advanced Heart Failure." *Texas Heart Institute Journal*, vol. 37, no. 3, 2010, pp. 284-290, www.ncbi.nlm.nih.gov/pmc/articles/PMC2879196. Accessed 16 Dec. 2016.

PULSE RATE

Category: Anatomy
Also known as: Heart rate
Anatomy or system affected: Blood, blood vessels, circulatory system, heart
Specialties and related fields: Anesthesiology, cardiology, critical care, emergency medicine, endocrinology, exercise physiology, family medicine, general surgery, internal medicine, neonatology, nursing, pediatrics, physical therapy, sports medicine, vascular medicine
Definition: The number of pulse beats per minute. The normal pulse rate in an average adult fluctuates with exercise, injury, illness, and emotional response.

STRUCTURE AND FUNCTIONS

Pulse rate is a measure of how many times the heart beats per minute. An average pulse rate for an adult is 70-72 beats per minute (bpm), but pulse rates from 60 to 100 are within the adult range of normal. In adults, a pulse rate below 60 bpm is termed bradycardia, while a rate above 100 bpm is termed tachycardia.

The surges of pressure passing through the arterial system are palpated by placing the index and middle fingers over a pulse point. The thumb should not be used, because it has a relatively large artery that may give a false reading of the examiner's own pulse. The fingers should exert light but firm pressure. The number of heartbeats is counted, and the pulse rate is expressed in number of beats per minute.

Pulse locations and their general uses include the radial artery (inner aspect of the wrist on the thumb side), used most commonly for routine assessment of adult pulse rates; femoral (in the groin), popliteal (behind the knee), posterior tibial (in the groove between the Achilles tendon and the tibia), and dorsalis pedis (on the instep of the foot), used for assessment of circulation in the legs; apical (at the left midclavicular line and the fifth intercostal space), used for infants and small children and for cardiovascular problems; and apical-radial (combination of apical and radial pulses), used for persons with cardiac arrhythmias.

An apical pulse is taken by listening to the heart with a stethoscope placed over the apex of the heart, which is located about three inches (7.5 centimeters) to the left of the midclavicular line. Taking an apical-radial pulse requires two persons, as one person counts the apical rate of the heart while the other person simultaneously palpates and counts the radial pulse for one full minute. All pulse points may be counted for thirty-second intervals and that number multiplied by two to arrive at the number of beats per minute. However, this method will give a false reading if the rhythm is irregular. The most accurate reading is obtained by counting the pulse for one full minute.

DISORDERS AND DISEASES

A variety of diseases and conditions affect cardiovascular function and thus influence pulse rate, including neurologic, cardiopulmonary, and renal disorders. Many factors aside from disease can influence the pulse as well. Fever, fear, anxiety, anger, and exercise will increase pulse rate, while rest and relaxation will decrease the number of beats per minute. Athletes often have a low resting pulse rate because their hearts pump very efficiently.

—*Jane C. Norman, PhD, RN, CNE*

See also Blood pressure; Cardiology; Cardiology, pediatric; Circulation; Diagnosis; Exercise physiology; Heart; Hypertension; Nursing; Physical examination; Signs and symptoms.

For Further Information:
"All about Heart Rate (Pulse)." *American Heart Association*, October 15, 2012.
Craven, Ruth F., Constance J. Hirnle, and Sharon Jensen. *Fundamentals of Nursing: Human Health and Function*. 7th ed. Philadelphia: Lippincott Williams & Wilkins, 2012.
Katz, Arnold M. *Physiology of the Heart*. 5th ed. Philadelphia: Lippincott Williams & Wilkins, 2010.
Malik, Marek, and A. John Camm, eds. *Heart Rate Variability*. New York: John Wiley & Sons, 1995.
Vorvick, Linda J., et al. "Pulse." *MedlinePlus*, March 22, 2013.

PYELONEPHRITIS

Category: Disease/Disorder
   Also known as: Kidney infection
Anatomy or system affected: Bladder, kidneys, ureters, urethra.
Specialties and related fields: Emergency medicine, family medicine, internal medicine, nephrology, obstetrics, urology
Definition: Inflammation of the kidney as the result of a bacterial infection in the bladder.

Key terms:
bacterial colonization: the presence of bacteria in an area that does not lead to infection
metabolites: the molecular breakdown products of a substance
renal: referring to the kidney
urinary catheter: a soft plastic drainage tube placed in the bladder to facilitate urination
vesicoureteral reflux: abnormal backflow of urine from the bladder into the ureter during urination, causing a predisposition to pyelonephritis
virulence: level of aggressiveness of an organism

CAUSES AND SYMPTOMS
The urinary tract consists of the kidneys, ureters, bladder, and urethra. The kidneys serve as filters that excrete unnecessary substances from the blood and retain essential ones. For example, the kidneys excrete excesses of water, electrolytes, or metabolites of drugs and other ingested substances that might otherwise build up to harmful levels in the body. Conversely, the kidneys can also preserve these substances when necessary. This is the case in dehydration, in which the water in the bloodstream is actively reabsorbed to prevent further losses.

The excess water and waste products filtered from the blood becomes urine, which drains from the kidneys through narrow tubes known as "ureters." These tubes connect the kidneys to the bladder, which is the storage reservoir for the urine. At the appropriate time, urine is released from the bladder and carried through the urethra, another small tube passing through the genitals, to exit the body.

Because of the differences in male and female anatomy, urinary tract infections (UTIs) arise more frequently in women. The female urethra is short, approximately four centimeters in length, and is located in close proximity to the vaginal and anal openings. In contrast, the male urethra travels the length of the penis and is distinctly separate from the anal opening.

Although harmless bacteria are normally found living in the vaginal area, it is typically bacteria from the bowel that cause UTIs. Given the proximity of the anal opening to the vagina, it is relatively easy for these bacteria to gain entry. Other factors that promote bacterial colonization of the vaginal and urethral openings include antibiotic use, genital infections, and use of contraceptives such as diaphragms. These bacteria may also be pushed into the bladder by pressure on the woman's urethra that occurs during sexual intercourse. Although the simple act of urination often serves to flush out these organisms, the number of bacteria, the virulence of the strain, and the individual's immune system are all important factors in whether an infection develops.

INFORMATION ON PYELONEPHRITIS

Causes: Spread of bacteria from bladder to kidney; may result from catheter contamination or obstruction from kidney stones, cancer, prostate enlargement or other anatomical abnormalities

Symptoms: Those associated with bladder infection (discomfort with urination, frequent urination, urgency), fever and chills, flank pain, nausea and vomiting, diarrhea

Duration: Ten to fourteen days

Treatments: Antibiotics (oral or intravenous), hospitalization, possibly surgery to remove obstruction

In men, the urethra passes through the prostate gland prior to entering the penis. The prostate gland typically enlarges with age and can encroach on the urethra, making drainage of urine more difficult. When urine is not drained completely from the bladder, any bacteria that have entered can proliferate, increasing the risk of infection. Therefore, men with prostate enlargement are predisposed to UTIs. Men who participate in anal intercourse are also at increased risk.

Other important risk factors for UTIs include pregnancy, neurologic diseases affecting bladder muscle function, presence of a urinary catheter, and (in children) the condition of vesicoureteral reflux.

In general, it is thought that pyelonephritis develops when bacteria present in the bladder are able to ascend upward toward the kidney. Often, the symptoms of a bladder infection, such as discomfort with urination, frequent urination, and sensation of an urgent need to urinate, precede such symptoms as fever, chills, pain in the mid back or sides, nausea, vomiting, and diarrhea. The latter symptoms are suggestive of pyelonephritis rather than simple bladder infection. Older individuals may develop confusion or disorientation.

TREATMENT AND THERAPY

The majority of patients with pyelonephritis respond well to antibiotic therapy. Usually, oral antibiotics are appropriate; however, in cases where vomiting precludes their use, intravenous (IV) antibiotics are used. In cases where patients are severely ill or dehydrated, hospitalization may be required. Treatment for ten to fourteen days is standard. There are typically no long-term consequences once the infection is treated.

Certain factors may complicate the treatment of pyelonephritis, requiring more aggressive antibiotic therapy, hospitalization, and possibly invasive procedures. Patients who have an abnormal urinary tract because of the presence of a catheter or other external drainage tube are more likely to harbor antibiotic-resistant organisms. Similarly, patients with diabetes or immune system disorders are at risk for resistant germs.

Patients with an obstruction in the urinary tract as a result of kidney stones, cancer, prostate enlargement, or other anatomical abnormalities may require surgical intervention to remove the blockage. It is difficult to eradicate the bacteria completely unless infected urine is removed by drainage.

Patients with underlying kidney diseases require more aggressive care to ensure no further loss of renal function. Pregnant women have a higher incidence of complications from pyelonephritis and typically require hospitalization. Antibiotics are also selected differently for these women to avoid harm to the fetus.

PERSPECTIVE AND PROSPECTS

The development of newer antibiotics that are highly active against bacteria responsible for most UTIs has made successful treatment of pyelonephritis straightforward. In addition, these antibiotics can achieve high levels in the bloodstream and kidneys when taken orally, making treatment at home rather than in the hospital safe and effective for many patients.

Procedures done with fiber-optic technology allow a urologist to extract an obstructing kidney stone without a surgical incision. Miniature cameras can be passed upward through the urethra and bladder and into the ureter, and miniature instruments can be used to remove the stone. In addition, specialized radiologists are able to pass a drainage tube directly into the kidney with X-ray guidance, without the need for an open surgical procedure. Both of these interventions are useful in cases of pyelonephritis complicated by obstruction.

Patients who experience frequent UTIs should use preventive measures such as copious fluid intake, urinating after intercourse, wiping "front to back" after urination, and urinating often throughout the day. Some women may require a prophylactic dose of antibiotic after intercourse.

A 2011 study funded by the National Center for Complementary and Alternative Medicine, part of the National Institutes of Health, found that, contrary to expectations, regular cranberry juice consumption failed to prevent UTI recurrence. The study was a double-blind, randomized, placebo-controlled trial conducted on otherwise healthy college-aged women and was the largest to test the efficacy of cranberry juice in preventing UTIs from recurring in this high-risk group.

—*Muneeza Khan, MD, FAAFP*

See also: Antibiotics; Bacterial infections; Kidney cancer; Kidney disorders; Kidneys; Nephritis; Nephrology; Nephrology, pediatric; Prostate enlargement; Stone removal; Stones; Urinary disorders; Urinary system; Urology, Urology, pediatric.

For Further Information:
Beers, Mark H., et al., editors. *The Merck Manual of Diagnosis and Therapy.* 18th ed., Merck Research Laboratories, 2006.
Longo, Dan Louis., et al., editors. *Harrison's Principles of Internal Medicine.* 18th ed., McGraw-Hill, 2012.
National Institute of Diabetes and Digestive and Kidney Diseases. "Kidney Infection (Pyelonephritis)." *NIDK,* www.niddk.nih.gov/health-information/urologic-diseases/kidney-infection-pyelonephritis.
National Kidney and Urologic Diseases Information Clearing House. "Cranberry Juice Fails to Prevent Recurrence of Urinary Tract Infections." *National Kidney and Urologic Diseases Information Clearinghouses: Urologic Diseases Research Update, Summer 2011,* Sept. 2011.
Parker, James N., and Philip M. Parker, editors. *The Official Patient's Sourcebook on Pyelonephritis.* ICON Group, 2007.
Savitsky, Diane. "Kidney Infection." *Health Library,* 26 Nov. 2012.
Shaikh, Nader, and Nina Tolkoff-Rubin. "Pyelonephritis: Kidney Infection." *National Institutes of Health: National Kidney and Urologic Diseases Information Clearinghouse (NKUDIC),* 11 June 2012.

Pyloric stenosis

Category: Disease/Disorder
Anatomy or system affected: Gastrointestinal system, stomach
Specialties and related fields: Gastroenterology, general surgery, pediatrics
Definition: An obstruction of the stomach in infancy caused by muscular hypertrophy of the gastric outlet.

CAUSES AND SYMPTOMS

The exact cause of pyloric stenosis is unknown. The condition is usually characterized by nonbilious projectile vomiting beginning at three weeks of age, although it may occur as early as the first week of life or as late as five months of age. The vomiting is progressive and leads to poor growth and dehydration. Initially, the vomit resembles the fluid that the infant ingested, but it may become brownish in later stages of the disease.

TREATMENT AND THERAPY

Pyloric stenosis is diagnosed through palpation of a small, firm mass, similar to the size and shape of an olive, in the mid-upper abdomen. This mass is not palpable in all infants with pyloric stenosis. In these cases, imaging procedures such as an upper gastrointestinal (GI) series or ultrasound of the upper abdomen can confirm the diagnosis.

The initial treatment of pyloric stenosis involves correction of dehydration with intravenous fluids. The surgical treatment is called a pyloromyotomy. After the infant is anesthetized, an incision is made in the right-upper abdomen, through which the pyloric mass is removed. The pyloric muscle is split down to the mucosa, or lining of the stomach. Postoperative vomiting is common and is probably caused by slow emptying of fluids from the stomach. The vomiting usually resolves, however, such that the infant may resume feeding within twenty-four hours after surgery, with advancement to regular feeding within two days. This operation is usually curative, with low mortality and recurrence rates.

PERSPECTIVE AND PROSPECTS

Pyloric stenosis was first described in 1788. Harald Hirschsprung coined the term "congenital hypertrophic pyloric stenosis" in 1888. At that time, approximately one-fourth of infants affected by pyloric stenosis died without treatment, while more than half of the infants with this condition died after surgery. A significant advance in the treatment of pyloric stenosis came in 1912 when Conrad Ramstedt reported performing a pyloromyotomy. The procedure that he described remains the standard treatment.

—*David A. Gremse, MD*

See also Birth defects; Congenital disorder; Dehydration; Failure to thrive; Gastroenterology; Gastroenterology, pediatric; Gastrointestinal disorders; Gastrointestinal system; Nausea and vomiting; Neonatology; Obstruction; Pediatrics; Surgery, pediatric.

For Further Information:
Kliegman, Robert and Waldo E. Nelson, eds. *Nelson Textbook of Pediatrics.* 19th ed. Philadelphia: Saunders/Elsevier, 2011.
Christian, Janet L., and Janet L. Greger. *Nutrition for Living.* 4th ed. Redwood City, Calif.: Benjamin/Cummings, 1994.
Cockburn, Forrester, et al. *Children's Medicine and Surgery.* New York: Oxford University Press, 1996.
Garrow, J. S., W. P. T. James, and A. Ralph, eds. *Human Nutrition and Dietetics.* 10th ed. repr. New York: Churchill Livingstone, 2004.
Kaneshiro, Neil K. "Pyloric Stenosis." *MedlinePlus,* August 2, 2011.
Keet, Albertus D. *The Pyloric Sphincteric Cylinder in Health and Disease.* New York: Springer, 2012.
Martin, Richard J., Avroy A. Fanaroff, and Michele C. Walsh, eds. *Fanaroff and Martin's Neonatal-Perinatal Medicine: Diseases of the Fetus and Infant.* 9th ed. St. Louis, Mo.: Mosby/Elsevier, 2011.
Smith, Nathalie. "Pyloric Stenosis." *Health Library,* September 26, 2012.

Q

QUADRIPLEGIA

Category: Disease/Disorder
Anatomy or system affected: Arms, legs, nervous system, spine
Specialties and related fields: Neurology
Definition: Devastating, permanent paralysis of all four extremities below the level of injury to the spinal cord.

CAUSES AND SYMPTOMS

Quadriplegia may result from spinal cord injury, especially in the area of the fifth to seventh cervical vertebrae. Such injury usually follows trauma or vertebral pressure on the soft tissue of the cord. Damage causes flaccidity in the arms and legs, as well as loss of power and sensation below the level of injury. Spinal cord injuries above the fifth cervical vertebra dramatically affect other body systems as well.

For example, cardiovascular complications result from a block in the sympathetic nervous system that allows the parasympathetic system to dominate. One possible complication is hypotension (blood pressure below 90/60) resulting from vasodilation, which allows blood to pool in the veins of the extremities and thereby slows the venous blood return to the heart. Another complication is low body temperature (96 degrees Fahrenheit or lower) from the inability of blood vessels to constrict efficiently, allowing constant close blood vessel contact with the body surface and consequent heat loss. Bradycardia (slow heart rate) may occur from stimulation of the heart by the vagus nerve and absence of the inhibiting effects of the sympathetic system. A decrease in peristalsis, the movement of food through the gastrointestinal system, results from various types of shock. Respiratory complications, a major cause of death, may occur from damage to the upper cervical cord. Autonomic dysreflexia may occur in injuries above the fourth thoracic vertebra, in which a severed connection between the brain and the spinal cord produces an exaggerated autonomic response to such stimuli as distended bladder, fecal impaction, infection, decubitus ulcers, or surgical manipulation. The key symptom of autonomic dysreflexia is hypertension (high blood pressure).

A complete physical and neurologic examination must assess remaining motor function and determine

> ### INFORMATION ON QUADRIPLEGIA
>
> **Causes:** Spinal cord injury
> **Symptoms:** Flaccidity in arms and legs, loss of power and sensation below level of injury; complications may include low blood pressure, low body temperature, slow heart rate, decreased peristalsis, respiratory problems
> **Duration:** Chronic
> **Treatments:** Immobilization of neck and spine, stabilization, steroids, glycopyrrolate, Foley catheter, diuretics, surgical fusion, aggressive respiratory therapy (often intubation and ventilator assistance)

if the cord injury is complete or partial. Detailed information about the trauma may help health care providers anticipate other related injuries. computed tomography (CT) scans can identify fractures, dislocations, subluxation, and blockage in the spinal cord. X-rays of the head, chest, and abdomen can rule out underlying injuries. Since this type of injury has such far-reaching physiologic effects, significant laboratory data assessing respiratory, hepatic (liver), and pancreatic functions are necessary to provide a baseline.

TREATMENT AND THERAPY

The treatment of quadriplegia begins at the scene of the accident, with immobilization of the neck and spine. At the hospital, methods of immobilization include insertion of Gardner Wells tongs or halo traction. A turning frame helps prevent pulmonary complications such as atelectasis (partial lung collapse), pneumonia, and pulmonary embolism; cardiovascular complications such as blood clot formation and orthostatic hypotension; and other complications such as kidney stones, muscle atrophy, decubitus ulcers, and infections.

After stabilization, therapy consists of steroids, intravenous glycopyrrolate to maintain the integrity of the gastrointestinal tract, insertion of a Foley catheter, and administration of a potent diuretic such as mannitol. This treatment regimen is followed for ten days to decrease spinal cord edema (swelling). Unchecked edema further compromises the blood supply to sensitive cord tissue, producing irreversible cord damage. Prevention of ascending cord edema preserves higher cord segments and maximum function in the upper extremities. Each cord segment preserved means greater potential for rehabilitation.

After ten days of therapy, surgical fusion stabilizes the unstable spine. Surgery must also remove bone fragments that can irritate the spinal cord and, in later stages, aggravate spasticity. Another necessary part of treatment is aggressive respiratory therapy that, in the intubated patient, includes instillation of three to five milliliters of normal saline solution and bagging the patient before thorough suctioning to remove secretions and prevent mucus plugs. In cervical cord injuries above the fifth vertebra, intubation and ventilator assistance are always necessary.

—Jane C. Norman, PhD, RN, CNE

See also Head and neck disorders; Hemiplegia; Laminectomy and spinal fusion; Nervous system; Neuralgia, neuritis, and neuropathy; Neuroimaging; Neurology; Neurology, pediatric; Paralysis; Paraplegia; Physical rehabilitation; Spinal cord disorders; Spine, vertebrae, and disks.

For Further Information:

Asbury, Arthur K., et al., eds. *Diseases of the Nervous System: Clinical Neuroscience and Therapeutic Principles.* 3d ed. New York: Cambridge University Press, 2002.
Berczeller, Peter H., and Mary F. Bezkor. *Medical Complications of Quadriplegia.* Chicago: Year Book Medical, 1986.
Christopher and Dana Reeve Foundation. "Paralysis Resource Center." *Christopher and Dana Reeve Foundation,* 2013.
Mayo Clinic. "Spinal Cord Injury." *Mayo Clinic,* October 22, 2011.
MedlinePlus. "Paralysis." *MedlinePlus,* August 9, 2013.
Rowland, Lewis P., ed. *Merritt's Textbook of Neurology.* 12th ed. Philadelphia: Lippincott Williams & Wilkins, 2010.
Smith, Nathalie. "Quadriplegia and Paraplegia." *Health Library,* March 15, 2013.
Victor, Maurice, and Allan H. Ropper. *Adams and Victor's Principles of Neurology.* 9th ed. New York: McGraw-Hill, 2009.

QUINSY

Category: Disease/Disorder
Also known as: Peritonsillar abscess
Anatomy or system affected: Glands, lungs, mouth, throat
Specialties and related fields: Otorhinolaryngology
Definition: An abscess usually forming in the peritonsillar space behind the tonsils.

CAUSES AND SYMPTOMS

Quinsy, also called peritonsillar abscess, is a rare disorder. Medical professionals most often diagnose the

> **INFORMATION ON QUINSY**
> **Causes:** Spread of bacterial infection (usually streptococci) after extreme tonsillitis
> **Symptoms:** Pus-filled tissues in throat, swollen tonsils, sometimes infection of palate and lungs, fever, chills, tender throat glands, painful swallowing, facial swelling, drooling, hoarseness, bad breath, earache, headache, fatigue; complications may include pneumonia, meningitis, heart inflammation, fluid surrounding lungs
> **Duration:** Acute, sometimes recurrent
> **Treatments:** Prevention through antibiotics, abscess drainage, tonsillectomy if needed

condition in young adults. Primarily after extreme tonsillitis, bacterial infections (usually streptococci) spread from one or both tonsils to adjacent tissues, which become pus-filled. In addition to the throat, the infection may cover the palate and extend to the lungs, potentially blocking the airway.

Patients develop a fever and tender throat glands. Some people experience chills. Because swollen tonsils shift and push the uvula aside, patients often are unable to open their mouths normally, a condition known as trismus, and swallowing is painful. Patients sometimes lean their heads in the direction of the abscess. Other symptoms include swelling of facial tissues, drooling, fatigue, earache, and headache. Some patients become hoarse and have foul breath.

Quinsy is often prevented because patients with tonsillitis are administered antibiotics and are monitored to stop infections from spreading. A person who has had tonsillitis and who develops symptoms of quinsy should consult health care professionals. Sore throats that do not heal with antibiotics or that become worse alert physicians to the possibility of quinsy.

Medical professionals evaluate patients for quinsy by examining the tonsils for swelling and abnormal reddening of the mouth, throat, and chest tissues. In some cases of quinsy, the tonsils may appear normal. Samples of aspirated abscess fluid are examined for bacteria. Ultrasound or computer imaging is used if patients cannot open their mouths.

TREATMENT AND THERAPY

Physicians are divided on the preferred treatment for quinsy. Surgical procedures involve draining pus from abscesses through incisions or needle aspiration. Studies have shown that incision drainage is effective at stopping quinsy and that needle aspiration is more likely to result in additional abscessing. Tonsillectomy specifically for quinsy is usually advised only if no other treatments are effective. Approximately 10 to 15 percent of patients undergoing treatment experience recurring quinsy.

Emergency surgery is necessary if quinsy affects breathing. Other possible complications include pneumonia, meningitis, heart inflammation (pericarditis), and fluid surrounding the lungs (pleural effusion). Rarely, quinsy patients develop endocarditis, a bacterial infection of the heart. Quinsy patients should seek medical care if they have chest pains, coughing, or breathing complications.

PERSPECTIVE AND PROSPECTS
The word "quinsy" is based on references made by the ancient Greeks to abscessed throats. As early as the fourteenth century, medical literature included details about the peritonsillar space. The term "quinsy" was appropriated after that time to describe sore throats and tonsils. Modern physicians disproved claims that President George Washington died from quinsy, as contemporary sources had claimed. Since the 1980s, researchers have been evaluating the most effective treatments for quinsy. The *Haemophilus influenzae* type b vaccine, first administered in 1987, has minimized quinsy occurrence.

—*Elizabeth D. Schafer, PhD*

See also Abscess drainage; Abscesses; Antibiotics; Bacterial infections; Otorhinolaryngology; Respiration; Sore throat; Strep throat; Tonsillectomy and adenoid removal; Tonsillitis; Tonsils.

For Further Information:
Ben-Joseph, Elana Pearl. "What Is a Peritonsillar Abscess?" *TeensHealth*. Nemours Foundation, May 2012.
Bluestone, Charles D., et al., eds. *Pediatric Otolaryngology*. 4th ed. 2 vols. Philadelphia: W. B. Saunders, 2003.
Gleeson, Michael, et al, ed. *Scott-Brown's Otolaryngology: Head and Neck Surgery*. 7th ed. Boston: Butterworth-Heinemann, 2008.
Litin, Scott C., ed. *Mayo Clinic Family Health Book*. 4th ed. New York: HarperResource, 2009.
Neff, Deanna M., and Michael Woods. "Peritonsillar Abscess." *Health Library*, Mar. 15, 2013.
Schwartz, Seth, et al. "Periotonsillar Abscess." *MedlinePlus*, Nov. 9, 2012.
Woodson, Gayle E. *Ear, Nose, and Throat Disorders in Primary Care*. Philadelphia: W. B. Saunders, 2001.

R

RABIES

Category: Disease/Disorder
Anatomy or system affected: Brain, muscles, musculoskeletal system, nervous system, psychic-emotional system
Specialties and related fields: Epidemiology, neurology, public health, virology
Definition: a virus that attacks the nerve cells and is most often transmitted by the bite of a rabid animal; control of the disease is accomplished through vaccination of pets and immediate immunization of humans if exposed to the disease; once symptoms occur in humans, the disease is nearly always fatal

Key terms:

anticoagulant: a chemical that blocks the clotting of blood; some anticoagulants stimulate internal bleeding when ingested by vampire bats and can be used as a method of extermination

epidemiology: the study of the maintenance and spread of disease in a population

fixed virus: a virus that has been repeatedly cultured in the laboratory so that it has lost its natural variation and is more predictable in experiments

passage: one of the culture steps in the production of a fixed virus

replication: the reproduction of a virus; many copies are made within a host cell, then released to infect other host cells

reservoir: the host species in which a parasite is maintained in each area and from which it may infect other species, initiating an epidemic

street virus: a virus derived directly from a natural source; a fixed virus is produced from a street virus by several passages through an artificial culture system

sylvatic rabies: rabies in wild animal populations (as opposed to rabies in domestic animals and pets)

CAUSES AND SYMPTOMS

Rabies is caused by a bullet-shaped virus that attacks warm-blooded animals, especially mammals. The virus can enter many types of mammal cells and cause them to produce and bud off new viruses. However, it is particularly adept at attacking nerve cells and glandular cells. This combination enhances the virus's chance of being transmitted to another host.

Dog bites are a potential source of rabies. Photo via iStock/YuriyGreen. [Used under license.]

The following events occur in an untreated human being after being bitten by a rabid animal. The bite introduces large amounts of saliva, which contains abundant rabies virus because of the virus's efficient growth in salivary glands. The virus enters muscle cells in the vicinity of the bite and replicates there. The new viruses then enter the nerve cells that carry signals from the brain and spinal cord to the muscle cells. They move along these nerve cells to the spinal cord, eventually making their way to the brain. The viruses replicate at certain sites as they ascend the nerve and spinal cord. In the brain, they replicate especially well in the centers that control emotions. Once established in the brain and spinal cord, the virus moves out of these organs along the nerves to most body organs. The salivary glands are favored targets in this migration.

As a result of its extensive migrations, the virus is present in many body tissues. Yet, the critical ones for the pathology and transmission of the disease are the brain and salivary glands, where the virus reproduces especially well. To understand this relationship between transmission and pathology, consider the dog or other animal that bit the human being described above. A sequence of events similar to that described for the human being has occurred in the animal. The viruses attacking the emotional centers of the animal's brain initiated the characteristic aggressive state in which it wandered, attacking anything it encountered. Viruses attacking the brain also stimulated the production and release of copious amounts of saliva, giving rise to another familiar symptom of rabies: frothing at the mouth. The viruses reproducing in the salivary glands and the excessive salivation assured that an abundance of the virus would be chewed into the wound.

A human victim's time sequence and pathology include an incubation period that may range from ten days to a year; in most victims, however, it is between two and eight weeks. During this time, the virus replicates in cells at the site of the bite and moves to the central nervous system. As the nervous system begins to be involved, generalized symptoms begin. These include fever, headaches, and nausea and last about a week. Neurologic symptoms then develop, including hyperactivity, seizures, and hallucinations. The throat sometimes becomes so sore and prone to spasms that the patient has trouble swallowing and fears choking while drinking. Another common name for rabies, hydrophobia (literally, fear of water), is based on this aspect of the disease. Paralysis and coma occur about a week after the neurologic symptoms, and death follows a few days later. Once the symptoms begin in a human being, the disease is nearly always fatal.

A similar sequence of events occurs in dogs, though the timing is somewhat different, and dogs occasionally recover. The aggressive stage described above is called the "furious stage" in animals. The gradual development of paralysis is called the "paralytic or dumb stage." Both phases may occur in dogs, or the furious stage may be bypassed. Still, death commonly occurs soon after symptoms begin.

Rabies in wildlife is called "sylvatic rabies," and the species of wildlife involved differ according to geographic area. Some species act as the virus's reservoir and as the source of rabies epidemics in humans or their pets. In the arctic regions of North America and Eurasia, arctic foxes and wolves are the most important hosts of sylvatic rabies. Red and gray foxes and skunks play important roles in spreading the disease in various parts of eastern Canada and the United States, as do raccoons. Some investigators believe that weasels and their relatives are important carriers in maintaining the virus in nature in many areas. However, they are not particularly important in the direct transfer of the virus to humans. Bats are common sources of rabies throughout the United States, but especially in the southern part of the country. They play a major role in rabies epidemiology in Mexico and Central and South America, where the disease often occurs in vampire bats.

In 2010, there were 6,153 cases in animals and only 2 cases of rabies in humans reported in the United States and Puerto Rico. Raccoons (36.5 percent), bats (23.2 percent), skunks (23.5 percent), and foxes (7 percent) were the most commonly infected animals. In 2010. 8 percent of rabies reports were for domestic species. Surprisingly, there were more cats than dogs reported with rabies, undoubtedly due to rabies vaccination programs for dogs.

Other mammals, both wild and domestic, are attacked by the virus. Still, they are not important in transmitting rabies between species or acting as reservoirs. Examples of these species are grazing and browsing animals such as cattle and deer, which seldom bite other animals and are not likely to pass the virus to other creatures. However, many of these animals die from rabies, and the economic and ecological impact of these deaths may be great.

The virus attacks these animals in the same manner as humans and dogs, showing similar symptoms. Rabid wild animals do not always suffer a furious stage. Raccoons, for example, often skip the furious stage and go directly

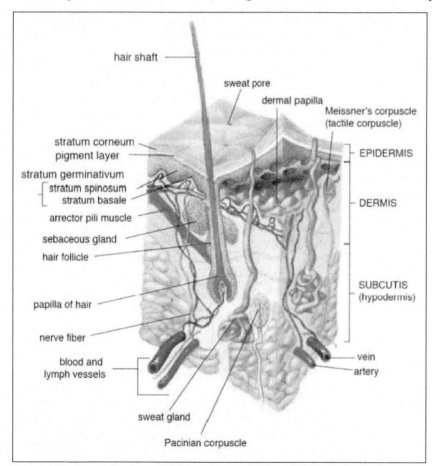

Anatomy of the human skin. Image by National Library Medicine, NIH. [Public domain.]

into the dumb stage. Early in this stage, they may lose their fear of humans and appear to be friendly. If left alone, they seldom attack, but humans who approach these "friendly" raccoons may be bitten and exposed to rabies. Many bat species also do not go through the furious stage; a bat suffering from dumb rabies is easily caught and may bite if handled, exposing the handler to rabies. Unlike humans, bats, skunks, raccoons, and other wildlife often survive the symptoms of rabies.

In addition to the disease it causes in humans and their pets, the rabies virus has negatively impacted human society. Rabies transmitted to cattle by vampire bats has had a devastating economic effect on the cattle industry in all of Latin America. Rabies in red foxes has occasionally negatively affected Canada's fur industry. In many parts of the world, wildlife populations may be periodically decimated by rabies epidemics, which sometimes reduces the population of a species of recreational importance to humans or one critical to the ecological stability of a region.

TREATMENT AND THERAPY
Active immunization by vaccination can be used after exposure to rabies because of the relatively long latency period of the virus. If a rabid animal has bitten a person, symptoms usually do not appear for two or more weeks. Prompt vaccination after the bite induces the production of antibodies that attack the virus and neutralize it before it reaches the central nervous system. Two other precautions are often taken. The wound is cleaned and treated with antiviral agents. Passive immunity is often produced by injecting antirabies antiserum into the victim.

The rabies vaccinations of early immunization series were numerous, extremely painful, and not always successful. Since the early twentieth century, it has been possible to determine whether the attacking animal was rabid and thus whether this painful treatment was necessary. The animal was sacrificed, and its brain was sectioned and stained. When treated this way, a rabid animal's brain cells often display Negri bodies, named for the scientist who first described them. They are the sites of production of new virus particles in the brain cell, and their presence indicates the need for vaccination of the victim. Even though the immunization sequence that was first developed was painful, the certain death that followed the onset of symptoms made immunization imperative if there was any possibility of rabies exposure.

Improved immunization sequences and rabies tests have been developed. These immunization sequences are refined and nearly infallible and require only three inoculations, and are no more painful than most shots. Tests using antibodies are more rapid and reliable at detecting the presence of the rabies virus than the Negri bodies test.

In contrast to the postexposure immunization described above, preexposure immunization is used to protect persons who might be exposed to rabies in their normal activities and protect pets from contracting rabies. Since the overwhelming majority of human rabies cases come from dog bites, pet vaccination is the most important part of the successful rabies control programs in developed countries. Laws requiring the immunization of pets against rabies and leash laws (which require that pets be controlled and not allowed to wander freely) have effectively reduced human rabies in these countries.

Because wildlife may harbor rabies, attempts have been made to control or eliminate the disease by killing (culling) or immunizing wildlife. Neither approach has been particularly successful, and troublesome side effects accompany the first. The purpose of culling members of host species is to reduce the host population below the point that will sustain the rabies virus's population. This method is based on the idea that each infected host must, on average, infect at least one other susceptible host before it dies for the parasite to persist in the population. The lower the host population, the lower the chance of one host meeting another, and thus the lower the probability of an infected host infecting other population members. Yet many of the methods of culling (trapping and poisoning, for example) are not species-specific, and members of other species are killed, sometimes in large numbers. Culling has also been ineffective in many cases. It is most successful in small, isolated areas with a low probability of reinvasion.

Instead of reducing the population size of the host, the goal of immunization is to increase the number of members that are immune. Oral immunization by scattering bait containing rabies vaccine has shown promising results in reducing rabies in foxes, coyotes, and raccoons.

An argument against immunization of wildlife to control human rabies is based on the success of the control programs and can be stated as follows. Immunization and regulation of pets, preexposure immunization for humans regularly exposed to rabies, and effective postexposure treatment have already minimized the incidence of human rabies in developed nations. Therefore, wildlife immunization is not necessary for the control of human rabies. In developing nations, where human rabies is still a serious disease, all the potential solutions strain available resources. However, the most cost-effective solution would be in use in developed countries. Most public health professionals agree that wildlife immunization might be an effective way to increase the population size of a wildlife species that is normally susceptible to rabies, if desirable.

In Latin America, vampire bats carry rabies. These bats deleteriously affect the cattle industry. Culling the bats has been attempted repeatedly, often unsuccessfully, and with serious side effects. For example, other bat species, some of which are important to insect control and the pollination of fruit trees, have been regular victims of indiscriminate attempts at vampire bat control by culling.

A more effective and less ecologically disruptive method for controlling vampire bats employs anticoagulants. These chemicals stimulate bleeding in the digestive tract of vampire bats that swallow them, resulting in death. The anticoagulant can be applied directly to the backs of the vampire bats. It will spread through the bat population when the bats groom one another at the roosting colony. Alternatively, an anticoagulant can be injected into a cow's rumen, the enlarged first chamber of its four-part stomach. The anticoagulant is then absorbed into the animal's blood and spread to vampire bats when they feed on the cattle.

Each method has reduced the number of vampire bat bites in cattle by 90 percent in test areas, but each has drawbacks. Direct application to these bats requires extensive netting or trapping, special equipment, and workers skilled in vampire bat identification. The rumen injection technique requires expensive equipment and workers experienced in handling large numbers of cattle. In developing countries, either combination can be difficult to finance.

Education is another important aspect of rabies control. While dogs are the most common source of human rabies, humans occasionally contract the disease after being bitten by a wild animal. In addition, there are potential avenues of transfer other than bites. These include skinning rabid animals, being licked by a rabid animal on broken skin, and breathing air infested with the rabies virus. All these alternative transmission mechanisms are exceptionally infrequent, but there are documented cases of aerial transmission to humans. For example, two men who were not bitten died of rabies contracted while exploring a bat cave in Texas. The rabies virus must be highly concentrated in

Rabies vaccines are often put into bait and distributed in the wild, sometimes via airdrop. Matchbox for scale. Photo by Izvora via Wikimedia Commons.

the air to be transmitted in this way. These concentrations probably occur only in caves occupied by many bats, and many of them must be carrying the rabies virus.

While educating spelunkers and hunters about these dangers would have a minimal effect on the incidence of rabies, as these transmission mechanisms are so infrequent, such educating could be of the utmost importance to an individual who is spared a rabies infection by the knowledge. Educating people, especially children, to leave animals acting in an unnatural fashion alone would significantly affect rabies incidence. Most wild animals that can be caught or approached closely are sick and may be suffering from dumb or paralytic rabies. They should be avoided and reported to the appropriate authorities, as should any dog or cat that behaves unnaturally. Educating the public about the importance of pet vaccination and control is the most important role of education in regulating rabies.

PERSPECTIVE AND PROSPECTS

Rabies in humans and their association with mad dog attacks have been known for more than two thousand years. Even though rabies has never caused epidemics accompanied by mass mortality like smallpox and bubonic plague, its frightful symptoms and ability to turn a loving family pet into a vicious animal have given the disease a terrifying and mysterious aura. As a result, cures and preventions have been sought throughout history.

In the late nineteenth century, Louis Pasteur and his associates performed many experiments. They isolated the rabies virus from a dog and injected it into rabbit brains. Pasteur called it a "street" virus because it was isolated directly from dogs in the street. The virus replicated in the rabbit's brain and could be transferred into another rabbit's brain, where it again replicated. The growth of the virus in one of the rabbit brains was called a "passage." A sequence of such passages resulted in a virus that had a more predictable and shorter incubation period. This virus was called a "fixed" virus because of its fixed incubation period. After a hundred such passages, the virus had lost much of its ability to infect dogs.

Pasteur then developed an immunization sequence that protected dogs from the street virus. He air-dried rabbit spinal cord tissue infected with the fixed virus for varying times. Pasteur developed a series of virus solutions, ranging from those that could not infect rabbits through those that could occasionally establish weak infections to those that were maximally infective. He then injected dogs daily for ten days, beginning with the noninfective preparation the first day and increasing the infectivity with each day's injection until,

---

INFORMATION ON RABIES

Causes: Viral infection usually transmitted by animal bite

Symptoms: Fever, headaches, nausea, neurologic symptoms (hyperactivity, seizures, hallucinations)

Duration: Several days to weeks; fatal if untreated

Treatments: Antiviral agents, antiserum

---

on the tenth day, he was injecting a highly infective virus. The dogs he treated were resistant to experimentally injected street viruses.

Pasteur was still refining his immunization system when a boy who had been attacked by a rabid dog was brought to him. Knowing that the latency period of the virus might allow time for the development of immunity before the symptoms appeared and aware of the almost certain fatal result if nothing was done, Pasteur treated the boy with the sequence that he had used on the dogs. The boy lived with no apparent side effects, and Pasteur's treatment became the standard for rabies. The modern treatment sequence is a refinement of Pasteur's. While the immunization sequence for rabies was not the first to be used successfully—smallpox immunization nearly a century earlier, Pasteur's work established the distinction—the possibility of immunization after exposure to diseases with long incubation periods.

Considerable work has been done on the epidemiology of rabies. Mathematical and computer models have been developed that attempt to predict the characteristics of the disease spread under different conditions and thus suggest means of controlling and preventing rabies epidemics. Arguments over the effectiveness of wildlife vaccination are partially based on such models. The usefulness of these models is not restricted to rabies epidemiology. Instead, it contributes to an understanding of epidemiology in general. Thus, research on rabies continues to enhance the control and prevention of that terrifying disease and add to the general knowledge base of medicine.

—Carl W. Hoagstrom, PhD

For Further Information:
Johnson, Shannon. "Rabies." Healthline, 14 Sept. 2021, www.healthline.com/health/rabies. Accessed 7 Apr. 2022.
Koury R., Warrington, S.J. "Rabies." StatPearls, 9 Nov. 2021, www.ncbi.nlm.nih.gov/books/NBK448076/. Accessed 7 Apr. 2022.
Newman, Tim. "What You Need to Know About Rabies." *MedicalNewsToday*, 29 Nov. 2021, www.medicalnewstoday.com/articles/rabies. Accessed 7 Apr. 2022.

Rabies. Centers for Disease Control and Prevention, 23 Sept. 2021, www.cdc.gov/rabies/index.html. Accessed 3 Dec. 2021.

Rabies. Mayo Clinic, 2 Nov. 2021, www.mayoclinic.org/diseases-conditions/rabies/symptoms-causes/syc-20351821. Accessed 7 Apr. 2022.

Rabies. Virginia Department of Health, Nov. 2018, www.vdh.virginia.gov/epidemiology/epidemiology-fact-sheets/rabies/. Accessed 7 Apr. 2022.

Rabies. World Health Organization, 17 May 2021, www.who.int/news-room/fact-sheets/detail/rabies. Accessed 7 Apr. 2022.

Rabies and Your Pet. American Veterinary Medical Association, n.d., www.avma.org/resources/public-health/rabies-and-your-pet. Accessed 7 Apr. 2022.

RADIATION SICKNESS

Category: Disease/Disorder

Anatomy or system affected: Gastrointestinal system, hair, skin, stomach

Specialties and related fields: Critical care, emergency medicine, occupational health, oncology, public health, radiology

Definition: An acute illness that occurs when an individual is exposed to a sudden, large dose of nuclear radiation or X rays.

CAUSES AND SYMPTOMS

Typical symptoms of radiation sickness are nausea, diarrhea, skin burns, internal bleeding, and severe anemia. The production of blood corpuscles in the bone marrow is inhibited, and the ability of the body to fight infection is reduced.

The severity of radiation sickness depends on the dose, which is commonly measured in units called rads (an acronym for radiation absorbed dose). For humans, a whole-body dose greater than six hundred rads is usually fatal. At 450 rads, there is a 50 percent survival rate. Below fifty rads, no symptoms of radiation sickness are observable, although the risk of cancer is somewhat higher than normal. Radiation therapy for cancer patients has typically been prescribed in total doses of about five thousand rads. Such large doses are not fatal for two reasons: first, only a small region of the body (the actual cancer site) is irradiated; and second, the therapy is given in smaller doses of about two hundred rads over a period of several weeks, so that the body has time to recover between treatments.

TREATMENT AND THERAPY

Once radiation damage occurs, little can be done to repair it directly. Immediate treatment involves washing the body with soap and lukewarm water to remove radioactive material, as well as monitoring of the levels

---

INFORMATION ON RADIATION SICKNESS

Causes: Exposure to sudden, large dose of nuclear radiation or X rays

Symptoms: Nausea, diarrhea, skin burns, internal bleeding, severe anemia

Duration: Acute

Treatments: Drug therapy, antibiotics, bone marrow transplantation

---

of radiation in the body. This monitoring continues throughout the course of treatment, which centers on whichever parts of the body have been affected and focuses on helping the body's natural processes of recovery. Vomiting and diarrhea can be controlled with drugs, while bacterial infections and wounds are treated with antibiotics. In extreme cases, bone marrow transplants can be performed to reestablish the formation of new blood cells. Donor cells are not likely to be rejected because the body's immune system has been inactivated temporarily by the radiation.

—*Hans G. Graetzer, PhD*

See also Biological and chemical weapons; Bone marrow transplantation; Burns and scalds; Carcinogens; Environmental diseases; Occupational health; Radiation therapy.

For Further Information:

Frigerio, Norman A. *Your Body and Radiation*. Washington, DC: US Atomic Energy Commission, 1966.

Hall, Eric J. *Radiation and Life*. 2d ed. New York: Pergamon Press, 1984.

Montemayor-Quellenberg, Marjorie, and Igor Puzanov. "Radiation Exposure." *Health Library*, 20 June 2013.

Ogura, Toyofumi. *Letters from the End of the World: A Firsthand Account of the Bombing of Hiroshima*. New York: Kodansha International, 2001.

Perez, Eric, et al. "Radiation Sickness." *MedlinePlus*, 1 Feb. 2013.

Prasad, Kedar N. *Handbook of Radiobiology*. Rev. 2d ed. Boca Raton, Fla.: CRC Press, 1995.

"Radiation Exposure." *MedlinePlus*, 26 Aug. 2013.

"Radiation Exposure and Cancer." *American Cancer Society*, 29 Mar. 2010.

"Understanding Radiation: Overview." *Environmental Protection Agency*, 23 Jan. 2013.

RADIATION THERAPY

Category: Treatment

Anatomy or system affected: All

Specialties and related fields: Nuclear medicine, oncology, radiology

Definition: The use of X-rays or radioactivity in the treatment of cancer patients, frequently in combination with surgery and chemotherapy.

Key terms:

brachytherapy, or sealed internal radiotherapy: therapy in which a small radioactive source in a container is implanted close to the cancer site, such as in the cervix or inside the chest cavity

computed tomography (CT) scanning: from the Greek word *tomos*, meaning "section"; the process of using X-rays to obtain a computer picture of an interior cross section from a patient's body

external beam radiotherapy (EBRT): therapy in which a machine outside of a patient emits beams of radiation toward a specific target on or inside the patient

gamma rays: penetrating radiation that comes from a radioactive source, such as cobalt 60

magnetic resonance imaging (MRI): a diagnostic technique using large magnets (not X-rays) to outline the shape and size of a tumor

metastasis: the spread of cancer cells from one part of the body to another

oncologist: a physician who specializes in the treatment of cancer

radiation dose: the amount of radiation absorbed, depending on the intensity of the source and the time of exposure; measured in units of rads or grays

tumor: an abnormal mass of tissue that may be malignant (growing larger) or benign (not spreading)

X-rays: penetrating radiation produced by means of a high-voltage machine; useful for both diagnosis and therapy of cancerous tissue

INDICATIONS AND PROCEDURES

When a person is diagnosed with cancer, three main methods of treatment may be used alone or in combination: surgery, radiation, and chemotherapy (drugs). Surgery and radiation are most useful if the cancer is a localized tumor whose shape and size can be determined. Radiation is the treatment of choice if the tumor is at an inoperable location, such as inside the brain, liver, or spine. In some cases, radiation is utilized with the goal to cure the cancer, such as when radiation is used following surgery in order to prevent recurrence of a malignant growth. In other cases, radiation is used with the purpose of palliating or alleviating the symptoms caused by the cancer, such as when cancer has spread to the bones and is causing pain there. While radiation therapy is most commonly utilized for cancer treatment, it may also be used for noncancerous conditions, such as keloids, heterotopic ossification, and trigeminal neuralgia.

The amount of energy absorbed in radiation therapy can be expressed quantitatively in a unit called a "gray." It was named after a British radiobiologist, Louis Harold Gray, who studied the biological effect of various ionizing radiations. One gray corresponds to the absorption of a fixed amount of radiation energy.

Before 1984, radiation doses were commonly measured in rads, which was an acronym for radiation absorbed dose. The conversion factor is "100 rads = 1 gray." Since most references continue to use the more familiar rad, it will be adopted here. For converting to grays, each rad value is divided by one hundred.

To develop a feel for typical dose levels in radiation therapy, it is helpful to remember two numbers for comparison: First, the maximum safe dose established by the Nuclear Regulatory Commission (NRC) for radiation exposure in the workplace is 5 rads per year; second, a lethal dose for 50 percent of humans, known as LD-50, is about 450 rads. LD-50 means that, statistically, 50 percent would die and 50 percent would recover from such a massive dose.

The numbers given above must be interpreted with care. For example, a dental X-ray gives a dose of about 2 rads. Four dental X-rays give a total exposure of 8 rads, exceeding the NRC yearly maximum of 5 rads. Only a small part of the body, however, perhaps 1 percent, is irradiated during a dental X-ray. Therefore, the radiation dose averaged over the whole body is only 1 percent of 8 rads. Another example is a patient with malignant cancer might be given twenty radiation treatment sessions of 250 rads each, for a total dose of 5,000 rads. Even though this far exceeds the LD-50 of 450 rads, it is not lethal because it is spread out over time. The patient may develop symptoms of radiation sickness, such as skin reddening, nausea, loss of hair, and blood changes depending on the treatment site, but the body has time to heal partially between radiation treatment sessions. The healing process can be compared to recovery from a serious burn injury, in which the skin and flesh repair themselves but permanent scars may be left behind. The present trend in radiology is to subdivide the total dose into more and smaller increments, reducing patient discomfort. In summary, the percentage of body treated and the time between radiation therapy sessions matter significantly in the efficacy and safety of radiation therapy.

There are two main types of radiation therapy: external beam radiotherapy (EBRT) and internal radiotherapy. The two differs in where the radiation is coming from. EBRT is a therapy in which a machine outside of a patient emits beams of radiation toward a specific target on or inside the patient. One of the most common machines that deliver EBRT is a medical particle accelerator, which can send out beams of X-rays, electrons, and/or other particles. The personnel and equipment costs to operate an accelerator, however, are too great for most hospitals. Also, patients may find the experience of being bombarded by the output beam from a large and noisy accelerator to be too traumatic. EBRT can also be delivered from a radioactive source, such as cobalt 60, which is created by irradiating ordinary cobalt in a research reactor. Because the radioactive form of cobalt emits gamma rays with a penetrating power that is equivalent to a 2-million-volt X-ray machine, it is useful for the treatment of deep internal cancers. The radioactive source must be kept in a thick lead shield. When a patient is to be treated, the source is positioned near the cancer site, and a small port is opened briefly to irradiate it. Sometimes, the cobalt source is moved around the patient so that the gamma rays enter the body from different angles, thus reducing the damage to healthy tissue lying above the cancer site. The irradiation procedure is done by remote control so that the radiation oncologist (a physician that uses radiotherapy for treatment) and other medical personnel will not be exposed.

In contrast to EBRT, brachytherapy or sealed internal radiotherapy utilizes radioactive substances "sealed" in needles, seeds, or other small devices that are placed in a specific body cavity or opening. The radiation from such sources only penetrates a few centimeters of tissue surrounding them, thus limiting damage to healthy cells farther from the sources. Such sources are common for treating cancers of the prostate, vagina, cervix, uterus, rectum, throat, larynx, and eyes. Depending on the specific cancer and the specific radioactive source, the source may be placed permanently to provide continuous treatment for a short time or may be removed shortly after placement. One problem with implanted sources is the radiation dose received by the physician during the surgery. Sometimes, it is possible to use "afterloading," in which a hollow tube or shell is positioned in the patient and radioactive material is loaded into it at a later time. There are also "unsealed" radioactive substances that are not contain in small containers. Such substances are known as "radiopharmaceuticals" that can travel through bloodstream or digestive system, with various half-lives and energies for different applications.

The various types of radiation, including X-rays, gamma rays, and particle beams, all produce damage in living tissue by the process of ionization. The radia-

Patient positioned on Varian TruBeam linear accelerator with restraining mask, to receive postoperative IMRT to primary tumour bed and neck for oropharyngeal cancer. Green lines are laser alignment beams. Photo by Michael Goodyear, via Wikimedia Commons.

tion strikes individual atoms and breaks the bonds that hold molecules together. The breakup of normal molecules produces positive and negative ions, which act as toxic chemicals. The internal structure of cells is disrupted so that they can no longer replicate themselves. Fortunately, cancer cells tend to be more sensitive to radiation damage than normal cells.

Cancer is the second leading cause of death for American women. Breast cancer is the second most common cancer for women, after skin cancers. Early detection and treatment are the keys to improving the chances for survival. A radicalmastectomy (breast removal) can be an emotionally traumatic experience. If the cancer is not too advanced, however, radiation therapy is an alternative. In some cases, daily treatment with external beam radiotherapy can be done on an outpatient basis, with only minor disruptions of schedule and decreased long-term disfigurement. For external beam radiotherapy, treatment is typically given daily on weekdays for five sessions a week, for however many weeks needed to complete the course of radiation treatment.

During treatment for any type of cancer, the radiation oncologist needs to determine whether the radiation therapy is shrinking the tumor. Therefore, computed tomography (CT) scanning or magnetic resonance imaging (MRI) can be used during and after treatment to monitor the size of the tumor. The radiation dose then can be adjusted to take into account the individual characteristics of various patients.

The goal of radiation therapy is to deliver a dose of several thousand rads to a cancer site while minimizing the damage to surrounding tissue and nearby organs. The shape of a malignant cancer may be a simple round lump, or it can be a complex group of nodules with tentacles extending through the flesh. For effective treatment, it is essential to determine the location and shape of the tumor as precisely as possible. An ordinary X-ray photograph is not very useful for diagnosing a tumor. The problem is a lack of contrast between a tumor and surrounding tissue, because there is very little difference in their densities. An X-ray of the head, for example, provides an excellent outline of the skull, but it cannot distinguish between tumor and brain material on the inside.

In the 1970s, a major advance in X-ray technology, computed tomography (CT) scanning, was developed in England; it is also referred to as a computed axial tomography (CAT) scan. CT scanning replaces the film of conventional X-rays with pictures on a computer screen. The sharpness and contrast obtained with CT scans are remarkable improvements over X-ray film. A radiation oncologist can view the computer display of a tumor from various angles and with different enlargements. The computer screen can be

photographed to provide a permanent record. The two scientists who developed the CT scan, Allan Cormack and Godfrey Hounsfield, shared the Nobel Prize in Physiology or Medicine in 1979. An entirely different method to determine the location and outline of an internal tumor is magnetic resonance imaging, (MRI). Instead of using X-rays, MRI utilizes the magnetic properties of hydrogen nuclei, which can be aligned by a very strong magnet. PET (positron emission tomography)-CT is an imaging scan that uses an injected radiopharmaceutical to show where very active cells, such as cancers, are located. CT, MRI and PET-CT scanning are all complex diagnostic procedures. To diagnose and treat a cancer, radiation oncologist, medical physicists, other physicians, and computer specialists must work together as a team. New techniques for obtaining and displaying information are under continuing development.

USES AND COMPLICATIONS

Before starting any radiation treatments, there are two main steps for any patient. First, the patient will see a radiation oncologist to assess the role of radiotherapy. In terms of cancer management, there are three main types: surgery, radiotherapy, and systemic therapy (including hormonal therapy, chemotherapy, and immunotherapy). Radiation therapy may be given alone or in combination with the others depending on many factors, such as tumor location, the age and overall health of the patient, and the extent and stage of the cancer. Thus, the role of radiotherapy must be first determined for any patient. Second, the patient will undergo a simulation session, also known as a "radiotherapy mapping session." During the simulation session, the radiation oncologist and the radiation therapists will determine the optimal treatment position (such as standing upright, lying on the back, or lying on the front) and, if using internal radiotherapy, the optimal treating device(s). To help position the patient properly each time so each radiotherapy session is consistent in providing the predicted amount of radiation to the target, sometimes immobilization devices (such as a body bean bag or a mask) and/or tiny tattoos in the form of dots on the patient's skin will be used. Additional scans, such as a CT, may be done at the simulation session to help visualize the target in the specific treatment position. After a simulation session, the actual radiotherapy session typically starts one to two weeks afterward given the making of a radiation treatment plan is complex.

The process of making a radiation treatment plan involves multiple individuals, including the radiation oncologist, medical physicist, and dosimetrist, in order to ensure a safe and effective radiation treatment plan. The plan is devised to ensure adequate radiation is going to the target. At the same time, the radiation dose to the patient's healthy organs, such as the lungs, heart, and liver, is minimized; the direction of entry for the beam of radiation should avoid passing through these sensitive organs. Furthermore, the radiation treatment has to make sure that the proper dose will be received at various depths below the skin. A plastic dummy to simulate the patient, called a "phantom," can be irradiated with detectors placed inside it to measure the dose. Also, the scattering of radiation and shielding effects by bones can be very complex and must be determined by computer calculations supplemented by careful measurements. The radiation pattern can be shaped with filters and baffles so that it will conform to the shape of the tumor as closely as possible, thereby allowing adequate target coverage.

Two final considerations in treatment planning for a patient are how the total radiation dose is to be subdivided and what the time interval between exposures should be. Prior research studies have looked at these questions for many types of cancers. The results of those studies are used to make national treatment recommendations for radiotherapy. Sometimes, the stamina of the patient and the urgency of the treatment may influence the radiation oncologist to make a decision if a choice is available.

The overall effectiveness of radiation therapy can be summarized approximately by the "half-half-half" rule. About half of all cancers are treated with radiation. Half of those patients are given a large enough dose to attempt a cure. (For the others, radiation is used simply for pain relief.) Finally, about half of those patients are actually cured by radiation. This success rate is encouraging, but there is always room for improvement.

The survival rate after radiation treatment varies greatly depending on the site of cancer in the body. For example, patients with localized cancer of the prostate and breast have five-year survival rates of nearly 100 percent. At the other end of the scale, patients with stomach or lung cancers that have spread and are at a much later stage typically have about a 5 percent survival at five years. Radiation therapy for ten different kinds of cancer—breast, cervix, larynx, prostate, uterus, bladder, testicle, tongue, mouth cancers, and Hodgkin disease—results in cure rates that are equal to or greater than those with surgery while preserving the organ function.

Any medical treatment, especially curative cancer treatment, has possible side effects and complications. This is also true for radiation therapy given both cancerous cells and its surrounding normal cells are harmed by the treatment. Radiation therapy is a "local" treatment given radiation only goes to a specific site where the radiation treatment team is aiming it. Thus, its side effects are mainly "local" as well. For ex-

ample, radiation treatment to the head may cause headache, dizziness, hair loss, while treatment to the intestines may cause nausea, vomiting, and diarrhea. The radiation treatment team is well-versed in the possible side effects and is therefore well-equipped to advise and help with any side effect or other concern.

Many people are apprehensive about the hazards of radiation with good reason. In the 1920s, some workers who were hired to apply radium paint to watch dials (to make them glow in the dark) developed cancer when they ingested radioactive material. At Hiroshima and Nagasaki, many people developed radiation sickness and died from the aftereffects of the atomic bombs dropped on those cities. For medical applications of radiation, regulatory agencies that are responsible for the general public must evaluate potential benefits and risks. Sometimes, sensationalized articles are published that present frightening scenarios of highly unlikely hazards. The perception of risk from low-level radioactive waste, for example, far exceeds the actual hazard. The advantages of radiation therapy would be lost if permits for hazardous waste storage were denied. The responsible use of any technology should balance concerns for safety with the benefits of that technology.

Ensuring the health and safety of medical personnel who administer radiation therapy to patients requires proper training. All workers must wear radiation monitors, which are checked regularly. Radiation areas have to be posted with warning signs. The nuclear medicine department at a hospital must keep an accurate inventory of radioactive materials. The shipment and disposal of radiopharmaceuticals are strictly regulated. Periodic on-site visits by Nuclear Regulatory Commission inspectors also are part of the licensing procedure. Careless overexposure of personnel must be avoided if the benefits of radiation therapy are to find continued acceptance by the medical profession and the general public.

PERSPECTIVE AND PROSPECTS

Radiation therapy most commonly makes use of X-rays or radioactivity. It is interesting to note that both types of radiation were discovered only a year apart in the 1890s. Wilhelm Röntgen, a German physicist, discovered X-rays in 1895. He received the Nobel Prize for his work in 1901, the first year in which the award was given. He used high voltage to accelerate an electron beam; when the electrons hit a metal target, they released a new kind of penetrating radiation. Röntgen made a now-famous X-ray photograph of his wife's hand that clearly showed the bones inside the flesh. The medical profession adopted X-rays with great enthusiasm, primarily for the diagnosis of broken bones, swallowed objects, and bullet or shrapnel fragments.

Radioactivity was first observed in 1896 by Henri Becquerel, in Paris. By chance, Becquerel had placed a uranium rock next to an unused photographic film that was still wrapped in its container. He was amazed to find that radiation from the uranium had penetrated the wrapping and had exposed the film inside. His discovery and follow-up experiments earned for him the Nobel Prize in 1905.

Marie Curie, a graduate student under Becquerel, became famous for isolating a new radioactive element from uranium ore, which she named radium. It emits radiation at a rate that is a million times greater than that of an equivalent weight of uranium. In her doctoral thesis in 1904, Curie described an experiment in which she placed a small capsule containing radium on her husband's arm. It produced a sore that took more than a month to heal. The hazards of handling radioactivity and the possibility of using it to destroy cancer cells were recognized quite early. The element radium is very rare on earth. In fact, the world's total supply is less than 1 kilogram. Only after the invention of nuclear particle accelerators and neutron sources in the 1930s was it possible to create artificial radioactive elements in substantial amounts.

Radiation therapy has since become a treatment of choice in oncology and in certain noncancerous diseases. Such treatment will likely remain necessary for some time to come given it is not reasonable to expect a cure for cancer soon because there are too many different types. Much has been accomplished, however, in the area of prevention. The strong correlation between lung cancer and smoking has received wide publicity, so many people have stopped, at least in the United States. Research with animals has linked cancer to certain food additives and industrial pollutants, leading to legal restrictions on their use. In addition to surgery, radiation, and chemotherapy, other treatment methods are under investigation. For example, one procedure involves blocking the blood supply from reaching a tumor so that the malignant cells die from lack of nutrients. Other researchers hope to use genetic engineering, trying to stimulate the body's immune system to produce specific antibodies that will fight against the cancer cells.

Within the field of radiation therapy, there continues to be much research and development. New studies are exploring different total radiation dose and how it is subdivided to identify a regimen that provides the same if not improved disease control while minimizing side effects, looking into combining radiation therapy with new treatments and drugs to increase their efficacy, and more. There is also an increased interest in utilizing proton for radiotherapy because the properties of proton allow for decreased radiation effect on surrounding healthy structures, and thus decreased side effects and complications. Though radiation therapy has come far since its discovery, there is still more to come.

—Kristin Hsieh, MD

See also: Cancer; Chemotherapy; Computed tomography (CT) scanning; Hair loss and baldness; Magnetic resonance imaging (MRI); Malignancy and metastasis; Nuclear medicine; Nuclear radiology; Oncology; Radiopharmaceuticals.

For Further Information:
Brown, G. I. *Invisible Rays: A History of Radioactivity*. Sutton, 2002.
Cameron, John R., James G. Skofronick, and Roderick M. Grant. *Medical Physics: Physics of the Body*. Medical Physics, 1992.
Hall, Eric J. *Radiation and Life*. 2nd ed., Pergamon Press, 1984.
Hendee, William R., Geoffrey S. Ibbott, and Eric G. Hendee. *Radiation Therapy Physics*. 3rd ed., John Wiley & Sons, 2005.
Laws, Priscilla W., and the Public Citizen Health Research Group. *The X-Ray Information Book*. Farrar, Straus and Giroux, 1983.
Puzanov, Igor. "Radiation Therapy-External." *Health Library*, 26 Sept. 2012.
Puzanov, Igor, and Michael Woods. "Radiation Therapy-Internal." *Health Library*, 30 May 2013.
"Radiation Therapy." *MedlinePlus*, 10 June 2013.
Saha, Gopal B. *Physics and Radiobiology of Nuclear Medicine*. 4th ed., Springer, 2013.
Sandler, Martin P., R. Edward Coleman, and James A. Patton, editors. *Diagnostic Nuclear Medicine*. 4th ed., Lippincott Williams & Wilkins, 2003.
Smith, F. A. *A Primer in Applied Radiation Physics*. World Scientific, 2000.
"Understanding Radiation Therapy: A Guide for Patients and Families." *American Cancer Society*, 24 Jan. 2013.

Radiculopathy

Category: Disease/Disorder
Also known as: Radiculoneuropathy, mononeuropathy, polyneuropathy, neuropathy, radiculitis
Anatomy or system affected: Musculoskeletal system, nerves, nervous system, spine
Specialties and related fields: Geriatrics and gerontology, neurology, nursing, orthopedics, osteopathic medicine, pathology, physical therapy, radiology, rheumatology, sports medicine
Definition: Pain distributed along a specific pathway resulting from irritation of a nerve root.
Key terms:
deep tendon reflex: a brisk contraction of a muscle responding to a sudden stretch produced by a sharp tap of a rubber hammer on a tendon insertion of a muscle

intervertebral disk: one of the fibrous disks found between adjacent spinal vertebrae

spinal nerves: pairs of nerves connected to the spinal cord and numbered according to the level at which they emerge from the cord; each spinal nerve attaches to the spinal cord by an anterior and a posterior root

spinal stenosis: a condition in which the diameter of the spinal canal is decreased and compromises the spinal cord and spinal nerve roots

vertebrae: a cylindrical bony mass that encompasses and protects the spinal column; collectively, thirty-three vertebrae separated by cartilaginous disks make up the vertebral column

CAUSES AND SYMPTOMS

The nervous system provides an avenue of signaling from the brain to the muscles. Each spinal nerve departing from the spinal cord is part of the peripheral nervous system. Any disruption at the spinal nerve or as it travels farther away from the spine will affect the signal, resulting in radiculopathy. The anatomic region or regions affected determine the severity of the involvement and the amount of function that may be lost.

Nerve root irritations resulting in radiculopathy include a variety of causes. Because of this, several classifications are used such as rate of onset, distribution pattern, or pathology. Compression from surrounding anatomic structures upon a spinal nerve root is a common cause of radiculopathy. It can originate from any level of the spine: the cervical, thoracic, or lumbar vertebral levels. Encroaching material causing the nerve root compression and irritation can be from the intervertebral disk or from vertebral bone. Causative factors of this compression include trauma or degeneration of the spine over time. With age, water content of the intervertebral disk decreases, resulting in the disk space becoming thinner. Over time, the spinal nerve roots potentially become compressed and entrapped, resulting in a condition called spinal stenosis. Spinal stenosis of the lumbar spine commonly produces radiculopathy in the legs and feet, whereas this condition in the cervical spine can produce similar symptoms in the arms and hands. Inflammation resulting from disk degeneration can compound this problem. Less common causes of radiculopathy are inherited disorders causing nerve root irritation. Some viruses such as herpes zoster infect spinal nerves and are revealed as a painful area of skin that is mainly supplied by a single spinal nerve called a dermatome.

Symptoms vary with each level of nerve root involved. Sensory changes such as tingling, prickling, and burning are some of the earlier signs of radiculopathy. When more than one nerve is affected,

---

INFORMATION ON RADICULOPATHY

Causes: Compression, infection, inflammation, inherited disorders, environmental toxins

Symptoms: Variable to each nerve root level; tingling, prickling, burning, glove-and-stocking distribution, weakness

Duration: Dependent on cause; short and long duration; can be permanent

Treatments: Physical therapy, medication, surgery

---

the sensory loss follows a distribution similar to a glove-and-stocking pattern as it encircles a limb. Over time, the nerve root irritation can cause further problems, including weakness of corresponding muscles called atrophy. Deep tendon reflexes-such as the Achilles tendon reflex or the biceps tendon reflex, involving the lumbar and cervical spine respectively-will be diminished or completely absent. This becomes a useful indication for the clinical diagnosis of nerve root irritation associated with radiculopathy.

TREATMENT AND THERAPY

Medical attention and treatment for radiculopathy at any level should not be delayed. Primary treatment is reducing and or eliminating the cause of the nerve irritation. Depending upon the severity, nonsurgical treatment is usually attempted initially, such as the use of epidural steroid injections, which are effective in decreasing the inflammation around the nerve root. Physical therapy is commonly used and proves effective for many cases of radiculopathy. This discipline utilizes techniques of spinal traction and mobilization, which helps decompress the nerve root.

Once symptoms have been stabilized, physical therapy introduces spinal stabilization exercises to aid in the prevention of future problems and reoccurrences. In the case of nerve root compression, surgery may be required to decompress the spinal nerve. One of the minimally invasive approaches is a microdiskectomy, which removes the portion of the disk that presses against the nerve root. The success rate of this surgery is high, and results are favorable because of the minimal recovery time. Frequently, there is immediate relief of the radiculopathy caused by a nerve root compression.

PERSPECTIVE AND PROSPECTS

Research is ongoing for the treatment of radiculopathy of any origin. Medications that address nerve pain have been developed, with additional clinical trials currently in progress. The development of other minimally invasive surgical procedures is also important to the medical specialties of orthopedic surgery and neurosurgery. Studies have shown, however, that long-term outcomes do not differ between those who undergo surgery and those who do not. The decision to undergo surgery is not a trivial one, and it is preferably made in consultation with several physicians.

—Jeffrey P. Larson, PT, ATC

See also Back pain; Nervous system; Neuralgia, neuritis, and neuropathy; Neuroimaging; Neurology; Neurology, pediatric; Neurosurgery; Numbness and tingling; Pain; Sciatica; Spinal cord disorders; Spine, vertebrae, and disks; Stenosis.

For Further Information:
Bogduk, N., and L. Twomey. *Clinical Anatomy of the Lumbar Spine.* 4th ed. New York: Elsevier/Churchill Livingstone, 2005.

Hoppenfeld, Stanley. *Physical Examination of the Spine and Extremities.* Norwalk, Conn.: Appleton-Century-Crofts, 1976.

Magee, David J. *Orthopedic Assessment.* 5th ed. Philadelphia: W. B. Saunders Elsevier, 2008.

Malone, T. R., T. McPoil, and A. J. Nitz. *Orthopedic and Sports Physical Therapy.* 3d ed. St. Louis: Mosby Year Books, 1997.

"NINDS Peripheral Neuropathy Information Page." *National Institute of Neurological Disorders and Stroke*, Sept. 19, 2012.

"Spinal Stenosis." *MedlinePlus*, May 14, 2013.

Stahl, Rebecca J., and Rimas Lukas. "Neuropathic Pain." *Health Library*, Mar. 15, 2013.

Umphred, Darcy A. *Neurological Rehabilitation.* 6th ed. St. Louis: Mosby, 2012.

RADIOLOGY. SEE IMAGING AND RADIOLOGY; NUCLEAR RADIOLOGY.

RADIOPHARMACEUTICALS

Category: Procedure
Anatomy or system affected: All
Specialties and related fields: Endocrinology, internal medicine, oncology, radiology
Definition: Imaging techniques involving radioactive chemical agents that are designed to localize in specific organs and emit radiation, which can be detected outside the body with a camera in order to provide visual images of the organ.

Key terms:
becquerel: the international unit of radioactivity, defined as a radioactive sample that is decaying at the rate of one disintegration per second

electron volt: a unit of energy defined as the energy acquired by an electron traveling through a potential difference of 1 volt

gamma camera: a type of radiation detection instrument that detects gamma rays external to the body and makes an image of the radionuclide distribution in body organs; also known as a scintillation camera

gamma ray: a type of electromagnetic radiation that has the same physical properties as X rays but is emitted by unstable nuclei in their decay process; gamma rays are capable of penetrating soft tissue, thereby allowing their detection outside the body to produce images of organs

half-life: the time required for one-half of the nuclei in a radioactive sample to decay

radioimmunotherapy: a cancer therapy using radionuclides; the radionuclides attach themselves to antibodies that tend to target cancer cells in the body, thus eradicating the cancer cells through selective irradiation

radionuclide: an unstable atomic nucleus that, in the process of decay, emits radiation; also referred to as a radioisotope

THE FUNDAMENTALS OF RADIOACTIVITY

All matter consists of atoms, which contain a central nucleus and tiny particles called electrons that revolve around the nucleus. Electrons carry a small negative charge, while the nucleus is made up of particles called neutrons, which have no charge, and protons, which carry a positive charge. Atoms are generally neutral, with the number of protons in the nucleus equaling the number of electrons. Most objects are made up of atoms in which the neutron and proton numbers in their nuclei are arranged in such a way that they are stable. If the proton number or the neutron number in the nucleus is altered, the atom may become unstable. Such unstable atoms are termed radioactive and tend to reach a stable state by emitting radiation. This process is referred to as radioactive decay, and the elemental atoms that emit radiation are called radioisotopes or radionuclides. All stable elements can be made into radioactive elements by either adding or removing neutrons or protons, a process known as the artificial production of radioactivity. The few naturally occurring radioisotopes, such as radon 222 and uranium 235, are not used in nuclear medicine.

Radioactivity was first discovered by the French scientist Antoine-Henri Becquerel in 1896, when he observed that a photographic plate sitting next to a uranium sample had darkened. Appropriately, the international unit of radioactivity was chosen to be the becquerel. Radioactivity is a property of unstable atomic nuclei, and the rate of decay cannot be affected by normal physical and chemical processes such as heat, pressure, or the presence of magnetic or electric fields. The nuclei in a radioactive sample do not decay spontaneously or all at once. Rather, they decay randomly at a rate that is characteristic of the given radioisotope. While it is impossible to tell when a particular nucleus will decay or disintegrate, the fraction of nuclei in a sample that will decay in a given time can be determined. The decay rate of a radioactive sample is usually expressed in terms of its half-life, the time required for one-half of the original sample nuclei to decay. Half-life is a characteristic property of a particular radionuclide. The half-lives of radioactive isotopes vary from a small fraction of a second to millions of years. For example, carbon 14 has a half-life of 5,730 years, while the half-life of iodine 123 is thirteen hours. Naturally occurring uranium 238 decays with a half-life of 4.5 billion years, which is the approximate age of Earth itself. Hence, at present there remains only half of the original uranium 238 that was formed when the earth was born.

Radionuclides emit three types of radiation: alpha particles, beta particles, and gamma rays. Alpha particles are positively charged ions containing two protons and two neutrons. Beta particles are either positively (positron) or negatively (electron) charged and have the same mass as an electron. In contrast, gamma rays are electromagnetic waves that have no mass or charge and are sometimes called photons. Because alpha particles are relatively massive, they can be totally absorbed by a sheet of paper. Beta particles can penetrate up to about a centimeter or so into an object, depending on their energy. On the other hand, gamma rays of moderate energy can easily penetrate through the body, as with x-rays. When radionuclides that emit gamma rays are administered to patients, the gamma rays exit the body and are captured by a scintillation camera, which produces an image. The desirable energy of the gamma rays for external detection and imaging with gamma cameras is generally in the range of 100 kilo-electron volts to 300 kilo-electron volts. The half-life of the radionuclide emitting the gamma rays should be long enough to allow its uptake by the organ of interest, then subsequent imaging with a gamma camera, and short enough so as not to irradiate the patient long after the image is obtained. Half-lives between three hours and three days are considered optimal for diagnostic purposes. When radionuclides are used for therapy, the half-life is generally required to be in the range of several days, and the preferred form of radiation consists of beta particles because they tend to deposit their energy near the disintegration site.

USES AND COMPLICATIONS

If the physician is interested in imaging a particular organ, drugs that take the radionuclide preferentially to that organ are necessary. This is achieved by chemically attaching the radionuclide to a pharmaceutical carrier. Once the radiopharmaceutical is localized in the organ, the gamma rays that it emits are detected by a gamma camera, which electronically displays an image that is representative of the radionuclide distribution. Such images are of substantial diagnostic value. Similarly, radionuclides attached to drugs that selectively target cancer cells can potentially deliver lethal doses of radiation to the cancer cells, a process called radioimmunotherapy. Hence, radiopharmaceuticals play an important role in medicine, providing new and promising avenues for diagnosis and therapy.

Radiopharmaceuticals are generally administered intravenously to patients. Blood flow to the organ of interest determines the fraction of the administered radioactivity that will be delivered. The ability of the organ to accumulate the circulating radiopharmaceutical is also an important determinant of the pathological condition of the organ. Such considerations are usually taken into account in developing appropriate pharmaceuticals.

Although many radionuclides are available, the most preferred one is called technetium 99m, an excited (metastable) state of technetium 99. This radionuclide is readily available, has a convenient half-life of six hours, and has very desirable radiation properties. Accordingly, many pharmaceuticals are labeled with this radionuclide for diagnostic nuclear medicine purposes. A few other radionuclides, such as thallium 201, iodine 123, gallium 67, and indium 111, can be used when technetium 99m compounds are not available.

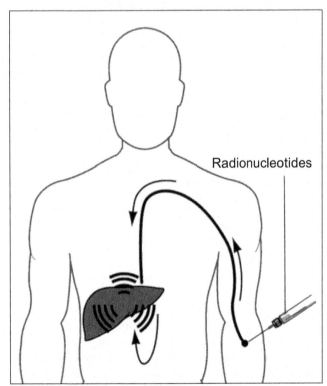

One use of radiopharmaceuticals is to deliver radioactivity to a target organ, such as the liver, that may otherwise be inaccessible to radiation treatment.
©EBSCO

The most widely used radiopharmaceutical for brain imaging is technetium 99m pertechnetate. The primary advantage of this chemical is that it is inexpensive and can be easily prepared. Other radiopharmaceuticals used for brain studies are technetium 99m diethylenetriamine-pentacetic acid (DTPA) and technetium 99m glucoheptonate. Brain imaging usually consists of a dynamic study immediately after bolus intravenous injection of the compound in which rapid sequential images are obtained as the radiopharmaceutical enters the brain. This is followed by a static image one hour later. When a brain lesion is suspected, a delayed static image is sometimes necessary three to four hours after an injection. These imaging techniques are valuable in detecting neoplastic tissue, inflammatory processes, infarction, Alzheimer's disease, and stroke. Another class of radiopharmaceuticals has also been developed to study brain function. These compounds, such as carbon 11 N-methylpiperone, use very short-lived radionuclides that need on-site radionuclide production facilities and require a sophisticated imaging system called a positron emission tomography (PET) scanning unit. Imaging of cerebrospinal fluid is performed using DTPA labeled with indium 111 after an intrathecal administration. Radiopharma- ceuticals for such administrations are tested carefully for their safety.

Lung imaging using radiopharmaceuticals is usually performed to study either pulmonary perfusion or ventilation. For perfusion studies, the radiopharmaceutical of choice is microaggregated albumin (MAA) labeled with technetium 99m. Ventilation studies are performed using the radioactive inert gas xenon 133. The patient breathes while the images are obtained with a gamma camera. These lung studies are used extensively to detect several conditions, including pulmonary embolism, asthma, bronchitis, tumors, inflammatory disease, congestive heart failure, and deep-vein thrombus.

Bone imaging with radiopharmaceuticals often provides earlier diagnosis and better detection of lesions than other radiographic procedures. Furthermore, the extent of metastatic disease may be determined using radionuclide imaging techniques. Other applications of bone imaging include determination of the viability of bone; detection of infections in prosthetic joints, necrosis, and infarction; and evaluation of fractures and bone pain. Bone-seeking compounds are usually similar to calcium or phosphates in their chemical behavior. Hence, diphosphonate labeled with technetium 99m and its analogs are the compounds of choice for this purpose.

Radionuclide imaging techniques play an important role in evaluating the function of the heart. Coronary artery perfusion is studied using thallium 201 chloride. The patient is asked to exercise on a treadmill, and the radionuclide is injected at peak stress. The patient continues to exercise for an additional minute, and redistribution of the thallium 201 within the myocardium occurs immediately after cessation of the exercise. Gamma camera images are obtained soon thereafter. Abnormal thallium distribution is the basis for the detection and diagnosis of stress-induced ischemia and permanent myocardial damage. Acute myocardial infarction can be detected using pyrophosphate labeled with technetium 99m within twenty-four to seventy-two hours after the onset of symptoms. Other radiopharmaceuticals using technetium 99m as a label are also under development. To evaluate ventricular function, the radiochemical is administered intravenously and images are obtained during the first pass of the radionuclide through the heart, lungs, and great vessels. An alternate technique for this purpose is to obtain images of the cardiac blood pool after the radiopharmaceutical has achieved equilibrium in the intravascular space. Such noninvasive studies are invaluable in the diagnosis of heart problems and in the management of patients with heart disease.

Evaluation of thyroid function using radioisotope techniques marked the beginning of the field of nuclear medicine. The element iodine is actively transported into the thyroid gland, where it is retained. Therefore, the readily available radioiodines iodine 131 and iodine 123 have been used for this purpose. Technetium 99m pertechnetate is sometimes used because of its low cost and favorable radiation characteristics. Thyroid uptake tests usually involve administration of a small dose of sodium iodide 131 in either liquid or capsule form and measurement of the radioiodine in the thyroid eighteen to twenty-four hours later. Significantly higher uptake compared to the normal value is a reflection of an overactive gland (hyperthyroidism). Conversely, a lower uptake indicates an underactive gland (hypothyroidism). Thyroid imaging is performed using either sodium iodide 123 or technetium 99m pertechnetate to detect cancer. Effective treatment of benign and malignant cancers, as well as hyperthyroidism, is accomplished by administering larger doses of iodine 131. Although the strong uptake of radioactive iodine by the thyroid gland is useful in nuclear medicine, uptake of iodine 131 in the thyroids of people living in nuclear-fallout zones, such as the one around the Chernobyl nuclear reactor, is a major concern. The risk from such exposure can be reduced by saturating the thyroid with nonradioactive iodine using orally administered doses of Lugol's iodine solution.

Radiopharmaceutical studies of kidneys are sometimes necessary to evaluate structural and functional abnormalities. Renal imaging is indicated to assess renal blood flow and the differential and quantitative functioning of natural or transplanted kidneys. Among the radiopharmaceuticals used for these studies are technetium-labeled glucoheptonate, 2,3-dimercaptosuccinic acid (DMSA), and DTPA. Iodine 123 hippurate is also employed for glomerular filtration studies.

Nuclear medicine techniques to image the liver and spleen are also available. Alcohol-related liver diseases can be readily diagnosed using liver images obtained after injection of technetium-labeled sulfur colloid. Primary liver cancers and metastases can also be detected, and the physiological functioning of transplanted livers can be assessed. Spleen imaging with technetium 99m sulfur colloid has been useful in detecting hepatomas, cysts, infarctions, and neoplasms. Gastrointestinal hemorrhaging and associated bleeding are identified by removing a small portion of the patient's red blood cells, labeling them with technetium 99m, and injecting the labeled cells back into the patient. Similarly, white blood cells labeled with indium 111 are used to image abscesses and inflammation. Radionuclide procedures also provide a method to assess digestive disorders and esophageal transit noninvasively. A variety of tumors can be diagnosed when gallium 67 citrate is used for imaging. This radionuclide is also used in studying patients with acquired immunodeficiency syndrome (AIDS).

Radiopharmaceuticals are also playing an important role in treating many functional disorders and cancers. As pointed out earlier, hyperthyroidism and thyroid carcinoma are best treated with iodine 131. Malignant pheochromocytomas and other neuroendocrine lesions can be treated with metaiodine 131 benzylguanidine. Gold 198 colloid has been used to assist in the therapy of peritoneal metastases and recurrent malignant ascites. Phosphorus 32 colloids are employed in treating malignant pericardial effusion associated with breast and lung carcinomas. Intra-arterial injection of phosphorus 32 colloid to treat inflammatory arthritis of bone joints is also common. The uncontrolled proliferation of bone marrow cells is checked by administering phosphorus 32 orthophosphate. Patients with advanced bone metastases and intractable bone pain are also often treated with single or multiple doses of phosphorus 32 orthophosphate. Other radionuclides that are useful for this purpose are strontium 89, rhenium 186, and yttrium 90.

The implementation of monoclonal antibodies labeled with suitable radionuclides to treat cancer has received considerable attention. This approach involves selecting an antibody that is directed against a tumor-specific antigen and labeling the antibody with an energetic beta particle-emitting radionuclide. If the tumor selectively concentrates these labeled antibodies, then it can be lethally irradiated without seriously affecting the normal tissues and organs. Thus far, however, clinical trials using this approach have met with limited success because of insufficient tumor uptake and bone marrow toxicity. Nevertheless, labeled antibodies are becoming useful in diagnosing a variety of primary and metastatic tumors.

PERSPECTIVE AND PROSPECTS
Although radioactivity was discovered in the late nineteenth century, application of radionuclides as biological tracers did not begin until 1924, when Georg von Hevesy used a bismuth radionuclide to study circulation in rabbits. In that same year, bismuth 214 was used in humans to measure the blood circulation time after injecting the radionuclide in one arm and then following the arrival of radioactivity in the other arm. The researchers found that it takes eighteen seconds in normal patients, and longer in patients with heart disease. The discovery of artificial radioactivity by Frédéric Joliot and Irène Joliot-Curie in 1934 led to the wider use of radionuclides as tracers. When Enrico Fermi artificially produced several radionuclides, Hevesy used phosphorus 32 to study phosphorus metabolism in rats. Such artificial production of radionuclides became possible after the pioneering work of Ernest Lawrence, who invented the cyclotron in 1929. Cyclotrons are still widely employed to produce a variety of radionuclides for medical use. The most commonly used one in nuclear medicine imaging is technetium 99m; this radionuclide is generated in the decay of another radionuclide called molybdenum 99, which was first produced by a cyclotron in 1938.

Radiopharmaceuticals and nuclear medicine took a major leap forward when technetium 99m, the radionuclide of choice for imaging, became readily available. Concurrent development of the scintillation camera by Hal Anger in 1958 advanced the field of nuclear medicine imaging. Radiolabeled compounds are also used extensively in biomedical research to trace biologically important molecules. The radioimmunoassay is another area in which labeled compounds are used to diagnose diseases; here, an antigen-antibody interaction is utilized. These procedures require only a trace amount of radioactivity, along with a blood sample of the patient.

Radiopharmaceutical imaging techniques have become important for the diagnosis and treatment of many diseases, and they will continue to play a major role in improving the quality of health care. Improvements in imaging instrumentation technology and the availability of computer technology to process the images are likely to further the accuracy of nuclear medicine images. Future developments in biotechnology should also assist in designing new pharmaceuticals that are more target-specific, thus further reducing the risks and enhancing both the diagnostic quality of the images and the therapeutic efficacy of radiolabeled compounds.

Another challenge for future research may include searching for new ways to create and manufacture radiopharma- ceuticals. In the early part of the twenty-first century, planned and unplanned closures of nuclear reactors created shortages of radiopharmaceutical materials in Europe; given this, one area of future research may be to find the means to develop these materials in other ways. In December, 2009, the Food and Drug Administration issued a ruling (effective December, 2011) on regulations about the manufacturing process of radiopharmaceuticals for PET scanning, designed to accommodate producers in commercial and nonprofit, academically oriented institutions.

—*Dandamudi V. Rao, PhD*

See also Angiography; Catheterization; Imaging and radiology; Invasive tests; Magnetic resonance imaging (MRI); Nuclear medicine; Nuclear radiology; Positron emission tomography (PET) scanning; Radiation therapy; Single photon emission computed tomography (SPECT).

For Further Information:
Cherry, Simon R., James A. Sorenson, and Michael E. Phelps. *Physics in Nuclear Medicine*. 4th ed. Philadelphia: Elsevier/Saunders, 2012.
Harbert, John C., William C. Eckelman, and Ronald D. Neumann, eds. *Nuclear Medicine: Diagnosis and Therapy*. New York: Thieme Medical, 1996.
Levin, Ken. "Imaging and Radiology." *MedlinePlus*, March 22, 2012.
MedlinePlus. "Nuclear Scans." *MedlinePlus*, May 8, 2013.
Mettler, Fred A., Jr., and Milton J. Guiberteau. *Essentials of Nuclear Medicine Imaging*. 6th ed. Philadelphia: Elsevier/Saunders, 2012.
Radiological Society of North America. "General Nuclear Medicine." *Radiology Info*, May 9, 2013.
Sandler, Martin P., R. Edward Coleman, and James A. Patton, eds. *Diagnostic Nuclear Medicine*. 4th ed. Philadelphia: Lippincott Williams & Wilkins, 2003.
Society of Nuclear Medicine and Molecular Imaging. "What Is Nuclear Medicine?" *SNMMI Resource Center: About Nuclear Medicine & Molecular Imaging*, 2013.

RAPE AND SEXUAL ASSAULT

Category: Disease/Disorder
Anatomy or system affected: Anus, genitals, mouth, psychic-emotional system
Specialties and related fields: Gynecology, psychiatry, public health, emergency medicine
Definition: A crime of violence in which a person is forced to submit to sexual acts.

Key terms:
date rape: a forced sexual act during a date
deoxyribonucleic acid (DNA): genetic material contained in cells, which can definitively identify an individual
incest: a sexual act between close relatives such as father-daughter or brother-sister
perpetrator: an individual who commits a crime
sexual harassment: physical behavior of a sexual nature that is aimed at a particular person or group of people, especially in the workplace or school
statutory rape: a sexual act with a child below the legal age of consent, even if the act is consensual

CAUSES AND SYMPTOMS

Rape is an act of violence; it is an expression of aggression and anger rather than a sexual motivation. A power imbalance usually exists, with the stronger of two individuals committing the assault. The typical victim of rape is a sixteen- to twenty-four-year-old woman; however, any male, female, or child can be raped. Sexual assault has a broader definition than rape. In addition to vaginal, anal, or oral penetration, sexual assault includes inappropriate touching as well as any physical contact, speech, or presentation of images that an individual finds objectionable. Many types of rape and sexual assault exist, including spousal, incest, child, elder, date, acquaintance, coworker, stranger, and same-gender. Cases of women raping women or men exist.

In the United States, the estimated lifetime prevalence of sexual assault is approximately 18 percent in females and 3 percent in males. The typical rapist is a twenty-five- to forty-four-year-old man who plans the attack and usually selects a woman of the same race. About 50 percent of the time, the victim knows the rapist through work, friends, family, or by living in the perpetrator's neighborhood. More than 50 percent of rapes occur in the victim's home. The rapist may break in or gain entry through a ruse, such as posing as a salesman. Compared with other men, rapists drink more heavily, begin having sexual experiences earlier, and are more likely to have been physically or sexually abused as children. Individuals who have been sexually assaulted as children are also more likely to be assaulted as adults. Many studies note that more than 50 percent of all physical and sexual assaults involve a perpetrator who was reported to have been drinking. Often, rape victims have also consumed alcohol before the incident (estimates run as high as 60 to 70 percent). Illegal drug use is a factor in many rapes. The perpetrator may be under the influence of drugs or administer them to the victim. Date rape occurs when a sexual assault occurs during a date. The rapist often gives the victim drugs or alcohol; the most common date rape drug is alcohol. Regardless of the circumstances, victims of sexual abuse are not at fault. For example, if the victim exhibits provocative behavior, the perpetrator should control his (or her) impulses. Most rapes are not reported to the police (80 to 90 percent by most estimates).

Immediately after a rape, the victim may exhibit the following symptoms: inappropriate behavior, confusion, crying, fear, nervousness, hostility, inappropriate laughter, sleep disturbances, anorexia, physical pain, and/or social withdrawal. Physical symptoms of rape include vaginal and rectal lacerations as well as injuries to other body parts. The presence of semen in the vagina or rectum, which can be subjected to DNA analysis for identification of the perpetrator, confirms the diagnosis of intercourse but not rape. Rape victims may suffer from posttraumatic stress syndrome, which may persist for years and have a marked impact on the victim's life. Following a rape, some victims abuse alcohol and/or drugs; some become suicidal. More than 50 percent of rape victims develop difficulties with interpersonal relationships (such as with a husband or other partner).

TREATMENT AND THERAPY

Following a rape, the victim should proceed directly to a hospital without changing clothes, showering, douching, or urinating, as these activities may destroy evidence. Often, rape victims are referred to specialized centers that provide focused care and make certain that proper procedures are followed, including preserving the "chain of evidence." Chain of evidence refers to the proper handling of evidence (semen, hair samples, and skin samples) from the time of collection throughout the legal process. Specimens collected for forensic evaluation include mucosal swabs, skin swabs, fingernail clippings, hair samples, blood samples, saliva samples, the victim's clothes, and semen samples, if available. Sperm may be detected up to 72 hours after an assault in vaginal swabs, up to 24 hours in anal swabs, and are rarely detected in oral swabs. A complete evaluation of the victim may take up to six hours. In female victims, areas that should be carefully evaluated include the breasts, perineum, vagina, anus, and rectum. Nongenital trauma is commonly seen on the victim's extremities, face, and/or neck, which may consist of bruising, abrasions, lacerations, and/or erythema. These are more likely to be present when the victim is examined within 72 hours of the assault, or if the perpetrator is a stranger. Colposcopy may be used to detect milder genital trauma and an ultraviolet (UV) light (ex: Wood's lamp) may assist in detecting semen on the skin. In male victims, areas of concern include the penis, scrotum, prostate, anus, and rectum.

Immediate care includes medical and surgical treatment of injuries, which may be significant. The vic-

> **INFORMATION ON RAPE AND SEXUAL ASSAULT**
>
> **Causes:** For perpetrators, impulsive and antisocial tendencies, alcohol, illegal drug use, history of sexual abuse as child
>
> **Symptoms:** For victims, vaginal and rectal tears, bruises, injury to other body parts
>
> **Duration:** For rapists, many are repeat offenders, who will attempt rape for decades
>
> **Treatments:** For perpetrators, psychological counseling, drug and alcohol rehabilitation, medication; for victims, medical, surgical, and psychiatric treatment

tim-and, if possible, the rapist-should be tested for sexually transmitted diseases (STDs). Minimal screening consists of testing for gonorrhea, chlamydia, trichomonas, bacterial vaginosis, and candidiasis. Necessity to screen for human immunodeficiency virus (HIV) hepatitis, and syphilis should be determined on an individual basis. Victims may opt out of testing for STDs if he/she consents to prophylactic treatment. Prophylactic treatment for STDs is recommended due to the poor follow-up visit rates. Postexposure Hepatitis B vaccination is considered adequate protection against Hepatitis B, unless the perpetrator is known to have Hepatitis B. Prophylactic antiviral medications are controversial after a sexual assault. The risk of HIV transmission after a single consensual episode of vaginal or anal intercourse is estimated to be 0.1-2 percent. Transmission after an assault is presumed to be higher, secondary to the trauma and bleeding. Risk and benefits should be discussed with the patient.

Pregnancy tests should be performed on any female of child-bearing age. If the possibility of exposure to pregnancy exists, then hormonal treatment can be administered to prevent that eventuality. Drug screening may also be performed to detect levels of alcohol, benzodiazepams (for example, the date rape drug, Rohypnol), gamma-hydroxy butyrate (GHB), or other common drugs of abuse.

In addition to treatment of the immediate physical and emotional trauma, follow-up care should be arranged. The victim may be in need of long-term counseling, psychiatric care, and psychiatric medication. Posttraumatic stress disorder (PTSD), depression, and anxiety are commonly seen in victims. Victims may avoid any future pelvic exams, which then puts them at higher risk for cervical cancer.

Child molesters, serial rapists, and violent rapists are often given long-term prison sentences. While in prison, they are offered treatment; however, treatment cannot be enforced. An evaluation of sex offenders incarcerated at Atascadero State Hospital in California reported that 80 percent of sex offenders never participated in any treatment. Occasionally, some child molesters and repeat offenders are given suspended sentences or paroled after a short prison sentence. Some of these offenders have committed further violent attacks, including murder of the rape victim. Sex offenders are required to register with local authorities so that their whereabouts can be made available to the public. Some states define a sexually violent predator as someone who commits a sexually violent crime and who has a mental abnormality or personality disorder. A number of researchers report a high level of success for rapists who undergo a treatment program. A standard premise for counseling and psychiatric care is that the rapist must admit that he or she has a problem for therapy to be successful.

PERSPECTIVE AND PROSPECTS

From the days of ancient Greece through the American colonial period, rape was deemed to be a capital offense. Rapists were subjected to a wide range of punishments, including beatings, castration, and execution. However, in colonial America, the rape of Native American women was not deemed to be a crime because the women were "Pagan and not Christian." Two centuries ago, rape was often not viewed as a type of physical assault; rather, it was deemed to be a serious property crime against the man to whom the woman belonged (her father or husband). The loss of virginity was a particularly serious matter. Under biblical law, if the father agreed, the rapist was required to marry his victim instead of receiving the civil penalty.

Anecdotal reports of rape during warfare have been described since antiquity-Greek, Roman, Persian, and Israelite armies reportedly engaged in rape. During the 1937 Nanking Massacre, it was reported that Japanese soldiers raped as many as 80,000 Chinese women over a six-week period. Anecdotally, by the end of World War II, Red Army soldiers were estimated to have raped approximately 2,000,000 German women and girls. During the 1994 Rwandan genocide, an estimated 500,000 women were raped. One study found that during Liberia's thirteen-year-long civil war, 92 percent of the women interviewed had experienced sexual assault. Even today, rape is being used as a weapon of war in the Democratic Republic of Congo (DRC) to humiliate, dominate, and instill fear in the civilians of a community.

The medical literature contains numerous analyses of rape and sexual assault. In August 2009, researchers at St. Paul's Hospital in Vancouver, British Columbia, published a study that evaluated the sexual assault of prostitutes. They found an "alarming rate" of violence against these women. They recommended that the following steps were crucial to stem violence against pros-

titutes: socio-legal policy reforms, improved access to housing and drug treatment, and scaled-up violence prevention efforts, including police-prostitute partnerships.

Although young adult women are the most frequent targets of sexual assault, physical abuse of older women has risen rapidly during the last decade. In October 2009, researchers with the Michigan State University Program in Emergency Medicine published a study comparing a group of postmenopausal victims of sexual assault with younger adult women (eighteen to thirty-nine years old). During the five-year study period, 1,917 adult sexual assault victims qualified for inclusion in the study; 84 percent of the victims were eighteen to thirty-nine years old, and 4 percent were postmenopausal women who were at least fifty years old. The 72 postmenopausal victims were more likely to be assaulted by a single perpetrator, usually a stranger (56 percent versus 32 percent); to be assaulted in their own home (74 percent versus 46 percent); and to have experienced more physical coercion (72 percent versus 36 percent). The younger women were more likely to have used alcohol or illicit drugs before the assault (53 percent versus 18 percent) and to have a history of sexual assault (51 percent versus 15 percent). Postmenopausal victims had a higher number of nongenital (2.3 percent versus 1.2 percent) as well as anal injuries (2.5 percent versus 1.8 percent). The authors concluded that postmenopausal women are not immune from sexual assault and that the epidemiology of sexual trauma in this age group is different from that of younger women.

Sexual harassment and assault are not uncommon at the workplace. A study published in August 2009, by the University of Southern Maine evaluated the frequency and impact of workplace sexual harassment on the health, work, and school outcomes on high school girls. They noted that sexual harassment has a significant impact on high school girls' connections to work and school; it not only taints their attitudes toward work but also threatens to undermine their commitment to school. They added that as a consequence of sexual harassment experienced at work, teenagers may have their career development or career potential impeded or threatened because of school absence and poor academic performance. In addition, they noted, the physical safety of working students may be at risk under these circumstances, which would create a need for teenagers to receive training to deal with sexual assault and other types of workplace violence.

As it is in adults, alcohol is a frequent component of adolescent peer-on-peer sexual aggression. A study published in September 2009 by the Institute for Research on Women and Gender, University of Michigan, examined the characteristics of adolescents involved in alcohol-related and nonalcohol-related sexual assault of peers. The researchers conducted a Web-based survey of 1,220 students (grades seven through twelve) and found that adolescents who reported alcohol-related and nonalcohol-related sexual aggression had higher levels of impulsivity and more extensive histories of dating, early sexual activity, and alcohol consumption than adolescents who did not assault. Furthermore, perpetrators of alcohol-related assault had higher levels of alcohol use in the past thirty days as well as more alcohol- or drug-related problems than perpetrators of nonalcohol-related assault.

A particularly heinous form of sexual assault is one on a child. In October 2009, investigators at the Crimes Against Children Research Center, University of New Hampshire, Durham, published a study that strove to obtain national estimates of exposure to the full spectrum of childhood violence, abuse, and crime. The researchers conducted a cross-sectional national telephone survey that involved 4,549 children up to age seventeen. The authors found that a clear majority (60.6 percent) of the children had either experienced or witnessed victimization in the previous year. Almost half (46.3 percent) had experienced a physical assault in the study year, almost 25 percent had experienced a property offense, about 10 percent had experienced a form of child maltreatment, 6.1 percent had experienced a sexual victimization, and about 25 percent had been a witness to violence or experienced another form of indirect victimization in the year (including 9.8 percent who had witnessed an intrafamily assault). About 10 percent had experienced a victimization-related injury. More than one-third (38.7 percent) had been exposed to two or more direct victimizations (10.9 percent had five or more, and 2.4 percent had 10 or more) during the study year.

A 2010-2011 survey of adolescents, between the ages of fourteen and twenty-one, revealed that 1 out of 10 adolescents had been the perpetrator of a sexual assault. An association was found with perpetrators and a higher exposure to violent X-rated media. Up to the age of seventeen, the majority of the perpetrators were male. Among those older than seventeen, females and males had an equal representation as perpetrators.

—Robin L. Wulffson, MD; updated by Elizabeth Lynn, MD

See also Addiction; Alcoholism; Club drugs; Depression; Domestic violence; Ethics; Intoxication; Psychiatric disorders; Psychiatry; Psychiatry, child and adolescent; Psychiatry, geriatric; Psychoanalysis; Stress

For Further Information:

American College of Obstetricians and Gynecologists. www.acog.org. The website of the nation's leading group of professionals providing health care for women.

Matsakis, Aphrodite. *The Rape Recovery Handbook: Step-by-Step Help for Survivors of Sexual Assault.* Oakland, CA: New Harbinger, 2003. A step-by-step program to help rape victims deal with the aftermath of an assault.
National Sex Offender Registry. www.family watchdog.us. A free service that allows users to locate registered sex offenders in their area by entering an address.
Reddington, Frances P., and Betsy Wright Kreisel, eds. *Sexual Assault: The Victims, the Perpetrators, and the Criminal Justice System.* Durham, NC: Carolina Academic Press, 2005. Provides a broad overview of sexual assault.
Seneski, Patty. *Color Atlas of Sexual Assault.* St. Louis: Mosby/Elsevier, 2007. A clinical resource for practitioners who treat sexually assaulted individuals.
Summerfeld, Leila Rae. *Beyond Our Control: Restructuring Your Life after Sexual Assault.* Grand Rapids, MI: Kregel, 2009. A personal chronicle of recovery from rape.
United Nations Human Rights: Rape: Weapon of War. www.ohchr.org/en/newsevents/pages/rapeweaponwar.aspx. The website of a United Nations organization that brings awareness to the violations of human rights.
Violence Against Women: State Resources. www.womens health.gov/violence/state. A listing of U.S. organizations by state, with program and contact information.
World Health Organization (WHO). www.who.int/en. The website of this international organization, which monitors human rights abuses including rape.

RECONSTRUCTIVE SURGERY. SEE PLASTIC SURGERY.

RECTAL POLYP REMOVAL. SEE COLORECTAL POLYP REMOVAL.

RECTAL SURGERY. SEE COLORECTAL SURGERY.

RAYNAUD'S PHENOMENON

Category: Disease/Disorder
Anatomy or system affected: Blood vessels, breasts, ears, feet, hands, mouth
Specialties and related fields: Family practice, vascular medicine
Definition: The reduction of circulation in the extremities, inducing a cold- or stress-induced color change
Key terms:
prostaglandin: a group of fatty acids that act as short-range signaling molecules and mediate a wide range of body functions
sympathetic nervous system: a branch of the autonomic system that mediates the "fight or flight" response
vasospasm: sudden, spontaneous constriction of blood vessels

CAUSES AND SYMPTOMS

Raynaud's phenomenon (RP) results from a sudden decrease in blood flow to the extremities, which occur most commonly in the fingers, but also can affect the toes, ears, nose, lips, and nipples. Blood vessel constriction (vasospasm) causes the sudden decrease in circulation. However, what drives vasospasm remains controversial, and many mechanisms have been proposed, but none can account for all cases of RP.

There are two types of RP: primary and secondary RP. The far more common and generally less severe primary RP occurs without an associated disease or an apparent cause (idiopathic). Secondary RP results from some other underlying disease. Diseases of connective tissue, eating disorders, certain drugs or occupations, infectious diseases, environmental conditions, and other miscellaneous effects can cause RP.

Five percent of the population in the United States has RP. In people with RP, exposure to cold causes the skin of the fingers or toes to whiten and feel cold and numb. Over time, the skin turns a bluish tint (cyanosis). Upon warming, the skin turns red and then normal, accompanied by swelling, tingling, and a kind of "pins and needles" feeling.

After experiencing repeated episodes of oxygen depletion, the skin of the extremities can become thin

Raynaud's phenomenon. Photo by MSM98, via Wikimedia Commons.

> **INFORMATION ON RAYNAUD'S PHENOMENON**
>
> **Causes:** Narrowing of small blood vessels that lead to the extremities
> **Symptoms:** Cold extremities; color changes in skin of extremities in response to cold or stress; numb, prickly feeling or stinging pain upon warming or relief of stress
> **Duration:** Usually presents early in life and tends to come and go, but lasts a lifetime
> **Treatments:** Avoiding triggers, medications, in severe cases surgery

and fragile. Ulcers can form and the nails of the hands and toes can deform. In very severe cases the fingers and toes and become gangrenous.

TREATMENT AND THERAPY

Although the above-mentioned symptoms can justify a diagnosis of RP, Doppler ultrasound tests can effectively assess the blood flow in the extremities, as can digital artery pressure tests.

In most cases, avoiding the cold or stresses that cause the attacks can suffice. Avoiding caffeine or other compounds known to cause blood vessel constriction (e.g., pseudoephedrine) can also help. For more severe cases of RP, medication may be required. Medicines used to treat RP include calcium channel blockers, angiotensin-converting enzyme (ACE) inhibitors, alpha-1 receptor blockers, angiotensin receptor blockers, the antidepressant fluoxetine (Prozac), sildenafil (Viagra), nitrates, and a topical cream called RayVa, which contains prostaglandin E1, a known dilator of blood vessels.

Alternative treatments include Gingko biloba extracts, acupuncture, laser therapy, and temperature biofeedback. All of these treatments have been shown to relieve RP symptoms to some degree in various studies.

In extremely severe cases, surgically cutting the sympathetic nerves to the extremities (sympathectomy) provides relief for some patients. In other cases grafting a vein into the extremity (bypass vein grafts) can greatly increase blood flow the hands, augment healing, and relieve symptoms.

—*Michael A. Buratovich, PhD*

See also Alternative medicine; Antihypertensives; Cutis marmorata telangiectatica congenita; Immunopathology; Neurology; Orthopedics; Rheumatology; Systemic sclerosis; Vascular medicine

For Further Information:
Laundry, Gregory J. "Current Medical and Surgical Management of Raynaud's Syndrome." *Journal of Vascular Surgery* 57, no. 6 (June, 2013): 1710-1716.
Porter, Steven B., and Peter Murray. "Raynaud Phenomenon." *Journal of Hand Surgery* 38A (February, 2013): 375-378.

RECREATIONAL THERAPY

Category: Specialty

INTRODUCTION

Recreational therapy (also known as therapeutic recreation) is a form of physical therapy that uses various forms of leisure activities and life skills to promote physical and mental well-being for people with illness or disability. Recreational therapists seek to enhance patients' physical and mental capabilities through activities that patients find stimulating, such as creating art, playing games, or engaging in sports or other physical activities such as dance. The type of prescribed activities varies according to the individual patient's interests and needs.

Recreational therapy is used to assist people suffering from a wide variety of physical, emotional, and mental impairments. For instance, recreational therapy can be used to help people recovering from conditions such as a heart attack or spinal cord injury, or to aid patients suffering from various forms of mental illness or developmental disabilities. It may also be useful in geriatric care to help stimulate the minds and bodies of elderly persons through activities that generate pleasure. Recreational therapy may be practiced in a wide variety of settings, including community, residential, medical, and clinical arenas.

BACKGROUND

Recreational therapy can be used to treat many different categories of health conditions. It is often prescribed for people who have recently suffered severe injuries such as quadriplegia (paralysis of both arms and both legs) or paraplegia (paralysis of the legs or lower body), for people suffering through chronic illnesses, or for patients who have mental impairments. In such situations, recreational therapy can assist in learning life skills to enable independent living or to bring greater pleasure to life through the reduction of anger, anxiety, depression, and stress.

To assist patients properly, recreational therapists, often working closely with occupational therapists, must assess the patients' current needs and long-term goals while evaluating and understanding their existing mental or physical limitations. For example, quadriplegic patients will often require therapy that will help them to live a more independent and, therefore, fulfilling life. This typically includes educating them on how to use adaptive equipment and providing them with therapy that enriches their mental and emotional well-being. Beyond teaching basic life skills, recreational therapists also seek to provide activities that can promote physical rejuvenation. This may include simple games that improve patients' cognitive and social functions while assisting with their psychological recovery. In the case of a quadriplegic who has severely limited physical motion, recreational therapists will also incorporate activities that the patient enjoys, such as listening to music or reading books, to improve his or her quality of life. In this sense, recreational therapy encompasses not just rehabilitation but also promotes psychological exercises intended to allow patients to address their suffering, accept their limitations, and embrace a fulfilling lifestyle moving forward.

Recreational therapy can offer many benefits. People who remain physically and mentally fit after an injury or who learn to adapt to new disabilities, tend to remain healthier and happier for longer periods than those who do not. Older patients who engage in various forms of stimulation provided through recreational therapy remain more physically active and tend to live healthier, more satisfying lives. Older patients who engage in recreational therapy combined with physical and occupational therapies are also more likely to live independently without assistance and take fewer medications.

OVERVIEW

Recreational therapy seeks to promote the ability of patients to enjoy levels of physical and mental activity that enable them to lead productive lives that are fulfilling.. Recreational therapy embraces a holistic view of health management. This often means assessing the needs of patients using a multidisciplinary approach that includes reviewing cognitive, emotional, physical, social, spiritual, and vocational needs and requirements. Based on assessment, the recreational therapist creates a plan of action that incorporates both the care needs and leisure interests of the patient. This plan may require the involvement of family to succeed. After establishing a course of action, the therapist will institute a series of benchmark goals while working with the patient to make sure he or she remains motivated to make progress toward achieving these goals.

Recreational therapists work in a variety of fields. They may apply their skills to aid in recovery from addiction, assist ongoing rehabilitation, work with people with developmental disabilities, or help promote improved mental health. They may also work with a wide type of clientele ranging from pediatric to geriatric patients. Typically, these types of therapists are employed by heath care agencies to work as in-house specialists at hospitals, clinics, health centers, hospices, schools, and adult day care programs. Increasingly, they are also being hired in private practice settings to assist with in-home treatment.

Recreational therapists provide many different services. A patient does not necessarily need to be sick to use this form of therapy. For instance, recreational therapists have assisted veterans returning from wars. In this capacity, they help provide social readjustment through either individual or group therapy. Therapists may also offer assistance with weight management, diabetes, hypertension, and pain management. Recreational therapy has also proven useful in enhancing self-esteem, reducing social isolation, promoting the immune system, and improving mental acuity and alertness. As a result, it can dramatically improve the quality of life of patients.

This form of therapy may take a variety of approaches, including wheelchair sports, yoga, stress management, animal assisted therapy, aquatics therapy, social skills training, and pet therapy. Such programs may use unconventional means to help patients. For instance, the US Veterans Health Administration used a fly-tying class. In addition to providing skills that can be used later to go fly-fishing, it has proven useful in enabling injured veterans to promote increased fine motor skills, develop muscle control, and help motivate them to complete tasks. Upon completion of the class, the veterans are taken on a fishing excursion, which provides them with the chance to socialize with other veterans and relax by catching fish in a calming environment. Similarly, a recreation therapist may play games with children that can simultaneously help with grip strength, cognitive function, and self-confidence. Therapists are also able to help patients self-monitor their health by learning to identify symptoms or other problems that may require intervention.

According to the US Bureau of Labor Statistics, in 2015, recreational therapists earned $45,890 per year, or $22.06 per hour on average. In this same year, there were roughly 18,600 people employed as recreational therapists in the United States, with this profession estimated to demonstrate a 12 percent growth rate between 2014 and 2024. Recreational therapy typically requires a bachelor's degree and certification to be employed in the field.

—*Eric Bullard;*
updated by Patricia Stanfill Edens, PhD, RN, LFACHE

For Further Information:
Austin, David R. *TherapeuticRecreation: Processes and Techniques.* 6th ed., Sagamore Publishing, 2009.
Cherniak, E. Paul, and Ariella R. Cherniak. "The Benefit of Pets and Animal-Assisted Therapy to the Health of Older Individuals." *Current Gerontologyand GeriatricsResearch*, vol. 2014, *National Center for BiotechnologyInformation*, www.ncbi.nlm. nih.gov/pmc/articles/PMC4248608/. Accessed 11 Jan. 2017.
"Definitions of Recreational Therapy." *TherapeuticRecreation Directory*, www.recreationtherapy.com/define.htm. Accessed 11 Jan. 2017.
Luu, Anna. "What Is Recreation Therapy and the Top 10 Activities That You Can Do." *AgeComfort.org*, 31 May 2013, www.agecom fort.org/what-is-recreation-therapy-and-the-top-10-activities-that-you-can-do/. Accessed 11 Jan. 2017.
Murray, Susan "Boon," and Anita Burton. "More than Fun and Games: Recreational Therapists Are Value-Adding Team Members." *Team Rehab Report*, Sept. 1997, pp. 31-5, www.wheelchairnet.org/WCN_ProdServ/Docs/TeamRehab/RR_97/9709art2.PDF. Accessed 11 Jan. 2017.
"Occupational Outlook Handbook: Recreational Therapists." *Bureau of LaborStatistics, United States Department of Labor*, www.bls.gov/ooh/healthcare/recreational-therapists.htm. Accessed 11 Jan. 2017.
"Recreational Therapy: Restoring Function, Recreating Lives." *VeteransHealth Administration*, www.va.gov/health/NewsFeatures/ 20110712a.asp. Accessed 11 Jan. 2017.
"The Recreational Therapy Professional." *Health Professions Network*, www.healthpronet.org/ahp_month/07_04.html. Accessed 11 Jan. 2017.
Skalko, Thomas K., et al. "Assessing Balance and Fall Efficacy in Community-Dwelling Older Adults: Evidence-Based Instruments for Use in Recreational Therapy Practice." *TherapeuticRecreation Journal*, vol. 47, no. 4, 2013, pp. 291-306.
Travers, Catherine, et al. "An Evaluation of Dog-assisted Therapy for Residents of Aged Care Facilities with Dementia." *Anthrozoös*, vol. 26, no. 2, 2013, pp. 213-25.

RECTUM

Category: Anatomy
Anatomy or system affected: Anus, gastrointestinal system, intestines
Specialties and related fields: Gastroenterology, internal medicine, oncology, proctology
Definition: The pouch at the end of the gastrointestinal tract that collects and stores food wastes just before defecation.

STRUCTURE AND FUNCTIONS
The rectum is the pouch at the end of the gastrointestinal tract, between the sigmoid colon and the anal canal. It is about 6 inches (15 centimeters) in length, dilated slightly at the end (the rectal ampulla), and lined by an orange-red tissue with mucous glands, much like the colon.

The rectum remains empty until just before defecation, when wastes pass into it from the colon. Three lateral folds in the rectum, called Houston's valves, hold the feces in place until a sufficient quantity is collected and the walls of the rectum are distended. Nerve receptors in the walls detect the stretching and prompt the urge to defecate. Waves of muscular contraction, known as peristaltic waves, move the feces into the anal canal and through the anus.

Defecation depends in part on a person's conscious relaxation of the anus in response to the defecation urge. If the urge is resisted, then the feces may return to the colon, where water may be absorbed from them. If defecation is postponed repeatedly, the feces may harden and cause constipation.

DISORDERS AND DISEASES

Like the anus, the rectum is subject to a variety of malformations caused by infection or injury. The rectum may develop an abscess-a cavity in its wall that is filled with pus-when bacteria infest a mucous gland. The abscess may open a channel, or fistula, to another part of the rectum, the anus, or an entirely different organ, such as the vagina; fistulas can also be the product of other diseases, such a diverticulitis or injury to the rectum. When the rectum is made to protrude through the anus and outside the body, usually from straining at stool, the condition is called rectal prolapse. Proctitis is inflammation of the rectal lining from a variety of infectious diseases, such as ulcerative colitis or a sexually transmitted disease.

About a quarter of colorectal cancers, the most common of the gastrointestinal tract, occur in the rectum, about equally in men and women. They are adenocarcinomas, growing in the lining of the rectum, and if untreated often spread to the liver or less commonly to the lungs and bones. Rectal cancer usually grows slowly and can be surgically removed.

—*Roger Smith, PhD*

See also Anus; Colon; Colorectal cancer; Colorectal polyp removal; Colorectal surgery; Constipation; Diarrhea and dysentery; Digestion; Gastroenterology; Gastroenterology, pediatric; Gastrointestinal disorders; Gastrointestinal system; Hemorrhoid banding and removal; Hemorrhoids; Hernia; Intestines; Peristalsis; Proctology.

For Further Information:
Ahuja, Nita, and Brenda S. Nettles. *Johns Hopkins Medicine Patients' Guide to Colon and Rectal Cancer.* Burlington, Ma.: Jones and Bartlett Learning, 2014.
Beers, Mark H., ed. *The Merck Manual of Medical Information: Second Home Edition.* London: Pocket Books, 2004.
Keshav, Satish. *The Gastrointestinal System at a Glance.* 2d ed. Oxford: Wiley-Blackwell, 2013.
Levin, Bernard, et al., eds. *American Cancer Society's Complete Guide to Colorectal Cancer.* Atlanta: American Cancer Society, 2006.
Parker, Steve. *The Human Body Book.* 2d ed. New York: Dorling Kindersley, 2013.
Thibodeau, Gary A., and Kevin T. Patton. *Structure and Function of the Human Body.* 14th ed. St. Louis, Mo.: Mosby/Elsevier, 2012.

REFLEXES, PRIMITIVE

Category: Development
Also known as: Newborn reflexes
Anatomy or system affected: All
Specialties and related fields: Family medicine, pediatrics, perinatology
Definition: Involuntary patterns of behavior that can be elicited in the newborn infant.
Key terms:
in utero: a Latin phrase meaning "in the uterus"; refers to the period of fetal development
subcortical centers of the brain: the parts of the brain that control and regulate basic physiological functions, including breathing, body temperature regulation, sleeping, and waking; these parts are contrasted with the cortex, where voluntary control of behavior originates

PHYSICAL AND PSYCHOLOGICAL FACTORS

Primitive reflexes range from very simple reactions such as the blinking and startle reflexes to more complex patterns of behavior such as the stepping and crawling reflexes. Primitive reflexes appear to be important for orienting the infant to its environment and for protecting it against potential threats to its safety. The reflexes are automatically elicited when an appropriate stimulus is present, such as liquid in the mouth or pressure on the bottom of the feet, and they take the same form on every occasion.

Several primitive reflexes exist for the head and face. Blinking is elicited when an object approaches the eye. This reflex functions to protect the eye from harm. The head-turning reflex is seen when an infant is placed face down on a soft surface such as a mattress. The infant will turn its head to one side to allow breathing to continue. Similarly, the defensive reaction reflex is seen when a cloth is placed over an infant's face. The infant will turn its head and make swiping movements with its arms in an attempt to clear away the obstruction. Rooting and sucking are two important reflexes of the face that assist in feeding. The rooting reflex is elicited when an object gently touches an infant's cheek; the infant will turn its mouth in the direction of the touch. Sucking is elicited whenever a nipple-sized object is placed in an infant's mouth.

The reflexes of the arms include the Moro reflex and the tonic neck reflex. The Moro reflex is seen when an infant's head is dropped slightly. The infant's legs and its arms, with hands extended, will spread wide, then come together in an embracing movement as the hands clench. This sequence of behaviors appears to be a defense against falling, as the reflexive response could allow the infant to grasp on to something. The Moro reflex is seen in other primates as well. The tonic neck reflex is seen when an infant, lying on its back, has its head turned to one side. The infant's arm on the same side will extend, and the other arm will move up to the back of its head, to assume a "fencing position." This reflex is also called the fencer's reflex.

The primitive reflex of the hand is the palmar or grasping reflex. If an object touches an infant's palm, then the hand will clench into a fist. If the object is small enough for the infant to get a grip on it, then the infant's grip will be strong enough to support its own weight. A newborn infant grasping an adult's fingers with both hands can be pulled to a sitting or standing position.

The swimmer's reflex is seen when an infant is lying on its stomach. If the infant is gently tapped along its side above the waist, then it will turn its torso in the direction of the touch. Another primitive reflex of the torso is the crawling reflex. If an infant is lying on its stomach and pressure is applied against the soles of its feet, then it will move its arms and legs in a crawling movement. This reflex may be a precursor for later voluntary crawling behavior.

Two reflexes of the legs also appear to prefigure later-developing motor behavior. If an infant is held upright under the arms and its feet are allowed to touch a surface, then the infant will demonstrate the standing reflex by straightening its legs and supporting some of its body weight. If the infant is then tilted forward and moved forward slightly, then it will make high stepping movements characteristic of the stepping reflex.

The plantar reflex is similar to the palmar reflex. If an infant's foot is stimulated with an object touching the sole just below the toes, then the toes will curl around the object as if to grasp it. The Babinski reflex is another reflex of the foot; if the outside edge of an infant's foot is gently stroked, then the toes will fan out. The Babinski reflex, unlike many of the other primitive reflexes, does not have an obvious function; the lack of a Babinski response, however, may indicate neurological dysfunction.

Some of the primitive reflexes, such as sucking and grasping, have been detected in utero. Most of the reflexes disappear within a few months after birth, although some primitive reflexes, such as blinking, persist throughout life. Still other reflexes, such as the crawling and walking reflexes and the defensive reaction, are later replaced by behaviors that are voluntarily controlled.

DISORDERS AND EFFECTS
Because the absence of primitive reflexes can indicate neurological damage, most infants are tested for some of the reflexes soon after birth. Reflexes of the face, hands, and feet are components of neurological examinations such as the Brazelton Neonatal Behavioral Assessment Scale.

Despite the fact that the primitive reflexes are involuntary, infants show variability in their reflexive responses. There are individual differences among infants, such that some infants may show stronger or weaker primitive reflexes than others. Within individual infants, there is variation in the strength with which the reflexes may be elicited on different occasions. The age of the infant, its state of arousal, and the interval since its last feeding are all factors that can affect an infant's reflexive responses.

PERSPECTIVE AND PROSPECTS
Traditionally, it was believed that primitive reflexes disappeared with brain development, as the higher centers of the brain took over some motor functions from the subcortical centers of the brain. Recent investigations of the stepping reflex, however, have shown that other factors can affect the development of the reflexes.

Esther Thelen and Linda B. Smith, in their book *A Dynamic Systems Approach to the Development of Cognition and Action* (5th ed., 2002), report that infants who no longer show the stepping reflex under typical circumstances do demonstrate stepping if their legs are submerged in water. Similarly, the stepping reflex can be suppressed in very young infants by adding weights to their legs. Another study, by Philip Zelazo, as described in an article found in *Developmental Psychobiology: The Significance of Infancy* (1976), provided infants with daily stepping practice and showed that under those conditions, the stepping reflex did not disappear. These findings suggest that experience, growth, and weight gain, as well as brain development, influence the developmental course of the primitive reflexes.

—*Virginia Slaughter, PhD*

See also Breast-feeding; Cognitive development; Developmental stages; Motor neuron diseases; Motor skill development; Neonatology.

For Further Information:
Behrman, Richard E., Robert M. Kliegman, and Hal B. Jenson, eds. *Nelson Textbook of Pediatrics.* 18th ed. Philadelphia: Saunders/Elsevier, 2007.
Berk, Laura E. *Child Development.* 8th ed. Boston: Pearson/Allyn & Bacon, 2009.
Brazelton, T. Berry, and J. Kevin Nugent, eds. *Neonatal Behavioral Assessment Scale.* 3d ed. New York: Cambridge UP, 1995.
Field, Tiffany. *Infancy.* Cambridge, Mass.: Harvard UP, 1991.
Goddard, Sally. *Reflexes, Learning And Behavior: A Window Into The Child's Mind: A Non-Invasive Approach to Solving Learning & Behavior Problems.* Eugene, Oregon: Fern Ridge Press, 2009.

Huether, Sue E. *Understanding Pathophysiology*. New York: Mosby, 2011.

Jarvis, Carolyn. *Physical Examination & Health Assessment*. New York: Saunders, 2011.

Nathanson, Laura Walther. *The Portable Pediatrician: A Practicing Pediatrician's Guide to Your Child's Growth, Development, Health, and Behavior from Birth to Age Five*. 2d ed. New York: HarperCollins, 2002.

Stanley, Jenna. "Reflex Action." *Parents* 73, no. 5 (May, 1998): 24-25.

Thelen, Esther, and Linda B. Smith. *A Dynamic Systems Approach to the Development of Cognition and Action*. 5th ed. Cambridge, Mass.: MIT Press, 2002.

REFRACTIVE EYE SURGERY

Category: Procedure

Also known as: Vision correction, laser-assisted in situ keratomileusis (LASIK), laser epithelial keratomileusis (LASEK), photorefractive keratectomy (PRK)

Anatomy or system affected: Eyes

Specialties and related fields: Ophthalmology

Definition: A surgical procedure that changes the way in which the eye refracts light, thus correcting vision disorders.

INDICATIONS AND PROCEDURES

When light rays enter the eye, the cornea and lens bend (refract) the rays to focus them on the retina. When the eye is shaped in such a way that light rays are not sharply focused on the retina, an error in refraction occurs. Refractive eye errors that can be alleviated or cured with surgery are myopia, hyperopia, and astigmatism. Myopia (nearsightedness) is caused by a cornea that is too sharply curved, causing light rays to focus in front of the retina rather than on it, resulting in blurry distance vision. With hyperopia (farsightedness), the cornea is too flat, so light rays focus beyond the retina rather than on it, causing blurred vision when viewing near objects. Astigmatism is caused by a cornea that is uneven, curving and flattening in different spots on the eye, which makes it difficult to see objects at any distance. It is estimated that ninety million people suffer one or more of these vision defects.

Laser-assisted in situ keratomileusis (LASIK) is the most common refractive surgery in use. By 2006, more than forty million of these surgeries had been performed in the United States. LASIK can be used if the patient is nearsighted, farsighted, and with or without astigmatism. The surgeon conducts an intensive eye examination prior to the surgery to determine whether the cornea needs to be flattened or curved, and in what specific area. Then anesthetic drops are used to numb the eye.

The surgeon uses a blade or a special cutting laser to cut a hinged flap about the size of a contact lens from the front of the eye. The flap is folded back to allow access to the tissue in the cornea that needs reshaping. After the tissue is properly shaped with another kind of laser called an excimer laser, the flap is folded back in place. Usually, no stitches are required. The procedure is painless and takes fifteen to twenty minutes, depending on the condition of the eye before surgery and whether both eyes are reshaped. Patients can usually leave the doctor's office within two hours. Postsurgery care involves the use of medicated eyedrops and wearing an eye shield at night. Healing is usually complete in five to seven days. The vision shows some immediate improvement, and, in about two to three months, most patients will have between 20/20 and 20/40 vision.

Laser epithelial keratomileusis (LASEK) is similar to LASIK up to the point of surgery. During a LASEK procedure, however, a thinner layer of the cornea is folded back. This is of particular benefit to people who have thinner-than-normal corneas. Also, people who work in jobs where there is a high risk of injury prefer LASEK. A thinner flap means less damage to the patient's vision should the flap be torn before it is healed. Healing is rapid, and full vision is recovered.

Photorefractive keratectomy (PRK) is used with patients who have a low-to-moderate degree of nearsightedness or farsightedness, or farsightedness with astigmatism. Unlike the LASEK procedure, to which it is very similar, with PRK the thin layer of the cornea is removed altogether. The surgeon then uses a laser to either flatten or curve the cornea, depending on the patient's need. A contact lens is placed on the raw cornea, to be worn as a bandage for three or four days. It takes the eye three to six months before vision improves completely. With PRK, the recommendation is to do only one eye at a time. It is the least used of the three procedures. Healing after the LASEK or LASIK methods is faster and involves less discomfort and scarring.

USES AND COMPLICATIONS

Some risks are associated with refractive surgery. Undercorrection occurs when too little tissue is removed from the eye, more often in treatments for nearsightedness. Another surgery to remove more tissue may be required. Overcorrection, when too much tissue is removed from the cornea, can occur when the eye moves during surgery. It is difficult to fix, and additional surgery may be needed to remedy the condition. Astigmatism can also be caused by uneven tissue removal.

Double vision, glare, and halos around bright lights are also risks of refractive surgery. These conditions can be greatly helped with eyedrops that contain cortisone, but sometimes a second surgery is needed. Cases of dry eyes, sometimes severe, also occur. Special plugs for tear ducts are used to prevent tears from draining away from the surface of the eyes, keeping them moist. Flaps folded back during surgery can sometimes become infected and tear and swell. The flap removed during PRK may also grow back abnormally.

PERSPECTIVE AND PROSPECTS

In 2002, the LASIK procedure was improved by a technique known as wavefront-guided LASIK. Wavefront sensors measure the acuity and quality of a patient's vision twenty-five times more accurately than previous testing methods. They record how the eye processes light and show unique distortions in each individual eye. This enables the surgeon to make a more precise cut.

Alternative refractive surgery procedures developed in recent years include conductive keratoplasty, which uses radio frequency (RF) energy instead of a laser to reshape the cornea, and phakic intraocular lenses (IOLs), which are essentially surgically implanted contact lenses that can correct severe myopia. These and other procedures widen the range of options for people seeking surgical vision correction.

The total cost of LASIK refractive eye surgery varies widely, but is generally between $1,000 and $2,500 per eye. Use of the wavefront technology adds another $500. Many insurance companies consider refractive eye surgery elective and will not pay for it. The Food and Drug Administration (FDA) urges people who are considering refractive eye surgery to check a doctor's credentials before the operation.

—*Billie M. Taylor, MSE, MLS*

See also Blurred vision; Eye infections and disorders; Eye surgery; Eyes; Laser use in surgery; Myopia; Ophthalmology; Optometry; Sense organs; Surgery, general; Vision; Vision disorders.

For Further Information:
Braham, Lewis. "Eye Surgery: It's Getting Sharper." *Business Week*, October 18, 2004, pp. 142-143.
Fiscbetti, Mark. "Clear Favorite." *Scientific American* 290 (May, 2004): 106-107.
"LASIK Eye Surgery." *Mayo Clinic*, November 4, 2011.
"LASIK-Laser Eye Surgery." *American Academy of Ophthalmology*, 2013.
Rapuano, Christopher J., ed. *Refractive Surgery*. San Francisco: American Academy of Ophthalmology, 2012.
Sunshine, Wendy Lyons, and Adam Martin. "Lasik Woes: Here's Help." *Health* 18, no. 1 (January/February, 2004): 50-54.

REITER'S SYNDROME

Category: Disease/Disorder
Anatomy or system affected: Eyes, gastrointestinal system, joints, mouth, skin, urinary system
Specialties and related fields: Dermatology, family medicine, gynecology, ophthalmology, orthopedics, urology
Definition: An autoimmune disorder with associated symptoms of arthritis, urethritis, conjunctivitis, and ulcerations of the skin and mouth.

CAUSES AND SYMPTOMS

Although the exact cause of Reiter's syndrome is unknown, the disease is associated with the entry of an infectious agent through the urinary or intestinal tract. Reiter's syndrome associated with sexual contact occurs primarily in men and is most often linked to the bacteria *Chlamydia trachomatis*. Dysenteric Reiter's syndrome is caused by other bacteria, particularly *Salmonella* or *Shigella*. Genetic factors may also play a vital role in causing the disease, as a large majority of patients with Reiter's syndrome have the gene *HLA-B27*, while other people do not.

After the onset of Reiter's syndrome, urethritis occurs within seven to fourteen days, typically followed by conjunctivitis and arthritis over the next several weeks. The urethritis is often accompanied by a burning sensation during urination and a mild discharge from the urethra or the genitals. Conjunctivitis occurs in approximately 40 percent of the victims and ranges from mild to very painful. The arthritis usually involves the spine and large joints of the lower extremities, producing significant swelling, redness, and pain. The disease is often accompanied by low-grade fever, watery growths on the skin, and lesions on the palms of the hands, soles of the feet, trunk, and mouth. In some cases, an inflammation of the iris known as iritis may occur.

TREATMENT AND THERAPY

Treatment for Reiter's syndrome includes taking anti-inflammatory drugs, such as aspirin, ibuprofen, indomethacin, or phenylbutazone, as well as cortisone injections. Tetracycline may help control associated urethritis, while cortisone drops can relieve conjunctivitis. Topical medications are used to treat skin lesions. Appointments with different specialists, including dermatologists, urologists, and ophthalmologists, may be necessary in order to treat specific symptoms of the disease. In about half of the victims, Reiter's syndrome resolves itself within three to six months.

In addition to medical therapy, physical therapy is often prescribed. Short periods of bed rest can reduce

INFORMATION ON REITER'S SYNDROME

Causes: Bacterial infection, usually transmitted through sexual contact; may be related to genetic factors

Symptoms: Urethritis (burning sensation during urination, mild urethral or genital discharge); conjunctivitis (mild to painful); arthritis of spine and lower extremities (swelling, redness, pain); low-grade fever; watery skin growths; lesions on palms, soles, trunk, and mouth; sometimes inflammation of iris

Duration: Three to six months

Treatments: Anti-inflammatory drugs (aspirin, ibuprofen, indomethacin, phenylbutazone), cortisone injections, tetracycline, topical medications for skin lesions, physical therapy, bed rest, occupational therapy

pain and inflammation. Exercises can increase joint mobility and improve muscle tone. Occupational therapy teaches victims how to place less stress on affected joints and how to better cope with painful symptoms by promoting positive attitudes. In rare cases that involve severe joint damage, orthopedic surgeons may need to reconstruct the joints.

PERSPECTIVE AND PROSPECTS

Reiter's syndrome was first diagnosed in a World War I soldier in 1916 by Hans Reiter, a German military physician. He described the disorder as inflammation of the joints, urinary tract, and eyes. It primarily affects males between the ages of twenty and forty. Approximately half of those who suffer one or two bouts with Reiter's syndrome never have another attack. Subsequent attacks beyond that can lead to joint deformity and permanent arthritis.

—*Alvin K. Benson, PhD*

See also Arthritis; Autoimmune disorders; Bacterial infections; Chlamydia; Conjunctivitis; Joints; Lesions; Men's health; Salmonella infection; Shigellosis; Urethritis.

For Further Information:
Mayo Clinc. "Reactive Arthritis." *Mayo Clinic*, March 5, 2011.
Parker, James N. and Phillip M. Parker *Reiter's Syndrome: A Medical Dictionary, Bibliography, and Annotated Research Guide to Internet References*. San Diego, Calif.: ICON Group, 2004.
Rosenfeld, Isadore. *Symptoms*. New York: Bantam Books, 1994.
Standring, Susan, et al., eds. *Gray's Anatomy*. 40th ed. New York: Churchill Livingstone/Elsevier, 2008.
Teitel, Ariel D. "Reactive Arthritis." *MedlinePlus*, June 15, 2012.
Teitel, Ariel D. "Reiter Syndrome-View of the Feet." *MedlinePlus*, June 15, 2012.
Toivanen, Auli, and Paavo Toivanen, eds. *Reactive Arthritis*. Boca Raton, Fla.: CRC Press, 1988.

RELAXATION

Category: Biopsychosocial
Anatomy or system affected: Body, mind, spirit
Specialties and related fields: Psychology, CAM, integrative medicine
Definition: A general term referring to a release of tension and restoration of equilibrium

Relaxation is recreation engaged in by people usually after working or participating in any other physically or mentally strenuous activity. Relaxation may take the form of simple downtime, in which one sleeps longer, reads a book, exercises, or travels. The term *relaxation* can also refer to a mental state of calmness and serenity, in which one is free from anxiety and stress. Stress is mental or emotional tension caused by difficult, unfavorable, or dangerous circumstances. A relaxed person generally experiences a slowed heartbeat and breathing rate, lowered blood pressure, reduced stress, and increased confidence for managing obstacles.

Many health providers emphasize the importance of regular relaxation, particularly for people whose jobs or personal lives cause them a great deal of stress. Stress has long been known to have negative effects on the heart, brain, and other areas of the body. Relaxation techniques such as meditation, breathing exercises, and physical activity can reduce stress and create a sense of general well-being in people. In these ways, relaxation plays an important role in human mental health.

BACKGROUND

People may find that they need to relax after becoming stressed by various activities or life situations. Stressors can be different for everyone. Many people report becoming stressed by certain aspects of their jobs, particularly being dissatisfied with their position within their work setting, having too much work to do, working under unfair or dangerous conditions, or being harassed or discriminated against by customers, coworkers or superiors.

Conditions in one's personal life can also cause stress. Marriage, divorce, the loss of a job, financial obligations, the death of a friend or relative, or moving to a new location can all cause people to feel stressed. In other cases, people can cause their own stress with the attitudes they take to adverse life situations. Consistently worrying about stories in the news, such as terrorism and natural disasters, can. Be the source of stress as well as focusing on the negative aspects of a situation rather than the positive ones.

Long-term stress can have detrimental effects on a person's health. Stress activates the nervous system's fight-or- flight response, which releases the hormone adrenaline into the body. Adrenaline raises heart rate and breathing rate, and causes sweating and muscle tension. This is a normal biological reaction to stress, and the human body can quickly calm itself after isolated stressful incidents. Stress over an extended period, however, can lead to significant health problems such as high blood pressure; irregular heartbeat, or arrhythmia; heart attacks; ulcers; headaches; and depression.

Health providers claim it is important for people to manage their stress in healthy ways to reduce their chances of developing more serious health complications. Leading a healthy lifestyle and maintaining a positive outlook on life can help reduce stress, and making time to relax both physically and mentally has also been shown to benefit one's overall health. For this reason, health providers recommend that people practice a number of relaxation techniques, or relax simply by slowing down the pace of their everyday lives, to recover from stressors.

METHODS FOR RELAXATION

Meditation is a relaxation technique in which people generally sit on the floor or in a comfortable place, close their eyes, breathe regularly. Linking the repetition of the mantra to one's breaths can aid in this concentration. The goal of meditating is to focus the mind on peaceful thoughts and forget about one's stress, thereby bringing about mental relaxation.

There are many different methods for practicing meditation, with roots linked in both Eastern and Western philosophy. It is important to find a type of meditation that most effectively allows relaxation to occur. Three generally accepted types of meditation are mantra meditation, mindfulness meditation, and spiritual meditation. Most modern meditation employs and combines techniques found in these types of meditation.

Mantra meditation involves the repetition of a mantra, either vocally or internally, as the focus of concentration. A mantra is a word or phrase that is used as the focal point of concentration. Spiritual meditation focuses on religious principles and the practice of this type of meditation varies depending on one's beliefs. The goal of spiritual meditation is to connect with a higher power or spiritual concept. Mindfulness meditation consists of focusing on being in the present moment involving a non-reactive internal awareness.

Related to meditation is another relaxation technique involving measured breathing. To relax by breathing, people should sit with their backs straight and inhale deeply through the nose, hold the breath, and then exhale through the mouth. Repeated cycles of deep inhalation and exhalation can reduce stress

by slowing one's heart rate and decreasing blood pressure.

Other relaxation methods require a person to conjure up mental images that play a role in stress reduction. In autogenic relaxation, people may imagine peaceful places while concentrating on relaxing each part of their body individually. Visualization is similar to autogenic relaxation but focuses more intensely on the mental image of a happy setting. People practicing visualization try to use most of their senses to feel as though they actually are at that setting. They imagine seeing the scenery, hearing its natural sounds, and feeling the wind or the sun on their bodies. Visualization may be accompanied by measured breathing.

Physical activity is another effective method for relaxation. Physiological changes that occur in the body during and after physical activity allow for mental relaxation to occur. Health providers praise regular exercise for its ability to produce endorphins and thereby reduce a person's stress and anxiety. Exercise has even been found to be an effective treatment for moderate depression. In addition to helping a person mentally relax, exercise can also lower body fat, strengthen muscles, and make the heart healthier.

Aerobic exercise, strength training, and yoga are all effective physical activities that help alleviate stress and allow for relaxation. Aerobic exercises can be practiced at any level of intensity in order to achieve a relaxed state. Some types of aerobic exercise include walking, jogging, biking and swimming. The term "runner's high" describes a state of mind achieved through the release of endorphins that cause the brain to experience a state of euphoria. Despite the name, this feeling can be achieved doing any aerobic exercise. Strength training involves the use or combination of free weights, body weight, and resistance bands to strengthen muscles. Similar to aerobic exercise, strength training releases endorphins. Strength training can be an effective method of increasing mobility and loosening tight muscles, which are both major stressors for people living sedentary lifestyles. Yoga is the practice of combining body positioning, mental concentration, and controlled breathing. There are numerous ways to practice yoga, different types may focus more on the physical components or the mental components. The goal is to achieve a state of mental and physical well-being.

Other methods of relaxation involve less devoted attention and consist simply of leisure activities. Some people relax by reading, which lets them temporarily forget their stressors. Others may relax by hiking in nature, driving in scenic locations, spending time with friends and family, taking vacations, cleaning, sleeping, playing musical instruments, or cooking. Certain foods contain substances that interact with the brain to produce feelings of well-being. Green tea, for instance, contains the chemical L-theanine, which can help relieve anxiety. The anti-inflammatory properties of honey can reduce anxiety and depression. The linalool contained in mangos, meanwhile, can decrease stress.

—Michael Ruth;
updated by Michael Moglia

For Further Information:
Casano, Tom. "20 Fun Ways to Relax on the Weekend." *Huffington Post*, 8 Sept. 2016, www.huffingtonpost.com/tom-casano/20-fun- ways-to-relax-on-t_b_8091420.html. Accessed 27 Dec. 2016.
"Causes of Stress." *WebMD*, www.webmd.com/balance/guide/causes-of-stress. Accessed 27 Dec. 2016.
"Exercise and Depression." *WebMD*, www.webmd.com/depression/guide/exercise-depression#1. Accessed 27 Dec. 2016.
Klein, Sarah. "10 Health Benefits of Relaxation." *Huffington Post*, 16 Apr. 2012, www.huffingtonpost.com/2014/08/14/stress- awareness-day-relaxation-benefits_n_1424820.html. Accessed 27 Dec. 2016.
Lebowitz, Shana. "40 Ways to Relax in 5 Minutes or Less." *Greatist*, 8 Mar. 2014, greatist.com/happiness/40-ways-relax-5-minutes-or-less. Accessed 27 Dec. 2016.
Moninger, Jeannette. "10 Relaxation Techniques That Zap Stress Fast." *WebMD*, www.webmd.com/balance/guide/blissing-out- 10-relaxation-techniques-reduce-stress-spot. Accessed 27 Dec. 2016.
"Relaxation Techniques: Try These Steps to Reduce Stress." *Mayo Clinic*, www.mayoclinic.org/healthy-lifestyle/stress-management/in-depth/relaxation-technique/art-20045368?pg=1. Accessed 27 Dec. 2016.
Shakeshaft, Jordan. "6 Breathing Exercises to Relax in 10 Minutes or Less." *Time*, 8 Oct. 2012, healthland.time.com/2012/10/08/6- breathing-exercises-to-relax-in-10-minutes-or-less/. Accessed 27 Dec. 2016.
"Stress Basics." *Mayo Clinic*, www.mayoclinic.org/healthy-lifestyle/stress-management/basics/stress-basics/hlv-20049495. Accessed 27 Dec. 2016.
"Exercising to Relax." Harvard Health, Harvard Health Publications, Feb. 2011, www.health.harvard.edu/staying-healthy/exercising- to-relax. Accessed 09 Sept. 2017.
Burke, Adam, et al. "Prevalence and Patterns of Use of Mantra, Mindfulness and Spiritual Meditation among Adults in the United States." BMC Complementary and Alternative Medicine, vol. 17, no. 1, 2017, doi:10.1186/s12906-017-1827-8.

REMINISCENCE THERAPY

Category: Procedure
Anatomy or system affected: Memory, psychological well being
Specialties and related fields: Gerontology, psychology
Definition: The use of life histories—written, oral, or both—to improve psychological well-being

OVERVIEW

At its most basic, *reminiscence therapy* involves listening to a patient and encouraging the individual to share his or her memories. The listener may ask directed questions to encourage further sharing. Reminiscence therapy is most beneficial in treating individuals with memory disorders such as dementia, as well as anxiety and depression, and may be useful as an alternative to drug therapies for challenging patients.

Persons benefit from knowing their experience is valued by others. Many times, older individuals feel marginalized. They may have mobility issues that prevent them from seeking out company, or they may be intimidated by technology—cell phones and computers, for example—and therefore feel isolated. Individuals with cognitive challenges such as dementia may find the modern world confusing and lonely. They often lose *short-term memory*—memory of what has happened very recently—and may feel disoriented and frightened. Such feelings of isolation often lead to depression. Caregivers may be older individuals' only source of companionship. By encouraging persons to share stories and actively listening to these tales, caregivers often can help these individuals to feel connected to the modern world.

Persons with dementia generally retain their earliest memories for the longest time. Reminiscence therapy has been found to be most beneficial to individuals with mild to moderate dementia. According to the Institute for Research and Innovation in Social Services (IRISS) in Scotland, several 2009 studies found that patients who participated in reminiscence therapy had better relationships with caregivers and families, had improved cognitive abilities and mood, functioned better, and had reduced symptoms of depression. A 2010 study in Taiwan found that aged persons without dementia also benefited from reminiscence therapy, according to IRISS. They were less depressed, more sociable, and generally in better mental health than individuals in the control group. The studies found no negative effects from reminiscence therapy.

Reminiscence therapy provides both *therapeutic*, or healing, benefits and pleasure. Recalling happier times reinforces the individual's connection to the world and may increase feelings of self-worth. Memories of difficult experiences such as loss or tragedy may help individuals process feelings and gain a better understanding of both events and themselves. Reminiscence therapy can improve cognitive ability among patients by providing stimulation.

WORKING WITH PATIENTS

Reminiscence therapy may be conducted one-on-one or in group settings with a therapist who facilitates discussion and encourages all participants to share stories. Reminiscence activities have an overall positive effect when conducted with groups of aged populations. Therapists may use items, such as photos, or play music to spark memories. At times, therapists may use one-on-one sessions to collect information and create a book of an individual's life history (*life story work*), which may further help a patient who struggles to maintain his or her identity as cognitive function fails. Such information also aids caregivers. For example, reminiscence therapy and life story work may reveal and document favorite or hated foods and activities such as hobbies and lifestyles—information that enables care homes and caregivers to provide appropriate opportunities. A patient who once enjoyed outdoor activities may benefit from regular walks outside, for instance. A person who once practiced needlepoint may be encouraged to try painting. Family members may even develop life stories for individuals as they prepare to move to care facilities to aid the transition and help the patient hold on to his or her identity. Both music therapy and reminiscence therapy are currently being used to increase aspects of wellbeing in older people, including those with memory diseases such as dementia, as alternatives to pharmacological treatments. There is growing evidence that combining these therapies in a focused way would provide unique wellbeing outcomes for this population.

Though sad memories of difficult times may bring tears, they can be therapeutic. Listeners must respect the memories and experiences of the patient and allow them to feel their emotions. Silence, too, is important—while at times a listener may need to ask questions or share appropriate stories, at other times it is best to sit in silence together.

Reminiscence may be encouraged at all times of the day, and nurses and other caregivers may be best positioned to facilitate such talk. Patients in care facilities might be open to talking about the past during meals, while receiving physical therapy, or while walking with assistance. Reminiscence also may be used as an aid to encouraging relationships with caregivers and developing friendships with other patients. This therapy may help patients transition from their home environment to an institutional setting or when moving between institutions. Caregivers such as nurses are encouraged to see patients as individuals (to see beyond the diagnosis) and be sensitive to their culture and background to deliver *person-centered care*, which focuses on treating patients with dignity and respect and ensuring they have personal choice and a sense of community and security. Reminiscence therapy has been shown to benefit both patients and caregivers.

For late-stage dementia patients, who often are unable to communicate well or to even speak, stimulation such as music is likely to trigger memories. By providing music associated with happy times or events, caregivers can improve patients' moods. This outcome may provide a long-lasting effect, because moods often last longer than memories.

Caregivers can provide reminiscence therapy by encouraging communication using many methods, including the following:

- *Ask open-ended questions.* How did you learn to paint? What were you doing when (the first astronauts went to space, World War II ended, etc.)?
- *Take cues from the patient's possessions.* Ask questions about photographs and souvenirs: Who are the people in the photo? Is this memento from a trip? What was it like?
- *Stimulate the senses.* Music, dancing, food, and smells, for example, may trigger memories.
- *Turn to literature.* Read an excerpt from a book set in an earlier time or an account of some event or activity from decades ago, and ask the individual to comment.

—*Josephine Campbell;*
updated by Geraldine Marrocco

For Further Information:
Fletcher, T. S. (2017). Factors that bring meaning to mementos created by elders. *Agingand Mental Health, 21*(6), 609-615. doi:10.1080/13607863.2016.1141284
Huntsman, Mark. "How Reminiscence Therapy Improves the Lives of Alzheimer's Patients." *Alzheimers.net.* A Place for Mom, Inc. 22 Apr. 2014. Web. 3 Feb. 2015. www.alzheimers.net/2014-04-22/reminiscence-therapy-improves-alzheimers/
Istvandity, L. (2017). Combining music and reminiscence therapy interventions for wellbeing in elderly populations: A systematic review. *Complementary Therapies in Clinical Practice, 28*, 18-25. doi:10.1016/j.ctcp.2017.03.003
Klever, Sandy. "Reminiscence Therapy: Finding Meaning in Memories." *Nursing* 43.4 (Apr. 2013): 36-37. Lippincott Williams & Wilkins. Web. 3 Feb. 2015. journals.lww.com/nursing/Fulltext/2013/ 04000/Reminiscence_therapy_Finding_ meaning_in_memories.11.aspx
"Supporting Those with Dementia: Reminiscence Therapy and Life Story Work." *IRISS.* The Institute for Research and Innovation in Social Services. May 2011. Web. 3 Feb. 2015. www.iriss. org.uk/resources/supporting-those-dementia-reminiscence- therapy-and-life-story-work
Watson, Karen Everett. "Reminiscence Therapy Benefits Residents." *Provider.* Provider. Jun. 2011. Web. 3 Feb. 2015. www.providermagazine.com/archives/archives-2011/Pages/0611/Reminiscence%20Therapy%20Benefits%20LTC%20Residents.aspx
"What Is Reminiscence Therapy?" *Dorset HealthCare.* Dorset HealthCare NHS Foundation Trust. Apr. 2009. Web. 3 Feb. 2015. www.dorsethealthcare.nhs.uk/WS-Dorset-HealthCare/Downloads/Managing%20Your%20Health/Therapy%20Infor mation%20Leaflets/L141-09 ReminiscenceTherapy.pdf
Derived from: "Reminiscence therapy." *Salem Press Encyclopedia of Health.* Salem Press.

RENAL FAILURE

Category: Disease/Disorder
Anatomy or system affected: Heart, immune system, kidneys
Specialties and related fields: Immunology, internal medicine, nephrology, pathology
Definition: A breakdown of kidney function that prevents the removal of waste materials from the body.

CAUSES AND SYMPTOMS

Renal failure, also called kidney failure, renal insufficiency, or end-stage renal disease (ESRD), can be defined as a decline in kidney function sufficient to result in the retention of metabolic waste material in the body. The loss of the ability of the kidneys to excrete waste material is often progressive, culminating in complete renal failure in untreated cases. Although kidney disease can occur at any age, most cases occur in adults, frequently as a complication of diabetes and/or hypertension.

There are three major causes of renal failure. The first, prerenal, results from obstruction of the renal artery because of vascular causes such as hypertension. The decreased blood flow to the kidney causes tissue destruction and loss of renal function. Prerenal causes may also be linked to liver disease and congestive heart failure. The second major cause of renal failure is a direct breakdown of kidney function as a result of inflammatory processes associated with infection. Certain drugs may also have toxic effects on kidney function. The third major cause of renal failure is postrenal, which refers to obstructions that block the flow of urine from the kidney.

The body cannot survive without at least one functioning kidney. As a consequence of renal failure, toxic metabolic wastes accumulate in the bloodstream, such as urea nitrogen produced in the metabolism of proteins. Renal failure also results in disturbances of electrolyte balance, associated with high levels of sodium, potassium, and other salts. Other complications include compromised cardiovascular function, pulmonary edema, gastrointestinal symptoms, chronic fatigue, and infections.

TREATMENT AND THERAPY

Acute renal failure can be treated effectively with hemodialysis and/or kidney transplantation. The hemodialysis machine has made it possible to extend the lives of many patients. This external device filters the blood as it traverses fluid-bathed semipermeable membrane filters that remove metabolic wastes while permitting the retention of essential blood components. Blood leaves the body and returns postfiltration through a

---

> ## INFORMATION ON RENAL FAILURE
>
> **Causes:** Obstruction of renal artery (from hypertension, liver disease, congestive heart failure), infection, certain drugs, obstruction of urine flow from kidney
> **Symptoms:** Accumulation of toxic metabolic wastes in bloodstream, electrolyte imbalance, cardiovascular problems, pulmonary edema, gastrointestinal symptoms, chronic fatigue, infections
> **Duration:** Acute or chronic and progressive
> **Treatments:** Hemodialysis, kidney transplantation

fistula or access joint inserted under the skin to link arterial and venous blood flow. Dialysis must be carried out on a regular basis and requires several hours.

The best treatment for renal failure is a kidney transplant. Sadly, there are not enough donor kidneys to meet the need; patients who do receive organ donations may wait for years before transplantation occurs. As of 2013, United Network for Organ Sharing data show that about one million people in the United States have ESRD and more than 95,000 are on the waiting list to receive a kidney donation. Research continues on an artificial kidney that would replicate the delicate filtering functions of the kidney's glomeruli. A study published in the journal *Nature Medicine* in April 2013 reported that scientists have been able to bioengineer working kidneys in rats. While the kidneys lacked the full function of normal kidneys and much more work needs to be done, the milestone represents a promising step towards the goal of creating fully functional artificial kidneys from the cells of patients in need of a transplant.

—*Sarah Crawford, PhD*

See also Dialysis; End-stage renal disease; Hemolytic uremic syndrome; Kidney cancer; Kidney disorders; Kidney transplantation; Kidneys; Nephritis; Nephrology; Nephrology, pediatric; Polycystic kidney disease; Transplantation.

For Further Information:
Aronoff, George. *Kidney Failure: The Facts*. New York: Oxford University Press, 1996.
Brenner, Barry M. et al., eds. *Brenner and Rector's The Kidney*. 9th ed. Philadelphia: Saunders/Elsevier, 2012.
HealthDay. "'Bioengineered' Kidneys Show Promise in Rat Study." *MedlinePlus*, April 15, 2013.
MedlinePlus. "Kidney Failure." *MedlinePlus*, May 20, 2013.
Mitch, William E., and Saulo Klahr, eds. *Handbook of Nutrition and the Kidney*. 6th ed. Philadelphia: Lippincott Williams & Wilkins, 2010.
Molitoris, Bruce A., and William Finn, eds. *Acute Renal Failure*. Philadelphia: W. B. Saunders, 2001.
Savitsky, Diane. "Kidney Failure." *Health Library*, October 31, 2012.

REPRODUCTIVE SYSTEM

Category: Anatomy

Anatomy or system affected: Abdomen, genitals, uterus

Specialties and related fields: Embryology, genetics, gynecology, obstetrics, proctology, urology

Definition: The organs of the female (the vagina, uterus, Fallopian tubes, ovaries, and mammary glands) and the male (the penis, testes, vas deferens, and prostate gland) that are necessary for the production of offspring.

Key terms:

bladder: the pouch in the abdominal cavity that collects urine until it can be eliminated from the body; while not a part of the reproductive system, it is located adjacent to the reproductive organs and is an important landmark

fertilization: the process in which the sperm head penetrates the ovum, resulting in the formation of an embryo

gametes: the reproductive cells in either sex (the sperm and the ova)

hormone: a chemical signal that is carried in the blood from its site of production to the area where it has an effect

menstrual cycle: the cycle of ovum development, hormone production, and menstruation in female primates; in humans, the average duration is about twenty-nine days

ovulation: the release of an ovum from its follicle in the ovary

ovum: the female gamete; a large spherical cell that carries the female's chromosomes

sperm: the male gamete; the mature sperm has an oval head that contains the male's chromosomes and a long tail that allows it to swim in fluid

STRUCTURE AND FUNCTIONS

The reproductive system in each sex includes the organs that produce the gametes, called the gonads, and those that transport the gametes. In addition, the female mammary glands are also considered reproductive organs since they produce milk to nourish the newborn, a critical step in survival of the species.

The male gonads are the testes, which are located within the scrotum, a pouch of skin and muscle that is suspended from the body wall. In the adult, each egg-shaped testis measures about 2.5 centimeters by 4.0 centimeters. Internally, the testes contain seminiferous tubules, hollow tubes in which the sperm develop. Besides the sperm cells, the seminiferous tubules also contain Sertoli cells, large cells in which the developing sperm are embedded. The Sertoli cells produce hormones, pass nutrients to the sperm, protect them from blood-borne toxins, and control their development. In spaces between adjacent seminiferous tubules are the interstitial cells of Leydig, which produce testosterone and other hormones.

Lying near each testis within the scrotum is the epididymis. Sperm undergo several stages of development within the testis, then move into the epididymis, where they proceed through further steps in maturation, including the development of the swimming ability that is necessary for fertilization of an ovum.

The narrow end of the epididymis is continuous with the long (45-centimeter) tubule called the vas deferens. The vas deferens leads upward from the epididymis and passes through a narrow ring of tissue, the inguinal canal, to enter the abdominal cavity. Within the abdominal cavity, the vas deferens loops over the top of the bladder, then turns downward to enter the prostate gland below the bladder. Near the end of the vas deferens, an enlarged area called the ampulla serves as a storage site for mature sperm.

Within the prostate gland, the vas deferens becomes a short segment of tubule known as the ejaculatory duct. The two ejaculatory ducts (one on each side) empty into the urethra, the tube that extends downward from the bladder. In the male, theurethra carries either semen or urine, but not both at the same time: A valve-like structure below the bladder prohibits urine outflow when semen is moving through the system. The urethra passes through the penis to open to the outside at the tip of the penis.

Besides the urethra, the penis contains three columns of erectile tissue, spongy material with a large blood supply. During sexual excitement, the blood flow into the erectile tissue increases while the outflow decreases; the accumulation of blood within the erectile tissue causes the penis to increase in both length and diameter, a process known as erection. Erection allows the penis to become stiff enough to be inserted into the female's vagina during intercourse. On the outside of the penis, the enlarged area at the tip, the glans penis, is well supplied with touch receptors that play a role in sexual excitement.

During intercourse, stimulation of the touch receptors on the penis results in ejaculation, the expulsion of semen from the male's body. During ejaculation, sperm move out of the vasa deferentia, through the ejaculatory ducts, and then through the urethra. This sperm movement is caused not by the swimming of the sperm but by the contractions of involuntary muscles in the walls of the tubules. As sperm pass through the tubules, they are mixed with fluid secreted by three glands: the prostate, located immediately below the bladder; the seminal vesicles, which open into the vas

The Male Reproductive System

Urinary bladder

Vas deferens

Pubis

Prostate gland

Erectile tissue

Urethra

Seminal vesicle

Glans penis

Epididymis

Testis

Scrotum

©EBSCO

deferens above the prostate; and the bulbourethral or Cowper's gland, which lies below the prostate and opens into the urethra. The fluid secreted by these glands contains chemicals and nutrients that will ensure the survival of the sperm within the female tract.

The female's vagina serves as the repository for sperm released during ejaculation and as the outlet for the fetus during childbirth. The outer opening of the vagina is located behind the urethra, which carries only urine and does not have a reproductive role in the female. Bartholin's and Skene's glands are located near the urethral and vaginal openings; these glands supply moisture and mucus to the female external genitals. The vaginal and urethral openings are located between folds of tissue, the labia majora and the labia minora. At the front junction of these folds is the clitoris, a small round structure containing many touch receptors; stimulation of the clitoris during intercourse is important in promoting sexual gratification in the female. The area that includes the labia, the vaginal and urethral openings, and the clitoris is known as the vulva.

Internally, the vagina consists of a recess with elastic walls and a large blood supply, but little sense of feeling since there are only sparse touch receptors. The vagina slants upward and slightly backward from its outer opening. Near its upper end is the cervix, the lowest portion of the uterus. The cervix consists of strong connective tissue and contains glands that secrete mucus. The cervix has a narrow passageway, the cervical canal, that opens into the main part of the uterus.

The uterus is about 7.5 centimeters long and 5.0 centimeters wide in the nonpregnant woman. The wall of the uterus is composed primarily of involuntary muscle controlled by nerves and hormones. The inner part of the uterus is hollow and is lined with a spongy layer of cells, the endometrium; the endometrium has a large blood supply and contains glands that secrete nutrients for the embryo during pregnancy. The endometrium undergoes growth during the menstrual cycle and is shed as the menstrual discharge if the woman does not become pregnant.

At either side of the upper end of the uterus are the oviducts, or Fallopian tubes, which are hollow tubes that open into the cavity of the uterus. The oviducts lead upward and sideways away from the uterus toward the ovaries, with their funnel-shaped ends adjacent, but not attached, to the ovaries.

The ovaries are the female gonads; they produce ova, the female gametes. Each 3-centimeter-long ovary contains thousands of follicles, spherical structures that each contain one ovum. Hormonal signals cause growth of some of the follicles during the menstrual cycle, and, as they grow, the ova within them mature. The follicles are also sites of production of the hormones estrogen and progesterone. In the middle of the menstrual cycle, one follicle will ovulate, releasing its ovum, which will enter the oviduct to be transported toward the uterus.

During intercourse, after sperm are deposited in the vagina, the sperm will swim in the fluids of the female tract, passing upward through the cervical canal, the uterus, and the oviducts. If an ovum is present in one of the oviducts, it may be fertilized by a sperm. The fertilized ovum will then move downward to the uterus, where it will attach to the endometrium and develop into an embryo. At birth, uterine muscle contractions will cause stretching of the cervical canal and movement of the fetus through the cervix and vagina.

Milk production (lactation) in the woman's breasts after childbirth will allow for the nourishment of the newborn. Milk is produced in glands within the breast; ducts carry the milk to openings in the nipple. In between the milk-producing glands are wedges of fat; it is the fat tissue that determines the size of the breast in the nonpregnant woman. Breast size is not related to milk-producing ability.

DISORDERS AND DISEASES

Abnormalities may exist in either the male or the female reproductive tract as a result of deviations during embryonic development, injury, or disease. Anatomical abnormalities in the reproductive system often can be corrected surgically.

In hypospadias, a problem during embryonic development of the male reproductive organs causes the urethral opening to be on the underside of the penis rather than at its tip. Hypospadias can occur independently or can be a sign of more serious problems. Urethral stricture or stenosis refers to a narrowing of the urethra; this can occur anywhere along its length, from the tip of the penis back to the prostate gland. Urethral stenosis causes difficulty in urination; it may be present from birth or result from later damage or infection. Cryptorchidism is the presence of one or both testes in the abdominal cavity instead of in the scrotum. In the male embryo, the testes begin development in the body cavity near the kidneys and then migrate into the scrotum during the last month or two before birth. In some male infants born with undescended testes, the testes will spontaneously move into the scrotum shortly after birth. If not, then the cryptorchidism must be corrected surgically, usually within the first year of life, in order to prevent later infertility and other complications.

In females, problems during embryonic development can also lead to malformed reproductive organs. The vagina may be present but may not have an outer opening, or conversely, the outer opening may lead to an abnormally shallow vagina. The uterus may be divided into two separate halves (bicornuate uterus), and the vagina may also show such a division. It is also possible for a normal uterus to have an abnormal placement in the abdomen: It may be tilted backward or bent forward at an atypical angle. Surprisingly, variations in the anatomy of the uterus often have little effect on fertility.

Malfunctions in embryonic development of the reproductive organs can lead to hermaphroditism, a rare condition in which an individual has a mixture of male and female reproductive organs. A hermaphrodite may be either a genetic male or a genetic female. Hormone treatment and surgery can usually assure a fulfilling sex life in adulthood for such individuals.

In inguinal hernia, the wall of the inguinal canal between the scrotum and abdominal cavity becomes weakened and stretched. A loop of the intestine may then become lodged in the canal, or the testis and epididymis may move upward to block the canal. The symptoms of inguinal hernia include pain during

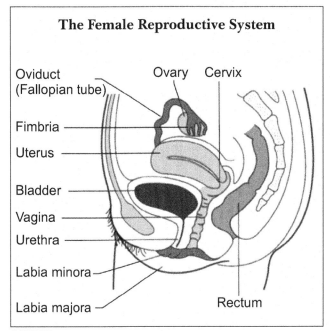

The Female Reproductive System

Oviduct (Fallopian tube)
Ovary
Cervix
Fimbria
Uterus
Bladder
Vagina
Urethra
Labia minora
Labia majora
Rectum

©EBSCO

movement, especially during the lifting of heavy objects, and the presence of a soft lump in the herniated area.

A varicocele is a group of enlarged blood vessels within the scrotum. Varicoceles are thought to arise because of impaired blood flow from the testis. Normally, the blood flowing through the scrotum maintains the temperature of the testes a few degrees below that of the rest of the body. When the blood flow out of the scrotum is reduced in the presence of a varicocele, the temperature in the testes tends to increase. This increased temperature can cause infertility, since sperm production requires a local temperature that is lower than the normal body temperature. Increased scrotal temperature can be the cause of infertility in other situations as well: the wearing of tight clothing, prolonged soaking in hot water, or during episodes of fever. Infertility in these situations is usually temporary and self-correcting.

In women, stretching of the pelvic area during childbirth sometimes leads to uterine prolapse, a condition in which the uterus sags into the vagina. Other causes of prolapse are developmental abnormalities, lifting heavy objects, and loss of muscle and tissue strength with aging. A prolapsed uterus is associated with pain during intercourse and may cause difficulty in urination. Temporary relief from a uterine prolapse can be achieved with the use of a pessary, a device worn in the vagina to support the uterus. Surgery to restore the supporting tissues in the pelvis may be necessary for long-term relief, but in some cases the uterus cannot be returned to its proper position and so must be removed, a process called hysterectomy.

In endometriosis, patches of endometrial tissue from the uterine lining attach to and grow on other organs in the pelvic cavity, affecting the shape and function of these organs. It is thought that the endometrium escapes into the pelvis through the oviducts during menstruation. The abnormally placed endometrial tissue can cause pain and infertility. Endometriosis can be treated with hormone therapy or with surgery to remove the endometrial patches. In more severe cases and when the woman does not wish to bear children in the future, the removal of the uterus may be required to control the invasion of other organs by the endometrial patches. The ovaries may also be removed in order to eliminate the source of hormones that produce the growth of the endometrium.

In polycystic ovary syndrome, one or both ovaries contain cysts that are formed from follicles that have failed to ovulate. Women with polycystic ovaries either do not menstruate or have irregular patterns of bleeding. Because ovulation does not occur, they are infertile. Another symptom of polycystic ovary syndrome is growth of hair in a male pattern on the face, neck, and chest; the hair growth is caused by certain hormones that are produced in abnormal amounts by the ovaries. Therapy usually involves hormone treatment in an attempt to establish ovulation and to prevent the deleterious effects of abnormal hormone levels on the body.

Both benign (nonspreading) and cancerous tumors may appear in the reproductive organs. Potential sites of tumor growth are the testes and prostate gland in the male and the ovaries, uterus, and breasts in the female. Only rarely do tumors cause pain, but they may be detected during routine self-examination of the testes or breasts or during a doctor's examination. Treatment usually begins with surgery to remove the tumor, and x-ray therapy or chemotherapy prevents further tumor growth. Hormone treatment can also be useful in controlling the growth of some reproductive tumors. The exact factors that cause tumors to form are not well understood, but a family history of such problems, abnormal hormone levels, and exposure to radiation, pollutants, and toxins have all been implicated.

Prostate tumors should not be confused with nodular prostatic hyperplasia, an increase in the size of the prostate gland that occurs in about 75 percent of men over sixty years old. The enlargement appears to be caused by dihydrotestosterone (DHT), a hormone related to testosterone; the prostate gland itself is one site of conversion of testosterone into DHT. Prostate enlargement is associated with difficulty during urination and ejaculation. It has traditionally been managed with surgery to remove the gland or to reduce its size. More recently, several drugs have been approved to reduce the production of DHT and either prevent

the progression of growth of the prostate or shrink the prostate in some individuals..

PERSPECTIVE AND PROSPECTS

Rituals involving alteration of the reproductive organs have been performed since ancient times. Castration (removal of the testes) has been carried out for various reasons. In early times, men who were guards of noble women were castrated to control their sexual activity. During the Renaissance, castration of boys was performed to produce singers who would retain their clear, high-pitched voices, since it is testosterone that causes the deepening of the voice at puberty. More recently, castration has been espoused as a "treatment" for habitual rapists: Some judges sentence convicted sex offenders to castration, despite the fact that many authorities believe that rape is a manifestation of violent tendencies, rather than the result of excessive sexual desire.

In the United States and elsewhere, it is common for boys to undergo circumcision, or the removal of the foreskin, a flap of tissue that covers the glans of the penis. Parents have their sons circumcised in order to conform to religious and cultural practices. In the United States, the procedure is usually performed shortly after the boy's birth, but in other cultures circumcision may occur during puberty rituals. One rationalization for performing circumcision is that removal of the foreskin helps to prevent the buildup of smegma, a thick secretion produced by glands located under the base of the foreskin. In fact, some studies have shown that circumcised boys are less likely to have urinary tract infections. There are no apparent effects of circumcision on sexual functioning. Researchers debate the advisability of circumcision, however, and the medical establishment has not established a definitive recommendation.

It is less well known that circumcision of women is practiced in some cultures. Indigenous groups who perform female circumcisionare found in the Pacific Islands, Asia, the Middle East, and Africa, and the practice has been carried to the United States by immigrants. The term *female circumcision* refers to three procedures that may be carried out singly or together. In simple circumcision, the flap of tissue covering the clitoris is removed. The entire visible part of the clitoris is removed in clitoridectomy. Infibulation is the sewing together of the labia to cover the vaginal opening, leaving only a small hole for the discharge of urine and menstrual fluid. A woman who has been infibulated cannot have intercourse or give birth; the tissue must be cut open to allow either of these events, after which the area may be sewn closed again.

Female circumcision may take place shortly after a girl's birth or at puberty, and it is performed for a variety of reasons. Infibulation is a means of enforcing female abstinence from sexual activity. A wish to control women's sexual desire is also given as a reason for performing simple circumcision and clitoridectomy. Also involved are the society's views of what the ideal female organs should look like. From a medical standpoint, female circumcision is of concern because of pain and discomfort caused by the development of scar tissue in the vulval area. It is not known how many women die from infection or bleeding following these procedures, which are usually performed by other women under less-than-sanitary conditions.

—*Marcia Watson-Whitmyre, PhD*

See also Abortion; Amenorrhea; Amniocentesis; Aphrodisiacs; Assisted reproductive technologies; Breast-feeding; Breasts, female; Candidiasis; Catheterization; Cervical, ovarian, and uterine cancers; Cervical procedures; Cesarean section; Childbirth; Childbirth complications; Chlamydia; Circumcision, female, and genital mutilation; Circumcision, male; Conception; Contraception; Culdocentesis; Cyst removal; Cysts; Dysmenorrhea; Ectopic pregnancy; Electrocauterization; Endocrine disorders; Endocrinology; Endometrial biopsy; Endometriosis; Episiotomy; Erectile dysfunction; Fistula repair; Gamete intrafallopian transfer (GIFT); Gender reassignment surgery; Genital disorders, female; Genital disorders, male; Glands; Gonorrhea; Gynecology; Herpes; Hormone therapy; Hormones; Hydroceles; Hypospadias repair and urethroplasty; Hysterectomy; In vitro fertilization; Infertility, female; Infertility, male; Laparoscopy; Masturbation; Menopause; Menorrhagia; Men's health; Menstruation; Miscarriage; Multiple births; Myomectomy; Obstetrics; Orchitis; Ovarian cysts; Ovaries; Pap test; Pelvic inflammatory disease (PID); Penile implant surgery; Pregnancy and gestation; Premature birth; Premenstrual syndrome (PMS); Prostate cancer; Prostate enlargement; Prostate gland; Prostate gland removal; Puberty and adolescence; Semen; Sexual differentiation; Sexual dysfunction; Sexuality; Sexually transmitted diseases (STDs); Sterilization; Stillbirth; Syphilis; Systems and organs; Testicles, undescended; Testicular cancer; Testicular surgery; Testicular torsion; Trichomoniasis; Tubal ligation; Ultrasonography; Uterus; Vasectomy; Warts; Women's health.

For Further Information:
Ammer, Christine. *The New A to Z of Women's Health: A Concise Encyclopedia.* 6th ed. New York: Checkmark Books, 2009.
Berek, Jonathan S., ed. *Berek and Novak's Gynecology.* 15th ed. Philadelphia: Lippincott Williams & Wilkins, 2012.
Jones, Richard E., and Kristin H. Lopez. *Human Reproductive Biology.* 4th ed. London: Academic Press, 2013.
Manassiev, Nikolai, and Malcolm I. Whitehead, eds. *Female Reproductive Health.* New York: Parthenon, 2004.
Marieb, Elaine N. *Essentials of Human Anatomy and Physiology.* 10th ed. San Francisco: Pearson/Benjamin Cummings, 2012.
Quilligan, Edward J., and Frederick P. Zuspan, eds. *Current Therapy in Obstetrics and Gynecology.* 5th ed. Philadelphia: W. B. Saunders, 2000.
Strauss, Jerome F., III, and Robert L. Barbieri, eds. *Yen and Jaffe's Reproductive Endocrinology: Physiology, Pathophysiology, and Clinical Management.* 6th ed. Philadelphia: Saunders/Elsevier, 2009.
Taguchi, Yosh, and Merrily Weisbord, eds. *Private Parts: An Owner's Guide to the Male Anatomy.* 3d ed. Toronto, Ont.: McClelland & Stewart, 2003.
Wade, L. "Learning from Female Genital Mutilation: Lessons from Thirty Years of Academic Discourse." *Ethnicities* 12, no. 1 (February, 2012): 26-49.

RESEARCH VS. ANIMAL RIGHTS. SEE ANIMAL RIGHTS VS. RESEARCH.

RESPIRATION

Category: Biology
Anatomy or system affected: Chest, lungs, muscles, musculoskeletal system, nose, respiratory system, throat
Specialties and related fields: Biochemistry, exercise physiology, otorhinolaryngology, pulmonary medicine, vascular medicine
Definition: A basic physiological process in which an organism takes in oxygen (which is utilized as a source of energy) and produces carbon dioxide (which is excreted as a waste product).
Key terms:
capillaries: the smallest and most numerous blood vessels in the cardiovascular system; these vessels connect the arteries to the veins and are where all exchange of oxygen and nutrients occurs
diffusion: the process in which substances move from an area of high concentration to an area of low concentration; given enough time, the concentration of the substance will be the same everywhere
hemoglobin: a special molecule, found only in red blood cells, that binds oxygen very efficiently in the lung and releases it to the tissues
partial pressure of a gas in a gas: the measure of the contribution of one gas of a mixture of gases to the total pressure pushing on the walls containing it; it is the pressure that would be exerted if all the other gases were removed from the container, leaving only the gas of interest
partial pressure of a gas in a liquid: the measure of how much of a gas dissolves into a liquid when the liquid is in contact with a gas mixture; if the gas and liquid are in contact long enough, the liquid is said to have the same partial pressure as the gas mixture; the absolute measure of the amount of gas in a liquid is the partial pressure multiplied by the ability of the gas to dissolve in liquid (solubility)
plasma: the fluid of blood in which the blood cells (white and red) are suspended
pressure: the measure of how much a gas or a liquid pushes on the walls of its container

THE MECHANICS OF RESPIRATION

The primary function of respiration is performed by the lungs and their associated tissues. Air must be breathed in through the mouth and nose through the larynx (voice box) into the main airway, the trachea (windpipe). Inside the chest, the trachea branches into the two main airways called bronchi, which in turn successively branch many times into small bronchi called bronchioles. These airways end in very small sacs called alveoli. These alveoli have a very thin membrane separating the air space from the blood in the capillaries. Oxygen (O_2) diffuses through the alveolar membrane across the capillary membrane and into the blood to be taken to all the tissues of the body. Tissues excrete carbon dioxide (CO_2) into the blood that is carried back to the lungs. Carbon dioxide diffuses from the blood into the alveoli and is carried back through the airways and out of the lungs with the exhaled air. The mouth and nose humidify dry air to ensure that the linings of the lower airways do not dry out. The main airway divides to supply the left and right lungs. These large airways are cylindrical. Their circular shape is maintained by C-shaped cartilage in the walls. The stiff walls prevent collapse of the airways and the loss of gases through the walls of these "conducting" airways. The airways branch repeatedly into smaller airways. As the airways become smaller, they have less cartilage, until, in the very smallest airways, the cartilage is absent. These thin airways, which are called respiratory bronchioles, have alveoli budding from their walls. Gases may diffuse through the walls of these airways. These bronchioles become alveolar ducts and then erupt into lobular sacs of alveoli. There are about 300 million alveoli in an individual's lungs, which provide about 70 square meters of extremely thin membrane through which most gas exchange occurs.

The lungs are elastic in nature and have a tendency to collapse. They do not because they adhere to the inside surface of the chest wall in much the same way that a moist suction cup adheres to a smooth surface. The two surfaces may slide against each other without separating. The chest wall has a tendency to expand because the rib cage and the muscles between the ribs (the intercostal muscles) tend to pull the chest out and up. The balance of these forces (elastic recoil and chest wall expansion) keeps the lungs slightly expanded at all times. Like balloons, the alveolar sacs have a tendency to collapse. The lungs produce a substance called surfactant that keeps the small air sacs from collapsing.

Air gets into and out of the lungs in the following way. The lungs expand, drawing air into them. The lungs adhere to the diaphragm in the same way that they adhere to the chest wall. When the muscles of the diaphragm contract, the lungs are pulled down. At the same time, the intercostal muscles contract slightly, making the chest wall rise up and out. These actions cause the lungs to expand. This expansion causes the pressure inside the lungs to decrease, sucking in air. When the intercostal muscles and diaphragm relax, the elasticity of the lungs causes them to deflate again to their resting state. This passive recoil of the lungs causes the pressure inside them to increase and pushes air out of the lungs.

The amount of air breathed in each breath is called the tidal volume. Each breath contains about 500 milliliters of air. Normally, a human being breathes in and out about twelve times in one minute. This results in about 6,000 milliliters of air being breathed each minute. Not all air that enters the mouth or nose reaches the area of the lung where gases are exchanged. About 150 milliliters of each breath stay in the larger airways. Therefore, 4,200 milliliters of air reach the alveolar space each minute. Since the chest wall and the chemical surfactant tend to keep the lungs partially inflated even after the breath is normally exhaled, additional air can be blown from the lungs, if one exhales consciously and forcefully. The volume of air blown out in this manner, which is called the expiratory reserve volume, is normally about 1,000 milliliters. Additional air can also be drawn into the lungs after a normal inspiration. This volume, the inspiratory reserve volume, is normally about 3,000 milliliters. The sum of the tidal, inspiratory reserve, and expiratory reserve volumes, which is called the vital capacity of the lungs, is about 4,500 milliliters. If these reserves are called into play, tidal volume can be increased almost tenfold. The breathing rate can also be increased at least twofold. Therefore, total alveolar ventilation can be as great as 120,000 milliliters per minute.

The oxygen that is drawn into the lungs diffuses into the blood, and carbon dioxide diffuses out of the blood into the alveolar spaces to be exhaled. Fresh air exerts a pressure (barometric pressure) of 760 millimeters of mercury (mmHg). Oxygen is 21 percent of air; therefore, it has a partial pressure of about 160 mmHg. It mixes with air in the lungs that has lost oxygen to the blood. This results in a reduction in the partial pressure to about 100 mmHg by the time the breathed air reaches the alveoli. Blood pumped by the right ventricle of the heart into the lungs to be oxygenated has only 40 mmHg of oxygen. Oxygen diffuses from an area of high concentration in the alveoli to the blood, which has a low concentration. This diffusion process is rapid enough that the partial pressure in the blood becomes equal to that of the alveoli before it courses one-half the distance through the lung capillary. Although the partial pressure is 100 mmHg, the amount of oxygen carried in blood fluids (plasma) is low. Therefore, without red blood cells containing hemoglobin, blood cannot carry much oxygen to the tissues.

Hemoglobin is a very efficient carrier of oxygen. Each molecule of hemoglobin can carry four molecules of oxygen. In the same way that a disposable diaper absorbs water, hemoglobin absorbs oxygen from the plasma, allowing more oxygen to diffuse into the blood from the alveoli. As hemoglobin absorbs oxygen, it turns from a bluish purple to red. Between partial pressures of 20 and 100 mmHg, hemoglobin can absorb a large amount of oxygen. Hemoglobin does have a maximum capacity for oxygen that is reached at about 100 mmHg. Hemoglobin is called saturated at this point, and it can hold no more even if the partial pressure of oxygen increases. Hemoglobin is filled to half capacity by the time the plasma partial pressure reaches 30 mmHg. When the partial pressure increases from 20 to 100 mmHg, the increase in the amount carried by the plasma is 2.1 milliliters of oxygen per liter of blood. With the same change in partial pressure, hemoglobin increases the amount of oxygen carried by approximately 150 milliliters per liter of blood. Blood can carry more than seventy times the amount that plasma alone can carry at this range of partial pressure. If the partial pressure does increase beyond 100 mmHg, little more oxygen is added to the blood. Oxygen is added to plasma in the dissolved form at a rate of 0.03 milliliters of oxygen per liter of plasma for each 1 mmHg change in the partial pressure.

Oxygen is carried to the tissues by the blood, where it is efficiently removed from hemoglobin. The partial pressure in the tissues is between 20 and 60 mmHg, depending upon the particular tissue and the rate at which the tissue uses oxygen. Inside the tissues, the partial pressure can be as low as 1 mmHg, providing a large difference to stimulate diffusion into the tissues. Oxygen is quickly absorbed by the tissue. Just as rapidly, carbon dioxide diffuses out of the cells and into the blood. There are also special ways in which the blood carries carbon dioxide to increase its capacity.

Carbon dioxide dissolves in plasma in much the same way that oxygen does, but supplemental mechanisms are required to carry the large amounts of carbon dioxide produced by the body. Carbon dioxide is also absorbed by red blood cells. It diffuses into the red blood cells, where it is changed in chemical form. Stimulated by an enzyme, carbonic anhydrase, carbon dioxide is combined with water and converted to a new chemical (the bicarbonate ion). The bicarbonate ion can attach to hemoglobin in this form. This, in effect, keeps the concentration of carbon dioxide in the plasma low, allowing more to diffuse. In the normal range of operation (40 to 50 mmHg), blood can absorb about 470 milliliters of carbon dioxide per liter of blood. With this large capacity, the partial pressure need change only a few mmHg to carry all the carbon dioxide that is produced by the tissues.

The anatomy of the lungs and the functioning of the respiratory system are well suited to meet most of the challenges that life presents. Exercise is a good example of how the respiratory system can handle a challenge. At rest, a fit young man breathes 6,000 milliliters of air per minute and uses about 250 milliliters of oxygen per minute to supply his body's needs. When exercising to his maximal capacity, the same individual may use as many as 4,000 milliliters of oxygen per minute. To supply this increased demand, the respiratory system must utilize all the reserve volumes discussed above and increase the breathing rate to a total of 120,000 milliliters of air per minute. The brain senses the movement of the arms and the legs. It also senses the greatly increased amount of carbon dioxide produced by the exercising muscles. In turn, the brain sends signals to the chest and diaphragm to breathe much deeper and faster.

Another example of the large reserve capacity of the human lungs is the ability to hold the breath. Since only a small amount of oxygen from each breath is used, a person can take a deep breath and hold it easily for nearly one minute. Some pearl divers can take a deep breath and swim underwater for four minutes or longer. The urge to breathe that one experiences while holding one's breath is produced when the brain senses the buildup of carbon dioxide and the decrease of oxygen in the blood.

The brain also uses its ability to sense the oxygen in the blood to adjust to unusual environments. At high altitudes, there is less oxygen in the air. With less oxygen in the air, less gets into the blood. The brain senses this condition and signals the respiratory system to breathe more air. Therefore, when one travels into the mountains, one will breathe slightly deeper and faster. One is not aware of the increased breathing until fairly high altitudes are reached (above 10,000 feet). If one begins to exercise, however, performing even mild exercise such as brisk walking, one will be very aware of breathing heavily. This situation is greatly intensified if the person has diseased lungs. With some severe lung diseases, even people living at low altitudes (sea level) have shortness of breath, and some need to breathe air supplemented with extra oxygen.

DISORDERS AND DISEASES

The major type of lung disease, which is called obstructive disease, has three subclasses. The first is general obstruction, a disease in which material is abnormally present in an airway. The second is disease in which the large airways are narrowed. The third is disease in which the small airways and alveoli are diseased.

The case of general airway obstruction is simple. The simplest form is one in which a foreign body such as food or part of a child's toy is lodged in a large airway, such as the trachea or a main bronchus. The Heimlich maneuver (standing behind the affected individual, clasping the hands in a fist just below the rib cage, and thrusting up and in with the fist) is very effective in dislodging food caught in the trachea or larynx. An object that is small enough (such as a peanut), however, can get farther into the lung, in which case special instruments or surgery are necessary to remove the object. Tumors can also grow into the opening of an airway and obstruct it. Severe cases of tonsillitis are examples of this type of obstruction. Surgery is sometimes necessary to remove such a tumor if it limits airflow.

Large-airway narrowing is another type of related airway obstructive disease. Asthma and bronchitis are examples of this type of disease. The walls of the trachea and larger bronchi become thickened and thus make the passageway for air smaller. In addition, the specialized muscle (smooth muscle) surrounding the large airways has a tendency to contract, making the opening in the airway even smaller. These conditions result in difficulty of breathing, particularly when inhaling. Relatively rapid airway narrowing caused by smooth muscle contraction is called an asthma attack. Irritants such as air pollution, tobacco smoke, and pollen can start an asthma attack. Exercise, particularly in cold weather, can also stimulate an attack in some asthmatics. Asthma attacks can last for hours and sometimes days. There are some drugs, frequently taken in an inhaled form, that help relieve the symptoms by relaxing the smooth muscle. Many cases of asthma, however, are resistant to these drugs. Some asthmatics have benefited from drugs that help decrease the frequency and severity of attacks. Asthma usually begins in childhood and has a tendency to run in families.

Chronic obstructive pulmonary disease is the term that characterizes obstructive disease of the smallest airways and alveoli. Emphysema and chronic bronchitis belong to this class of lung disease. Emphysema consists of enlargement of the smallest bronchioles and the alveolar sacs. The walls of the alveoli disappear, and with them the capillaries. Therefore, the area previously used to exchange oxygen and carbon dioxide is lost. Since the air sacs are enlarged, the oxygen must travel farther to diffuse into the blood. Emphysema can be indicated by chest X rays and pulmonary function tests but cannot be definitely identified until after death. Emphysema is frequently associated with chronic bronchitis. Chronic bronchitis is charac-

terized by enlargement of the mucous glands and by excessive mucus (sputum) production in the bronchial tree. The enlargement of the mucous glands alone can increase the resistance to airflow. Bronchitis is considered chronic when mucus is produced for three months of the year for at least two years.

The sputum can be very thick and may form into plugs to completely block off areas of the lung from airflow. Chronic obstructive pulmonary disease is generally a combination of both emphysema and chronic bronchitis of varying degrees. Persistent cough with expectoration is a normal symptom of this lung disease. With the destruction of airways and alveoli, some of the elastic recoil of the lungs is lost. As a result, exhalation is very laborious. Excess air is left in the lungs at the end of the exhalation, causing the chests of sufferers to be enlarged. Chronic obstructive disease is commonly found in long-term smokers.

Restrictive lung disease is another major classification of lung diseases. The main general feature of this class is primary changes in respiratory system tissues that restrict the movement of the lungs and thus respiration. Cystic fibrosis is the primary example of this disease. Cystic fibrosis appears to be caused by a malfunction of the immune system that produces a thick scarlike substance in the walls of the alveoli. The walls of the alveoli become thick and very stiff (fibrous). In some cases, the scar tissue grows across the small airway opening and closes off the airway. These closed air pockets are called cysts. The stiffness of the airways increases the elastic recoil of the lungs, making it very difficult to inhale.

PERSPECTIVE AND PROSPECTS

Hippocrates (c. 460-c. 370 BCE) recognized the breathing of air as an important function. He believed, however, that the function of breathing was to cool the generator of heat, the heart. Aristotle (384-322 BCE) believed that air was breathed into the arteries, which carried it in the gaseous form to the rest of the body. Galen (129-c. 199 CE) transformed medicine from a hypothetical (philosophical) science into an experimental science by performing the first experiments on animals. He found that the arteries did not contain air, and he deduced that a quality of air (oxygen had not yet been discovered), not air itself, was important to life. In the seventeenth century, William Harvey discovered that blood circulated from arteries to veins in both the lung and the rest of the body, and oxygen was identified at the end of the eighteenth century by Joseph Priestly. Claude Bernard described the union of oxygen and hemoglobin at the end of the nineteenth century.

Many major technological advances have been made. Machines have been developed to assist and in some cases completely take over the function of respiration. Respirators can assist patients who have difficulty breathing on their own. Victims of poliomyelitis whose muscles for respiration are no longer functional, as well as paralyzed patients, have been greatly helped by respirators. Respirators maintain breathing during surgery when the patient receives general anesthesia. They also assist premature babies whose lungs are not fully developed. Scientists can now make the chemical surfactant that helps keep the lungs open. Premature babies frequently do not make enough surfactant; therefore, administration of synthetic surfactant can be lifesaving. Some machines can completely assume the function of the lung. These machines, called extracorporeal membrane oxygenators, can do the job of both the heart and the lungs. They are used in heart transplantation operations. They are also used to function in the place of severely damaged lungs of newborns until those lungs can repair themselves.

Knowledge of the functioning of the respiratory system has allowed humans to function in unusual environments. Humans are able to travel to high altitudes (for example, the top of Mount Everest) with the assistance of supplemental oxygen. Travel into outer space, where there is no oxygen, is now possible because an atmosphere can be created that is suitable for long-term living in space. Experimental work is being performed with the breathing of special liquids instead of air. Success with liquid breathing may allow humans to exist in different environments, such as the deep sea, and may also have therapeutic value.

—*J. Timothy O'Neill, PhD*

See also Acute respiratory distress syndrome (ARDS); Asbestos exposure; Aspergillosis; Asthma; Avian influenza; Blood and blood disorders; Bronchi; Bronchitis; Cardiopulmonary resuscitation (CPR); Choking; Chronic obstructive pulmonary disease (COPD); Circulation; Critical care; Critical care, pediatric; Cyanosis; Cystic fibrosis; Diaphragm; Drowning; Emergency medicine; Emergency medicine, pediatric; Emphysema; Exercise physiology; Heimlich maneuver; Hyperbaric oxygen therapy; Hyperventilation; Hypoxia; Lung cancer; Lung surgery; Lungs; Otorhinolaryngology; Oxygen therapy; Pneumothorax; Pulmonary diseases; Pulmonary hypertension; Pulmonary medicine; Pulmonary medicine, pediatric; Respiratory distress syndrome; Resuscitation; Severe acute respiratory syndrome (SARS); Sleep apnea; Tonsillitis; Tracheostomy; Tumors; Wheezing.

For Further Information:
Kittredge, Mary. *The Respiratory System*. Edited by Dale C. Garell. Philadelphia: Chelsea House, 2000.
Levitzky, Michael G. *Pulmonary Physiology*. 7th ed. New York: McGraw-Hill Medical, 2007.
Mason, Robert J., et al., eds. *Murray and Nadel's Textbook of Respiratory Medicine*. 5th ed. Philadelphia: Saunders/Elsevier, 2010.
McLafferty, Ella. Carolyn Johnston. Charles Hendry. Alistair Farley. "Respiratory System Part 1: Pulmonary Ventilation." *Nursing Standard*. 27.22 (2013): 40-47. Print.
Parker, Steve. *The Lungs and Breathing*. Rev. ed. New York: Franklin Watts, 1991.
"Respiratory System Overview." *MedlinePlus*. August 2, 2011.
"The Respiratory System." *National Heart, Lung, and Blood Institute*. July 17, 2012.
Ware, Lorraine B., and Michael A. Matthay. "The Acute Respiratory Distress Syndrome." *New England Journal of Medicine* 342, no. 18 (May 4, 2000): 1334-1349.
"What Are the Signs and Symptoms of Cystic Fibrosis?" *National Heart, Lung, and Blood Institute*. June 1, 2011.
West, John B. *Pulmonary Pathophysiology: The Essentials*. 7th ed. Philadelphia: Wolters Kluwer/Lippincott Williams & Wilkins, 2008.

RESPIRATORY DISEASES. SEE PULMONARY DISEASES; RESPIRATION; SPECIFIC DISEASES.

RESPIRATORY DISTRESS SYNDROME

Category: Disease/Disorder
Also known as: Premature lungs, pulmonary immaturity, hyaline membrane disease, surfactant deficiency syndrome
Anatomy or system affected: Heart, lungs
Specialties and related fields: Neonatology, pediatrics, pulmonary medicine
Definition: A deficiency of surfactant in the neonatal lungs, causing generalized alveolar collapse leading to respiratory failure.
Key terms:
air bronchograms: a term used in radiology to describe the presence of air in the terminal bronchi that does not reach the alveoli because they are collapsed
alveoli: the small air sacs in the lungs where gas exchange occurs
endotracheal intubation: the placement of a plastic tube in the trachea to deliver a combination of oxygen and air under pressure to the lungs
mechanical ventilation: the delivery by mechanical means of air and oxygen to the lungs under fine control of pressure and inspiratory/expiratory times by electronic and mechanical equipment
prematurity: the status of being born before thirty-seven weeks of gestation
respiratory failure: the inability of the lungs to perform adequate gas exchange, resulting in insufficient oxygen absorption and carbon dioxide elimination to sustain life
reticulogranular pattern: a term used in radiology to describe a lack of air in the alveoli
surfactant: a mixture of phospholipid and protein substances produced by cells lining the alveoli that reduces surface tension and prevents their collapse

CAUSES AND SYMPTOMS

Respiratory distress syndrome (RDS) is a condition observed mainly in premature infants and children born to diabetic patients. It is also known as premature lungs, pulmonary immaturity, hyaline membrane disease, and surfactant deficiency syndrome. In 1959, researchers discovered that surfactant deficiency is the cause of RDS in premature infants; this discovery has been the basis for treatment since that time.

The main symptom is a rapid respiratory rate involving the use of accessory muscles to increase the amount of air taken into the lungs. The forceful closure of the vocal cords while contracting the abdominal muscles and diaphragm causes a particular grunting sound. The premature rib cage is very flexible, and affected infants must use extra effort to maintain expanded lungs.

A diagnosis of RDS is made on a clinical basis, including a history of premature delivery and the symptoms listed above. A chest x-ray is also useful; in RDS, a reticulogranular pattern and air bronchograms are observed together with a whited-out appearance in the lung fields. Respiratory function is determined by measuring the amount of oxygen and carbon dioxide in the arterial blood. The samples are obtained using a catheter inserted in an arterial vessel and analyzed in a blood gas machine. In newborns, the catheter is usually placed in one of the umbilical arteries, but samples from radial, posterior tibial, or dorsal pedis arteries are acceptable for analysis. Respiratory failure is defined as the inability of the lungs to perform adequate gas exchange, resulting in insufficient oxygen absorption and carbon dioxide elimination to sustain life.

TREATMENT AND THERAPY

Initially, the treatment for RDS was nonspecific. Physicians used various methods to maintain open airways and waited until the infant's lungs matured on their own. The treatment of RDS was one of the main areas of research that helped in the development of the subspecialty of neonatology.

At present, the pregnant patient who is in imminent danger of delivering a child prematurely, between twenty-four and thirty-six weeks of gestation, is given antenatal steroids. The use of prenatal steroids has been associated with accelerated maturity of the lungs in infants born prematurely. Once a premature infant is born, endotracheal intubation, mechanical ventilation, and natural or artificial surfactants are used in order to maintain open airways and to prevent the development of atelectasis, the defective expansion of the alveoli.

Mechanical ventilation became a standard of care across the United States in teaching institutions. It has helped decrease mortality rates for premature infants

---

INFORMATION ON RESPIRATORY DISTRESS SYNDROME

Causes: Premature birth, surfactant deficiency, mother with diabetes
Symptoms: Rapid respiration, grunting sound
Duration: Acute
Treatments: For pregnant woman at risk, antenatal steroids; for newborn, endotracheal intubation, mechanical ventilation, natural or artificial surfactants

---

and has evolved into a fine art assisted by advanced technology. Mechanical ventilation uses a variety of techniques to maximize lung expansion and to minimize the damage to lung tissues caused by high concentration of oxygen and pressures. Pressure, volume, and high-frequency ventilators are among the current equipment available to neonatologists for use with infants suffering from RDS.

In 1980, a report was published concerning the use of bovine surfactant mixed with saline solution administered endotracheally in infants with RDS. This treatment offered significant improvement in the outcome of this disease. Natural surfactants have been extracted from the lung tissues of calves and pigs, and surfactant has even been harvested from amniotic fluid in humans. The main difference between natural and artificial surfactants is the presence of surfactant-associated proteins. Surfactant-associated proteins function as dispersing agents for the lipid components that line the internal surface of the alveoli, thus preventing the collapse of these air sacs. Artificial surfactants are pure chemicals mixed in the laboratory without surfactant-associated proteins; other chemical substances are used as dispersing agents.

At least seven different types of surfactant have been tested in humans in clinical trials; controversy still exists regarding the proper timing of surfactant replacement, either as prophylaxis or as a rescue treatment. In addition, concern remains about the possible increased incidence of two major complications, pulmonary hemorrhage and intraventricular hemorrhage, in premature infants with RDS following the use of surfactant treatment.

Overall, the use of surfactants and mechanical ventilation has decreased mortality and complications in premature infants, but the number of patients with long-term complications, such as chronic lung disease with oxygen dependency, has increased considerably.

PERSPECTIVE AND PROSPECTS

In 1960, the infant son of John Fitzgerald Kennedy, then president-elect of the United States, died of respiratory distress syndrome. Since then, significant advances in the understanding and treatment of this condition have been made, but the elimination of this disease will be achieved only when premature births are prevented. Until then, RDS will continue to exist in nurseries everywhere.

—*Fortunato Perez-Benavides, MD*

See also Acute respiratory distress syndrome (ARDS); Critical care; Critical care, pediatric; Cyanosis; Lungs; Multiple births; Premature birth; Pulmonary diseases; Pulmonary medicine; Pulmonary medicine, pediatric; Respiration; Wheezing.

For Further Information:

Bradford, Nikki. *Your Premature Baby: The First Five Years.* Toronto, Ont.: Firefly Books, 2003.

Martin, Richard J., Avroy A. Fanaroff, and Michele C. Walsh, eds. *Fanaroff and Martin's Neonatal-Perinatal Medicine: Diseases of the Fetus and Infant.* 9th ed. 2 vols. Philadelphia: Mosby/Elsevier, 2011.

Rosenbaum, Laurie. "Respiratory Distress Syndrome in Newborns." *Health Library,* September 10, 2012.

Turner, Joan, Gwendolyn J. McDonald, and Nanci L. Larter, eds. *Handbook of Adult and Pediatric Respiratory Home Care.* St. Louis, Mo.: Mosby, 1994.

West, John B. *Pulmonary Pathophysiology: The Essentials.* 8th ed. Philadelphia: Wolters Kluwer/Lippincott Williams & Wilkins, 2012.

"What Is Respiratory Distress Syndrome?" *National Heart, Lung, and Blood Institute,* January 24, 2012.

Restless legs syndrome

Category: Disease/Disorder

Also known as: Periodic limb movement

Anatomy or system affected: Brain, muscles, musculoskeletal system, nervous system, psychic-emotional system

Specialties and related fields: Neurology, psychiatry, psychology, sleep medicine

Definition: A sensorimotor disorder characterized by uncomfortable and even painful sensations in the limbs, especially the legs, when at rest or trying to sleep.

Key terms:

akathisia: an unpleasant sensation of "inner" restlessness that compels the patient to move or walk

dopaminergic: related to the brain's neurotransmitter dopamine, which plays a role in such processes as mood, movement, and psychological functioning

neurotransmitter: a chemical messenger that transmits a neural impulse between neurons

Parkinson's disease: a movement disorder characterized by decreased levels of brain dopamine

substantia nigra: a midbrain structure that plays a role in movement, reward, and addiction

diurnal: of or during the day; daily

CAUSES AND SYMPTOMS

Patients with restless legs syndrome complain about unpleasant sensations, especially in the evening or at night, that drive them to move their limbs in order to alleviate the discomfort. There is diurnal pattern of worsened symptoms at night. Patients typically describe an inability to tolerate sitting, lying, or remaining still for even short periods of time, accompanied by an intense urge to walk, run, or move about.

There are two types of restless legs syndrome: primary and secondary. The idiopathic cause of restless legs syndrome is due to central nervous system (CNS) iron deficiency (especially in the brain's substantia nigra) leading to dopamine defects, CNS hypersensitivity and arousal, disrupted circadian rhythm, and genetic predisposition via an autosomal dominant inheritance. Several of the secondary causes include iron deficiency, end-stage renal disease, diabetes mellitus, rheumatic disease, venous insufficiency, peripheral neuropathy, folate or magnesium deficiency, amyloidosis, lumbosacral radiculopathy, fibromyalgia, celiac disease, and some medications (tricarboxylic acids [TCAs], neuroleptics, selective serotonin reuptake inhibitors [SSRIs], and diphenhydramine).

The condition appears to be relatively common, with an estimated prevalence in the general population of up to 15 percent. Hereditary restless legs syndrome tends to occur in ages less than 45. Polymorphisms in genes including BTBD9 and MEIS1 are associated with restless legs syndrome.

Although excessive leg movements can be demonstrated during a sleep study test (nocturnal polysomnography), restless legs syndrome is diagnosed by history where all five criteria's need to be met. First, the patient experiences a compelling urge to move the legs (or affected body parts) as a result of unpleasant and uncontrollable sensations. Second, the unpleasant sensations and urge to move the legs worsen during the evening or at night and can significantly interfere with relaxation and sleep and they also appear at rest or during periods of sleep inactivity. Third, the urge to move the lower extremities may partially or completely be relieved by movement or stretching the legs and as the activity continues, the symptoms are mild or absent. Fourth, the urge to move the lower extremities is worse during the evenings and make it impossible to sleep leading to fatigue during the day. Fifth, the presence of these symptoms are not attributed to other behavior conditions, such as tardive dyskinesia, leg cramps, muscle spasms, or discomfort from the position. In addition, patients reporting symptoms of restless legs syndrome should undergo toxicology studies, as well as have their iron, electrolyte, and

INFORMATION ON RESTLESS LEGS SYNDROME

Causes: Unknown, though likely involves abnormalities in brain's dopaminergic system

Symptoms: Evening or nighttime "inner" restlessness (akathisia), discomfort, pain, and/or need to move limbs or walk

Duration: Varies from episodic to chronic

Treatments: Dopaminergics, benzodiazepines, opioids, anticonvulsants; lifestyle modifications (decreasing the use of caffeine, alcohol, and tobacco, especially starting in afternoon)

medication levels checked to rule out other causes. Comorbid psychiatric disorders must also be identified.

The symptoms and sensations of restless legs syndrome are typically depicted in negative terms: "fidgety," "creepy crawlies," "insect crawlies," "painful," and "electric," among other descriptors. Most report that these sensations can become so intense that they must "jiggle" or "shake," before ultimately resorting to getting up and walking. Spouses may also complain that patients move their limbs while asleep, thus disturbing the quality of sleep for both partners.

Restless legs syndrome is not limited to the evening hours, bedtime, or sleeping, nor is it necessarily limited to the lower extremities. It can involve an inability to tolerate confinement or immobility—at any time of the day—on airplanes, buses, and cars, as well as in meetings, in movie theaters, and during medical testing, such as magnetic resonance imaging (MRI) or computed tomography (CT) scanning. It can also involve, in more severe cases, other areas of the body, including the hips, upper back, shoulders, and arms. Patients report that it is difficult or impossible to ignore the negative sensations, which adversely affect not only sleep but also daily activities.

TREATMENT AND THERAPY

Difficulties arise when attempting to treat restless legs syndrome, as the disorder appears to involve multiple brain processes. Avoidance of caffeine, antidepressants, antipsychotics, dopamine-blocking antiemetics, and centrally acting antihistamines can help with the treatment. Shortened daily dialysis in renal failure patients, iron replacement therapy, exercise, massage, and heat can all alleviate the symptoms. The mainstay of medical therapy today consists of daily low-dose dopamine agonists (dopaminergics), the most popular of which are ropinirole, pramipexole, rotigotine, and cabergoline that reduce the symptoms and improve sleep quality. Rotigotine transdermal patch is well-tolerated and has low risk of clinically significant

augmentation of restless legs syndrome. Pramipexole has shown to improve the symptoms of patients with primary moderate-to-severe restless leg syndrome and maybe better than ropinirole. The side effects of ropinirole and pramipexole are representative of the dopamine agonists as a class: headaches, nausea, insomnia, "sleep attacks," and problems related to impulse control (gambling, drinking, shopping, hypersexuality). Using alpha2-delta calcium-channel ligand (gabapentin or pregabalin) should be considered for the initial treatment of those patients who have severe sleep disturbance, comorbid insomnia, anxiety, pain, or a previous history of an impulse control disorder (ICD). Drug treatments are effective from one to five years with possible adverse effects reducing their compliance. Patients should also be taught to engage in good sleep hygiene (obtain sufficient hours of rest, have a regular time to retire and awaken), avoid exercising too close to bedtime, avoid taking aggravating medications, and take ferrous sulfate supplements if iron studies show this to be warranted.

PERSPECTIVE AND PROSPECTS

Restless legs syndrome is an underappreciated disorder that causes millions of people a great deal of distress and misery. Health care is beginning to take this problem seriously as a complex disorder with a significant morbidity resulting from chronic interruption of sleep and daily activities. This condition can be a disabling diagnosis, which can be managed with a team of nurses, primary care physician, neurologist, physical therapist, and pharmacist. Doing daily exercise in bed, keeping up with one's mental health and obtaining consultations on drugs used to treat restless legs syndrome can prevent this disorder's high morbidity.

—Vaidehi Patel, MS, MS-III

See also: Lower extremities; Muscle sprains, spasms, and disorders; Muscles; Nervous system; Neuralgia, neuritis, and neuropathy; Neurology; Neurology, pediatric; Sleep; Sleep disorders; Upper extremities.

For Further Information:

Allen, Richard P., and Merrill M. Mitler. "Restless Legs Syndrome (RLS) and Sleep." *National Sleep Foundation*, 2011.

Badash, Michelle, and Michael Woods. "Restless Legs Syndrome." *Health Library*, 15 Mar. 2013.

Buchfuhrer, Mark J., Wayne Hening, and Clete Kushida. *Restless Legs Syndrome: Coping with Your Sleepless Nights.* Demos, 2007.

Guo, S., J. Huang, H. Jiang, et al. "Restless Legs Syndrome: From Pathophysiology to Clinical Diagnosis and Management." *Frontiers in Aging Neuroscience*, vol. 9, 2017, p. 171.

Maheswaran, Murali, and Clete A. Kushida. "Restless Legs Syndrome in Children." *Medscape General Medicine*, vol. 8, no. 20 June 2006, p. 79.

Mansur A., P. R. Castillo, F. Rocha Cabrero, et al. "Restless Legs Syndrome." *StatPearls*, 12 Dec. 2021.

Pratt, D. P. "Restless Legs Syndrome/Willis-Ekbom Disease and Periodic Limb Movements: A Comprehensive Review of Epidemiology, Pathophysiology, Diagnosis and Treatment Considerations." *Current Rheumatology Reviews*, vol. 12, no. 2, 2016, pp. 91-112.

"Restless Legs." *MedlinePlus*, 5 Mar. 2013.

"Restless Legs Syndrome Fact Sheet." *National Institute of Neurological Disorders and Stroke*, 25 Nov. 2011.

Trotti, L. M., and D. B. Rye. "Restless Legs Syndrome." *Handbook of Clinical Neurology*, vol. 100, 2011, pp. 661-73, doi:10.1016/B978-0-444-52014-2.00047-1, PMID: 21496614.

RESUSCITATION

Category: Procedure

Anatomy or system affected: Brain, chest, circulatory system, heart, lungs, respiratory system

Specialties and related fields: Critical care, emergency medicine

Definition: The physical act of reviving a person in cardiac or respiratory arrest, which involves such techniques as artificial respiration, chest compressions, and defibrillation.

Key terms:

advanced cardiac life support (ACLS): a variety of life support procedures provided by trained medical personnel, including the administration of drugs and electrical defibrillation

arrhythmia: a heart rhythm that is abnormal in either speed or force; arrhythmias do not always lead to a heart attack

basic life support (BLS): a variety of life-support procedures, including rescue breathing and chest compressions, often given to a heart attack victim by the first person responding to a patient; public training in such procedures is available from the Red Cross and the American Heart Association

cardiopulmonary resuscitation (CPR): a method of producing some breathing and circulation of blood to a patient in cardiac arrest using chest compressions and artificial ventilation

defibrillation: the application of electrical energy through the chest in order to correct abnormal heart function and restore a normal heart rhythm

electrocardiogram (EKG) monitor: a machine which records the electrical activity of the heart onto a monitor and paper strip, which is then used by medically trained personnel to determine further treatment

PHYSIOLOGY OF RESPIRATION AND CIRCULATION

Every cell in the human body needs a constant and steady supply of oxygen. The delivery of oxygen is possible only through a continuous movement of oxygen-rich blood, with the heart and lungs working efficiently together. To survive, the body must have a functioning heart and lungs, or an outside force that makes both organs function artificially. Two major life-threatening conditions include respiratory arrest (cessation of breathing) and cardiac arrest (cessation of heartbeat). Death is certain unless something is done to put oxygen into the blood and circulate it throughout the body. Cardiopulmonary resuscitation (CPR) is the artificial action of putting oxygen into the lungs and making the heart pump blood throughout the body. By understanding the anatomy and physiology of the heart and lungs, and their entire systems, it is easier to see how CPR can help a person who is not breathing and whose heart is not pumping blood.

The respiratory system. This system has many parts, from the nose down to the smallest sacs of the lungs. After air is taken in through the nose or mouth, it moves farther down into the throat (pharynx), past the larynx (voice box) and the trachea (windpipe). Next, the inhaled air goes through specialized tubes called bronchi, one connected to each lung. From this larger tube, the air passage narrows into smaller tubes called bronchioles. The bronchioles become smaller and end at the air sacs, called alveoli. Alveoli are actually millions of tiny air sacs that allow oxygen to move into the bloodstream and carbon dioxide to be removed from the blood and exhaled. The alveoli are hollow and surrounded by a very thin, specialized membrane that is only one or two cells thick. This transfer of needed oxygen, along with the removal of the carbon dioxide waste products, happens through the small capillaries surrounding the alveoli. In the blood, oxygen attaches to the hemoglobin found in red blood cells, and, in return, carbon dioxide crosses back into the lungs in order to be exhaled.

It is this carbon dioxide buildup in the blood that stimulates how deep and how often one breathes. An area of the brain called the medulla is considered the body's respiratory center because it is responsible for sending electrical signals to the chest muscles that control breathing. A check-and-balance system monitors the amount of carbon dioxide in the bloodstream. When the level increases, the rate and depth of respirations also increase so that the excess amount can be exhaled.

The brain sends messages via the nerves to the muscles of the ribs. In addition to smaller muscles between each rib, the neck and shoulder muscles must also help during breathing. The diaphragm, a large, sheetlike muscle that separates the chest from the abdominal organs, also plays a major role in inspiration and expiration. The diaphragm extends from front to back by attaching to the lower part of the ribs. During inhalation, the muscles raise the ribs up and forward while the diaphragm moves downward toward the abdominal cavity, thus making room for the lungs to expand. As a result, the pressure inside the lungs becomes less than that of the surrounding air. It is this difference in air pressure, not an actual sucking in of air, that causes air to move into the lungs. The act of exhaling occurs when these muscles relax, causing the ribs to move back down and the diaphragm to rise. The size of the chest cavity decreases, the elastic nature of the lungs causes them to become smaller, and air moves out of the lungs.

The circulatory system. Life cannot be sustained simply by air moving in and out of the lungs. Once the oxygen moves from the tiny air sacs in the lungs and across into the bloodstream, it must be moved to every cell in the body. This transportation is possible because of the circulation of blood within the many vessels. At the center of this circulatory system, the heart acts as the pump, pushing blood out through the large arteries and the smaller arterioles and capillaries. After reaching the capillaries, the oxygen is delivered to the cells, and waste products such as carbon dioxide are picked up. The capillaries branch into larger venules and then into even larger veins. The major veins, from all areas of the body, return blood to the heart that is no longer rich in oxygen. Instead, it contains carbon dioxide that needs to be removed. It is this lack of oxygen that makes the blood in veins appear bluish, whereas the oxygen-rich blood found in arteries is more red in color.

The heart is responsible for sending out oxygen-carrying blood to all body tissues and moving carbon dioxide-rich blood to the lungs so that it can be exhaled. The right side of the heart is responsible for receiving blood that no longer has enough oxygen, called deoxygenated blood. The blood is next pumped through the bottom half of the heart (right ventricle) into a specialized artery called the pulmonary artery and then into each lung. Although the term "arteries" is usually reserved for vessels carrying blood with high levels of oxygen, there is one exception: The pulmonary artery does not carry oxygen-rich blood. The blood then flows into smaller capillaries surrounding the alveoli in the lungs, where it exchanges carbon dioxide for oxygen. On the return trip to the left side of the heart, after leaving the lungs, the oxygenated blood moves through the pulmonary veins. Blood then travels from the left upper portion of the heart (left atrium) to the left ventricle, which is the major muscle of the heart responsible for pumping blood to all the cells of the body.

In summary, the right side of the heart carries deoxygenated blood from the body to the lungs. The left side of the heart receives the oxygenated blood from the lungs and pumps it throughout the body. The huge network of connections in the circulatory system, from the heart all the way out to the tips of the toes and returning to the heart, makes up a closed system that must not have any large leaks, which occur during bleeding.

INDICATIONS AND PROCEDURES

It might seem that whether the heart is functioning is not a matter of yes or no, black or white. However, there are many gray areas that represent a heart that is beating but not working in a manner that will support life. These gray areas include many types of abnormal beats, known as arrhythmias, or abnormal rhythms. If the heart is beating too fast (tachycardia) or extremely slowly (bradycardia), then it cannot supply body tissues with needed oxygenated blood. A constant and even pressure of blood flow must also be maintained.

The amount of pressure inside the circulatory system varies. Blood pressure is measured as systolic pressure over diastolic pressure. In a blood pressure reading of 120/70, the top number, 120, indicates the amount of pressure on the walls of the vessels when the heart is beating (contracting). The bottom number, 70, reflects the amount of pressure on the vessel walls between beats when the heart is at rest. In cases when both numbers are extremely low or high, the system is not working properly and urgent measures must be taken to identify and fix the problem.

When either the circulatory or the respiratory system is not able to perform properly, the entire body suffers quickly. Without oxygenated blood, brain damage begins within four to six minutes. While sitting, the human heart pumps sixty to one hundred times each minute, moving about 5.5 liters of blood throughout the body every minute. The average 150-pound man has a total of about 6.75 liters of blood that must be kept constantly moving. The heart acts like a pump because it is a special muscle with its own electrical system. Much the same way as a light switch turns on a light bulb, the heart pumps because an electrical message at the top of the heart, in the sinoatrial (S-A) node, makes the entire heart muscle contract. This natural pacemaker keeps the heart beating when all things are in proper working order. If the heart stops beating correctly or the lungs do not work, however, the person will die unless resuscitation is started.

Resuscitation means making the heart pump blood and getting oxygen into and out of the lungs. In an example of the most severe case, a person is found not breathing and without a pulse. Cardiopulmonary resuscitation (CPR) courses teach that the first step is to open the airway and be sure that nothing is blocking the flow of air in and out of the lungs. If a blockage is found, it must be removed immediately. If the person is not breathing, the rescuer must breathe for him or her. Artificial respiration, or mouth-to-mouth ventilation, in which one individual breathes air into another's mouth, will force oxygen-containing air into the lungs so that it can be picked up in the bloodstream and transported to body cells. Pinching the patient's nose and blowing into the mouth forces air into the lungs in much the same way as taking a deep breath. Yet this artificial breathing alone is not enough. The oxygen put into the lungs must be moved around the body, which can only be done through circulating blood.

To move the blood through the circulatory system, something must be done to make the heart pump. This can be accomplished through chest compressions. Since the heart lies between the breastbone (sternum) and the spine, it is surrounded by hard, bony structures. By pressing in the correct position, with sufficient pressure and depth, the heart muscle can be squeezed. This squeezing action will result in blood being forced out of the heart and onto its path around the body. The oxygen blown into the lungs will be picked up by the passing blood and moved out to necessary areas of the body.

Even with the use of proper techniques, however, cardiopulmonary resuscitation should only be a temporary measure for a person who has no pulse and who is not breathing. CPR is only a momentary first-aid measure. Yet this procedure is a vital one: Until further medical assistance can be given, it is extremely important that oxygen circulate in the patient's body.

CPR is usually done by the first responder who finds the victim. This form of resuscitation is known as basic life support (BLS). The administration of BLS is the step just before advanced cardiac life support (ACLS), which offers additional treatment measures given by medically trained personnel. ACLS is given by emergency medical technicians (EMTs), paramedics responding in ambulances, or other health care professionals. While continuing CPR, the medical team will start advanced care before or during the drive to a hospital emergency department.

To provide the proper treatment, paramedics must determine the electrical activity of the heart. The heart's rhythm is recorded on an electrocardiograph (ECG or EKG) machine, which helps the medical team find the cause of the problem. The portable ECG machine, which is commonly called a cardiac monitor,

displays the electrical activity in the heart. When the electrical impulses are not producing a rhythmic beating pattern, various treatment procedures may follow, depending on how the heart is pumping or if it is working at all. It is possible to correct a heart that has an irregular beat caused by abnormal electrical activity. A total lack of electrical activity in the heart is called asystole and is recorded on the monitor as a flat line. The ACLS team can attempt to adjust the abnormal electrical signal but usually cannot mechanically restart a heart that has no electrical impulses. Other heart problems produce other types of tracings on the monitor. In one type of arrhythmia called ventricular fibrillation, the heart has a rapid, chaotic electrical activity that does not allow the heart to beat; the patient will stop breathing and will have no pulse. In this case, CPR is needed to reduce brain damage caused by decreased oxygen to cells, while paramedics and other health care professionals begin advanced life support in an attempt to reverse the dying process.

Many different protocols exist on how ACLS treatment should progress, and the following is merely one example. In 2005, the American Heart Association made changes in CPR, BLS, and ACLS protocols. The medics may use an electrical machine known as a defibrillator to deliver electrical shocks through the chest and toward the heart in the hope of correcting the rhythm. A single electric shock is given, followed by CPR. A needle and special catheter are placed in a vein to start intravenous (IV) fluids, in which medications can be given to travel to the heart through the veins. A high concentration of oxygen is delivered through a tube inserted through the mouth or nose and passed into the upper part of the lung so that artificial ventilation can aid in the movement of concentrated oxygen. Adrenaline (also known as epinephrine) is given through the IV; this drug will increase the blood flow to the heart and brain by narrowing other vessels and will also increase the heart rate and blood pressure. CPR is continued for two minutes, then a brief pause occurs for another single electric shock. CPR resumes immediately.

Studies of actual resuscitation processes have demonstrated that CPR was often stopped while personnel prepared medications or prepared to defibrillate. These pauses caused the absence of blood flow and oxygen for prolonged periods of time. This observation led to the new guidelines. Single shocks are given, rather than the previous three shocks of increasing voltage. CPR is given continuously except during the actual shock.

The next drug given may be amiodarone, which helps to calm a heart that is beating too fast or erratically. If the irregular rhythm has still not been corrected, then sodium bicarbonate may given to reduce the acids produced in the body because of the lack of oxygen. This entire scenario is repeated until the heart is beating in a manner that will sustain life or it is determined by a physician that the person cannot be resuscitated.

Other drugs that are used for specific heart problems include atropine, lidocaine, vasopressin, procainamide, verapamil, dopamine, and adenosine. All these drugs target specific problems during a cardiac episode. For individuals who are successfully resuscitated and are stable but unresponsive on arrival at the hospital, induced hypothermia is recommended for the first twenty-four hours to improve brain functioning.

When the heart slows or weakens to the point that it is barely beating, life can be artificially maintained in a few cases by using a cardiac pacing unit to create an artificial heartbeat electrically, a procedure called cardiac pacing. This artificial heartbeat may be sufficient until a permanent pacemaker can be implanted.

PERSPECTIVE AND PROSPECTS

Over the years, huge advances have been made in resuscitation measures. More lives have been saved by the training of medical personnel to administer advanced life support before a patient reaches the hospital. Lifesaving drugs and defibrillation have greatly decreased the death rate for heart attack victims and cardiac patients. With the continued training of emergency medical technicians, the survival rate can improve as a result of earlier and more aggressive medical treatment.

Medical treatment could be avoided entirely, however, if more preventive health measures were implemented. With continued research identifying risk factors, the public can be educated about how to prevent conditions that lead to heart attacks. Among the known risk factors are cigarette smoking, hypertension (high blood pressure), high cholesterol and triglycerides, lack of exercise, excess weight and improper nutrition, stress, and diabetes mellitus. Three risk factors cannot be changed: predisposing heredity, gender (men are more likely to have heart attacks), and increasing age.

With further research, the first group of risk factors may be addressed in society through extensive education, but heart attack rates cannot be curbed unless people change their lifestyles. An understanding of heredity, gender, and age risk factors can bring changes in these rates only through further research into their relationship to heart attacks.

Until people are willing to change their lifestyles, early recognition of the warning signs of a heart attack may be the easiest method of increasing survival rates. A heart attack occurs when the heart muscle itself does not receive enough oxygen. The heart muscle has its own blood supply through the coronary arteries. The blood supply to the heart may be reduced by a clot or by a narrowing in the coronary arteries. The warning signals of a heart attack include a squeezing tightness or pressure in the chest; pain in either arm, neck, jaw, or between the shoulder blades; sweating; nausea; weakness; and shortness of breath. People with diabetes and women may have milder or different symptoms. Too often, people deny that they could be suffering a heart attack, with many believing that the pain is heartburn or indigestion. If medical attention is sought immediately, however, severe damage can often be reduced or stopped. Special drugs such as streptokinase or tissue plasminogen activator (TPA) can dissolve clots that interfere with blood flow, while surgical techniques such as coronary artery bypass surgery (CABG) or angioplasty can open clogged arteries. Heart transplants offer a solution for patients with extensive heart damage. Research continues to decrease the rejection rates for heart transplants. Medications are being developed to decrease the buildup of plaque in arteries. The fields of genetics and gene therapy hold many keys to the prevention and treatment of heart disease.

It is important to note that all medically trained personnel, from the EMT to the emergency medicine physician, must be able to perform life-support measures. Unless patients have given appropriate do-not-resuscitate (DNR) orders, they will receive some form of the previously mentioned procedures. A living will is a legal document that directs medical personnel in the level of care an individual wishes to have. For example, a person with advanced cancer may want to not be placed on a breathing machine. Those wishes are to be communicated through a living will. Without this document, health care providers are mandated by law to provide lifesaving measures. Future resuscitation measures will be influenced by ethical questions regarding when to sustain life.

Bystander CPR (initiation of CPR by the first person to find a cardiac arrest victim) is a vital component in the chain of survival between BLS and ACLS. It has been recognized, however, that very few people are willing to perform mouth-to-mouth rescue breathing, a vital component of success for CPR. Therefore, it has been acknowledged that it is better to at least open the victim's airway by extending the neck and doing chest compressions alone versus doing nothing at all. The layperson will no longer be taught to check for a pulse before initiating CPR. Checking for a pulse was removed from the recommendations because it was demonstrated that laypersons could not be taught to reliably check for a pulse. Instead, they will be taught to look and examine for "signs of circulation," which include breathing, coughing, or chest movements, before starting CPR. Another recommendation for BLS was to train nonmedical professionals such as police, firefighters, security officers, and others exposed to large populations in the use of the automated external defibrillator (AED). The AED has two pads that, when applied to the chest of the cardiac victim, analyze the electrical heart activity. The AED then administers the electrical shock (defibrillation) necessary to restart a heart if the cause of cardiac arrest was ventricular fibrillation, the most common arrhythmia of cardiac arrest. Bystander CPR and early defibrillation by the AED have been shown to do more to reduce morbidity and mortality from cardiac arrest than all current therapies for cardiac arrest combined.

—*Maxine M. Urton, PhD; Laurence Katz, MD; updated by Amy Webb Bull, DSN, APN*

See also Arrhythmias; Bypass surgery; Cardiac arrest; Cardiopulmonary resuscitation (CPR); Choking; Circulation; Critical care; Critical care, pediatric; Defibrillation; Drowning; Electrocardiography (ECG or EKG); Emergency medicine; Ethics; First aid; Heart; Heart attack; Heimlich maneuver; Hyperbaric oxygen therapy; Lungs; Malpractice; Pacemaker implantation; Paramedics; Pulmonary medicine; Pulmonary medicine, pediatric; Respiration; Thrombolytic therapy and TPA; Tracheostomy.

For Further Information:
"Cardiopulmonary Resuscitation (CPR): First Aid." *Mayo Clinic*, February 7, 2012.
Cayley, William E., Jr. "2005 AHA Guidelines for CPR and Emergency Cardiac Care." *American Family Physician* 73, no. 9 (May 1, 2006): 1645.
"CPR." *American Heart Association*, 2013.
Hamilton, Glenn C., et al. *Emergency Medicine: An Approach to Clinical Problem-Solving*. 2d ed. New York: W. B. Saunders, 2003.
Henry, Mark C., and Edward R. Stapleton. *EMT: Prehospital Care*. Rev. 4th ed. St. Louis, Mo.: Mosby/Elsevier, 2012.
Tintinalli, Judith E., ed. *Emergency Medicine: A Comprehensive Study Guide*. 7th ed. New York: McGraw-Hill, 2011.
Torpy, Janet M., Cassio Lynm, and Richard M. Glass. "Cardiopulmonary Resuscitation." *JAMA* 304, no. 13 (October 6, 2010): 1514.
White, Roger D. "2005 American Heart Association Guidelines for Cardiopulmonary Resuscitation: Physiologic and Educational Rationale for Changes." *Mayo Clinic Proceedings* 81, no. 6 (2006): 736-740.

Retina

Category: Anatomy
Anatomy or system affected: Eye
Specialties and related fields: Ophthalmology, retina specialist
Definition: A multilayer of exquisitely organized neurons that line the back of the eye designed to con-

vert photons into neural impulses that travel along the visual pathways to the visual cortex.

The retina is the innermost layer of the eye, and it works to capture light in the form of photons and relay a neural signal to the brain regarding the incoming light beam. Before reaching the retina, light must pass through the ocular media, which consists of the tear film, cornea, anterior and posterior chambers, crystalline lens, and the vitreous body—these structures serve unique purposes, such as providing nutrients to the eye, focusing rays of light, and clearing the eye of any foreign bodies.

BACKGROUND
Description. The retina (roughly 0.5 mm thick) forms the inner layer of the eye and is composed of several layers. The innermost layer consists of photoreceptors, which are specialized cells responsible for capturing incoming light photons. As light reaches the photoreceptor layer of the retina, a pigment in the photoreceptors undergoes a conformational change and releases a chemical substance, known as a neurotransmitter. This begins the signaling cascade to the brain representing the information pertaining to the current visual stimulus.

Rodsand Cones. Photoreceptors come in two main types: rods and cones. There are approximately 92 million rods in the photoreceptor layer, which are saturated at natural light intensities and are unable to discriminate between colors. Their high sensitivity to light renders them effective for night vision. In contrast, cone photoreceptors come in three varieties, distinguished by their unique structural and functional properties. Each of these subsets has a specific inclination towards a particular wavelength of light; they consist of the long (maximum absorption in the red light range), medium (maximum absorption in the green light range), and short (maximum absorption in the blue light range) wavelength cones. Cones only account for about 5% of the total photoreceptors in the retina, but are heavily gathered in an area of the retina called the *fovea*, an area devoid of blood vessels with the highest concentration of cones, allowing for high spatial acuity and color discrimination. (Overall, the retina is fed by two main blood supplies: the central retinal artery and the choroidal blood vessels—they account for 20-30% and 65-85% of blood flow, respectively.)

Light and Phototransduction. As light travels through the eye and reaches the retina layer, the photons from the incoming light beam strike the photoreceptors and commence a series of chemical, structural, and physical changes that allow for propagation of a nerve impulse—a process known as *phototransduction*. Both rods and cones contain different photopigments, the membrane protein responsible for capturing light photons and thereby initiating a phototransduction cascade. Rods contain the photopigment known as *rhodopsin*, while the cone photopigment is known as *opsin*. The subtle structural difference between these two photopigments forms the basis for divergent light and color sensitivities (as well as overall function) between rods and cones.

As photons reach the photoreceptors, they are "captured" by either a rod or a cone photopigment. The photopigment subsequently undergoes a structural change, causing a signaling cascade within the photoreceptor. This, in return, causes the release of a chemical—known as a neurotransmitter—that begins transducing a signal to the brain regarding the incoming light stimulus. After being physically transformed by the incoming photon, the photopigments must return to their original conformation in order to remain continually responsive to light and maintain high fidelity neural transmission to the brain. Through this mechanism, the brain is able to interpret information presented in the current visual field.

OVERVIEW

The retina is regarded as the layer of the eye with photoreceptive qualities. The composition of the retina (which measures roughly 0.5 mm thick) is that of a vascular membrane with a network of cell layers. When light waves enter the eye, they are transformed by the eye into neural impulses. The primary function of the retina is to translate the waves of light it receives into nerve or neural impulses. These are, in turn, transmitted to the brain, and the sense of sight is manifested.

How does the physiology of vision occur through the retina? An image is formed on the retina. In order for this image to be perceived by the body as a visual entity, the photosensitive cells of the retina must come into play. The rods and cones function as transmitters of nervous signals. The millions of rods and cones, perceiving light differently, are concentrated in specific areas. The *macula* is a small yellow-pigmented area bearing a high concentration of cones. The *fovea* is a small section at the center of the macula, and it contains the highest density of cones in the retina. The center of the fovea, known as the *foveal pit*, is 200 microns—a fifth of a millimeter—in diameter and exhibits an even higher degree of specialization.

The propensity of the cones and rods to detect light and translate it into color can be attributed to the photosensitive chemicals (pigments) that they contain. Rods and cones possess rhodopsin and opsin respectively; upon interaction with light, these chemicals go through a cycle to culminate in a nerve impulse. Altogether, this creates a visual stimulus. Rods are associated with night vision, given their ability to pick up low or dim levels of light. In contrast, cones are associated with daylight vision and color. Pigments picking up primary colors of red, blue, and green are found in cones. Accordingly, there are three different kinds of pigment, each with variable color sensitivity.

Neural Pathways. The visual pathway begins with the rods and cones that serve to send the impulses. These impulses reach bipolar cells, followed by ganglion cells connected to the optic nerve. Horizontal and amacrine cells are vertically oriented neurons that act by transmitting signals over the retina. The optic nerve is a central circular region of the retina that measures approximately 2 x 1.5 mm across. It contains the ganglion cell axons directing signals out to the brain. Once the brain receives these nerve impulses, it is able to translate them into the sense of sight.

COLOR BLINDNESS

Color blindness occurs when a person is lacking pigments connected with the particular color. When someone cannot distinguish red or green, for instance, this is usually due to an insufficient supply of the pigments most sensitive to red or green light.

RETINAL DISORDERS

Given its delicate nature, the retina is prone to significant damage and degeneration in various conditions. Retinal disorders primarily result when the macula nerve tissue is affected. Macular pucker (scar tissue) and macular hole are some notable manifestations. To cite another prominent example, age-related macular degeneration is a leading cause of blindness worldwide, which results from degeneration and lipid deposition behind the retina (in the layer known as the retinal pigmented epithelium). These changes cause fluid to seep in behind the fovea and damage the overlying cone photoreceptors, thereby compromising central vision. Moreover, in diabetic retinopathy, the blood vessels supplying the eye become severely compromised, with uncontrolled proliferation and leakage into the retina. Retinoblastoma is a cancer of the retina found most frequently in children. Moreover, retinitis pigmentosa is a hereditary disease whereby the rods of the peripheral retina undergo significant degeneration, leading to impaired night vision. Finally, when the retina becomes detached from the back of the eye (i.e., retinal detachment), the retina membrane separates from the layers that support it; this often warrants immediate surgery for sight preservation.

—*Nicholas Koen, Derrick Cheng and Ariel Choi*

For Further Information:
Dubuc, Bruno. "Photoreceptors." *The Brain from Top to Bottom*. Sept. 2002. Web. 9 May 2016.

Hubel, David. "The Eye." *Eye, Brain, and Vision*. n.d. Web. 9 May 2016.

Jacob, Stanley; Francone, Clarice Ashworth; and Lossow, Walter J. *Structure and Function in Man*. London: Elsevier Health Sciences, 1982. Print.

Kapit, Wynne, and Elson, Lawrence M. *The Anatomy Coloring Book*. 2nd edition. U.S.A.: Addison- Wesley Educational Publishers, Inc., 1993. Print.

Kolb, Helga. "How the Retina Works." *American Scientist*. 91.1 (2003):28. Web. 9 May 2016.

Kolb, Helga. "Simple Anatomy of the Retina." Webvision: The Organization of the Retina and Visual System. In: Kolb H, Fernandez E, Nelson R, editors. Salt Lake City (UT): University of Utah Health Sciences Center. Web. Published 1 May 2005. Updated 31 Jan 2012. 10 Sept 2017.

National Eye Institute. "Facts About Retinal Detachment." *National Eye Institute*. Department of Health and Human Services. Oct. 2009. Web. 9 May 2016.

Prasad, Sashank; Rizzo, Joseph.
"Modern-Neuro-Ophthalmology: Anatomy & Physiology of the Human Visual System." Feb. 2016.

"The Eye." *Kellogg Eye Center*. University of Michigan Kellogg Eye Center, 2015. Web. 9 May 2016.

U.S. National Library of Medicine. "Retina." 3 May 2016. Web. 9 May 2016.

U.S. National Library of Medicine. "Retinal Disorders." 10 July 2014. Web. 9 May 2016.

RETINAL DETACHMENT

Category: Disease/Disorder

INTRODUCTION

The retina is a thin film of tissue that sits in the back of the eye. It is attached to an underlying layer of cells known as the retinal pigmented epithelium (RPE), responsible for absorbing excess light and providing key nutritional support to the retinal neurons. The retina is responsible for translating light information into chemical and electrical signals, which travel through multiple layers of neurons, the optic nerve, the thalamus, and visual cortex in the brain. As a result, a tear or detachment in the retinal film can cause the loss of vision. Annual incidence of retinal detachment (RD) is approximately 1 in 10,000. Average age of presentation is approximately 60.

There are three main types of RD. *Rhegmatogenous* (from the Greek word *rhegma*, meaning "break") detachments are the most common and occur when a tear or hole forms in the retina. This opening allows fluid from the inside of the eye to seep in between and separate the retina and the RPE. *Tractional* detachments are less common, but occur when scar tissue forms on the retinal surface. This scar tissue contracts and pulls the retina away from the RPE. Additionally, the vitreous gel that fills the inside of the eye can

clump and become sticky with age, allowing it to pull on the retina. *Exudative* detachments typically occur in the setting of inflammation, cancer, or other diseases that promote fluid or blood exudation in the eye. While there are no tears, excess fluid may separate the retina and RPE, causing a retinal detachment.

There are also varying degrees of RD severity. In minor detachments or tears, the vitreous gel filling the inside of the eye may cause traction on the retina and cause small tears that do not significantly affect vision. In larger, more severe detachments, vital areas of the retina including the macula (vision center) may become separated and require urgent medical attention.

BRIEF HISTORY

The first diagnosis of a retinal tear was made in 1953 by Ernst Adolf Coccius, following the invention of the ophthalmoscope in 1950. Early approaches to treatment focused on rest and ocular immobilization using molds, weights, binding, and atropine. Surgical techniques emphasized vitreous and subretinal fluid removal.

A Swiss ophthalmologist by the name of Jules Gonin developed the first approach towards repairing the torn retina, using cauterization (burning) to bind the retinal tear to the underlying retinal pigment epithelium and choroid (retinal blood supply). An alternative approach using cryotherapy was developed soon afterwards. Over the past half-century, approaches to retinal detachment treatment have seen remarkable growth and have significantly improved vision restoration rates.

RISK FACTORS, CAUSES, AND SYMPTOMS

There are a variety of risk factors that promote retinal detachments. In patients with nearsightedness (myopia), for example, the eye is elongated and the focal point of light lies in front of the retina. This stretched configuration increases the risk of a tear or detachment of the retina. Other risk factors include age, cataract surgery, malignant hypertension, prior history of vitreous or retinal diseases and detachments, a family history of retinal detachments, ocular trauma (including a history of eye surgery), and diabetes, which can cause prolonged vascular damage, scarring, and tractional detachment.

Patients suffering from an acute retinal detachment often report a sudden onset of flashing lights or floaters—symptoms that appear due to the vitreous gel clumping together and putting tension on the retina. Other symptoms may include transient loss of vision, especially at the periphery, that may gradually spread towards the center with the progression of detachment. If left untreated, chances of recovery fall significantly, as the retina is starved of vital nutrients or oxygen.

TREATMENT AND SURGICAL OVERVIEW

There are varying degrees of retinal detachment, and treatment methods vary depending on the physician. However, the vast majority of retinal tears and detachments require surgical intervention. Notably, only those detachments that are identified and treated early will spare the patient's vision; once the detachment expands over the fovea, permanent vision loss is all but inevitable. For this reason, prompt referral to an ophthalmologist for surgical repair is essential. Surgical procedures may include:

Photocoagulation/Cryotherapy: Photocoagulation and cryotherapy are commonly used to treat small retinal tears. These procedures involve the use of a laser or freezing probe to form a small scar around the tear, sealing the retinal flap to the underlying tissue and preventing the leakage of fluid into the subretinal space. While treatment is almost always successful, this technique may promote the development of new breaks in other locations or cause re-detachment by forming excess scar tissue.

Scleral Buckling: Scleral buckles provide one of the most common surgical procedures for RD repair. They are flexible bands (similar to rubber bands) typically reserved for more severe retinal detachments. During this more invasive procedure, ophthalmologists place the buckle around the outside of the eye. This band applies pressure to the eye and reduces the distance between the retina and the underlying RPE/choroid, which often promotes re-attachment and allows excess fluid to drain from the subretinal space. This procedure is often combined with photo- or cryotherapy to prevent the retina from detaching after the operation.

Pneumatic Retinopexy: Rheumatic retinoplexy involves the injection of a gas or oil bubble into the eye. When positioned correctly, this bubble applies pressure to the retina, pressing it against the back of the eye and allowing for resorption of subretinal fluid. Typically, this surgical approach also includes photocoagulation or cryotherapy to prevent re-detachment. Post-operative care may require the patient to lie in specific positions depending on the location of the detachment to allow the bubble to press against the retina. After the retina heals, the bubble is often left in the patient to naturally dissolve or can be removed in a separate procedure.

Vitrectomy(Pars Plana Vitrectomyor 3-Port Vitrectomy): Vitrectomy is the removal of the vitreous gel that fills the inside of the eye. Typically, this involves the formation of three ports that the ophthalmologist uses to illuminate the space, remove the vitreous, and refill the cavity with saline. This technique is often used during scleral buckling and pneumatic retinoplexy procedures to reduce post-operative scarring and traction.

PERSPECTIVE AND PROSPECTS

Retinal detachment repair is fairly well understood and has a success rate of 80-90%. However, re-detachment may occur in some patients due to excessive scarring or delayed treatment. While some patients have a full recovery, patients with more severe detachments may experience a permanent reduction in visual acuity or may not recover for several months. Current research revolves around identifying further risk factors, improving pharmacological management and post-operative care, and the development of new surgical techniques that may improve visual acuity for patients with severe detachments and reduce risk of re-detachment.

—Derrick Cheng, Nicholas Koen and Ariel Choi; updated by Geraldine Marrocco

For Further Information:

Fisher SK, Lewis GP, Linberg KA, et al. Cellular Remodeling in Mammalian Retina Induced by Retinal Detachment. 2005 May 1 [Updated 2007 Jul 3]. In: Kolb H, Fernandez E, Nelson R, editors. Webvision: The Organization of the Retina and Visual System [Internet]. Salt Lake City (UT): University of Utah Health Sciences Center; 1995-. Available from: www.ncbi.nlm.nih. gov/books/NBK11552

Kang, Hyong Kwon, and A J Luff. anagement of Retinal Detachment: A Guide for Non-Ophthalmologists. BMJ: British Medical Journal 336.7655 (2008): 1235 240. PMC. Web. 10 Sept. 2017.

Besharse, Joseph C., and Dean Bok. *The Retinaand Its Disorders*. Academic Press, 2011. Print.

Clark, Antony, et al. "Risk for Retinal Detachment After Phacoemulsification." Archives of Ophthalmology 130.7 (2012): 882 8. Print.

Fineman, Mitchell S., and Allen C. Ho. Retina. Philadelphia: Wolters Kluwer Health/Lippincott Williams & Wilkins, 2012. Print.

Kreissig, Ingrid, ed. Primary Retinal Detachment: Options for Repair. Heidelberg: Springer, 2005. Print.

Pournaras, Constantin, et al. "Surgical and Visual Outcome for Recurrent Retinal Detachment Surgery." Journal of Ophthalmology 2014 (2014): 1. Web. 8 Jan. 2016.

Rogers, Adam H., and Jay S. Duker. Retina. Philadelphia: Mosby Elsevier, 2008. Print.

Soubrane, Gise, and Gabriel Coscas. "Pathogenesis of Serous Detachment of the Retina and Pigment Epithelium." Retina (2013): 618 3. Print.

Yorston, D., and S. Jalali. "Retinal Detachment in Developing Countries." Eye 16.4 (2002): 353 8. Print.

RETROVIRUSES

Category: Disease/Disorder
Anatomy or system affected: All
Specialties and related fields: Biochemistry, genetics, oncology, pathology, public health, virology
Definition: ribonucleic acid (RNA) viruses that replicate by synthesizing a double-stranded deoxyribonu-

cleic acid (DNA) molecule that integrates into the host genome; they infect virtually all animals and sometimes cause serious diseases, including cancer

Key terms:

capsid: a virally encoded protein that surrounds and protects the viral RNA genome

envelope: a lipid bilayer membrane that surrounds the retrovirus particle

glycoprotein: a protein to which is attached one or more sugar molecules

integrase: a virally encoded enzyme that catalyzes the integration of viral double-stranded DNA into the host genome

matrix: the layer of virally encoded protein that surrounds the viral capsid

nucleoprotein: a virally encoded protein that is directly associated with the viral nucleic acid

oncogene: a gene or DNA segment that can cause cancer

oncogenic: having the potential to cause cancer, as in oncogenic retroviruses

positive-sense RNA (+RNA): an RNA molecule that can serve as a template for protein synthesis

reverse transcriptase: an enzyme that synthesizes double-stranded DNA from single-stranded RNA

src: a gene found in Rous Sarcoma Virus that confers on the virus the ability to transform normal cells into cancer cells

tRNA: an RNA molecule that attaches to an amino acid and interacts with the ribosome during protein synthesis; in retroviruses, it serves as a primer for reverse transcriptase

BIOLOGY OF RETROVIRUSES

Retroviruses are members of the viral family Retroviridae. They are enveloped, positive sense (+) ribonucleic acid (RNA) viruses about 100 nanometers in diameter that replicate within the host's cytoplasm through a double-stranded deoxyribonucleic acid (DNA) intermediate that is integrated into the host genome. In addition to the +RNA, a cellular tRNA hydrogen-bonded to the +RNA serves as a primer for reverse transcriptase.

The viral RNA genome, associated nucleoprotein, reverse transcriptase, and integrase surround a protein capsid. Immediately external to the capsid is the matrix protein. The outer layer of the retrovirus is a lipid bilayer envelope derived from the host's plasma membrane that is acquired as the virus emerges from the host cell. Within the envelope are two glycoproteins encoded by the virus genome and serve as plasma membrane attachment sites during entry into the cell.

The retrovirus genome consists of two, seven kilobase to 11 kilobase +RNA molecules that code for only a few proteins, including *gag*, which codes for the matrix, capsid, and nucleoprotein; *pol*, which codes for reverse transcriptase, RNAse, integrase, and a protease; and *env*, which codes for the envelope glycoproteins.

The retrovirus binds to plasma membrane receptors via the viral envelope glycoproteins. When the retrovirus enters the cell, the viral RNA is released along with its reverse transcriptase. A double-stranded DNA is synthesized from the +RNA using viral reverse transcriptase. Integrase catalyzes the incorporation of the double-stranded DNA molecule into the host genome. When integrated, the viral DNA is referred to as a provirus and replicates with the host genome. Host RNA polymerase transcribes the viral genes, making copies of the viral genome and mRNA molecules translated into viral proteins. Viral RNA and proteins are assembled into new viral particles that emerge from the plasma membrane by budding.

Some retroviruses such as Rous sarcoma virus (RSV), feline leukemia virus (FLV), and mouse mammary tumor virus (MMTV) can induce tumors in their host species. More than twenty-five cancer-causing (oncogenic) retroviruses have been isolated. The retrovirus gains oncogenic potential when it inadvertently acquires a eukaryotic gene during infection. Although the eukaryotic gene may not be oncogenic when first acquired, after several generations, it may mutate or otherwise become altered, transforming it into one that is oncogenic. Retroviruses such as FLV that do not carry an oncogene can still transform by disrupting the function of a normal gene by integrating within it or by integrating next to it so that the neighboring gene can use the viral promoter, resulting in gene overexpression and cellular proliferation.

PERSPECTIVE AND PROSPECTS

The study of retroviruses dates to 1910 with the work of Peyton Rous, who discovered that certain sarcomas in chickens are caused by an agent later identified as a virus. The virus was later named Rous sarcoma virus. In 1970, the laboratories of Howard Temin and David Baltimore independently discovered that certain RNA viruses have an enzyme, now known as reverse transcriptase, that permits the viruses to reverse transcribe their RNA genomes into double-stranded DNA. In the early 1970s, the laboratory of J. Michael Bishop and Harold Varmus demonstrated that the Rous sarcoma virus has a gene, now known as *src*, responsible for transforming normal cells into tumor cells. Uninfected cells, including human cells, have a normal *src* gene related to the viral *src* gene. In the past, an RSV infected a chicken and incorporated the host *src* gene into its genome. The *src* gene acquired by the virus became altered over time so that it now causes cancer when an RSV infects a chicken cell.

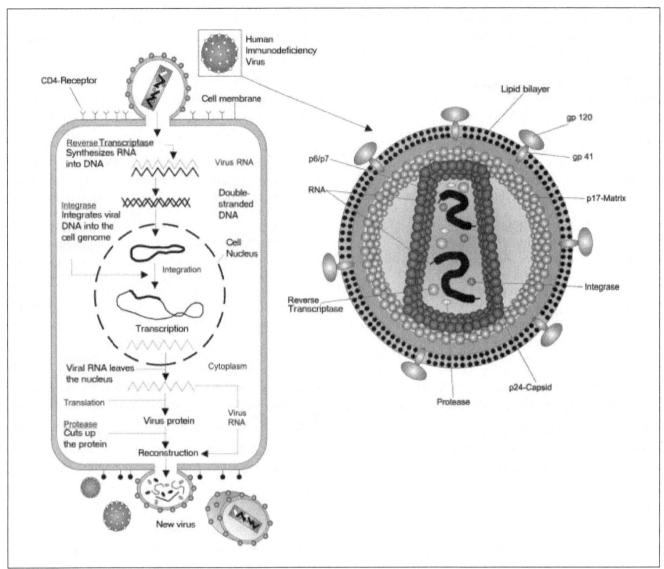

HIV retrovirus schematic of cell infection, virus production, and virus structure. Image by Raul654, via Wikimedia Commons.

There are many examples of retroviruses, including the human T-cell leukemia virus (HTLV), the first pathogenic human retrovirus discovered in 1980 by Bernard J. Poiesz, Robert Gallo, and their colleagues at the National Institutes of Health and by Mitsuaki Yoshida in Japan. Human immunodeficiency virus (HIV), which causes acquired immunodeficiency syndrome (AIDS), is also a retrovirus; it was discovered in 1983 by Luc Montagnier, Françoise Barré-Sinoussi, and their colleagues at the Pasteur Institute in France.

Since reverse transcriptase does not have the proof-reading activities associated with DNA polymerase, retroviruses mutate and evolve more rapidly than DNA viruses, making the development of drugs and vaccines difficult.

Recombinant retroviruses are often used as vectors for genetic engineering. Retroviruses that are modified by removing the genes that make them harmful and replacing them with normal eukaryotic genes can deliver a normal copy of a gene to a defective cell. The DNA copy of the recombinant retrovirus can integrate into the host genome and genetically modify the cell.

—*Charles L. Vigue, PhD*

For Further Information:

Bodine, David M. "Retrovirus." *National Institutes of Health: National Human Genome Research Institute*, n.d., www.genome.gov/genetics-glossary/Retrovirus. Accessed 8 Apr. 2022.

Boskey, Elizabeth. "How a Retrovirus or RNA Virus Works." *VeryWellHealth*, 23 Jul. 2020, www.verywellhealth.com/hiv-is-a-retrovirus-what-does-that-mean-3132822. Accessed 8 Apr. 2022.

"Retroviruses." *YouTube*, uploaded by Beverly Biology, 26 Jun. 2016, www.youtube.com/watch?v=EGfMRVBDxaY.

Retroviruses that May Cause Human Illness. Minnesota Department of Health, n.d., www.health.state.mn.us/diseases/retrovirus/index.html. Accessed 8 Apr. 2022.

Schulman, Jill Seladi. "What is a Retrovirus?" *Healthline*, 1 Mar. 2019, www.healthline.com/health/what-is-a-retrovirus. Accessed 8 Apr. 2022.

REYE'S SYNDROME

Category: Disease/Disorder
Anatomy or system affected: Brain, circulatory system, heart, kidneys, liver, nervous system, urinary system
Specialties and related fields: Emergency medicine, internal medicine, neurology, pediatrics
Definition: A somewhat rare, noncontagious disease of the liver and central nervous system that strikes individuals under the age of eighteen.

CAUSES AND SYMPTOMS

The exact cause of Reye syndrome has not been determined, but the majority of patients develop the disease while recovering from a mild viral illness, such as chickenpox, influenza, or a minor respiratory illness. It is theorized that the virus combines with another unknown substance or substances in the body to produce a damaging poison. Reye syndrome usually occurs in children between four and twelve years of age. For reasons not well understood, the taking of salicylates, such as aspirin, during viral illnesses may precipitate the development of this potentially fatal illness.

The first symptom of the disease is a sudden onset of vomiting, then high fever, headache, and drowsiness. Blood sugar levels drop, while blood ammonia and acidity levels increase. As the disease progresses, alternating states of excitation and confused sleepiness may occur, as well as convulsions and a loss of consciousness. In the final stages of the disease, damage occurs to the liver, kidneys, and brain. The liver swells and develops large amounts of fat deposits. The brain cells swell and pressure builds in the skull, followed by coma, permanent brain damage, and, in some cases, death.

Reye syndrome is often mistaken for a number of other disorders, including meningitis, encephalitis, diabetic shock, or poisoning, potentially complicating the early diagnosis that is crucial for treating this condition.

TREATMENT AND THERAPY

There is no known cure for Reye syndrome. Early recognition and specialized care may be lifesaving. If a child begins to exhibit symptoms of Reye syndrome shortly after a viral illness, then competent medical care must be sought immediately. Treatment consists of helping the victim survive the first few days of the

---

INFORMATION ON REYE'S SYNDROME

Causes: Unclear; likely related to mild viral infection and possibly aspirin use
Symptoms: Sudden onset of vomiting, high fever, headache, drowsiness, alternating excitation and confused sleepiness, convulsions, loss of consciousness
Duration: Acute
Treatments: Fluids, glucose, and other nutrients; medications (mannitol); surgery to reduce pressure in skull

---

illness through intake of fluids, glucose, and other nutrients. If the patient survives the first three or four days, the symptoms usually subside and recovery follows. The degree of recovery, however, depends upon the degree of brain swelling of the patient during the illness. Some children suffer permanent brain damage.

Medication, such as mannitol, or surgery will reduce the pressure within the skull if it reaches dangerous levels. Although it has not been proven that aspirin causes or promotes Reye's syndrome, based on a variety of medical studies, it is recommended that aspirin not be given to children with viral infections, especially chickenpox and influenza. With few exceptions, acetaminophen or ibuprofen are safe alternatives.

PERSPECTIVE AND PROSPECTS

Reye syndrome was first described by an Australian pathologist, R. D. K. Reye, in 1963. In the early 1980s, approximately 50 percent of the cases were fatal, but improved diagnosis and treatment of the disease had reduced that number to less than 10 percent by 2006.

—Alvin K. Benson, PhD;
updated by Lenela Glass-Godwin, MWS

See also Brain damage; Chickenpox; Influenza; Pediatrics; Viral infections.

For Further Information:
Badash, Michelle. "Reye's Syndrome." *Health Library*, November 26, 2012.
Bhutta, Adnan T. "Reye's Syndrome: Down but Not Out." *Southern Medical Journal* 96, no. 1 (January 1, 2003): 43-46.
Parker, James N. and Phillip M. Parker.*Reye's Syndrome: A Medical Dictionary, Bibliography, and Annotated Research Guide to Internet References*. ICON Group, 2007.
Kliegman, Robert and Waldo E. Nelson, eds. *Nelson Textbook of Pediatrics*. 19th ed. Philadelphia: Saunders/Elsevier, 2011.
Taubman, Bruce. *Your Child's Symptoms: A Parent's Guide to Understanding Pediatric Medicine*. New York: Simon & Schuster, 1992.
Woolf, Alan D., et al., eds. *The Children's Hospital Guide to Your Child's Health and Development*. Cambridge, Mass.: Perseus, 2002.

RH FACTOR

Category: Biology
Anatomy or system affected: Blood, immune system
Specialties and related fields: Embryology, genetics, hematology, neonatology, obstetrics, serology
Definition: Also called the Rhesus factor; an important chemical sometimes found on the surface of red blood cells in humans, the presence or absence of which can complicate pregnancy and blood transfusions.

Key terms:

agglutination: a clumping of blood cells caused by antibodies joining with antigens on the cell surfaces

antibody: a protein made by B lymphocytes that is found in blood; a specific antibody binds with a specific antigen

antigen: a substance that is capable of causing an immune response if it is foreign to the body that it enters; antigens may be free or located on cell surfaces

antisera: the fluid portion of blood that contains specific antibodies

blood type: a blood classification group based on the presence or absence of certain antigens on red blood cells

serum: the fluid part of blood without red blood cells and clotting factors

transfusion: the injection of whole blood or its parts into the bloodstream

STRUCTURE AND FUNCTIONS

Blood replacement in emergency or surgery can be critical: blood loss exceeding 40 percent can lead to a condition called shock in which the heart cannot pump efficiently, resulting in death. In the search for human blood replacements, scientists have found that animal blood is not compatible. More important, they have discovered that even blood from different humans does not always mix. Sometimes the red blood cells will agglutinate, or settle out of the plasma in clumps. Consequently, these red blood cells are destroyed by the body, and jaundice and death may follow. To prevent this reaction, human blood must be classified into types and cross-matched. The two most important general groupings are the ABO and Rh types.

Human blood is classified into types according to the antigens that might be present on the red blood cells as a result of heredity. Antigens are usually large, complex molecules made of protein alone, protein with attached carbohydrates, or lipids with attached fatty acids and alcohol. They may be free molecules, as in the case of toxins released by invading bacteria, or they may be located on a cell's surface and serve to la-

bel or mark the cell. The markers attached to cell surfaces identify the cell as "self" or "foreign." Such antigens are the basis of blood types.

Karl Landsteiner showed that there are four major blood types, based on two antigens that might be present or missing. He called the markers A and B. People with both markers on their cells are called type AB, people with one of the two are type A or type B, and those without either marker were originally called C but later changed to O. Landsteiner's system of classifying blood according to the presence of the A and B antigens is now termed the ABO system. Landsteiner demonstrated the chemistry of the antigens and the antibodies by mixing blood from himself and coworkers in his laboratory and observing that some combinations agglutinated.

Rh Incompatibility

First pregnancy

Rh-negative mother

Rh-positive baby

During childbirth, the baby's blood enters the mother's circulation, causing antibodies to form against Rh-positive blood.

Second pregnancy

Antibodies

Rh-positive baby

If a second baby is Rh positive, these antibodies may cross the placenta and destroy the baby's red blood cells.

The next major breakthrough came with Philip Levine and Rufus Stetson's study of the blood of a woman whose fetus had died six weeks before birth. The mother's immune system had produced antibodies against the Rh factors on the blood cells of her developing child. She was Rh negative while her child was positive, having inherited an Rh-positive gene from the father. The positive blood of the child caused the mother's immune system to react. The importance of the discovery was twofold. It not only explained why some babies suffered from an immune reaction in their mothers but also showed that blood transfusions could be typed as ABO compatible and still fail if the Rh factor was not considered.

The term *Rh factor* came about because of a misunderstanding. Working independently and believing that they had found the same factor first in their laboratory animals, Landsteiner and Alexander Wiener claimed discovery and named the Rh antigen after the rhesus monkey. They injected the monkey blood into rabbits, and the rabbits developed antibodies against the foreign factor. Hypothesizing that closely related primates might share the factor, the rabbit antibodies in a serum were then mixed with samples of human blood. Further work verified that there was indeed a new important human factor, but it differed from the one in monkeys. By this time, however, it was too late to change the misleading name. To clear up the confusion, the factor in humans kept the name of Rh factor, while the monkey antigen was labeled the LW factor.

Even if it is inappropriately named, the Rh factor is an important discovery. People with the marker on their blood cells are Rh positive, while people without it are Rh negative. Rh-negative people can give blood to people who are positive if all other antigens such as those found in the ABO types are compatible. If the reverse is attempted, however, the Rh-negative person will develop antibodies against the Rh marker. Clumping of the red blood cells will occur, and illness and death are likely.

Discovery of the presence of these markers was the key to understanding both the blood types and what happens in immune responses. When a foreign protein or antigen enters the body, antibodies are produced by the immune system and released into the blood and lymph. These antibodies are specific in the sense that a particular antibody will only combine with a particular antigen. (If a particular antigen is present on a person's own blood cells, the individual would not normally produce and carry antibodies for this molecule; otherwise, the antibodies would attack the person's own blood cells.) The antibodies fasten the cells together in what is called agglutination. Agglutinated cells are destroyed by white blood cells.

Combining the ABO and Rh systems, a person could be A+, A-, AB+, AB-, B+, B-, O+, or O-. Because an AB+ individual has A, B, and Rh antigens and no antibodies against them, this person can receive blood from all others. An O- individual has no antigens and is a universal donor, assuming that the O- person has no other important antigen differences from other, more rare types. The importance of the ABO and Rh systems is shown by the standard practice of hospitals in typing and sorting by these systems.

Unlike the ABO types, Rh-negative blood does not normally contain antibodies for positive blood unless the person has been previously exposed (sensitized) to positive blood. The A and B antibodies are developed early in people because A and B antigens are common in the environment. They are found not only on red blood cells but also in milk, colostrum, saliva, and other body fluids. Should a transfusion of Rh-positive blood be given to an Rh-negative person, the negative blood produces the antibody, which will have a violent reaction with the next similar transfusion.

The Rh factor is inherited, as are all blood types. A person inherits one gene involving the factor from each parent. If the person inherits two genes (DD) for the factor, it will be present on the red blood cells. If a person inherits one gene for the factor and one that does not produce it (Dd), the individual will still be Rh positive. If a person inherits two recessive genes (dd), that person will be Rh negative. Consequently, the gene for production of the Rh factor is called dominant; the other gene is recessive.

The original Rh factor can also be called the D factor. Additional investigation has shown that the entire Rh factor is not a single factor caused by one pair of genes; rather, at least three pairs of genes may be involved. Antisera have been found not only for the most reactive D antigen but also for four other factors. The situation can be explained by imagining Rh to be determined by a combination of three genes, which are probably closely linked on the same chromosome. Ronald Fisher labeled the genes C, c, D, d, E, and e. An Rh gene complex could then be any of these combinations: CDE, CDe, CdE, Cde, cdE, cDe, cde, or cDE. An individual would have two of these complexes, one from each parent. The number of different Rh types then reaches sixty-four.

To illustrate, a person with CDe/cdE would test Rh positive using standard anti-D sera because of the D gene; so would people with any combination of C, c, E, and e with at least one D. Nevertheless, the other nearby genes can cause agglutination problems. Each of them, except d, produces an antigen on the red blood cells. The antigens cause antisera to form in human blood that recognizes them as foreign. One can also choose to think of the situation as having eight different alleles for Rh.

Then a single symbol can stand for each combination: r = cde, r' = Cde, r" = CdE, r_y = cdE, R_0 = cDe, R_1 = CDe, R_2 = cDE, and R_Z = CDE. Any r is an Rh-negative combination in the classic sense, and any R is Rh positive. Additional discoveries of new Rh antisera have caused some investigators to hypothesize about the possibility of more than thirty antigens, some that are variant forms of the above and some that require more genes.

A 1948 paper by R. R. Race, A. E. Mourant, Sylvia D. Lawler, and Ruth Sanger reported that R_1r (or CDe/cde) is the most common Rh blood gene combination in England, at about 33 percent of those tested. The R_1R_1 (or CDe/CDe) combination follows at 16.6 percent, rr (or cde/cde) at 15.8 percent, R_1R_2 (or CDe/cDE) at 12.9 percent, R_2r (or cDE/cde) at 12.8 percent, and R_2R_2 (or cDE/cDE) at 2.7 percent. All the other combinations total about 6 percent.

Rh has turned out to be quite complex. Nevertheless, the system can be understood and applied at a very basic and useful level of Rh positive or Rh negative, which involves consideration of the very reactive D antigen on the blood cells. In that case, the Rh symbol is often labeled *RhO*.

DISORDERS AND DISEASES

The discovery of the ABO system allowed transfusions to proceed with some confidence of success during World War I. Still, some transfusions produced problems, and some minor independent blood-type systems (MNS, P) were discovered. Clearly, people were members of more than one blood-type system. The additional discovery of the highly reactive Rh factor or D antigen was critical for safe transfusions.

Another immediate application of the discovery was in the area of childbirth. Rh incompatibility explained why some babies either died at birth or were born in serious trouble. The attack of the mother's antibodies on the fetal blood cells can lead to various forms of hemolytic disease of newborns, or erythroblastosis fetalis. Incompatibility between mother and child is also one of the causes of spontaneous miscarriage early in pregnancy. Knowing the existence of the Rh factor has saved countless infants.

Recall that the Rh factor is inherited. If an Rh-negative woman (dd) marries an Rh-positive man (DD or Dd), the child may be Rh positive. During pregnancy, there is no direct blood flow from mother to child because red blood cells cannot cross the placenta. At some time during the pregnancy or at birth, however, blood will probably mix, and the mother will then be sensitized. She then will form antibodies against the Rh factor. Many of these antibodies are of the IgG type

and are smaller than A or B antibodies (IgM). The small IgG antibodies can cross the placenta into the blood of the fetus. The first Rh-positive child usually escapes harm by being born, but a second positive child will be in great danger, as the mother's preformed antibodies will cross the placenta and attack the red blood cells of the fetus. Blood cells are likely to be broken open, releasing hemoglobin. The fetus will become anemic and jaundiced and may suffer brain damage or be stillborn.

The occurrence of erythroblastosis fetalis can be prevented if an Rh-negative mother is given an injection of rhesus gamma globulin (RhoGAM) within seventy-two hours of the delivery of her first Rh-positive child. This approach was developed by C. A. Clark, P. M. Sheppard, and others working at Liverpool University. The gamma globulin destroys the fetal blood cells in the mother and prevents the production of antibodies that would affect the next positive child. Miscarriages or abortions of Rh-positive pregnancies count as an exposure to the antigen and can cause the mother's immune system to react. Therefore, these events also require the injection to protect future children. Also, any Rh-negative woman accidentally given a transfusion of positive blood would be in danger herself, as would the fetuses in any of her future pregnancies.

Amniocentesis, a sampling of fluid from the sac around the developing fetus, can reveal such difficulties as Rh incompatibility. An Rh-negative woman can also be given a series of blood tests (Rh titers) during her pregnancy. If the tests show that the antibodies are increasing in number, intrauterine transfusion of negative blood may be attempted. Moreover, if the child is nearing full term, delivery may be induced to prevent the blood of the fetus from being completely destroyed. If the child is born with signs of circulatory problems, a blood transfusion can help.

Anthony Smith notes that the ABO type has an effect on trouble with Rh during pregnancy. If the mother is Rh negative, the child is positive, and their ABO types are also incompatible, then the Rh reaction is diminished. The reason may be that the mother already has antibodies against incompatible ABO types. When the red blood cells leak into the mother's circulatory system, they are immediately destroyed by already-existing maternal ABO antibodies before any antibodies against Rh factor can be formed.

Some interesting associations with Rh have been discovered but are not yet understood. Typhoid, mumps, mononucleosis, and viral meningitis are more common in Rh-negative people. Viral diseases tend to be more common in the nonantigenic types of both the ABO and Rh systems (O and Rh negative).

PERSPECTIVE AND PROSPECTS

Few successful blood transfusions took place before 1900. In that year, Karl Landsteiner discovered that there are different types of blood. Some would mix, while others would clump. He and his coworkers identified four major human blood groups: A, B, AB, and O. Even so, eight years passed before the first transfusion using Landsteiner's ABO types was attempted. Transfusions became more likely to succeed. People could be typed by the antigens on their blood cells, and donors could be matched with the patient. Yet sometimes the transfusions still did not work as predicted. In 1930, Landsteiner won the Nobel Prize in Physiology or Medicine for his discovery of ABO blood types.

Landsteiner and Philip Levine discovered the MNS types in 1927; these are not important in transfusions but are of great help in cases of doubtful paternity. When beginning his own work, Levine agreed with Landsteiner not to study new blood groups, as Landsteiner had reserved that project for himself. Nevertheless, in 1939, Levine and Rufus E. Stetson published a report showing that the blood of a mother with a stillborn child was able to react hemolytically with 80 out of 104 ABO-compatible donors. They correctly concluded that the mother's blood lacked an antigen that many others had: an unknown marker that was independent of the known ABO, MNS, and P blood groups. Levine and Stetson had correctly analyzed the problem but did not name their new antigen. Clearly, they had discovered what would be called the Rh factor.

Less than a year later, Landsteiner and Alexander Wiener immunized rabbits and guinea pigs with the blood of the monkey *Macacus rhesus*. They found that the resulting rabbit serum agglutinated not only the rhesus monkey blood but also about 85 percent of blood samples from people in New York City. They called these people Rh positive and the remaining 15 percent Rh negative. Wiener and H. R. Peters attempted to show that the Rh antibody in the rabbits was the same as that found in the serum of people who had suffered incompatible transfusion reactions not explained by ABO blood typing.

A bitter exchange ensued between Levine and Wiener about who had discovered the Rh factor. This was resolved when it was shown that the antigen on the rhesus monkey cells was not the same as the human Rh factor. Unfortunately, the name Rh was too well established to be changed by this time. To avoid further confusion, Levine suggested that the factor in the monkeys be called the LW factor after Landsteiner and Wiener. Despite this controversy, R. R. Race and Ruth Sanger called the discovery of the Rh factor the most

important event in blood-group science since the discovery of the ABO system forty years before.

Soon, different investigators were able to derive sera with different antibodies for the Rh factor. Clearly, the Rh factor was not simply a single antigen. In 1943, Ronald Fisher studied the different antisera that had been developed and proposed that eight different Rh gene complexes were involved.

The existence of the Rh factor is useful in other ways. In addition to transfusions, another application of blood typing (including the presence or absence of the Rh factor) is in criminology. Blood left at the scene of a crime can be powerful evidence against a suspect. Blood types can also eliminate individuals as possible fathers in paternity suits. For example, if both parents are Rh negative, the child cannot be Rh positive. A more complete typing of the blood would allow further strong evidence. Such typing does not prove paternity, however; it only shows whether paternity is possible.

Blood typing also allows anthropologists to develop theories about the relationships among various human groups and how people may have migrated. The breakdown between being Rh positive or negative varies among the races. The Basques, a group of people near the Bay of Biscay between Spain and France, are only 64 percent positive, while about 85 percent of the Caucasian population in general is Rh positive. Races other than Caucasian are generally nearly 100 percent Rh positive. According to Sir Peter Medawar, however, the advantages of being one type or another are obscure. Why there are so many different blood types remains an interesting question.

The discoveries of the ABO types and the Rh factor stand as fundamental achievements in medical science. Even though many other types continue to be uncovered, ABO and Rh determinations remain the most basic steps in matching blood for many purposes, especially for safe transfusions.

—Paul R. Boehlke, PhD

See also Amniocentesis; Blood and blood disorders; Blood banks; Blood testing; Embryology; Genetic counseling; Genetics and inheritance; Hematology; Hematology, pediatric; Hemolytic disease of the newborn; Neonatology; Obstetrics; Perinatology; Phlebotomy; Pregnancy and gestation; Transfusion.

For Further Information:
Alan, Rick, Andrea Chisholm, and Brian Randall. "Rh Incompatibility and Isoimmunization." *Health Library*, March 18, 2013.
Bibel, Debra Jan, ed. *Milestones in Immunology: A Historical Exploration.* New York: Springer, 1988.
Jandl, James H. *Blood: Textbook of Hematology.* 2d ed. Boston: Little, Brown, 1996.

Martin, Richard J., Avroy A. Fanaroff, and Michele C. Walsh, eds. *Fanaroff and Martin's Neonatal-Perinatal Medicine: Diseases of the Fetus and Infant.* 2 vols. 9th ed. St. Louis: Mosby/Elsevier, 2011.

Moore, Keith L., T. V. N. Persaud, and Mark G. Torchia. *The Developing Human: Clinically Oriented Embryology.* 9th ed. Philadelphia: Saunders/Elsevier, 2013.

Page, Jake. *Blood: The River of Life.* Washington, DC: US News Books, 1981.

Race, R. R., A. E. Mourant, Sylvia D. Lawler, and Ruth Sanger. "The Rh Chromosome Frequencies in England." *Blood* 3, no. 6 (June 1948): 689-695.

"Rh Factor Blood Test." *Mayo Clinic,* June 16, 2012.

Rodak, Bernadette F., George A. Fritsma, and Elaine M. Keohane, eds. *Hematology: Clinical Principles and Applications.* 4th ed. St. Louis, Mo.: Saunders/Elsevier, 2012.

Starr, Douglas P. *Blood: An Epic History of Medicine and Commerce.* New York: Alfred A. Knopf, 1998.

RHEUMATIC FEVER

Category: Disease/Disorder
Anatomy or system affected: Heart
Specialties and related fields: Cardiology, family medicine, immunology, pediatrics
Definition: An inflammatory disease of the heart that may follow certain streptococcal infections.
Key terms:
B hemolytic streptococci: streptococcal bacteria that secrete an enzyme capable of dissolving red blood cells
pharyngitis: inflammation of the pharynx (throat), which is sometimes associated with streptococcal infection
polyarthritis: pain and inflammation in multiple joints
rheumatic heart disease: damage to heart muscle or valves because of rheumatic fever
rheumatic nodules: accumulations of white cells in soft tissue or over bony areas in patients with rheumatic fever

CAUSES AND SYMPTOMS

Rheumatic fever is an inflammatory disease affecting the heart that may follow infection by the bacterium *Streptococcus pyogenes*. The streptococci constitute a large number of gram-positive cocci, some of which are pathogens. They were originally classified in the 1930s, by Rebecca Lancefield, into groups based on characteristics of carbohydrates and proteins in their cell walls. *S. pyogenes* is the sole species of streptococcus in group A. Group A streptococcus (GAS) causes a wide array of illnesses, most notably pharyngitis (causing strep throat) and impetigo. The most serious complication associated with infection by specific strains of *S. pyogenes* is rheumatic fever.

INFORMATION ON RHEUMATIC FEVER

Causes: Bacterial infection
Symptoms: Severe joint pain, fever, abdominal pain, chest pain, heart palpitations, transient circular skin lesions
Duration: Acute
Treatments: Bed rest, increased fluid intake, limited physical activity, steroids or other anti-inflammatory drugs

---

Rheumatic fever is an autoimmune phenomenon. Certain proteins on specific strains of GAS contain segments that cross-react with body tissues, frequently heart muscle and valves, as well as other tissues in the body. This cross-reactivity between two similar foreign materials (i.e., cardiac tissue and GAS surface polysaccharides) is called "molecular mimicry." This cross-reactivity results in inflammation and possible tissue damage. The most specific S. *pyogenes* protein to induce molecular mimicry is the M-protein. Since the immune reaction occurs over a period of weeks to months, the onset of rheumatic fever may be considerably removed from the initial GAS infection.

Acute rheumatic fever has two primary presentations, either as an acute febrile illness or as a neurologic illness, both occurring after recovery from a GAS infection. The most common GAS infection presentation is strep throat, a.k.a. strep pharyngitis. Those from tropical regions have a higher prevalence of developing rheumatic fever after GAS infection presenting as the skin infection, streptococcal pyoderma, a.k.a. impetigo.

The acute febrile form of rheumatic fever is the most common. It develops within one to five weeks (typically within two to three weeks) after GAS infection recovery. The earliest manifestation of the disease is often a fever accompanied by a severe "migratory" polyarthritis that predominantly involves large joints like the knees, ankles, elbows, and wrists. Carditis, which is inflammation of the heart tissues, can sometimes present with chest pain and heart palpitations. The prominent complication of this carditis is heart valve dysfunction, often leading to mitral valve regurgitation or aortic valve regurgitation. While these are not typically acute symptomatic processes, valvular regurgitation can lead to the chronic development of heart failure over the course of the patient's life. However, severe initial insults can cause a rapid deterioration via acute congestive heart failure as well as potential electrical heart block. These are the most feared complications of rheumatic heart disease.

A rare eruption often associated with rheumatic carditis is a skin rash called "erythema marginatum," which is a transient, pinkish-red, non-itchy, circular lesion with sharp outer edges that mainly affect the trunk and sometimes limbs. Rheumatic nodules are also rare, typically associated with severe rheumatic carditis, and are usually symmetric and non-painful. They most commonly affect the elbows, as well as other joints and tendons, along the spine, and even on the head.

The less common neurologic illness sequela of rheumatic fever typically develops within two to six months after GAS infection. Fever and joint manifestations are usually absent. Instead, Sydenham's chorea, which is the exhibition of irregular, often asymmetric, abrupt, involuntary, nonrhythmic body movements is the predominant finding. It is often accompanied by emotional changes, embarrassment regarding the condition, or obsessive-compulsive disorder (OCD). In severe cases, the patient may become incapacitated.

While there is no specific diagnostic test for rheumatic fever, the combination of clinical symptoms may suggest its onset, particularly if there was a recent sore throat. The Jones Criteria groups various manifestations to yield a high predictive probability in correctly diagnosing rheumatic fever. The production of serum antibodies against streptococcal antigens is also indicative of rheumatic fever.

Most of the time, the symptoms subside with bed rest. Mild cases generally last three or four weeks, while more severe cases may last several months. A single bout with rheumatic fever may be followed by recurrent episodes with additional infections by B hemolytic streptococci.

TREATMENT AND THERAPY
The goals of treatment for acute rheumatic fever are to provide relief from symptoms, to eradicate GAS infection if present, prophylaxis against further infection, and providing education to the patient and care givers about prevention and anticipatory guidance. Because the illness represents an autoimmune reaction to an earlier streptococcal infection, antibiotic treatment is of limited value, however streptococci may persist in the upper respiratory tract even if throat cultures are negative, making eradication with antibiotics prudent. Penicillin or similar antibiotics may be administered for their prophylactic value, preventing further streptococcal infection and recurrence of the illness during the recovery period. Those with impetigo also require antibiotic therapy.

Bed rest and restriction of activities is recommended during the course of the illness. The patient should receive large amounts of fluids. Anti-inflammatory medications may be administered in response to severe polyarthritis or valvular inflammation. The duration of such inflammation is generally no more than two weeks.

Repeated infections with streptococci may trigger additional episodes of rheumatic fever, so antibiotics may be administered on a regular basis. While not all streptococcal infections trigger rheumatic fever, any previous cardiac episode is likely to be repeated after an additional streptococcal infection, often resulting in greater damage. For this reason, prophylactic antibiotic treatment may be long term.

If rheumatic heart disease has resulted in permanent damage to heart tissue, additional therapies may be necessary. Initial assessment and periodic clinical and echocardiographic evaluations with frequency based on severity of valvular disease are warranted throughout life. Often, such damage may not be apparent for years. Thickening or scarring of the heart valves, particularly the mitral and aortic valves, may necessitate valve replacement at some point in the future. There is no therapy that slows the progression of valvular damage in the setting of rheumatic fever.

PERSPECTIVE AND PROSPECTS
Thomas Sydenham, called the "English Hippocrates," in 1685 provided the first description of what was probably rheumatic fever. He also described what has become known as Sydenham's chorea, now known to be symptomatic of rheumatic fever. In 1797, London doctor Matthew Baillie noted the damage to heart valves among patients suffering from the illness. The association of rheumatic fever with bacterial infection, however, was not established until well into the twentieth century.

In part this delay resulted from the inability to isolate an organism either from the diseased heart or from blood of patients with rheumatic fever. In 1928, Homer Swift, a New York physician, suggested that rheumatic fever was an immunologic response following streptococcal infections. A few years later, the role of serologic group A, B hemolytic streptococci as the actual agent associated with the disease was established by Alvin Coburn.

A decline in the incidence of rheumatic fever in the United States began in the first decades of the twentieth century. The reason is unclear in this period before antibiotics; the decrease may have been attributable in part to the presence of less virulent strains of the bacteria. With the introduction of penicillin in the 1940s as an effective treatment for streptococcal infections, the incidence of acute rheumatic fever continued its decline. Nonetheless, by the late 1940s, rheumatic fever and rheumatic heart disease accounted for more than half of schoolchildren with cardiovascular problems in the United States.

A resurgence of the disease was first noted in the 1980s. The reasons remain unclear. Since different strains of streptococci differ in their ability to induce rheumatic fever, it is suspected that the increase may have resulted from the introduction of new bacterial strains into the population. The disease has also been seen to cluster in families, suggesting that a genetic predisposition may exist in the general population which contributes to the rise in numbers of cases. Fortunately, the streptococci have not yet established the widespread resistance to antibiotics seen among other bacteria, and rheumatic fever as a sequela to streptococcal pharyngitis may be prevented with proper treatment.

—*Michael Raghunath, MD*

See also: Antibiotics; Arrhythmias; Bacterial infections; Cardiology; Cardiology, pediatric; Childhood infectious diseases; Endocarditis; Fever; Heart; Heart disease; Heart failure; Heart transplantation; Heart valve replacement; Pharyngitis; Sore throat; Strep throat; Streptococcal infections.

For Further Information:
English, Peter C. *Rheumatic Fever in America and Britain: A Biological, Epidemiological, and Medical History*. Rutgers UP, 1999.
Gewitz, Michael H., et al. "Revision of the Jones Criteria for the Diagnosis of Acute Rheumatic Fever in the Era of Doppler Echocardiography: A Scientific Statement from the American Heart Association." *Circulation*, vol. 131, no. 20, 2015, pp. 1806-18, doi:10.1161/CIR.0000000000000205.
Kasper, D. L., A. S. Fauci, S. L. Hauser, et al. *Harrison's Principles of Internal Medicine*. 19th ed., McGraw Hill Education, 2015.
Kiple, Kenneth F., editor. *The Cambridge World History of Human Disease*. Cambridge UP, 1999.
McCance, Kathryn L., and Sue M. Huether. *Pathophysiology: The Biologic Basis for Disease in Adults and Children*. 6th ed., Mosby/Elsevier, 2010.
Murray, Patrick R., Ken S. Rosenthal, and Michael A. Pfaller. *Medical Microbiology*. 7th ed., Mosby/Elsevier, 2013.
Parks, Tom, et al. "Streptococcal Skin Infection and Rheumatic Heart Disease." *Current Opinion in Infectious Diseases*, vol. 25, no. 2, 2012, pp. 145-53, doi:10.1097/QCO.0b013e3283511d27.
"Rheumatic Fever." *Health Library*, 15 Mar. 2013.
"Rheumatic Fever." *Mayo Clinic*, 21 Jan. 2011.
Steeg, Carl N., Christine A. Walsh, and Julie S. Glickstein. "Rheumatic Fever: No Cause for Complacence." *Patient Care*, vol. 34, no. 14, 30 July 2000, pp. 40-61.
Woolf, Alan D., et al., editors. *The Children's Hospital Guide to Your Child's Health and Development*. Perseus, 2002.

RHEUMATOID ARTHRITIS

Category: Disease/Disorder
Also known as: Rheumatism
Anatomy or system affected: Heart, immune system, musculoskeletal system, respiratory system
Specialties and related fields: Geriatrics and gerontology, immunology, orthopedics, rheumatology
Definition: A chronic, systemic, and inflammatory autoimmune disease that affects the synovial membranes of joints and other organs in the body.

Key terms:
autoimmune: relating to an immune response by the body against itself
erythrocyte sedimentation rate: a screening test for active inflammation in the body
metacarpophalangeal: referring to the joints of the fingers closest to the body or knuckles
proximal interphalangeal: referring to the middle joints of the fingers
rheumatoid factor: an antibody found in the blood that identifies an inflammatory process
rheumatoid nodule: a small hard growth under the skin of the hands and elbows that may be present in those with rheumatoid arthritis
Sjögren's syndrome: dry eyes and mouth that are related to rheumatoid arthritis
symmetric: occurring on both sides of the body at the same time
synovial membrane: a sac in a joint space filled with synovial fluid that reduces friction during joint movement
white blood cell: a component of the blood that indicates an infective or inflammatory process occurring in the body

CAUSES AND SYMPTOMS

Most experts believe that rheumatoid arthritis (RA) results from stress on the body that triggers an autoimmune response characterized by chronic inflammation, swelling, and pain in joint spaces as cartilage erodes and bony cysts cause deformities in the joints, and joint motion is lost. Specific genes associated with the immune system increase the possibility of developing RA.

Initially, persons with RA may have general, vague complaints such as fatigue, weakness, weight loss, anorexia, low-grade fever, and tingling in the hands and feet during the weeks or months after some traumatic physical event in their life. Joint stiffness lessens as the day progresses but may recur after inactivity and worsen after strenuous activity. Although all joints may

---

INFORMATION ON RHEUMATOID ARTHRITIS

Causes: Autoimmune response, possibly resulting from stress on body, genetic factors
Symptoms: Chronic inflammation, swelling, and pain in joint spaces; morning stiffness; fatigue; weakness; weight loss; anorexia, low-grade fever; tingling in hands and feet
Duration: Chronic
Treatments: NSAIDs (aspirin, ibuprofen, naproxen), DMARDs (methotrexate, hydroxychloroquine, sulfasalazine, gold salts, minocycline, azothiaprine, cyclosporine, leflunomide), glucocorticoids, surgical repair

Normal joints vs those affected by arthritis. Image via Wikimedia Commons. [Public domain.]

be affected, the proximal interphalangeal or metacarpophalangeal joints and joints of the wrists, knees, ankles, and toes are most often affected. Rheumatoid nodules may appear on the hands and elbows. Sjögren's syndrome may also be present. There is also potential for renal, cardiovascular, pulmonary, neurological, and ophthalmological involvement. RA is a disease of remissions and exacerbations and should be monitored regularly.

Diagnosis of RA involves identifying at least one painful or swollen joint that has been that way for at least six weeks and a variety of blood tests intended to identify autoimmune disease. These tests may measure rheumatoid factor, anticitrullinated protein antibodies, erythrocyte sedimentation rate, and C-reactive protein. Radiologists take x-rays to identify erosions, bony calcifications, and narrowing in affected joints.

TREATMENT AND THERAPY

The goals of rheumatoid arthritis treatment are to reduce inflammation and pain, slow disease progression, improve function, and maintain quality of life. The three main categories of medication used in treating RA are nonsteroidal anti-inflammatory drugs (NSAIDs), disease-modifying antirheumatic drugs (DMARDs), glucocorticoids, biologic agents, and JAK inhibitors. RA medications have analgesic, anti-inflammatory, cytotoxic, and immunosuppressive effects.

NSAIDs such as aspirin, ibuprofen, naproxen, and more powerful prescription NSAIDs, like meloxicam, nabumetone, celecoxib, piroxicam, and indomethacin, reduce joint pain and swelling but do nothing to slow the progression of RA. These drugs quell inflammation by preventing the synthesis of prostaglandins, small molecules that promote inflammation. Additionally, NSAIDs relieve pain. Unfortunately, NSAIDs cause stomach ulcers, diminished kidney function, and increased heart attack risk with routine use. Therefore, NSAIDs are not long-term solutions for rheumatoid arthritis.

DMARDS, which include methotrexate, hydroxychloroquine, sulfasalazine, gold salts, azathioprine, cyclosporine, and leflunomide, slow the progression of RA. Methotrexate, even at low doses, decreases symptoms, limits joint damage, and improves outcomes. This drug interferes with single-carbon transfer reactions used to synthesize the building blocks for deoxyribonucleic acid (DNA) and ribonucleic acid (RNA). Unfortunately, methotrexate can cause substantial gastrointestinal distress and liver and kidney damage. Some patients tolerate it well, but others do not, and it is contraindicated during pregnancy. Hydroxychloroquine is an antimalaria medication that suppresses inflammation by unknown mechanisms. It is moderately effective for patients with mild RA and is usually well tolerated. Hydroxychloroquine causes nausea and retinopathy and is not safe during pregnancy. Patients on this drug should see their eye doctor routinely.

Sulfasalazine prevents joint erosions in RNA patients. It takes two to three months before it starts to work. This drug is commonly combined with methotrexate or hydroxychloroquine. Sulfasalazine causes nausea, appetite loss, and rash, but it is safe to take during pregnancy. Gold salts include *Myochrysine, Solganal*, and others, and these drugs decrease inflammation in joints by unknown means.

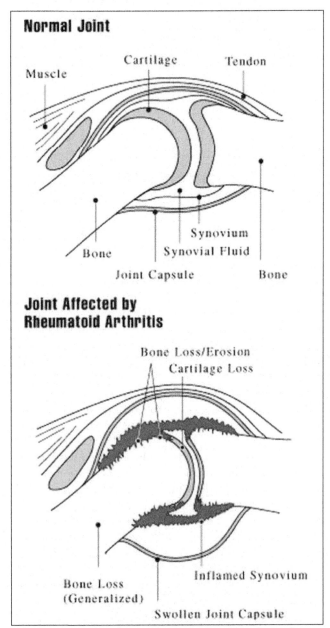

Normal Joint

Muscle

Cartilage

Tendon

Bone

Synovium

Synovial Fluid

Joint Capsule

Bone

Joint Affected by Rheumatoid Arthritis

Bone Loss/Erosion

Cartilage Loss

Bone Loss (Generalized)

Inflamed Synovium

Swollen Joint Capsule

A diagram showing how rheumatoid arthritis affects a joint. Image via Wikimedia Commons. [Public domain.]

These medications cause pulmonary fibrosis and sensitivity to light. The availability of better-tolerated options limits the utility of gold salts. Azathioprine is effective for RA patients whose disease extends beyond their joints. This drug is another DNA/RNA building block inhibitor, and it is safe for pregnant women. Azathioprine causes upset stomach, liver damage, and bone marrow suppression. It also increases the risk of developing lymphoma. Cyclosporine inhibits T-cell activation and diminishes joint erosion in RA patients. Cyclosporine is not safe for pregnant women and causes high blood pressure and kidney damage. Leflunomide also inhibits the synthesis of DNA and RNA building blocks, effectively limiting RA symptoms and joint damage. Diarrhea commonly afflicts those who take leflunomide, as does hair loss, liver damage, rash, bone marrow suppression, and neuropathy. Leflunomide is also poisonous to an unborn baby, and future mothers and fathers should avoid this drug altogether.

Glucocorticoids are effective for rapidly reducing joint inflammation. Short-term courses of oral corticosteroids provide effective bridge therapy before the effects of a DMARD appear. Prednisone reduces joint and bone erosion. However, most clinicians do not prescribe them for long periods due to the extensive number of side effects corticosteroids cause. Injections of corticosteroids into the joints or interarticular injections relieve inflamed rheumatoid joints. Unfortunately, high-dose corticosteroid injections accelerate cartilage destruction. Therefore, low-dose triamcinolone or methylprednisolone remain better options for RA patients.

Biologic disease response modifiers are a newer class of drugs targeting areas of the immune system that cause joint and tissue damage. The two main biologic agents include tumor necrosis factor-alpha (TNF-a) inhibitors and interleukin-6 (IL-6) inhibitors. TNF-a is a cytokine that promotes inflammation, and inhibiting TNF- a activity effectively quells inflammation. Five TNF inhibitors are Food and Drug Administration (FDA)-approved for RA treatment and include adalimumab, certolizumab pegol, etanercept, golimumab, and infliximab. These drugs are monoclonal antibodies that bind to TNF-a and render it innocuous. These drugs relieve RA symptoms and limit joint destruction more effectively than methotrexate alone. TNF inhibitors work faster than conventional DMARDs. Some patients report substantial improvement after the first dose. Combining a TNF-a inhibitor with methotrexate has synergistic beneficial effects. TNF-a inhibitors increase the risk of infections, particularly tuberculosis and lymphomas. Because they come in injector pens for subcutaneous injections, healthcare providers can easily teach patients to administer

Hand X-ray of a person who has rheumatoid arthritis. Photo by Dr. Martin Steinhoff, via Wikimedia Commons.

their medication at home, increasing the convenience of these drugs.

IL-6 is another proinflammatory cytokine, and preventing IL-6 from binding to its receptor diminishes joint inflammation and RA progression. Two IL-6 inhibitors, tocilizumab, and sarilumab, effectively treat RA in patients who failed to achieve satisfaction with other treatments. The adverse effects of IL-6 inhibitors include infusion reactions, high blood pressure, low white blood cell counts, liver damage, and high blood lipid levels. Severe infections and hypersensitivity reactions can occur.

Other biologics that treat RA include the T-cell costimulation blocker abatacept and the anti-CD20 B-cell depleting monoclonal antibody rituximab. Both these agents treat RA patients who failed with other anti-RA drugs. Rituximab steeply increases the risk of various infections. Abatacept increases blood pressure, causes headaches, dizziness, and, rarely, allergic reactions. It also increases the risk of serious infections.

JAK inhibitors inhibit an intracellular enzyme called "Janus kinase" that transduces activating signals within immune cells. JAK inhibitors constrain cytokine and growth factor signaling. These drugs are available in the United States for use in RA and include tofacitinib, baricitinib, and upadacitinib. These oral medications cause diarrhea, upper respiratory tract infections, headaches, and high blood pressure. Liver damage may occur with high blood lipids, low white blood cell numbers, and an increased risk of infections and cancers.

Research has shown that fish oils containing omega-3 fatty acids may also decrease inflammation in joints. Fish oils containing omega-3 fatty acids may also decrease inflammation in joints.

Education for the management of RA includes isometric exercise, stress control, methods to protect joint integrity, and support groups that assist individuals and their families in maintaining independence and planning for care during exacerbations of RA. Surgical interventions to repair damaged joints and joint replacement are also part of RA therapy.

PERSPECTIVE AND PROSPECTS

More than two million Americans have rheumatoid arthritis, most of them women. The peak onset for RA is among people in their sixties. Juvenile rheumatoid arthritis occurs in children younger than sixteen years of age. Research has indicated a possible link between infections and the development of rheumatoid arthritis.

—*Michael A. Buratovich, PhD*

For Further Information:
"Drugs for Rheumatoid Arthritis." *Medical Letter on Drugs and Therapeutics*, vol. 60, no. 1552, 2018, pp. 123-28.
Krause, Megan L, and Ashima Makol. "Management of Rheumatoid Arthritis during Pregnancy: Challenges and Solutions." *Open Access Rheumatology: Research and Reviews.* vol. 8, 2016, pp. 23-36, doi:10.2147/OARRR.S85340.
Healthline Editorial Team. "Everything You Want to Know About Rheumatoid Arthritis." *Healthline*, 23 Nov. 2021, www.healthline.com/health/rheumatoid-arthritis. Accessed 5 Apr. 2022.
Rheumatoid Arthritis. American College of Rheumatology, Dec. 2021, www.rheumatology.org/I-Am-A/Patient-Caregiver/Diseases-Conditions/Rheumatoid-Arthritis. *Accessed 5 Apr. 2022.*
Rheumatoid Arthritis. National Institute of Arthritis, and Musculoskeletal, and Skin Diseases, Sept. 2019, www.niams.nih.gov/health-topics/rheumatoid-arthritis. *Accessed 5 Apr. 2022.*
Rheumatoid Arthritis. The Centers for Disease Control and Prevention, 27 Jul. 2020, www.cdc.gov/arthritis/basics/rheumatoid-arthritis.html. Accessed 5 Apr. 2022.
Rheumatoid Arthritis of the Foot and Ankle. OrthoInfo, Sept. 2017, orthoinfo.aaos.org/en/diseases—conditions/rheumatoid-arthritis-of-the-foot-and-ankle. Accessed 5 Apr. 2022.

RHEUMATOLOGY

Category: Specialty
Anatomy or system affected: Bones, hands, hips, immune system, joints, knees, legs, musculoskeletal system
Specialties and related fields: Geriatrics and gerontology, immunology, orthopedics, pharmacology
Definition: The field of medicine concerned with the diagnosis and treatment of joint inflammation and bone or joint destruction and with the surgical repair of damaged joints.

Key terms:
acute: referring to a disease process of sudden onset
arthritis: joint inflammation
capillary exudate: a group of substances secreted by the capillaries as part of the inflammatory process
chronic: referring to a lingering disease process
joint: the conjunction of two or more bones

SCIENCE AND PROFESSION

Rheumatology is concerned with the major diseases of bones and joints: arthritis, osteoarthritis, other arthritic disorders such as gouty arthritis, and ankylosing spondylitis, among a host of others.

The onset of rheumatoid arthritis is usually in middle age. It strikes three times as many women as men. To understand the disease, it is necessary to understand the body's skeletal system-the bones and bone structures, as well as the tissues between and around bones and joints.

There are 206 bones in the human body. Some function as support mechanisms that hold the body erect and support the weight, such as the spine and the bones of the hips and legs. Some bones form defensive "cages" that protect body organs, such as the skull and the ribs. Some bones are involved in movement, specifically the bones in the spine, shoulders, arms, hands, hips, legs, and feet.

Bones are composed of three main sections. The tough membranous tissue that covers the bone, the periosteum, contains the blood vessels that nourish bone cells and the nerve fibers that sense pain and pressure. The outer layer of the bone itself is called compact bone; it forms the hard exterior. Inside is a spongy inner structure called cancellous (chambered) bone. Cancellous bone contains the marrow that manufactures blood cells, and it also stores fat cells.

When bones meet, the structure formed is called a joint, or articulation. Some joints are fixed, such as the ribs and the bones of the skull; they are called fibrous joints because a tough, fibrous adhesive material connects them, prohibiting movement and maintaining the integrity of the protective cage.

Some joints are capable of motion. Moving joints are of two types: synovial joints and cartilaginous joints. An example of the latter is the spine, where each vertebra is connected to its neighbor by a spinal disk made of cartilage. Cartilaginous joints are capable of movement, but they have nowhere near the mobility of the synovial joints, so called because they are filled with synovial fluid, a liquid resembling the white of an egg.

There are six kinds of synovial joints: ball-and-socket, ellipsoidal, hinge, pivot, saddle, and gliding joints. Ball-and-socket joints are found in the shoulders and hips. In these joints, a long bone-the femur in the leg and the humerus in the arm-end with a ball-shaped structure that fits neatly into a round, concave socket. Ball-and-socket joints are capable of the widest range of movement. Ellipsoidal joints are modifications of the ball-and-socket structures, where the bones are not round but oval. They are found in the wrists and ankles. The elbows and knees are hinge joints, which permit only bending and extending motions, up and down or side to side, as with a common door hinge. In pivot joints, one bone contains a small cup or arch that accepts a point of another bone, permitting it to rotate on its axis. The two bones at the top of the spine, which govern the range of motion of the head, are examples. A saddle joint consists of two bones, shaped rather like saddles; they fit snugly into each other and allow a wide range of movement. The joint connecting the thumb to the rest of the hand is the only saddle joint in the human body. The bones of gliding joints are almost flat; their surfaces slide over one another, permitting limited motion forward and back or from side to side. Some of the wrist bones are gliding joints.

The synovial joints are the most intricate and mobile of all the joints, and they are also the most prone to disease. The synovial joint capsule is a complex structure that encloses the moving bones and other tissues. It consists of the capsular ligament, which forms the joint capsule; the joint cavity, an open space between bones that allows free mobility; and the synovial membrane, a thin, smooth tissue that secretes synovial fluid. The synovial fluid fills the joint cavity and lubricates bone surfaces. Bones do not actually rub against each other; they are too rough and would become abraded. They are separated by a covering of smooth, white tissue called articular cartilage that permits smooth movement and absorbs impact. Just outside the joint capsule are bursae, small pouches that store synovial fluid.

In rheumatoid arthritis, the first signs of disease are pain and inflammation in the synovial joint capsule. This initial manifestation may be attributable to a number of factors, such as bacterial infection or injury.

The hand of an elderly patient suffering from severe rheumatoid arthritis. Rheumatologists diagnose and treat such joint inflammation. Photo by James Heilman, MD, via Wikimedia Commons.

The reasons that an acute episode of pain and inflammation in the synovial joints progresses to chronic rheumatoid arthritis are unknown. It is suspected that genetic factors may be involved; the disease often runs in families. Blood components called rheumatoid factors are present in the majority of rheumatoid arthritis patients. The role of these factors in the development of disease, however, is unclear because rheumatoid factors are also found in people who do not develop rheumatoid arthritis.

In some patients, rheumatoid arthritis is relatively benign, with pain and inflammation that can be controlled by medication and other support techniques. In other patients, the disease progresses to devastating bone deformities and complete loss of mobility in the affected joints. How this degeneration occurs is related to a disruption in the body's normal reaction to infection or injury. Pain and inflammation are protective mechanisms with which the body attempts to compensate for a disease or disorder. The following sequence of events is what normally occurs when a synovial joint is damaged by infection, physical injury, or a toxic substance.

Tissue injury-from trauma or infection-causes the release of chemical mediators from surrounding cells. These chemicals include prostaglandins, leukotrienes, histamine, serotonin, and bradykinin. Collectively, they cause the local blood vessels to enlarge (vasodilate), increasing blood flow to the affected area and causing redness and heat.

Ordinarily, the capillaries, the tiny blood vessels that supply nutrients to the cells, have openings in their walls so small that only tiny bits of matter can get through. During inflammation, they become more permeable; that is, the openings in the capillary walls enlarge so that the capillaries can deliver larger substances to the affected area. This group of substances forms the capillary exudate, and it flows copiously into the affected area, causing swelling. The exudate consists of lymphocytes, which produce antibodies to fight infection; neutrophils; and macrophages, specialized white blood cells that facilitate the removal of tissue debris, dead cells, and other material. These white blood cells can also release other substances, such as superoxide, an agent used by white blood cells to kill bacteria but which can also damage healthy tissue. Another is interleukin-1, an agent that promotes healing and stimulates lymphocytes to produce antibodies. The spread of inflammation is prevented by a third agent released by the white blood cells, fibrinogen, which effectively closes off the area of inflammation.

In normal situations, the agent causing the inflammation is neutralized, the capillaries return to their normal size, certain white blood cells remove the protective shield, and the healing process begins. In rheumatoid arthritis, the orderly process that begins with pain and inflammation and ends with healing is disrupted by various events. Instead of neutralizing the trauma, the anti-inflammatory phase can set off a chain of events that makes the condition progressively worse.

Why this disruption occurs is not yet known, but four major theories have been suggested. The first is the theory of genetic predisposition to the disease, a factor which may or may not relate to the other three. The second theory is that rheumatoid arthritis is an immune-complex disease. Ordinarily, when the body fights an infectious microorganism that has invaded the body, lymphocytes produce antibodies that combine with the antigens characteristic of the microorganism. This antigen/antibody combination is the immune complex, and it is removed by other white blood cells. In this theory, the process is altered. Instead of being removed by white blood cells, the immune complex lodges in the synovial membrane and causes continuing inflammation. Capillaries continue to release exudate, whose constituents cause cell proliferation, thickening of the synovial membrane, and destruction of articular cartilage and bone tissue.

The autoimmune theory is similar, but in this case the causative agent is not a foreign substance but something natural within the body. For example, if a specific protein released by a gland finds its way into a joint, it may be regarded as a foreign, infective agent. Thus it will set off an immune response and cause inflammation, initiating the same process described above.

The fourth theory links rheumatoid arthritis to viral or bacterial infection. It has been noted that fever, malaise, and enlarged lymph nodes-common symptoms of infection-are often seen in patients with rheumatoid arthritis. Furthermore, rheumatoid arthritis sometimes occurs simultaneously with bacterial pneumonia, tuberculosis, hepatitis, and sexually transmitted diseases, as well as with diseases caused by viruses, such as mumps and measles.

The progress of rheumatoid arthritis is variable. In some patients, it is characterized by occasional flare-ups (episodes of acute pain and inflammation) and periods of remission (times when the patient is relatively comfortable). In others, the disease causes progressive, insidious destruction of the joint and may involve other organs of the body. Articular cartilage may be destroyed, and the joint may become immobilized, an extremely painful condition. The bones in the joint may fuse together, becoming one solid mass. The bones may also become dislocated. In about 30 to 35 percent of patients, rheumatoid nodules develop.

These hard, solid lumps usually occur at the elbows but may also be found at the knees, ankles, and feet. In advanced cases, nodules may be discovered in the heart muscle, the lungs, and other organs where they could impair organ function.

The diagnosis of rheumatoid arthritis has been codified by the American Rheumatism Foundation. This organization lists seven symptoms and suggests that the presence of any four should confirm the diagnosis of rheumatoid arthritis (although patients with two or more of the symptoms should not be excluded). The seven symptoms are morning stiffness lasting an hour or more; arthritis in three or more joints; arthritis in hands, fingers, or wrists; arthritis occurring symmetrically (for example, in both hands, elbows, or knees); rheumatoid nodules; the presence of rheumatoid factor; and x-ray evidence of bone deterioration.

DIAGNOSTIC AND TREATMENT TECHNIQUES

Once a patient is suspected of having rheumatoid arthritis, the physician may wish to conduct further laboratory tests to assess the severity of the disease and, from that analysis, develop a treatment regimen. In addition to testing for rheumatoid factor, the physician will check the patient's erythrocyte (red blood cell) sedimentation rate (ESR). This test helps to determine the presence of inflammatory activity. Another blood test looks for C-reactive protein (CRP). CRP also indicates inflammatory activity; levels rise during an acute attack and fall during a period of remission. Synovial fluid is analyzed to discover changes that occur during inflammation. For example, during inflammatory episodes, the color of the fluid becomes significantly darker, turning yellow or green. Ordinarily quite clear and viscous, it becomes cloudy and thinner in consistency. Many more tests are available to the physician to help him or her evaluate the severity of the disease, including an analysis of the various substances involved in the immune process.

There is no cure for rheumatoid arthritis, but most patients can be helped with the therapies available. In spite of treatment, however, 5 to 10 percent will eventually be disabled by bone deterioration and destruction.

Treatment depends on the severity of the condition. The regimen can simply involve rest and immobilization of the affected joint, or it may include any of a wide range of medications, from aspirin to potent, often toxic compounds. In advanced cases, joint deformity may be so severe as to require surgery and/or prosthetic implants.

The goals of therapy are to relieve pain, reduce inflammation, and maintain the function of the joint. Ideally, the physician would also like to halt the progress of the disease. Some medications in use today promise to slow or stop the progress of the disease, but nothing is available to cure it.

For the relief of pain, the physician has a large number of medications available, many of which will also reduce inflammation. These include a group of drugs called nonsteroidal anti-inflammatory drugs (NSAIDs). NSAIDs as a class include the salicylates, such as aspirin, ibuprofen, acetaminophen, and at least twenty other drugs currently in use in the United States.

Far and away the largest number of patients with rheumatoid arthritis are being treated with NSAIDs. Many of the NSAIDs are perfectly safe when used in lower doses. At the high doses often required to control the pain of rheumatoid arthritis, however, they can cause significant adverse reactions. A significant percentage of patients given some NSAIDs develop side effects severe enough to warrant stopping the drug. Many develop gastrointestinal (GI) problems ranging from stomachaches to bleeding ulcers, which can be fatal.

One of the ways in which NSAIDs work is to reduce the production of prostaglandins, substances released in the capillary exudate that are partially responsible for the inflammatory process. At the inflamed synovial joint, this attribute of NSAIDs is a desirable one. In the stomach, however, NSAIDs can cause problems. One of the prostaglandins helps to protect the stomach lining from damage by the organ's highly acid contents. NSAIDs can remove this protection, allowing stomach acids to attack the lining, causing irritation and inflammation. Therefore, some physicians prescribe an NSAID with a prostaglandin analog, such as misoprostol, in the hope of avoiding or reducing GI distress. Misoprostol has problems of its own, however, such as causing severe diarrhea in some patients.

For the patient with severe rheumatoid arthritis-defined as painful, debilitating illness that does not respond to NSAIDs and is progressing to deformity-the available medications are both more potent and more toxic. A group of agents called disease-modifying drugs promise to reduce the degenerative processes in rheumatoid arthritis. These drugs include gold compounds, D-penicillamine, drugs used to treat malaria, and sulfasalazine. They appear to alter the course of rheumatoid arthritis, but they do not relieve pain or inflammation, so they must be given with NSAIDs. They all have a high potential for toxicity and must be used carefully, with constant monitoring, to avoid serious side effects.

In some cases, physicians find it necessary to prescribe corticosteroids to patients with rheumatoid arthritis. These drugs present a problem, because rheumatoid arthritis is a lifelong condition, and toxicity and physical changes often occur with long-term steroid therapy. Sometimes corticosteroids are given as short-term therapy to achieve a rapid reduction of inflammation. In this case, there is a danger of a severe rebound reaction when the drug is stopped. A corticosteroid may be administered as an injection into the joint, which is an effective short-term procedure to bring fast relief of pain and inflammation in an acute situation.

Immunosuppressive therapy is sometimes prescribed for patients with rheumatoid arthritis. Immunosuppressive agents have the potential to be highly toxic, and their use is reserved for patients who have not responded to other treatments.

Exercise and physical therapy are useful to the patient with rheumatoid arthritis. During acute inflammation, passive exercise within pain limits, with the limb manipulated by another person or the patient, will help keep the joint mobile and prevent muscle tightening. After the inflammation has subsided, active exercise is recommended to maintain muscle mass and mobility, but the activity should never be strenuous or fatiguing.

Flexion contracture, a condition in which the muscles that move the joint become stiff and shortened, may respond to exercise. If the contracture has become established, however, then more intensive exercise, splinting, or orthopedic treatment may be necessary.

Orthopedic surgery to correct fused or dislocated joints can be performed on any joint in the body, and in some cases, a fused or badly deteriorated joint can be replaced with an implant of metal and/or plastic (arthroplasty). The two most successful implant procedures are total replacement of the hip or knee. When a hip is replaced, the surgeon reveals the joint where the ball of the femur nests in the socket of the acetabulum, a cavity in the hipbone. The ball of the femur is replaced by a metal or plastic ball attached to a shaft that is anchored inside the femur. The socket is replaced as well, usually with a plastic cup that is anchored into the hipbone. The implant can give the patient instant relief from pain and restore mobility. The length of time that the hip replacement will last varies, but many patients receive years of relief from a single operation. A similar procedure is used to replace the hinge joint of the knee, and, although knee replacement is not as successful as hip replacement, it has helped many patients.

PERSPECTIVE AND PROSPECTS

Rheumatoid arthritis afflicts about 1 percent of all populations. While the disease is not life-threatening, it is one of the most significant crippling disorders in the world. Most patients can be treated successfully by medication, exercise, and other support measures. The disease is progressive in most patients. After ten years,

80 percent of patients will have some degree of deformity, ranging from minor destruction of bone and cartilage to complete fusion of the joint.

Some patients medicate themselves with over-the-counter painkillers and rarely, if ever, see a physician. It is to be expected that, in these patients, the disease is mild, with acute episodes occurring only sporadically. The majority of patients with moderate-to-severe rheumatoid arthritis are seen by physicians.

Currently, there is no perfect therapy for rheumatoid arthritis, in the sense that there is no one agent or family of agents that promises to be safe and effective in all patients. The danger of significant adverse reactions exists with most drugs that are effective, particularly in those patients who require high doses to control the pain and inflammation of the most severe forms of the disease.

Pharmaceutical science continues to search for new medications that will relieve pain and inflammation without damaging side effects. New drugs that will stop the progress of the disease safely and effectively are also sought. There is also the hope that rheumatoid arthritis will be curable or preventable one day.

Orthopedic surgeons continue to improve the techniques for alleviating the effects of bone and joint destruction that occur in some patients. New prosthetic appliances are designed and produced constantly in an effort to widen the range of joint replacement procedures.

—*C. Richard Falcon*

See also Aging; Aging: Extended care; Arthritis; Arthroplasty; Arthroscopy; Autoimmune disorders; Behçet's disease; Bone disorders; Bones and the skeleton; Bursitis; Geriatrics and gerontology; Gout; Hydrotherapy; Inflammation; Joints; Juvenile rheumatoid arthritis; Lyme disease; Orthopedic surgery; Orthopedics; Orthopedics, pediatric; Osteoarthritis; Osteonecrosis; Physical examination; Rheumatic fever; Rheumatoid arthritis; Spondylitis; Sports medicine.

For Further Information:
American College of Rheumatology. *American College of Rheumatology*, 2013.
Isenberg, David A., et al., eds. *Oxford Textbook of Rheumatology.* 3d ed. New York: Oxford University Press, 2004.
Lahita, Robert G. *Rheumatoid Arthritis: Everything You Need to Know.* Rev. ed. New York: Avery, 2004.
Litin, Scott C., ed. *Mayo Clinic Family Health Book.* 4th ed. New York: HarperResource, 2009.
Mayo Clinic. *Mayo Clinic on Arthritis.* New York: HarperCollins, 2005.
MedlinePlus. "Rheumatoid Arthritis." *MedlinePlus*, August 26, 2013.
Parker, James N., and Philip M. Parker, eds. *The 2002 Official Patient's Sourcebook on Rheumatoid Arthritis.* San Diego, Calif.: Icon Health, 2002..
Shlotzhauer, Tammi L., and James L. McGuire. *Living with Rheumatoid Arthritis.* 2d ed. Baltimore: Johns Hopkins University Press, 2003.
Sutton, Amy L., ed. *Arthritis Sourcebook: Basic Consumer Health Information About Osteoarthritis, Rheumatoid Arthritis, Other Rheumatic Disorders, Infectious Forms of Arthritis, and Diseases with Symptoms Linked to Arthritis.* 3d ed. Detroit, Mich.: Omnigraphics, 2012.
Yung, Raymond L."What Is a Rheumatologist?" *American College of Rheumatology*, August, 2012..

RHINITIS

Category: Disease/Disorder
Also known as: Runny nose, hay fever, nasal allergies
Anatomy or system affected: Nose, respiratory system, throat
Specialties and related fields: Family medicine, immunology, otorhinolaryngology, pediatrics
Definition: A discharge from the nose caused by inflammation of the internal nasal structures.
Key terms:
allergic rhinitis: acute or seasonal nasal stuffiness and sneezing that follows the exposure to allergens such as pollen or animal dander; hay fever is one form of allergic rhinitis
nonallergic rhinitis: acute nasal stuffiness produced as a result of the common cold or flu
postnasal drip: the discharge of nasal mucus into the back of the throat

CAUSES AND SYMPTOMS
Rhinitis can have a variety of causes, including infection by a rhinovirus or certain bacteria and exposure to cold air or nasal allergens. Foreign bodies in the nose and certain structural deformities can also cause rhinitis.

When the nasal symptoms are due to allergies, the condition is called allergic rhinitis. A partial list of allergens that can produce allergic rhinitis includes pollen, dust, molds, wool, feathers, tobacco smoke, airborne environmental pollutants, strong odors, spicy foods, and animal dander.

When the nasal symptoms are not due to allergies, the condition is called nonallergic rhinitis or nonallergic vasomotor rhinitis. Nonallergic rhinitis can be caused by a viral or bacterial infection, exposure to cold air, structural deformities, certain endocrine disorders such as hypothyroidism, or emotional stress; it is occasionally observed during the first trimester of pregnancy. Nonallergic rhinitis usually begins with a feeling of irritation in the nose or throat. The irritation is followed by sneezing and mucus discharge as the nasal air passageways become more obstructed.

Atrophic rhinitis, a chronic form of nonallergic rhinitis, is a condition often seen first at puberty; because there is a genetic component, the condition tends to run in families. The causes of atrophic rhinitis are not fully understood, although deficiencies in iron and vitamins A and D may contribute. In this condition, the moist, pink, thick lining of the inside of the nose is replaced by a thin crusty surface that can be foul smelling. Although the nasal cavity is wide open, people often complain of a feeling of stuffiness. The condition is sometimes accompanied by nosebleeds.

Nasal dripping and/or sneezing can be seen with all the forms of rhinitis. The discharge can be clear and watery or thicker and more viscous. It can be colorless; if there is a color, it is often white or less often green or yellow. Postnasal drip is when the discharge is into the back of the throat, a condition that can result in a dry, usually nonproductive cough.

TREATMENT AND THERAPY
The treatment for rhinitis is an attempt to manage symptoms. The most effective treatment for allergic rhinitis is to remove the source of the irritation. In the home, keeping the windows closed, using an air conditioner, and filtering the circulating air can reduce allergen exposure. Saline irrigation can also be used to reduce the nasal symptoms. When symptoms persist despite these efforts, treatment focuses on minimizing the allergic response. This can be done using antihistamines, steroids, or antileukotrienes.

When the body encounters an allergen, the white blood cells produce antibodies, which then promote the release of compounds called mediators. Histamine is perhaps the best known of these mediators. The mediators trigger the nasal symptoms. Most of the drugs used to treat allergic rhinitis are designed to inhibit the actions of the mediators. Antihistamines block the action of histamine and so significantly reduce swelling and discharge. Likewise, antileukotrienes work by blocking leukotrienes, another immune system mediator. The mechanism by which nasal steroids (usually given in the form of a spray) work is less clear, but they can provide temporary relief.

When the symptoms do not respond well to the above treatments, immunotherapy is required. For this treatment, it is necessary to determine the allergens to which the person is sensitive. This can be accomplished in a variety of ways, although skin or blood testing are the most common. Once the specific allergen has been identified, the immune system can be desensitized through carefully administered challenges, which in effect raise the tolerance level necessary to produce the nasal symptoms.

If the cause of nonallergic rhinitis was exposure to cold air, then going into a warmer environment will

INFORMATION ON RHINITIS
Causes: Irritants, infections, cold air
Symptoms: Stiffness or irritation in nose often accompanied by mucus discharge
Duration: Usually acute but can be chronic
Treatments: Removal of irritation, resolution of infection, antihistamines, nasal steroids

usually eliminate the symptoms. If the cause is the common cold or the flu, then symptoms are sometimes relieved by decongestants and/or antihistamines. Some of these drugs are available over the counter, while others require a prescription. Unless there is a primary or secondary bacterial infection accompanying the rhinitis, antibiotics are not effective. Drinking lots of fluids, getting bed rest, and breathing humidified air can reduce the discomfort. With any viral or bacterial infection (especially H1N1 influenza infections), a medical professional should be consulted immediately if breathing becomes a problem. Muscle aching and the general feeling of malaise that accompanies nonallergic rhinitis can often be relieved by over-the-counter medications such as aspirin or ibuprofen.

Atrophic rhinitis can be treated be irrigating the nose with saline. If a bacterial infection is present, then antibiotics are indicated. The crusting can be treated by irrigation with nasal douches. In severe cases, atrophic rhinitis is treated by Young's operation, a surgical procedure that reduces the size of the nasal cavity.

When the cause of the rhinitis is a foreign body or structural deformity, removing the foreign body or surgically changing the internal structure of the nose often eliminates the symptoms.

PERSPECTIVE AND PROSPECTS
Considerable financial and personal costs are associated with rhinitis, since it is such a common condition. Because rhinitis is so common, considerable effort is going into completely understanding this disease. As a result, new treatments with fewer side effects should become available.

—*David Hornung, PhD*

See also Allergies; Antihistamines; Common cold; Decongestants; Ear infections and disorders; Hay fever; Influenza; Multiple chemical sensitivity syndrome; Nasal polyp removal; Nasopharyngeal disorders; Otorhinolaryngology; Rhinoviruses; Sinusitis; Sneezing.

For Further Information:
Baraniuk, James N., and Dennis Shusterman, eds. *Nonallergic Rhinitis*. New York: Informa Healthcare, 2007.
Busse, William W., and Stephen T. Holgate, eds. *Asthma and Rhinitis*. Hoboken, N.J.: Wiley-Blackwell, 2000.

Carson-DeWitt, Rosalyn. "Allergic Rhinitis." *Health Library*, October 31, 2012.

Henochowicz, Stuart I. "Allergic Rhinitis." *MedlinePlus*, June 17, 2012.

Henochowicz, Stuart I. "Vasomotor Rhinitis." *MedlinePlus*, June 17, 2012.

Scadding, Glenis K., and Wytske J. Hokkens. *Rhinitis*. Albuquerque, N.Mex.: Health Press, 2007.

RHINOPLASTY AND SUBMUCOUS RESECTION

Category: Procedures
Anatomy or system affected: Nose
Specialties and related fields: General surgery, otorhinolaryngology, plastic surgery
Definition: Surgical procedures that correct cosmetic and health problems related to the nose.
Key terms:

cartilage: white, fibrous connective tissue attached to the articular surfaces of bones

inspired air: air that is breathed in

pharynx: the part of the respiratory-digestive passage that extends from the nasal cavity to the larynx (voice box)

INDICATIONS AND PROCEDURES

The nose, in addition to being an important organ for breathing and smelling, is cosmetically significant because of its prominence on the face. Hence, surgery to improve the nose may be medically necessary or an elective procedure to enhance facial appearance (cosmetic surgery). In modern society, the latter type of nasal surgery is the most common. Nasal surgery, however, usually involves both. Before examining rhinoplasty and submucous resection, it is useful briefly to denote the function of the nose, its anatomy, and its interconnections with the body's respiratory and olfactory systems.

Air breathed in enters the nose through the nostrils, which are separated by a wall of cartilage and bone called the nasal septum. In most cases, the septum produces two nostrils of similar size. In some cases, however, injury or heredity causes the septum to become thickened on one side or to exhibit ridges or bumps. In a minor case of deviated septum, the irregularity may make one nostril smaller than the other and can affect breathing and sinus drainage adversely during colds. In very severe cases, it can obstruct and irritate the nose enough so that relatively permanent nasal tissue swelling requires chronic, uncomfortable breathing through the mouth.

In most individuals, inspired air passes into two nasal passages which lead into the upper part of the throat. They allow the air to pass through the pharynx and trachea (windpipe) to reach the lungs. Each nasal passage is lined with a soft, moist mucous membrane which is covered with fine cilia (hairs) that catch dust and other particles and keep them from reaching the lungs. The nose and the nasal passages also raise the temperature of inspired air before it enters the lungs. Furthermore, the nose plays a large part in the sense of taste, as shown by the inability of people with severe colds to taste food.

Submucous resection is performed when the nasal septum is so distorted that it causes discomfort to the patient, especially chronic nasal pain, the need for continuous and uncomfortable mouth breathing, or repeated and prolonged colds. In these cases, the septum is reshaped in order to cure the problem, allowing the patient to breathe normally again through the nose. Septum resection may be accomplished with fine scissors, a scalpel, and/or bone rasps.

Cosmetic nose alterations are collectively referred to as rhinoplasty. The most common procedures correct prominent bumps, bulbousness, drooping tip, and overly large or small size. Text on cosmetic surgery of the nose include descriptive terms that graphically identify the surgical problems encountered in rhinoplasty, such as "saddle nose," "short nose," "pig nose," and "hook nose." Rhinoplasty is also used to repair damage caused by accidents and cancer. Furthermore, it is an essential part of repairing a deviated nasal septum, which can greatly impair the breathing of afflicted individuals if left untreated.

Most often, nasal surgery is performed by use of intranasal incisions. The nasal skin is temporarily freed and pulled back from underlying bone and cartilage. Then, this hard framework is altered by partial removal, rearrangement, augmentation with synthetic materials, or bone and cartilage grafts from various parts of the patient's body. The site in the nose and the shape of the grafts used depend on the procedure to be carried out. Once all necessary procedures have been completed on cartilage and bone, the skin is redraped over them. In some cases, especially where nose size is to be reduced, portions of the soft tissues of the nose are removed.

After nasal surgery-whether rhinoplasty, submucous resection, or some combination of techniques is used-the nostrils are packed with sterile gauze to prevent bleeding and to support the nasal mucosa during its initial healing, as incisions are usually sutured only minimally and with resorbable suture materials. The packing is often removed after several days. A nasal splint is also used in many cases. It provides external support and aid in maintaining nasal recontouring. The splint also protects the altered nose from damage during the several weeks usually required for most swelling to subside. After the removal of the splint, it takes at least several months for normal feeling and final nose shape to be attained as postsurgical swelling subsides entirely.

USES AND COMPLICATIONS
Nasal surgery can be done under local or general anesthesia in a hospital or in a surgeon's office. Hospitalization and general anesthesia are most often used, although frequently they are not needed. Most reconstructive surgeons prefer these operative conditions for the patient's sake and because they allow easier physical manipulation of the patient.

Most procedures attempted are quite safe and uncomplicated. Occasional problems include excessive bleeding, internal scarring of nasal mucosa, recurring airway obstruction, and unexpected contour irregularities. Infections after nasal surgery are rare except in cases where cartilaginous nasal implants are used. The incidence of infection may increase, however, as surgeons add forehead and chin alteration to rhinoplasty to optimize the overall cosmetic results.

Overall, nasal surgery is straightforward and has few real risks. Patients should be aware, however, that the procedure can fail to yield a chosen cosmetic improvement and that airway obstruction can be generated by the process or can recur after repair.

PERSPECTIVE AND PROSPECTS
Among the exciting advances being made in rhinoplasty and submucous resection are the replacement of deficient nostril parts and septa with cartilage from other body parts or with synthetic materials. It is projected by some doctors that implants obtained from other individuals will eventually be used to repair function and appearance in individuals whose noses are irreversibly damaged by accidents and cancer.

Another aspect of importance to cosmetic nasal surgery is the growing realization that the chin, forehead, and other parts of the face are important to the appearance of the nose. This has led some surgeons performing nose recontouring to expend much effort toward examining these features and designing complementary surgical procedures to achieve good results.

—*Sanford S. Singer, PhD*

See also Facial transplantation; Nasal polyp removal; Nasopharyngeal disorders; Otorhinolaryngology; Plastic surgery.

For Further Information:
Dutton, Jay M. "Rhinoplasty Overview." *American Rhinologic Society*, July 2011.
Elsahy, Nabil. *Plastic and Reconstructive Surgery of the Nose.* New York: Elsevier, 2000.
Ferrari, Mario. *PDxMD Ear, Nose, and Throat Disorders.* Philadelphia: PDxMD, 2003.
Gruber, Ronald P., and George C. Peck, eds. *Rhinoplasty: State of the Art.* St. Louis, Mo.: Mosby Year Book, 1993.
Jewet, Brian, Shan R. Baker, and Sam Nacify, eds. *Principles of Aesthetic Nasal Reconstruction.* St. Louis, Mo.: Mosby, 2002.
"Rhinoplasty." *Health Library*, September 10, 2012.
"Rhinoplasty." *Mayo Clinic*, March 1, 2011.

RHINOVIRUSES

Category: Disease/Disorder
Anatomy or system affected: Cells, chest, lungs, nose, respiratory system, throat
Specialties and related fields: Biochemistry, biotechnology, cytology, epidemiology, genetics, histology, immunology, otorhinolaryngology, pathology, preventive medicine, public health, serology, virology
Definition: Disease-causing agents that are responsible for more common colds than any other respiratory virus.

Key terms
antigen: a proteinaceous, membrane-bound, cell surface component that stimulates the production of antibodies, which subsequently provoke an immune response
endothelial cell: cells that line blood and lymph vessels
Enterovirus: a genus of viruses similar to rhinoviruses
leukocyte: a white blood cell
picornavirus: the family of viruses that includes the *Enterovirus* and *Rhinovirus* genera
receptor: a membrane-bound protein that normally mediates interactions between the cell in which it is bound and specific, external signals, such as hormones
serotype: a group of viruses that can be characterized by common cell surface antigens

CAUSES AND SYMPTOMS
Rhinoviruses have been identified as the virus most often responsible for the common cold. Rhinoviruses have also been implicated in complications of asthma. Rhinoviruses are transmitted through sneezing and coughing, which expels droplets of moisture laden with virus. Once introduced into the respiratory system, the virus enters cells by interfacing with the intercellular adhesion molecule-1 (ICAM-1) receptor. As its name implies, ICAM-1 provides adhesion between endothelial cells and leukocytes after injury or stress, but it also facilitates the entry of rhinoviruses into cells, where they can replicate. The subsequent immune response is responsible for most of the symptoms of the common cold.

Colds occur more often in winter than in other seasons, although they can occur year-round. This sea-

INFORMATION ON RHINOVIRUSES

Causes: Transmitted through sneezing and coughing

Symptoms: Sneezing, coughing, nasal and sinus drainage, congestion, fluid in the ears, headache, fever; in more severe cases, wheezing and pneumonia

Duration: Approximately seven days for infection; two or more weeks for symptoms

Treatments: Zinc lozenges, rest; preventive measures (handwashing with soap or antiseptic such as alcohol-based sanitizer, disinfection of surfaces commonly touched by people, covering coughs and sneezes with tissue or article of clothing)

sonal effect is thought to be the result of an increase in time spent in closer contact with other people who may carry a rhinovirus.

TREATMENT AND THERAPY

No cure exists for the treatment of rhinoviruses once contracted, and no vaccine exists to inoculate against infection with rhinoviruses. However, many strategies exist for reducing the transmission of viruses between infected individuals. Traditional home remedies such as chicken soup, bed rest, and drinking a lot of fluids may increase the comfort level of the sufferer, but they do not shorten the course of the disease. Additionally, while vitamin C and echinacea may help reduce cold symptoms and the length of the cold, there has not been extensive evidence as to their helpfulness in preventing or getting rid of a cold. Antibiotics are not effective against rhinoviruses. Preventive measures are the best methods for reducing infection rate, including breast-feeding of infants and frequent handwashing. Increased vitamin D levels may also be associated with a lowered risk of infection.

Studies conducted on the use of zinc lozenges as a treatment for the common cold have produced mixed results. In test tubes, positively charged zinc inhibits processing of viral proteins by several different mechanisms. One analysis of previous studies suggested that differences in effectiveness of zinc lozenges could be explained by the ligand or ligands bound to the zinc. Zinc lozenges with only one ligand, such as zinc acetate or zinc gluconate lozenges, were observed to be more effective in reducing cold duration than were zinc lozenges with more ligands, though even they were not effective in all studies. The ineffectiveness of intranasal zinc application was hypothesized to result from an electrical potential difference of 60 to 120 millivolts between the nose and mouth, which results in repulsion of charged particles such as ionized zinc.

There are ninety-nine known serotypes of rhinoviruses. This variety of cell surface antigens makes the development of a vaccine that is effective against multiple rhinoviruses difficult. In the first decade of the twenty-first century, a region of a rhinoviral protein called VP4 was shown to be very common between the different serotypes. Future efforts to synthesize a vaccine may focus on this common element.

PERSPECTIVE AND PROSPECTS

The common cold has been known for millenia and was first given this name in the sixteenth century. Evidence exists across cultures demonstrating knowledge of the cold, extending as back as far as ancient Egypt. In the eighteenth century, Benjamin Franklin's *Definition of a Cold* (1773) demonstrated insightful speculation about the airborne nature of cold transmission and suggested methods for preventing the disease.

The Rhinovirus was first isolated in 1956 and during successive decades was identified as the virus best associated with the common cold. As technology improved, so did detection and identification of different viruses that could be responsible for the common cold. Simple culturing methods gave way to reverse transcriptase polymerase chain reaction (RT-PCR) assays, which were more sensitive in detecting and characterizing specific rhinoviruses. In various campaigns to find a treatment for the common cold, antiviral drugs and interferon have been shown to be effective in protecting against rhinoviruses, though attempts to translate these results into a treatment have not been successful.

The Common Cold Research Unit (CCRU), originally established in Great Britain at the outset of World War II as the Harvard Hospital, operated from 1946 to 1989 and was devoted to researching the causes of the common cold as well as possible treatments for the disease. It was there that coronaviruses, which can also be responsible for causing the common cold, were first isolated in 1965.

—*Andrew J. Reinhart, MS*

See also Antihistamines; Bronchitis; Common cold; Coughing; Decongestants; Nasopharyngeal disorders; Noroviruses; Otorhinolarnygology; Pneumonia; Rhinitis; Sinusitis; Sneezing; Sore throat; Viral infections.

For Further Information:
Carson-DeWitt, Rosalyn, and Brian Randall. "Common Cold." *Health Library*, Jan. 9, 2013.
"Common Cold." *MedlinePlus*, Apr. 23, 2013.
"Common Colds: Protect Yourself and Others." *Centers for Disease Control and Prevention*, Mar. 11, 2013.
Eccles, Ronald, and Olaf Weber, eds. *Common Cold.* Birkhäuser Advances in Infectious Diseases. Basel, Switzerland: Birkhäuser Basel, 2009.
"Rhinovirus Infections." *HealthyChildren.org*. American Academy of Pediatrics, May 11, 2013.

Tyrrell, David, and Michael Fielder, *Cold Wars: The Fight Against the Common Cold*. New York: Oxford University Press, 2002.

Yin-Murphy, Marguerite, and Jeffrey W. Almond. "Picornaviruses-Classification and Antigenic Types." In *Medical Microbiology*, edited by Samuel Baron. Galveston: University of Texas Medical Branch, 1996.

RICKETS

Category: Disease/Disorder
Anatomy or system affected: Bones, musculoskeletal system, teeth
Specialties and related fields: Nutrition, orthopedics, osteopathic medicine, pediatrics
Definition: A disorder involving the softening and weakening of a child's bones, primarily caused by lack of vitamin D and/or lack of calcium or phosphate.

CAUSES AND SYMPTOMS

Rickets is a relatively rare bone disease that most frequently afflicts children. It is the result of insufficient or inefficient absorption of vitamin D in the body, which causes a progressive softening and weakening of the bone. Certain physical conditions can reduce digestion or absorption of fats and may also diminish vitamin D absorption by the intestines. The loss of calcium and phosphate from the bone eventually causes destruction of the supportive bone matrix. In adult deficiency, demineralization (osteomalacia) may occur in the spine, pelvis, and lower extremities, causing osteoporosis (an adult disorder causing brittle bones).

Symptoms of rickets may include pain or tenderness of the long bones and pelvis, skeletal deformities such as bowlegs, bumps in the rib cage (rachitic rosary), spinal and pelvic deformities (including kyphosis or scoliosis), pigeon breast, an asymmetrical or

Bowed legs is a sign of a skeletal deformation that is a classic effect of rickets. ©EBSCO

odd-shaped skull, increased tendency toward fractures, dental deformities and cavities, night fevers, muscle cramps, impaired growth, decreased muscle tone and growth, and general weakness and restlessness.

Hereditary rickets is a sex-linked vitamin D-resistant disorder that occurs when the kidney is unable to retain phosphate. Rickets may also occur in children with liver or biliary disorders, when vitamin D and fats are inadequately absorbed.

TREATMENT AND THERAPY

Uncomplicated infantile rickets can be cured with a daily replacement of deficient calcium, phosphorous, and vitamin D. Clinical testing reveals improvement after one week. Dietary sources of vitamin D include fish, liver, and processed milk. In addition, moderate exposure to sunlight is therapeutic. Skeletal deformities can be corrected with good posture or body braces; in some cases, surgery may be necessary. If rickets is not corrected in children, short stature and skeletal deformities may become permanent.

—John Alan Ross, PhD

INFORMATION ON RICKETS

Causes: Vitamin D, calcium, or phosphate deficiency; hereditary factors
Symptoms: Pain or tenderness in long bones and pelvis, skeletal deformities (bowlegs, bumps in ribcage), spinal and pelvic deformities (scoliosis), odd-shaped skull, increased tendency toward fractures, dental deformities, night fevers, muscle cramps, impaired growth, decreased muscle tone and growth, general weakness
Duration: Short-term to chronic
Treatments: Dietary supplements, moderate exposure to sunlight

See also Bone disorders; Bones and the skeleton; Bowlegs; Fracture and dislocation; Growth; Lower extremities; Malabsorption; Malnutrition; Nutrition; Orthopedics; Orthopedics, pediatric; Osteonecrosis; Osteoporosis; Scoliosis; Spinal cord disorders; Spine, vertebrae, and disks; Vitamins and minerals.

For Further Information:

Alan, Rick, and Michael Woods. "Rickets." *Health Library*, Feb. 25, 2013.

Ballard, Carol. *Bones*. Rev. ed. Chicago: Heinemann Library, 2002.

Bentley, George, and Robert B. Greer, eds. *Orthopaedics*. 4th ed. Oxford, England: Linacre House, 1993.

Currey, John D. *Bones: Structures and Mechanics*. 2d ed. Princeton, N.J.: Princeton University Press, 2006.

"Hereditary Hypophosphatemic Rickets." *Genetics Home Reference*, Sept. 2010.

Icon Health. *Rickets: A Medical Dictionary, Bibliography, and Annotated Research Guide to Internet References*. San Diego, Calif.: Author, 2004.

Kaneshiro, Neil K., and David Zieve. "Rickets." *MedlinePlus*, Aug. 1, 2012.

"Rickets." *MedlinePlus*, June 29, 2012.

Tortora, Gerard J., and Bryan Derrickson. *Principles of Anatomy and Physiology*. 13th ed. Hoboken, N.J.: John Wiley & Sons, 2012.

Wenger, Dennis R., and Mercer Rang. *The Art and Practice of Children's Orthopaedics*. New York: Raven Press, 1993.

RINGWORM

Category: Disease/Disorder
Also known as: Tinea
Anatomy or system affected: Skin
Specialties and related fields: Dermatology, family medicine
Definition: A group of fungal diseases caused by several species of dermatophytes and characterized by itching, scaling, and sometimes painful lesions.

CAUSES AND SYMPTOMS

Ringworm is a skin disease characterized by itching and redness. Despite its name, it is caused by a fungal infection, not a worm. The skin in areas affected with ringworm often contains round lesions that are colored red, have scaly borders, and contain normal-appearing skin in their centers. Alternatively, the lesions can simply be scaly, red patches with no clearly defined shape. Typically, these lesions are relatively small, approximately 1 inch in their largest dimension. Complications of ringworm include spread to the scalp, hair, or nails of the fingers or toes.

The lesions of ringworm are caused by species of fungi that are members of the genus *Trichophyton*. The most common pathogen is *Trichophyton rubrum*. Ringworm appears on exposed areas of the body, often on the face and arms. Cats are the most common means

INFORMATION ON RINGWORM

Causes: Fungal infection
Symptoms: Itching, scaling, sometimes painful lesions
Duration: Approximately one month
Treatments: Topical skin creams, antifungal medications

of transmitting the *Trichophyton* pathogen from one person to another.

Examination of scrapings from skin lesions is used to diagnose ringworm. Species of *Trichophyton* can be tentatively identified by their microscopic structure. Culturing material from a skin lesion provides a definitive diagnosis.

TREATMENT AND THERAPY

The treatment of ringworm involves both the patient and any carriers. The patient can be treated effectively with any of several creams applied to the skin that are available without a prescription. Their use should be continued for one to two weeks after the skin lesions have cleared. Other drugs are available but require a physician's prescription. They are used for more extensive lesions or when fingernails or toenails are involved. Body ringworm usually responds within four weeks of treatment. The carrier should be identified and treated. Avoiding contact with infected household pets or clothing that has been worn by an infected person can prevent ringworm.

PERSPECTIVE AND PROSPECTS

Tinea species cause infections in other parts of the body: tinea capitis on the scalp, tinea pedis on the feet, and tinea cruris in the groin region. Ringworm must be differentiated from several other diseases that also cause round skin lesions: psoriasis, syphilis, pityriasis rosea, and systemic lupus erythematosus. The lesions of psoriasis usually appear on the elbow, knees, and scalp. Syphilis lesions usually appear on the mucous membranes of the genitals or on the palms of the hands or soles of the feet. Although pityriasis rosea often begins with a single round lesion, many more usually follow. The classic skin lesion of lupus is butterfly-shaped and covers the nose and cheeks. The presence of a cat or other domestic pet is often an important element in establishing a diagnosis of ringworm.

—*L. Fleming Fallon, Jr., MD, PhD, MPH*

See also Athlete's foot; Dermatology; Dermatology, pediatric; Fungal infections; Itching; Pityriasis rosea; Psoriasis; Rashes; Skin; Skin disorders; Syphilis; Systemic lupus erythematosus (SLE); Zoonoses.

For Further Information:
Badash, Michelle. "Ringworm." *Health Library*, September 10, 2012.
Berman, Kevin. "Ringworm." *MedlinePlus*, May 24, 2011.
Burns, Tony, et al., eds. *Rook's Textbook of Dermatology*. 8th ed. 4 vols. Hoboken, N.J.: Wiley-Blackwell, 2010.
Goldsmith, Lowell A., Gerald S. Lazarus, and Michael D. Tharp. *Adult and Pediatric Dermatology: A Color Guide to Diagnosis and Treatment*. Philadelphia: F. A. Davis, 1997.
Lamberg, Lynne. *Skin Disorders*. Philadelphia: Chelsea House, 2001.
Mackie, Rona M. *Clinical Dermatology*. 5th ed. New York: Oxford University Press, 2003.
MedlinePlus. "Tinea Infections." *MedlinePlus*, April 11, 2013.
Middlemiss, Prisca. *What's That Rash? How to Identify and Treat Childhood Rashes*. London: Hamlyn, 2002.
Turkington, Carol, and Jeffrey S. Dover. *The Encyclopedia of Skin and Skin Disorders*. 3d ed. New York: Facts On File, 2007.
Weedon, David and Geoffrey Strutton. *Weedon's Skin Pathology*. 3d ed. repr. New York: Churchill Livingstone/Elsevier, 2011.

ROCKY MOUNTAIN SPOTTED FEVER

Category: Disease/Disorder
Anatomy or system affected: Blood vessels, brain, circulatory system, kidneys, nervous system, skin
Specialties and related fields: Dermatology, emergency medicine, epidemiology, family medicine, internal medicine
Definition: An acute febrile illness caused by *Rickettsia rickettsii*.

CAUSES AND SYMPTOMS

In 1906, a young Ohio-born physician, Howard Taylor Ricketts, went to Montana to study the cause of "spotted fever." Through his efforts, Rocky Mountain spotted fever became the first tickborne infection to be recognized in North America. For the first half of the twentieth century, the disease was found mostly in the western United States, but since then the majority of the cases have been in the south Atlantic and south-central states. *Dermacentor andersoni* (Rocky Mountain wood tick) and *D. variabilis* (American dog tick) have been the two dominant tick species serving as vectors in the west and south, respectively.

Following the bite of an infected tick, rickettsia are transmitted through the skin into the lymphatic system and small blood vessels. Once in the bloodstream, they invade endothelial cells. The rickettsia multiply intracellularly by binary fission and spread to adjacent endothelial cells, injuring and killing their cellular hosts, which results in widespread vascular damage.

The incubation period or time from tick bite to illness is usually about seven days. The illness begins

> **INFORMATION ON**
> **ROCKY MOUNTAIN SPOTTED FEVER**
> **Causes:** Bite of infected tick
> **Symptoms:** Fever, headache, myalgias, characteristic rash, shock, abdominal pain, neurological problems
> **Duration:** Incubation period of about seven days
> **Treatments:** Antibiotic (doxycycline); preventive measures (light-colored clothing, insecticides and repellants, careful removal of ticks)

with fever, often greater than 102 degrees Fahrenheit, accompanied by headache and myalgias (muscle pain). The classic rash usually begins on the third day, starting on the wrists and ankles and spreading to the trunk. The palms and soles are often involved. The rash begins as small blanching macules and progresses to petechiae. Shock, abdominal pain, and neurological problems may mimic other diseases, making the correct diagnosis more difficult. Specific laboratory confirmation can be obtained by measuring antibodies two to three weeks later.

TREATMENT AND THERAPY

Doxycycline, a tetracycline antibiotic, is the treatment of choice for both children and adults. Therapy with doxycycline should be started immediately if Rocky Mountain spotted fever is suspected, as delays in therapy are associated with poor outcomes. Prevention can be accomplished by measures to prevent tick bites, such as wearing light-colored clothing and using insecticides and repellants on clothing and skin. Careful removal of ticks from individuals and their dogs before injection of rickettsia can occur will also prevent the disease.

PERSPECTIVE AND PROSPECTS

Rocky Mountain spotted fever is spreading into new geographic locations with the acquisition of new tick vectors. It is also no longer a rural disease and has been found in urban parks. Prompt treatment with doxycycline has reduced the mortality rate from more than 80 percent in the pre-antibiotic era to less than 1 percent. Early diagnostic tests are lacking but are needed, as the majority of Rocky Mountain spotted fever cases are incorrectly diagnosed upon the first visit to a doctor. Thus far, researchers have been unable to develop a protective vaccine.

—*H. Bradford Hawley, MD*

See also Antibiotics; Bacterial infections; Bacteriology; Lice, mites, and ticks; Lyme disease; Plague; Rashes; Shigellosis; Tularemia; Typhus.

For Further Information:

Badash, Michelle, and Michael K. Mansour. "Rocky Mountain Spotted Fever." *Health Library*, May 20, 2013.

Chen, Luke F., and Daniel J. Sexton. "What's New in Rocky Mountain Spotted Fever?" *Infectious Disease Clinics of North America* 22 (2008): 415-432.

Dugdale, David C. III, Jatin M. Vyas, and David Zieve." Rocky Mountain Spotted Fever." *MedlinePlus*, June 9, 2011.

Margolis, Lynn, and Betsy Palmer Eldridge. "What a Revelation Any Science Is!" *ASM News* 71 (2005): 65-70.

"Rocky Mountain Spotted Fever." *Centers for Disease Control and Prevention*, Apr. 30, 2012.

"Rocky Mountain Spotted Fever." *National Institute of Allergy and Infectious Diseases*, Jan. 28, 2011.

"Tick Bites." *MedlinePlus*, Apr. 29, 2013.

Walker, David H. "*Rickettsia rickettsii* and Other Spotted Fever Group Rickettsiae (Rocky Mountain Spotted Fever and Other Spotted Fevers)." In *Principles and Practice of Infectious Diseases*, edited by Gerald L. Mandell, John F. Bennett, and Raphael Dolin. 7th ed. Philadelphia: Churchill Livingstone/Elsevier, 2009.

ROOT CANAL TREATMENT

Category: Procedure
Anatomy or system affected: Gums, mouth, teeth
Specialties and related fields: Dentistry
Definition: The removal of irreparably damaged tooth pulp and its replacement with inert materials.

INDICATIONS AND PROCEDURES

At the center of every tooth is soft pulp tissue. Among its main components are blood vessels that nourish teeth, sensory nerves, and supportive connective tissue. Tooth fractures or deep dental caries (cavities) irreparably damage this pulp. When this happens, root canal treatment is rendered. All dentists can carry out this procedure, but specialists who limit their practice to such efforts-endodontists- are the most skilled. The symptoms that often require root canal treatment are steady throbbing pain and sensitivity to pressure on or tapping of the tooth. Because pulp disease is associated with bacterial infection, gum abscesses may occur in extreme cases.

Root canal therapy is carried out when upon examination the pulp is found to be irreversibly damaged. A local anesthetic is administered by injection to desensitize the area. The tooth is then opened by drilling an access channel. Then, the pulp is removed from the center and from the tooth root portions-the root canals-that it also fills. Next, the pulp chamber and root canals are cleaned and reshaped by drilling and with specialized endodontic files. Lastly, the canals are filled with inert materials such as gutta-percha (a rubber-like substance), and a temporary filling is put in place. At a later time, when it is clear that the proce-

dure has been successful, a permanent filling or an artificial crown is substituted.

Antibacterial medicine may be directly administered in the tooth itself during the procedure, and antibiotic medication may be prescribed for follow-up care.

USES AND COMPLICATIONS

Root canal therapy prolongs the life of teeth by creating a tooth that retains much of its strength over time. Without pulp, however, the blood supply and support of the tooth are reduced. Hence, teeth that have undergone root canal treatment are likely to become brittle and susceptible to fracture. Other possible risks associated with root canal treatments include recurrent abscess, nerve damage, pain, swelling, and infection; those risks are greater in patients with preexisting systemic conditions such as bleeding disorders, circulatory conditions, or immune system disorders, and those who smoke.

The success of root canal therapy is about 90 percent. Nevertheless, it can produce later complications, including fine, virtually undetectable canal fractures that may allow the entry of bacteria; imperfectly filled canals can have the same result. In such cases, repeated root canal therapy may be needed or the tooth may require extraction. These problems, although relatively uncommon, occur because of the nature of this delicate surgery. For example, it is not possible to view the surgical site directly. Rather, the site is approximated by x-ray pictures taken at each treatment stage.

PERSPECTIVE AND PROSPECTS

Root canal treatment has improved markedly in recent years, and further advances are expected, such as better surgical tools and filling materials and an enhanced ability to evaluate the success of the procedure.

Artificial crown
Cement seal
Filling paste
Points
Gums

Root canal treatment may become necessary when the dental pulp is damaged; the pulp is removed and replaced with artificial material, and a crown is fitted. ©EBSCO

In addition, efforts to preserve and/or regenerate damaged tooth pulp are ongoing.

—Sanford S. Singer, PhD

See also Dental diseases; Dentistry; Endodontic disease; Gum disease; Oral and maxillofacial surgery; Periodontal surgery; Periodontitis; Teeth; Tooth extraction; Toothache.

For Further Information:

A.D.A.M. Medical Encyclopedia. "Root Canal." *MedlinePlus*, February 22, 2012.

Connecticut Consumer Health Information Network. "Your Dental Health: A Guide for Patients and Families." *UConn Health Center*, November 27, 2012.

Chwistek, Marcin, ed. "Root Canal Treatment." *Health Library*, March 15, 2013.

Klatell, Jack, Andrew Kaplan, and Gray Williams, Jr., eds. *The Mount Sinai Medical Center Family Guide to Dental Health*. New York: Macmillan, 1991.

Langlais, Robert P., and Craig S. Miller. *Color Atlas of Common Oral Diseases*. 4th ed. Philadelphia: Lippincott Williams & Wilkins, 2009.

"Myths about Root Canals and Root Canal Pain." *American Association of Endodontists*, 2013.

"Root Canals." *American Association of Endodontists*, 2013.

Smith, Rebecca W. *The Columbia University School of Dental and Oral Surgery's Guide to Family Dental Care*. New York: W. W. Norton, 1997.

Taintor, Jerry F., and Mary Jane Taintor. *The Complete Guide to Better Dental Care*. New York: Checkmark Books, 1999.

Whitworth, John M. *Rational Root Canal Treatment in Practice*. Chicago: Quintessence, 2002.

ROSACEA

Category: Disease/Disorder
Also known as: Acne rosacea, adult acne, rhinophyma
Anatomy or system affected: Nose, skin
Specialties and related fields: Dermatology
Definition: A chronic inflammation and redness of the face that usually affects people between the ages of thirty and fifty; it is more common in women but is more severe in men.

CAUSES AND SYMPTOMS

Guy de Chauliac, a French surgeon, first described rosacea medically in the fourteenth century, attributing the condition to the excessive consumption of alcoholic drinks. It is now known that although alcohol may exacerbate the condition, rosacea can develop in individuals who have never consumed alcohol. While the actual cause is unknown, rosacea is more common in fair-skinned people who flush easily and those whose family members have had the condition.

The most common triggers for this flushing are hot drinks, caffeine, alcohol, spicy foods, cosmetics, stress,

---

INFORMATION ON ROSACEA

Causes: Unknown; worsened by hot drinks, alcohol, spicy foods, stress, sunlight, extreme heat or cold
Symptoms: Facial redness; slight swelling; pimples, pustules, and prominent facial pores on nose, forehead, and chin
Duration: Chronic
Treatments: Oral and topical antibiotics, avoidance of triggers

---

exercise, sunlight, wind exposure, and extreme heat or cold. There is no cure for rosacea, but it can be treated.

Untreated, rosacea may progress from facial redness to slight swelling, pimples, pustules, and prominent facial pores on the nose, mid-forehead, and chin. In some patients, particularly in men, the oil glands enlarge, causing a bulbous, enlarged red nose and puffy cheeks. Thick bumps can develop on the lower half of the nose and nearby cheeks. This stage is known as rhinophyma, a condition made famous by actor W. C. Fields with his red, bulbous nose. Rhinophyma can be extremely disfiguring, and its mistaken association with alcoholism can cause embarrassment and affect self-esteem.

TREATMENT AND THERAPY

Rosacea and rhinophyma cannot be cured, but the symptoms can be lessened or even eliminated. Oral and topical antibiotics and avoidance of triggers are the primary ways in which rosacea is managed. Eyelid washing and prescription medication may be recommended for patients whose eyes are affected.

Rhinophyma is usually treated with surgery. The excess tissue that has developed can be removed with a scalpel or a laser or through electrosurgery.

—Lisa M. Sardinia, PhD

See also Acne; Dermatology; Rashes; Skin; Skin disorders.

For Further Information:

Brownstein, Arlen, and Donna Shoemaker. *Rosacea: Your Self-Help Guide*. Oakland, Calif.: New Harbinger, 2001.

Hall, John C., and Gordon C. Sauer. *Sauer's Manual of Skin Diseases*. 10th ed. Philadelphia: Lippincott Williams & Wilkins, 2010.

Hellwig, Jennifer, and Purvee S. Shah. "Rosacea." *Health Library*, September 10, 2012.

Mackie, Rona M. *Clinical Dermatology*. 5th ed. New York: Oxford University Press, 2003.

Parker, James N., and Philip M. Parker, eds. *The Official Patient's Sourcebook on Acne Rosacea*. San Diego, Calif.: Icon Health, 2002.

Plewig, Gerd, and Albert M. Kligmanerd. *Acne and Rosacea*. 3d rev. ed. New York: Springer, 2000.

"Questions and Answers about Rosacea." *National Institute of Arthritis and Musculoskeletal and Skin Diseases*, October, 2012.

"Rosacea." *American Academy of Dermatology*, 2013.

Rosacea.org. www.rosacea.org.

Turkington, Carol, and Jeffrey S. Dover. *The Encyclopedia of Skin and Skin Disorders*. 3d ed. New York: Facts On File, 2007.

ROSEOLA

Category: Disease/Disorder
Also known as: Roseola infantum, exanthem subitum, sixth disease
Anatomy or system affected: Abdomen, arms, brain, immune system, legs, skin
Specialties and related fields: Family medicine, pediatrics
Definition: A disease characterized by a mild fever and a rash that mostly affects young children.

CAUSES AND SYMPTOMS

Roseola is caused by the human herpesvirus 6, to which most children have been exposed by age four. Immunity passed from mother to fetus usually protects infants from contracting roseola before they are six months old. Although the precise period of time during which patients are contagious is unknown, health professionals have determined that the virus incubates for as many as ten days after exposure. Patients usually are contagious only during the fever phase of roseola.

A child with roseola develops a fever that can reach 106 degrees Fahrenheit and persist for two to five days. The lymph glands in the throat may become swollen, and upper respiratory congestion may occur. Some children appear agitated, while others do not behave in an ill manner and continue normal activities. Lethargy, lack of appetite, and diarrhea may accompany the fever. The fever occasionally causes febrile seizures as the brain reacts to sudden and extreme temperature changes. Approximately 5 to 15 percent of roseola patients experience these convul-

INFORMATION ON ROSEOLA

Causes: Herpesvirus infection
Symptoms: Red or pink rash, high fever, swollen lymph nodes, lethargy, lack of appetite, diarrhea, sometimes febrile seizures
Duration: A few weeks
Treatments: Alleviation of symptoms; may include baths, acetaminophen and ibuprofen, adequate fluid intake, isolation during fever stage

sions, which last several minutes and usually are not harmful.

When the fever ceases, a red or pink rash appears on most patients' bodies and remains for several hours to three days. When pressed, the rash blanches. It does not blister, cause pain, or itch. Occasionally, a roseola patient is feverish and never develops a rash or has a rash without a preceding fever. A rash may appear prematurely during the fever phase or be delayed until after the fever has subsided. Some children infected with roseola never display any symptoms. Rarely, roseola can precede encephalitis and aseptic meningitis.

TREATMENT AND THERAPY

Treatment for roseola consists of methods to soothe symptoms. Pediatricians recommend baths and the use of acetaminophen and ibuprofen, if the child is old enough, to lower the fever. Health professionals also advise patients to drink fluids to prevent dehydration. The patient should be isolated until the fever is gone.

A child who has convulsions should be examined by medical professionals immediately. Patients with dark purple rashes should also be seen by physicians, as should children whose rashes do not blanch when touched or remain more than several days. Blisters and itchy or painful rashes also demand professional attention. Children with roseola who seem unusually sick should also be taken for examination, as should children with prolonged fevers that do not improve with medication and baths.

Most patients recover fully. Although the resulting antibodies are present in most adults, roseola can be reactivated if the immune system is weakened.

PERSPECTIVE AND PROSPECTS

Roseola has been referred to in medical literature since the mid-nineteenth century. Early twentieth century investigators unsuccessfully attempted to identify the disease's pathogen. By 1988, medical professionals determined that the herpesvirus 6 causes roseola. Two strains, A and B, have been identified, with strain B causing most roseola cases in children. The herpesvirus 7 has been linked to cases occurring in older patients.

—*Elizabeth D. Schafer, PhD*

See also Blisters; Childhood infectious diseases; Fever; Herpes; Pediatrics; Rashes; Viral infections.

For Further Information:
Gershon, Anne A., Samuel L. Katz, and Peter J. Hotez, eds. *Krugman's Infectious Diseases of Children*. 11th ed. Philadelphia: Mosby, 2004.

Grossman, Leigh B., ed. *Infection Control in the Child Care Center and Preschool*. 8th ed. Charlottesville, Va.: Silverchair Science, 2012.

Hoekelman, Robert A., ed. *Primary Pediatric Care*. 4th ed. St. Louis, Mo.: Mosby, 2001.

Parker, James N., and Phillip M. Parker. *Roseola: A Medical Dictionary, Bibliography, and Annotated Research Guide to Internet References.* San Diego, Calif.: Icon Health, 2004.
"Roseola." *Health Library*, November 26, 2012.
"Roseola." *MedlinePlus*, August 2, 2011.

ROTATOR CUFF SURGERY

Category: Procedure
Anatomy or system affected: Musculoskeletal system, arms, joints, muscles, tendons
Specialties and related fields: General surgery, orthopedics, rheumatology, sports medicine, physical therapy
Definition: The surgical correction of a muscle and/or tendon tear within the shoulder.

INDICATIONS AND PROCEDURES

The shoulder, considered to be a ball and socket joint, is the most flexible joint in the human body. Because of its structure, the shoulder has a wide range of motion; however, this also predisposes the shoulder to a very high risk of injury. To counter this risk, the shoulder is stabilized by a group of four muscles, collectively known as the rotator cuff: the subscapularis, the supraspinatus, the infraspinatus, and the teres minor.

The signs and symptoms of rotator cuff injuries include point tenderness in the joint around the region of the humeral head deep within the deltoid muscle, pain and stiffness within the shoulder region within a day of participating in activities that involve shoulder movements, and difficulty in producing overhead motions involving the upper arm. Pain often occurs at night because of sleeping positions that put excess pressure on the joint. Occasionally, a clicking noise can be heard emanating from the joint upon movement or the patient may experience a "sticking point" when shoulder movements are attempted. Injuries to the rotator cuff can mimic other common shoulder region problems, including bursitis (inflammation of a bursa, a soft, fluid-filled sac that helps cushion surfaces that glide over one another) and tendinitis (inflammation of a tendon). Injuries to the rotator cuff include impingement and tears.

Impingement occurs when the rotator cuff tendons are pinched because of a narrowing of the space between the acromion (shoulder blade) process and the rotator cuff. This narrowing commonly occurs with aging, but it can also be traumatically induced. Sports that commonly put excess stress on the rotator cuff include baseball, swimming, and tennis. Besides a traumatic injury, chronic impingement of the rotator cuff tendons can cause partial or complete tears. To evaluate the extent of shoulder dysfunction, the physician will conduct a physical examination to determine range of motion and use diagnostic imaging procedures such as x-rays, an arthrogram (an x-ray after a tracer dye has been injected into the shoulder), magnetic resonance imaging (MRI), and ultrasound. Nonsurgical interventions include rest, ice immediately following an injury or heat twenty-four hours afterward, painkillers, anti-inflammatory medications, and physical therapy.

Rotator cuff surgery is usually recommended when there is little improvement in shoulder function or pain reduction after a course of noninvasive therapies. Surgery to correct rotator cuff tears is more successful if the procedure is performed within three months of the date of injury. If the shoulder is surgically treated later there is a complication of the torn tendons retracting away from each other increasing the difficulty of the surgery and decreasing the chances of a satisfactory outcome. Surgery can be a classic open procedure, requiring a 2- to 3-inch incision in the shoulder, or less traumatic arthroscopy, which requires only a small incision, half an inch or less, just large enough to accommodate the instruments and a video camera apparatus. Occasionally, the surgeon will use a combination of the open procedure and arthroscopy. Either general anesthesia, in which the patient is asleep, or local anesthesia, in which the region is "frozen" but the patient is awake, can be used for the procedure. An interscalene block may also be used to remove all sensation from the extremity, but limb sensation returns shortly after surgery. With local anesthesia, a light sedative may also be used to put the patient at ease, but not asleep. Acromioplasty reduces the impingement of the rotator cuff tendons. In this procedure, a portion of the bone underneath the acromion is shaved to give the tendons more room to move and prevent them from becoming pinched. This process is often included in rotator cuff surgical repairs. In rotator cuff repairs, the torn tendons are reattached to the humerus (upper arm bone). The open surgical procedure requires a relatively large incision through the shoulder as well as cutting through the deltoid muscle. Any scar tissue that has formed is removed, and a small ridge is cut into the top of the humerus. Small holes are drilled into the bone, and the tendons are sutured to the bone using these holes as anchors. The surgeon will also correct any other problems encountered, such as removing bone spurs, shaving down the acromion, or freeing up ligaments that may be pressing against the tendons.

During arthroscopic surgery, the majority of these additional procedures are still able to be performed. After the small incision is made into the shoulder, a thin tube is inserted. This tube contains the surgical instruments as well as a video camera that is used to guide the repair procedure. Arthroscopic surgery is becoming more common and is preferred for small to larger tears, as it limits the amount of surgical intervention, reduces surgical risks, and quickens recovery time. If more extensive damage is discovered, then the surgeon may elect to combine the arthroscopic procedure with open surgery. However, arthroscopic tear repair has advanced tremendously, to the point that tears previously thought to be irreparable or too extensive are now being completed with arthroscopy.

USES AND COMPLICATIONS
The varying outcomes from rotator cuff surgery range from almost full recovery to no improvement at all. The degree of recovery is dependent upon the extent of damage to the rotator cuff as well as patient compliance with physical therapy after surgery. If the tendon has been torn for a long time, then it may not be reparable.

As with all surgical procedures, the patient may have an adverse reaction to the anesthesia. This risk is greater if the person is obese or has a cardiovascular, pulmonary, or metabolic condition. Surgical incisions always have the risk of infection, but this risk is minimized with the arthroscopic procedure because of the small incision size and the relatively short operative time (one to two hours). In rare instances, there is also the risk of nerve damage resulting in partial paralysis or temporary numbness at the incision area.

After surgery, the recovering arm will be put in a sling with a small shock-absorbing pillow placed behind the elbow. Extreme care should be taken with shoulder movements for the first three months following surgery. Reaching and lifting objects above the head should be avoided during this period. Passive range of motion exercises, in which the arm is moved by the physical therapist, should be started as soon as possible to prevent scar tissue formation and resultant stiffness. Exercises should be done several times a day so that within two to three weeks, the range of motion (flexibility) of the repaired shoulder should be equivalent to that of the uninjured shoulder. After six weeks, more advanced exercises are recommended to strengthen the rotator cuff as well as the surrounding shoulder muscles. Full recovery and rehabilitation from rotator cuff surgery can take up to a year.

—*Bonita L. Marks, PhD*

See also: Arthritis; Arthroplasty; Arthroscopy; Bones and the skeleton; Bursitis; Joints; Muscle sprains, spasms, and disorders; Muscles; Orthopedic surgery; Orthopedics; Rheumatology; Sports medicine; Tendinitis; Upper extremities.

For Further Information:
Codsi, Michael Howe, Chris R. "Shoulder Conditions: Diagnosis and Treatment Guideline." *Physical Medical and RehabilitationClinics of North America* 2015; 26(3): 467-489. doi:10.1016/j.pmr. 2015.04.007.
Lo, I. K., and S. S. Burkhart. "Current Concepts in Arthroscopic Rotator Cuff Repair." *American Journal of Sports Medicine* 1, no. 2 (2003): 308-324.
Matsen, Frederick A., and Steven B. Lippitt. *Shoulder Surgery: Principles and Procedures*. Philadelphia: W. B. Saunders, 2003.
Pfeiffer, Ronald P., and Brent C. Mangus. *Concepts of Athletic Training*. 6th ed. Sudbury, Mass.: Jones and Bartlett, 2012.
Rockwood, Charles A., Frederick A. Matsen, and Michael Wirth. *The Shoulder*. 4th ed. 2 vols. St. Louis, Mo.: Saunders/Elsevier, 2009.
"Rotator Cuff Repair." *Health Library*, March 18, 2013.
"Rotator Cuff Repair." *MedlinePlus*, June 30, 2011.
Williams, G. R., and M. Kelley. "Management of Rotator Cuff and Impingement Injuries in the Athlete." *Journal of Athletic Training* 35, no. 3 (2000): 300-315.
Yamaguchi, K., et al. "Transitioning to Arthroscopic Rotator Cuff Repair: The Pros and Cons." *Journal of Bone & Joint Surgery, American Volume* 85, no. 1 (2003): 144-156.
Lewis, Sarah, "Rotator Cuff Surgery." *Healthgrades Operating Company, Inc.* 2017 www.healthgrades.com/procedures/rotator-cuff-surgeryAccessed 9-16-2017.
Pile, JC. Evaluating postoperative fever: A focused approach. Cleveland Clinic Journal of Medicine. 2006;73 (Suppl 1):S62. ccjm.org/content/73/Suppl_1/S62.full.pdf,
Rotator Cuff Repair. MedlinePlus, a service of the National Library of Medicine National Institutes of Health. www.nlm.nih. gov/medlineplus/ency/article/007207.htm.
Rotator Cuff Tears. American Academy of Orthopedic Surgeons. orthoinfo.aaos.org/topic.cfm?topic=A00064.
Rotator Cuff Tears: Surgery and Exercise. Cleveland Clinic. my.clevelandclinic.org/disorders/rotator_cuff/hic_rotator_cuff_tears_surgery_and_exercise.asp.
Rotator Cuff Tears: Surgical Treatment Options. American Academy of Orthopedic Surgeons. orthoinfo.aaos.org/topic.cfm? topic=A00406.
Shoulder Problems. National Institute of Arthritis and Musculoskeletal and Skin Diseases. www.niams.nih.gov/Health_Info/Shoulder_Problems/.
Shoulder Surgery. American Academy of Orthopedic Surgeons. orthoinfo.aaos.org/topic.cfm?topic=a00066.

ROTAVIRUS

Category: Disease/Disorder
Also known as: Sporadic or severe viral gastroenteritis, rotaviral enteritis, infantile diarrhea, winter diarrhea
Anatomy or system affected: Gastrointestinal system
Specialties and related fields: Epidemiology, gastroenterology, pediatrics, virology
Definition: A virus with a characteristic wheel-like appearance when viewed under an electronic microscope that causes viral gastroenteritis in children worldwide.

CAUSES AND SYMPTOMS

Rotavirus is classified into groups A through G, with group A responsible for gastroenteritis in children. Adults can also contract the virus but will experience milder symptoms. The virus is very contagious, with oral-fecal transmission occurring through ingestion of contaminated water or food or contact with an infected surface such as a toy or hand. Airborne infection is rare. In temperate climates, the disease occurs more often in the cooler months, from late autumn to early spring, with year-round infection present in tropical climates. Almost all children have been infected more than once by the time they are four years old.

Symptoms are manifested after two days from the initial exposure and include severe watery diarrhea, vomiting, nausea, and fever, with the gastroenteritis lasting from three to ten days. Dehydration may result if fluids are not adequately replenished. Symptoms of severe dehydration include dry mouth, dry skin, sunken eyes, no tears when crying, lethargy, irritability, and reduced or no wet diapers over three hours. A physician should be notified if symptoms of severe dehydration are observed. Because the virus is highly contagious, epidemic outbreaks may be seen in child-care centers.

TREATMENT AND THERAPY

Clinical diagnosis is made from detection of the virus antigen in a stool sample. Detection of rotavirus is also possible with an electron microscope or tissue culture. Treatment involves drinking plenty of fluids to prevent dehydration. Antidiarrheal medication should not be given to children unless prescribed by a doctor. Hospitalization may be required for intravenous (IV) fluid rehydration if severe dehydration occurs. Immunity develops after repeat infections, with subsequent infections exhibiting less severe symptoms. The virus may survive on hard surfaces for years. Diligent hand washing and disinfection of surfaces with a diluted bleach solution or 70 percent alcohol may help slow the spread of the virus.

INFORMATION ON ROTAVIRUS

Causes: Viral infection transmitted through contaminated food or water, fecal-oral contamination, or contact with contaminated surface

Symptoms: Severe watery diarrhea, vomiting, nausea, fever

Duration: Three to ten days

Treatments: Fluids to prevent dehydration, prevention through handwashing and disinfection of surfaces

---

PERSPECTIVE AND PROSPECTS

Rotavirus was discovered in 1973 from intestinal biopsies of children diagnosed with winter vomiting disease. The name is derived from the Latin word *rota*, which means "wheel." In February, 2006, the U.S. Food and Drug Administration (FDA) approved a live, oral vaccine for use in children. In 2009, the World Health Organization, which estimates that rotavirus kills about 527,000 people annually, recommended that the vaccine be made a routine part of national immunization programs around the world.

—*Susan E. Thomas, MLS*

See also Childhood infectious diseases; Dehydration; Diarrhea and dysentery; Food poisoning; Gastroenteritis; Gastroenterology; Gastroenterology, pediatric; Gastrointestinal disorders; Gastrointestinal system; Intestinal disorders; Intestines; Nausea and vomiting; Noroviruses; Pediatrics; Viral infections.

For Further Information:

Aronson, Susan S., and Timothy R. Shope, eds. *Managing Infectious Diseases in Child Care and Schools: A Quick Reference Guide*. Elk Grove Village, Ill.: American Academy of Pediatrics, 2005.

Kohnle, Diana. "Rotavirus." *Health Library*, February 20, 2013.

"Rotavirus." *Centers for Disease Control and Prevention*, October 28, 2010.

"Rotavirus." *Mayo Clinic*, March 27, 2013.

"Rotavirus." *World Health Organization*, October, 2011.

Heymann, David L., ed. *Control of Communicable Diseases Manual*. 19th ed. Washington, DC: American Public Health Association, 2008.

Matson, David O. "Rotaviruses." In *Principles and Practice of Pediatric Infectious Diseases*, edited by Sarah S. Long, Larry K. Pickering, and Charles G. Prober. 3d ed. Philadelphia: Churchill Livingstone/Elsevier, 2008.

ROUNDWORMS

Category: Disease/Disorder

Anatomy or system affected: Blood vessels, circulatory system, gastrointestinal system, intestines, lungs, lymphatic system

Specialties and related fields: Environmental health, epidemiology, public health

Definition: Worm-shaped animals that act as parasites of plants and animals.

Key terms:

cuticle: the protective noncellular outer covering of an animal

intermediate host: an animal or plant in which nonadult life stages of endoparasites occur

primary host: an organism in which adult endoparasites are found and can reproduce

CAUSES AND SYMPTOMS

Roundworms are tube-shaped animals in the phylum Nemotoda. They are a highly diverse group, numbering twelve thousand named species, but some taxonomists suggest that fifty thousand more species have yet to be discovered and named. Roundworms occur from the tropics to the tundra and are found in virtually all habitats. Most are free-living animals, but some are parasites of plants and animals. At least fifty are important internal parasites of humans.

Structurally and organizationally, roundworms are very simple animals; most are composed of fewer than one thousand cells. The circular, long body of a roundworm is covered by a tough, protective cuticle. Inside is a tubular digestive tract and simplified nervous system. Its reproductive system is capable of producing enormous numbers of eggs.

Ascaris lumbricoides is a common intestinal parasite of humans and also one of the largest of the nematodes, with a length of 30 centimeters or more. A female can produce two hundred thousand eggs per day for several months, which are secreted into intestinal fluids and voided with the feces. If the eggs are ingested, then they pass through the stomach and into the digestive system and hatch in the intestines. The juveniles burrow through the intestinal wall and are carried via the circulatory system to the lungs. They are reswallowed and returned to the intestines via the esophagus, where they mature. Large numbers of juveniles in the lungs can produce a severe pneumonia, while heavy infestations of adults can cause malnutrition and intestinal blockages.

More than half a billion people in tropical regions may be infected by hookworms, which feed on the blood contents of the gut rather than intestinal fluids. Hookworm life cycles differ from that of *Ascaris lumbricoides*, in that eggs hatch on the ground and juveniles burrow into the skin of the feet or hands and are carried via the blood to the lungs. From the lungs, the juveniles migrate to the pharynx and are then carried to the intestines, where they cause serious blood and tissue damage including anemia and malnutrition.

Pinworms are the most common of the parasitic roundworms. Infection by the human pinworm, *Enterobius vermicularis*, occurs when a female pinworm deposits its eggs at night in the perianal region, causing irritation. Scratching lodges eggs under the fingernails which, if put in the mouth, cause infection or reinfection.

A number of roundworm parasites have an intermediate host in their life cycle. For example, *Trichinella spiralis*, the trichina worm, which causes trichinosis in humans, has two hosts in its life cycle; humans are the primary hosts, while pigs are the intermediate hosts. Juveniles lodge in the muscle tissue of pigs as calcified

---

> ### INFORMATION ON ROUNDWORMS
>
> **Causes:** Parasitic infection transmitted through skin exposure or ingestion
> **Symptoms:** Depends on type; may include severe pneumonia, malnutrition, intestinal blockages, anemia, itching, elephantiasis, severe pain, and sometimes death
> **Duration:** Often chronic
> **Treatments:** Species-specific drugs

---

cysts. If contaminated meat is ingested by humans, then the juveniles hatch and migrate into the intestines. Infection with trichina worms produces severe pain and sometimes death as juveniles and adults burrow through body tissues.

The most spectacular of the roundworm parasites is the dracunculoid guinea worm (*Dracunculus medinensis*), which lives in connective tissue and may reach 2 to 3 feet in length. A female discharges its eggs directly into standing water through an ulcerated sore in a human's skin, often on the feet. The larvae are eaten by freshwater copepods (water fleas) called *Cyclops* and embed in their tissues. Larvae gain entry to humans when a human drinks water containing the nearly microscopic *Cyclops*, thus beginning the life cycle again.

The filaroid roundworm parasites such as *Wuchereria bancrofti* of Africa and Asia are spread by means of a blood-feeding arthropod vector. All eight species of filaroids live in lymph nodes and associated ducts and feed on lymph. The female produces larvae, called microfilariae, which are carried to the skin via the circulatory system. Blood-feeding insects suck up blood containing the larvae, which are injected into another person during the next blood meal. Heavy infestations of male and female worms block the lymph vessels, which enlarge to produce the condition called elephantiasis.

TREATMENT AND THERAPY

Parasitic roundworm infection continues to be a global medical health problem of great concern, especially in the warmer regions of the world. Modern medicine has greatly reduced the pathologies associated with heavy parasitic infections, which can be detected by blood or stool samples, and treatment with species-specific drugs can very effectively eliminate most species. The best prevention method remains adequate sanitation and access to clean water.

—Dwight G. Smith, PhD

See also Elephantiasis; Insect-borne diseases; Intestinal disorders; Intestines; Parasitic diseases; Pinworms; Trichinosis; Tropical medicine; Worms; Zoonoses.

For Further Information:
"Parasites." *Centers for Disease Control and Prevention*, April 19, 2013.
"Parasitic Roundworm Diseases." *National Institute of Allergy and Infectious Diseases*, June 10, 2011.
Parker, Philip M., and James N. Parker. *Roundworms: A Medical Dictionary, Bibliography, and Annotated Research Guide to Internet References*. San Diego, Calif.: Icon Health, 2004.
Roberts, Larry S., and John Janovy, Jr., eds. *Gerald D. Schmidt and Larry S. Roberts' Foundations of Parasitology*. 8th ed. Boston: McGraw-Hill Higher Education, 2010.
Ruppert, Edward E., Richard S. Fox, and Robert D. Barnes. *Invertebrate Zoology: A Functional Evolutionary Approach*. 7th ed. Belmont, Calif.: Thomson-Brooks/Cole, 2004.

RUBELLA

Category: Disease/Disorder
Also known as: German measles
Anatomy or system affected: Joints, lymphatic system, nervous system, skin
Specialties and related fields: Family medicine, pediatrics
Definition: An acute, contagious childhood disease caused by a virus and characterized by a rash.
Key terms:
arthralgia: pain in a joint or joints
arthritis: inflammation of a joint or joints
congenital: present at birth; having to do with a fetus carried by a pregnant woman

CAUSES AND SYMPTOMS

Rubella can be either acquired, infecting both children and adults, or congenital, infecting a fetus before birth. Acquired rubella is typically a mild disease with few complications. The incubation period is usually sixteen to eighteen days, but it can last fourteen to twenty-one days. For children, the first symptom is typically a rash that is small, red, and spotty. It starts on the face and behind the ears and spreads downward in the next one or two days. This rash is much milder than the rash of measles. In adults, the rash is preceded by symptoms that include a low-grade fever, headache, loss of appetite, mildly red eyes, a stuffy nose, a sore throat, coughing, and lymph node enlargement in the neck. Typically, this enlargement occurs behind the ears and in the back of the neck.

Complications of rubella are more common in adults, particularly in young women. The most common complications are arthralgia and arthritis. These joint manifestations can occur in any time from when the rash subsides to several weeks later. Rarer complications include effects on the blood, the heart, and the nervous system.

INFORMATION ON RUBELLA

Causes: Viral infection, congenital transmission
Symptoms: Small, red, and spotty rash; low-grade fever; headache; appetite loss; mildly red eyes; stuffy nose; sore throat; coughing; lymph node enlargement in neck
Duration: Acute
Treatments: Alleviation of symptoms

Congenital rubella is associated with multiple birth defects in the infant. The most common manifestations of congenital rubella affect three areas: growth, the blood, and the central nervous system. The effects on growth include prematurity and intrauterine growth retardation. The effects on the blood include thrombocytopenia (a decrease in platelets), anemia, and an enlarged liver and spleen. The effects on the central nervous system include microcephaly (a small head), deafness, eye damage (including cataracts and retinal damage), intellectual disabilities, and behavioral disorders. Whether these effects of congenital rubella are manifested depends on the timing of the infection during pregnancy and the severity of the infection. Some newborns may appear normal at delivery and develop manifestations during their first five years of life.

The diagnosis of acquired rubella primarily hangs on the clinical symptoms, such as a rash and lymph node enlargement in the back of the neck. The diagnosis of congenital rubella may be confused with other congenital or perinatal infections, such as syphilis, toxoplasmosis, herpes simplex, and cytomegalovirus (CMV). These congenital infections can all lead to intrauterine growth retardation, deafness, intellectual disabilities, and thrombocytopenia.

TREATMENT AND THERAPY

Infants with congenital rubella must be viewed as having a continually evolving disease, since there is no present method to stop or decrease the replication of the rubella virus in the infected newborn. No antiviral medications or antibody preparations have been found to be of therapeutic benefit in children with congenital rubella. Thus, therapy is supportive and requires a multidisciplinary approach. Hearing disabilities require testing, which involves special equipment for infants. If hearing loss is found, support for the child's language and communication development must take place; specially designed educational programs are available. A full eye examination should be performed by an ophthalmologist.

Acquired rubella infection is fairly benign, and its management usually involves allowing the virus to run its course. Since the greatest damage done by rubella virus is to a developing fetus, the management of rubella should focus on prevention of infection in women of childbearing age. Because acquired rubella infection is commonly asymptomatic or subclinical, the only adequate way to prevent this disease and its effects on the fetus is immunization.

A vaccine is available and has been shown to produce an excellent immune response. Two doses of rubella vaccine are recommended, given as the combined vaccine known as measles, mumps, and rubella (MMR). The first dose is given to a child at twelve to fifteen months of age. The second dose should be given prior to the child's entry into school. The vaccine should also be given to adult women who have not received the vaccine previously.

Although it is not recommended that the vaccine be given to pregnant women because of the theoretical risk of inducing congenital rubella, no infants whose mothers were vaccinated during pregnancy have shown congenital defects. Rubella vaccine should not be given after the administration of antibody preparations. The vaccine also should not be given to immunosuppressed patients unless recommended by a doctor. The side effects of the vaccine, occurring in about 10 percent of children, include fever, a rash, and lymph node enlargement. Adult women are prone to developing arthralgia after receiving the rubella vaccine. Other, very rare complications of the vaccine have also occurred.

PERSPECTIVE AND PROSPECTS

Since the introduction of the rubella vaccine in the United States in 1969, rubella and the associated congenital rubella syndrome have been virtually eliminated from the Western Hemisphere, signaling the success of the Unites States' immunization program. Nearly 58,000 cases of rubella were reported in the United States in 1969; by 1999 that number had fallen to 272; no endemic case of rubella has been reported in the Americas since 2009. However, rubella continues to be a health problem in developing countries in other parts of the world, with the World Health Organization reporting an estimated 110,000 babies born each year with congenital rubella syndrome.

—Peter D. Reuman, MD, MPH

See also Birth defects; Cataracts; Childhood infectious diseases; Congenital disorders; Eyes; Fever; Hearing loss; Immunization and vaccination; Intellectual disability; Joints; Measles; Mumps; Rashes; Viral infections; Vision disorders.

For Further Information:

Beers, Mark H., et al., eds. *The Merck Manual of Diagnosis and Therapy.* 18th ed. Whitehouse Station, N.J.: Merck Research Laboratories, 2006.

Behrman, Richard E., Robert M. Kliegman, and Hal B. Jenson, eds. *Nelson Textbook of Pediatrics.* 19th ed. Philadelphia: Saunders/Elsevier, 2011.

Bellenir, Karen, and Peter D. Dresser, eds. *Contagious and Noncontagious Infectious Diseases Sourcebook.* Detroit, Mich.: Omnigraphics, 1996.

Carson-DeWitt, Rosalyn. "Rubella." *Health Library,* September 27, 2012.

Martin, Richard J., Avroy A. Fanaroff, and Michele C. Walsh, eds. *Fanaroff and Martin's Neonatal-Perinatal Medicine: Diseases of the Fetus and Infant.* 2 vols. 9th ed. Philadelphia: Mosby/Elsevier, 2011.

Middlemiss, Prisca. *What's That Rash? How to Identify and Treat Childhood Rashes.* London: Hamlyn, 2002.

"Rubella." *World Health Organization,* July, 2012.

Shaw, Michael, ed. *Everything You Need to Know About Diseases.* Springhouse, Pa.: Springhouse Press, 1996.

Woolf, Alan D., et al., eds. *The Children's Hospital Guide to Your Child's Health and Development.* Cambridge, Mass.: Perseus, 2002.

RUBINSTEIN-TAYBI SYNDROME

Category: Disease/Disorder
Also known as: Broad thumb-hallux syndrome
Anatomy or system affected: Bones, ears, eyes, feet, genitals, hands, head, heart, mouth, nose, teeth
Specialties and related fields: Cardiology, dentistry, genetics, neurology, ophthalmology, orthopedics, pediatrics, speech pathology
Definition: A syndrome typically characterized by small skeletal stature, intellectual disability, and large thumbs and toes.

CAUSES AND SYMPTOMS

Medical investigators have linked Rubinstein-Taybi syndrome to a mutation of the CREB-binding protein (CREBBP) gene on chromosome 16. Studies estimate

---

INFORMATION ON RUBINSTEIN-TAYBI SYNDROME

Causes: Genetic mutation
Symptoms: Intellectual disabilities, poor motor skill development, small body size, small head, large thumbs and big toes, long nose, tiny mouth, wide-set eyes with sagging eyelids; misshapen ears; bunched teeth; undescended testicles; excessive body hair
Duration: Lifelong
Treatments: Physical, behavioral, and occupational therapies; surgical correction of knees, testicles, eyes, teeth; medications or surgeries for various complications; antibiotics for related infections; institutionalization and constant monitoring

an occurrence rate ranging from 1 to 3 cases per 100,000 people, with a higher incidence in institutions. The syndrome hinders physical and intellectual development. Patients are intellectually disabled, and they do not develop motor skills at normal rates.

Body size, particularly of the head, is much smaller than that attained by typical children because growth is stunted. Most patients have thumbs and/or big toes that are unusually large and have flat tips. Sometimes, the big toes are separated from the smaller toes, which are grouped closely together.

A patient's face often bears distinctive characteristics, including a long nose, a tiny mouth, and far-apart eyes with sagging eyelids and extended eyelashes. The patient sometimes squints. The ears are frequently misshapen. Inside the mouth, the teeth are bunched together on steep palates. In males, the testes usually do not descend. Both genders often grow more body hair than do normal children.

TREATMENT AND THERAPY

Medical care for Rubinstein-Taybi syndrome includes various physical, behavioral, and occupational therapies to treat specific problems. Speech therapy helps patients learn to communicate. Corrective shoes or surgery may be necessary to aid walking if toe size and placement interfere with movement. The knees and testicles may also require surgical adjustment. Eye surgery may be necessary if eyeglasses do not resolve vision flaws. Dentistry corrects faulty bites.

Patients sometimes suffer seizures, brain tumors, and heart, lung, or digestive complications and require appropriate medications or surgeries. Antibiotics mitigate urinary tract infections, ear infections, and kidney problems related to this syndrome. Patients are vulnerable to heart or breathing problems while anesthetized. Many require institutional- ization and constant monitoring because they experience sleeping and eating difficulties. Individuals with this syndrome can attain average life spans if they do not suffer serious physical problems or infections.

PERSPECTIVE AND PROSPECTS

Greek physicians J. Michail, J. Matsoukas, and S. Theodorou reported a case in 1957 of a child with the traits of this syndrome. Unaware of that publication, in the late 1950s Jack H. Rubinstein and Hooshang Taybi observed distinctive characteristics in seven patients. Taybi delivered their joint paper at the 1962 Society for Pediatric Radiology meeting. The next year, they published a 1963 article outlining this syndrome. In the early twenty-first century, medical researchers continued genetic investigations for this syndrome.

—Elizabeth D. Schafer, PhD

See also Birth defects; Congenital disorders; Embryology; Genetic diseases; Intellectual disability; Neonatology; Pediatrics.

For Further Information:
Rubinstein-Taybi Syndrome. www.rubinstein-taybi.org.
Rubinstein, Jack H., and Hooshang Taybi. "Broad Thumbs and Toes and Facial Abnormalities: A Possible Mental Retardation Syndrome." *American Journal of Diseases of Children* 105 (1963): 588-608.
"Rubinstein-Taybi Syndrome." *MedlinePlus*, August 4, 2011.
"Rubinstein-Taybi Syndrome; Williams Syndrome." *American Journal of Medical Genetics* Supplement 6. New York: Wiley-Liss, 1990.
Taybi, Hooshang. *Handbook of Syndromes and Metabolic Disorders: Radiologic and Clinical Manifestations*. St. Louis, Mo.: Mosby, 1998.
Wiley, Susan, et al. "Rubinstein-Taybi Syndrome Medical Guidelines." *American Journal of Medical Genetics* 119A, no. 2 (June 1, 2003): 101-110.

S

SAFETY ISSUES FOR CHILDREN

Category: Procedures
Anatomy or system affected: All
Specialties and related fields: Critical care, emergency medicine, family medicine, pediatrics, sports medicine
Definition: Measures taken to prevent accidents among children.

THE IMPORTANCE OF SAFETY MEASURES

Each year in the United States, approximately 1 million children receive medical care as a result of unintentional injury. Of these, about forty thousand to fifty thousand suffer permanent damage and about four thousand die. The first years of a child's life are the most dangerous: Unintentional injuries are the primary cause of death in children up to the age of five.

Cribs can pose serious health threats to babies; the government issued guidelines regarding the dimensions and spacing between slats and prohibited drop-side rail cribs.

Sudden Infant Death Syndrome (SIDS) in apparently normal babies between ages of two weeks and six months has greatly declined since the American Academy of Pediatrics (AAP) in 1992 recommended that babies should be placed on their backs to sleep unless otherwise indicated by their pediatrician. However, in 2011, the AAP expanded the guidelines for infant sleep safety and SIDS risk reduction as sleep-related deaths from other causes (other than sleep position) have increased. The following information for parents on safe sleep environment is from those guidelines:

- Always place your baby on his or her back for every sleep time.
- Always use a firm sleep surface. Car seats and other sitting devices are not recommended for routine sleep.
- The baby should sleep in the same room as the parents, but not in the same bed (room-sharing without bed-sharing).
- Keep soft objects or loose bedding out of the crib. This includes pillows, blankets, and bumper pads.
- Wedges and positioners should not be used.
- Pregnant woman should receive regular prenatal care.
- Don't smoke during pregnancy or after birth.
- Breastfeeding is recommended.
- Offer a pacifier at nap time and bedtime.
- Avoid covering the infant's head or overheating.
- Do not use home monitors or commercial devices marketed to reduce the risk of SIDS.
- Infants should receive all recommended vaccinations.
- Supervised, awake tummy time is recommended daily to facilitate development and minimize the occurrence of positional plagiocephaly (flat heads).

Foresight, common sense, and vigilance are required to prevent injuries to children, particularly those under the age of two, who do not communicate verbally. Between the ages of two and four, although a child has a sense of cause and effect (a boy who kicks a ball knows that it may roll into the street), the child is unable to consider the outside effects (a car could hit him if he runs into the street after the ball).

Basic information in case an emergency occurs should be accessible in all homes with children. The phone number of the family physician, the nearest hospital and emergency service, and the local poison control center should be posted adjacent to the phone. When caregivers are employed, they should be given transportation fare, copies of children's medical cards, the doctor's phone number, and the phone number where the parents can be reached. For optimum communication, parents should travel with a cellular phone. The number of a relative to contact in the event of an emergency occurring to the parents should be included as well.

SAFETY IN THE HOME

All parents should develop a childproofing plan before a newborn arrives and modify it when the baby begins to crawl and walk. Hazards change with age. The Consumer Product Safety Commission urges families to do a room-by-room check of their house. The best way to do this is to put oneself in the place of the child, getting down on one's hands and knees and imagining what would be interesting or constitute an obstacle.

Equipment: Surprisingly, almost as many children are injured or die from using objects designed for their use as from automobile accidents. In the United States, accidents related to playing with toys send 120,000 children to the emergency room annually. Most standards for baby equipment went into effect in the early 1970s, so extra caution must be exercised with equipment manufactured prior to that date.

Baby walkers, which are involved in more than twenty-eight thousand injuries annually, are not approved by the American Academy of Pediatrics. Tripping is the most common cause of injury; it can be prevented by using a walker with at least six wheels and a base wider than the seat height. Walkers can also fall down stairs.

Falls from high chairs send around seven thousand infants to the hospital a year. High chairs should have a safety strap and a wide base to prevent tipping. Cantilevered high chairs that hook to a table are unstable. They should lock to the table and be attached only if the table is strong enough to support them.

Despite standards to ensure safe cribs, up to 30 million potentially dangerous cribs are in use in the United States, and approximately fifty babies suffocate or strangle in cribs annually. Cribs more than twenty-five years old are the most hazardous because the slats are too wide. Moreover, they may have lead-based paint. Even newer cribs with decorative cutouts can trap a baby's head. In addition, corner posts can catch clothing, resulting in strangulation.

The first safety measure is to ensure that crib slats are spaced no more than 2.375 inches apart and that corner posts extend no more than .0625 inch above the railing. Cribs should never be placed next to a wall lamp, electrical outlet, window, radiator, or vent. To prevent the possibility of suffocation, puffy gear such as large stuffed animals, adult pillows, or comforters should not be used in cribs until a child reaches one year of age. Securely fastened bumpers, however, may be used until the baby is able to stand (and thus able to climb on them to exit the crib).

Bunkbeds pose a similar threat as cribs. To safeguard these beds, wooden bars should be added to ensure that any spaces, such as those between the guardrail and the bed frame or cutouts in the headboard and footboard, do not exceed 3 inches.

Portable playpens may have faulty latches that can cause the enclosure to collapse, trapping a child's head in the top rails. Latches on a playpen should click audibly, signifying that they are securely locked. Also, the side of a mesh playpen should never be left lowered, as an infant can be trapped in the slack mesh.

The Consumer Product Safety Commission's hotline provides information about specific models of a child's equipment that are hazardous and repair information from manufacturers.

Windows: Children aged five and younger are most likely to fall from windows because they are mobile but

Cribs can pose serious health threats to babies; the government issues guidelines regarding dimensions and spacing between slats. Photo via iStock/Image Source. [Used under license.]

do not comprehend the danger of an open window. In the United States, about fifteen thousand children aged ten and younger are injured annually from window falls, with three-quarters of the accidents happening in the spring and summer. Surprisingly, the majority of falls occur when children play on furniture adjacent to an open window and topple out as a result of losing their balance, rather than because they leaned against the window.

The following safeguard measures are recommended, and in some U.S. cities required, for any household with young children. All windows from the second floor up must have window guards. Each guard should have a quick-release mechanism for swift exit in case of a fire. Screens do not support a child's weight, so windows should be opened at the top rather than the bottom; if they are opened on the bottom, they should not be wide enough to allow a child to fit through them. Above all, furniture should not be placed under a window. Drapery and blind cords should be secured so that a child is unable to play with them.

Electrical outlets: The most important safety procedure is to cover unused electrical outlets with a safety plug. In wet areas, such as the kitchen or the bathroom, a ground-fault circuit interrupter can be installed in outlets to prevent electrocution if an appliance comes in contact with water. Tempting electrical appliances such as hair dryers should be unplugged and stored out of reach of a child when not in use.

Household furniture: If toddlers are in the house, any standing object such as bookcases, dressers, desks, or a television stand may tip onto a child, who may be tempted to climb on it or any open drawers. To diminish the hazard of household furniture, angle braces or anchors should be used to secure any potentially unstable items, such as bookcases or china hutches, to a wall. Heavy furniture must rest flat on the floor; gliders should be removed. Television sets should be mounted above a child's reach or set far back from the edge on a very low piece of furniture.

Furniture poses many unsuspected threats to safety. For example, bean bag chairs are hazardous because a toddler can unzip the chair, inhale the foam pellets, and suffocate. If such a chair must be in the house, it should have a permanent seam or sealed zipper. Automatic locks on furniture that is big enough to climb into, such as certain types of chests, should be replaced with safety locks.

A recliner is another unsuspected hazard, as openings of 5 inches or more between the footrest and the seat can trap a child's head. Hammocks are dangerous as well if they do not have spreader bars at each end to hold the netting apart to prevent entrapment of a child's limbs or head.

Tablecloths and placemats should not be used, as a child can grab them and spill hot food or heavy items. Drawers within a child's grasp should have automatic safety latches to prevent spilling sharp items such as knives.

Rugs on slippery areas, such as linoleum tile or the bathroom floor, should be stabilized with nonskid backing. Any edge that could cut a child, such as on a table, should be covered with padding; heat-resistant padding is available for hearths. Glass tables should not be used. All breakable items should be kept on high shelves.

Stairs: If young children are in the home, safety gates should be installed at both the top and bottom of the stairs. Stair gates should have a straight top edge and be filled with a rigid mesh screen containing slats less than 4.25 inches apart. According to the Consumer Product Safety Commission, accordion gates made before February, 1985, are unacceptable, as the openings are wide enough to trap a child's head. The V-shaped openings at the gate's top edge should be no more than 1.5 inches wide. All gates should be at least 32 inches high.

Hardware: Mounted gates securely attached to a solid structure, such as a stair post or wall, should be used at the top of the stairs rather than an expanding-pressure gate, which can be dislodged by the weight of a toddler. Gates should be removed as soon as a child attempts to climb over them.

OUTDOOR SAFETY MEASURES

Summer is a fun time for many children, but most parents are unaware that hospital emergency room staff call May through August "the trauma season." Long daylight hours, no school, and more outdoor activities add up to increased opportunity for accidents. Prevention consists of three facets: supervision, education (of both parents and child), and safeguarding.

Playgrounds: Shockingly, more than 200,000 injuries occur annually on playgrounds to children aged fourteen or younger in the United States. While most parents assume that a playground is safe simply because it is designed for children, in truth, there are no mandatory safety standards for this equipment. More than half of playground injuries result from a fall onto a hard surface, including asphalt, concrete, and even grass and dirt. A significantly higher risk for serious injury is associated with a fall of more than 4 feet for preschoolers or more than 8 feet for school-age children. One problem is that most parents are unaware that playground equipment is specifically designed for one of two age groups: two to five years old or five to twelve years old. To address this issue, equipment made after 1994 is supposed to be marked with a sign indicating its intended age group.

To optimize safety on playgrounds, children should use a playground covered with pea gravel, sand, chips, rubber, or a soft synthetic surface. This protective surface should extend at least 6 feet around slides and twice the height of the swings in front and back to create a safety fall zone. Playgrounds should be checked for sharp edges, loose joints, and protruding hardware, such as unclosed "S" hooks. Swings that are not at least 2 feet apart and 2.5 feet lower than the swing support should be avoided. Platforms and ramps are usable only if they have guardrails. Above all, a toddler should play on equipment lower than 4 feet high, while a school-age child should be restricted to structures 8 feet high or lower.

Drowning: Drowning is known as the "silent death" since young children do not scream or splash while drowning. Each year in the United States, one thousand children aged fourteen and younger drown, while four thousand more are treated for near-drowning injuries. Of these, 20 percent end up with permanent neurological damage. More than three hundred children aged four and younger drown in residential pools annually. Accidents in children ages five and older tend to occur in lakes or oceans as well as in pools, and they tend to occur as a result of "horsing around."

The American Red Cross and the National Safe Kids Campaign issued guidelines to optimize safety near water. The most important rule is that a pool should be enclosed with a four-sided fence at least 5 feet high that is filled with vertical bars 3.5 inches apart or less. The gate should be self-locking and self-closing, with the latch out of reach of children.

Parents and caregivers should know cardiopulmonary resuscitation (CPR), and the CPR instructions should be posted near the pool. Basic life-saving equipment, including a pole, rope, and flotation device, should be next to the pool. Many parents also keep a phone near the pool. In addition, children who cannot swim should wear an approved flotation device that has a collar to keep the head upright and the face out of the water.

Children should never have access to the pool while unsupervised, which includes exiting the back door while a parent is on the phone. Once discovered, the pool is a fascinating place. Caregivers should be mindful of this, as drowning happens in a matter of minutes. Toys and floats that attract young children should be kept away from the pool when not in use, and furniture that enables climbing over a pool fence should be moved to a different location. A toddler should be taught repeatedly not to go near the pool without a parent. Many parents install a motion-sensing device that sounds an alarm if something has fallen into the water.

Hot tubs are dangerous for young children; children under the age of four years should not be allowed in them. Most parents are unaware that hot tubs and spas manufactured prior to 1987 have strong suction that could injure a child; children should be cautioned to keep their head above water and their hair tied up and to sit away from a drain. The water temperature should not exceed 104 degrees Fahrenheit.

Animals and insects: Children, especially babies, are more likely to be bitten by pets than are adults. Animals should never be left alone with infants. Any animal bite that breaks the skin, no matter how minor, necessitates a visit to the pediatrician.

Shrubbery should be trimmed, since it is a breeding ground for disease-carrying rodents and ticks. In areas with a high frequency of Lyme disease, such as New Jersey and Connecticut, children should be checked and bathed daily, especially if they have been outdoors or around animals. The health department and certain medical centers test ticks for Lyme disease. The tick must be alive and in a plastic container. Ticks removed within twenty-four hours usually do not transmit disease. To prevent infection, the tick should be removed gently with tweezers. The area around the bite should be squeezed, so that pus is pushed outward, and then sterilized.

Sports injuries: Protecting our children during sports and recreational activities is of paramount importance as more than 2.6 million children under age nineteen are treated in the emergency department for injuries that result from such activities. Prevention of such injuries can be accomplished through using the right well-fitted protective gear for the sport, such as helmets, wrist guards, and knee and elbow pads. Children should also practice well enough before being involved in any competitive sport by gradually increasing their physical fitness in appropriate environmental conditions, with close attention to proper hydration and diet.

SAFETY IN THE CAR

Child passenger anticipatory safety guidance has become the main focus over the past decade as motor vehicle accidents are the leading cause of death in children four years and above. In 2011 the American Academy of Pediatrics (AAP) issued a policy statement with recommendations for best child restraints in the car from birth to adolescence. All infants and toddlers should ride in a rear-facing car safety seat (CSS) in the rear seat until the age of two years or reach the highest weight or height as per manufacturer recommendations. Children over two years of age or who outgrow a CSS should use a forward-facing CSS with a harness as long as possible and up to the highest weight or height as per manufacturer recommendations. Those children whose weight or height are above a forward-facing CSS should use a belt-positioning booster seat until the vehicle lap and shoulder seatbelt fits properly. All children younger than thirteen years of age should be restrained in the rear seats.

MEDICAL EMERGENCIES

Burns: Experts consider the kitchen to be the most dangerous room in the home for children. A burn may occur when a hot pan or liquid falls on a child or when a child presses hands against an oven door or pulls a pan off the stove. The insulation on oven doors may wear out and cause second-degree and third-degree burns, even when the oven is at a relatively low temperature.

To prevent such injuries, the following precautions should be instituted. Above all, the child should be placed at a safe remove from the potential source of burns. Counter space should be well organized and spacious, so that a hot pan placed there is far enough from the edge to prevent it from falling off. Pots should be placed on the back burners, with their handles turned toward the rear, so a child cannot reach them. In addition, stove knobs may be removed or covered when the stove is not in use if they are especially accessible or tempting to a child.

The oven door, and the window in particular, should be checked to ensure that it is not hot enough to cause even a slight burn. The manufacturer or a repair company should be called immediately if it is too hot. Several working fire extinguishers should be readily available, and smoke detectors should be installed outside sleeping areas and tested regularly.

To prevent scald burns from hot water, the temperature on water heaters should be set to a maximum of 120 degrees Fahrenheit. In addition, a parent should always test the water before putting a child in the bathtub.

If a child is burned, the immediate goal is to prevent heat from penetrating deeper into the skin. Clothing, which retains heat, must be removed from the burned area immediately. If fabric is stuck to the skin, it should not be pulled away, as this can tear the skin, but cut away as best as possible. A physician should remove the remainder.

Cold water should be applied to the burn at once until the pain subsides and the skin is no longer hot to the touch, usually at least five minutes. Nothing else should be applied to the area, including ice cubes, which may cause frostbite, and butter, grease, or ointment, which may impel the heat deeper into the skin.

If the burn is not oozing, a sterile gauze dressing should be applied, taking care not to break blisters or remove any skin. Medical attention should be sought immediately if the burn is on a child six months old or younger or if the burn affects a child's eyes, face, mouth, hands, feet, or genitals. In addition, blisters, oozing, severe pain, dizziness, and breathing problems are all reasons to seek medical attention.

Choking: Choking is the most common cause of accidental death in children under age one. Choking is life-threatening if a child swallows an object that blocks the flow of air to the lungs. The child will be unable to talk, and his or her face will turn blue. A child who is coughing should not be interrupted, as this strong natural reflex may dislodge the object.

Parents must be familiar with the emergency medical procedures for choking; approved first-aid courses are sponsored by the American Heart Association and the American Red Cross. The Heimlich maneuver is not recommended for infants; rather, they are to be turned face down on the forearm or lap and administered rapid blows between the shoulder blades. If this fails, the infant is turned on the back and four rapid chest thrusts over the breastbone are given with only two fingers. If all else fails, mouth-to-mouth or mouth-to-nose respiration should be performed.

Items that can be swallowed should be kept away from babies, including marbles, coins, safety pins, and small refrigerator magnets. Particular caution must be exercised with toys. Hazards include rattles less than 1.625 inches across, eyes or ribbons that come off stuffed animals, balloons, and small parts of toys that break off. Toys labeled for ages three and younger must meet federal guidelines requiring they have no small parts. Young children can choke on certain foods. Those foods to be avoided include peanuts, candy, whole grapes, or any hard, smooth food that must be chewed with a grinding motion.

Drawstrings in clothing pose a hazard, as they can strangle a child if the drawstring is caught on a slide, school bus door, or handrail. Drawstrings should not be worn at the neck. If they are at the waist of a garment, then knots should be untied, as they may catch on objects. A child should not use playgrounds while wearing clothing with drawstrings. In 1994, the Consumer Product Safety Commission asked clothing manufacturers to remove drawstrings from the hoods of children's garments; hand-knit or secondhand clothing still poses a risk.

Poisoning: Ironically, although most parents are aware of the poisonous hazard posed by cleaning products, they do not consider the toxicity of household plants. For example, ivy, geraniums, and philodendrons are poisonous if ingested. In addition, many plants in the yard are toxic. A poison control center can provide names of hazardous plants in a particular region.

The poison control center should be called immediately if a child ingests a toxic substance. The number of the regional center is listed on the inside cover of the telephone book and should be posted next to the phone. The parent should report what was ingested, how much, and, if it is a plant, the common and botanical name. Syrup of ipecac to induce vomiting should be readily available, but it should not be administered until instructions are received from the poison control center, since in some cases vomiting causes more harm. If a child gets poison in the eyes or on the skin, the area should be flushed immediately with lukewarm water for a period of fifteen minutes as the poison control center is being called.

To prevent the ingestion of poisons, safety locks should be installed on low-level cabinets containing cleaning products and on the medicine chest. Over-the-counter and prescription medicines, soaps, cosmetics, and shampoos are all potentially toxic if ingested by a child. Many people are unaware that vitamins consumed in a sufficient quantity can cause an overdose reaction. Shampoo and soap in the tub should be kept out of a child's reach. Many parents opt to keep medicines and vitamins, as well as sharp items such as razors, in a separate, high, and locked place.

Many automobile and building products are poisonous as well as flammable; they should be kept in locked metal cabinets away from children. In addition, lawn products, such as fertilizer and weed killer, should be kept in a locked area away from toddlers.

Lead poisoning: Lead poisoning constituted one of the most underrated afflictions of children until education efforts raised awareness. In the late 1990s, about 1 million children in the United States had elevated blood lead levels. Any building constructed before 1978, the year that lead paint was banned, probably has lead in the paint. This puts a child at risk, especially if the paint is chipped or sanded or renovations are being done. Lead is also found in pipes, which were made entirely of lead in the United States until the 1950s; lead was used to fuse copper pipes until 1986.

Safety measures include determining if lead paint exists in the home or soil. The local department of health may be contacted for further information. Repainting a home built prior to 1977 is recommended. Even if an area has been covered with nonleaded paint, precautions should be taken when children are not in the house. Chipped and peeling paint should be removed with a wet cloth. If extensive peeling has occurred, the area should be sanded and painted over. Guidelines for the removal of lead paint are available from the National Association of Homebuilders.

Tap water should be run for ninety seconds before using it, as water that has been standing in the pipes has a higher concentration of lead. Cold water should be used for drinking and cooking, as it is less likely to leach lead. High-phosphate detergents are recommended for cleaning.

All infants should be tested for lead, no matter how safe the home is. The Centers for Disease Control and Prevention (CDC) and the American Academy of Pediatrics (AAP) recommend that babies be tested at ages one and two, the ages when they are most likely to put objects that may be covered with lead dust into their mouths. Risk factors for lead exposure in children include living in cities; being poor, African American, or Hispanic; or living in areas where houses were built prior to 1950. Parents should remain alert to any possible exposure, even if their children are not considered at risk.

Teenage work: Every year about 70 teens die from work injuries in the United States. Another 70,000 get hurt badly enough that they go to a hospital emergency room. There are many federal and state regulatory rules regarding teenage work. The Fair Labor Standards Act (FLSA) provides restrictions on the types of jobs and the number of hours that teenagers can work. Such regulations are less strict for farm work, and teenagers are permitted to perform any job at any age on their family farm. The FLSA also provides certain exemptions for nonagricultural jobs in parent-owned businesses.

Teenagers' work experience is a great opportunity for parents and teenagers to learn about the occupational safety of the selected work that teenagers can do. Teenage workers and their parents should ask about the safety and healthfulness of the workplace environment, the appropriateness of the work's time schedule, and the use of appropriate safety measures while on the job (e.g., respiratory protection for teenage hospital volunteers, helmets for bicycle delivery workers, safety shoes for slippery floors).

—Lee Williams;
updated by Emad Hanna, MD, MSc

See also Accidents; Allergies; Bites and stings; Bleeding; Burns and scalds; Choking; Concussion; Critical care; Critical care, pediatric; Drowning; Electrical shock; Emergency medicine; Emergency medicine, pediatric; Emergency rooms; First aid; Food poisoning; Fracture and dislocation; Frostbite; Hives; Insect-borne diseases; Lead poisoning; Lice, mites, and ticks; Mercury poisoning; Poisoning; Poisonous plants; Snakebites; Sunburn; Zoonoses

For Further Information:
American Academy of Pediatrics. "AAP Expands Guidelines for Infant Sleep Safety and SIDS Risk Reduction." www.aap.org/en-us/about-the-aap/aap-press-room/pages/AAP-Expands-Guidelines-for-Infant-Sleep-Safety-and-SIDS-Risk-Reduction.aspx. This link provides details regarding expanded guidelines for infant sleep safety.

American Academy of Pediatrics. "Children's Health Topics: Safety and First Aid." www.aap.org/healthtopics/safety.cfm. Includes links to information on such topics as car safety, water safety, and injury prevention.

Bentz, Ric, and Christine Allison. *Street Smarts for Kids: What Parents Must Know to Keep Their Children Safe.* New York: Fawcett Books, 1999. Detective Bentz of the Kenosha, Wisconsin, Police Department, and Allison, a children's writer, have compiled an outstanding tool for parents and caretakers concerning child safety. They cover topics such as pedophiles, child abductors, and cyberspace safety threats and identify certain characteristics in children that might make them vulnerable to strangers.

Centers for Disease Control and Prevention. "Sports Injuries: The Reality." www.cdc.gov/safechild/sports_Injuries/index.html.

Committee on Injury, Violence, and Poison Prevention. "Policy Statement-Child Passenger Safety." *Pediatrics.* March 21, 2011. pediatrics.aappublications.org/content/early/2011/03/ 21/peds.2011-0213.full.pdf

Department of Labor. "Young Worker Toolkit." www.youthrules.dol.gov/support/toolkit/index.htm. This is an excellent website that provides information by age about jobs that can be done at different teenagers

Department of Labor. "Exemptions from Child Labor Rules in Non-Agriculture." www.dol.gov/elaws/esa/flsa/cl/exemptions.asp.

Information for parents about sleep safety: www.healthychildren.org/English/ages-stages/baby/sleep/Pages/Preventing-SIDS.aspx

Kattwinkel, John, et al., eds. *Textbook of Neonatal Resuscitation.* 5th ed. Elk Grove Village, IL: American Academy of Pediatrics, 2006. An invaluable guide that provides a practical, step-by-step guide for the resuscitation of both premature and full-term neonates.

Lanky, Vicki. *Baby Proofing Basics: How to Keep Your Child Safe.* 2nd ed. Minnetonka, MN: Book Peddlers, 2002. An excellent guide that contains childproofing tips for every room in the house as well as for outdoors, backyard, beach, camping, hiking, and travel of all kinds. Covers topics such as safety at playtime, mealtime, and holidays; dealing safely with pets; and poisoning dangers.

Litin, Scott C., ed. *Mayo Clinic Family Health Book.* 4th ed. New York: HarperResource, 2009. Perhaps the best general medical text for the layperson, this book covers the entire medical field and includes an excellent section on first aid and emergency care.

Priven, Joshua, David Borgenicht, and Sarah Jordan. *The Worst-Case Scenario Survival Handbook: Parenting.* New York: Scholastic, 2004. A humorous but helpful guide to surviving numerous parenting scenarios, which covers first aid and babyproofing one's house.

Rubenstein H., S.H. Sternbach, and M.R. Pollack. "Protecting the Health and Safety of Working Teenagers." *American Family Physician* 60, no. 2 (1999): 575-580.

Shelov, Steven P., et al. *Caring for Your Baby and Young Child: Birth to Age Five.* 5th ed. New York: Bantam Books, 2009. Offers a comprehensive discussion of the accidents that commonly occur with young children, accident-prevention techniques for the home and outdoors, and emergency measures to enact if an accident does take place.

Theurer, W.M., and A.K. Bhavsar. "Prevention of Unintentional Childhood Injury." *American Family Physician* 87, no. 7 (2013): 502-509.

SAFETY ISSUES FOR OLDER ADULTS

Category: Procedures
Anatomy or system affected: All
Specialties and related fields: Critical care, emergency medicine, family medicine, geriatrics and gerontology
Definition: Measures taken to prevent accidents among older adults.

THE IMPORTANCE OF SAFETY MEASURES

The age-related changes that older people experience often alter what constitutes a risk to their safety. The family home environment can be dangerous for an older person, not because the aspects of the house have changed, but because of the change in the physical abilities of the older person. Older people with intact cognitive abilities may choose to take the risk of staying in their familiar home environments with full knowledge of the increased risk. The dilemma for others, especially health providers, is defining what constitutes an acceptable level of risk for the older adult.

Older adults may experience mobility problems that pose a threat to safety. Falls are much more serious with advanced age because bones and tissues do not heal as quickly or completely as in youth.

Unintentional injuries (accidents) are the sixth leading cause of death in people over sixty-five years of age. The death rate is 51 per 100,000 people for those sixty-five to seventy-four years of age, rises to 104 per 100,000 for those aged seventy-five to eighty-four, and reaches a high of 256 per 100,000 for those who are eighty-five years of age or older. In the over-eighty-five age group, accidental injury is the fifth-leading cause of death. Generally speaking, injuries cost the United States between $75 billion and $100 billion each year. In 2015, the direct adjusted medical cost of falls came to $50 billion, comprising a significant portion of resource allocation for the cost of treating those injuries. Accidents are usually viewed as random events over which individuals have little or no control. Many other types of injuries are preventable, and safety enhancement may decrease the number of serious outcomes.

FALLS

Falls account for a considerable number of deaths and injuries among older people. Falls are the leading cause of fatal and nonfatal injuries in the older population. Previous studies from 2000 found that 46 percent of fatal falls are due to traumatic brain injury. Falls are not an uncommon event for older people; approximately one-third of noninstitutionalized older adults report a fall each year. One-half of the people who report falls experience multiple falls. Although

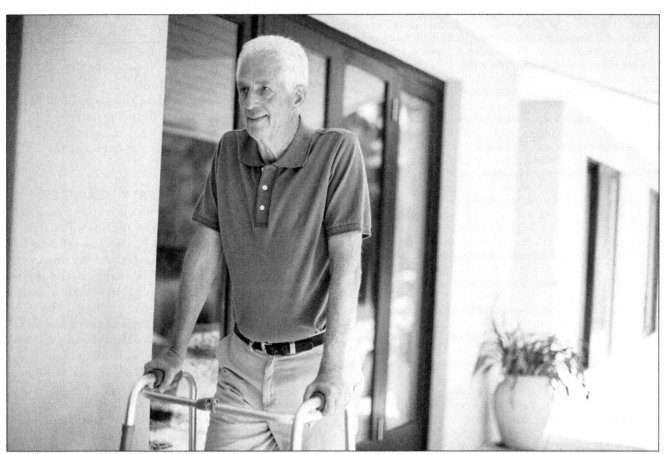

The elderly may experience mobility problems that pose a threat to safety. Falls are much more serious with advanced age because bones and tissues do not heal as quickly or completely as in youth. Photo via iStock/shapecharge. [Used under license.]

falls are a common occurrence, they are not always dangerous: Only 11 percent result in a serious injury, and an estimated 1 percent result in hip fractures. The number of hip fractures yearly in the United States (200,000) is substantial and serious. They lead to death in 12 percent to 20 percent of cases and account for 2 percent of the mortality rate in the United States. More than 40 percent of deaths from falls occur in the home. Stairs account for a large proportion of falls, many occurring because the older individual misses the last step. Falling injuries account for 40 percent of nursing home admissions; however, more than 20 percent of all fatal falls occur in the nursing home setting. Over the past decade, mortality from falls in older adults has risen impressively, with about 42,100 older adults dying from unintentional fall injuries in 2020.

Falls among older adults may be caused by a variety of factors: physical frailty, pathological states, psychological stress, drug interactions, and multiple environmental hazards. The risks of falling increase with the following: increasing age, the number of chronic diseases present, the number and type of medications being taken, cognitive impairment, and physical disability. The risk of falling is often associated more with the intake of some types of medications (antidepressants,

sedatives, or vasodilators) than with medical conditions. Most doctors provide older patients with information concerning the effects of drugs that they may be taking, including the risk of a drop in blood pressure related to these medications. Instruction concerning how to decrease the effects of orthostatic hypotension, a condition in which blood pressure drops upon standing, is an example of how to instruct patients to be more aware of what may result in a fall. They may be instructed to dangle their feet before getting out of bed or rising slowly from seated or reclining positions to prevent falls due to orthostatic hypotension.

Falls may cause bruises, abrasions, pain, swelling, or fractures. Changes in cognitive function related to pressure from edema or blood clots within the brain may also be evidenced. Psychological damage resulting from falls is subtler. An older person who sustains little or no injury in a fall may delay or avoid discussing it in order to avoid embarrassment or risk of being viewed as less competent. Falls may also prompt changes in behavior, such as decreased thoroughness in housekeeping tasks or discussion of fears of living alone. Changes in grooming, dress, and personal appearance may also be observed. Increased fear of venturing out into the neighborhood may lead to a decreased ability to meet the daily requirements of shopping and food preparation. Affected individuals may further decrease other activities, resulting in their becoming increasingly sessile. This leads to a relative reduction in physical fitness, impacting their quality of life and increases the risk of future falls.

Falls are better prevented than treated. People aged seventy-five and older who fall are four to five times more likely than those aged between sixty-five to seventy-four to be admitted to a long-term care facility for a year or longer. Because quality of life is as important as length of life, limiting activity in the hope that falls will not occur is the least acceptable method of prevention. A more realistic approach is to modify the environment. Although cost may be a limiting factor, many alterations can be implemented that are both acceptable to the older person and minimal in expense. Many environmental modifications are relatively easy to perform.

Many falls occur in the bathroom. Nonslip bath mats and adhesive-backed, nonskid strips in the bathtub or shower are important safety measures. Grab bars may be placed at critical locations near the bathtub and toilet to lend support. Railings may be installed on stairways for support. A piece of fabric, a knob, or some other marker can be attached to the rail to indicate the level of the top and bottom steps.

Other steps can be taken to prevent falls in older adults. Regular exercise, focusing on leg strength and improving balance, can prevent falls as these physical attributes diminish greatly with age. The Centers for Disease Control and Prevention (CDC) maintains that Tai Chi programs are especially conducive to improving these weaker areas. Reviewing medications with a physician or pharmacist may help to identify medications causing side effects such as dizziness and drowsiness. Yearly eye exams and updating eyeglasses to maximize vision are also helpful.

The need for light increases with age. An environment can be illuminated at a safe level by increasing either the number of lights or the intensity of the lightbulbs. Adequate illumination that does not cause shadows, which may cause problems with perception, is extremely important in high hazard areas, such as stairways and stair landings. Night-lights or lighted switches enable those who get up at night to orient themselves more easily within the environment and minimize the risk of falling. The removal of obstructions and obstacles can also help increase the safety of the home. Among the objects that may cause elderly people to trip are extension cords and long phone cords, low furniture, carpet edges, and throw rugs. These can easily be removed from high-traffic areas or taped down to minimize the risk of causing injury.

TRAFFIC INJURIES

In modern societies, an important rite of passage for adolescents is to receive a driver's license. Driving an automobile is viewed as the first step toward adult life because it fosters independence. On the other hand, driving a car also calls for a sense of responsibility to others who share the roads. Many roads are crowded, and traffic moves at a rapid and sometimes confusing rate. Drivers must be physically and mentally alert to handle the hazards of the roads. Older people with impaired physical capabilities must make a choice between continuing to drive, and therefore maintaining their independence, or taking measures to increase safety for themselves and others on the road.

Traffic injuries in the older population are divided into two categories: pedestrian injuries and vehicle-related injuries. Older people are more at risk for injury at street intersections than anywhere else, both as pedestrians and as drivers or passengers in an automobile. As pedestrians, many older people are at risk because of an inability to cross the street in the time allotted between changes in the traffic lights. Factors that may influence pedestrian injuries are curb height, driver error, and physical and cognitive impairment of the older pedestrian.

A major problem for older drivers is motor vehicle accidents, in which the risk for injury in these crashes increases dramatically with age. The majority of such accidents take place in daylight, on good roads, and with no alcohol involvement. Older people experience a higher mortality rate with less severe injuries in vehicle crashes; the risk of death is three times greater for a seventy-year-old person than for a twenty-year-old person. The major factor that influences the high susceptibility of involvement in traffic injuries may be the decreased skill of the older person in operating an automobile. This change in skill level may be caused by age-related changes, such as decreased visual acuity or a slower neurological response time.

Citations for traffic violations, such as failure to yield right-of-way and failure to obey traffic signs, increase after the age of sixty. Although older adults have lower accident rates and fewer traffic violation citations than those under twenty-five years of age, older people have an increased risk of fatality in traffic accidents. One group of older adults at increased risk for vehicle-related injury is those who are experiencing the early signs and symptoms of dementia. The American Association for Retired Persons (AARP) operates special classes in driver education to help older adults cope with age-related changes that affect their driving abilities.

SAFETY CONSIDERATIONS

Safety is a major concern when assessing living conditions. Many older adults live in unsafe housing.

Relatively minor nuisances—such as excessive clutter, loose flooring or floor coverings, poor lighting, and unstable stairs—can pose safety risks for the older adult. Financial constraints may prompt older adults to settle for living in less desirable areas. Other safety concerns are related to the older adult's physical or mental functioning. People who have trouble walking or climbing stairs are prime examples of those at risk as the result of impaired physical functioning. People who are forgetful or who wander off and get lost pose a significant risk to themselves and others as the result of impaired mental function.

It may be necessary to observe older adults actually moving about in their environment to locate any potential problems. If the older person uses an assistive device, such as a cane, walker, or wheelchair, the environment may require further modifications. Ramps may need to be installed, or living arrangements may need to be changed to accommodate the need for special access.

Most older people prefer to stay in their own homes in familiar communities for as long as possible. As people get older, they often fear that they may have to leave home for health reasons. Such fears are realistic because acute and chronic health problems associated with aging often dictate at least temporary changes in environment, leading older adults to reside in places they do not prefer. Their desire to stay at home challenges the health care system to study their special needs and devise solutions that will accommodate them in the most acceptable way.

Older individuals who live alone are well-advised to learn how to summon emergency help and to make home adaptations to compensate for decreased mobility and dexterity. Cognitive impairments often present a more serious threat to safety than physical impairment. People who know they are having problems are likely to call for help and remain safely in the home until help arrives. However, individuals with impaired judgment may present a hazard to themselves, as well as to their neighbors, through such behavior as forgetting to turn off the stove. In isolated instances, a choice may be made to preserve such a person's autonomy at the risk of serious injury; however, few would agree that the impaired older person has a right to put others at risk of serious injury.

Medication usage is another important factor to consider when evaluating whether or not an older person can safely remain at home alone. Sometimes the deciding factor in whether a cognitively impaired individual can remain at home alone is the nature of the medication regimen. Some individuals must have regular medication to maintain health. There are various systems to help people with cognitive impairment take their medicines. Avoiding polypharmacy and simplify-

ing medication regimen is an important step that providers always need to consider. Preparing and labeling medications for each day is one strategy for simplifying medication administration. Medication calendars, which show each type of pill with its time of administration and which have a space for marking when the pill is taken, are useful to individuals with early memory impairment. Functionally impaired individuals who want to stay at home but require assistance or supervision with activities of daily living are often helped by paraprofessional personnel.

It is always wise, and strongly recommended, for the elderly or anyone with any cognitive concerns, to bring someone with them—close friend or relative—for medical appointments. There are significant limitations to what is printed on a medication label such as knowing which medications have been discontinued.

It is clear that injuries in the older population are costly both financially and in terms of independence. By preventing the most common causes of injury, adjusting medications, and altering acceptable aspects of an older person's lifestyle, the risk of such injuries can be decreased. These changes will hopefully result in fewer injuries and a greater quality of life.

—*Yuji Yamada, MD*

See also: Accidents; Aging; Aging: Extended care; Alzheimer's disease; Assisted living facilities; Balance disorders; Critical care; Deafness; Death and dying; Dementias; Emergency medicine; Emergency rooms; First aid; Fracture and dislocation; Geriatrics and gerontology; Hip fracture repair; Hip replacement; Home care; Hospice; Memory loss; Nursing; Osteoporosis; Pick's disease; Psychiatry, geriatric.

For Further Information:
Beerman, Susan, and Judith Rappaport-Musson. *Eldercare 911: The Caregiver's Complete Handbook for Making Decisions.* Rev. ed., Prometheus Books, 2008. A practical guide for elder care. Includes topics such as locating services, managing medications, understanding benefits, choosing a nursing home, coping with memory loss, hiring and handling in-home help, helping a parent who refuses help, and recognizing signs of elder abuse.
Gill, T. M., C. S. Williams, J. T. Robison, and M. E. Tinetti. "A Population-Based Study of Environmental Hazards in the Homes of Older Persons." *American Journal of Public Health*, vol. 89, no. 4, 1999, pp. 535-56. An environmental assessment was completed in the homes of one thousand persons seventy-two years and older. Weighted prevalence rates were calculated for each of the potential hazards and subsequently compared among subgroups of participants.
Lachman, M. E., et al. "Fear of Falling and Activity Restriction: The Survey of Activities and Fear of Falling in the Elderly (SAFE)." *Journals of Gerontology Series B-Psychological Sciences and Social Sciences*, vol. 53B, no. 1, 1998, pp. 43-50. A new instrument was developed to assess the role of fear of falling in activity restriction. The instrument assesses fear of falling during performance of eleven activities, and it gathers information about participation in these activities as well as the extent to which fear is a source of activity restriction.

Lachs, Mark S. "Caring for Mom and Dad: Can Your Parent Live Alone?" *Prevention*, vol. 50, no. 10, Oct. 1998, pp. 155-57. Information on how to develop a care plan for an aging parent who is having problems with activities of daily living.

Lisak, Janet M., and Marlene Morgan. *The Safe Home Checkout: A Professional Guide to Safe Independent Living.* 2nd ed., Geriatric Environments for Living and Learning, 1997. Covers safety measures for older buildings, accident prevention, and self-help devices for the disabled. Includes bibliographical references.

Litin, Scott C., editor. *Mayo Clinic Family Health Book.* 4th ed., Harper Resource, 2009. Perhaps the best general medical text for the layperson, this book covers the entire medical field and includes an excellent section on first aid and emergency care.

Stenchever, Morton A. *Health Care for the Older Woman.* Chapman and Hall, 1996. A reference that provides medical practitioners and students with comprehensive, current information specific to the care of middle-aged and advanced-aged women. It covers health maintenance issues, including diet, exercise, safety, psychological and psychosocial problems, social problems, and grief and loss.

Warner, Mark L. *Complete Guide to Alzheimer's—Proofing Your Home.* Rev. ed., Purdue UP, 2000. An excellent guide that details how to create a home environment for elderly patients with Alzheimer's and related dementia. Covers both interior and exterior spaces, discussing problems and solutions associated with specific areas, such as the kitchen, the bathroom, corridors, and patios and decks.

SALMONELLA INFECTION

Category: Disease/Disorder
Anatomy or system affected: Blood, gastrointestinal system
Specialties and related fields: Bacteriology, family medicine, gastroenterology, pediatrics, public health
Definition: a broad spectrum of clinical diseases caused by many types of *Salmonella* bacteria
Key terms:
asymptomatic: without symptoms
bacteremia: the presence of bacteria in the blood, which is usually associated with chills and fever
gastroenteritis: infection of the gastrointestinal tract, usually accompanied by nausea, vomiting, diarrhea, and abdominal pains
typhoid fever: a particular disease syndrome most often associated with infection by *Salmonella typhi* but occasionally caused by other types of *Salmonella* bacteria

CAUSES AND SYMPTOMS

Salmonella are a group of bacteria that cause enteric or typhoid fever. All types can cause gastrointestinal, blood, and various local infections. All types of *Salmonella* can be carried in the gastrointestinal tract without symptoms after recovery from infection.

The clinical disease caused by *Salmonella* depends on the type of bacteria, the number of organisms ingested, and the age and immune status of the person infected. Infection with *Salmonella* can occur with the ingestion of one or 100 million organisms. Increasing the dosage of bacteria decreases the incubation period and increases the severity of the resulting disease. After ingestion, the bacteria adhere to and invade the gastrointestinal tract. In the intestinal tract wall, *Salmonella* survive and multiply in immune cells and then enter the bloodstream, where they proceed to any area of the body. Young infants and people with immune deficiencies and hemolytic anemia are at increased risk for severe and complicated infections.

Typhoid fever or enteric fever is very rare in the United States, causing less than five hundred cases per year; it is primarily seen in people coming from developing countries. Classically, this disease is caused by *Salmonella typhi* bacteria, but other types of *Salmonella* can also cause it. During the first week of illness, symptoms include progressively increasing fever with an associated headache, muscle aches, abdominal pains, and lethargy. In the second week, the heart rate decreases, the liver, and spleen enlarge, small red bumps form on the trunk, and the patient becomes stuporous. During the third to fourth week, intestinal bleeding and perforation are common. The fever begins to remit in the fifth to sixth week of illness. Diarrhea usually starts in the first week and resolves within six weeks. Without treatment, death can occur from gastrointestinal bleeding and perforation. Infants tend to have much more severe diseases than older children.

Salmonellosis caused by nontyphoid *Salmonella* is more common in the United States, causing about fifty thousand cases per year. The major reservoir of nontyphoid *Salmonella* is the gastrointestinal tract of many animals, including mammals, reptiles, birds, and insects. Farm animals and pet reptiles commonly carry *Salmonella*. Some antibiotic resistance is caused by the use of antibiotics in animal feeds. *Salmonella* can be isolated from 50 percent of chicken, 16 percent of pork, 5 percent of beef, and 40 percent of frozen eggs in retail stores. Contaminated eggs and milk products are common sources of human infection.

Gastroenteritis is the most common disease caused by nontyphoid *Salmonella*. The incubation period for this disease is about one day, ranging from six hours to three days. Symptoms include nausea, vomiting, and abdominal pain. Diarrhea typically contains blood and white cells. Usually, symptoms disappear in less than a week in healthy children. Still, symptoms may persist for several weeks in young infants and children with immune deficiencies.

Bacteremia can occur in 1 to 5 percent of patients with *Salmonella* gastroenteritis. Bacteremia is generally associated with fever, chills, and toxicity in the older child but may be asymptomatic in the infant. Children with an increased risk of bacteremia include those with acquired immunodeficiency syndrome (AIDS) or other immune deficiencies and hemolytic anemias such as sickle cell disease.

Bacteremia can lead to infection of almost any organ. Children with sickle cell anemia are more prone to bone infections and meningitis. *Salmonella* may localize to areas of the body that have received trauma or contain damaged tissue or a foreign body. Meningitis, inflammation of the covering of the spine and brain, is primarily seen as a complication of bacteremia in infants. Meningitis has a 50 percent death rate, and residual developmental and hearing defects are commonly found in survivors. Patients who have persistent bacteremia should be evaluated for heart infection.

The diagnosis of *Salmonella* infection is best made by culturing stool and blood samples. With enteric fever, it is important to culture multiple sites multiple times. The clinical laboratory must perform antibiotic susceptibility testing routinely to guide therapy. Other bacterial causes of gastroenteritis can be confused with *Salmonella* infection.

TREATMENT AND THERAPY
Treatment for gastroenteritis usually does not require antibiotics. Antibiotics do not speed the resolution of disease but instead lead to prolonged excretion of *Salmonella*. Therapy primarily focuses on correcting fluid and salt abnormalities and general supportive care. However, if the patient has indications of sepsis, shock, or chills, then antibiotics should be administered.

Scanning electron micrograph showing Salmonella typhimurum invading cultured human cells. Photo via Wikimedia Commons. [Public domain.]

Infants under three months of age and children with immune deficiencies should also be treated with antibiotics. Ampicillin is usually used as the initial treatment in uncomplicated cases, and third-generation cephalosporin antibiotics are used in severe and complicated cases. Over 20 percent of nontyphoid *Salmonella* in the United States is resistant to ampicillin and other antibiotics. Antibiotic treatment should last ten days to two weeks in children with bacteremia and four to six weeks with bone infection or meningitis. Local infections may require surgical drainage.

Typhoid fever is treated for a minimum of two weeks. It is important to perform susceptibility testing for the possibility of resistance so that the physician can choose proper antibiotic therapy. Healthcare providers should treat chronic carriers of *Salmonella typhi* with antibiotics. If eradication is unsuccessful, the patient should seek a surgical assessment of the biliary tract.

Prevention of the spread of *Salmonella* requires several public health procedures. Proper sewage disposal, water purification, and chlorination are essential public health measures. Hand washing is critical to the prevention of transmission. *Salmonella* carriers should be excluded from food preparation and childcare settings. Hospitalized infants and children should be isolated. In developing countries, the promotion of prolonged breastfeeding also reduces the infection rate.

There are two typhoid vaccines commercially available in the United States. The first is an oral, live attenuated vaccine requiring four doses for one week and a booster every five years. The second is a parenteral capsular polysaccharide vaccine given as a single intramuscular injection and a booster every two years. The vaccines are 50 to 80 percent protective. The live attenuated vaccine should not be given to patients who are pregnant, taking antibiotics, or immunocompromised, such as persons with the human immunodeficiency virus (HIV).

PERSPECTIVE AND PROSPECTS

Salmonella was identified as the cause of typhoid fever in 1880 and was first cultured in 1884. Since 1920, improvements in sanitation, water supplies, and sewage disposal have resulted in a marked decrease in typhoid fever in the United States. In 1920, 36,000 cases were reported; after 1965, the number of cases per year has rarely exceeded 500. Since then, the number of cases has remained fairly constant because of the importation of disease by tourists, immigrants, and migrant laborers. About 62 percent of *Salmonella typhi* infections are acquired through foreign travel. Direct person-to-person transmission is rare except in the homosexual population.

> **INFORMATION ON SALMONELLA INFECTION**
>
> **Causes:** Bacterial infection transmitted through ingestion or exposure to infected animals
> **Symptoms:** Fever, headache, muscle aches, abdominal pain, lethargy, diarrhea, vomiting
> **Duration:** Six hours to three days
> **Treatments:** Correction of fluid and salt abnormalities, supportive care

Recent research is focused on public health. Measures to decrease food contamination such as improved cleanliness, decreased use of antibiotics in animal feeds, and food irradiation, decrease human transmission. Research into alternate vaccines with fewer side effects and improved immune response is underway.

Nontyphoid *Salmonella* causes one-half million infections per year in the United States. One-third of these infections are in children less than five years of age, and 40 percent are in adults over thirty years of age.

—*Peter D. Reuman, MD, MPH*

For Further Information:
Brazier, Yvette. "All You Need to Know About *Salmonella*." *MedicalNewsToday*, 12 Mar. 2020, www.medicalnewstoday.com/articles/160942. Accessed 5 Apr. 2022.
Bush, Larry M. "Salmonella Infections." *Merck Manual Consumer Version*, Feb. 2020, www.merckmanuals.com/home/infections/bacterial-infections-gram-negative-bacteria/salmonella-infections. Accessed 5 Apr. 2022.
Dodd, Christine, E. R., et al., editors. *Foodborne Diseases*. 3rd ed., Academic Press, 2017.
Grünberg, Walter. "Salmonellosis in Animals." *Merck Manual Veterinary Manual*, Oct. 2020, www.merckvetmanual.com/digestive-system/salmonellosis/salmonellosis-in-animals. Accessed 5 Apr. 2022.
Salmonella. The Centers for Disease Control and Prevention, 2 Feb. 2022, www.cdc.gov/salmonella/index.html. Accessed 5 Apr.
Salmonella. Washington State Department of Health, n.d., doh.wa.gov/you-and-your-family/illness-and-disease-z/salmonella. Accessed 5 Apr. 2022.

SARCOIDOSIS

Category: Disease/Disorder
Also known as: Besnier-Boeck disease, Schaumann's syndrome, Lofgren syndrome (acute sarcoidosis)
Anatomy or system affected: Brain, chest, circulatory system, eyes, heart, immune system, joints, kidneys, lungs, lymphatic system, nerves, nervous system, respiratory system, skin, spleen

Specialties and related fields: Bacteriology, cardiology, dermatology, genetics, immunology, internal medicine, nephrology, neurology, ophthalmology, optometry, pulmonary medicine, radiology, rheumatology, serology, toxicology, virology

Definition: An inflammatory disease of unknown cause characterized by noncaseating granulomas, that affect multiple systems, especially the lungs, lymph nodes, skin, and eyes. This disease is thought to be the result of a dysregulated immune response to an infectious agent or environmental factor. If severe, sarcoidosis is treated with corticosteroids.

Key terms:

cytokine: a small, regulatory protein of the immune system that mediates cell interactions

fibrosis: the development of scar tissue consisting of excess fibrous connective tissue

fluorodeoxyglucose-positron emission tomography (FDG-PET): a molecular imaging method in which radioactive sugar is injected into the body; the sugar accumulates in tissues with hypermetabolism and is detected by its positron emission

granuloma: a clump of cells, or nodule, in the immune system

immune system: a body system that protects the body from foreign substances by identifying and destroying them; includes the thymus, bone marrow, and lymph tissues

lymphocyte: a white blood cell that produces antibodies

macrophage: a white blood cell that engulfs foreign substances and stimulates other immune cells

noncaseating: not causing tissue death and a resulting cheeselike appearance of tissue

CAUSES AND SYMPTOMS

Sarcoidosis, an inflammatory disease of unknown cause, affects multiple organs and systems in the body. Most commonly affected are the lungs, lymph nodes, skin, and eyes. Other organs and systems that can be involved include the liver, spleen, bone, joints, heart, muscle, and central nervous system. Sarcoidosis is thought to be the result of an unusual immune reaction to an environmental antigen, such as a bacterium, fungus, or environmental toxin. Sarcoidosis is characterized by the presence of noncaseating granulomas in the affected tissues. These granulomas are ball-shaped clusters of immune cells consisting of macrophage and epitheloid cells encircled by lymphocytes. A granuloma begins when certain types of lymphocytes interact with antigen-presenting cells. Macrophages that have engulfed antigens are chronically stimulated by cytokines, differentiate into epitheliod cells, and fuse to form multinucleated giant cells. If a granuloma persists for an extended period of time, then fibroblasts and collagen encase the ball of cells. This

INFORMATION ON SARCOIDOSIS

Causes: Unknown; dysregulated immune system response to pathogen or environmental toxin
Symptoms: Fatigue, cough, inflammation, granulomas
Duration: Years; may resolve without treatment or persist
Treatments: Corticosteroids

eventually leads to fibrosis, or permanent scarring, which can lead to organ impairment.

The incidence of sarcoidosis varies greatly by ethnic group, indicating a genetic component to sarcoidosis. In the United States, 40 in 100,000 African Americans develop sarcoidosis, while 5 in 100,000 Caucasians develop it. In Sweden, the incidence is 64 in 100,000. In general, more women develop sarcoidois than do men. Sarcoidosis can occur at any age, but the average age when it is detected is between twenty and forty years.

The initial symptoms of sarcoidosis may include coughs, wheezing, chest discomfort, night chills, and weight loss. Many patients learn that they have sarcoidosis when a routine chest X ray shows abnormalities. Most if not all of the symptoms of sarcoidosis are not unique to the disease, so diagnosis involves ruling out other conditions, such as an infection. Typical first signs of sarcoidosis include skin lesions, problems with the lungs (such as decreased lung function), and enlarged lymph nodes. A bronchoscopy may be performed to inspect the bronchial tubes and to obtain a tissue for biopsy. A positive biopsy would reveal a large number of white blood cells, general inflammation, and the presence of granulomas. Gallium-67 scans may be used, in which the radioactive element gallium-67 is injected and accumulates in areas of inflammation, infection, or rapid cell division. More recently, the more sensitive FDG-PET scan, which uses the radioactive sugar FDG instead of gallium, is being used for some patients. Patients with sarcoidosis in the eyes have redness in the eyes, photophobia, and blurred vision.

TREATMENT AND THERAPY

An estimated 60 to 70 percent of cases of sarcoidosis will resolve within one to two years. For severe sarcoidosis, corticosteroids, such as prednisone, are given to reduce inflammation. Since steroids can have severe side effects, treatment may not be given unless organs are impaired. Some 20 to 30 percent of patients will develop a chronic condition of persistent sarcoidosis that damages organs as a result of fibrosis. It is estimated that in 5 to 10 percent of patients, sarcoidosis will be the cause of death, usually from lung fibrosis resulting in respiratory failure or from cardiac or neurological complications.

PERSPECTIVE AND PROSPECTS

The skin lesions of sarcoidosis were first recognized in 1869 by English dermatologist Jonathan Hutchinson. In 1897, Caesar Boeck independently described the skin lesions using the term "sarcoidosis," meaning "fleshlike condition." The multiple system involvement was recognized by Jörgen Schaumann in 1915, the same time that Alexander Bittorf described lung lesions of the condition. In 1941, Morten A. Kveim, a Norwegian physician, developed a test for sarcoidosis that involved injecting lymph node tissue from a confirmed sarcoidois patient into the skin of a person suspected of having sarcoidosis. If granulomas developed at the injection site four to six weeks later, then the test was positive for sarcoidosis. In 1954, Louis Siltzbach modified the test to inject tissue from the spleen of sarcoidosis patients. If the patient was receiving steroid treatment, then the granulomas might not develop, leading to a false negative on the test. The Kveim test is no longer used to diagnose sarcoidosis, largely because of the lack of commercially available Kveim reagent and its replacement by other diagnostic methods, such as bronchoscopy. A promising new development in the treatment of extensive sarcoidosis is the use of FDG-PET to monitor a patient's response to drug therapy. FDG-PET is more sensitive than the conventional gallium method. Research into the genetics of sarcoidosis indicates likely multiple genetic factors. A predisposition to developing sarcoidosis is associated with *HLA-DQ* and *HLA-DR* genes.

—*Susan J. Karcher, PhD*

See also Autoimmune disorders; Corticosteroids; Eye infections and disorders; Eyes; Immune system; Immunology; Lesions; Lungs; Lymphatic system; Pulmonary diseases; Pulmonary medicine; Skin; Skin disorders.

For Further Information:
Culver, Daniel A., Mary Jane Thomassen, and Mani S. Kavuru. "Pulmonary Sarcoidosis: New Genetic Clues and Ongoing Treatment Controversies." *Cleveland Clinic Journal of Medicine* 71, no. 2 (2004): 88-106. Discusses genetics.
Iannuzzi, Michael C., Benjamin A. Rybicki, and Alvin S. Teirstein. "Medical Progress: Sarcoidosis." *New England Journal of Medicine* 357, no. 21 (2007): 2153-2165. A review.
Smith, C. Christopher, Jess Mandel, and Booker Bush. "Less Is More." *New England Journal of Medicine* 344, no. 14 (2001): 1079-1082. Difficulty of sarcoidosis diagnosis.

SARCOMA

Category: Disease/Disorder
Anatomy or system affected: Arms, back, bones, cells, joints, legs, muscles

Specialties and related fields: Cytology, general surgery, genetics, histology, oncology, pathology
Definition: A malignant tumor that develops in connective tissues of the body and can occur in children or adults.
Key terms:
mesenchyme: tissue that develops into connective and skeletal tissues, including blood and lymph.
systemic therapies: any type of cancer treatment that targets the entire body
targeted therapies: A type of treatment that identifies and attacks specific types of cancer cells with less harm to normal cells.

CAUSES AND SYMPTOMS

Sarcomas are a rare, poorly understood group of human cancers. Although the incidence of sarcomas is far lower than for the more common types of human malignancy, the disease is no less devastating to afflicted individuals and their families. *Sarcoma* comes from the Greek term for "fleshy growth." It refers to the fact that sarcomas are malignant tumors that arise in connective tissues of the body. In the embryo, connective tissue arises from primitive cells called the "mesenchyme." During embryogenesis, the mesenchymal tissues differentiate to form the many specialized connective tissues found in the body. Malignant tumors may arise in any of these connective tissue types. Cancers arising in fatty tissue are called liposarcomas; smooth muscle tumors are leiomyosarcomas; cancers in developing skeletal muscle are rhabdomyosarcomas; and angiosarcomas affect the blood or lymph vessels. Other types of sarcomas include:

• Fibrosarcoma, occurs in fibroblasts;
• Synovial sarcomas occur in the joints;
• Neurofibrosarcoma is a malignancy of cells surrounding the nerves;
• Osteosarcoma occurs in bone tissue; and
• Chondrosarcoma occurs in cartilage.

Gastrointestinal stromal tumors (GISTs) are a rare type of stomach cancer. Ewing's sarcoma IEwing's sarcoma represents a family of childhood malignancies occurring in very primitive cells of bone tissue and is one of the most common forms of bone cancer in children, exceeded only by osteosarcomas. Finally, Kaposi's sarcoma IKaposi's sarcoma is a rare sarcoma caused by infection by human herpesvirus 8. While it is a rare disease in the general population, occurring primarily among Jewish men of Mediterranean origin, it represents the most common malignancy in patients with acquired immunodeficiency syndrome (AIDS). Kaposi's sarcoma seems to result from the expression of a viral gene that activates growth regulatory genes in infected cells.

Although there are many types of sarcomas, they share common features, including cellular characteristics, symptoms, and treatment approaches. However, the causes of sarcoma appear to be diverse and poorly understood. Sarcomas have been linked to environmental exposure to toxic chemicals. Genetic links have been identified in families with hereditary predispositions to cancer, including Li-Fraumeni syndrome, which results from an inherited mutation in the *p53* tumor suppressor gene, and neurofibromatosis (Von Recklinghausen's disease), which involves an inherited mutation in the tumor suppressor gene called *NF1*. Many sarcomas contain genetic chromosomal rearrangements called "translocations". These chromosomal rearrangements create novel growth control genes similar to those observed in leukemias and lymphomas. These genetic similarities suggest common features in the pathways by which these malignancies arise. For example, the Ewing's sarcoma family of tumors (ESFT) contains a translocation between chromosomes 11 and 22, resulting in uncontrolled expression of certain oncogenes and their products, including growth factors and kinases.

TREATMENT AND THERAPY
According to the American Society of Clinical Oncology (ASCO), the three primary interventions to treat sarcoma include surgery, radiation therapy, and systemic therapies. However, since there are over fifty types of sarcomas, each with its unique pathophysiology, treatment will vary. Management options depend on multiple aspects, such as the type, stage, grade of sarcoma, and the patient's overall health.

When the sarcoma is removed surgically, the goal is to excise enough normal tissue surrounding the tumor to obtain a clean margin. Surgical resection is the best method to ensure no tumor cells remain in the area. Patients with a very large tumor involving the arm or leg's major nerves and blood vessels may require surgical amputation.

Radiation therapy is often prescribed before or after surgery. When radiation is used before surgery, its purpose is to shrink the tumor so that the surgeon may more easily remove it. Radiation treatment may make it possible to lessen the severity of the surgery. Postsurgical radiation is used to remove any remaining cancer cells.

There are several systemic medications prescribed to treat different types of sarcomas. Chemotherapy may be used alone or in combination. Some chemotherapies used to treat sarcoma include doxorubicin (Adriamycin), epirubicin (Ellence), and ifosfamide (Ifex). Chemotherapy is used when a sarcoma has metastasized.

INFORMATION ON SARCOMA

Causes: May include environmental exposure to toxic chemicals, genetic predisposition, genetic translocations, viral infection
Symptoms: Malignant tumors in conective tissue; wide-ranging
Duration: Chronic
Treatments: Surgery, radiation, chemotherapy

Medication that targets cancer's specific genes, proteins, or tissue environment are known as "targeted therapies." Drugs such as imatinib (Gleevec), pazopanib (Votrient), and tazemetostat (Tazverik) contribute to reducing cancer growth and increasing patient survival.

—*Robert Koch, DNSc, RN, OCN*

See also: Bone cancer; Bone disorders; Bone grafting; Bones and the skeleton; Cancer; Carcinogens; Chemotherapy; Connective tissue; Ewing's sarcoma; Kaposi's sarcoma; Muscle sprains, spasms, and disorders; Muscles; Neurofibromatosis; Oncology; Orthopedic surgery; Orthopedics; Orthopedics, pediatric; Radiation therapy.

For Further Information:
Grisham, J. "What's New in Sarcoma Treatment? MSK Researchers Are Leading Many Innovative Clinical Trials." *Memorial Sloan Kettering Cancer Center*, 30 Sept. 2020, www.mskcc.org/news/what-s-new-sarcoma-treatment-msk-researchers-are-leading-many- innovative-clinical-trials.
MacGill, M. "What You Should Know About Sarcoma." *Medical News Today*, 21 Aug. 2021, www.medicalnewstoday.com/articles/301762.
McMillin, M. "Sarcoma." *WebMD*, 24 Sept. 2022, www.webmd.com/cancer/sarcoma.
"Sarcomas of Specific Organs." *Cancer.net*, 12 Jul. 2019, cancer.net/cancer-types/sarcomas-specific-organs.
"Sarcomas, Soft Tissue—Introduction." *Cancer.net*, 16 Apr. 2021, www.cancer.net/cancer-types/sarcomas-soft-tissue/introduction.
"Soft Tissue Sarcoma—Patient Version." *National Cancer Institute*, 2022, www.cancer.gov/types/soft-tissue-sarcoma.

SARS. See Severe acute respiratory syndrome (SARS).

Scabies

Category: Disease/Disorder
Anatomy or system affected: Skin
Specialties and related fields: Dermatology, family medicine
Definition: Skin infestation by mites, causing a rash and severe itching.

CAUSES AND SYMPTOMS

The human scabies mite *Sarcoptes scabiei*, a small arachnid, approximately 0.4 millimeter long, produces intense pruritus (itching) and a red rash. Though scabies is most commonly noted on the fingers and hands, almost any skin surface can be affected. After fertilization, the female mite burrows into the upper layer of the host's skin and deposits several eggs. Upon hatching, the young migrate to the surface, where they mature; this life cycle lasts three to four weeks. In most cases, an affected human host will have an average of eleven adult females. The elderly and immunocompromised patients are susceptible to a more severe, widespread variant called Norwegian scabies. In cases of Norwegian scabies, a human host may carry more than two million adult females.

A patient with scabies generally complains of severe itching, and the skin may be inflamed from scratching. Examination with a magnifying lens reveals characteristic burrows several millimeters in length, especially in the spaces between the fingers. A skin scraping aids in the diagnosis, producing a specimen for microscopic viewing which reveals the adult mite, eggs, or feces.

TREATMENT AND THERAPY

The treatment of scabies is straightforward. Clothing and bed linen should be washed in hot water. Shoes or other articles that cannot be washed may be sealed in a plastic bag for a week; this kills the mites, which need a human host to survive for more than a few days. Patients are treated with a 5 percent preparation of permethrin applied from head to foot (sparing the mouth and eyes) and left on overnight. An alternative treatment is lindane, which is less commonly used because of the risk of nerve toxicity in children. With either treatment, the medication is rinsed off in the morning shower. A single dose of oral ivermectin may be used alone or in combination with topical agents to treat difficult cases. Rapid diagnosis and treatment decrease the chance of the mites spreading to other individuals.

—*Louis B. Jacques, MD*

See also Dermatology; Itching; Lice, mites, and ticks; Parasitic diseases; Rashes; Skin; Skin disorders.

For Further Information:
Chosidow, Oliver. "Scabies and Pediculosis." *The Lancet* 355, no. 9206 (March 4, 2000): 819-826.
Gach, J. E., and A. Heagerty. "Crusted Scabies Looking Like Psoriasis." *The Lancet* 356, no. 9230 (August 19, 2000): 650.
Haag, M. L., S. J. Brozena, and N. A. Fenske. "Attack of the Scabies: What to Do When an Outbreak Occurs." *Geriatrics* 48 (October, 1993): 45-46, 51-53.
Levy, Sandra. "The Scourge of Scabies: Some Ways to Treat It." *Drug Topics* 144, no. 22 (November 20, 2000): 56.
Sheorey, Harsha, John Walker, and Beverly Ann Biggs. *Clinical Parasitology.* Melbourne, Vic.: University of Melbourne Press, 2003.
Stewart, Kay B. "Combating Infection: Stopping the Itch of Scabies and Lice." *Nursing* 30, no. 7 (July, 2000): 30-31.
Turkington, Carol, and Jeffrey S. Dover. *The Encyclopedia of Skin and Skin Disorders.* 3d ed. New York: Facts On File, 2007.
Weedon, David. *Skin Pathology.* 3d ed. New York: Churchill Livingstone/Elsevier, 2010.

SCALDS. SEE BURNS AND SCALDS.

SCARLET FEVER

Category: Disease/Disorder
Also known as: Scarlatina
Anatomy or system affected: Immune system, skin
Specialties and related fields: Bacteriology, family medicine, internal medicine, pediatrics
Definition: An acute, contagious childhood disease caused by bacterial infection.

CAUSES AND SYMPTOMS

The streptococci constitute a large number of gram-positive cocci, some of which are pathogens. They were originally classified, in the 1930s, by Rebecca Lancefield, into groups based on characteristics of carbohydrates and proteins in their cell walls. The bacteria, *Streptococcus pyogenes,* is the sole species of streptococcus in group A. Group A streptococcus (GAS) causes a wide array of illnesses, most notably pharyngitis (causing strep throat), impetigo, and rheumatic fever. In addition, *S. pyogenes,* causes scarlet fever (which is also known as scarlatina).

The bacteria produce pyrogenic exotoxins A, B, and C, formerly known as erythrogenic toxins, or scarlet fever toxins. These pyrogenic exotoxin-producing strains of GAS are sometimes associated with unusually severe invasive infections including necrotizing fasciitis and streptococcal toxic shock syndrome. Historically, scarlet fever has been associated with toxin A-producing streptococcal strains, but by the late twentieth century there was a prevalence of toxins B and C. Nevertheless, a resurgence of toxin A-producing streptococci has also been observed.

The GAS bacteria are spread by inhalation of air that has been contaminated by the coughing or sneezing of an infected person. Touching your face without washing your hands after contact with contaminated surfaces can also be a source of infection. After exposure, the incubation period is between two and four days. The disease is characterized by a sore throat, fever, and rash; it may follow throat infections and, occasionally, wound infection and septicemia (blood poisoning).

Typically, by the first or second day of GAS illness, the scarlet fever rash may erupt. It is made up of tiny papules that start on the upper trunk that spreads to the extremities, typically sparing the palms and soles. It gives the skin a characteristic "sandpaper" feel when touched. The rash may be accentuated linearly on the skin folds, such as opposite the elbow and the inguinal area. They are called "Pastia's lines." The face may be flushed, with a pale area around the mouth. The mucous membranes of the mouth, throat, and tongue may be covered with a yellowish-white coat. When scraped off, the tongue reveals a "strawberry" red, raw, glazed surface with swollen-appearing papillae. A simultaneous pharyngitis may also occur, commonly known as strep throat.

After the fever and rash subside, desquamation of the skin starts on the face, and spreads to the trunk and then to the hands and feet. Large sheaths of skin may shed in a glove-like and stocking-like distribution, exposing more tender layers, especially at the tips of the fingers and toes. This desquamation may last anywhere from four to eight weeks with minimal, to no long-term scarring. Beau's lines, which are transverse nail grooves, may appear several weeks after skin signs of scarlet fever have cleared.

TREATMENT AND THERAPY

The goals of treatment for scarlet fever are to eradicate GAS infection, reduction of potential complications, and providing education to the patient and caregivers about prevention and anticipatory guidance. Scarlet fever with pharyngitis can predispose to acute rheumatic fever, a feared complication of GAS pharyngitis, which damages the heart valves and worsens over time

Presence of a scarlatiniform rash should prompt treatment. Antibiotic stewardship calls for appropriate use of antibiotics only for people who need them; to avoid unnecessary use of antibiotics in people with nonbacterial illnesses, and to narrow the spectrum of the antibiotic to one that will be most effective for that particular bacterium. Antibiotic treatment for pharyn-

---

> **INFORMATION ON SCARLET FEVER**
>
> **Causes:** Bacterial infection
> **Symptoms:** Sore throat, fever, rash, flushed face (resembling sunburn with goosebumps), pale area around mouth
> **Duration:** Acute
> **Treatments:** Antibiotics, alleviation of symptoms

---

gitis, with or without scarlatiniform rash, is reserved for people who have symptomatic pharyngitis, are negative for viral features (i.e., runny nose, red eyes, cough, hoarseness, etc.), and who also have a positive rapid antigen test or culture for GAS. The Centor criteria is a risk-stratification scoring system used to help guide providers appropriately obtain rapid antigen tests or throat cultures.

For patients with no allergy to penicillin medications, treatment of GAS infection can be with penicillin or amoxicillin. Those with a mild penicillin allergy can use an antibiotic from the drug class of cephalosporins, which are cousins of penicillin. Alternatives for those who are severely allergic to penicillin include macrolides like clindamycin or azithromycin. Penicillin or similar antibiotics may be administered for their prophylactic value, preventing further streptococcal infection and recurrence of the illness during the recovery period.

In mild cases, recovery takes two to three days. To decrease its contagious effect, isolation for the patient for the first twenty-four hours is recommended. A child with scarlet fever should rest and be given plenty of fluids and antipyretics (fever-reducing agents), such as acetaminophen, to reduce discomfort.

PERSPECTIVE AND PROSPECTS

Scarlet fever was first clearly distinguished from measles and other rash-producing diseases in 1860. Fifty years later, Russian scientists associated its cause to streptococcus, a hemolytic microorganism (one that destroys red blood cells). In 1924, George and Gladys Dick isolated the rash-causing substance in the medium used to grow hemolytic streptococci. They applied it to susceptible individuals in an attempt to establish immunity in them, but the technique was not successful. The loss of human life as a result of scarlet fever continued until the development of antibiotics in the 1940s. For an unknown reason, the incidence of the disease had declined drastically by the end of the twentieth century.

—Michael Raghunath, MD

See also: Antibiotics; Bacterial infections; Childhood infectious diseases; Fever; Pediatrics; Rashes; Septicemia; Streptococcal infections.

For Further Information:

Behrman, Richard E., Robert M. Kliegman, and Hal B. Jenson, editors. *Nelson Textbook of Pediatrics*. 18th ed., Saunders/Elsevier, 2007. Text covering all medical and surgical disorders in children with authoritative information on genetics, endocrinology, etiology, epidemiology, pathology, pathophysiology, clinical manifestations, diagnosis, prevention, treatment, and prognosis.

ESCMID Sore Throat Guideline Group, et al. "Guideline for the Management of Acute Sore Throat." *Clinical Microbiology and Infection*, vol. 18, suppl. 1, 2012, pp. 1-28, doi:10.1111/j.1469-0691.2012.03766.x.

Habif, Thomas P. *Clinical Dermatology: A Color Guide to Diagnosis and Therapy*. 4th ed., Mosby, 2004.

Icon Health. *Scarlet Fever: A Medical Dictionary, Bibliography, and Annotated Research Guide to Internet References*. Icon Health, 2004. Designed for physicians, medical students, researchers, and patients.

Kasper, D. L., A. S. Fauci, S. L. Hauser, et al. *Harrison's Principles of Internal Medicine*. 19th ed., McGraw Hill Education.

Kimball, Chad T. *Childhood Diseases and Disorders Sourcebook: Basic Consumer Health Information About Medical Problems Often Encountered in Pre-adolescent Children*. Omnigraphics, 2003. Offers basic facts about common childhood illnesses as well as cancer, sickle cell disease, diabetes, and other chronic conditions in children. Discusses frequently used diagnostic tests, surgeries, and medications.

Leikin, Jerrold B., and Martin S. Lipsky, editors. *American Medical Association Complete Medical Encyclopedia*. Random House Reference, 2003. A concise presentation of numerous medical terms and illnesses. A good general reference.

Professional Guide to Diseases. 9th ed., Lippincott Williams & Wilkins, 2008. This book covers more than six hundred disorders, organized by body system. Each disease entry is complete in itself, defining the disease and describing signs and symptoms, causes and complications, and relevant diagnostic tests.

Shulman, Stanford T., et al. "Clinical Practice Guideline for the Diagnosis and Management of Group A Streptococcal Pharyngitis: 2012 Update by the Infectious Diseases Society of America." *Clinical Infectious Diseases*, vol. 55, no. 10, 2012, pp. e86-102, doi:10.1093/cid/cis629.

Woolf, Alan D., et al., editors. *The Children's Hospital Guide to Your Child's Health and Development*. Perseus, 2002. An authoritative and comprehensive guide to children's health, providing a guide to every common illness or condition that affects children and a carefully designed emergency section.

SCHISTOSOMIASIS

Category: Disease/Disorder

Also known as: Bilharziasis, Katayama fever, swimmers' itch

Anatomy or system affected: Bladder, blood, blood vessels, circulatory system, lungs, urinary system

Specialties and related fields: Environmental health, internal medicine, public health

Definition: A human disease caused by infection by one of several endoparasites of blood flukes.

Key terms:

bilharziasis: an alternative and more regionalized name for schistosomiasis

blood fluke: a parasitic flatworm that belongs to the class Trematoda and subclass Digenia within the phylum Platyhelminthes

cercaria: the tailed swimming larvae of blood flukes

intermediate host: an animal or plant that harbors a development stage in the life cycle of a parasite

primary host: an animal or plant in which adult parasites occur

CAUSES AND SYMPTOMS

Schistosomiasis is a parasitic disease of humans that is prevalent in tropical and subtropical regions of the world. Also called bilharziasis, the disease is caused by blood flukes of the family Schistosomatidae. Five species of blood flukes have been identified as causing schistosomiasis, including *Schistosoma mansoni*, which is widespread across central Africa but also occurs in New World tropics; *S. japanicum* and *S. mekongi* of the Pacific region and a number of African countries; *S. intercalatum*, which occurs widely in Africa; and *S. haematobium* in Portugal, Turkey, and across North Africa. All schistosomes are trematode flukes that belong to the phylum of flatworms called the Platyhelminthes.

Unlike many internal parasites of humans, schistosomes exist as separate male and female individuals. The male *S. mansoni* is about 6 to 10 millimeters in length and has a ventral groove within which the somewhat longer but considerably thinner female resides. The two remain together permanently, paired throughout life.

The life cycle of blood flukes involves two human hosts and an intermediate host, which is a species of freshwater snail. Reproduction occurs in the first human host. The female deposits its eggs in small veins of the intestinal wall or the wall of the urinary bladder, depending on the *Schistosoma* species. The eggs work through the intestinal wall and into the lumen, to be carried away and eliminated with the host's feces or in the urine.

If human waste is deposited on land, then the *Schistosoma* eggs dry and decompose. If it is dropped in freshwater, however, then the eggs hatch, releasing ciliated larvae called miracidium that swim about in search of certain species of freshwater snails. The miracidium burrows into the snail and undergoes asexual reproduction, producing one or two generations of immobile sporocysts. The second generation of sporocysts transform into tailed larvae called cercaria that burrow out of the snail and into the water. The cercaria can survive about forty-eight hours in the water as they swim about in search of a second human host.

Human infection occurs if the swimming cercaria encounter someone wading, bathing, swimming, or walking in shallow water. The cercaria attach to the skin by oral and ventral suckers, discard their tails, and use a combination of muscles and enzymes to bore through the skin and enter the dermal blood vessels as larval forms called schistosomules. Within the blood vessels, schistosomules are carried throughout the circulatory system, eventually arriv-

ing in the pulmonary capillaries of the lungs, where they transfer to systemic vessels that carry them to the portal veins. There, they mature and pair, a female lodging in the gynecophoric canal of a male. Together for life, the pair migrates through the circulatory system to the mesenteric veins of the lining mucosa or to the vesicular veins and begin to produce eggs. A noted departure from this life cycle is seen in *S. haematobium*, which lodges in the walls of the urinary bladder instead of the intestinal veins and voids its eggs into the urine.

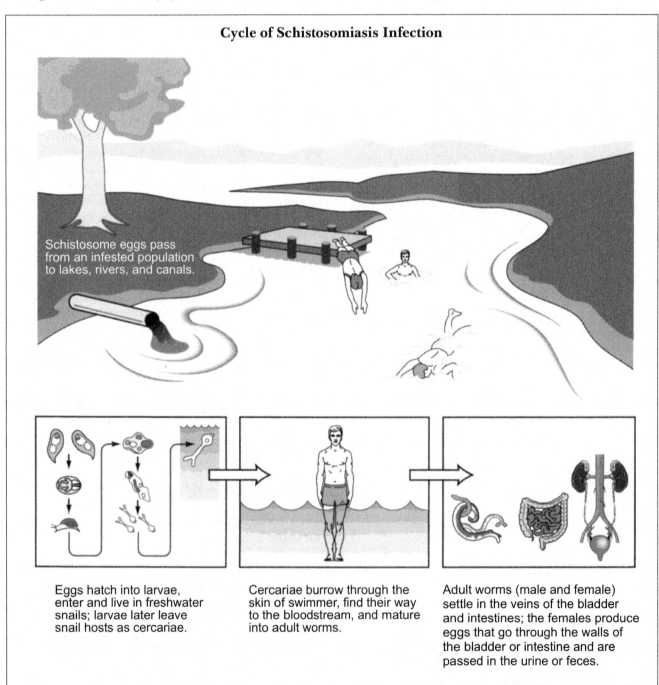

Cycle of Schistosomiasis Infection

Schistosome eggs pass from an infested population to lakes, rivers, and canals.

Eggs hatch into larvae, enter and live in freshwater snails; larvae later leave snail hosts as cercariae.

Cercariae burrow through the skin of swimmer, find their way to the bloodstream, and mature into adult worms.

Adult worms (male and female) settle in the veins of the bladder and intestines; the females produce eggs that go through the walls of the bladder or intestine and are passed in the urine or feces.

The first symptoms of schistosomiasis infection are typically a rash or itchiness that occurs at and around the entry site of the cercaria. These symptoms gradually disappear, but within one to two months additional flulike symptoms such as fever, chills, and muscle aches become evident. These symptoms are typically produced by immunological reaction to the eggs rather than infestation by the blood flukes. Heavy infestations may result in enlargement of the lymph nodes, spleen, and liver; dysuria and hematuria; abdominal pain; and diarrhea.

Pathophysiological injury resulting from schistosomiasis infection may include inflammation, necrosis, and fibrosis produced by the lodging and movement of the eggs in the walls of the intestines and bladder. Movement of the schistosomules in the lungs may also cause respiratory problems.

Some flukes of the Schistosomatidae family cause a condition called swimmers' itch. The blood flukes that cause swimmers' itch are actually parasites of birds and mammals other than humans. The intense "itching" irritation occurs when aquatic cercaria of these species mistakenly try to penetrate into the skin of people who are wading or swimming. The cercaria lodge within the skin and die, producing the intense itching sensations characteristic of swimmers' itch.

TREATMENT AND THERAPY
Schistosoma infections are diagnosed by blood tests that reveal the presence of eggs or chemicals released by the blood parasites. Infections are treated with a battery of safe and effective drugs, including praziquantel, oxamniquine, and metrifonate. The last medication is an effective treatment for urinary schistosomiasis caused by *S. haematobium*.

PERSPECTIVE AND PROSPECTS
Schistosomiasis is an ancient parasitic disease that has plagued humans for centuries. Schistosome eggs have been found in mummies five thousand years old from the upper kingdom of ancient Egypt. Today, schistosomiasis continues to be a debilitating and sometimes fatal disease of humans. It is endemic in the warmer pantropics of the world and in regions where bathing and other sanitation facilities are lacking, including sub-Saharan Africa, the Nile River Valley region, central and northern South America, a number of Caribbean islands, Southeast Asia, the Philippines, Japan, and much of the Middle East. Schistosomiasis also poses a threat to tourists that visit these areas. Schistosomiasis blood flukes do not occur naturally in the United States, but recent immigrants may be infected.

Worldwide, current estimates of infection rates suggest a minimum of two hundred million to three hundred million or more humans infected by one of the

---

INFORMATION ON SCHISTOSOMIASIS

Causes: Parasitic infection with blood flukes through skin exposure
Symptoms: Rash and itchiness at entry site; flulike symptoms (fever, chills, muscle aches); enlargement of lymph nodes, spleen, and liver; dysuria and hematuria; abdominal pain; diarrhea
Duration: Often chronic
Treatments: Medications (praziquantel, oxamniquine, metrifonate)

Schistosoma species of blood flukes, which translates into roughly one in every twenty-five to thirty persons. At this rate of infection, schistosomiasis, along with malaria and hookworm, remains one of the three worst parasitic diseases of humans.

—*Dwight G. Smith, PhD*

See also Parasitic diseases; Tropical medicine; Worms; Zoonoses.

For Further Information:
Mahmoud, Adel A. F., ed. *Schistosomiasis*. River Edge, N.J.: World Scientific, 2001. A general but comprehensive treatment.
Parsonnet, Julie, ed. *Microbes and Malignancy: Infection as a Cause of Human Cancers*. New York: Oxford University Press, 1999. A series of papers presented by experts that explores the relationships between parasitic infections and origin of various human cancers.
Rollinson, David, and Andrew J. G. Simpson, eds. *The Biology of Schistosomes: From Genes to Latrines*. London: Academic Press, 1987. An excellent introduction to the biology, ecology, and epidemiology of *Schistosoma* infections of humans.
Secor, W. Evan, and Daniel G. Colley, eds. *Schistosomiasis*. New York: Springer, 2005. Covers genetics, the host-schistosome interaction with larvae and adult worms, the host immune response to eggs, and public health concerns.
Stephenson, Lani S., ed. *Schistosomiasis and Malnutrition*. Ithaca, N.Y.: Cornell University Press, 1986. This work explores the relationship between blood flukes and malnutrition.
World Health Organization. *The Control of Schistosomiasis: Second Report of the WHO Expert Committee*. Geneva: Author, 1993. Good account of the history of the efforts to control *Schistosoma* infections of humans.

SCHIZOPHRENIA

Category: Disease/Disorder
Anatomy or system affected: Brain, psychic-emotional system
Specialties and related fields: Psychiatry

Definition: A condition characterized by disordered thinking and odd perceptions that cause dysfunction in major activities, sometimes including withdrawal from the world, delusions, and hallucinations.

Key terms:

delusions: a false view or belief of what is real

genetic cause: something that is handed down through the genes

hallucinations: a false or distorted perception of objects or events

hereditary: something that is passed down from generation to generation through the genes

CAUSES AND SYMPTOMS

Schizophrenia is a disorder affecting the brain and mind. Eugen Bleuler (1857-1939), a Swiss psychiatrist, first named the disease in a 1908 paper that he wrote titled "Dementia Praecox: Or, The Group of Schizophrenias." In 1911, he published a book with the same title describing the disease in more detail. Bleuler served as the head of an eight hundred-bed mental hospital in Switzerland and treated the worst and most chronic cases. Beginning in 1896, he embarked on a project to understand the inner world of the mentally ill. He developed work therapy programs for his patients, and he visited them and talked to them almost every day. Bleuler insisted that the hospital staff show the same kind of dedication and support for his clients that he did.

Bleuler's discoveries challenged the traditional view of the causes and treatment of the disease. The traditional view, based on the work of the great German psychiatrist Emil Kraepelin (1856-1926), held that dementia, as it was called, always got worse and that the patient's mind continued to degenerate until death. Kraepelin suggested that the disease, which he called "dementia praecox," was hereditary and was the result of a poisonous substance that destroyed brain cells. Bleuler's investigation of living victims led him to reject this view. Instead, he argued, continuing deterioration does not always take place because the disease can stop or go into remission at any time. The disease does not always follow a downhill course. Bleuler's views promised more hope for patients suffering from schizophrenia.

The word *schizophrenia* can roughly be translated to mean "split mind." This does not mean, however, individuals with schizophrenia have two personalities or two minds. Instead, it refers to how individuals with schizophrenia do not always experience the world as it is. Instead, the world can be one way in their mind and another way in what is going on around them.

The symptoms of schizophrenia are better known than the cause. Diagnosis is based on a characteristic set of symptoms that must last for at least several months. The "psychotic symptoms" include a break with reality, hallucinations, delusions, or evidence of thought disorder. These symptoms are referred to as positive symptoms because they are so readily available. Negative symptoms, which are less readily observed, include withdrawal from society, the inability to show emotion or to feel pleasure or pain, total apathy, and lack of facial expression. A person with negative symptoms might be found simply sitting and staring blankly at the world, no matter what is happening. Schizophrenia can take many forms. Among the most frequent are those that display acute symptoms under the following labels. Melancholia includes depression and hypochondriacal delusions, with the patient claiming to be physically very ill but having no appropriate symptoms. Schizophrenia can also be catatonic, in which patients become immobile and seem fixed in one rigid position for long periods of time. Delusional states can be accompanied by hallucinations. These hallucinations frequently involve hearing voices, which often scream and shout abusive and derogatory language at the patient or make outrageous demands. The delusions can also be visual and involve perceptions of frightening monsters or aliens sent to do harm to the afflicted person.

Disconnected speech patterns, broken sentences, excessive body movement, and purposeless activity usually accompany the symptoms noted above. Victims of the disease also suffer through states of extreme anger and hostility. Cursing and outbursts of uncontrolled rage can result from relatively insignificant causes, such as someone looking at them "in the wrong way." Many times, anniversaries of important life experiences, such as the death of a parent or the birthday of a parent or of the patient, can set off positive and negative symptoms. Hallucinations and mania can also follow traumatic events such as childbirth or combat experiences during war.

The paranoid form of schizophrenia is the only one that develops later in life, usually between the ages of thirty and thirty-five. It is a chronic form, meaning that patients suffering from it usually become worse. Paranoid schizophrenia is characterized by a feeling of suspiciousness of everyone and everything, hallucinations, and delusions of persecution or grandiosity. This form becomes so bad that many victims eventually commit suicide simply to escape their tormentors. Others turn on their alleged tormentors and kill them, or at least someone who seems to be responsible for their terrible condition.

Another chronic form of the disease includes Hebephrenic Schizophrenia. In this case, patients suffer disordered thinking and frequent episodes of incoherent uttering of incomprehensible sounds or words. The victims move quickly from periods of great excitement to equally exhausting periods of desperate depression. They frequently have absurd, bizarre delusions such as perceived sex metamorphosis, identification with god-like creatures, or experiences of being born again and again, literally, and in a sense that is not tied to spiritual or religious practices.

Individuals suffering from "simple" schizophrenia exhibit constant feelings of dissatisfaction with everything in their lives or a complete feeling of indifference to anything that happens. They are usually isolated and estranged from their families or any other human beings. Patients with these symptoms tend to live as recluses with barely any interest in society, in work, or even in eating or in talking to anyone else.

There are several forms of schizophrenia. Each form presents at different points in the aging, or maturation, process. Most often the disease develops during late adolescence but the exception is the paranoid form. Men show signs of schizophrenia earlier than women, usually by age eighteen or nineteen. It is unusual for signs of the disorder to appear in males after age twenty. In women, symptoms may not appear until the early twenties and sometimes are not evident until age thirty. Occasionally, there are signs in childhood. People who later develop schizophrenia tended to be withdrawn and isolated as children and were often made fun of by others. Not all withdrawn children develop schizophrenia, however, and there is no way to predict who will and who will not develop it.

Schizophrenia is a genetic disease. Individuals with the disease are very likely to have relatives—mothers, fathers, brothers, sisters, cousins, grandmothers, or grandfathers—with the disorder. Surveys indicate that 1 percent of all people have the diagnosis. A person with one parent who has the disease is ten times more likely to develop schizophrenia than a member of the general public. Thirty-nine percent of people who have both parents afflicted with the disease will also develop schizophrenia.

As to why the disease develops later in life rather than at birth, investigators provide the following information. First, the brain develops more slowly than other organs and does not stop developing until late adolescence. Many genetic diseases of the central nervous system remain dormant until later in life (e.g., Huntington's chorea).

In 2003, researchers announced that they had discovered clues suggesting a specific gene as the cause of schizophrenia. The gene is known as "dysbindin," and it is involved in the operation of the synapses, the points where one neuron wires itself to another. The team found that genetic variations in the dysbindin gene were more common among schizophrenic patients. Medical research is increasingly pinpointing regions, or loci, within chromosomes that contain ge-

---

INFORMATION ON SCHIZOPHRENIA

Causes: Genetic factors
Symptoms: Varies; may include withdrawal, delusions, hallucinations, thought disorders, inability to show emotion or feel pleasure or pain, total apathy, lack of facial expression, depression, mania, paranoia
Duration: Typically chronic
Treatments: Psychotherapy, drug therapy

---

netic mutations, a task that has proven difficult in years past. Since the human genome sequence has become available, however, research groups have started to focus on the same handful of loci, suggesting that they could be seeing a true signal for the disease. The gene dysbindin has been located in these limited chromosomal regions. Moreover, Icelandic researchers have discovered a gene called "neuregulin-1." Mutations in this gene are highly correlated with schizophrenia in about 15 percent of Icelandic patients. The next step for the research teams will be to examine whether both genes might work together in the regulation of synapses and to see if other scientists can replicate and confirm the initial findings.

TREATMENT AND THERAPY

Since the 1950s, many medications have been developed that are effective in treating the symptoms of schizophrenia. Psychotherapy can also be effective and beneficial to many patients. Drugs can be used to treat both positive and negative symptoms. Antipsychotic medications are commonly categorized into two classes. First-generation antipsychotics (FGAs) were developed in the 1950s, while Second-generation antipsychotics (SGAs) emerged in the 1980s. Each class is considered to have a distinct side-effect profile, although there is considerable overlap between them. FGAs are mainly associated with dry mouth, sedation, and extrapyramidal symptoms, which are movement disorders characterized by repetitive, involuntary muscle movements, restlessness, or an inability to initiate movement. Neuroleptic malignant syndrome is a rare but serious adverse effect. Some, such as Haldol, Mellaril, Prolixin, Navane, Stelazine, and Thorazine, are used to treat positive symptoms. Clozapine and Risperidone can be used for both positive and negative symptoms. These medications work by blocking the production of excess dopamine, which may cause the positive symptoms, or by stimulating the production of the neurotransmitter, which reduces negative symptoms. Clozapine blocks both dopamine and serotonin, which apparently makes it more effective than any of the other drugs. These drugs are nonaddictive and do not provide a high or euphoric effect of any kind.

Unfortunately, these drugs are associated with significant side effects. The most significant side effect, from the point of view of the patient, is tardive dyskinesia (TD). This problem emerges after many years of use. TD is characterized by involuntary movement of muscles, frequent lip-smacking, facial grimaces, and constant rocking back and forth of the arms and the body. It is completely uncontrollable.

Dystonias can also result from use of this class of medications. Symptoms include the abrupt stiffening of muscles, a sudden contraction of muscles in the arms, neck, and face. Most of these effects can be controlled or reversed with antihistamines. Some patients receiving medication suffer effects similar to those movements associated with Parkinson's disease. They suffer from the slowing of movements in their arms and legs, tremors, and muscle spasms. Their faces seem frozen into a sad, masklike expression. These effects can be treated with medication.

Another potential side effect of antipsychotics is akathisia, a feeling developed by many patients that they cannot sit still. Akathisia may respond to benzodiazepines (diazepam, alprazolam, etc.). Some side effects can be severe or embarrassing and patients cite them as the primary reason for not taking their medication.

A shift towards the use of SGAs was partly driven by their lower risk of extrapyramidal symptoms and other adverse side effects. The pharmacology of SGAs is diverse (based on action at several types of receptors) with associated heterogeneity in effects and harms; nevertheless, this class is more prone than FGAs to some adverse effects including weight gain, elevated lipid, and prolactin levels, and development of metabolic syndrome. This risk profile has led to great concern, because of the known associations between weight gain and obesity with diabetes, dyslipidemia, and hypertension, all of which are leading risk factors for future cardiovascular morbidity and mortality.

Many patients report great value in family or rehabilitation therapy. These therapies are not intended to cure the disease or to "fix" the family. Instead, they are aimed at helping families learn how to live with mentally ill family members. Family support is important for victims of schizophrenia because they usually are unable to live on their own. Therapy can also help family members understand and deal with their frustration and the constant pain that results from knowing that a family member is very ill and probably will not improve much. Rehabilitation therapy is an attempt to teach patients the social skills that they need to survive in society.

The results of treatment are not always as successful as the patient or family hope for, even with medication and therapy. Approximately 5 percent of people with schizophrenia commit suicide rather than trying to continue living with the disease.

PERSPECTIVE AND PROSPECTS

Hope for improving the treatment of schizophrenia rests mainly on the continuing development of new drugs. Several studies suggest that psychotherapy directed at improving social skills and reducing stress can help many people with the disease improve the quality of their lives. It is known that stress-related emotions lead to increases in delusions, hallucinations, social withdrawal, and apathy. Therapists can help patients find ways of dealing with stress and living in communities. They encourage their patients to deal with feelings of hostility, rage, and distrust of other people. Family therapy can teach all members of a family how to live with a mentally ill family member. Such therapy, along with medication, can produce marvelous results.

If patients with schizophrenia perceive their social support in a positive way, they are more likely to obtain and cooperate with treatment, reducing rigidity and improving symptoms. Patients diagnosed with schizophrenia who lived with their families, received individual therapy, and took their medications showed far fewer recurrences of acute symptoms than did a group that did not experience the same level of support. For individuals who received therapy but lived alone or with nonfamily members, symptoms of schizophrenia worsened. People living alone usually had more severe symptoms to start out with and found it difficult to find housing, food, or clothing, even with therapy.

—*Shuba Samuel, PhD*

See also: Anxiety; Bipolar disorders; Depression; Hallucinations; Hypochondriasis; Paranoia; Psychiatric disorders; Psychiatry; Psychiatry, child and adolescent; Psychoanalysis; Psychosis; Suicide.

For Further Information:
Barlow, D. H., editor. *Clinical Handbook of Psychological Disorders: A Step-by-Step Treatment Manual*. Guilford Publications, 2021. This collection defines and describes psychological disorders and uses case histories as illustrations for treatment.
The Brain & Behavior Research Foundation, www.bbrfoundation.org/faq/frequently-asked-questions-about-schizophrenia. One section of the site, "Disorders and Conditions," provides excellent information on a range of mental health disorders, including schizophrenia. Site also covers updated research and provides personal stories.
"First and Second-Generation Antipsychotics for Children and Young Adults—Comparative Effectiveness Review Update." *Effective Health Care Program*. Agency for Healthcare Research and Quality, Apr. 2020, effectivehealthcare.ahrq.gov/products/antipsychotics-children-update/research-protocol.

Gorman, Jack M. *The New Psychiatry: The Essential Guide to State-of-the-Art Therapy, Medication, and Emotional Health.* St. Martin's Press, 1996. A well-written, easy-to-understand book by a doctor and researcher that provides the latest information concerning the development of new medications, treatments, and therapies. Valuable information on the new antipsychotic drugs, how they work, and what their possible side effects are.

Gottesman, Irving I. *Schizophrenia Genesis: The Origins of Madness.* W. H. Freeman, 1991. The author, a leading researcher into the genetic causes of schizophrenia, describes recent discoveries on the origins of the disease. He also evaluates different treatments and the many kinds of counseling and therapeutic techniques.

Johnstone, Eve C., et al. *Schizophrenia: Concepts and Clinical Management.* Cambridge UP, 1999. Written in conjunction with colleagues from Edinburgh, Eve Johnstone's book is a useful summary of current knowledge. The suggestion that psychosis can be thought of as occurring along three dimensions—positive, negative, and disorganized—with distinct pathological mechanisms, is well argued but probably still falls short of being an accepted theory.

Miller, R., and S. E. Mason. *Diagnosis: Schizophrenia.* Columbia UP, 2011. Written by professionals to discuss a wide range of issues that impact schizophrenic patients, including hospitalization, rehabilitation, medication, coping skills, social services, and clinical research.

Schizophrenia.com, www.schizophrenia.com. A website of a nonprofit organization dedicated to providing support and information for individuals with schizophrenia, and their caregivers. Volunteers supporting the site include researchers, professors, scientists, family advocates, and people who have schizophrenia.

Sheehan, Susan. *Is There No Place on Earth for Me?* Houghton Mifflin, 1982. A book that provides an accurate, compassionate view of the course of chronic schizophrenia, including the many difficulties faced by victims of the disease. Describes the ineffective care available for many patients in public facilities.

Torrey, E. Fuller. *Surviving Schizophrenia: A Family Manual.* 7th ed., Collins, 2019. Perhaps the best single book on the topic, by a leading medical researcher and advocate of more humane care for the mentally ill. Describes the latest research into the origins of the illness and provides useful information and evaluations of the newest drugs and best forms of treatment.

SCIATICA

Category: Disease/Disorder
Anatomy or system affected: Back, hips, legs, nerves, nervous system, spine
Specialties and related fields: Family medicine, internal medicine, neurology
Definition: Painful inflammation of one of the sciatic nerves.

CAUSES AND SYMPTOMS

The two sciatic nerves are the largest nerves in the body. One runs from the spine down the left leg, the other

---

> **INFORMATION ON SCIATICA**
>
> **Causes:** Vitamin deficiencies, arthritic inflammation in lower spine, prolonged constipation, tumors, slipped disk, pregnancy
> **Symptoms:** Shooting pain down sciatic nerve and extending into hip, thigh, and back portion of leg
> **Duration:** Acute to chronic
> **Treatments:** Surgery, heat application, medications, physical therapy

down the right leg; they supply the tissues of the thigh, lower leg, and foot. The roots of the sciatic nerves are in the lower spinal column. It is here that difficulty is most likely to occur. Inflammation of these nerves is most often caused by a pinching of one or more spinal nerve roots between the vertebrae of the lower back.

Sciatica is characterized by shooting pain down the sciatic nerve and extending into the hip, the thigh, and the back portion of the leg. The pain may occur in all these points at once or skip about from point to point. Sciatica often begins with a long period of intermittent, mild low back pain. Suddenly, however, the slightest movement, such as lifting a weight or merely bending over, may bring about intense sciatic pain.

A mild case of sciatica can be brought on by vitamin deficiencies or by arthritic inflammation in the lower spine. Prolonged constipation can build pressure on the nerve and cause sciatic pain. Occasionally, a tumor may develop near the nerve and press on it. Sometimes, a herniated, or slipped, disk at the level where the nerve roots emerge in the low back may protrude and press on the nerve, thereby causing sciatica.

TREATMENT AND THERAPY

If the sciatic nerve is being compromised, surgery may be indicated. More than 50 percent of patients with sciatica, however, recover on their own in six weeks. In the acute stage, rest is essential. Heat may give temporary relief from pain. The type of medication used depends on the cause of the sciatica. Ultimately, a therapeutic exercise program to develop stabilizing strength and endurance in the trunk muscles is essential for functional recovery.

—*Genevieve Slomski, PhD*

See also Back pain; Lower extremities; Nervous system; Neuralgia, neuritis, and neuropathy; Neurology; Slipped disk.

For Further Information:

Brown, Mark D., and Björn L. Rydevik, eds. *Causes and Cure of Low Back Pain and Sciatica.* Philadelphia: W. B. Saunders, 1991. Discusses the etiology and treatment of low back pain and sciatica. Includes bibliographical references.

Fishman, Loren, and Carol Ardman. *Back Pain: How to Relieve and Cure Low Back Pain and Sciatica*. New York: W. W. Norton, 1999. Discusses the mechanisms of backache and offers some treatment options. Includes bibliographical references and an index.

Gillette, Robert D. "A Practical Approach to the Patient with Back Pain." *American Family Physician* 53, no. 2 (February 1, 1996): 670-678. When treatment is based on a specific diagnosis, when patients are followed proactively to recovery, and when psychosocial factors receive appropriate attention, then the management of back pain will probably be effective.

Hooper, Paul D. *Preventing Low Back Pain*. Baltimore: Williams & Wilkins, 1992. Discusses such topics as the prevention of backache and its treatment, including chiropractic. Includes bibliographical references and an index.

SCID. SEE SEVERE COMBINED IMMUNODEFICIENCY SYNDROME (SCID).

SCLERODERMA

Category: Disease/Disorder
Also known as: Systemic sclerosis, CREST syndrome
Anatomy or system affected: Blood vessels, circulatory system, gastrointestinal system, hands, heart, immune system, joints, kidneys, lungs
Specialties and related fields: Dermatology, gastroenterology, immunology, rheumatology
Definition: A rare autoimmune connective tissue disorder affecting various organs.

CAUSES AND SYMPTOMS

Scleroderma is a connective tissue disease characterized by fibrosis and hardening of the skin and internal organs. The word "scleroderma" is derived from the Greek *sclero*, meaning "hard," and *derma*, meaning "skin." This disease affects roughly 300,000 persons in the United States, with women being affected four times more than men. The disease affects persons between the ages of twenty and fifty.

It is believed that scleroderma is autoimmune in origin. The exact cause of the disease is yet to be discovered, but an overproduction of collagen has been observed in skin biopsies of patients with scleroderma. Two types of the disease have been recognized: localized scleroderma and systemic sclerosis. The localized form of the disease is more common in children and can affect small areas of the skin or muscle or can be widespread, manifesting as morphea and/or linear scleroderma. Morphea affects the skin, with gradually enlarging inflammatory plaques or patches; they may regress spontaneously over time and typically last for months to years. The skin over the lesions appears

---

INFORMATION ON SCLERODERMA

Causes: Unknown, probably autoimmune; may be related to overproduction of collagen
Symptoms: Fibrosis and hardening of skin and internal organs; may include inflammatory plaques or patches, ivory or yellow skin lesions, limb shortening, limited joint mobility, Raynaud's phenomenon, swelling of hands and feet, difficulty swallowing, heartburn
Duration: Chronic
Treatments: Alleviation of symptoms; may include calcium-channel blockers, NSAIDs, antacids and antireflux medications, cyclophosphamide, penicillamine, corticosteroids, topical cortisone ointment, plastic surgery, physical and occupational therapy

---

firm to hard, and the lesions themselves are ivory or yellow in color. Linear scleroderma usually affects a limb or the forehead and, if present early in childhood, can result in permanent limb shortening. This type may also affect the muscles and joints, causing limited joint mobility.

Systemic sclerosis, on the other hand, is a more widespread disease that affects multiple organs, such as the skin, esophagus, gastrointestinal tract, muscles, joints, blood vessels, heart, kidneys, lungs, and other internal organs. This disease usually manifests in adults, with symptoms of at least one or more of the following: Raynaud's phenomenon (extreme sensitivity of the extremities to cold temperatures, with a tingling sensation and the limb turning blue, red, or white upon exposure to cold); thickening of the skin with a leathery, shiny appearance (sclerodactyly); fibrosis and thickening of the joints with decreased mobility; swelling of the hands and feet, with pain and stiffness of the joints; and orofacial abnormalities from thickening of the skin. Some patients may experience symptoms of esophageal, heart, lung, or kidney disease. Systemic sclerosis should always be suspected in every case of difficulty swallowing and heartburn, especially if seen in a middle-aged woman. Patients may complain of nonspecific problems, such as bloating of the abdomen, weight loss, fatigue, generalized weakness, diarrhea, constipation, shortness of breath, and vague aching of joints and muscles. They may also exhibit dryness and redness of the conjunctiva and mucous membranes (Sjögren's syndrome or keratoconjunctivitis sicca).

Some patients experience the CREST syndrome, which is an acronym for *c*alcinosis, *R*aynaud's phenomenon, *e*sophageal dysmotility, *s*clerodactyly, and vascular *t*elangiectasia. Another form of the disease is localized cutaneous systemic sclerosis, which affects mainly the skin of the hands, face, feet and forearms, with Raynaud's phenomenon being the primary symptom.

Diagnosis of the disease is difficult, especially in the initial stages, as the symptoms are common to a variety of immunologically mediated diseases such as rheumatoid arthritis, Sjögren's syndrome, and systemic lupus erythematosus (SLE). The diagnosis is mainly based on clinical findings, an elevated erythrocyte sedimentation rate (ESR), and a skin biopsy showing elevated collagen levels. Sometimes, a positive antinuclear antibody test and a positive rheumatoid factor test may be seen. About 30 percent of patients are positive for the Scl-70 antibody, which is highly specific for the disease. X rays and lung function tests are used to determine the extent of the disease.

Those with the systemic form are prone to various complications, including heart failure, kidney failure, respiratory problems, and intestinal malabsorption.

TREATMENT AND THERAPY

As of the beginning of the twenty-first century, no cure for scleroderma had been found. Each symptom, however, can be treated effectively, and the quality of life can be greatly improved if the disease is detected early in its course. The disease is primarily managed by rheumatologists and dermatologists, owing to the severity of its course and the difficulty of diagnosis. Calcium-channel blockers are used to decrease the symptoms caused by Raynaud's phenomenon, joint pain and stiffness can be treated with nonsteroidal anti-inflammatory drugs (NSAIDs), esophageal dysmotility and subsequent heartburn is treated with antacids and antireflux measures, lung inflammation and fibrosis can be treated with cyclophosphamide, and heart failure and renal failure are treated appropriately with drugs. Penicillamine and corticosteroids are used to treat the fibrosis seen in the disease. In addition, physical and occupational therapy is instituted to improve joint mobility.

Morphea or localized scleroderma can be managed by the application of cortisone ointment to the lesions. This will not reverse or treat the disease completely, but it appears to slow the progression and provide symptomatic relief. Patients are also advised to use sunscreen lotions and moisturizers to soften the skin and prevent sunburn. Plastic surgery may be employed to correct serious deformities.

PERSPECTIVE AND PROSPECTS

Scleroderma is an individual disease, with each patient exhibiting different aspects. This makes diagnosis even more difficult and complicated. Scleroderma is not contagious, and it is not believed to be heritable. It is thought that certain people are inherently more susceptible to the disease, and they develop it only if

environmental or physical trigger factors, such as stress, are activated. Prognosis of the localized form of scleroderma is good, with the lesions resolving spontaneously, and the five-year survival rate for those with systemic disease is 80 to 85 percent. Presently, many clinical trials are being conducted for such treatments as the use of stem cells as a "rebooting" mechanism, alpha interferon, ultraviolet therapy, and even psychotherapy. These approaches appear promising and aim to at least improve the quality of life of patients with scleroderma, if not cure the disease.

—*Rashmi Ramasubbaiah, MD
and Venkat Raghavan Tirumala, MD, MHA*

See also Autoimmune disorders; Collagen; Connective tissue; Dermatology; Dermatology, pediatric; Dermatopathology; Immune system; Immunology; Neurofibromatosis; Rheumatoid arthritis; Rheumatology; Sjögren's syndrome; Skin; Skin disorders; Systemic lupus erythematosus (SLE).

For Further Information:
Brown, Michael. *Scleroderma: A New Role for Patients and Families.* 2d ed. Los Angeles: Scleroderma Press, 2002.
Frazier, Margeret Schell, and Jeanette Wist Drzymkowski. *Essentials of Human Diseases and Conditions.* 4th ed. St. Louis, Mo.: Saunders/Elsevier, 2009.
Kasper, Dennis L., et al., eds. *Harrison's Principles of Internal Medicine.* 16th ed. New York: McGraw-Hill, 2005.
Mayes, Maureen D. *The Scleroderma Book: A Guide for Patients and Families.* 2d ed. New York: Oxford University Press, 2005.
Rakel, Robert E., ed. *Textbook of Family Practice.* 6th ed. Philadelphia: W. B. Saunders, 2002.
Tapley, Donald F., et al., eds. *The Columbia University College of Physicians and Surgeons Complete Home Medical Guide.* Rev. 3d ed. New York: Crown, 1995.

SCOLIOSIS

Category: Disease/Disorder
Anatomy or system affected: Back, bones, musculoskeletal system, spine
Specialties and related fields: Orthopedics, physical therapy
Definition: Abnormal curvature of the spine, often progressive, which can result in severe deformity and associated medical problems.
Key terms:
adolescent scoliosis: curvature of the spine that is diagnosed in the early stages of puberty
Cobb angle: the commonly used measure of the degree of spinal curvature; the angle created by perpendiculars to the top of the first and bottom of the last vertebrae in a curve
idiopathic: referring to a medical condition with no known cause

skeletal or bone age: a measurement of age based on a comparison by an X ray of the bone structure in the left hand with the standards of the Gruelich and Pyle Atlas

spine: the combined spinal cord and the spinal column, a structure central to erect posture and the complex nervous communications system of the body

vertebra (pl. *vertebrae*): the individual bones that are stacked upon one another to form the vertebral column, or spine

CAUSES AND SYMPTOMS

Of all the structures making up the human body, the spine is second only to the closely associated brain in its centrality to human characteristics. Two distinct aspects of human life are deeply involved in the correct functioning of the spine. First, the spinal column protects the spinal cord, which carries out critical message-carrying functions in the body. Second, the spinal column also holds the body erect, a distinctly primate feature. An abnormal curvature of the skeletal structure of the spinal (or vertebral) column is known as scoliosis.

The usual term for the spine, the backbone, is completely misleading. If one really had a backbone, one would be unable to bend, nod, or stretch. The normal spine consists of approximately thirty-three separate bones whose very name, vertebrae, is derived from the Latin verb "to turn." Furthermore, it is essential to know that the normal spine takes the form of four separate curves. Each of these curves is associated with a distinct set of vertebrae. At the very top of the spine are the cervical vertebrae. In the chest area are found the thoracic vertebrae, which support the body when one leans backward and which are the sites of attachment of the twelve pairs of ribs. The largest of the vertebrae, which support the upper body weight, are called lumbar, from the Latin for "loin." At the very base of the spine are two sets of small vertebrae called the sacrum and coccyx.

Although these curves are a vital part of a healthy spine, they are not always obvious because one usually sees people from the front or rear, so that the spine appears straight. If one looks at a person with good posture from the side, however, the gently S-shaped curve of the spine is clearly visible. Deformities involving abnormal spinal curvature toward the front or back are well known, but they are not called scoliosis. The side-to-side curvature of scoliosis is referred to as a lateral curve.

As important as the bones are, the vertebral spine is a much more complicated structure. Along its entire length is a surrounding complex of ligaments and muscles making it possible for the body to bend and straighten again. Within the vertebral column are rub-bery cylinders of cartilage called disks. These disks absorb shocks, relieving the body from the countless pressures of movement. With this array of closely balanced mechanisms and associated forces, it is no wonder that the curvature of the spine is a complex subject for diagnosis and treatment.

Scoliosis can result from a number of different causes. While a birth defect, an accident, poliomyelitis, or muscular dystrophy can all result in lateral curvature, the cause is unknown in the majority of cases. Some authorities believe that 80 percent of all scoliosis cases have no known cause. The technical term for this important class of malady is "idiopathic scoliosis." Within this general subdivision, three separate forms are recognized, based on the age of the patient at the onset of the curvature.

The adolescent form of scoliosis, which is usually recognized between ten and thirteen years of age, is by

Scoliosis

far the most common form. A brief look, however, at infantile (birth to three years) and juvenile (four to ten years) scoliosis will help to illustrate the difficulty faced by researchers in this area and the enormous problems yet to be solved. (All these age groupings refer to the age at which the deformity is first noted, not the age at which the curvature began.)

When the scoliosis is recognized in the youngest range, it is more common in males, with one study giving a 3:2 ratio. By contrast, in the far more common adolescent condition one finds a striking shift to females, who are three times more likely to be affected. While it is often observed that infantile idiopathic scoliosis corrects itself (that is, it spontaneously resolves), this natural remission is rarely observed when the diagnosis is made later. More fascinating but puzzling is the noted absence of the infantile conditions in the United States and Canada, while its occurrence is well documented in Great Britain and France. J. I. P. James, who studied scoliosis extensively at the University of Edinburgh for many years, reported this form to be as common in Europe as the adolescent variety is worldwide. At a subtler level of research, one finds that 90 percent of the curves in infants are formed to the left, whereas 90 percent of those in adolescent girls lie to the right.

It is small wonder that James's collaborator, Ruth Wynne-Davies, calls the cause of infantile scoliosis "multifactorial" and states, "The exact cause in each individual is likely to be different." Wynne-Davies has made important studies of the influence of heredity in producing scoliosis. She, like many others, sees infantile idiopathic scoliosis in a different class from the adolescent variety.

The juvenile condition is likely to be related closely to adolescent scoliosis. As before, there is marked evidence of hereditary influence. In this age range, males and females share equally in the likelihood of being diagnosed. The chance of significant progression of the curvature is so variable that close watching of the patient is the single point of common agreement among specialists. There is concern among parents, patients, and practitioners alike over the excessive use of X rays for diagnosis.

Some research suggests intriguing clues about the cause of scoliosis from unexpected sources. For example, studies at the University of Rochester suggest that in scoliosis patients there may be significant differences in the side of the brain that processes sound. In most people, the left hemisphere of the brain hears and understands phonetic sound as in language, but those people with scoliosis seem much more likely to use both sides or the right side of the brain for these functions. It may be possible that a simple listening test can determine who is at risk for spinal curvature.

INFORMATION ON SCOLIOSIS

Causes: Unknown in most cases; may include birth defects, injury, poliomyelitis, muscular dystrophy
Symptoms: Deformity of spine, curved back, impaired movement
Duration: Chronic
Treatments: Corrective devices (e.g., braces), surgery, exercise, physical therapy

---

A dozen different types of curves associated with scoliosis have been identified, but four major classes are of greatest frequency and concern. In the chest area, one finds the most common of all curve patterns, the right thoracic curve. It is possible for this condition to progress rapidly. Early treatment is essential. As the curve develops, the ribs on the right side shift and create a deformity which not only is unattractive but also can squeeze the heart and lungs; this so-called rib hump can result in serious cardiopulmonary difficulties.

A similar, but gentler, curve is the thoracolumbar curve. It begins in the same region of the thoracic vertebrae and ends farther down the back, in the lumbar region. The twist may be either right or left and is generally less deforming in its appearance. A lumbar curve is found far down in that region of the back, producing a twist in the hips. In pregnant women and other adults, this twist often causes severe back pain.

The three curves described thus far are single, or C-shaped, curves. The double major curve is an S-shaped curve and is the most common of that type. Curvature begins in the thoracic or chest area and is complemented by a second curve in the opposite direction found in the lumbar region. To some extent, the two curves offset each other and the scoliosis is less deforming. The double major curve can progress and become the source of a rib hump.

These and the other less common curves demand an accurate description beyond their location. John Cobb searched for such an important tool and developed the widely used Cobb angle measurement. His suggestion was to relate the top of the first and the bottom of the last vertebrae of a curve by determining the angle formed by the intersection of lines perpendicular to them. It is not difficult, using an X ray of the spine, to draw lines above and below the vertebrae, construct the required perpendiculars, and measure the angle of their intersection. This technique allows physicians to communicate accurately and have a useful measure with which to note the progression, remission, or stabilization of the patient's scoliosis. In addition to degree of curvature, the complex structure of the spine shows rotation in scoliosis. The rotation causes the pedicles or indentations of the vertebrae to shift closer to the midline drawn on the X ray. The relative shift is described as a rotation of +1, +2, and so on.

TREATMENT AND THERAPY

Scoliosis can result from many different causes, each of which demands treatment, as well as the idiopathic variety under discussion. Since there is no known cause, prevention is impossible, and since there are enormous difficulties in predicting the course of the disease, the most that can be achieved is satisfactory correction.

A diagnostic examination for scoliosis demands specific attention to accurate family history. Particularly important is information concerning the first recognition and previous treatment of the condition. Then a detailed evaluation of the nature and extent of the curvature must be made. The examining physician should make certain that the patient is standing straight with the knees unflexed. A simple plumb line is used to examine the patient's back to determine any curvature in the spine. Then the forward bending test is conducted. This observation is considered one of the most reliable diagnostic tools. Various forms of curvature, including scoliosis, can be seen by the trained observer. When viewed at eye level from both front and back, one side of the thoracic or lumbar regions is higher. An accurate measurement of the degree of difference can be made with a level. The use of X-ray photographs also forms a vital part of the diagnostic data.

Even with the best diagnostic skill, training, and experience, the decision concerning the treatment of scoliosis is hardly straightforward. One important consideration is the patient's bone age. Because people grow and mature at such different rates, chronological age may not correspond well to the degree of maturity of that person's skeleton. Many clues are used to determine the bone age, including the degree of fusion observed in the individual vertebra or the bony pelvic girdle. A catalog of X rays of hands is available and provides a useful measure of the bone age. The central concern is that curvature is more likely to progress if the growth and development of the patient's skeleton is still incomplete.

The treatment of scoliosis varies from none at all to extensive surgical procedures. In general, treatment is undertaken for the prevention of further curvature or for the correction of the curvature already present. Some treatments, such as exercise, are of benefit to the patient in general but are seen as having no prospect of arresting or correcting the spinal curvature. Research has also suggested that copper in the diet may play a key role in scoliosis treatment. These studies were carried out with chickens, which show scoliosis very similar to that found in humans, but much remains to be learned about these and similar studies on rabbits, salmon, and quail before much confidence can be placed in the applicability of the data to human treatment or prevention.

Of all the methods proposed, the use of braces and casts is certainly the oldest and the most common. The many modifications of design and material used in braces over the centuries have had the central purpose of forcing the spine to become straight. The evolution of the brace has reached the point of an active or kinetic apparatus called the Milwaukee brace, developed by Walter Blount and Albert Schmidt. It is a carefully designed assembly of a molded plastic pelvic girdle and three metal bars which keep the wearer erect and allow a neck ring to be attached. The neck ring and its associated axillary sling keep the torso balanced and prevent listing to the right or left.

In order for the Milwaukee brace (or any modified versions of it) to be effective, it must be worn day and night and until the growth period of the patient has been completed. It is also imperative that exercise be carried out on a daily basis. There are many advantages of the modern brace over older systems. For example, it can be removed for showering and swimming, and much greater activity is allowed. The one serious drawback is that a patient must not expect correction of the scoliosis. The value of the brace is that it can, with good use and exercise, maintain the already present curvature and prevent further progression.

Only in certain cases will braces be of benefit to the patient. With curves of 40 or 50 degrees, pain that does not respond to treatment, or the failure of the brace to stop the curve's progression, surgery is the most reasonable approach. Surgery can offer some degree of correction, but it is important to recognize that only a partial correction is possible. Even with the safest techniques, pressure must be applied to the spine, creating a serious risk of damage to the spinal cord. Most authorities estimate reasonable correction to be about 60 percent.

Once it is agreed that surgery is the proper route of treatment, a wide range of methods are available. The most common, and generally considered the safest, method is the Harrington rod technique. The incision is from the back (as opposed to front or side entries), and metal hooks are inserted at the highest and lowest points in the curve. These hooks hold metal rods used to straighten the spine and then to hold it in place. Small chips of bone are then taken from the hip or ribs and inserted between especially prepared vertebrae. In a period of six to eight months, solid bone will grow and fuse the vertebrae, giving a solid bone mass of a single elongated vertebra. After the surgery, the patient is usually placed in a brace or cast for four to six months.

The success of the Harrington rod technique has inspired several modifications, such as using two rods to achieve more balance and greater correction. With a patient who has unusually soft bones, a system of wires is used to hold the rods in place. This method is considered superior because the normal hooks might break off. Several variants of the wire technique are also available. Some surgeons thread the wires through the neural canal, and others drill small holes to avoid coming near to the spinal cord.

Another technique which is growing in popularity avoids the use of a Harrington rod. Many small wires are attached through the neural canal and twisted around two thin rods, one on either side of the curvature. This Luque method provides greater stability, and usually there is no need to wear a cast after surgery. These advantages must be balanced, however, against a significantly greater risk of paralysis and a smaller amount of room for new bone growth in fusion.

Another modern technique which is showing some success involves placing small electrodes near the spine and transmitting tiny electrical impulses to nerve endings periodically during sleep. This electronic bracing, or electrosurface stimulation, appears to stop scoliosis curves from progressing in about 80 percent of the cases studied. These devices have about the same limitations as do conventional braces-that is, curves of greater than 40 degrees, curves treated after the end of bone growth, and certain types of lumbar curves will fail to benefit from this treatment.

PERSPECTIVE AND PROSPECTS
One finds the beginning of serious study of the spine in the writings of Hippocrates (c. 460-c. 370 BCE). He described the curves of both the normal and the abnormal spine. He may not have been as clear in his description of scoliosis as with those of the clubfoot or epilepsy, but he was well aware of the difficulty of its treatment and recognized its possible relationship to pulmonary disease. Another celebrated physician of antiquity, Galen (129-c.199 CE), first suggested the medical term for this deformity, scoliosis, in the late years of the second century. Among the complications faced by early medical science were the inadequate methods and equipment available for making subtle diagnoses. Thus it was not until the sixteenth century that Ambrose Pare carefully described the various types of spinal curves. He also noted for the first time that scoliosis is largely a condition of children.

Over the centuries, many men and women added to the array of methods and instruments as well as the store of knowledge and thoughtful speculation about scoliosis. Many possible causes were presented on the basis of observation and research. Many approaches to the treatment of these deformities were described and tested. Yet, despite all this research, scientists are just beginning to appreciate the complexity of the problem of scoliosis.

—*K. Thomas Finley, PhD*

See also Back pain; Birth defects; Bone disorders; Bones and the skeleton; Braces, orthopedic; Casts and splints; Muscular dystrophy; Orthopedic surgery; Orthopedics; Orthopedics, pediatric; Pediatrics; Poliomyelitis; Puberty and adolescence; Spinal disorders; Spine, vertebrae, and disks.

For Further Information:
Eisenpreis, Bettijane. *Coping with Scoliosis*. New York: Rosen, 1999. Designed for students in grades seven to ten, this clearly written and well-organized book looks at the patterns of spinal curvature, treatment options, and emotional effects of this condition.
Griesse, Rosalie. *The Crooked Shall Be Made Straight*. Atlanta: John Knox Press, 1979. While this book does not pretend to offer specific medical information concerning scoliosis, it contains valuable insights for those facing the painful task of fighting this crippling malady. A truly inspiring story.
National Scoliosis Foundation. www.scoliosis.org. Provides updated medical research information, physician referrals, and community support.
Neuwirth, Michael, and Kevin Osborn. 2d ed. *The Scoliosis Sourcebook*. New York: McGraw-Hill, 2001. Origins of the disease, early detection and treatment, the pros and cons of braces, and surgery preparation are topics covered. Also includes a comprehensive list of scoliosis organizations and associations.
Parker, James N., and Philip M. Parker, eds. *The 2002 Official Patient's Sourcebook on Scoliosis*. San Diego, Calif.: Icon Health, 2002. Draws from public, academic, government, and peer-reviewed research to provide a wide-ranging handbook for patients with scoliosis.
Schommer, Nancy. *Stopping Scoliosis: The Whole Family Guide to Diagnosis and Treatment*. Rev. ed. New York: Putnam, 2002. One of the best books written for the layperson that is devoted to the discussion of a medical problem. Includes many references to other information, specialists, and organizations concerned with the study and treatment of scoliosis.

SCOPE OF PRACTICE

Category: Health care system

INTRODUCTION
Scope of practice refers to the range of responsibilities and functions that a particular group of professionals are legally allowed to do within their professional license. Although the term scope of practice can be used in reference to almost any profession, it is most often used in discussions of health care.

For health-care professionals, scope of practice is addressed mainly by law at the state level. These laws are designed by the state in question and create the framework within which the medical services in the state are delivered to the public. These laws determine the professions that are allowed to offer particular services, the settings in which these services can be provided, and the boundaries of professional activities offered by professionals.

OVERVIEW

Scope of practice controls what professionals-such as physicians and therapists-are allowed to do, and sets parameters that prevent health-care workers from engaging in activities that are considered beyond their knowledge and expertise. For example, scope of practice prevents nurses from performing the work of physicians, dental hygienists from doing the work of dentists, psychiatrists from doing the work of general internists, and so on.

Scope of practices control the delivery of medical services and provide a layer of protection to the public, whose members may not understand the education, professional credentialing, and experience required to perform in a particular discipline. The legal guidelines developed by states are often referred to as *practice acts*.

DEVELOPMENT

Although some exceptions exist, state governments are responsible for developing and managing the scope of practice statutes that apply within their boundaries. Dedicated licensing boards are responsible for developing these statutes. These boards are comprised of both members of the profession in question and representatives of the public. The state governor typically appoints licensing board members, and individuals are generally chosen based on their understanding of the education, professional credentialing, and experience needed to offer trustworthy services in a particular discipline.

In addition to creating and enforcing practice acts, licensing boards set the rules and policies that concretely define the behavior of health-care professionals. These rules and policies communicate the intentions of the practice acts and outline what members of the profession are allowed to do.

Because this process is individualized by state, laws and regulations may vary from one state to another. For example, some states may give more latitude to individual professionals, while others may more closely manage their services.

—Marie Keenan;
updated by Patricia Edens

For Further Information:

Christian, Sharon, Catherine Dower. "Scope of Practice Laws in Health Care: Exploring New Approaches for California." *Chcf.org*. California Healthcare Foundation. Web. 16 Nov. 2015. www.chcf.org/publications/2008/03/scope-of-practice- laws-in-health-care-exploring-new-approaches-for-california

McCarty, Michael N., Esq. "The Lawful Scope of Practice of Medical Assistants: 2012 Update." *AMT Events*. American Medical Technologists. June 2012. Web. 16 Nov. 2015. www.american medtech.org/portals/0/pdf/news/scopeofpracticearticle_june %202012.pdf

White, Debbie, et al. "Nursing Scope of Practice: Descriptions and Challenges." *NursingLeadership* 21, no. 1: 2008. Ontario Nurses' Association. Web. 16 Nov. 2015. local70. ona.org/documents/File/pdf/NursingScopeof Practice.pdf

"Why Consumers Need to be Involved in Scope of Practice Reform." *NCSBN.org*. National Council of State Boards of Nursing. Web. 16 Nov. 2015. www.ncsbn.org/Why_consumers_need _to_be_involved.pdf

Derived from: "Scope of Practice." *Salem Press Encyclopedia of Health*. Salem Press.

SCREENING

Category: Procedure
Anatomy or system affected: All
Specialties and related fields: Epidemiology, preventive medicine, public health
Definition: Procedures that are used to detect a potential disease or condition in individuals who have no known signs or symptoms of that disease or condition.

Key terms:

mass screening: screening for all individuals in a defined area or population

multiple or multiphasic screening: a type of screening procedure that uses a variety of tests during the same screening visit

predictive value: the probability in a screening test that a person with a positive test result truly has the disease and a person with a negative test result actually does not have the disease

prescriptive screening: a type of screening procedure that is used for early detection, in presumptively healthy individuals, of disease that can be controlled better if treated early in its natural history

reliability: the ability of a screening test to give consistent results when the test is performed more than once on the same individual under the same conditions

sensitivity: the ability of a screening test to identify correctly those who have a particular disease

specificity: the ability of a screening test to identify correctly those who do not have a particular disease *validity*: the ability of a screening test to measure what it is supposed to measure

yield: the number or proportion of cases of a previously unrecognized disease that is diagnosed and brought to treatment as the result of a screening program

INDICATIONS AND PROCEDURES

In its natural course, a disease usually starts asymptomatically, gradually develops symptoms, and becomes severe when no treatment is given. If the disease can be identified early, especially before it shows any signs or symptoms, then treatment can be initiated early. Early or prompt treatment usually produces a better and more effective cure for a disease. Treatment at the early stage of a disease also has a lower cost than treatment for a disease at its late stages.

The most effective way to detect diseases before they develop symptoms is through screening. Screening is the application of a test or procedure to detect a potential disease or condition in individuals who have no known signs or symptoms of that disease or condition. For example, some people are unaware that they have a high cholesterol level, which can increase the risk for the development of cardiovascular disease. Through screening for cholesterol levels, these individuals can be identified, and proper dietary consultation, exercise prescription, and treatment can be followed to decrease the risk for cardiovascular disease. Screening tests use criteria to classify people according to the likelihood of disease. Screening is just an initial examination. Individuals with positive results from a screening test are required to have a secondary diagnostic examination, which is often more comprehensive and in depth, to confirm the positive finding from their screening test.

Screening tests can be classified into three categories: mass, multiple or multiphasic, and prescriptive. Mass screening means the screening of all individuals in a defined area or population. Multiple or multiphasic screening involves the use of a variety of tests or procedures during the same screening visit. Prescriptive screening is the early detection in presumptively healthy individuals of disease that can be controlled better if treated early in its natural history. From a public health perspective, the following factors are of importance to consider before implementing a screening program. The disease or condition should be a major medical problem. Effective treatment should be available for the disease discovered from the screening test. Follow-up diagnosis and treatment should be available to individuals with positive results from the screening test. The disease should have identifiable early and latent stages. An effective test or examination for the disease should be available. The test or procedure used in screening should be acceptable to the general population. The natural history of the disease should be adequately understood. Policies, procedures, and threshold levels on tests should be determined in advance to clarify who should be referred for further diagnosis and possible treatment. The process should be simple enough to encourage large groups of people to participate. Finally, screening should be done as a regular and ongoing process, not as an occasional activity. Based on these considerations, screening is not necessarily available or suitable for every disease.

Accuracy and effectiveness are important for a screening test; they are evaluated by the characteristics of validity, predictive value, reliability, and yield. The validity of a test means how well the test actually measures what it is supposed to measure. Validity has two components: sensitivity and specificity. Sensitivity is defined as the ability of a test to identify correctly those who have the disease, while specificity is defined as the ability of a test to identify correctly those who do not have the disease. Both sensitivity and specificity are determined by comparing the results obtained from the screening test with the results derived from some definitive diagnostic procedure. Sensitivity is calculated as the proportion of subjects with the disease who have a positive screening test (true positive). Specificity is calculated as the proportion of subjects without the disease who have a negative screening test (true negative). If a screening test has a low sensitivity, then it could misclassify healthy individuals as disease cases (false positive). If a screening test has a low specificity, then it could fail to identify individuals with the disease (false negative). Thus, high levels of sensitivity and specificity are the foundation for the accuracy of a screening test, although it is impossible to have 100 percent of both sensitivity and specificity in practice.

The ability of a screening test to predict the presence or absence of the disease indicates the quality of the test. The predictive value of a screening test is influenced by the sensitivity and specificity of the test as well as the prevalence of the disease, which means how common the disease is in populations. The higher the prevalence of a disease in a population, the more likely a positive test will represent a true positive; the lower the prevalence of a disease in a population, the more likely a positive test will represent a false positive. The predictive value of a screening test can be measured as either positive or negative. The predictive value of a positive test is the probability that individuals with a positive test actually have the disease. On the other hand, the predictive value of a negative test is the probability that individuals who have a negative result from a screening test do not have the disease. Thus, along with sensitivity and specificity, a high level of predictive value is also desirable for an effective screening test. In comparison, sensitivity and specificity are calculated from the screening test results of the diseased or nondiseased individuals, while predictive value depends on the proportion of diseased individuals in the population.

Reliability, also called precision, is another important characteristic of a screening test. A reliable screening test is one that gives consistent results when the test is performed more than once on the same individual under the same conditions. Two common factors affect the consistency of results: the variation of the method used in a screening test and the variation between different observers. These variations usually can be reduced by standardization of procedures or protocols used in a screening test, by training the observers of a screening test, by using more than one observer at the same time with each making independent observations, and by quality control measures, such as periodic checks.

The yield of a screening program is defined as the number or proportion of cases of a previously unrecognized disease that are diagnosed and brought to treatment as a result of the screening program. Several factors can affect the yield of a screening program. If a screening test has a low sensitivity, and therefore identifies only a portion of the diseased individuals, then the yield of the screening test could be poor. If the prevalence of the disease being screened for is low, then the yield of the test could be low even though the sensitivity of the test is high. Using multiphasic screening approaches often increases the cost-effectiveness of a screening program and results in a high level of yield. Frequency of screening is another factor influencing the yield of a screening program. The optimal interval between screenings should be determined by a particular disease's natural course-how long it takes to develop from its first detectability of symptoms-and by different individuals with different risk factors. For example, certain cancers may need to be screened more frequently in older individuals than in younger individuals. The yield of a screening program can also be affected by the proportion of the population participating in the program. Low participation rates could turn out low yields. To increase participation rates in a disease screening program, the population needs to be educated about the disease, including information about the fact that the disease is understood as a serious threat to health, that all individuals are vulnerable to the disease, that the method of the screening test is safe, and so on. The cost of a screening test can also have a significant effect on the participation rate.

Screening is usually concerned with chronic illness. Based on the individuals' ages, gender, occupation, overall health status, lifestyle, and medical and family history, physicians may prescribe specific screening tests. Mass screening programs may be carried out in communities to detect common diseases such as hypertension, high blood cholesterol, type 2 diabetes, breast cancer, colorectal cancer, prostate cancer, and osteoporosis.

USES AND COMPLICATIONS

Some diseases are good candidates for screening. For example, data from the National Health and Nutrition Examination Survey showed that 24 percent of the adult population in the United States had high blood pressure, or hypertension. Almost one in every three African Americans was hypertensive. More than one-third of the individuals with hypertension were unaware of their condition, since hypertension is usually asymptomatic. Hypertension is defined as a blood pressure reading of 140/90 millimeters of mercury (mmHg) or higher. The higher the blood pressure, the higher is the chance of developing hypertension complications, such as coronary heart disease, stroke, renal dysfunction, and sudden death. The treatment of hypertension is very effective. Reduction in blood pressure through treatment can significantly decrease the risk for stroke, coronary heart disease, renal disease, and sudden death. Screening is the best way to detect hypertensive individuals without symptoms. The common method of screening for hypertension is sphygmomanometry that measures cuff pressures. Ambulatory blood pressure monitoring is an alternative method, which uses an automated sphygmomanometer that records blood pressure at frequent intervals over twenty-four hours. Although ambulatory blood pressure monitoring is more accurate, it is also more expensive and impractical, thus, it is not as commonly used as sphygmomanometry. As the benefit of the screening is evident and the risk of sphygmomanometry is nearly none, it is recommended that every adult should be screened for hypertension.

High blood cholesterol is another common condition that is asymptomatic but increases the risk of coronary heart disease and stroke. More than 37 percent of people in the United States have blood cholesterol levels higher than the normal range. Cholesterol comes from food or is produced in the body. When there is too much cholesterol in the blood, it builds up in the walls of the arteries and hardens them, so that the arteries become narrowed and blood flow to the heart or the brain is slowed down or blocked, resulting in coronary heart disease or stroke. Since high cholesterol is asymptomatic, many people are unaware that their level is too high. Cholesterol screening is performed using a blood test after a fourteen-hour fast. This test includes measurements of total cholesterol: both low-density lipoproteins (LDLs), or "bad" cholesterol, the main source of cholesterol buildup and blockage in the arteries, and high-density lipoproteins (HDLs), or "good" cholesterol, which helps keep cholesterol from building up in the arteries. Triglyceride, another form of fat in the blood, may be checked at the same time. A healthy individual should have a total cholesterol level less than 200 milligrams per deciliter, an LDL level less than 100 milligrams per deciliter, and an HDL level greater than 45 milligrams per deciliter. The normal triglyceride level is less than 200 milligrams per deciliter. Individuals aged twenty years or older are recommended to have their cholesterol level checked every five years. Cholesterol screening can raise awareness of high blood cholesterol, so that individuals can modify their lifestyle by consuming less saturated fat and engaging in more physical activity and drug treatment can be initiated, if necessary, to prevent heart disease and stroke. The American Heart Association recommends mass screening for high cholesterol at worksites to identify high-risk populations of middle-aged men and women and in communities targeting low-income, low-education, and minority groups who are often underrepresented in other voluntary screenings.

The number of people with type 2 diabetes is increasing in the United States as a result of the high prevalence of obesity. Complications of diabetes are severe, such as increased risks for cardiovascular disease, kidney failure, blindness, and amputation of the legs. Many people with diabetes are undiagnosed. The natural history of diabetes includes an asymptomatic preclinical phase. The length of this preclinical phase varies and may last ten years or longer. Screening tests can detect diabetes in the preclinical phase. Different tests have been used for diabetes screening: the two-hour postload plasma glucose test, the fasting plasma glucose test, and the test of hemoglobin A1c. The third test has been proposed as a standard reference for diagnosing diabetes. Research studies showed that after diabetes was detected during its preclinical phase, interventions, such as aggressive control of hypertension and cholesterol levels and use of aspirin during the preclinical phase, could reduce the risk of cardiovascular disease. The benefit of tight control of blood sugar levels during the preclinical phase, however, was unclear or minimal. Overall, screening for diabetes has been controversial. The most important gap in the understanding of screening is the lack of information on the added benefits of starting various interventions and treatments earlier, during the preclinical period, compared with at clinical detection.

More than 215,000 women are diagnosed with breast cancer every year in the United States. Approximately one in every eight women will develop breast cancer during her lifetime. Breast cancer is the second

leading cause of cancer death in women. Early detection and effective treatment can reduce the number of women who die from breast cancer. Three approaches are considered for screening for breast cancer: breast self-examination (BSE), X-ray mammography, and clinical breast examination. The sensitivity of BSE and clinical breast examination is unclear, but the sensitivity of mammography is relatively high. The American Cancer Society recommends screening with mammography every one to two years, with annual clinical breast examinations beginning at the age of forty and annual mammography with clinical breast examinations beginning at the age of fifty.

Prostate cancer is the most common cancer and the second leading cause of cancer death in men in the United States. After fifty, the risk of prostate cancer increases with age. African American men have a higher risk for prostate cancer. The principal screening tests for prostate cancer are the digital rectal examination, a blood test of serum tumor markers called prostate-specific antigen (PSA), and transrectal ultrasound. The reference standard for these tests is pathologic confirmation of malignant disease in tissue obtained by biopsy or surgical resection. Because biopsies are not generally performed on patients with negative screening test results, the sensitivity and specificity of screening tests for prostate cancer cannot be determined with certainty. The American Cancer Society recommends an annual digital rectal examination for prostate cancer beginning at age forty. It recommends an annual measurement of serum tumor markers for average men aged fifty and older; however, this measurement should begin at age forty for African American men and those with a family history of prostate cancer. The natural history of prostate cancer is still poorly understood, and there is no direct evidence that prostate cancer screening decreases mortality. The cost associated with the screening tests for prostate cancer is another concern. Thus, screening for prostate cancer remains controversial.

Colorectal cancer is the second most common form of cancer, as well as one of the leading causes of death from cancer in the United States. Since it is asymptomatic at its early stage, about 60 percent of patients with colorectal cancer have regional or distant metastases at the time of diagnosis. The principal screening tests for detecting colorectal cancer are fecal occult blood testing, sigmoidoscopy, and digital rectal examination. Less frequently used screening tests include barium enema and colonoscopy, which have been advocated primarily for high-risk groups, such as persons with a family history of hereditary syndromes associated with a high risk of colon cancer. Screening for colorectal cancer is recommended for men and women aged fifty years and older with annual fecal occult blood testing, sigmoidoscopy, or both. There is good evidence that periodic fecal occult blood testing reduces mortality for colorectal cancer, and there is fair evidence that sigmoidoscopy alone or in combination with the fecal occult blood testing reduces mortality. There is no direct evidence, however, that colonoscopy or barium enemas reduce mortality. The digital rectal examination is of limited value as a screening test for colorectal cancer. The examining finger, which is only seven to eight centimeters long, has limited access even to the rectal mucosa, which is usually eleven centimeters in length. Thus, a negative digital rectal examination performed by a physician provides little reassurance that the patient is free of colorectal cancer.

It is estimated that in the United States 1.3 million people experience a fracture each year as a result of osteoporosis, or fragile bones. Osteoporosis can progress painlessly until a bone breaks. Over half of all postmenopausal women will develop a spontaneous fracture as a result of osteoporosis. Hip fractures and vertebral deformities, two common consequences of osteoporosis, can result in significant pain, disability, decreased functional independence, and death. Low bone density is strongly associated with an increased risk of fracture. The World Health Organization (WHO) defines osteoporosis as a bone mineral density of 2.5 or more standard deviations below the mean of healthy young adult women. A number of tests are available to measure bone density, including conventional skeletal radiographs, quantitated computed tomography, single photon absorptiometry, dual photon absorptiometry, and dual energy X-ray absorptiometry. The correlations among different bone density devices are low. Dual energy X-ray absorptiometry is considered the gold standard because it is the most extensively validated test against fracture outcomes. The likelihood of being diagnosed with osteoporosis depends on the number of tested sites, which include the forearm, hip, spine, or heel. Because women over age sixty-five have a significantly increased risk of osteoporosis, routine screening in this population is recommended. For women aged sixty to sixty-four, screening may be needed if they have risk factors, such as low body weight, family history, smoking, and removal of the ovaries before age forty-five. The screening intervals should be two years for women aged sixty-five years and older and five years for women younger than sixty-five. Once osteoporosis is diagnosed, changing lifestyle, such as an increase in dietary calcium and vitamin D intake, weight-bearing exercise, and smoking cessation, along with drug treatment, can help prevent fractures.

Other common screening procedures include those meant to detect cervical cancer, testicular cancer, skin cancer, carotid artery stenosis, peripheral arterial disease, abdominal aortic aneurysm, thyroid disease, iron deficiency anemia, sexually transmitted diseases, visual impairment, hearing impairment, phenylketonuria (PKU), Down syndrome, dementia, and depression.

PERSPECTIVE AND PROSPECTS

By the middle of the twentieth century, infectious diseases were gradually replaced by chronic diseases as the leading causes of death in developed countries such as the United States. This transition occurred as a result of improvement in living standards and nutritional status, the prevention of infectious diseases through immunization, and increased life expectancy. Hence, prevention of chronic disease became an important task in public health and medicine practices in developed countries. In 1951, the United States multi-sponsored Commission on Chronic Illness organized the Conference on Preventive Aspects of Chronic Diseases and advocated screening for diseases. Since then, more and more screening tests and procedures have become available for different diseases and conditions because of development in medical technologies.

At the beginning of the twenty-first century, however, chronic diseases were still the leading cause of death in developed countries as well as some developing countries. The most important chronic diseases that contribute to mortality are heart disease, cancer, and stroke. Many aspects of screening for these chronic diseases remain unclear. For some diseases, no tests or no effective tests are available, such as for lung cancer. For other conditions, powerful methods of detection exist but no effective treatments are available, such as for human immunodeficiency virus (HIV). Many screening procedures still lack evidence to support their effectiveness or justification for the balance between benefit, harm, and cost. Therefore, further investigations, epidemiological studies, development of low-cost and effective screening methods, and increases in participation in screening through health education are the future challenges.

—*Kimberly Y. Z. Forrest, PhD*

See also Acquired immunodeficiency syndrome (AIDS); Anemia; Apgar score; Biostatistics; Blood testing; Breast cancer; Cancer; Cervical, ovarian, and uterine cancers; Chlamydia; Cholesterol; Chorionic villus sampling; Colonoscopy and sigmoidoscopy; Colorectal cancer; Colorectal polyp removal; Diabetes mellitus; Diagnosis; Disease; Down syndrome; Epidemiology; Genetic counseling; Genetic diseases; Genetics and inheritance; Genomics; Glaucoma; Gonorrhea; Hearing tests; Heart disease; Hepatitis; Human immunodeficiency virus (HIV); Human papillomavirus (HPV); Hypertension; Laboratory tests; Mammography; Niemann-Pick disease; Noninvasive tests; Pap sampling; Phenylketonuria (PKU); Physical examination; Pregnancy and gestation; Preventive medicine; Prostate cancer; Rh factor; Sexually transmitted diseases (STDs); Sickle cell disease; Skin cancer; Spina bifida; Syphilis; Tay-Sachs disease; Testicular cancer; Thyroid disorders; Ultrasonography; Vision disorders; Well-baby examinations.

For Further Information:

Holland, Walter W., and Susie Stewart. *Screening in Disease Prevention: What Works?* Seattle: Radcliffe, 2005. This book discusses different issues in screening for diseases in children, adults, and the elderly.

Snow, Vincenza, ed. *Screening for Diseases: Prevention in Primary Care.* Philadelphia: American College of Physicians, 2004. This book summarizes research findings of screening for major diseases, such as breast cancer, prostate cancer, colorectal cancer, hypertension, type 2 diabetes, and osteoporosis.

Thorner, Robert M., and Quentin R. Remein. *Principles and Procedures in the Evaluation of Screening for Disease.* Washington, DC: Government Printing Office, 1961. This classic monograph provides guidelines and methods for evaluating the effectiveness of screening programs.

U.S. Preventive Services Task Force. *Guide to Clinical Preventive Services.* Washington, DC: Agency for Healthcare Research and Quality, 2006. Offers guidelines for physicians, students in health fields, and the general public on the use of clinical preventive services. Contains detailed screening information for various health conditions.

Scurvy

Category: Disease/Disorder

Anatomy or system affected: Blood vessels, eyes, gums, kidneys, muscles, teeth

Specialties and related fields: Nutrition, preventive medicine

Definition: An illness that results from a deficiency of vitamin C (ascorbic acid) in the diet.

CAUSES AND SYMPTOMS

Scurvy is a disease characterized by hemorrhages in body tissue, muscular pain, tender gums, physical exhaustion, and vision disorders, especially night blindness. In advanced cases, teeth fall out, and complications with kidney or intestinal functions may lead to death. The disease at one time was common among sailors who went on long ocean voyages where their diet did not include fruits and vegetables containing vitamin C. Also, the populations of cities under siege and prisoners with very restricted diets often suffered from scurvy. During the American Civil War in the 1860s, scurvy was reported as a problem among the troops.

TREATMENT AND THERAPY

A causal connection between scurvy and a person's diet had been suspected for a long time, but the particular

---

> **INFORMATION ON SCURVY**
>
> **Causes:** Vitamin C deficiency
> **Symptoms:** Hemorrhaging, muscle pain, tender gums, exhaustion, visual disorders (especially night blindness), tooth loss
> **Duration:** Chronic
> **Treatments:** Synthetic or natural vitamin C

missing nutrient was not known until the work of a Scottish physician, James Lind, in the 1750s. Lind experimented on six pairs of patients who had scurvy symptoms, giving them one of six different acidic diet supplements: vinegar, seawater, sulfuric acid solution, apple cider, garlic and mustard seed, or two oranges and a lemon. He found that the men who ate the citrus fruit improved rapidly, the ones who drank the cider recovered slowly, and the others showed no improvement. The British navy adopted a requirement for lemon juice aboard its ships in 1795, which virtually eliminated scurvy. Subsequently, lemons were replaced by limes, which led to the nickname Limeys for British sailors.

The essential nutrient in citrus fruits, now known as vitamin C, was first identified in 1932 by C. G. King and W. A. Waugh at the University of Pittsburgh. Its scientific name is ascorbic acid, which means "without scurvy." Synthetic vitamin C is identical to the naturally occurring variety, in both its composition and its physiological effect. Vitamin C is essential for the formation and repair of collagen, which is a primary component of blood vessels. It is also necessary for the synthesis of hormones that control the rate of metabolism in the body.

PERSPECTIVE AND PROSPECTS

During the nineteenth century, medical research by the so-called microbe hunters had firmly established that bacteria are the cause of numerous diseases that are transmitted from person to person. Some illnesses, however, were shown to be completely unrelated to bacteria but rather attributable to dietary deficiencies. Among these disorders are beriberi, rickets, anemia, and scurvy. They have been almost totally eradicated as people have learned that a healthy diet must include fruits, vegetables, whole grain foods, and vitamin supplements.

—*Hans G. Graetzer, PhD*

See also Malnutrition; Nutrition; Vitamins and minerals.

For Further Information:

Consumer Guide, editors of. *Complete Book of Vitamins and Minerals.* Lincolnwood, Ill.: Publications International, 1996.

Kasper, Dennis L., et al., eds. *Harrison's Principles of Internal Medicine*. 16th ed. New York: McGraw-Hill, 2005.
"Medicine and Surgery, History: Nutrition." In *The New Encyclopaedia Britannica*. 15th ed. Chicago: Encyclopædia Britannica, 2002.

SEASONAL AFFECTIVE DISORDER

Category: Disease/Disorder
Also known as: Recurrent major depression with seasonal pattern
Anatomy or system affected: Nervous system, psychic-emotional system
Specialties and related fields: Psychiatry
Definition: A subtype of depression characterized by seasonal fluctuation.
Key terms:
hypersomnia: a condition in which sleep periods are excessively long
major depressive episode: a group of symptoms that include depressed mood and a loss of interest or pleasure that must be identified before a psychiatric disorder of depression can be diagnosed
phototherapy: light therapy first introduced in 1984 to treat seasonal affective disorder

CAUSES AND SYMPTOMS

For a person to be diagnosed with seasonal affective disorder, the criteria for a major depressive episode as defined in the *Diagnostic and Statistical Manual of Mental Disorders: DSM-V* (5th ed., 2013) must be met. These criteria include having a depressed mood for most of the day, nearly every day, for a two-week period. Signs of a depressed mood can include reports of feeling sad, empty, or tearful. In addition, loss of interest or pleasure in almost all activities for most of the day, nearly every day, for at least two weeks can be part of a major depressive episode. If either of these two criteria is identified, then the patient must show four or more of the following symptoms: significant weight loss when not dieting or weight gain of more than 5 percent of body weight within a month, insomnia or hypersomnia nearly every day, psychomotor agitation or retardation nearly every day, fatigue or loss of energy nearly every day, feelings of worthlessness or inappropriate guilt, diminished ability to think or concentrate, and recurrent thoughts of death or suicide ideation. If the patient has experienced two recurrent major depressive episodes in the last two years that demonstrate temporal relationship to season, then a diagnosis of seasonal affective disorder can be made.

In addition to the *DSM-V* criteria for major depressive episode, a person with seasonal affective disorder may experience several other symptoms. Anxiety is a common symptom of depression and affects as many as 90 percent of all persons with depression. The depressed person often loses interest in sexual activities, and female patients may experience abnormal menstruation. About two-thirds of all depressed patients contemplate suicide, and approximately 10 to 15 percent complete suicide. It should be noted that some depressed persons do not complain of mood disturbance even as they are withdrawing from family, friends, and activities. The majority of depressed persons complain about reduced energy and difficulty finishing tasks. Thus, they become impaired at school or work and lack the motivation to begin new projects.

Seasonal patterns of depression can also be identified among patients who have bipolar disorder. In this disorder, the patient experiences both major depressive episodes and elated moods. When a patient shows an elevated, expansive, or irritable mood that is excessive and impairs daily functioning, then a manic episode can be diagnosed. The elevated mood is euphoric and leads the person to engage in excessive behaviors that demonstrate poor judgment. These patients have an unlimited amount of energy and continue their activities without the need for sleep or rest. If a person experiences both manic episodes and recurrent major depressive episodes during certain seasons of the year, then the patient has a bipolar disorder with a seasonal pattern.

The causes of seasonal affective disorder are not well understood, but they probably involve dysfunction in a number of hormones and neurotransmitters, genetic influences, and personality. The seasonal mood changes have led to particular interest in studying the circadian rhythms of these individuals. Many studies have found that the circadian rhythms of persons with seasonal affective disorder are phase-delayed relative to the sleep-wake cycle. Seasonal affective disorder is considered an abnormal response to seasonal changes in length of the day and appears related to the photoperiod between sunrise and sunset. The hormone melatonin, which helps to regulate sleep-wake cycles, has been implicated. Melatonin is secreted by the pineal gland in response to darkness and is suppressed by bright light that enters through the retinal-central nervous system pathway. Genetic studies have shown that between 35 and 69 percent of persons with seasonal affective disorder have a family history of depression, and 7 to 37 percent have a family member who had seasonal depression.

Seasonal affective disorder is diagnosed following a clinical interview with the patient in order to identify the *DSM-V* criteria. The patient provides self-reports of possible symptoms, and the interviewer observes the person for any signs of depression that could fulfill the diagnostic requirements. In addition, seasonal affective disorder may not occur in isolation. Individuals may also suffer from other mental health problems, such as substance use disorders. Therefore, in addition to diagnosing seasonal affective disorder, the diagnostic process should also focus on ruling out other conditions that may demand additional or specialized treatment.

TREATMENT AND THERAPY

Phototherapy or light therapy involves exposing the patient to a bright light and is the dominant treatment for this disorder. The individual sits in front of a specific type of therapeutic light source for approximately one to two hours, usually in the morning each day. Light visors with a light source built into the brim also may be used for treatment. Light therapy can be challenging for some individuals because they must build time into their schedules to be exposed to the light. Future treatments in this area are likely to seek ways of better integrating exposure to light into the environment and activities of those affected. Light visors were a step in this direction, and other convenient methods can be expected.

Other treatment methods that help with major depressive disorder have been found to help with seasonal affective disorder. Cognitive behavior therapy (CBT) and antidepressant medication are often used in conjunction with phototherapy. Serotoninergic antidepressants are most often used to augment light therapy.

PERSPECTIVE AND PROSPECTS

Prevalence rates point to the fact that winter seasonal affective disorder is more common than any other seasonal pattern. Evidence exists that people living in northern climates have a higher incidence of the disorder than do those living at other latitudes. Individuals with seasonal affective disorder typically experience depression as the amount of daylight decreases with advancing winter. Women have been found to represent at least 75 percent of patients with seasonal depression, being two to four times as likely than men to

develop this problem. Most individuals who will develop this problem do so in their twenties and thirties. The rates of newly diagnosed seasonal affective disorder tend to decrease during the fifties and markedly decrease after age sixty-five. Understanding these age-related trends is likely to be a focus of future research that may perhaps uncover new understandings of the etiology of and treatment for the disorder.

—*Kendi Tang, DO*

See also: Antianxiety drugs; Antidepressants; Anxiety; Bipolar disorders; Depression; Emotions: Biochemical causes and effects; Light therapy; Pharmacology; Psychiatric disorders; Psychiatry; Sleep; Sleep disorders; Suicide.

For Further Information:
Lee, T. "Seasonal Affective Disorder." *Clinical Psychology: Science and Practice*, vol. 5, 1998, pp. 275-90.
Partonen, Timo, and Andres Magnusson, editors. *Seasonal Affective Disorder: Practice and Research*. 2nd ed., Oxford University Press, 2010.
Rosenthal, Norman E. *Winter Blues: Everything You Need to Know to Beat Seasonal Affective Disorder*. Guilford Press, 2006.
"Seasonal Affective Disorder (SAD)." *American Psychiatric Association*, www.psychiatry.org/patients-families/depression/seasonal-affective-disorder. Accessed 27 Jan. 2022.
Young, M., and P. Meaden. "Which Environmental Variables Are Related to the Onset of Seasonal Affective Disorder?" *Journal of Abnormal Psychology*, vol. 106, 1997, pp. 554-62.

SEIZURES

Category: Disease/Disorder
Anatomy or system affected: Brain, head, muscles, musculoskeletal system, nerves, nervous system
Specialties and related fields: Neurology, pediatrics
Definition: Asynchronous, paroxysmal discharges of neurons in the brain that result in body movements, unusual sensations, altered perceptions, and/or hallucinations that interfere with normal function and behavior.
Key terms:
aura: the initial event signaling the beginning of a seizure
clonic: referring to the alternate contraction and relaxation of muscles
convulsion: an involuntary contraction of the body musculature, tonic or clonic, that can be of either cerebral or spinal origin
epilepsy: a chronic brain disorder of various causes, characterized by recurrent seizures resulting from the excessive discharge of cerebral neurons
seizure: an unsynchronized, paroxysmal discharge of neurons in the brain that results in body

movements, unusual sensations, altered perceptions, hallucinations, or various mixtures of such symptoms; also called an ictus

tonic: characterized by tension or contraction, especially muscular tension

CAUSES AND SYMPTOMS

Seizures can be divided into two fundamental groups-partial and generalized. In partial seizures, the abnormal discharge of neurons usually arises in a portion of one hemisphere and may spread to other parts of the brain during a seizure. Generalized seizures, however, have no evidence of localized onset; the clinical manifestations and abnormal electrical discharge give no indication of the locus of onset of the abnormality, if such a locus exists.

Partial seizures are divided into three groups: simple partial seizures, complex partial seizures, and partial seizures secondarily generalized. Simple partial seizures are associated with the preservation of consciousness and unilateral hemispheric involvement. The area of seizure may spread until the entire side is involved. This type of seizure, with motor, sensory, or autonomic signs, was originally called Jacksonian epilepsy. Complex partial seizures are associated with alteration or loss of consciousness and bilateral hemispheric involvement. A partial seizure secondarily generalized is a generalized tonic-clonic seizure that proceeds directly from either a simple partial seizure or a complex partial seizure. The distinction between simple partial seizures and complex partial seizures is clarified by the observation that neurologic problems that are confined to one hemisphere, such as a unilateral cerebral stroke, generally spare consciousness, whereas bilateral cerebral (or brain stem) involvement causes alteration of consciousness.

If there is no evidence of localized onset, then the attack is a generalized seizure. Generalized seizures are more heterogeneous than partial seizures. The generalized seizures include generalized tonic-clonic (grand mal), absence (petit mal), atonic, myoclonic, clonic, and tonic seizures.

Tonic-clonic seizure is a common seizure pattern with sudden loss of consciousness, tonic contraction of muscles, loss of postural control, and a cry caused by contraction of respiratory muscles forcing exhalation. This is followed by a generalized contraction of the muscles of the four extremities. After two to five minutes of unconsciousness and the cessation of clonic contractions, the individual gradually regains consciousness. Fecal and urinary incontinence, as well as biting of the tongue, may occur. The individual does not remember the event and may not be completely functional for several days.

The absence seizure usually begins in childhood or early adolescence, and in many cases individuals outgrow the condition. Although unresponsiveness is the rule, motionlessness occurs in less than 10 percent of absence attacks; in fact, phenomena such as mild clonic motion and increased or decreased postural tone may accompany such attacks. Absence seizures are generally brief, usually lasting less than ten seconds and very rarely longer than forty-five seconds. The attacks are not associated with auras, hallucinations, or other symptoms characteristic of partial seizures, generalized tonic-clonic seizures, or infantile spasms. Individuals exhibiting these seizures are normal except for the seizures, but the seizures may occur as frequently as one hundred times a day.

Atonic seizures are characterized by a sudden loss of muscle tone. Myoclonic seizures are sudden and brief contractions of a single group of muscles or of the entire body. The patients fall but do not lose consciousness. Clonic and tonic seizures are characterized by alternation of contraction and relaxation and by contraction, respectively.

Infantile spasms are generalized seizures occurring in the first year of life. These are synchronous contractions of the muscles of the neck, trunk, and arms. About 90 percent of infants experiencing these attacks are mentally deficient.

Seizures may be further subdivided into epileptic (those involving recurrent seizures) and nonepileptic. The term "nonepileptic seizure," however, is somewhat problematic. For example, a seizure caused by hypoglycemia (low blood sugar) may not be considered an epileptic attack by some because it is a transient event easily corrected by metabolic manipulation. Of the organic nonepileptic seizures, the most common are of cardiovascular origin; others are caused by transient cerebral ischemia, movement disorders, toxic or metabolic problems, sleep disorders, and even headaches. Nonepileptic attacks may also be of nonorganic or psychiatric origin, such as with hysteria and schizo-

---

INFORMATION ON SEIZURES

Causes: Often unknown; may include hypoglycemia, cardiovascular disorders, TIAs, movement disorders, toxic substances, metabolic disorders, sleep disorders, headaches, brain tumors, progressive neurological disease, fever, infection

Symptoms: Uncontrolled body movements, unusual sensations, altered perceptions, hallucinations that interfere with normal function and behavior

Duration: Acute to chronic

Treatments: Drug therapy, neurosurgery

phrenia, in which case they are called psychogenic seizures or pseudoseizures.

Attempts to find a cause for the sudden abnormal discharge of cerebral neurons has not been possible in all types of seizure activity. In some cases, a brain tumor, scar tissue remaining from trauma to the brain, or a progressive neurological disease may be responsible. In the great majority of cases, however, no pathologic basis for the seizures is evident, either during life or at autopsy. The latter type of seizure has been classified as "idiopathic." In certain circumstances, for example, fever, infection, or hyperglycemia, the response may include seizure. In many instances, these events are isolated and do not recur, and for this reason they are not categorized as epilepsy.

The cause of a seizure is related to the age of onset of the first attack. When seizures begin in the neonatal and infant period, the most likely causes are perinatal anoxia (a deficiency of oxygen), congenital brain defects, meningitis, birth injuries, or other metabolic problems, such as hypoglycemia or hypercalcemia (excessive calcium). Less common causes of seizures in young children include toxins such as lead poisoning, as well as rare degenerative diseases. In older children or adults, although metabolic or degenerative processes must be considered, other causes become more probable.

Head trauma accounts for the origin of many partial epileptic seizures in young adults, whereas brain tumors and vascular diseases are the major cause of such seizures in later life. Brain tumor is not a common cause of epilepsy in children, since 60 to 70 percent of brain tumors in children are located in the posterior fossa. Arteriosclerotic cerebrovascular disease is the most common cause of seizures in patients over the age of fifty. In about 4 percent of patients with brain infarction and 10 percent of those with intracerebral hemorrhage, seizures accompany the stroke; an additional 3 percent of patients who experience a stroke have recurrent seizures in later life, presumably generated by the cerebral scar.

Most idiopathic seizure activity appears to have its origin in an inherited propensity to cerebral dysrhythmia. Although there is a high incidence of electroencephalographic (EEG) abnormalities in close relatives of persons with recurrent seizures, not all family members have clinical seizures. In general, genetic factors are particularly important when recurrent seizures begin in childhood and decrease in importance with age.

In most studies of early seizures predicting future epilepsy, the conditions that are associated with high risk include a depressed skull fracture, an acute intracerebral hematoma, post-traumatic amnesia lasting more than twenty-four hours, and the presence of tears in the dura mater of the brain or focal neurologic signs.

Generalized tonic-clonic seizures sometimes develop during the course of chronic intoxication with alcohol or barbiturates, almost always in association with withdrawal or reduction of the drugs. How long a period of chronic drug intoxication or abuse must last to produce seizures upon withdrawal is uncertain, but such patients often give a history of many years (sometimes decades) of drug dependence. Usually, the patients experience one or more seizures or short bursts of two to six seizures over a period of hours. An episode of alcohol withdrawal rarely precipitates more than a single burst of convulsions, while convulsions may recur for several days after barbiturate withdrawal. Studies have shown that among those who have had withdrawal seizures without other evidence of neurological damage, seizures almost always occurred during the seven-hour to forty-eight-hour period following cessation of drinking. With alcohol withdrawal seizures, tremor, anorexia, and insomnia follow the seizure in perhaps 20 to 30 percent of cases. Delirium tremens is a less frequent event.

TREATMENT AND THERAPY
Prior to treatment, it is necessary for the physician to conduct a thorough investigation of the patient to identify any remediable cause of the seizures. This investigation would include metabolic diseases, endocrine system disturbances, cerebral tumors, abscess of the brain, or meningitis.

Persons who have recurrent convulsions controlled by medications can participate in sports and lead a relatively normal life; most countries will permit a person to drive an automobile if he or she has experienced no seizures for six months to one year. If seizures are uncontrolled, however, then automobile driving, swimming, the operation of unguarded machinery, and ladder climbing are not advised.

Drug therapy varies with the type of seizure presented. In the case of recurrent seizures, it generally consists of at least two to four years of daily medication. Careful neurologic examinations every four to six months, monitoring of seizure frequency correlated with drug blood level, and serial EEGs about once a year are also required. If there is a change in seizure frequency despite adequate drug blood levels, if there are focal neurologic signs or signs of increased intracranial pressure, or if evidence of focal changes on EEGs develop, further evaluation, including a computed tomography (CT) scan, is necessary. A small brain tumor may not be apparent even on a CT scan at the time of the initial evaluation, particularly in a patient with adult-onset epilepsy or in an older child or adolescent with partial seizures without a documented specific cause.

Absence seizures present less urgency. The patient rarely seeks medical advice until repeated episodes have occurred. Early treatment and prevention or reduction of repeated seizures can be beneficial. The drugs of choice for absence epilepsy are ethosuximide or valproate sodium. Medication is generally discontinued after two to four seizure-free years, depending on the presence or absence of generalized tonic-clonic seizures and the results of the EEGs. After the medication is discontinued, and after follow-up for fifteen to twenty-three years, there is about a 12 percent incidence of recurrence.

If the seizure process is strong enough to require more than one drug, multiple drug administration needs to be maintained. The aim of the treatment is to achieve the best possible seizure control with the least amount of side effects. This goal may necessitate a compromise in patients with resistant seizures; such patients may prefer having an occasional seizure to being continuously sedated or unsteady. This is particularly true with patients who experience partial seizures that are not excessively disruptive.

The side effects of drugs may cause impairment of liver function in susceptible individuals. Thus, periodic monitoring of the patient's complete blood count and platelet count is necessary, as are liver function tests. This monitoring is done more frequently at the onset of therapy or after an upward adjustment of dosage.

The selection of specific drugs to be used for the prevention and control of seizures depends on the type of seizure. The most commonly used drugs include phenytoin, carbamazepine, phenobarbital, primidone, ethosuximide, methsuximide, clonazepam, valproate sodium, and trimethadione.

The pharmacokinetics and side effects of these drugs in infants and children differ somewhat from those observed in older children and adults. Absorption, plasma-protein binding, and metabolism are subject to age-specific variations. Younger children usually require a higher dose per kilogram to maintain a therapeutic blood level than do adults. Some of the classic signs of toxicity to the medications that are seen in adults may not be obvious in children.

If the seizures are related to a lesion in the brain, neurosurgical treatment is indicated. Surgery is the obvious form of treatment for demonstrable structural lesions such as cysts lying in accessible areas of the cerebral hemispheres. In a more restricted sense, surgical therapy is considered in patients without a mass lesion when the seizures are unresponsive to drug treatment and the patient has a consistent, electrophysiologically demonstrable focus emanating from, for example, a scar. Specific surgical treatments vary from case to case.

Up to 80 percent of properly selected patients have been found to benefit to some extent from surgical removal of the focal lesion. In some cases of intractable seizures associated with behavior disorders and hemiplegia of childhood, removal of a damaged cerebral hemisphere has been found to control the intractable seizures and improve the behavior disorder without causing further neurological deficit.

PERSPECTIVE AND PROSPECTS

In the twentieth century, major developments were made in diagnosis and therapy. In 1929, Hans Berger recorded the first human electroencephalogram. Descriptions of EEG patterns and their correlation with clinical absences, partial seizures, and generalized tonic-clonic seizures led to important developments in classification and treatment. Special EEG recordings with activation techniques, depth recordings, and long-term recordings for patients with intractable seizures became available to aid in the diagnosis and medical management of patients and in the selection of candidates for possible neurosurgical treatment.

Prolonged EEG recording by telemetry (the transmission of data electronically to a distant location) and ambulatory monitoring became helpful in making a diagnosis in patients who have brief spells of uncertain type. Electrical activity at the time of the attack can be documented. Videotaping with split-screen EEG recording and patient observation allows excellent correlation between the clinical and EEG manifestations, which aids in the classification and determination of appropriate therapy in difficult clinical problems. In those patients with intractable epilepsy, prolonged recording can document the frequency of seizures and correlation with anticonvulsive drug blood levels.

Radiological advances and CT scans in the 1970s, and later positron emission tomography (PET) scans, improved diagnostic skill in delineating potentially remediable lesions in patients with seizures.

During the twentieth century, many other medications became available for patients with seizures. The use of the operating microscope and technical advances in microsurgical techniques refined surgical treatments and improved the outlook for patients with structural lesions such as brain tumors, vascular malformations, and scars.

—Genevieve Slomski, PhD

See also Addiction; Alcoholism; Arteriosclerosis; Batten's disease; Bites and stings; Brain; Brain damage; Brain disorders; Brain tumors; Electroencephalography (EEG); Epilepsy; Hallucinations; Head and neck disorders; Headaches; Hypoglycemia; Ischemia; Lead poisoning; Neuralgia, neuritis, and neuropathy; Neuroimaging; Neurology; Neurology, pediatric; Preeclampsia and eclampsia; Rabies; Schizophrenia; Sleep disorders; Snakebites; Strokes; Tetanus; Transient ischemic attacks (TIAs); Tumors.

For Further Information:

Bloom, Floyd E., M. Flint Beal, and David J. Kupfer, eds. *The Dana Guide to Brain Health.* New York: Dana Press, 2006. An easy-to-understand health guide to the brain from neuroscience, neurology, and psychiatry perspectives. More than seventy psychiatric and neurological disorders, their diagnoses, and their treatments are covered.

Delanty, Norman, ed. *Seizures: Medical Causes and Management.* Totowa, N.J.: Humana Press, 2002. Designed for health care personnel. Reviews seizures caused by fever and systemic infection, medications, alcohol or drugs, and environmental toxins.

Freeman, John M., Eileen P. G. Vining, and Diana J. Pillas. *Seizures and Epilepsy in Childhood: A Guide.* 3d ed. Baltimore: Johns Hopkins University Press, 2002. Designed for parents, an overall guide to the symptoms, diagnosis, and treatment of children with epilepsy. Third edition includes new chapters on alternative therapies and medicines, routine health care, insurance issues, and research resources.

Levy, René H., et al., eds. *Antiepileptic Drugs.* 5th ed. Philadelphia: Lippincott Williams & Wilkins, 2002. This useful work offers a quantitative analysis and interpretation of the drugs most often used in the treatment of recurrent seizures.

Rowan, A. James, and John R. Gates, eds. *Non-epileptic Seizures.* 2d ed. Boston: Butterworth-Heinemann, 2000. This book draws together a multidisciplinary perspective on knowledge of paroxysmal events that suggest a diagnosis of epilepsy but that are not of epileptic origin.

Solomon, Gail, Henn Kutt, and Fred Plum. *Clinical Management of Seizures.* 2d ed. Philadelphia: W. B. Saunders, 1983. Offers comprehensive treatment of seizures. After a brief historical perspective, the authors discuss the physiology, chemistry, and pharmacology of seizures; their classification; epidemiology and predisposing factors; treatment; and special management problems. Contains numerous charts, graphs, and illustrations.

Weaver, Donald F. *Epilepsy and Seizures: Everything You Need to Know.* Toronto, Ont.: Firefly Books, 2001. A lay guide covering research advances, history of the disease, different types, the mechanisms, diagnosis and treatment, and special situations, such as epilepsy in pregnant women, children, and the elderly.

SELF-MEDICATION

Category: Treatment

Also known as: Self-treatment, medications management

Anatomy or system affected: All

Specialties and related fields: All

Definition: Self-administration of drugs without the direction or supervision of a physician.

Key terms:

compliance: taking drugs as directed by a physician; completing therapeutic activities in proper fashion, as directed by a health care provider

drug interactions: the chemical effects of taking drugs in combination, where the effects will reduce, magnify, or alter the desired effects of the drug

illicit drugs: drugs that are illegal to possess, have addiction potential, and lack approved medical uses

over-the-counter drugs: pharmaceutical products, vitamins, herbal remedies, and other medicines that can be purchased by anyone, without a doctor's prescription

palliative care: care that decreases the suffering associated with health conditions by reducing the severity of symptoms, but does not provide a cure

prescription drugs: medicines that can be obtained only with the prescription of a doctor

INDICATIONS AND PROCEDURES

Every day, millions of people take medicinal drugs. Usually this is because they are experiencing symptoms, want to experience a particular feeling, or want to prevent a problem from developing and have information leading them to believe that the drug is the answer. For some, this occurs under the direction of a physician through the use of prescription medications. For others, this occurs through self-medication as a form of treatment. Most popularly, there are those who, through advertisements or personal experience, have learned that certain over-the-counter medications or popular legal drugs (such as cigarettes or alcohol) can be used to alleviate symptoms, provide palliative care, or cause certain symptoms or feelings. Others, via self-knowledge or guidance from alternative medicine specialists, will use teas, herbal remedies, and vitamins to achieve these same goals. Similarly, others may use illicit drugs to self-medicate in order to adjust their mood, physical feelings, or other abilities. For these individuals, it may be that they have didactic knowledge about drug properties or have learned about drug effects through their experience with drugs. Relatedly, even those receiving prescribed drugs may abuse those drugs by using them in ways unapproved by their doctor. This may be due to judgments that they need more or less of the drug or need to mix it with something else to get the desired effect(s). Together, access to drugs, knowledge of dosages and drug effects, and having a culture that encourages use of medicinal remedies and drugs all contribute to self-medication.

USES AND COMPLICATIONS

Drug interactions can be a danger of self-medication. When individuals mix different medicines, legal drugs, or illegal drugs, there is a risk that they may cause themselves harm. Some drug interactions can cause medicinal drugs to be less effective for treating the condition needing attention. Others can lead to substantial discomfort or more serious conditions such as seizures or death. Similar problems can come from mixing certain medicinal substances and herbal remedies with each other or with certain foods. As such, anyone using self-medication as a treatment strategy should learn as much as possible about the drug(s) they are taking. Persons who self-medicate in addition to taking prescription drugs should inform their physicians of the nonprescription drugs they are taking.

Another problem of self-medication as a style of treatment is that unsupervised medical problems can often worsen without proper care. Using alcohol, cigarettes, or marijuana to alleviate conditions such as anxiety or depression may provide relief in the short term, but in the long term such use may worsen the mood problems and lead to substance abuse or dependence. Similarly, taking an antacid or laxative can be helpful for minor gastrointestinal problems, but prolonged use of such drugs can result in dangerous physical conditions not getting much-needed medical attention. Therefore, the limits of self-medication as a strategy must be known.

PERSPECTIVE AND PROSPECTS

More than 30 percent of individuals living in the United States use an over-the-counter drug in any two-day period. It is estimated that 54 percent of three-year-olds receive over-the-counter drugs in any thirty-day period. Elderly adults use 25 percent of all over-the-counter drugs. Research also shows that 70 to 95 percent of all illnesses are managed without physician assistance. Additionally, over-the-counter drugs, herbal remedies, legal drugs, and illicit drugs constitute multibillion-dollar industries. Given these trends, self-medication as a treatment strategy is likely to continue. Increases can be expected as well because it is becoming easier to gain knowledge about how to use drugs safely. Furthermore, the practice of self-medication has the potential to decrease health care costs substantially by reducing the need for health care services, conserving valuable physician time.

The presence of self-medication as a positive force, however, must be balanced against problems such as a lack of compliance with medication regimens and the use of illicit and legal drugs to manage untreated mental and physical illnesses. When people do not take medicines as directed or fail to get proper medical treatment, problems can worsen. Work in the health care field therefore will need to address the longer-term problems that can develop as a result of these types of practices. Such investments may require increased time from service providers for purposes such as assessment and diagnosis, so as to uncover the hidden illnesses causing individuals to look for medicinal help in the first place. Additionally, barriers to treatment will have to be brought down so as to allow individuals who need medical and other health care to get the help they deserve.

—*Nancy A. Piotrowski, PhD*

See also Addiction; Alcoholism; Alternative medicine; Antioxidants; Ergogenic aids; Herbal medicine; Internet medicine; Marijuana; Over-the-counter medications; Pain management; Palliative medicine; Pharmacology; Pharmacy; Prescription drug abuse; Side effects; Smoking; Substance abuse; Supplements; Vitamins and minerals; Weight loss medications.

For Further Information:
Chamberlain, Logan V. *What the Labels Won't Tell You: A Consumer's Guide to Herbal Supplements*. Loveland, Colo.: Interweave Press, 1998.
Gorman, Jack M. *The Essential Guide to Psychiatric Drugs*. 4th ed. New York: St. Martin's Press, 2007.
Graedon, Joe, and Teresa Graedon. *Dangerous Drug Interactions: How to Protect Yourself from Harmful Drug/Drug, Drug/Food, Drug/Vitamin Combinations*. Rev. ed. New York: St. Martin's Press, 1999.
Griffith, H. Winter. *Complete Guide to Prescription and Nonprescription Drugs*. Revised and updated by Stephen Moore. New York: Penguin Group, 2010.
Silverman, Harold M. *The Pill Book*. 13th ed. New York: Bantam Books, 2008.
Vandeputte, Charles. *Alcohol, Medications, and Older Adults: A Guide for Families and Other Caregivers*. St. Paul, Minn.: Johnson Institute, 1991.

SEMEN

Category: Biology
Also known as: Ejaculate
Anatomy or system affected: Genitals, glands, reproductive system
Specialties and related fields: Urology
Definition: The fluid ejaculated by the male at orgasm, consisting of sperm and secretions from accessory glands.

STRUCTURE AND FUNCTIONS

Semen is released from the male reproductive system during ejaculation. It is a milky white, sticky fluid of 2 to 5 milliliters with an alkaline pH (7.2-7.8). It consists of spermatozoa (sperm) produced in the testes plus secretions of accessory glands: paired seminal vesicles that lie on the posterior surface of the bladder, the singular prostate gland that surrounds the urethra, and paired bulbourethral glands that lie just inferior to the prostate.

Sperm comprises only 5 percent of the semen, with 20 to 150 million sperm per milliliter. Seminal fluid contributes about 60 percent of the volume and contains high levels of fructose used by the sperm as an energy source. Seminal fluid also contains prostaglandins that stimulate smooth muscle contraction. This helps propel the semen through the urethra for release and aids in movement of sperm upward in the female reproductive tract. Two proteins, semenogelin I and II, inhibit sperm motility and protect the semen in the male urethra. The semenogelins cause the semen to form a temporary coagulate when deposited in the vagina. After fifteen to thirty minutes, the coagulum dissolves.

The prostate contributes about 30 percent of semen volume as a milky, slightly acidic fluid. It is high in citrate used as a nutrient by the sperm, plus several enzymes, including a protease called prostate-specific antigen (PSA). PSA hydrolyzes the semenogelins and helps to activate the motility of sperm. Prostatic fluid also contains seminalplasmin, an antibiotic active against *Escherichia coli (E. coli)* and several other bacteria that can cause urinary tract infections. The bulbourethral glands produce a thick, alkaline mucus that contributes only about 5 percent of semen volume. It is secreted in advance of ejaculation in order to neutralize any residual acidity from urine in the urethra. It also acts as a lubricant on the head of the penis to aid in vaginal penetration.

DISORDERS AND DISEASES
Disorders relating to semen involve pathologies of the individual glands. Infertility occurs in approximately 15 percent of males when there is a sperm count less than 20 million per milliliter, low sperm motility, or high levels of abnormal sperm. Decreased counts may be a result of testicular tumors, trauma, radiation, or infection with mumps virus. Infertility can also occur with autoimmunity when antibodies that bind to sperm are produced. Testicular cancer usually requires surgical removal of the testis. Semen can also transmit sexually transmitted infections, including human immunodeficiency virus (HIV).

Prostate hypertrophy, noncancerous enlargement of the prostate, occurs frequently in men over the age of fifty. It causes partial urethral obstruction, resulting in urinary hesitation, frequent urination, and possible painful urination. It may be treated with medication or corrected surgically. Prostate cancer occurs in one of every six men in their lifetime. Treatments include surgery, radiation, or hormonal therapy. Serum PSA increases in prostate cancer, and monitoring of PSA levels is important.

—*Ralph R. Meyer, PhD*

See also Conception; Contraception; Erectile dysfunction; Genital disorders, male; Glands; Infertility, male; Masturbation; Men's health; Orchitis; Penile implant surgery; Prostate cancer; Prostate enlargement; Prostate gland; Prostate gland

removal; Puberty and adolescence; Reproductive system; Sexual dysfunction; Sexuality; Sexually transmitted diseases (STDs); Sterilization; Testicles, undescended; Testicular cancer; Testicular surgery; Testicular torsion; Vas deferens; Vasectomy.

For Further Information:
Lilja, Hans, David Ulmert, and Andrew J. Vickers, "Prostate-Specific Antigen and Prostate Cancer: Prediction, Detection, and Monitoring." *Nature Reviews Cancer* 8 (2008): 268-278.
Marieb, Elaine N., and Katja Hoehn. *Human Anatomy and Physiology*. 8th ed. San Francisco: Pearson-Benjamin Cummings, 2009.
Poiani, Aldo. "Complexity of Seminal Fluid: A Review." *Behaviorial Ecology and Sociobiology* 60, no. 3 (2006): 289-310.

SENSE ORGANS

Category: Anatomy
Anatomy or system affected: Ears, eyes, gastrointestinal system, mouth, nerves, nervous system, nose, skin
Specialties and related fields: Audiology, dentistry, dermatology, neurology, ophthalmology, optometry, otorhinolaryngology
Definition: Specialized structures anatomically suited to a particular sense-the eyes for vision, the nose for smell (olfaction), the taste buds for taste, the ears for hearing and balance, and the skin for such cutaneous sensations as warmth, cold, light touch, deep pressure, and pain.
Key terms:
chemoreception: sensitivity to chemical stimuli
cochlear: referring to the parts of the ear concerned with hearing
cutaneous: occurring within the skin
photoreception: sensitivity to light
retina: the light-sensitive part of the eye
stimulus: anything capable of producing a response
vestibular: referring to the parts of the ear concerned with balance

STRUCTURE AND FUNCTIONS
The sense organs of the body include the cutaneous sense organs, the organs of chemical reception, the organs of vision or sight, and the organs of hearing and balance. The skin is the major organ of sensation for touch, pressure, cold, warmth, and pain; the nasal epithelium and taste buds are the major organs of chemoreception; the eyes are the major organs of vision or sight; and the ears are the major organs of both hearing and balance.

There are five types of cutaneous receptors within the skin, each with a different type of sensory nerve ending and each with a different spatial pattern of distribution. Free (naked) nerve endings are sensitive to pain and are widely distributed over the body's skin surface, especially at the base of each hair. Overstimulation of any type of nerve ending also results in a sensation of pain, but these nerve endings are so exposed that any stimulation at all is felt as an overstimulation. All the remaining cutaneous receptors are encapsulated in one of several types of end organs. Of these, the end bulbs of Krause are sensitive to cold; they are most numerous around the conjunctiva of the eye and along the glans of the penis and the glans of the clitoris.

The Pacinian corpuscles each contain a single central nerve fiber, enclosed in many concentric layers of semitransparent tissue resembling the bulb of an onion. These structures, which are about 2 to 4 millimeters in diameter, are sensitive to deep pressure and are distributed throughout the skin, principally within the dermal papillae. They are most numerous on the palm of the hand, the sole of the foot, and the insides of many joints such as the front of the elbow or the back of the knee. The tactile (Meissner's) corpuscles each consist of an oval, bulblike swelling in which the nerve endings run around in spiral patterns at right angles to the long axis. Meissner's corpuscles are sensitive to light touch and are most numerous along the fingertips (and the hand in general), the tongue and lips, parts of the eye, and the skin of the mammary nipple or papilla. The corpuscles of Ruffini are enclosed in connective tissue sheaths perpendicular to the nerve that serves them. The axons of this nerve branch repeatedly within the corpuscle and these branches intertwine, each ending in a tiny knob. Corpuscles of Ruffini are sensitive to warmth and are very numerous over the fingertips, the forearm, and the skin of the face. The evidence to associate particular nerve endings with particular sensations (such as the Meissner's corpuscles with light touch) comes largely from patterns of spatial distribution: The areas of the body most sensitive to touch are also those with the highest densities of Meissner's corpuscles.

Neuromuscular spindles occur in most voluntary muscles and are sensitive to the state of contraction or relaxation of the muscle fibers. The spindle consists of a muscle fiber or small bundle of such fibers, around which are wrapped several turns of infrequently branching sensory nerve endings. The tendons of many muscles also frequently contain neurotendinous spindles, encapsulated structures in which a bundle of tendon fibers receive branched nerve endings. These nerve endings branch slightly just before reaching the tendon fibers but then lose their sheaths and branch profusely within the tendon. These neurotendinous spindles act as stretch receptors, sensitive to the state of stretching of the tendon.

Chemoreceptors of the body include those tissues sensitive to certain chemicals. The carotid body, a swelling within the carotid artery of the neck, contains tissue sensitive to the carbon dioxide or acid content of the blood; it stimulates the breathing reflex when the carbon dioxide level is too high. The taste buds of the tongue are sensitive to the taste of a variety of chemical substances present in moderate concentrations. Each taste bud contains gustatory cells along with nonsensitive supporting (sustentacular) cells. Experimental evidence points to four basic types of taste sensations: sweet (like sugar), bitter (like quinine), sour (like vinegar or citric acid), and salty (like sodium chloride). Sensitivity to each of these four basic tastes has its own characteristic pattern of distribution over the tongue and palate.

The nasal epithelium is responsible for olfaction, or smell, which is a sensitivity to chemical substances in much smaller concentrations. Most of the nasal epithelium is associated with the nose and the nasal passages, but a small part of this epithelium has become attached instead to the roof of the mouth, where it forms the vomeronasal (Jacobsohn's) organ, which "smells" the contents of the mouth (mostly food). The nasal epithelium is structurally unusual in that the cell bodies of the sensory cells originate within the epithelium and their nerve endings (axons) migrate inwardly to the brain, through the cribriform plate, forming the first cranial nerve or olfactory nerve. All other sensory nerves in the body grow outward from the central nervous system, and their cell bodies are located where their growth began.

Attempts have been made to classify smells according to a scheme similar to the bitter-sweet-sour-salty system used for tastes, but there are many more basic smells than there are tastes-lists vary from seven to twenty to more than ninety-and there is no general agreement on any of these schemes.

The eyes are the body's principal visual receptors. (Some evidence also exists of the brain's own ability to sense daily changes in the level of light intensity, especially in the pineal body.) The primary parts of the eye include the eyelids, cornea, lens, ciliary body, iris diaphragm, pupil, aqueous humor, vitreous humor, retina, choroid coat, scleroid coat, and optic nerve. The eyelids protect the front of the eye and prevent injury to the eye by closing. The cornea is the transparent covering of the front of the eye; the lens is the transparent, almost spherical body that focuses rays of incoming light onto the retina; and the ciliary body is a largely connective tissue structure (also containing some muscle tissue) that supports the lens. The colored part of the ciliary body is the iris diaphragm; muscle fibers within the iris diaphragm adjust the size of the pupil for different brightness levels of light. The opening in the middle of the iris diaphragm is called the pupil. The aqueous humor is the watery fluid in front of the lens, while the vitreous humor is the thick, jellylike fluid behind the lens.

The light-sensitive portion of the eye is the retina. It is almost spherical in shape and consists of two layers: a sensory layer on the inside (closer to the front) and a pigment layer surrounding and behind the sensory layer. Within the sensory layer are contained both the rods, which are sensitive to finer details, and the cones, which are sensitive to colors. The eye's most sensitive area is called the area centralis; it is centered upon a depression called the fovea. The choroid coat is the connective tissue layer immediately surrounding the retina, which is continuous with the pia mater that surrounds the brain. The scleroid coat is the stronger connective tissue layer that surrounds the choroid coat; it is continuous with the dura mater surrounding the brain. The optic nerve fibers originate from the sensory layer of the retina, where they converge toward a spot called the blind spot, marking the place where the nerve fibers turn inward toward the brain. A majority of the optic nerve fibers cross over to the opposite side of the brain via the optic chiasma, but a small proportion of the fibers remains on the same side without crossing over. Experiments on the physiology of vision have led researchers to conclude that there are three separate types of color receptors (cones) in the retina, sensitive principally to red, green, and blue regions of the spectrum. All other color sensations can be simulated experimentally in people with normal vision by a suitable combination of red, green, and blue stimuli.

The ears are special sense organs devoted to the two distinct functions of hearing and balance. The ear may be divided anatomically into outer, middle, and inner portions or functionally into a cochlear portion for hearing and a vestibular portion for balance. The outer (external) ear consists of a flap called the pinna (or external ear flap) and a tubelike cavity called the external acoustic meatus. Within the external ear, sound impulses exist as waves of compressed or decompressed (rarefied) air, forming a series of longitudinal waves that vibrate in the same direction in which they are transmitted. The tympanic membrane (eardrum) is a vibrating membrane that marks the boundary between the outer and middle ears.

The middle ear consists of a cavity containing three tiny bones, the auditory ossicles. Within the middle ear, the vibrations of the tympanic membrane set up a series of vibrations within these tiny bones. The three auditory ossicles are called the malleus (hammer), incus (anvil), and stapes (stirrup). The malleus gets its name from its hammerlike shape, which includes a long handle (the manubrium) extending across the

tympanic membrane. The incus, the second of the auditory ossicles, rests against the malleus at one end and the stapes at the other. The stapes is shaped like a stirrup, in which the foot is placed when riding a horse. The flat base of the stapes is called the footplate, in analogy to the corresponding part of a stirrup; this footplate rests against the fenestra ovalis of the inner ear. The opening in the stapes is penetrated by an artery called the stapedial artery. The cavity of the middle ear connects to the pharynx by means of a tube, the pharyngotympanic or Eustachian tube.

The inner ear is entirely housed within the petrosal bone. It can be divided into cochlear (hearing) and vestibular (balance) portions. The cochlear portion of the inner ear begins with two windows, the fenestra ovalis (oval window) and fenestra rotundum (round window), communicating between the middle ear and the inner ear. Behind the fenestra ovalis lies a vestibule, filled with a fluid called perilymph and extending into a long scala vestibuli. Behind the fenestra rotundum lies another long tube, the scala tympani, also filled with perilymph and running parallel to the scala vestibuli. Between these two tubes lies a third, the scala media or cochlear duct, filled with a different fluid called endolymph. Together, the three are prolonged into a spiral coil called the cochlea (Latin for "snail"), which has a bit more than three complete turns. At the end of this coil, the scala media ends, and the scala vestibuli and scala tympani join with one another by means of an intervening loop called the helicotrema. The basilar membrane separates the scala tympani and the cochlear duct. The spiral organ (organ of Corti) runs within the cochlear duct along the basilar membrane, not far beneath a tectorial membrane that is suspended within the cochlear duct.

The outer ear receives vibrations that travel through the air and transmits these vibrations to the tympanic membrane. In the middle ear, the vibrations of the tympanic membrane are transmitted through the malleus, incus, and stapes to the oval window. These vibrations are transmitted through the perilymph of the inner ear (vestibular portion), where they cause vibrations of the basilar membrane. The vibrating basilar membrane causes vibrations within the endolymph and also in the tectorial membrane, but the tectorial membrane is less flexible than the basilar membrane, creating regions of greater and lesser pressure within the endolymph. The hair cells of the spiral organ are sensitive to these pressure differences and send out nerve impulses to the brain, where they are interpreted as sounds.

The vestibular portion of the inner ear includes two interconnected chambers called the sacculus and the utriculus, both filled with endolymph. The sacculus has a downward extension called the lagena, and it also connects into the scala media of the cochlear portion of the ear. From the utriculus emerge three semicircular ducts, approximately at right angles to one another, all filled with endolymph: an anterior vertical duct, a posterior vertical duct, and a horizontal duct. Each semicircular duct runs through a bony semicircular canal, filled with perilymph. Each duct has a bulblike swelling, the ampulla, at one end. Each ampulla has a patch, or macula, of sensory structures called neuromasts, which are sensitive to movements in fluids such as endolymph. Other maculae, or patches of neuromasts, are located in the sacculus, the utriculus, and the lagena.

The vestibular portion of the inner ear is sensitive to movements and especially to acceleration. Normally, this acceleration is caused by gravity, but nonlinear movements (such as the swerving of a fast-moving vehicle around a curve) may also result in accelerations that cause fluid movements within the semicircular canals. These movements are perceived by the sensitive hair cells (neuromasts) within each ampulla. Spinning around or other sudden acceleration causes temporary dizziness (vertigo) and a consequent loss of balance.

DISORDERS AND DISEASES
Several types of medical specialists deal with problems of the various sense organs: Ophthalmologists deal with diseases of the eye; otorhinolaryngologists deal with diseases of the ears (oto-), nose (rhino-), and throat (larynx); and neurologists deal with all the senses. All these specialists first conduct diagnostic tests in order to detect any sensory malfunction and to determine the probable cause; they then provide whatever treatment may be available for each condition.

The ability to distinguish tastes diminishes gradually with age in older persons as the number of gustatory cells declines, but complete loss of taste is rare. Persons with diminished taste are at greater risk for accidental poisoning. Except for the decline of taste among the elderly, other defects of smell or taste are rare and are usually indicative of more serious neurological problems such as brain damage or nerve damage. The inability to smell is a rare condition known as anosmia. Loss of cutaneous sensations, even over a small portion of the body, is usually indicative of nerve damage.

Disorders of the eye range from easily correctable vision problems to total blindness. Impaired function of one or more of the three types of color receptors results in one of the several types of color blindness. The most common type, red-green color blindness, is inherited as a sex-linked recessive trait and is thus more common in men than in women. Blindness may result from various defects or injuries: A defective lens or cornea may limit vision to large objects, and a defective retina may limit perception to light and darkness only. Total blindness results if the optic nerve is damaged or missing. More common visual defects include myopia (nearsightedness), hyperopia (farsightedness), and astigmatism (differences in vision along different axes), all of which can be corrected with glasses or contact lenses or by surgical procedures. A failure of the mechanism that drains fluid from the interior of the eyeball may result in a buildup of ocular pressure, a condition known as glaucoma. In times past, when treatment for glaucoma was not readily available, most cases resulted in permanent blindness. Glaucoma can now be treated, however, either surgically or with drugs. Several changes occur to the lens of the eye in older individuals. As the lens becomes more rigid with advancing age, reading and other near-vision tasks become more difficult, a condition known as presbyopia. Also frequent among older people are cataracts, tiny opaque grains that cloud up the lens and reduce the ability to see clearly. Untreated cataracts may eventually result in blindness, but various forms of treatment are available to prevent this from occurring.

Diseases of the ear should always be treated as serious. Tinnitus, or ringing in the ears, can result from damage to the hair cells of the organ of Corti. Damage to the auditory nerve can result in deafness. Upper respiratory infections can travel up the Eustachian tube and cause a common childhood infection of the middle ear known as otitis media. Infections of the vestibular portion of the inner ear can result in recurrent or permanent dizziness (vertigo) because the inflamed cells transmit impulses that the body wrongly interprets as resulting from accelerations in unusual directions. Some plant poisons (or the drugs derived from them, such as ipecac) can also impair the function of the inner ear and result in sensations of dizziness, often followed by nausea and by the vomiting of the plant containing the poison. This reaction may have evolved as an adaptive response to possible poisons; the same reaction also results in vomiting in other situations that cause unusual accelerations in the vestibular portion of the inner ear, as in the case of seasickness or other motion sickness.

PERSPECTIVE AND PROSPECTS
The many biblical references to deafness and blindness show that ancient civilizations were concerned about the proper functioning of the sense organs. The Greek philosopher Aristotle, also considered the greatest biologist of antiquity, enumerated five senses: touch, hearing, taste, smell, and sight. Detailed anatomical descriptions of the sense organs were made during the Renaissance by Bartolommeo Eustachio (or Eustachius) (1520-1574), after whom the Eustachian

tube is named; by Giulio Casserio (1552?-1616); and by Andreas Vesalius (1514-1564), whose superbly illustrated texts set new standards for art as well as science. Further discoveries were made by such anatomists as Alfonso Corti (1822-1876), who first described the detailed internal structure of the inner ear. The detailed cellular structure of the retina was first elucidated by the Nobel Prize-winning anatomist and histologist Santiago Ramón y Cajal (1852-1934). Other anatomists who expanded the understanding of the microscopic anatomy of sensory structures include Abraham Vater (1684-1751), Filippo Pacini (1812-1883), Georg Meissner (1829-1905), and Jan Evangelista Purkinje (1787-1869).

—*Eli C. Minkoff, PhD*

See also Appetite loss; Aromatherapy; Astigmatism; Audiology; Cataract surgery; Cataracts; Deafness; Dermatology; Ear surgery; Ears; Earwax; Eye surgery; Eyes; Hearing; Hearing loss; Microscopy, slitlamp; Myopia; Nasal polyp removal; Nasopharyngeal disorders; Nervous system; Numbness and tingling; Ophthalmology; Optometry; Otorhinolaryngology; Skin; Skin disorders; Smell; Synesthia; Systems and organs; Taste; Tinnitus; Touch; Vision; Vision disorders.

For Further Information:

Agur, Anne M. R., and Arthur F. Dalley. *Grant's Atlas of Anatomy*. 12th ed. Philadelphia: Wolters Kluwer Health/Lippincott Williams & Wilkins, 2009. This text contains many excellent, detailed illustrations.

Ferrari, Mario. *PDxMD Ear, Nose, and Throat Disorders*. Philadelphia: PDxMD, 2003. A clinical yet accessible reference text that provides a comprehensive list of disorders, with a summary of the condition, background, diagnosis, treatment, outcomes, prevention, and resources.

Møller, Aage R. *Sensory Systems: Anatomy, Physiology, and Pathophysiology*. Boston: Academic Press, 2003. An excellent text that describes how human sensory systems function, with comparisons of the five senses and detailed descriptions of the functions of each of them. Also covers how sensory information is processed in the brain to provide the basis for communication and for the perception of one's surroundings.

Riordan-Eva, Paul, and John P. Whitcher. *Vaughan and Asbury's General Ophthalmology*. 17th ed. New York: Lange Medical Books/McGraw-Hill, 2007. A clinical text that provides a range of information about the eye.

Rosse, Cornelius, and Penelope Gaddum-Rosse. *Hollinshead's Textbook of Anatomy*. 5th ed. Philadelphia: Lippincott-Raven, 1997. A very thorough, modern, detailed reference with good descriptions and illustrations.

Standring, Susan, et al., eds. *Gray's Anatomy*. 40th ed. New York: Churchill Livingstone/Elsevier, 2008. A great classic with the most thorough descriptions. The excellent color illustrations offer realistic detail in most cases and well-selected highlights in a few cases.

Sutton, Amy L., ed. *Eye Care Sourcebook: Basic Consumer Health Information About Eye Care and Eye Disorders*. 3d ed. Detroit, Mich.: Omnigraphics, 2008. A complete guide to eye care that includes such topics as eye anatomy, preventive vision care, refractive disorders and eye diseases, current research and clinical trials, and a list of organizations.

Wertenbaker, Lael T. *The Eye: Window to the World*. Reprint. New York: Scribner, 1984. Easy to read and understand, with good illustrations. Written for a popular audience.

SEPARATION ANXIETY

Category: Development
Anatomy or system affected: Psychic-emotional system
Specialties and related fields: Psychiatry, psychology
Definition: Common distress shown at the departure of a caregiver when a child is between ten to eighteen months of age and which may extend throughout the preschool years.

PHYSICAL AND PSYCHOLOGICAL FACTORS

Infants are often wary or even fearful when someone other than the usual caregiver approaches them or tries to touch or carry them. This may be partly attributable to anticipation of separation. Furthermore, in the second year of life, negative reactions to strangers may compound toddlers' concerns about separation from the caregiver.

Self-initiated separations and those that are brief, in familiar settings, and explained by the departing caregiver are less likely to elicit distress. Factors that do not seem to be related to separation distress are gender, birth order, and experience within the normal range for a given culture and economic class. Usually, separation anxiety subsides by about three years of age.

DISORDERS AND EFFECTS

Researchers used to think that the intensity of separation distress was an index of the strength of the attachment bond. However, the child's reaction during reunion with the caregiver is a better indicator of the security of attachment.

Child psychiatrists have described an uncommon disorder (with a prevalence of 4 percent) called separation anxiety disorder. This disorder must be distinguished from many other types of disorders that children may have. Because a child is anxious does not mean that separation anxiety disorder is present. The disorder may develop in early childhood for no apparent reason or may develop after a life stress such as the death of a relative or a change in school or neighborhood. Children with this disorder show excessive anxiety about separation from the caregiver or home that is more characteristic of younger children and therefore developmentally inappropriate. Separation anxiety disorder is typically long-lasting and causes significant disruption to functioning, such as school avoidance, excessive worry about losing caregivers, and fear of being left alone.

A relationship may exist between very strong and long-lasting separation anxiety as an infant and separation anxiety disorder in later life, but infant distress about separation is very common, almost universal, and is usually relatively short-lived. Thus, there is usually little reason to be concerned about separation anxiety in infancy.

—George A. Morgan, PhD,
and Robert J. Harmon, MD;
updated by Nancy A. Piotrowski, PhD

See also Anxiety; Bonding; Developmental stages; Emotions: Biomedical causes and effects; Phobias; Psychiatry, child and adolescent.

For Further Information:
Berk, Laura E. *Child Development*. 8th ed. Boston: Pearson/Allyn & Bacon, 2009.
Caplan, Theresa. *The First Twelve Months of Life: Your Baby's Growth Month by Month*. New York: Bantam, 1995.
Craig, Grace J., Marguerite D. Kermis, and Nancy Digdon. *Children Today*. 2d ed. Toronto, Ont.: Prentice Hall, 2002.
Leach, Penelope. *Your Baby and Child: From Birth to Age Five*. London: Dorling Kindersley, 2003.
Mooney, Carol Garhart. *Theories of Childhood: An Introduction to Dewey, Montessori, Erikson, Piaget, and Vygotsky*. St. Paul, Minn.: Redleaf Press, 2000.

SEPTICEMIA

Category: Disease/Disorder
Also known as: Blood poisoning, bacteremia
Anatomy or system affected: Blood, circulatory system, pulmonary system, renal system
Specialties and related fields: Hematology, internal medicine, serology, critical care
Definition: Life-threatening, systemic infection of the blood with pathogens from an infection in a part of the body; if untreated can lead to sepsis, which characteristically causes fever, chills, increased heart rate, rapid breathing, and gastrointestinal symptoms such as nausea, vomiting, and diarrhea.

Key terms:
antibacterial therapy: treatment for patients with septicemia, typically initiated with a combination of broad-antibiotics when the infecting organism is unknown based on originating source on infection and common microbes in the specific community/hospital; when cultures define the causative microbe(s) therapy is tailored to the most specific and effective antibiotic regimen
bacteria: microorganisms with a wide variety of biochemical, often pathogenic, properties
bacteremia: the presence of bacteria in the blood, also referred to as blood poisoning or septicemia
sepsis: a systemic inflammatory response due to rapid multiplication of bacteria in the blood; often causes fever, rapid heart rate and breathing, altered mental status, increased white blood, cells and organ damage
septic shock: a type of sepsis with increased mortality that is characterized by dangerously low blood pressures leading to tissue and organ damage
septic shock treatment: the immediate treatment of septic shock, including the use of antibiotics, intravenous fluid replacement, and pharmacological agents to increase blood pressure (vasopressors).

CAUSES AND SYMPTOMS

The presence of bacteria in the bloodstream is known as "septicemia," "bacteremia," or "blood poisoning." The bacteria can come from a multitude of sources including open wounds, pneumonia, and abdominal and urinary tract infections. If the bacteria are not removed by the immune system, rapid proliferation of the bacteria can occur. Large amounts of these pathogens along with the presence of their toxins in the blood can lead to a systemic inflammatory condition called "sepsis." Sepsis is a serious medical condition that requires prompt medical intervention. A person who has septicemia and whom sepsis develops will become seriously ill, often with a high fever, chills, rapid heart rate and breathing, altered mental status, and an elevated white blood cell count. Skin rashes may occur, and sometimes the skin becomes unusually warm. In many cases, especially when large amounts of toxins are produced by the circulating bacteria, the person passes into a state of septic shock, which is a type of sepsis where blood pressure drastically drops and can lead to organ damage.

Bacteria in the bloodstream can cause damage to the body both directly and indirectly through an exaggerated inflammatory response. Directly, the bacteria can seed organs such as the brain, bone, and heart, resulting in complications from local proliferation and direct tissue and organ damage. Systemically, the bacteria also trigger intravascular activation of inflammatory systems. Blood vessels become leaky and dilate, reducing blood pressure and decreasing the amount of oxygen and nutrients delivered to vital organs. This systemic response can also cause increased coagulation or blood clotting throughout the body and shifts in metabolic states such hyperglycemia and acidosis. These direct and indirect systems, which combine with stress-generated endocrine responses, produce a sequence of metabolic events, the end stage of which is systemic vascular collapse, traditionally called "septic shock."

Septic shock is a dangerous condition in which there is a dramatic drop in blood pressure (shock) as a result of septicemia, leading to decreased tissue perfusion and organ damage. Septic shock symptoms vary with the extent and site of major tissue damage and are usually preceded by signs of severe infection, including respiratory distress and poor renal function. Septic shock symptoms are similar to those for sepsis (fever, increased heart rate and respiratory rate, altered mental status), with additional symptoms including cold hands and feet, often with blue-purple coloration caused by poor blood flow; and markedly reduced blood pressure in which systolic blood pressure is less than 90 millimeters of mercury. There may also be vomiting and diarrhea, and a decrease in urine output often suggests the presence of an acute kidney injury and risk of renal failure. Cardiorespiratory failure may also occur.

The classic septic shock syndrome results primarily from the sequence of events triggered by bacteremia; however, the exact mechanism by which bacteria causes shock is still unclear. Currently, it is believed that molecular patterns on bacteria are recognized by our immune system and binding of immune cells to these molecular patterns initiates a cascade of inflammatory events, including release of proinflammatory factors. These proinflammatory factors lead to leakage of fluid from blood vessels and a reduction in the ability of the vessels to constrict, leading to a severe drop in blood pressure. Furthermore, these inflammatory factors promote clotting of blood in the smallest blood vessels and activation of stress hormones that increase blood sugar levels. Together, these inflammatory responses seriously interfere with tissue circulation, causing cell death and tissue necrosis. Consequently, organ damage occurs especially to tissues in the kidneys, heart, and lungs. In septic shock, the low blood pressure is typically unresponsive to adequate volume replacement and drugs to increase blood pressure are often needed. Morbidity and mortality associated with septic shock are high: about two-thirds of patients die.

Septicemia and septic shock can precipitate multiple organ failure. As the patient becomes hypermetabolic and febrile with progressive failure of one or more organs, the mortality rate can be as high as 90 percent. Populations particularly susceptible to developing septicemia, sepsis, and septic shock are those who are hospitalized, immunocompromised, have artificial heart valves or joints, and injection drug users. Typical patients that develop sepsis are those that are hospitalized with major disorders such as diabetes mellitus, cancer, or cirrhosis and who have a focus of infection somewhere in the body (often the intestines or urinary tract). Progression to septic shock is especially likely for people who have immunodeficiency disorders or are taking immunosuppressant drugs for cancer or an

---

INFORMATION ON SEPTICEMIA

Causes: Systemic bacterial infection
Symptoms: Fever, chills, pain, headache, nausea, rapid breathing, clouding of consciousness, rashes, jaundice, diarrhea
Duration: Acute
Treatments: Antibiotics (penicillin, chloramphenicol, ampicillin, neomycin); surgery (debridement, drainage); fluid replacement; oxygen therapy

---

inappropriate antibiotic treatment. Newborn infants are also particularly at risk if septicemia develops.

TREATMENT AND THERAPY
A presumptive diagnosis of septicemia is often made clinically based on historical, physical, and laboratory data, even in the absence of proof. The setting in which the episode is occurring should be evaluated promptly. Crucial to appropriate initial treatment decision making are the background history, which may help to define the type of host-defense defect present, and prior blood culture data, which might predict the infecting organism. The physical examination should be quick and thorough, searching for the septic source as well as signs that might indicate progression to shock.

A diagnosis can be confirmed, and the infective bacteria identified by growing a culture of the organisms from a blood sample. Several laboratory tests are often helpful in the evaluation of a potentially septic patient. In general, patients with fever should be considered septic until proven otherwise, and therapy should always be initiated for high-risk febrile patients in advance of a microbiologic confirmation of septicemia.

Common microorganisms that enter the bloodstream when the body's defenses break down include staphylococci from boils, abscesses, and wounds; streptococci from the tonsils, throat, or cuts; and pneumococci from the lungs. Other invaders of the bloodstream include the gonococci, the typhoid bacilli in typhoid fever, and *Escherichia coli (E. coli)* in bowel infections. All these bacteria may be detected by taking a blood culture.

Initial treatment for septicemia includes broad-spectrum antimicrobial therapy and identification and control of the source of the infection. Antibacterial therapy should be started as soon as septicemia is suspected, ideally within one hour after recognition of the septicemia. It is normally started by intravenous infusion of antibiotic drugs and glucose and/or saline solution. The source of infection is sought immediately and should be removed if suspected, including catheters and tubes. Abscesses that are present should be surgically removed. Surgical debridement (removal) and drainage of septic foci are especially important, and all severe localized infections should be widely debrided and drained. Rates of mortality are much lower if the source of infection is recognized and treated promptly.

Broad antibacterial coverage is typically initiated with a combination of antibiotics, especially when the infecting organism is unknown. Selection of antibiotics when the infecting organism is unknown is based on the site of infection, location of patient (hospital, nursing home, community), the patient's medical history, and local susceptibility to antimicrobial agents. When cultures define the causative microbe(s), antimicrobial therapy can be narrowed to only target the microbe of interest. Penicillin is usually used to combat staphylococcic, streptococcic, pneumococcic, and gonococcic infections; chloramphenicol and ampicillin are used against typhoid and paratyphoid infections; and neomycin is used against *E. coli* infections. Extreme care must be taken with the administration of chloramphenicol and neomycin because of their toxic side effects.

Antibiotics limit the microbiological complications of bacteremia, but other metabolic events, whether initiated by or independent of bacterial proliferation, may still produce substantial morbidity and mortality. Therefore, therapy in addition to antibiotics is recommended to counter this metabolic sequence.

Septic shock requires immediate treatment, including the use of antibiotics and surgery, rapid fluid replacement by infusion, and the maintenance of urine flow to prevent the effects of renal failure. Other measures must also be taken to raise the blood pressure and to promote a better supply of important nutrients to tissues, such as through intravenous infusion of vasopressors and oxygen therapy. The use of anti-inflammatory drugs is under active investigation.

PERSPECTIVE AND PROSPECTS

Most febrile patients lacking other signs of severe septicemia will usually do well. Such patients usually respond quickly to fluid administration, antibacterial therapy, and drainage of the primary focus of infection. The presence of septic shock, however, dramatically increases morbidity and mortality. Even when the inciting infection is localized, shock is associated with at least 30 to 40 percent mortality. A favorable outcome in a patient in severe shock depends early aggressive medical intervention and the skill of management in the intensive care unit. Early diagnosis and therapy of severely septic patients will greatly decrease the morbidity and mortality of these individuals. The best means of preventing septicemia is preventing unnecessary use of antibiotics, limiting use and duration of central venous catheters and tubes, increasing adherence to infection control protocols.

Infections most commonly occur in the hospital setting, where many infected patients become bacteremic. About 1 in 25 of all hospital patients develop an infection during hospitalization. This means that the number of patients at risk of developing septic shock is large. The clinician must be familiar with the manifestations and differential diagnosis of the patient who appears to suffer from sepsis and septic shock and must have in mind rapid, comprehensive diagnostic and therapeutic plans of action. It is important to develop the concept of a preshock phase of septic shock predicated on identifying a subgroup of infected patients more likely than others to develop shock. In such patients, fluids should be proactively administered, and broad antibiotic coverage started early. Rapid treatment with antibiotics and fluid replacement before shock develops undoubtedly prevents some of the morbidity and mortality associated with septicemia.

—*Risa Kiernan, MS, OMS-III*

See also: Antibiotics; Bacterial infections; Bacteriology; *E. coli* infection; Infection; Poisoning; Shock; Staphylococcal infections; Streptococcal infections; Typhoid fever; Toxicology.

For Further Information:
Brant, E. B., C. W. Seymour, and D. C. Angus. "Sepsis and Septic Shock." *Harrison's Principles of Internal Medicine*, edited by J. Loscalzo, A. Fauci, D. Kasper, et al., 21st ed., McGraw Hill, 2022. Comprehensive textbook on foundations of internal medicine with a clear, up-to-date chapter on the pathophysiology and management of sepsis and septic shock.

Goldman, Lee, and Dennis Ausiello, editors. *Cecil Textbook of Medicine*. 23rd ed., Saunders/Elsevier, 2007. An excellent, concise presentation of the topic. It is recommended that the reader have a good science background, especially in biology.

Litin, Scott C., editor. *Mayo Clinic Family Health Book*. 4th ed., HarperResource, 2009. Good presentation of blood; concentrates on illnesses, both causes and treatments.

Mosby's Medical Dictionary. 8th ed., Mosby/Elsevier, 2009. Offers a basic presentation of medical terms and concepts.

Rodak, Bernadette, editor. *Hematology: Clinical Principles and Applications*. 3rd ed., Saunders/Elsevier, 2007. A comprehensive textbook covering all aspects of hematology and hemostasis.

Strand, Calvin L., and Jonas A. Shulman. *Bloodstream Infections: Laboratory Detection and Clinical Considerations*. American Society of Clinical Pathologists, 1988. A technical monograph reviewing the concepts and factors important in the selection and development of optimal blood culture systems for the detection of septicemia.

Wilson, Michael, Brian Henderson, and Rod McNab. *Bacterial Disease Mechanisms: An Introduction to Cellular Microbiology*. Cambridge UP, 2002. Basing their discussion on research advances in microbiology, molecular biology, and cell biology, the authors describe the interactions that exist between bacteria and human cells both in health and during infection.

Zucker-Franklin, D., et al. *Atlas of Blood Cells: Function and Pathology*. 3rd ed., Lea & Febiger, 2003. Great pictorial presentation of blood components in different stages of function and disease.

SEROLOGY

Category: Specialty
Anatomy or system affected: Blood, immune system
Specialties and related fields: Bacteriology, cytology, hematology, immunology, microbiology, oncology, pathology, preventive medicine, public health, virology
Definition: The study of serum, the liquid portion of blood, the testing of which is used in blood typing, vaccination, diagnosis, and therapy.
Key terms:

antibody: a protein substance produced by lymphocytes in response to an antigen in order to combat bacterial, viral, chemical, or other invasive agents in the body

antigen: a chemical substance often on a bacterial or viral surface, containing antigenic determinants that initiate the body's immune response

antigenic determinant: a molecule on the surface of a cell or microorganism that is specific for evoking an immune response

bacteria: microscopic single-celled organisms that exist throughout the environment

host: the body of the person or animal infected

immunoglobulin: antibody; the globulin fraction of serum protein

microorganism: any bacterium, virus, or other minute organism; some are harmless in the body or are involved in essential body processes, while others are harmful and cause disease

pathogen: any disease-causing microorganism, such as bacteria, viruses, yeasts, fungi, and spirochetes

seronegative: the test result seen when blood does not contain the specific antibody or antigen being sought and the particular antigen-antibody reaction is not present

seropositive: the test result seen when blood contains the specific antibody or antigen being sought and the particular antigen-antibody reaction is present

SCIENCE AND PROFESSION

The term "serology" comes from the Latin *sero* (serum, a blood liquid) and *ology* (the study of). Many serologic testing procedures have been developed to determine the amounts of specific antibodies the individual has circulating in his or her bloodstream. These tests can help the physician diagnose disease conditions and develop appropriate treatment regimens. To understand serological testing in relation to blood typing and immunity-two major uses of serology-it is necessary to understand the structure and nature of blood cells and the workings of the human immune system.

The surface of red blood cells contains antigenic determinants that define the individual's blood group. There are more than twenty blood grouping systems; the most common, the ABO system, identifies individuals as being in A, B, AB, or O groups, depending on the antigenic determinant present on their red blood cells. The red blood cells of people in the A group are covered with A antigen, in the B group with B antigen, and in the AB group with both antigens. Red blood cells in the O group have neither A nor B antigens. The antigenic determinant causes the body to produce antibodies against other blood types. For example, if an individual's red blood cells are coated with A antigen, the body will produce antibodies against B antigen. Therefore, if a person with A blood is given B blood cells, these cells will be regarded as foreign, and the body's anti-B antibodies will dissolve them, leading to a severe, life-threatening hemolytic reaction.

All the blood groups in the ABO system are also classified as either negative or positive for Rh factor, another antigen found on the red blood cells, and so named because a similar antigen was first found in rhesus monkeys. About 85 percent of the population is Rh positive; that is, these individuals have Rh antigens on their red blood cells. If an Rh-negative person is given Rh-positive blood, he or she may tolerate the first transfusion, but a severe, even fatal, reaction can occur if a second is given. Furthermore, if an Rh-negative woman becomes pregnant with an Rh-positive baby, she may be exposed to Rh-positive red blood cells and may develop anti-Rh antibodies. This reaction may be of no significance for the first baby, but if a subsequent baby is also Rh-positive, the mother's antibodies will attack and dissolve the red blood cells of the fetus and may cause intrauterine anemia, heart failure, or miscarriage.

As on the red blood cells, there are antigenic determinants on the surfaces of invading microorganisms that trigger the body's immune process: When a virus, bacterium, or other infective agent enters the body, the immune system recognizes the invader as foreign. Once the organism is recognized as an enemy, the body begins to respond with the host-defense mechanism, an intricate process that not only destroys the offending pathogen but also protects against future infection by it.

Two factors determine whether an organism is antigenic and thus will trigger the immune response. First, there must be antigenic determinants present on the organism's surface that the body identifies as foreign, or nonself. Second, the organism must be large enough to carry antigenic determinants on its surface. Antigenic determinants are large molecules; the more there are on the organism's surface, the greater the antigenicity.

Antigens induce the production of certain white blood cells called lymphocytes. There are two basic types of lymphocytes involved in the immune process. One is the T cell, which originates in the bone marrow and travels to the thymus gland, where it becomes specialized for its immune function. The other lymphocyte is the B cell, which originates in the bone marrow and develops fully in the lymph system. T cells and B cells each develop into cells specialized for specific tasks in the immune process.

About 70 percent of T cells become helper-inducer cells, which have various functions. They promote the production of B cells, support B-cell activity, and increase the production of macrophages (cells that destroy foreign substances and dead cells). They also become "memory cells" capable of recognizing a pathogen to which the body has been exposed. If the particular pathogen reenters the body, the memory cells trigger the immune system to synthesize antibodies against it. T cells also become "killer" T cells that attack pathogens directly.

B cells produce the antibodies that are detected in seropositive blood tests. Antibodies, also called immunoglobulins, are rings, chains, or Y-shaped proteins that are carried in blood plasma. There are five groups of immunoglobulins involved in the immune system: IgG, IgA, IgM, IgD, and IgE. IgG makes up about 80 percent of all immunoglobulins and is found in tissue fluid and plasma. Its major function is to combat bacteria and viruses and to neutralize poisonous substances. IgA (13 percent) is found in the secretions of seromucous glands in the nose, gastrointestinal tract, eyes, and lungs. It also combats bacteria and viruses. IgM (6 percent) is found in blood plasma. It reacts with antigens during the first exposure to the disease organism. IgD (less than 1 percent) is found on the surface of most B cells. Its activities are not fully understood, but it is thought to be involved in the production of antibodies. IgE (less than 1 percent) is bound to mast cells found in connective tissue. It promotes allergic reactions.

Antibodies work in two ways-by direct attack on an antigen and by activating a protein complex called a complement. In direct attack, there are four ways in which antibodies destroy antigens: agglutination, which causes antigens to clump together; precipitation, which causes antigens to form insoluble substances; neutralization, which prevents antigens from producing toxic substances; and lysis, which causes the cell walls of antigens to rupture.

The activation of a complement causes three main activities: chemotaxis, which attracts macrophages and other white blood cells to the area, where they can eliminate the pathogens that are present; opsonization, which alters the structure of the antigen cell wall, making it easier for macrophages to engulf and destroy it; and inflammation, a process that helps to prevent the spread of pathogens.

Like T cells, some B cells become memory cells that help prevent reinfection by recognizing and destroying a pathogen that they have previously encountered.

DIAGNOSTIC AND TREATMENT TECHNIQUES

The major use for seronegative-seropositive testing is in blood typing. The patient's blood type is recorded as part of his or her medical history and is required for a blood transfusion to ensure that the patient receives blood from a compatible donor. Blood typing is an activity conducted in, or readily available to, virtually every medical facility. A major example is the Coomb's test, which detects antibodies on red blood cells in the bloodstream and establishes whether the patient has sensitized cells. This information is helpful in cross-matching donor and patient blood and in the diagnosis of hemolytic anemia.

Another important aspect of serologic testing is to determine the immune status of an individual-that is, whether a person or a local population is immune to a specific disease or is susceptible and therefore should be vaccinated. Such tests are geared to the identification of antibodies that protect against certain diseases. These antibodies are created by exposure to the disease-causing microorganism as a result of infection by the organism itself; vaccination, in which a modified form of the microorganism is used to trigger the body's immune response; or immunity that is acquired by a newborn baby from a mother, an immune state that lasts only a few months. A test that comes back seronegative or with very low antibody levels indicates that the patient is not immune to a given disease. A test that comes back seropositive indicates that the patient has circulating antibodies characteristic of a specific disease and that, if the amount of antibodies is high enough, the patient is immune to the disease.

A good example of immune status determination is the testing for hepatitis B surface antigen among health care workers. Hepatitis B is a blood-borne disease that can be transmitted when infected blood or other body fluids enter the bloodstream of another person. Transmission often occurs among health care workers because they are often exposed to the blood and body fluids of patients during operating procedures, dental procedures, or even when the nurse or other health care worker draws blood and is inadvertently stuck with the needle. Tests show that health care workers are seropositive for hepatitis B surface antigen at rates far above the general population. For example, 25 percent of surgeons and dentists become seropositive after five to ten years in practice. These tests prove that some health care workers are at high risk for contracting hepatitis B from their patients. Therefore, routine vaccination is recommended for those health care workers who are likely to be exposed to the blood and body fluids of patients carrying the hepatitis B virus.

Seronegative-seropositive testing can also reveal whether a person who has been vaccinated against a certain disease has achieved immunity (has "seroconverted" and developed antibodies in response to the antigen), whether the individual has not achieved immunity, or whether the individual has achieved immunity and then lost it.

No vaccine is 100 percent effective, but the better ones induce an immune response in 90 to 98 percent of individuals. For example, measles vaccine is about 95 percent effective. This means that most of the children who have received it are immune to measles, but 5 percent or so remain susceptible.

A few vaccines produce lifelong immunity. With most, however, the amount of antibody diminishes after time, and the vaccination must be repeated to maintain immunity. In other words, the patient is given a "booster" shot. In the late 1980s, many children who had received measles vaccine and who had seroconverted were found to be seronegative: They had lost their immunity to measles. This finding suggested that the measles vaccine conveyed an immunity that could diminish with time. Therefore, medical authorities and public health organizations revised their recommendations for mass vaccination against measles. Instead of only one vaccination of the infant at twelve to fifteen months of age, the protocol now recommends repeating the vaccination at a later date.

Serologic tests are used in virtually all branches of medicine. One group of seronegative-seropositive tests is used to detect fetal abnormalities. Another group, autoantibody tests, detects such diseases as autoimmune hepatitis, thyroiditis, and systemic lupus erythematosus (SLE). One example is testing for rheumatoid factor, an antibody that appears in the blood of adult patients with rheumatoid arthritis. Its presence will help the physician make a diagnosis and determine a course of treatment for a patient with joint inflammation. Similarly, specific antibodies will indicate specific disease conditions. A patient with lupus has antinuclear antibody (ANA). Rheumatic fever diagnosis requires evidence of the bacteria *Streptococcus pyogenes*. Syphilis patients have antibodies to the spirochete *Treponema pallidum*. Patients with mononucleosis are seropositive for heterophile antibodies.

Viral, bacterial, and fungal tests detect antibodies or antigens developed in response to infection. These include the antistreptolysin-O test for streptococcal antibodies, the febrile agglutination test to detect diseases caused by salmonella, and the latex particle agglutination (LPA) tests for antigens of other bacteria. Also in this group are the hepatitis-B surface and core antigen tests, which are used to screen blood donors as well as to identify persons who have been exposed to hepatitis B. Fungal serology tests are used to detect various fungal infections. The fluorescent treponemal antibody absorption test is used to diagnose syphilis.

Serologic tests called general humoral tests are used to detect and diagnose various bodily dysfunctions. Another group called the general cellular tests includes the lymphocyte transformation test to determine whether transplant donors and recipients are compatible. In this group, the terminal deoxynucleotidyl transferase test is used to diagnose leukemias and lymphomas, as well as to monitor the progress of treatment. In cancer therapy, the carcinoembryonic antigen test (CEA) is used to gauge the response of certain cancers to treatment or to detect the recurrence of certain cancers.

A major new field for serology is emerging with monoclonal antibody research. In this science, antibodies can be manufactured in the laboratory. Instead of injecting a patient with modified antigen and inducing the body to create antibodies to it (as in vaccination), physicians can provide the patient with the antibodies themselves. Because these antibodies are absolutely identical to their parent protein or cell and to one another, they are not subject to the variables present in antibodies produced by other methods. They have properties that make them ideal for treating certain diseases.

Once the analysis of tissue identifies a specific antigen, it may be possible to program monoclonal antibodies to search out and destroy them. It is also possible to link the antibodies to chemotherapeutic agents. Thus, monoclonal antibodies can not only target specific antigens but also bring medication to the specific tissues where it is required. In cancer therapy, these qualities promise to improve the efficiency of treatment greatly. With monoclonal antibodies, cancer-destroying drugs can be brought directly to the cancer cell and can destroy it without harming other body tissues, thus reducing the severity of side effects from chemotherapy.

PERSPECTIVE AND PROSPECTS
The science of serology and serological testing for antibodies and antigens in the body have become mainstays of modern medical diagnosis and treatment for a wide range of diseases. Virtually every individual in

the industrialized world and most members of the developing world urban populations undergo serologic testing as part of their regular medical routine.

Serological testing is part of every hospital workup, almost every routine medical examination, every blood transfusion, all transplant procedures, many diagnostic procedures, and many treatment regimens. It is the basis for most epidemiological studies that enumerate the extent of susceptibility to individual diseases in various populations and hence directs the development of immunization programs. It is an integral part of vaccine production and is critical in the development of new vaccines. With the development of monoclonal antibody research, serology enters a new era where the possibilities of improved serologic testing and therapeutic modalities seem almost unlimited.

Serological testing and therapy, so far, have been based on the manipulation and modification of living organisms. It is theoretically possible to develop vaccines and therapeutic agents that are completely synthetic in structure. This science promises greater specificity and efficacy, both for vaccines and for disease treatment.

—*C. Richard Falcon*

See also Anemia; Antibodies; Blood and blood disorders; Blood testing; Cholesterol; Cytology; Cytopathology; Diagnosis; Dialysis; Fluids and electrolytes; Forensic pathology; Hematology; Hematology, pediatric; Hemophilia; Hodgkin's disease; Host-defense mechanisms; Hypercholesterolemia; Hyperlipidemia; Hypoglycemia; Immune system; Immunization and vaccination; Immunology; Immunopathology; Jaundice; Laboratory tests; Leukemia; Malaria; Pathology; Phlebotomy; Plasma; Rh factor; Septicemia; Sickle cell anemia; Thalassemia; Transfusion.

For Further Information:

Bryant, Neville J. *An Introduction to Immunohematology.* 3d ed. Philadelphia: W. B. Saunders, 1994. This book was written as a background text for laboratory personnel and students. Somewhat technical, but the writing is clear and the author covers the subject well.

Chase, Allan. *Magic Shots.* New York: William Morrow, 1982. An excellent history of immunization that covers ancient medical practice and describes the work of such early pioneers as Edward Jenner and Louis Pasteur. Details the major discoveries that have taken place in the twentieth century, such as the development of the polio vaccine and the eradication of smallpox.

Griffith, H. Winter. *Complete Guide to Medical Tests.* Tucson, Ariz.: Fisher Books, 1988. A complete compendium of all tests used in hospitals and other medical facilities. All current seronegative-seropositive tests are described and categorized according to their diagnostic and therapeutic uses.

———. *Complete Guide to Symptoms, Illness, and Surgery.* Revised and updated by Stephen Moore and Kenneth Yoder. Rev. 4th ed. New York: Perigee, 2000. Covers more than five hundred diseases and disorders and includes information about diagnostic tests that involve serology.

Litin, Scott C., ed. *Mayo Clinic Family Health Book.* 4th ed. New York: HarperResource, 2009. A superior medical reference for the general reader which gives a good presentation of blood.

Turgeon, Mary Louise. *Immunology and Serology in Laboratory Medicine.* 4th ed. St. Louis, Mo.: Mosby/Elsevier, 2009. A good introductory clinical text that details methodologies, clinical applications, and interpretations of basic serology.

Widmann, Frances K., and Carol Ann Itatani. *An Introduction to Clinical Immunology and Serology.* 2d ed. Philadelphia: F. A. Davis, 1998. Discusses immunology, immunopathology, and serologic testing methods. Includes bibliographical references and an index.

SEROTONIN

Category: Biology
Also known as: 5-hydroxytryptamine (5-HT)
Anatomy or system affected: Nervous, muscular
Specialties and related fields: Neurology, biochemistry, psychology
Definition: A neurotransmitter synthesized in the brain and gastrointestinal tract that seems to be involved with various functions including appetite, digestion, memory, mood and social behavior, sexual desire, and sleep

Key terms:

5-HT receptor agonists: substances that bind to 5-HT receptors preventing the action of serotonin

enteramine: the original name used for serotonin

neurotransmitter: a substance in the body that carries the nerve signal from one nerve cell to another or to a muscle

sudden infant death syndrome (*SIDS*): the death of child less than one year of age due to unknown factors

STRUCTURE AND FUNCTIONS

Serotonin, scientifically known as 5-hydroxytryptamine (5-HT), is a neurotransmitter, which is a substance in the body that carries the nerve signal from one nerve cell to another or to a muscle. Serotonin, when released by an axon, travels across the synapse or neuromuscular junction, binds to its receptor in its target cell and stimulates a nerve impulse in the target cell. Along with adrenaline and dopamine, serotonin is one of several monoamine neurotransmitters. Serotonin is synthesized in the brain and gastrointestinal tract.

Serotonin or 5-HT is synthesized when a hydroxyl group (OH) is transferred to tryptophan, an amino acid, by the enzyme tryptophan hydroxylase. Between 80 and 90 percent of the body's serotonin is synthesized in the gastrointestinal tract, but it is also found throughout the body in the central nervous system and in platelets.

Serotonin is believed to be involved in various functions including appetite, digestion, memory, mood and social behavior, sexual desire, and sleep. Research has found a relationship between mood and serotonin. Serotonin can also stimulate blood clot formation as it is synthesized by the platelets. Scientists believed that low levels of serotonin caused depression; however, studies have not been able to confirm serotonin's relationship to depression. Researchers working with mice that cannot synthesize serotonin have found no signs of depression in the animals, though the mice did display compulsive and aggressive behavior. It is possible that depression causes a reduction in serotonin production. Other possible reasons for the apparent connection between mood and serotonin include low tryptophan levels, a failure or lack of receptor sites, failure of serotonin to reach receptor sites, and reduced brain cell regeneration.

Men and women appear to react differently to changes in serotonin levels. A 2007 study in the journal *Biological Psychiatry* indicated that men with reduced levels of serotonin in the brain became impulsive while women developed a poorer mood and increased caution. Other studies seem to indicate that the interaction of serotonin and hormones may affect women during menopause, the postpartum period, and the premenstrual period-times when hormone levels fluctuate.

DISORDERS AND DISEASES

It is thought that a deficiency in serotonin may play a role in sudden infant death syndrome (SIDS). Mutant mice that synthesize lower levels of serotonin exhibit many SIDS characteristics including low heart rate and early death.

Humans with depression and mouse models of depression show a low level of a protein that assists in serotonin's function in the brain. Various drugs can alter the level of serotonin. Medications known as selective serotonin reuptake inhibitors (SSRIs) also known as serotonin-specific reuptake inhibitors or serotonergic antidepressants are prescribed to treat depression and anxiety because they have been found to increase extracellular serotonin levels. Like other neurotransmitters, serotonin is reabsorbed by the body after it has relayed a neural impulse. SSRIs hinder this reabsorption process, boosting serotonin levels. Some research suggests that high levels of serotonin improve transmission between brain cells, which improves one's mood. Other drugs that increase serotonin levels have been used clinically to treat migraine headaches and nausea.

Some substances, including dietary supplements such as St. John's wort, various medications and illicit drugs can overstimulate serotonin receptors. Carcinoid tumors which are often found in the gastrointestinal tract may cause high levels of serotonin. High serotonin may lead to a potentially life-threatening condition known as serotonin syndrome. Symptoms of this condition include agitation, confusion, diarrhea, headaches, increased heart rate and blood pressure, loss of muscle coordination, muscle rigidity, pupil dilation, shivering, and sweating.

Some research indicates that serotonin levels may be increased without medications. Possible methods include eating high protein foods that increase one's level of tryptophan, exercising, light, such as that used in treating seasonal affective disorder, and psychotherapy.

Drugs that bind to serotonin receptors, the 5-HT receptor agonists, can decrease the effects of serotonin. These drugs are often prescribed to reduce nausea from chemotherapy and radiation therapy. They are also used to treat migraine headaches.

PERSPECTIVE AND PROSPECTS

Serotonin was first discovered during the 1930s by Vittorio Erspamer who first isolated the molecule from stomach cells while studying intestinal smooth muscles cells. When incubated with intestines, the molecule stimulated intestinal smooth muscle contraction. Since the compound was an amine, Erspamer named the compound enteramine. In 1948, Irvine Page, Maurice Rapport, and Arda Green at the Cleveland Clinic discovered a blood derived compound that was a vasoconstrictor. Hence, they called it serotonin. By 1952, serotonin and enteramine were shown to be the same compound.

While studying neurotransmitters in mussels, Betty Mack Twarog was unable to identify the neurotransmitter that regulated muscle relaxation in the mollusks. After she read the Cleveland Clinic researchers' paper on serotonin, she became intrigued, but the paper only addressed serotonin in mammals. About that time, Erspamer found enteramine in octopus salivary glands, and soon after this discovery, enteramine was identified as serotonin. Twarog obtained a sample of serotonin and soon confirmed her suspicions that the neurotransmitter in the mussels was serotonin. She later worked at the Cleveland Clinic and confirmed her theory that serotonin was also found in the brain. The work of these researchers was instrumental in the development of the field of neuroscience, which is the study of the nervous system.

—*Josephine Campbell;*
updated by Charles L. Vigue, PhD

For Further Information:
Bouchez, Colette. "Serotonin: 9 Questions and Answers." *WebMD*. WebMD, LLC. 19 Mar. 2015. www.webmd.com/depression/features/serotonin

McIntosh, James. "What Is Serotonin? What Does Serotonin Do?" *MNT*. MediLexicon International Ltd. Web. 19 Mar. 2015. www.medicalnewstoday.com/articles/232248.php

McIntosh, James. Serotonin: Facts, What Does Serotonin Do? Medical News Today, April 29, 2016. www.medicalnewstoday. com/kc/serotonin-facts-232248

Nauert, Rick. "Mice Study Suggests Lack of Serotonin Not Behind Depression." *Psych Central*. Psych Central. 28 Aug. 2014. Web. 20 Mar. 2015. psychcentral.com/news/2014/08/28/mice- study-suggests-lack-of-serotonin-not-behind-depression/74206.html

Whitaker-Azmitia, Patricia Mack. "The Discovery of Serotonin and Its Role in Neuroscience." *Nature*. Nature Publishing Group. 1999. Web. 20 Mar. 2015. www.nature.com/npp/journal/v21/n1s/full/1395355a.html

SEVERE ACUTE RESPIRATORY SYNDROME (SARS)

Category: Disease/Disorder

Anatomy or system affected: Immune system, lungs, respiratory system

Specialties and related fields: Critical care, emergency medicine, epidemiology, internal medicine, microbiology, public health, pulmonary medicine, virology

Definition: A newly recognized type of pneumonia, caused by a novel coronavirus, that may progress to respiratory failure and death.

Key terms:

coronavirus: a single-stranded ribonucleic acid (RNA) virus with a spherical shape and helical nucleocapsid surrounded by an envelope with a crown of glycoprotein spikes

electron microscopy: an imaging technique in which magnetically directed electrons in a vacuum tube are absorbed and deflected by structures, thus forming an image on a screen with very high resolution

Koch's postulates: criteria for judging whether given bacteria cause a given disease, including that the bacteria must be present in every case, that they must be isolated from the host and grown in pure culture, that the disease must be reproduced when the culture is inoculated into a healthy susceptible host, and that the bacteria must be recoverable from the experimentally infected host

tissue culture: a diagnostic method in which cells from plant or animal tissues bathed in sustaining liquid solution form a monolayer on a container that can be inoculated and observed for deterioration or destruction by replicating viruses

CAUSES AND SYMPTOMS

SARS first received worldwide attention in February, 2003, after a Chinese physician from Guangdong Province and twelve other guests at a hotel in Hong Kong became ill. Subsequent investigation of cases traced the illness back to November, 2002, when a businessman from Guangdong Province developed the new disease and soon died. Using electron microscopy, molecular techniques, and tissue cultures, researchers have identified a coronavirus in a variety of specimens from patients with SARS. Glycoprotein spikes on the outside of the envelope surrounding the viral capsid give the appearance of a crown, or corona, and make possible the identification by electron microscopy. The virus was cultured from lung and kidney specimens obtained at autopsy of the Chinese physician using African green monkey kidney cells. Pure cultures of the coronavirus have been inoculated into monkeys, producing pneumonia. With Koch's postulates fulfilled, researchers are confident that the coronavirus is the causative agent.

Human studies have revealed antibodies to this coronavirus only in SARS patients, suggesting that this is a new type of infection. Similar studies in animals have shown that SARS antibodies are present in wild animals, including the masked palm civet, raccoon dog, and ferret badger. While these animals have been found to host the SARS coronavirus, a 2006 study suggested that the natural reservoir host of SARS is likely the horseshoe bat. The crowded, unclean markets of Guangdong Province, which sell wild animals for human consumption, may have provided the opportunity for the virus to infect humans.

After an incubation period of two to sixteen days after exposure, patients develop fever, chills and rigors, myalgia (muscle pain), cough, headache, and dizziness. Less common symptoms are sputum production, sore throat, nausea and vomiting, and diarrhea. Radiographs and high-resolution computed tomography (CT) scans of the chest show ground-glass opacities and unilateral or bilateral air-space consolidation. Laboratory findings early in the illness often include lymphopenia, thrombocytopenia, and a variety of serum enzyme (lactate dehydrogenase, creatinine kinase, and alanine aminotransferase) elevations distinguish-

---

**INFORMATION ON
SEVERE ACUTE RESPIRATORY SYNDROME (SARS)**

Causes: Coronavirus infection transmitted through contact with infected humans or animals

Symptoms: Severe pneumonia, with respiratory failure, fever, chills and rigors, muscle pain, coughing, headache, dizziness

Duration: Acute, sometimes fatal

Treatments: Supportive measures, corticosteroids, isolation ing SARS from pneumonia caused by usual bacterial pathogens.

SARS is often progressive in severity and is highly infective, especially for family members and health care workers. During the 2003 outbreak, the disease spread to many countries, with more than eight thousand cases and nine hundred deaths worldwide. The overall mortality rate was about 5 percent. Researchers wondered whether this respiratory illness would follow the seasonal pattern of similar viral illnesses, such as influenza. A SARS case diagnosed in Guangdong Province in January, 2004, led the Chinese government to order the mass slaughter of civets and rats in the hope of containing the disease.

Besides the livestock and human tolls, SARS inflicted economic and political damage. During the outbreak months in 2003, Asian countries saw a financial loss of roughly $28 billion. For the first time, the World Health Organization (WHO) issued an advisory suggesting that travelers avoid parts of the world infected with SARS. North American-based airlines cut 10 percent of their flights to Asia, resulting in a 60 percent drop in tourism. In Canada, China, and the United States, sporting events, public gatherings, film productions, religious services, and parades were canceled because of fears concerning SARS. An interesting footnote to the SARS legacy occurred in June, 2006, when Chinese researchers revealed that at least one of the reported SARS deaths in China during April, 2003, was actually the result of H5N1 avian influenza; raising the possibility that other cases and deaths attributed to SARS may have actually been human cases of H5N1 bird flu and that the Chinese government covered up the possibility that two pathogens were creating simultaneous outbreaks in order to avoid further economic disruption.

TREATMENT AND THERAPY

No specific diagnostic test for SARS is available, hampering early diagnosis and treatment. SARS cases can be suspected but not reliably distinguished from other types of pneumonia. Thus far, no antiviral agent has been found to be active against the SARS virus, and initial empiric therapy with antibacterial and antiviral agents has been directed at other pathogens that cause pneumonia that is indistinguishable from SARS.

Supportive measures directed toward respiratory failure, often provided in an intensive care unit, are the mainstays of SARS therapy. In some cases of progressive pneumonia with respiratory failure, corticosteroid therapy has been used. Because of the alarming infectivity and spread of SARS, precautions against airborne droplets (respirators) and direct contact (gowns and gloves) are recommended. Despite such measures, spread has occurred, probably because of improper techniques used by inadequately trained personnel.

PERSPECTIVE AND PROSPECTS

A coronavirus was first cultured from an adult patient with a common cold in 1965. It is now recognized that coronaviruses may cause up to 30 percent of common colds, but before SARS coronaviruses rarely produced pneumonia. These viruses also cause disease in a wide variety of animals, but usually in only one species. It is unclear how the SARS agent jumped from animals to humans. Furthermore, while some wild animals have been identified as having prior infection by the virus, the natural host remains uncertain. A more complete understanding of these issues will improve the chances of eliminating the disease from humans. Fortunately, only a few cases of SARS have been reported in the first few years of the twenty-first century, and these cases have been in laboratory workers or individuals directly exposed to civet cats. Since the 2002-2003 epidemic, human-to-human spread has ceased.

Extraordinarily rapid research has already produced sequencing of the SARS coronavirus genome. With this knowledge, molecular diagnostic techniques have been developed and should produce rapid and accurate diagnostic tests that will be widely available. Thousands of antiviral agents are being tested for activity against the virus, and new antivirals are being developed. Vaccines are available for some animal coronaviruses, and a SARS vaccine may be developed. In the meantime, there is hope that infection control and quarantine measures will be able to limit the spread of SARS.

—H. Bradford Hawley, MD;
updated by Randall L. Milstein, PhD

See also Coronaviruses; Emerging infectious diseases; Environmental diseases; Environmental health; Epidemics and pandemics; Epidemiology; Microbiology; Pneumonia; Pulmonary diseases; Pulmonary medicine; Viral infections; Zoonoses.

For Further Information:
Kleinman, Arthur, and James L. Watson, eds. *SARS in China: Prelude to Pandemic?* Stanford, Calif.: Stanford University Press, 2006.
Ksiazek, Thomas G., et al. "A Novel Coronavirus Associated with Severe Acute Respiratory Syndrome." *New England Journal of Medicine* 348 (May 15, 2003): 1953-1966.
Lee, Nelson, et al. "A Major Outbreak of Severe Acute Respiratory Syndrome in Hong Kong." *New England Journal of Medicine* 348 (May 15, 2003): 1986-1994.
McIntosh, Kenneth, and Stanley Perlman. "Coronaviruses, Including Severe Acute Respiratory Syndrome (SARS)-Associated Coronavirus." In *Mandell, Douglas, and Bennett's Principles and Practice of Infectious Diseases*, 7th ed., edited by Gerald L. Mandell, John F. Bennett, and Raphael Dolin. New York: Churchill Livingstone/Elsevier, 2010.
Wang, Lin-Fa, et al. "Review of Bats and SARS." *Emerging Infectious Diseases* 12 (December, 2006): 1834-1840.

SEVERE COMBINED IMMUNODEFICIENCY SYNDROME (SCID)

Category: Disease/Disorder
Also known as: Bubble boy disease
Anatomy or system affected: Immune system
Specialties and related fields: Biotechnology, genetics, immunology, pediatrics
Definition: A syndrome in which the immune system cannot produce T and B cells, resulting in catastrophic failure of the immune system. The underlying cause is a mutation in one of several key genes. Without specialized treatment involving tissue transplantation from a donor, death typically occurs.

Key terms:

B cell: a lymphocyte that synthesizes immunoglobulins (antibodies)

graft-versus-host disease (GVHD): a condition that occurs when transplanted organs or cells are recognized by the host's immune system as invaders, resulting in the donor cells being attacked by the host's immune system

leukemia: any of a variety of types of cancer involving the blood or bone marrow

reservoir: the host species in which a parasite is maintained in each area and from which it may infect other species, initiating an epidemic

T cell: a lymphocyte responsible for cell-mediated immune responses, including graft rejection

X-linked gene: a gene located on the X chromosome

CAUSES AND SYMPTOMS

Severe combined immunodeficiency syndrome (SCID) is a genetic defect in which one of several genes involved in the immune system has a mutation that either prevents gene expression or causes the production of faulty products. The most common cause of SCID, accounting for about half of cases, is mutations in the X-linked gene *IL2RG*, which codes for the third chain of the interleukin-2 (IL-2) receptor and a part of several other interleukin receptors. Interleukin receptors are proteins embedded in the plasma membrane of cells in the immune system that interact with interleukin molecules, carrying necessary immune system signals. This type of SCID is called "X-linked combined immunodeficiency" (XCID). The faulty interleukin receptors prevent the development of T cells and natural killer (NK) cells, both of which are required to prevent infections successfully. Because XCID is an X-linked defect, it is much more common in males.

The remaining cases of SCID are attributable to mutations in many different genes, with new defects being discovered every year. The genes involved range from those that code for proteins that interact with

> ### INFORMATION ON SEVERE COMBINED IMMUNODEFICIENCY SYNDROME (SCID)
>
> **Causes:** Various genetic defects
> **Symptoms:** Repeated, persistent infections that are unresponsive to standard treatments; may include meningitis, septic arthritis, opportunistic infections, graft-versus-host disease (GVHD)
> **Duration:** Chronic
> **Treatments:** Bone marrow transplantation, hormonal therapy, gene therapy

interleukin receptors and enzymes involved in purine metabolism to genes that code for enzymes involved in antigen receptor production. In addition, a variety of lesser-known defects and some genetic disorders show some, but not all, of SCID symptoms.

The most common of the remaining defects, accounting for about 20 percent of cases, is a deficiency in the enzyme adenosine deaminase (ADA), which is involved in purine degradation. Nucleotides are the building blocks of nucleic acids like deoxyribonucleic acid (DNA) and ribonucleic acid (RNA). These building blocks consist of phosphate, a five-carbon sugar, and a base. Nucleotides have a functional lifetime, and cells either degrade them into simpler components to either excrete or recycle them. ADA degrades the purine adenosine into inosine. The absence of functional ADA causes a form of SCID called ADA SCID. Without ADA activity, a subunit of DNA, deoxyadenosine triphosphate or dATP, accumulates to toxic levels. dATP inhibits the enzyme ribonucleotide reductase, the enzyme responsible for making DNA subunits in the cell. Low levels of other deoxyribonucleotides (dNTPs) prevent lymphocytes from making DNA and proliferating in response to an infection or disease. No T or B cells are produced. Deficiency in another enzyme, purine nucleoside phosphorylase (PNP), although much rarer, acts similarly.

Regardless of the underlying causes, symptoms are similar for most types of SCID. The overwhelming clinical symptom is problems with repeated, persistent infections that do not respond to standard treatment. Severe infections such as meningitis or septic arthritis may occur. Infections with opportunistic pathogens such as *Pneumocystis jirovecii* also frequently occur. Symptoms of (GVHD) may occur in infants because of lymphocytes received from the mother or in patients following blood transfusion. A chest X-ray typically shows a lack of a thymic shadow, indicating that the thymus has not developed properly. There is often a family history of immunodeficiency and infant deaths caused by severe infection.

David Vetter, a child born in 1971 with severe combined immunodeficiency (SCID). Photo by CNX OpenStax, via Wikimedia Commons.

TREATMENT AND THERAPY

Prenatal diagnosis is possible and is recommended in families with a history of SCID or similar problems. Left untreated, most infants die within the first year, so rapid identification of the symptoms is crucial. If SCID is detected early enough, several treatment options are available, even potential prenatal treatment.

For most SCID cases, bone marrow transplantation is the standard treatment. To prevent GVHD, either the marrow must come from an identical twin or be depleted of T cells before transplantation. Although a close genetic match has the highest success rate, unmatched and T cell-depleted marrow can be used if matched marrow is unavailable. A more than 90 percent survival rate has been accomplished when the marrow is from a parent or full sibling. It has typically been routine to use chemotherapy to kill the recipient's bone marrow before transplanting donor marrow. However, this is unnecessary (and seems to lower the survival rate) because the recipient has no T cells to cause rejection.

When transplantation is successful, donor stem cells in the marrow populate the recipient's marrow and establish a functioning immune system. Unfortunately, some residual GVHD may occur, and T-cell function seems to diminish over time in many cases, despite apparent initial success. The reasons for the latter problem are unknown.

Although transplantation may also work for ADA SCID, an alternative is polyethylene glycol (PEG)-bovine ADA replacement therapy. Attachment of PEG to the enzyme reduces its recognition by the immune system and prevents its degradation by plasma-based enzymes. PEG-ADA circulates throughout the blood, degrading adenosine and its metabolites, preventing their accumulation. This treatment must be administered on an ongoing basis by frequent intravenous injections of PEG-ADA to maintain appropriate enzyme levels. While PEG ADA does not enter cells, it does degrade those molecules that build up in cells and spill into the bloodstream. More than 150 patients worldwide have received PEG-ADA treatment.

It is usually administered weekly or twice a week by intramuscular injections. PEG-ADA treatment seems to be well tolerated and confers clinical benefits after the first month of therapy. Unfortunately, PEG-ADA is not always available and is extremely expensive; bone marrow transplantation is the only option in some cases.

Still in the experimental stage is gene therapy to replace the defective genes. Experiments on this approach began in the early 1990s. Although the first attempts at curing ADA SCID showed partial success, the patients still required continued treatment with PEG-ADA. Since then, efforts have focused on better ways to insert the correct genes into the patient's stem cells. Stem cells from the bone marrow must be isolated, treated, and returned to the patient.

The most promising results came from experiments begun in 1999 involving gene therapy for XCID. Following the procedure, the infants developed normal immune systems. Unfortunately, by the summer of 2002, one of the boys developed leukemia, and another developed it by the end of the same year. The apparent cause of the leukemia was the insertion of the gene at the wrong location, a concern expressed early in the discussion of gene therapy for this disease. Some trials ceased as a result. Gene therapy still holds great promise, but more work is needed to ensure its long-term safety and effectiveness.

—*Bryan Ness, PhD*

For Further Information:
Genetics and Immune Disorder. Stanford Children's Health, n.d., www.stanfordchildrens.org/en/topic/default?id= genetics-and-immune-disorders-134-122. Accessed 8 Apr. 2022.
Severe Combined Immune Deficiency and Combined Immune Deficiency. Immune Deficiency Foundation, n.d., primaryimmune.org/node/291. Accessed 8 Apr. 2022.
Severe Combined Immunodeficiency (SCID) in Children. Stanford Children's Health, n.d., www.stanfordchildrens.org/en/topic/default?id=severe-combined-immunodeficiency-scid-90-P01706. Accessed 8 Apr. 2022.
Severe Combined Immunodeficiency. American Academy of Allergy, Asthma, and Immunology, n.d., www.aaaai.org/Conditions-Treatments/Primary-Immunodeficiency-Disease/severe-combined-immunodeficiency. Accessed 8 Apr. 2022.
Severe Combined Immunodeficiency Syndrome (SCID). National Institute of Allergy and Infectious Diseases, 4 Apr. 2019, www.niaid.nih.gov/diseases-conditions/severe-combined-immunodeficiency-scid. Accessed 8 Apr. 2022.
X-linked severe combined immunodeficiency. MedlinePlus, 18 Mar. 2022, medlineplus.gov/genetics/condition/x-linked-severe-combined-immunodeficiency/. Accessed 8 Apr. 2022.

SEXUAL DIFFERENTIATION

Category: Biology
Anatomy or system affected: Endocrine system, genitals, glands, reproductive system, uterus
Specialties and related fields: Embryology, endocrinology, genetics, gynecology, urology
Definition: The process by which an embryo becomes male or female under the influence of genetic and hormonal factors.

Key terms:

differentiation: the process of gradual remodeling of tissues in the embryo or fetus; in this context, the process of formation of the male or female reproductive organs

external genitalia: in the male, the penis and scrotum; in the female, the clitoris, the vaginal opening, and the folds (labia) around it

gender identity: the mental view of oneself as a girl or woman or as a boy or man

gonad: the internal organ in either sex that produces the reproductive cells (ova and sperm): the ovary in the female and the testis in the male

hormone: a chemical that is produced by a gland in the body and secreted into the blood; hormones act as coordinating signals

hormone receptor: a molecule contained in or on a cell that allows it to respond to a hormone; if receptors are not present, the hormone will have no effect

Müllerian ducts: the pair of tubes in the early embryo that will develop into the internal female organs (uterus, oviducts, and upper vagina)

urethra: the tube that drains the bladder; in the male, the urethra passes through the penis and carries sperm during ejaculation, while in the female, the urethra opens in front of the vagina but does not have a reproductive function

Wolffian ducts: the pair of tubes in the early embryo that will develop into the internal male organs (the epididymis, vas deferens, and seminal vesicles)

X and Y chromosomes: the chromosomes that determine genetic sex; females carry an XX pair, and males carry an XY pair

FUNDAMENTALS

The chromosomal sex of a human is determined at the time of conception, when the ovum from the mother is fertilized by a single sperm from the father. All ova (eggs) produced by a female contain one chromosome, denoted X. Sperm from the male can carry either an X or a Y chromosome. The Y chromosome is smaller than the X and contains fewer genetic codes. Men normally produce equal numbers of X- and Y-bearing sperm. The type of chromosome carried by the one sperm that fertilizes the ovum will determine the sex of the embryo. A Y-bearing sperm joining with the ovum will result in an embryo with one X and one Y; this embryo will develop as a male. If the ovum is fertilized with an X-bearing sperm, the embryo will have two X's and will develop as a female.

Although the genetic sex is determined at conception, male and female embryos initially look alike, both internally and externally. For the first seven weeks of development, each human embryo has the anatomical potential to develop in either a male or a female direction: This period is referred to as the sexually indifferent stage. Internally, the gonads, which lie in the kidney region, cannot yet be identified as ovaries or testes. The other internal reproductive organs are represented in every embryo by two pairs of ducts: the Müllerian ducts, which will later develop in the female but will be lost in the male; and the Wolffian ducts, which will later develop in the male but will regress in the female. Externally, male and female embryos possess the same rudimentary genital organs, which will later be remodeled to become either male or female genitalia.

The first organ to differentiate in the embryo is the gonad. Starting at about seven weeks of development in a male embryo, the cells within the gonad are reorganized to form a testis. This reorganization is brought about by the presence of the Y chromosome, which contains the codes for the production of a substance called testis-determining factor (TDF). The chemical nature of TDF has not yet been determined, but its existence is clear from experimental evidence. TDF acts on the gonad to cause it to become a testis. In the absence of a Y chromosome and TDF in a female embryo, the gonad develops into an ovary at about twelve weeks of development. If an individual has only one X chromosome (a condition known as Turner syndrome), the gonads will develop into ovaries, but these ovaries will not contain ova and so the person will be infertile.

The development of the other reproductive organs is not directly determined by the X and Y chromosomes, but rather by hormones secreted by the gonads. In the male, the fetal testes begin to produce testosterone by the tenth week of development, and this testosterone acts on the Wolffian duct system to cause it to develop into the epididymis, vas deferens, and seminal vesicles. The Müllerian duct system in the male regresses under the influence of another hormone from the testes, called Müllerian-inhibiting hormone (MIH). In the female, MIH is not produced, and the Müllerian ducts develop into the oviducts, uterus, and upper part of the vagina. The Wolffian ducts in the female regress in the absence of testosterone. Normal female development does not, at this stage, re-

quire any hormone produced by the ovaries, but instead occurs spontaneously in the absence of testicular hormones. Thus, the presence or absence of the Y chromosome determines which type of gonad develops, and the presence or absence of gonadal hormones determines which type of internal reproductive organs develop.

Similarly, the development of the external genitalia is hormonally directed. In the male, testosterone is converted by the action of the enzyme 5-alpha-reductase to 5-alpha-dihydrotestosterone (DHT). DHT acts on the undifferentiated external genital tissue, causing it to take on a male appearance: A pea-shaped structure (the genital tubercle) at the front of the crotch area grows to become the penis, a slitlike opening (the urethral groove) is enclosed within the penis to become the urethra when two folds behind the genital tubercle fuse together, and two swellings on the sides of the urethral groove become enlarged as the scrotum. In the female, it is the absence of DHT that causes development in the female direction: The genital tubercle remains as the relatively small clitoris; the folds do not fuse, allowing the urethral groove to remain as an open area where the vagina and urethral openings are located; and the swellings that become the scrotum in the male remain separated as the labia in the female.

Hormones also cause sexual differentiation of the brain, but the mechanism is not fully understood in humans. The most obvious result of brain differentiation is the difference in adult hormone production patterns. In the adult male, hormone production is relatively constant from day to day, and this results in constant production of sperm in the testes. In the female, hormone production changes in a monthly cycle that is associated with ovum maturation and ovulation. The difference in the pattern of hormone release in adult males and females appears to be attributable to hormonal programming of the fetal brain. Animal studies indicate that the development of the male pattern results from exposure of the fetal brain to testosterone or one of its derivatives. The female pattern of development is prevalent when testosterone is absent. In humans, testosterone also affects brain differentiation, but the effect appears to be less permanent than in animals.

It is not known for sure if there is any direct influence of the chromosomes or prenatal hormones on male and female behavior. Most researchers agree that human behavior is heavily influenced by social and cultural factors, so the importance of prenatal programming is difficult to assess. Indeed, it appears that gender identity, the internal view of oneself as male or female, is so heavily influenced by learning that a child with a disorder of sexual differentiation can be success-

2612 • Sexual differentiation

fully reared in the gender that is opposite to that of the chromosomes. For example, a child born with female-appearing genitalia, but with XY chromosomes and internal testes, can be reared as a girl and will firmly adhere to this identity even if some masculinization occurs at the time of puberty.

DISORDERS AND DISEASES

Disorders of sexual differentiation result from errors in the signaling systems that normally direct male and female anatomical development. There are several different classes of these disorders, some of which result in a mixture of male and female reproductive organs. These disorders are rare, with the number of documented cases numbering only in the hundreds for most types.

True hermaphrodites are defined as individuals who possess both ovarian and testicular gonadal tissue. There may be one ovary and one testis, two gonads in which ovarian and testicular tissue are combined (ovotestes), or an ovotestis on one side and a normal ovary or testis on the other. True hermaphroditism can result from several distinct genetic anomalies. Some hermaphrodites have been shown to be chimeras: individuals that develop from the fusion of two separate embryos at an early stage. These individuals possess two distinct cell populations, one with an XX pair of chromosomes and one with XY. It is thought that expression of both of these chromosome pairs leads to the mixture of ovarian and testicular tissue seen in true hermaphrodites. A similar condition is mosaicism, in which the mixture of XX and XY cells is caused by errors of chromosome replication in a single early embryo. Other true hermaphrodites are neither chimeras nor mosaics; they appear to have a normal pair of XX or XY chromosomes, but on closer examination, one of the chromosomes is found to have a defect. For example, a Y chromosome may be missing a tiny piece, or an X chromosome may contain a portion of a Y.

There is much variation in the anatomical features of true hermaphrodites. One basic guideline is that the effects of the presence of testicular tissue are local. Thus, a true hermaphrodite with a testis on the left side and an ovary on the right will have Wolffian duct-derived (male) organs on the left side but Müllerian duct-derived (female) organs on the right. The external appearance depends on the relative levels of estrogen and testosterone but might include a typical male penis along with enlarged breasts. There are documented cases of ovulation and even pregnancy in true hermaphrodites. Successful sperm production appears to be less frequent than ovulation, and sperm production and ovulation are not seen in the same individual.

Pseudohermaphrodites are individuals whose external reproductive organs do not match their gonadal sex. Male pseudohermaphrodites have testes but external organs that appear to be female; female pseudohermaphrodites have ovaries and varying degrees of external male development.

Female pseudohermaphroditism has only one basic cause: the exposure of an XX fetus to masculinizing hormones. These hormones might come from the fetus itself, as in certain disorders involving the adrenal gland, or synthetic hormones given to a pregnant woman may have a masculinizing effect on a female fetus. The extent of masculinization depends on the timing of the hormone exposure, with earlier exposure leading to more extensive malelike appearance of the external genitalia, including fusion of the urethral folds and enlargement of the clitoris. The internal organs are normal female.

Male pseudohermaphroditism arises from a wide variety of causes. There may be failure of testosterone production, or the reproductive organs may lack testosterone receptors, causing them to fail to respond to the hormone. Because of the hormonal abnormalities, the Wolffian duct organs may fail to develop, and the external genitalia will appear female to some extent. If MIH production is normal, internal female organs will not be present. The appearance at puberty is variable, depending on the exact hormonal deficiency. Some individuals undergo the typical male responses of increased muscle mass, deepening of the voice, and growth of beard and chest hair; others do not. Most male pseudohermaphrodites are infertile because of the hormonal problems.

Treatment of disorders of sexual development depends on the exact symptoms and their cause, but the prevailing overall philosophy is to attempt to produce an individual who will be able to function sexually as an adult, even if that means sacrificing fertility and rearing the child in the sex opposite to that of the chromosomes. Early diagnosis is a key, since most authorities agree that gender identity is irrevocably set by the age of eighteen to twenty-four months. After that time, few physicians would be willing to try to alter the individual's gender identity from that which has already been established.

For true hermaphrodites, the choice of sex for rearing usually depends on the predominant appearance of the external genitalia. If the genital tubercle has remained small, like a clitoris, the decision is usually for a female sex assignment; if the tubercle appears more penislike, the individual can be reared as a male. Usually, the gonadal tissue that does not correspond to the sex of rearing will be removed, to prevent the production of hormones that would interfere with the desired appearance. Appropriate hormone treatment and surgery can enhance the body form of the chosen sex. For example, testosterone treatment will cause beard growth, and estrogen treatment will cause breast development.

In the case of female pseudohermaphrodites, most can successfully be reared as girls. Surgical alteration of the external genitalia and hormone treatment to correct the original problem may be necessary. Assuming early diagnosis and treatment, most female pseudohermaphrodites will be fertile as adults.

Similarly, hormonal treatment of male pseudohermaphrodites who do not produce testosterone can allow these individuals to be reared as boys, even if they are not fertile later. There is no treatment, however, that will allow a male pseudohermaphrodite who is unresponsive to testosterone to develop a male appearance; these individuals are usually reared as girls, with female pubertal development induced by estrogen treatment.

A fascinating form of male pseudohermaphroditism is seen in the *guevedoces* (meaning "penis at twelve") of the Dominican Republic. In this island nation, the extensive intermarriage of related individuals has produced a population in which a certain genetic defect is seen in relatively high numbers. This genetic defect results in absence of the 5-alpha-reductase enzyme necessary to convert testosterone to DHT. Affected individuals are born with external genitalia that appear more female than male. The internal reproductive organs, which are stimulated by testosterone rather than by DHT, are normal for a male, although the testes may remain in the body cavity instead of descending into a scrotum. Female internal organs are absent, since MIH production is normal. Traditionally, these individuals were reared as girls until the time of puberty, when growth of the penis occurred under the influence of increasing levels of testosterone. (Although the penis would enlarge, the opening of the urethra would remain misplaced for a male, being on the bottom of or behind the penis, a condition known as hypospadias.) At this time, these individuals would make a transition to a male gender identity and sex role. Although initially reared as female, the *guevedoces* were typically heterosexual as adult males, participating in sexual activity with females. Physicians and psychologists have been puzzled by the fact that the *guevedoces* could switch their gender identity at such an advanced age, in the face of evidence suggesting that this should be impossible. This traditional switch of sex role at puberty is no longer seen, since most *guevedoces* are now diagnosed at birth and reared as males from the start.

PERSPECTIVE AND PROSPECTS

Anatomical descriptions of people with disorders of sexual development are found in writings beginning in the pre-Christian era. The word "hermaphrodite" itself derives from the Greek myth about Hermaphroditos, the son of Hermes and Aphrodite, whose body was permanently merged with that of a nymph in a loving embrace. The myth probably arose from a desire to explain the existence of hermaphrodites.

Although the existence of hermaphrodites was known long ago, there was no understanding of the mechanism of sexual differentiation until modern times. During the nineteenth century, embryological studies firmly established the concept that the early human embryo is sexually indifferent anatomically. In the twentieth century, genetic and hormonal studies revealed the controlling factors in male and female development.

It was in the 1920s that the X and Y chromosomes were first discovered and recognized to be important in sex determination. Since the 1960s, researchers have had the ability to pinpoint the exact chromosome sites associated with many disorders of sexual differentiation. Ongoing efforts deal with the identification of the TDF coded by the Y chromosome and the mechanism by which TDF causes testicular development.

The nature of the hormonal control of sexual differentiation was determined by experiments such as those performed on rabbit embryos by A. Jost in the 1940s and 1950s. Jost systematically removed or transplanted embryonic testes and ovaries, and treated the embryos with estrogen and testosterone, in order to demonstrate the importance of hormones from the testis on the development of the internal and external reproductive organs.

Jost's conclusions for rabbits were confirmed in humans by studying individuals with disorders of sexual differentiation caused by genetic factors. Additional confirmation came from observations of the offspring of pregnant women treated with synthetic hormones as a possible preventive for miscarriage. Such treatment was later found to be ineffective in preventing miscarriage, but worse, the treated women often gave birth to masculinized female fetuses. It is now recognized that synthetic hormones in oral birth control pills can also masculinize female fetuses.

Discovery of the causes of true hermaphroditism and pseudohermaphroditism have allowed physicians to make important distinctions between these disorders, with a clear physical cause and manifestation, and the psychological disorders of sexuality that were previously confused with them. For example, until the middle of the twentieth century, the term "hermaphrodite" was used to refer not only to people with a mixture of male and female reproductive organs but also to those with a psychological confusion of gender identity. The latter individuals are now called transsexuals; they identify themselves by the gender that does not conform to the gender indicated by their reproductive organs. Transsexuals possess a complete set of normal reproductive organs and have no known chromosomal or hormonal abnormality. Another behavior is transvestism, which refers to the wearing of clothing of the opposite gender. Many transvestites are male heterosexuals who engage in this behavior to achieve sexual arousal; like transsexuals, transvestites have normal anatomy, chromosomes, and hormones. Finally, homosexual orientation is now considered to be a personality trait, rather than a disorder. Homosexuals are sexually and romantically attracted to individuals of the same gender; their reproductive organs, chromosomes, and hormone levels are the same as those of heterosexuals.

—*Marcia Watson-Whitmyre, PhD*

See also Embryology; Gender identity disorder; Gender reassignment surgery; Genetics and inheritance; Hermaphroditism and pseudohermaphroditism; Hormones; Men's health; Reproductive system; Sexual dysfunction; Sexuality; Women's health.

For Further Information:

Henry, Helen L., and Anthony W. Norman, eds. *Encyclopedia of Hormones.* 3 vols. Boston: Academic Press, 2003. A comprehensive overview of the role of hormones, the major physiological systems in which they operate, and the biological consequences of an excess or deficiency of a particular hormone.

Kronenberg, Henry M., et al., eds. *Williams Textbook of Endocrinology.* 11th ed. Philadelphia: Saunders/Elsevier, 2008. Discusses normal sexual differentiation and then covers all the known disorders, including appearance, chromosomes, hormone levels, fertility, and treatment.

Moore, Keith L., and T. V. N. Persaud. *The Developing Human.* 8th ed. Philadelphia: Saunders/Elsevier, 2008. An outstanding textbook on human embryonic development, with specific information about the causes of congenital malformations and common defects occurring in each of the body's systems.

Morland, Iain, ed. *Intersex and After.* Durham, N.C.: Duke University Press, 2009. Scholars explore what it means for people born with ambiguous genitalia-intersexed persons-for theories of gender. Examines "the ethics of medical treatment and the repercussions of intersex surgery," showing "how biology, activism, law, morality, and ethics have a shared interest in the relationship between intersexuality and the meaning of sex, gender, and sexuality."

Simpson, Joe Leigh, and Sherman Elias. *Genetics in Obstetrics and Gynecology.* 3d ed. Philadelphia: W. B. Saunders, 2003. Deals with the genetic basis of disorders of sexual differentiation and provides a detailed, technical account of the results of various genetic defects.

SEXUAL DYSFUNCTION

Category: Disease/Disorder
Anatomy or system affected: Genitals, psychic-emotional system, reproductive system
Specialties and related fields: Endocrinology, gynecology, psychiatry, psychology, urology
Definition: Impotence is the persistent inability of a man to achieve and maintain an erection adequate for penetration and sexual intercourse; frigidity is the disinterest in sex, usually applied to women, because of inadequate or unpleasurable sensation during intercourse.

Key terms:
corpora cavernosa: two passageways in the penis containing spongy reservoirs of tissue and blood vessels
etiology: the science of causes or origins, especially of diseases
neuropathy: malfunction of the nerves
organic disease: a disease caused or accompanied by an alteration in the structure of the tissues or organs
psychogenic: psychologic in origin

CAUSES AND SYMPTOMS

It is evident from the term "performance anxiety" that sexual anxiety is more easily recognized when it involves performance (that is, erections and orgasms) than when it involves subjective arousal. The most extreme example of this way of thinking is the familiar notion that women do not experience performance anxiety because it is only men who have to perform. When researchers searched for a corresponding term that refers not to performance but to subjectively felt arousal, they devised the oxymoronic-sounding term "pleasure anxiety." Performance anxiety refers to the fear of not being able to perform, while pleasure anxiety refers to the fear of feeling pleasure. Sex therapists have traditionally been much more concerned with the fear of not being able to perform.

To explain this blind spot in the field, it is clear that, historically, lack of desire has been considered a female disorder, whereas lack of performance has been considered a male disorder. From the male-identified point of view, the failure to perform is relatively understandable; it is often treated with humor, sympathy, or indulgence. Traditionally, however, the same indulgence has not been extended toward a woman when she cannot fulfill the role expected of her.

If there are any doubts that "frigidity" is a more accusatory term than "impotence," "impotence" as a diagnostic term retains its currency, whereas "frigidity" has largely been dropped. Researchers William H. Masters and Virginia E. Johnson were the first authorities to drop the term, and as a result of their influence it is rarely used in the field of sex therapy and research. It is still used, however, in the psychoanalytic literature.

The category of "inhibited sexual desire" in the American Psychiatric Association's *Diagnostic and Statistical Manual of Mental Disorders: DSM-III* (3d ed., 1980) indicated the difficulty in finding a nonjudgmental means of referring to the lack of erotic arousal: The term "inhibition" implies that the conditions for desire are present but that desire is being withheld. One of the implied accusations in the term "frigidity" is that the woman who does not experience erotic arousal is a cold, unfeeling, or withholding person. The work group on psychosexual disorders for the revision of the DSM-III-R published in 1987 first recognized this difficulty and recommended that "inhibited sexual desire" be renamed "hypoactive sexual desire disorder," arguing that this more awkward term is necessary because it reflects greater neutrality in terms of etiology.

In the 1970s researchers noted that the diagnosis of low sexual desire among couples seeking help with sexual dysfunction increased from approximately one-third of couples in the early 1970s to more than one-half of couples by the early 1980s. Men as well as women were identified with low sexual desire, or frigidity. Most of the knowledge of the causes of low sexual desire is based on clinical experience, rather than on more empirical and objective research. It has become clear that there is no single cause for low sexual desire. Rather, many cases involve several causal factors working simultaneously.

Virtually every standard work on sexual dysfunction lists religious orthodoxy as a major cause of sexual dysfunction. Some patients suffer from low sexual desire because they essentially lack the capacity for play (the obsessive-compulsive personality). Specific sexual phobias or aversions also may cause low sexual desire. Low-desire men almost uniformly have some degree of aversion to the vagina and female genitals. Women who have been sexually molested as children, or raped as adults, often have specific aversion reactions.

Some patients fear that if they allow themselves to feel any sexual desire at all, they will lose all control over themselves and begin acting out sexually in ways that would have disastrous consequences. Fear of pregnancy is often a "masked" cause of low sexual desire among women. Depression, hormonal issues, the side effects of medication, relationship problems, lack of attraction to one's partner, fear of closeness, and an inability to fuse feelings of love and sexual desire are among the many causes of low sexual desire in both men and women.

With regard to impotence, although the exact number is not known, it has been estimated that there are approximately ten million men in the United States

---

INFORMATION ON SEXUAL DYSFUNCTION

Causes: Stress, psychological factors, injury, hormonal disorders, disease, substance abuse, chronic kidney failure, spinal cord malfunction, history of sexual abuse

Symptoms: Impotence, inhibited sexual desire

Duration: Acute to chronic

Treatments: Behavior therapy, psychotherapy, medications, vacuum tumescence devices, surgical reconstruction

---

suffering from impotence. In the past, it was thought that psychogenic causes accounted for 90 percent of impotence, with only 10 percent attributable to medical or postsurgical diseases, so-called physical or organic impotence. As medical knowledge increased, in the early 1990s it was estimated that medical or organic causes accounted for 50 to 70 percent of all patients suffering from impotence.

Until the 1980s, it was difficult to determine whether any given patient was impotent as a result of psychogenic causes or physical, organic ones. The availability of blood tests to measure hormone levels and of penile tumescence sleep laboratory testing now allows for accurate determination of the true cause of impotence in patients. Yet even when it is attributable to organic causes, impotence has significant psychological implications.

Impotence can be defined as the persistent inability to attain and maintain a rigid penis adequate for penetration and successful completion of intercourse. There are two types of impotence: primary and secondary. Primary impotence is the term used to describe the male who has never been able to achieve an erection adequate for sexual intercourse. This is a relatively rare condition. Except in very unusual circumstances that might have involved a surgical procedure on the penis during childhood, primary impotence is not caused by any physical defect but instead has a psychologic basis. Men with primary impotence are most often found to have had a severely repressive childhood. These patients generally exhibit considerable conflict in their relationships with women and have hostile or fearful attitudes toward females.

The majority of men with impotence have secondary impotence; that is, at one time in their lives they were capable of full erections and intercourse but have subsequently lost that ability. In the 1980s, other medical terms for impotence came into common use, such as "erectile dysfunction." As in the case of "frigidity," the word "impotence" has had negative connotations.

Diabetes mellitus is a rather common organic medical problem accounting for impotence in many men. It has been estimated that 50 percent of men who have had diabetes for twenty years become impotent. It is thought that diabetes results in impotence by causing neuropathy or malfunction of the nerves, as well as narrowing of the blood vessels. Arteriosclerosis, or hardening of the arteries, causes a narrowing of the blood vessels. Many patients who have arteriosclerosis involving the aorta or smaller blood vessels that supply blood to the penis will experience impotence.

Chronic kidney failure, cirrhosis (chronic liver disease), neurological diseases such as Parkinson's disease and multiple sclerosis, malfunction of the spinal cord (such as spina bifida or spinal cord injury), and low levels of testosterone are also frequent organic causes of impotence. Masters and Johnson have stated that alcoholism is the second most common cause of impotence. Pelvic fractures and trauma, radiation therapy, radical pelvic surgery (including removal of the prostate, bladder, or rectum), and aortic aneurysm repair can cause nerve and blood vessel injuries that can result in impotence and/or problems with ejaculation. Penile cancer, Peyronie's disease (curvature of the penis as a result of scar tissue formation), and priapism (prolonged erection of the penis) are also causes of organic impotence. It has been reported that prescription drugs may account for 25 percent of patients with impotence. By far the most common group of drugs resulting in impotence are those taken for treatment of hypertension, or high blood pressure.

TREATMENT AND THERAPY

There are several difficulties inherent in devising a treatment program for low sexual desire. While most of the behavioral exercises devised by Masters and Johnson may enhance arousal and orgasm, they often fail in increasing sexual desire or motivation, since they were not designed to deal specifically with low sexual desire. A second problem is that many cases of low sexual desire not only are quite complex but are diverse in apparent etiology and maintenance factors as well. Each case of low desire must be examined on its own terms, and treatment must be tailored to the specific needs of the individual.

Behavior therapy and social learning theory contributed most of the effective techniques that constituted sex therapy in the 1980s. Other therapeutic approaches, however, have been used as adjunct techniques or proposed alternatives. One broad-spectrum approach attempts to integrate interventions from many theoretical orientations into a comprehensive treatment program, while remaining sensitive to the need to fine-tune the program to the individual.

The first step in this broad-spectrum approach is experiential/sensory awareness. Many patients with low sexual desire are unable to verbalize their feelings and are often unaware of their responses to situations involving sexual stimulation. The goal of this phase of therapy is to help patients recognize, using bodily cues, when they are experiencing feelings of anxiety, pleasure, anger, or disgust.

The second stage is the insight phase of therapy, in which patients, with the help of the therapist, attempt to learn and understand what is causing and maintaining their low desire. Frequently, patients with low sexual desire have misconceptions and self-defeating attitudes about the cause of the problem. Patients are helped to reformulate attitudes about the cause of the problem in a way that is conducive to therapeutic change.

The third stage, the cognitive phase of therapy, is designed to alter irrational thoughts that inhibit sexual desire. Patients are helped to identify self-statements that interfere with sexual desire. They are helped to accept the general assumption that their emotional reactions can be directly influenced by their expectations, labels, and self-statements. Patients are taught that unrealistic or irrational beliefs may be the main cause of their emotional reactions and that they can change these unrealistic attitudes. With change, patients can reevaluate specific situations more realistically and can reduce negative emotional reactions that cause low desire.

The final element of this treatment program consists of behavioral interventions. Behavioral assignments are used throughout the therapy process and include basic sex therapy as well as other sexual and nonsexual behavior procedures. Behavioral interventions are used to help patients change nonsexual behaviors that may be helping to cause or maintain the sexual difficulty. Assertiveness training, communication training, and skill training in negotiation are examples of such behavioral interventions.

The treatment of psychogenic impotence includes supportive psychotherapy and behavior-oriented tasks. If, during the course of evaluation, symptoms of depression such as loss of libido and appetite or sleep difficulties are present without a physical basis, the patient is often treated with an antidepressant medication. As mental depression lessens, sexual interest and potency will often return. Depression is the most common mental disorder detected when impotent patients undergo psychological studies.

There are certain causes of organic impotence that may be reversible with appropriate therapy. The alcoholic patient, for example, may regain his potency if his drinking problem can be resolved. The heavy cigarette smoker may similarly experience improvement in his general health and regain erections following cessation of smoking. Patients with newly discovered diabetes mellitus and high blood sugars may regain their erections following control of their diabetes with insulin, diet, or oral medications. This improvement will not be seen, however, in those individuals with long-standing diabetes who lose their erections.

Treatment programs for organic impotence are geared toward the problems of each individual and are often age-dependent. From 1980 to 1990, there were major advances not only in the diagnosis but also in the treatment of erectile insufficiency; moreover, many of those major treatment advances were nonsurgical. As a result of these nonsurgical advances and their positive rate of success, men often are encouraged to begin their treatment program with the most conservative technique possible. It has been estimated that approximately 90 percent of patients with erectile insufficiency are adequately treated with one of the following (conservative) medical programs: oral medication, self-injection, and vacuum tumescence devices.

Often the first step to medical management of erectile dysfunction is oral medication. Generally, these medications cause smooth muscle relaxation, thereby enhancing the blood flow into the penis. The drug Viagra (sildenafil), introduced in 1998, allows sufficient blood flow for an erection over a four- to five-hour period. Viagra boasted a success rate of almost 80 percent and was immediately in great demand. Dangerous side effects were noted, however, when sildenafil is used in conjunction with nitroglycerin or long-acting nitrates in any form. These nitrate medications in combination with sildenafil produce significant blood pressure drops and are dangerous, especially to patients with compromised cardiac status. Soon after its introduction, concerns arose over the misuse of Viagra to enhance sexual performance instead of to treat impotence. Drugs similar to sildenafil, which are classified as phosphodiesterase V (PDE V) inhibitors, are new to the market. These drugs facilitate erectile function by stimulating the relaxation of smooth muscle tissue in the erectile bodies of the penis. This relaxation allows rapid blood flow into the penis and facilitates erectile function in men with erectile dysfunction. Additional drugs, including tadalafil (Cialis) and vardenafil (Levitra), have been approved for the treatment of erectile dysfunction in certain markets. Other agents, including apomorphine (Uprima), will stimulate central nervous system functions, providing improved erectile function. Uprima, which has been approved by the FDA Advisory Panel, is the first agent to act on the central nervous system to improve erectile dysfunction. Medications to increase sexual desire are also being investigated by various pharmaceutical companies in conjunction with the Food and Drug Administration (FDA).

Penile injection with drugs is a treatment for male impotence that was popularized in 1982 by Ronald Virag of Paris. Penile injection with vasoactive compounds to effect an erection, however, had not yet been approved by the FDA in the United States by the late 1990s. Thus patients were required to sign a legal release of liability if this method of treatment was chosen.

In the 1990s, there were approximately eighty thousand males using self-injection therapy (for the treatment of erectile impotence) in the United States. This method of treatment has gained much international acceptance and continues to be the focus of much clinical and laboratory research. This technique is relatively painless and quick, producing results in ten to twenty minutes. Treatment is initiated by administering a test dose of the medication. During this initial stage of treatment, the medication dosage level is adjusted. The patient is then taught the injection technique, given instructions on how to care for the medication and equipment, and given an assessment of erectile response. This method is considered simple, safe, and highly successful (with a success rate of approximately 75 to 80 percent). The major complications are priapism and penile scarring, which occurs in 1 to 2 percent of cases.

Another nonsurgical option available is vacuum tumescence therapy. This device enables the patient to attain penile enlargement and rigidity by inducing blood flow into the penile shaft. Once the blood flow is induced by the creation of a vacuum, it is trapped by the use of an occlusive device applied at the base of the penis. Although it produces a successful erection in approximately 75 percent of cases, the vacuum tumescence device and the accompanying obstructing rubber occlusive device prevent the ejaculate from being expelled in most cases.

Many men with erectile dysfunction are best treated by surgical reconstruction. This group represents approximately 10 percent of the entire impotent population. Penile revascularization is one option. The patients who are best treated with penile revascularization are typically men under fifty years of age. Generally, these men are nonsmoking, healthy individuals whose potency problems are caused by a single lesion or injury. The purpose of penile revascularization is to channel more blood into the corpora cavernosa and thereby increase the corpora cavernosa pressure. Pressure can be increased by a variety of methods, including bypass artery-to-artery, bypass artery-to-vein, or closure of specific leaking areas in the corpora cavernosa.

Although available since the mid-1930s, penile prosthetics made their greatest strides after the introduction of synthetic materials (plastics) in the 1950s. Since then, major changes in design, function, and surgical technique have evolved. The prosthetics available by the late twentieth century were of three basic varieties: simple rods, flexible rods, and hydraulic devices (one-piece, two-piece, and multicomponent). Once implanted, prosthetics give the patient a return to "normal erectile dynamics." Although the tumescence-detumescence cycle is a result of the patient's prosthesis, sensation, satisfaction, and often even ejaculation remain as they were prior to surgery.

PERSPECTIVE AND PROSPECTS

Anthropologists have found that impotence (erectile dysfunction) and frigidity (inhibited or low sexual desire) have been observed in both primitive and highly developed societies. During most of human history, it was taken for granted that women attain sexual gratification in the same manner as men. Little attention was paid to the failures.

One of the most significant social changes affecting attitudes toward these sexual dysfunctions has been the altered status of women in contemporary society. During the Victorian era, whether they worked or not, women were legally the wards of men and had virtually no civil rights. Many of the Victorian attitudes toward sex-fears, prejudices, taboos, and superstitions-remained powerful influences into the late twentieth century.

Researchers, however, have learned that they cannot understand the problem of impotence in women by comparing it with impotence in men, since the dynamics as well as the treatments for each disorder differ greatly. With the women's movement and the Masters and Johnson research into human sexuality, the archaic terms "impotence" and "frigidity" were called into question. More gender-neutral terms were used, and, particularly in the case of erectile insufficiency, organic as opposed to psychogenic etiologies were acknowledged. By the late twentieth century, erectile insufficiency had become a disorder more often treated by urologists than by psychiatrists.

With this changing attitude toward these sexual dysfunctions among the medical community as well as the public at large, more research was devoted to treating the problems effectively and to reassuring the patients. Age-old stereotypes came under attack, such as the notion that performance anxiety affects only men and that frigidity or low sexual desire is a disorder that affects only women. As more organic etiologies for both erectile dysfunction and low sexual desire are acknowledged, patients feel increasingly comfortable seeking medical attention, and the stigma of sexual dysfunction being purely psychological is slowly beginning to vanish.

—*Genevieve Slomski, PhD*

See also Alcoholism; Anxiety; Aphrodisiacs; Arteriosclerosis; Cirrhosis; Diabetes mellitus; Erectile dysfunction; Genital disorders, female; Genital disorders, male; Hormones; Hypertension; Menopause; Men's health; Multiple sclerosis; Parkinson's disease; Prostate cancer; Psychiatry; Psychiatry, geriatric; Psychosomatic disorders; Renal failure; Sexuality; Spina bifida; Stress; Urinary disorders; Women's health.

For Further Information:
Crooks, Robert, and Karla Baur. *Our Sexuality*. 10th ed. Belmont, Calif.: Wadsworth, 2010. A college textbook that covers the span of human sexuality, including topics such as sexual health, dysfunction, and recent research.
Daniluk, Judith C. *Women's Sexuality Across the Life Span: Challenging Myths, Creating Meanings*. New York: Guilford Press, 1998. Examines how women experience sexuality from childhood through old age, with a focus on the complex interaction of psychological, social, cultural, and biological influences on the creation of individual sexual meanings.
Ellsworth, Pamela, and Bob Stanley. *One Hundred Questions and Answers About Erectile Dysfunction*. 2d ed. Sudbury, Mass.: Jones and Bartlett, 2008. A patient-oriented guide that cover basic questions about the condition such as causes, symptoms, and diagnosis; available treatments and how to choose among them; and ways of coping with common emotional and physical difficulties associated with the diagnosis and treatment.
Kaplan, Helen Singer. *The Sexual Desire Disorders: Dysfunctional Regulation of Sexual Motivation*. New York: Brunner/Mazel, 1995. This book provides current thinking on disorders of sexual desire and directions for contemporary treatment.
Miller, Karl E. "Treatment of Antidepressant-Associated Sexual Dysfunction." *American Family Physician* 61, no. 12 (June 15, 2000): 3728. Many classes of antidepressants, including the selective serotonin reuptake inhibitors (SSRIs), can impair sexual function. Michelson and associates evaluated the effectiveness of buspirone and amantadine in the treatment of sexual dysfunction associated with fluoxetine use.
Parker, James N., and Philip M. Parker, eds. *The Official Patient's Sourcebook on Impotence*. San Diego, Calif.: Icon Health, 2002. Draws from public, academic, government, and peer-reviewed research to provide a wide-ranging handbook for patients with impotence.
Phillips, Nancy A. "Female Sexual Dysfunction: Evaluation and Treatment." *American Family Physician* 62, no. 1 (July 1, 2000): 127-136. Sexual dysfunction includes desire, arousal, orgasmic, and sex pain disorders. Basic treatment strategies, which may be successfully provided by primary care physicians for most sexual dysfunctions, are discussed.
Taguchi, Yosh, and Merrily Weisbord, eds. *Private Parts: An Owner's Guide to the Male Anatomy*. 3d ed. Toronto, Ont.: McClelland & Stewart, 2003. A guide to male genital and sexual health, covering topics such as prostate trouble, erectile dysfunction, infertility, cancer, sexually transmitted diseases, vasectomies, and artificial insemination.

SEXUAL REASSIGNMENT

Category: Procedure
Key terms:

cisgender: a person whose sense of gender identity corresponds to the designation given at birth

feminizing genitoplasty: male-to-female surgical procedures including penectomy, orchiectomy, and vaginoplasty

gender: the properties of organisms based on their reproductive roles

genderdysphoria: discomfort or anxiety that arises with discontent with one's biological sex, with desire for another sex's physical characteristics and role

intersex: genitalia that are not absolutely identifiable as either male or female

masculinizing vaginoplasty: female-to-male surgical procedures including metoidioplasty and phalloplasty

trans man: a person born female who has transitioned to male

trans woman: a person born male who has transitioned to female

transition: the process of assuming the sexual identity that is congruent with one's own private and subjective experience; this process may or may not include medical assistance such as cross-gender hormone replacement or surgery

transgender: an umbrella term for anyone whose sense of gender identity does not correspond to the designation given at birth (gender-variant people); includes transsexual people

transsexual: one who wishes to assume a sexual identity different from that assigned at birth, or someone who has undergone surgery to change the sexual organs; pertains to sexual characteristics but not necessarily to sexual activities

INDICATIONS

At or before birth a baby's sex is assigned based on the child's external genitalia. When a child's genitals are ambiguous, sometimes called intersex, generally a sex is assigned based on the sex that appears to be predominant. Even in the absence of ambiguity and even well before puberty, some people feel a gender identity that differs from the sex that was biologically assigned. The unease that this disparity evokes is called gender dysphoria.

People whose gender identity differs from their anatomic sex are transgender people, sometimes known as transgendered. When a woman feels that the sex she was assigned at birth is not who she is, she may either dress and act as a man or elect to undergo surgery known as female-to-male reassignment to bring her body more into line with her sexual identity; a man

whose sexual identity is female may identify as female or undergo male-to-female surgical procedures. When people transition from one sex to another, they are considered transsexual. The process of sexual reassignment is known as gender-confirmation surgery or sex-reconstruction surgery.

Although many transgendered people report that they felt gender dysphoria in childhood, one study found that most do not disclose these feelings to their families until later in their teens. Living with such unspoken disparity is hard, and mental illness rates are higher in the transgendered than in the cisgendered. In addition, transgendered people are often targets of violence—which may be self-inflicted. According to a 2010 study, transgender people attempt suicide at a rate 25 times higher than do the cisgendered. Childhood can be a time of trial for anyone. For the transgendered, support from the family is particularly important yet is available only for the fortunate. It is noteworthy that mental health has been shown to improve in young transgendered people who transition surgically.

PROCEDURES

People who experience gender dysphoria may elect to undergo sex-reassignment surgery (SRS, also called by a variety of terms including gender-reassignment surgery, gender-affirming surgery, sex-realignment surgery, sex-reconstruction surgery, or gender-confirmation surgery). The procedure (singular or several) seeks to alter physical appearance and existing sexual organs to more closely resemble those of the gender with which the transgendered person identifies.

In 1931 Berlin Dora Richter had the first known vaginoplasty, which consisted simply of removing the penis; other such surgeries followed suit. The limits of this disfigurement soon became apparent, and surgeons began to develop more complex and, for the patient, satisfying SRS procedures. The process was technically complex, but also hampered by reluctance on the part of many medical practitioners, in effect, to fix that which wasn't broken. Over time, however, the medical community and families of the transgendered began to be convinced that, to the afflicted, gender dysphoria is all too real and, in fact, might be capable of being 'fixed'.

As demand for the surgeries continued, a 1992 study found that 98.5% of those undergoing male-to-female surgeries, and 99% of those who underwent female-to-male surgeries, did not regret their decisions. It may be preferable, when possible, to transit earlier in life, prior to puberty, as trans people may experience considerable distress as their bodies begin to show characteristics that they feel are alien. Transgender surgery in people past puberty is also complicated by the difference in pubic bones between the sexes, as to accommodate childbirth a biological woman's pelvis is wider and larger and set at a more obtuse angle than a man's. Many variations in surgical procedures have been tried and are as yet being devised. Although most transgender surgeries go as planned, surgeons are human and surgical mishaps do occasionally occur. Even when all goes as planned SRS is in almost every case a lifetime commitment that before being undertaken must be thoroughly considered and understood. With or without surgery, hormone-replacement therapy has its own impacts, some of which are noted below.

MALE-TO-FEMALE SRS

Any procedure to construct a vagina is called vaginoplasty (including surgical reconstruction following removal of growths or to correct prolapse or congenital defects). Genital reconstruction for trans women often involves surgical inversion of the penis to construct a vagina. Inversion techniques using segments of the sigmoid colon or small intestine rather than the penis may produce a better semblance to genitals of cisgender women. Skin flaps from the penis and scrotum, sometimes in combination with a urethral flap, or nongenital skin grafts from other body parts may also be used. The neovagina may be lined with skin from the inferior pedicle or abdomen. The urethra is shortened and reoriented.

Ancillary procedures to more closely align with cisgender women include removal of testes (orchiectomy) and, if not inverted, penis (penectomy).

Trans women may choose aesthetic procedures such as breast augmentation and hair implants, and surgeries to feminize their facial contours.

Complications. Sex differences in pubic architecture, noted above, can make it difficult to allow sufficient septal thickness between the rectal wall and the neovagina; resultant weakness can cause fistula (tearing). When a vagina has been constructed, without sufficient post-surgical dilation the inner skin graft can shrink or collapse. In shortening the urethra, stricture (narrowing) may occur but is usually reparable.

FEMALE-TO-MALE SRS

Genital reconstruction for trans men entails formation of a penis through phalloplasty or metoidioplasty. Phalloplasty involves extending the urethra with a tubed flap of tissue from another part of the body. During a second surgery, an erectile prosthesis may be implanted.

For metoidioplasty (sometimes known as metaoidioplasty), provision of testosterone gradually enlarges the clitoris to the point where it can be removed from the labia minora and lowered to the position occupied by the penis. Erectile tissue in the enlarged clitoris functions normally, as the clitoris develops from the same embryonic tissue as does the penis. The urethra need not be extended for metoidioplasty and thus is less expensive and has fewer complications, but then standing urination is no longer an option.

Technically, metoidioplasty is less complex and less expensive than phalloplasty. But, once recovered from surgery, people who have undergone phalloplasty are often more able to complete sexual penetration. This may be in part because the enlarged clitoris may not be capable of attaining the rigidity of a penis.

Medically assisted transition for trans men may include mastectomy and further surgical shaping of a male-contoured chest. Trans men may also undergo hysterectomy and removal of ovaries and Fallopian tubes (salpingo-oophorectomy).

Complications. Because the urethra of a trans man must be lengthened significantly, complications are more likely to occur. Postoperatively, about a quarter of patients in one study who had had their urethrae elongated had transient swelling that caused some urine dribbling, but this subsided without medical intervention. Trans men who had had the urethra extended had small changes of strictures, or narrowing of the urethra, or of a fistula, or hole in the urethra, needing minor repair. Chest surgery to remove breasts will leave scarring. The nipples may have reduced sensation, and their placement may be asymmetrical.

HRT EFFECTS

For transitions accompanied by hormones (hormone-replacement therapy), trans men will probably use testosterone in one of its forms, be it injectable, topically as a cream or gel, applied via patch, or by a pellet subcutaneously inserted; trans women may block their testosterone with an antiandrogen, commonly called a "t-blocker", while receiving estrogen and progesterone.

Although hormones have effects in everyone, often we overlook or minimize them. Sex hormones are the same for men and women, but their ratios differ across genders as well as being affected by time. Receiving hormones from the identified sex can ease the path of transition, but the unaccustomed influx can also rock one's psychic boat.

Some generalities apply. For trans men, previously unexperienced testosterone levels can affect the emotions, pushing anger up the roster of options. For trans women, as breasts develop they may not only be tender, but may leak milky fluid as well. Testosterone may cause hair to sprout in unexpected and perhaps inconvenient places, or familial baldness may wreak havoc on the hairline. For anyone receiving cross-gender HRT, acne may be worse this second time around and may even appear in places never before afflicted. Finally, when produced by hormones from a whole new quadrant, sexual desire may feel bafflingly unfamiliar.

PERSPECTIVE AND PROSPECTS

Regardless of age, most people feel that they belong to a particular gender. Is that feeling of gender determined by the shape of our sex organs or by chemicals such as enzymes and hormones? If not, what causes it?

Because despite individual variations the structure of male and female brains varies slightly, some have questioned whether the brains of transgender people are more like their gender identities than their assigned gender. When Spanish investigators in one small study made MRI investigations of brains of a small number of female-to-male and male-to-female people, both before and after cross-sex hormonal treatment, results indicated that even before being treated the brains of transgendered people were in some ways more resembled the brains of their identified gender than those of their assigned gender. Subcortical areas, which tend to be thinner in men, were relatively thin in female-to-male subjects, while male-to-female subjects showed thinner right-hemisphere cortices, more characteristic of female brains. After hormonal treatment, these effects became more evident. But these researchers believe it an oversimplification to say that one sex is improperly housed in a body of the wrong sex. Instead, they propose that transgender people have transsexual brains.

The idea that being transgendered arises from hormonal imbalance has been debunked. A recent study in young people who do not identify with their assigned sex showed congruence between natally assigned sex and hormonal status; in other words, their sex hormones were in alignment with their anatomical sex. So if someone assigned to be female at birth because of possessing female genitalia has the same mix of estrogen, progesterone, and testosterone as did her mother, yet feels and has always felt male, it is not because of hormones.

Has a transgender gene been found? The short answer at this time is no. As embryos we all start as both genders with two sets of undeveloped (or ambiguous) gonads. Around the sixth week of development one of two things happens. Either a gene turns on and the female organs fade away, or that gene is silent and the female organs flourish; in either case the male organs do the converse. In most cases, that is. Mutations in engaged genes or chromosomes may subvert the process. Other mishaps may occur; receptors may not bind the sex hormones that should dock there, enzymes that ignite sex characteristics may misfire, a

hormonal cascade may be torrential or constrained. From without, drugs and chemicals not intended for fetal acquaintance may find their way in and wreak changes. How these and other potentialities are timed and interact cannot but introduce uncertainties.

Not everyone considers sexuality a polarity of male or female; black to white encompasses an infinity of shades. The term transgender includes not only people whose gender identity differs from their assigned sex, but also those occupying various places along the spectrum of one sex to its opposite; bigender, pangender, agender. To be transgendered (the sex that one is) is not the same as sexual orientation (the sex that one prefers sexually); it differs as well from intersexed, which describes people born with ambiguous sex organs. Being transgendered may be more congruent with one's identity as heterosexual, homosexual, bisexual, asexual, or any variant. Or maybe it deserves a category of its own. But there is nothing physiologically wrong; there is nothing to 'cure'. (It is well to be mindful that, while transitioning to one's gender identity may solve one big problem, others may stubbornly persist.) All the same, the courage and openness of people like Caitlin Jenner, Chaz Bono, and Chelsea Manning has helped to bring awareness of the gender-atypical experience to the gender-typical population.

Although the mysteries behind our differences are yet to be unraveled, in the end only we can decide who we are.

—*Jackie Dial, PhD*

See also: Gender; Gender dysphoria; Gender reassignment; Genitoplasty; Orchiectomy; Penectomy; Sex realignment; Transgender; Vaginoplasty

For Further Information:
Lewis, Ricki. "Is Transgender Identity Inherited?" *DNAScience Blog*, March 2, 2017. Web August 27, 2017. blogs.plos.org/ dnascience/2017/03/02/is-transgender-identity-inherited/
Olson, Johanna et al. "Baseline Physiologic and Psychosocial Characteristics of Transgender Youth Seeking Care for Gender Dysphoria." *Journal of Adolescent Health*, October 2015, 57:4: 374-380. Web August 10, 2017. www.jahonline.org/article/S1054-139X(15)00216-5/fulltext
Rogers, Ashley Lauren. "Eight Things That Really Happen When Transgender People Start Hormone Therapy." *Cosmopolitan*, September 29, 2015. Web August 14, 2017. www.cosmopolitan.com/sex-love/news/a46391/things-that-really-happen- when-trans-people-start-hormone-therapy/
Russo, Francine. "Is There Something Unique about the Transgender Brain?" *Scientific American*, January 1, 2016. Web August 10, 2017. www.scientificamerican.com/article/is-there-something- unique-about-the-transgender-brain/
Wanjek, Christopher. "Being Transgender Has Nothing to Do with Hormonal Imbalance." *LiveScience*, July 23, 2015. Web August10, 2017. www.livescience.com/51652 -transgender-youth-dont-have-hormonal-imbalance.html

SEXUALITY

Category: Biology
Anatomy or system affected: Genitals, psychic-emotional system, reproductive system
Specialties and related fields: Family medicine, genetics, gynecology, internal medicine, obstetrics, pediatrics, psychiatry, psychology
Definition: A complex, multidimensional, umbrella term referring to the identification of masculine and feminine gender, qualities associated with each gender, capacities for erotic stimulation, behaviors causing erotic stimulation, the biology of reproduction, and fundamental elements of individual personality and personal identity that relate to these; sexuality has procreative, recreational, and relational dimensions.

Key terms:

bisexuality: the capacity to be sexually attracted to and aroused by both genders; the term also implies a significant and consistent capacity for such arousal and does not refer to occasional attraction to or activity with both genders

celibacy: originally meaning "unmarried," it also refers to the willful or circumstantial refraining from sexual intercourse and, by implication, erotic behavior; though sometimes misconstrued, celibates are no less sexual than noncelibates

erogenous zones: bodily areas that are especially sensitive to touch, leading to sexual arousal; although a dozen or so such zones are common (e.g., the clitoral glans and labia, penile glans and shaft, breasts, buttocks, inner thighs), these zones can differ from person to person

erotic: referring to sensory perceptions that are sensual (gratifying or pleasurable) and sexual; the context in which they occur will determine whether the perceptions become erotic (e.g., breast and testicle examinations are typically not erotic, while caressing these same body parts in romantic settings typically is)

gender: strictly speaking, the behavioral and social aspects of being either a girl/woman or a boy/man; the term is more loosely used to refer to the biological and physical aspects of being male or female as well

gender identity: a person's inner sense and feeling of maleness/masculinity or femaleness/femininity, or both; it implies that one clearly identifies with one gender more than the other, although some people identify with both genders equally or near equally

gender role: behaviors and self-presentations that are associated with being a boy/man or a girl/woman and that one uses to identify or recognize others as a boy/man or a girl/woman; the term also implies the sociocultural expectations of boys/men and girls/women

heterosexual: being principally attracted to and aroused by a person of the opposite gender; a synonymous term, "straight," refers to persons of either gender who are primarily heterosexual

homophobia: obsessive fear of and anxiety about gay people and their social and sexual activities; while several causes of homophobia are known, the most common is a homophobe's private, often unconscious fear and doubt about his or her own sexuality and sense of sexual adequacy

homosexual: a clinical term referring to being principally attracted to and aroused by persons of one's own gender; two synonymous terms are "gay," which can refer to someone of any gender, and "lesbian," which refers only to girls/women; note that the term has fallen largely out of favor and is considered offensive by many members of the community because of its history of being used to pathologize

HISTORICAL OVERVIEW

Sexuality is usually manifested and experienced as an orientation toward and attraction to people of the same gender, the opposite gender, or both. Sexual orientation is also referred to as "sexual preference." However, the term "preference" can imply that sexual attraction and orientation are chosen and voluntary, that one can will oneself to find another person sexually appealing. In fact, most research suggests the opposite: People find themselves attracted to an individual or a particular gender without having thought about that attraction or having consciously willed it. The attraction and orientation are not chosen. People can wish not to be attracted in the ways they are, and they may choose not to act on these feelings, but the attraction felt and experienced is outside voluntary control. An individual plagued with unwanted feelings of sexual attraction must choose how to cope with the feelings, from acting on them directly, to carrying on despite them, to pretending that the feelings are not there.

The historical evidence suggests that the prevailing belief in most societies was that people had either a gay or a heterosexual orientation, regardless of what caused people to be attracted to their own or the opposite gender, sexual orientation was "either-or." In the twentieth century, most social scientists and sex researchers came to think about sexual orientation as lying on a continuum marked by degrees of likelihood of finding one's own or the opposite gender attractive. Sexologist Alfred C. Kinsey and his associates published their landmark works, *Sexual Behavior in the Human Male* in 1948 and *Sexual Behavior in the Human Female* in 1953, in which they used a continuum of sexual orientation to quantify a range of attraction, from those who found only members of the opposite gender attractive (whom they defined as "heterosexual") to those who found only members of the same gender attractive (whom they defined as "homosexual," although the term is no longer in widespread clinical use, and in 1973, the American Psychiatric Association removed the diagnosis of "homosexuality" from its *Diagnostic and Statistical Manual*). Between the two extremes were the majority of people, who find both genders attractive and arousing in varying degrees—and thus are defined as "bisexual."

In determining sexual orientation, researchers once focused on the gender of sex partners, which also was the criterion on which laypersons generally focused. If a male usually had female partners, they would consider him heterosexual; if a female usually had female partners, they would consider her "homosexual." Yet sexual orientation, how one is attracted by and toward others, is more accurately considered to be primarily the subjective experience of how one feels inside, not the overt behavior that one demonstrates outside.

Research has shown that, in any given individual, there can be a large discrepancy between the gender of one's actual partners and the gender to which one is more attracted and drawn. Social and cultural circumstances often affect, even determine, whether one will behave the way one feels. People primarily attracted to opposite-gender persons may be influenced to have and even pursue same-gender partners by particular religious beliefs, certain restricted environments (such as prison), or the sense that this behavior is or is not permissible. Orientation is better understood in the minds and feelings of persons themselves: which gender attracts, how often, and how much. Personal histories that include procreating children, marriage, gay-oriented activities, and bisexual experimentation should not be used to identify sexual orientation.

Although many studies followed the early work of Kinsey, most experts continued to respect and refer to Kinsey and his colleagues' observations about sexuality and sexual orientation. Conducting research in this field remains difficult. Different studies use different survey tools, and not all are equally reliable. In addition, many people will not candidly or honestly discuss their sexual attitudes, attractions, or behaviors. Nevertheless, the best estimates that rely and build on the Kinsey group's previous work suggest that about 10 percent of the population in Western countries is primarily gay or lesbian and that an additional 10 percent of the population is primarily bisexual. (There is less research available on non-Western nations, and much of what is available is methodologically less reliable.) However, far more important than the numbers is the reality that gay, lesbian, and bisexual orientations are neither unusual nor peculiar. This remains true even though heterosexuality is the more common

pattern, most of the time—a finding true for all societies ever studied. Yet a minority pattern of attraction cannot be considered abnormal simply based on numbers.

Expert and lay opinions about how sexual orientation develops differ, often considerably. Yet expert, if not lay, opinions do converge about when it develops: at about age four or five, which is a year to two earlier than when experts believe an individual's personal traits and characteristics emerge intact as an identifiable personality. Because erotic behavior and erogenous stimuli do not usually become an important part of one's personal world until puberty begins (the developmental marker used to interpret when childhood ends and adolescence begins), many do not learn what their orientation is until late adolescence or even well into adulthood. People who eventually come to have nearly exclusive heterosexual fantasies, attractions, and sexual affiliations often have had earlier, adolescent gay experiences. Likewise, people who eventually discover that their orientation is strongly gay have often married, borne children, and had long periods of gratifying heterosexual dating experiences.

Most people eventually identify their orientation, at least implicitly, in terms of direction and strength. Direction refers to the direction of sexual orientation toward one's own or one's opposite gender. Strength refers to the degree of exclusivity associated with the direction of one's orientation: attracted only by the same or opposite gender, sometimes attracted by each, always attracted to each.

Bidirectional orientation is the least researched and least understood sexual orientation. As in other orientations, bisexual encounters, even if gratifying, do not in themselves mean that someone is bisexually oriented and therefore bisexual. All sexual orientation is internal, not behavioral.

While learning about their sexual selves and their accompanying orientation, some people engage in experimental bisexual behavior. With limited access to the gender toward which they are more predominantly or exclusively oriented, some become sexually active with the gender toward which they are not oriented but which is more available. Some are sexually active with both genders for money. Some are sexually stimulated and aroused regardless of gender. (William H. Masters and Virginia E. Johnson, among the leading sex researchers and sex educators of all time, label this group "ambisexual.") Some indicate that they have a definite orientation toward sexual activity with both genders. Among this last group, some report having long-term, one-gender relationships that followed long-term, other-gender relationships, and others report having concurrent sexual relationships with partners of both genders.

Although descriptions of active bisexuality are readily available in the research, the sheer variety of patterns substantially challenges research-based understandings of how sexual orientation originates and develops. What is known is that people with bisexual orientations are neither poorer nor better psychologically adjusted than others and that bisexuality, while poorly understood, reflects a comfortable and fulfilling sexual life and identity for a significant percentage of the general population.

In recent years there has been growing acknowledgment that asexuality exists on a spectrum. Asexual people—also known informally within the community as "Aces"—may desire emotionally intimate relationships despite having little interest in having sex.

THEORIES OF SEXUAL ORIENTATION

No other area of sexuality has generated more interest, theory, or research than orientation and how it originates. No one theory stands alone as proven, and not-yet-explained data shake the foundations of even the most useful theories. Nevertheless, scientific inquiry has disproven many earlier theories. The most promising theories fall into several categories, some of which can overlap to a degree: genetic, hormonal, psychodynamic, parental, familial, behavioral, societal, and cultural.

The first significant study of genetic causality for sexual orientation was published in 1952. The research compared one group of male identical twins with one group of male fraternal twins. In both groups, one twin was known to be oriented to other males. Reasonably assuming that both twins of a pair would be exposed to essentially the same environments, the study counted how many second twins, whose sexual orientations were unknown at the start of the study, were also gay. If the rate of same-sex attraction for twins was higher among the group of identical twins than in the group of fraternal twins, it would be evidence that genetic makeup, which is virtually the same between identical twins, was the main cause of sexual orientation.

Twelve percent of fraternal twins who were gay had a gay twin. Because male fraternal twins are genetically as similar and dissimilar as any pair of brothers, and the rate of same-sex attraction among the fraternal set was close to the rates that the Kinsey group found in the general population, the results were initially considered a breakthrough. However, the study also showed that the twin of every known gay person in the identical set was also gay. One hundred percent concordance rates are rare in studies of identical twins (even studies that might compare heights or weights between identical twins would not achieve 100 percent concordance) and are almost nonexistent in all other

social groups on any variable ever studied. This particular study and its unique finding needed replication to be believed. Two later studies, published in 1968 and 1976, had quite different results. The view that sexual orientation was principally a product of genetic conditions and variability was abandoned. However, most researchers still believe genetics provides contributory influence.

Investigating the role that hormonal factors play in sexual orientation divides research on animals and research on humans. Studies clearly show that altering prenatal hormone exposure leads to same-sex behavior in at least several animal species. Several studies have had findings that link prenatal exposure to specific sexual orientation outcomes among humans. For example, females who were exposed to male hormones (androgens), especially testosterone, were more likely to develop lesbian orientations; males with Kleinfelter's syndrome, a chromosomal abnormality marked by a deficiency in androgens, are known to develop gay orientations at a greater frequency than the population average.

Other research on humans has shown different hormone levels between gay adults and heterosexuals. Some studies have found lower testosterone in gay males; some have found higher levels of estrogens (though present in both sexes, they are usually considered female hormones) in gay males, and other studies have found both. At least one study found higher blood testosterone in gay females than heterosexual females.

While this evidence seems illuminating on the surface, it is far from conclusive. First, although many studies show different hormone levels between heterosexual and gay persons, several studies have also found hormone levels to be the same in both groups. Second, administering sex hormones to adults does not affect their orientation in any way. Third, prenatal overexposure or underexposure to sex hormones is relatively rare. It would not account for the differences in orientation observed in the general adult population, nor is it beyond reason to view cases of abnormal hormonal prenatal environments as extraordinary and unrepresentative of how sexual orientation usually develops. Fourth, while animal studies often describe processes in particular species that are readily analogous to processes in humans, this does not seem to be the case with human sexuality in general or human sexual orientation in particular.

What seems clear is that there is no one-to-one link between sex hormones and sexual orientation. Prenatal hormones, which are known to influence brain development in many ways, may indirectly predispose individuals toward adapting certain adult sexual behavioral patterns of greater or lesser bisexuality.

Psychodynamic explanations focus on the nature of parent-child relationships and how parents encourage or discourage the growth of their children. Although early studies showed gay males reared in homes where mothers were dominant and overprotective, and fathers were weak, passive, or emotionally uninvolved, those findings have since been largely debunked. Overall, research outcomes from psychodynamic, parental, and familial studies lack cohesive evidence that being gay or of any orientation results from poor parent-child relationships or dysfunctional family environments.

Behavioral, societal, and cultural theories assume that orientation is primarily learned as people become culturally assimilated and psychologically conditioned (rewarded and punished) for specific sexual feelings, thoughts, and behaviors. Therefore, in an environment where homoerotic feelings were accepted and valued, people would be more likely to develop same-sex, and perhaps bisexual, orientations. In an environment where homophobic attitudes were considered the norm, homoerotic feelings would more likely be abandoned. While these theories have utility in explaining certain sociological phenomena, such as atypical gender role behavior, they seem to have less utility in explaining how orientation develops in the majority of the population.

PERSPECTIVE AND PROSPECTS

Although answers to the question of how orientation develops are complex, researchers Alan P. Bell, Martin S. Weinberg, and S. K. Hammersmith published the two-volume work *Sexual Preference: Its Development in Men and Women* (1981) in an attempt to reveal the causal chain of sexual orientation development in more than thirteen hundred adult gay, heterosexual, and bisexual men and women. They based their findings on lengthy face-to-face interviews with every person in their study and on a sophisticated and reliable statistical technique called "path analysis."

Bell, Weinberg, and Hammersmith's research represents an extensive data collection. Many experts still consider at least some of their findings to be conclusive. These results show that sexual orientation is strongly established in most people by late adolescence and that sexual feelings rarely undergo directional changes in adulthood.

Although their study was methodologically well planned and statistically sound, Bell, Weinberg, and Hammersmith could not find solid support for any prevailing theories about the causality of sexual orientation. Some theories explain some of the observed data, and some theories seem to enhance understanding of the origins of sexual orientation in some elements of the population. Still, no theory or combination of theories explains all the data.

If this research has moved medical science along to some degree, it also serves to remind everyone, professional and nonprofessional alike, that the very complexity of human experience and how humans develop their identity warrants caution if it is ever to be accurately understood. The evidence is not complete. It is known that some aspects of the theories of the origins of sexual orientation are true and that others are false.

Learning one's sexual orientation is a complex process requiring self-observation, self-reflection, and self-recollection. People discover what they like and who they like, the content and orientation of their sexual fantasies, and which gender feels closer to their sexual identity as persons (rather than the gender role that they feel a societal obligation to play). It is their own experiences of what is and is not sexually gratifying that teaches people how they are oriented sexually.

—*Mari Rich*

See also: Aphrodisiacs; Erectile dysfunction; Gender identity disorder; Gender reassignment surgery; Hormones; Masturbation; Men's health; Precocious puberty; Psychiatry; Psychiatry, child and adolescent; Psychiatry, geriatric; Psychoanalysis; Puberty and adolescence; Reproductive system; Sexual differentiation; Sexual dysfunction; Sexually transmitted diseases (STDs); Women's health.

For Further Information:

Berzon, Betty. *Permanent Partners: Building Gay and Lesbian Relationships That Last*. Rev. ed., Plume, 2004. A practical, realistic guide for same-gender partners in primary relationships. Berzon addresses the main conflict and confusing areas of relationships typically experienced by gay and lesbian couples.

Bogaert, A. F., and M. N. Skorska. "A Short Review of Biological Research on the Development of Sexual Orientation." *Hormones and Behavior*, vol. 119, 2020, p. 104659, doi.org/10.1016/j.yhbeh.2019.104659. The authors review biological research on the development of sexual orientation.

Byer, Curtis O., Louis W. Shainberg, and Grace Galliano. *Dimensions of Human Sexuality*. 6th ed., McGraw-Hill, 2002. An excellent, thorough, well-organized textbook on all areas of sexuality, with highlighted topics of special interest.

Corinna, Heather. *S.E.X.: The All-You-Need-to-Know Progressive Sexuality Guide to Get You Through High School and College*. Marlowe, 2007. A candid discussion of sex and sexuality for teenagers and young adults. Topics include anatomy, sexual orientation and sexual identity, relationships, safer-sex practices, sexual abuse and rape, pregnancy and contraception, and sexually transmitted diseases, including HIV.

Dibble, Suzanne L., and Patricia A. Robertson. *Lesbian Health 101: A Clinician's Guide*. UCSF Nursing Press, 2010. The first comprehensive textbook on lesbian health for clinicians and students. Helpful to general readers as well. It also provides insight into women's health in general.

Fairchild, Betty, and Nancy Hayward. *Now That You Know: A Parent's Guide to Understanding Their Gay and Lesbian Children*. 3rd ed., Harcourt Brace, 1998. A standard and compassionate reference for families with gay sons or lesbian daughters. Discusses the nature of homosexuality, counsels parents on how to respond supportively to gay and lesbian children, and informs parents on the pressing health and emotional issues that affect gays and lesbians.

GLAAD Media Reference Guide. 11th ed. GLAAD, 1 Mar. 2022, www.glaad.org/reference/. Accessed 5 Mar. 2022.

Katz, Jonathan Ned. *The Invention of Heterosexuality*. U of Chicago P, 2007. Using the now well-known premise of homosexuality as socially constructed, Katz, in this classic work, explores heterosexuality as a social construct.

Masters, William H., Virginia E. Johnson, and Robert C. Kolodny. *Human Sexuality*. 5th ed., HarperCollins College, 1995. A well-organized, highly readable textbook covering biological, psychological, social, cultural, ethical, and religious perspectives on human sexuality.

Strong, Bryan, et al. *Human Sexuality: Diversity in Contemporary America*. 6th ed., McGraw-Hill, 2008. Excellent coverage of human sexuality and the differences and similarities across ethnicities, cultures, genders, and sexual orientations.

SEXUALLY TRANSMITTED DISEASES (STDs)

Category: Disease/Disorder
Also known as: Venereal diseases, Sexually transmitted infections (STIs)
Key terms:

antibody: a protein found in the blood and produced by the immune system in response to contact of the body with a foreign substance
asymptomatic: an infection without any symptoms
bacteria: microscopic single-celled organisms that multiply using simple division; bacteria are found everywhere, and most are beneficial - only a few species cause disease
immunity: the capacity to resist a disease caused by an infectious agent
infertility: the inability to produce offspring by a person during their childbearing years though they have been having sex without contraception for twelve months
inflammation: a response of the body to tissue damage caused by injury or infection and characterized by redness, pain, heat, and swelling
latent: lying hidden or undeveloped within a person; unrevealed
pelvic inflammatory disease (PID): an extensive bacterial infection of the pelvic organs, such as the uterus, cervix, Fallopian tubes, and ovaries
protozoan: a single-celled organism that is more closely related to animals than are bacteria; only a few

drugs are available that will kill protozoa without harming their animal hosts
virus: a noncellular particle of protein and nucleic acid; viruses, which can reproduce only inside cells, usually cause damage to their hosts by killing the cells they enter

CAUSES AND SYMPTOMS

Sexually transmitted diseases, or STDs (formerly called venereal diseases), have plagued humankind for centuries. The most prevalent, serious STDs are syphilis, gonorrhea, nongonococcal urethritis, trichomoniasis, genital herpes, genital warts, viral hepatitis, and HIV/AIDS. Others, troublesome but not as serious, include lice, scabies, and vaginal yeast infections.

They are passed on from one person to another mostly by sexual contact. However, some of these diseases may be acquired indirectly through contaminated objects or blood. In addition, nearly all these diseases can be passed on from an infected mother to her fetus, which may cause congenital disabilities, severe and damaging infections, or even death. A person can acquire several STDs simultaneously, and since recovery from an STD does not confer immunity, a person can get them again and again. Many of these diseases are asymptomatic, which allows them to spread and cause serious complications before a victim is aware of being infected. Finally, some STDs are treatable, and some are not.

Syphilis is caused by *Treponema pallidum*. This bacterium normally infects the vagina or cervix. Still, it can also enter through a cut on the mouth or other parts of the skin. Once inside, the bacteria grow at the entry site, then spread throughout the body through the lymph and blood vessels. The symptoms of syphilis are caused by the efforts of the patient's immune response to fight off the infection.

The disease occurs in three stages: primary, secondary, and tertiary. There also may be latent stages in between each stage where the person infected is asymptomatic. In primary syphilis, a flat, firm, painless, red sore called a chancre appears at the entry site two to ten weeks after infection. Secondary syphilis is characterized by a red rash that appears two to ten weeks after the disappearance of the primary lesion. The rash will disappear in a few weeks. Forty percent of patients will progress to the tertiary stage without treatment within three to ten years. Tertiary syphilis is characterized by the formation of severe lesions called gummas on the skin, bones, or internal organs. Gummas on the spinal cord, brain, or heart can lead to seizures, insanity, or death. Almost all pregnant women with untreated primary or secondary syphilis will transmit the bacteria through the placenta to the developing baby, who will develop congenital syphilis. Many babies with congenital syphilis are spontaneously aborted or still-born. Many others are born with characteristic congenital disabilities, secondary or tertiary syphilis, or neurological damage and may die shortly after birth.

Gonorrhea is caused by the *Neisseria gonorrhoeae* bacterium (also known as gonococcus). The bacterium infects the cervix, vagina, or urethra in females. Between 20 and 80 percent of women infected with gonococcus are asymptomatic or show only mild symptoms. Symptoms include burning or high frequency of urination, vaginal discharge, fever, and abdominal pain. In 20 to 30 percent of untreated women, gonococcus will spread to the Fallopian tubes and cause pelvic inflammatory disease (PID), leading to infertility. Infected mothers can transmit the bacteria to their babies as they pass through the birth canal, causing ophthalmia neonatorum, a type of conjunctivitis (inflammation of the eye) that can cause blindness if untreated.

Most nongonococcal urethritis (NGU) cases are caused by *Chlamydia trachomatis* types *d* through *k*. This bacterium infects the cervix or urethra in females. The symptoms of chlamydia infection are often mild and go unnoticed. Women are either asymptomatic or experience mild cervicitis (inflammation of the cervix) or urethritis. Complications include PID and infertility in females. Infants born to mothers with cervicitis can develop eye (inclusion conjunctivitis) or lung (infant pneumonia) infections.

Trichomoniasis is caused by the protozoan *Trichomonas vaginalis*. The organism can infect the vulva, vagina, and cervix in women. In both sexes, the disease is often mild or asymptomatic. Women may suffer from severe vaginitis, which includes a tender, red, and itchy genital area and a profuse, frothy, foul-smelling, greenish-yellow discharge. Newborns may acquire the infection from an infected mother during delivery.

Most genital herpes infections are caused by herpes simplex virus type 2, but some are caused by herpes simplex virus type 1. The virus infects the cervix, vulva, vagina, or perineum in females. Two to seven days after infection, painful blisters appear in the genital area that ulcerate, crust over, and disappear in a few weeks.

Herpes viruses are unique in that they can remain latent in the nerves and cause a recurrent infection in the future. Fever, stress, sunlight, or local trauma may trigger the virus to reactivate and cause recurrent infection. The virus can be transmitted from an infected mother to her baby either congenitally, through the placenta, or neonatally, as the baby passes through the birth canal. In congenital or neonatal herpes, the virus can infect all body parts. The death rate is high, and survivors commonly have long-term neurological damage and recurrent infections.

INFORMATION ON SEXUALLY TRANSMITTED DISEASES (STDs)

Causes: Infection through sexual contact; also from contaminated blood or from infected mother to fetus
Symptoms: Varies; may include skin lesions or rash in genital area, itching, abdominal pain, painful urination, vaginal or penile discharge, birth defects, infertility
Duration: Acute to chronic with recurrent episodes
Treatments: Antibiotics, antiviral agents

Viral hepatitis is also an STD. At least three variants of the virus-hepatitis A virus (HAV), HBV, and HCV-are known to be transmitted sexually. HBV is the form most commonly transmitted sexually. Vaccines are available to immunize persons at risk for HAV and HBV.

Genital warts are caused by human papillomaviruses (HPVs). They are found on women's vagina, cervix, perineum, and anus. An obstetrician/gynecologist can remove warts, but the infection remains for the patient's life. HPV infection seems to increase a woman's risk for cervical cancer. FDA approved three vaccines: *Gardasil, Cervarix,* and *Gardasil 9.* All these vaccines vaccinate against HPV 16 and 18. Gardasil protects against two other strains, and *Gardasil 9* protects against nine total strains. As of 2017, Gardasil 9 is the only available HPV vaccine in the United States.

AIDS is caused by the human immunodeficiency virus (HIV). This virus is acquired through sexual contact, intravenous drug use, and blood transfusions. HIV infects and inactivates the T helper cells needed by the immune system to respond to and fight off infections. Without T helper cells, the immune system eventually becomes nonfunctional. The affected person becomes susceptible to every type of infection possible. Two-thirds of all AIDS patients get pneumonia caused by *Pneumocystis jirovecii.* Other common diseases associated with AIDS patients are tuberculosis and other mycobacterial infections, viral infections caused by cytomegalovirus and herpesviruses, fungal infections, cancers such as Kaposi's sarcoma and neurological disorders. HIV can also be transmitted from an infected mother to her baby through the placenta. Virtually every person infected with HIV will eventually die of AIDS.

TREATMENT AND THERAPY
Healthcare providers can diagnose sexually transmitted diseases in several ways. One way is by observing the symptoms and case history of the patient. Syphilis,

gonorrhea, chlamydia, and trichomoniasis organisms all have unique shapes that a doctor can recognize. Characteristic sores or symptoms can lead a doctor to suspect a particular disease. A scraping from a lesion or an unusual discharge can be examined to identify the infecting organism under a microscope.

All organisms that cause STDs can be grown in the laboratory. Since these organisms are not normally present in humans, isolation of the organism from the body signifies that a microorganism has infected the body. For those STDs with mild symptoms or no symptoms, a doctor can try to grow the organism in the laboratory from samples taken from appropriate sites on the body. Finally, many blood tests have been developed to test whether a person has specific antibodies in their blood that bind to one of these organisms. The presence of antibodies to an organism implies that one has been or is currently infected with that organism. In many cases, doctors will use several of these methods to confirm a diagnosis of an STD.

Specific treatment recommendations for each sexually transmitted disease are subject to periodic revision. Current recommendations are reviewed by the Centers for Disease Control and published in the *Morbidity and Mortality Weekly Report* every three or four years. Physicians need to review these recommendations to prescribe the best method for treating STDs. All bacterial and protozoal STDs can be treated and cured with antibiotics. It is important to seek early diagnosis and treatment of these diseases for three reasons: First, to prevent the disease from spreading; second, to prevent the various complications associated with the diseases; and third, to prevent the infection of infants by pregnant mothers. There is no cure for STDs caused by viruses; there are only drugs that slow the progress of the infection.

Syphilis is commonly treated with penicillin G or erythromycin, doxycycline, or ceftriaxone. In most patients receiving appropriate therapy during primary or secondary syphilis, the active disease is totally and permanently arrested. Treatment during the latent stage stops the development of symptoms of the tertiary stage. There is no successful treatment for patients with tertiary syphilis. A combination of an intramuscular injection of ceftriaxone and a seven-day course of oral doxycycline are the agents used to treat gonorrhea. Quinolones, such as ciprofloxacin and the macrolide azithromycin, are other antibiotics that can be an effective treatment for gonococcal infections. Doxycycline or azithromycin are used to treat NGU caused by chlamydia, and trichomoniasis is treated with metronidazole or tinidazole.

Genital herpes is treated with antiviral agents such as oral acyclovir, valacyclovir, or famciclovir for seven to ten days. The topical application of acyclovir helps reduce the duration of primary but not recurrent infections. Using oral acyclovir to suppress recurrent infections may cause more severe and more frequent infections once the therapy has stopped. Neonatal herpes is treated with intravenous acyclovir, which can reduce the severity of the infection but cannot reverse any herpes-related neurological damage or prevent recurrent infections. Genital warts can be removed by chemicals, freezing, electrocautery, or laser therapy. Antiviral drugs are useful in treating some STDs: acyclovir, valacyclovir, or famciclovir for genital herpes and interferon-a2b (mainly in younger people) or oral antiviral medications (tenofovir, entecavir, lamivudine, adefovir or telbivudine) for hepatitis B virus. These medications slow the progress of the disease in some persons, but they do not cure it. Antiretroviral therapy (ART) is recommended for all HIV-infected individuals regardless of CD4 cell count since it helps decrease viral load. It decreases serious adverse outcomes of HIV, including death. Pre-exposure prophylaxis (PrEP) medicines are given to people at high risk of getting HIV, such as *Truvada*. Post-exposure prophylaxis (PEP) medications are given to those who do not have HIV but have been exposed to HIV within 72 hours.

As with any disease, prevention is the most desirable way to control STDs. Except for viral hepatitis and HPV, there are no vaccines for STDs. However, many potential vaccines have been developed and tested, but none is satisfactory for general and routine use. Therefore, behaviors resulting in disease avoidance are the only means of preventing most STDs. The only 100 percent effective way to prevent a sexually transmitted disease is abstinence. Abstinence means to refrain voluntarily from engaging in sexual activity. Since many of these diseases spread through sexual activity other than intercourse, abstinence must include all sexual activity.

Choosing to exercise one's sexuality within a monogamous relationship for life can also help prevent sexually transmitted diseases. The use of a condom or any other barrier method is only somewhat helpful in preventing STDs. Prevention of transmission of STDs from infected mothers to their babies involves early diagnosis and treatment of the mothers before birth and preventive medication of the babies after birth. In the past, ophthalmia neonatorum was the cause of blindness for half of the children admitted to schools for the blind. Therefore, the government made it mandatory to treat all newborns' eyes with silver nitrate, tetracycline, or erythromycin, to prevent this disease. The instillation of silver nitrate in babies' eyes does not prevent chlamydia eye infections, so babies born to mothers with chlamydia need additional antibiotic treatment. Prevention of neonatal herpes may involve delivery by cesarean section to avoid infection of the child as it passes through the birth canal. Preventing the spread of AIDS includes screening blood supplies, organ donors, and semen donors and avoiding contact with infected body fluids through sexual contact, blood transfusions, or intravenous drug use.

Control of STDs in a population is complex since it is both a medical and a social problem. First, it is important that those who contract a sexually transmitted disease receive early diagnosis and adequate treatment to prevent further spread of the disease, serious complications, and infection of infants. Unfortunately, because many STDs are asymptomatic, people often do not know they have the disease and have no reason to seek treatment—many persons contract STDs from asymptomatic carriers. In addition, social stigma or embarrassment reduces the motivation of a victim to seek prompt medical care. Adequate treatment of STD victims is difficult if they do not want to return for subsequent treatment or will not take all their medication.

Not only does the person with an STD need to be treated, but all the sexual contacts of that person need to be contacted, tested, and treated. Public health officials interview victims of STDs to determine the names and addresses of contacts and then try to find and treat the contacts. Treating someone's sexual contact is difficult if a victim does not remember who their contacts are, if they do not want to discuss their sexual activity, or if the contacts do not want to be bothered by the health department. In addition, many private physicians do not report STDs to the public health department; therefore, in many cases, the sources of STDs are never interviewed. People often contract several STDs simultaneously, so detection of one STD should routinely instigate testing for other STDs.

A reduction in risky sexual behavior, such as unprotected sex, would aid in the control of STDs. Effective education to change sexual behavior must be predicated upon the motivation and cognitive development of the student. One-third of all cases involve teenagers and young adults; sexual activity in this age group is rising, and members of this group are more likely to have multiple sex partners. Prostitution for money or drugs also increases the incidence of STDs. Other control measures include the development of vaccines for these diseases, mandatory reporting of all STDs, and education of the population regarding the dangers and risks involved in acquiring these diseases.

PERSPECTIVE AND PROSPECTS

Syphilis was first recognized at the end of the fifteenth century in Europe. It rapidly reached epidemic proportions and was called the "great pox." Gonorrhea was described and given its present name by the Greek physician Galen in 150 CE. From the fifteenth century to the eighteenth century, there was much confusion about the nature of syphilis and gonorrhea. Many people thought they were at different stages of the same disease. In 1767, an English physician named John Hunter inoculated himself with a urethral discharge from a patient with gonorrhea to determine whether they were one disease or two. Unfortunately, that patient also had syphilis, so when Hunter developed symptoms of both gonorrhea and syphilis, he concluded they were a single disease. Not until 1838 physicians proved that they were two different diseases. Traditionally, 95 percent of all cases of sexually transmitted diseases were either syphilis or gonorrhea. However, since the late twentieth century, there has been a dramatic increase in several other sexually transmitted diseases, such as genital herpes, NGU, AIDS, genital warts, and trichomoniasis.

The rise in the incidence of STDs is of epidemic proportions. Worldwide in the 1990s, about 250 million new cases of STDs occurred annually. In the United States, about 12 million new cases, including 3 million in teenagers, occur annually. By 1997, chlamydia had become the most frequently diagnosed STD in the United States, estimated at more than 4 million annually. Other STDs with high incidence included gonorrhea (1.3 million new cases annually) and genital herpes (0.5 million annually). Because there is no cure for genital herpes, it may be present in 20 percent of Americans.

As of 2002, about 1 million North Americans were HIV-positive; only a portion of these had AIDS. By the late twentieth century, the U.S. government announced that the incidence of new cases of AIDS, about 56,000 at that time, had begun to decline. A decline in the number of persons dying from AIDS was also announced. It is estimated that there are 3 to 5 million new cases of NGU per year. One in five couples in the United States is infertile. Much of that infertility is caused by the complications associated with STDs, with chlamydial infection being the primary preventable cause of sterility in women. In the United States, it is estimated that 25 percent of all women are infected with trichomoniasis, and more than 20 million people are infected with *herpes simplex virus type 2*. Although most STDs can be controlled, the incidence of many of the diseases is still quite high; thus, STDs present a social and medical problem. An increase in education concerning the signs and risks of these diseases, a reduction in promiscuity, and the development of vaccines would help control these destructive and fast-spreading diseases.

IMPACT ON WOMEN

STDs are a major public health concern in the United States, especially among women. For various reasons, women are more commonly affected by STDs than men are. Women's anatomy puts them at a higher risk for STDs based on the delicate lining of the vagina. However, women are less likely to have obvious symptoms than men. Women are more likely to seek treatment; therefore, there is more record of women experiencing STDs. STDs in women can also lead to greater issues such as infertility. They have the chance of passing the infection or illness to their baby. Women are more likely to contract HPV, the leading cause of cervical cancer. Luckily women are more likely to seek treatment from their doctors for these conditions. Parents of young women should give their daughters the vaccine to prevent HPV. It is extremely important to educate young girls about how STDs are transmitted, to help them learn how to engage in safe sexual activity.

—*Vicki J. Isola, PhD, Armand M. Karow, PhD, Stephanie Marie Ong, RN, Kimberly Ortiz-Hartman, PsyD, LMFT*

For Further Information:

10 Ways STDs Impact Women Differently from Men. Centers for Disease Control and Prevention, 14 Mar. 2019, www.cdc.gov/std/health-disparities/stds-women-042011.pdf . Accessed 5 Apr. 2022.
Condom Fact Sheet in Brief. Centers for Disease Control and Prevention, 4 Mar. 2019, www.cdc.gov/condomeffectiveness/brief.html. Accessed 5 Apr. 2022.
Felman, Adam. "What You Need to Know About Sexually Transmitted Infections." *MedicalNewsToday*, 25 Sept. 2020, www.medicalnewstoday.com/articles/sexually-transmitted-diseases. Accessed 5 Apr. 2022.
"PEP (Post-Exposure Prophylaxis). Centers for Disease Control and Prevention, 25 May 2021, www.cdc.gov/hiv/basics/pep.html.
Sexually Transmitted Disease. MedlinePlus, 19 Nov. 2021, medlineplus.gov/sexuallytransmitteddiseases.html. Accessed 5 Apr. 2022.
Sexually Transmitted Infections. World Health Organization, 22 Nov. 2021, www.who.int/news-room/fact-sheets/detail/sexually-transmitted-infections-(stis)#:~:text=Of%20these%2C%204%20are%20currently,vaginal%2C%20anal%20and%20oral%20sex. Accessed 5 Apr. 2022.
Sharkey, Lauren. "Everything You Need to Know About Sexually Transmitted Diseases." *Healthline*, 21 Jan. 2022, www.healthline.com/health/sexually-transmitted-diseases. Accessed 5 Apr. 2022.

SHAKING. SEE TREMORS.

SHIGELLOSIS

Category: Disease/Disorder
Anatomy or system affected: Bladder, gastrointestinal system, intestines, kidneys, stomach, urinary tract

Specialties and related fields: Bacteriology, critical care, infectious disease, internal medicine, hematology, microbiology, nephrology, public health, urology
Definition: an acute bacterial infection attacks the lining of the intestines, resulting in diarrhea, fever, and stomach cramps
Key terms:
endothelial cells: the main type of cell found in the inside lining of blood vessels, lymph vessels, and the heart
gastroenteritis: inflammation of the stomach and intestines, typically resulting from bacterial toxins or viral infection and causing vomiting and diarrhea
ischemia: an inadequate blood supply to an organ or part of the body
mucosae: an epithelial layer rich in mucous glands that lines body cavities and passages (as of the gastrointestinal or respiratory tract) that communicate directly or indirectly with the outside of the body
Shiga toxin: a toxin that inhibits protein synthesis in host cells produced by the bacterium *Shigella* dysenteriae, or a similar one produced by E. coli, that causes dysentery in humans
virulent: The ability of an agent of infection to produce disease

CAUSES

Shigella is a gram-negative, rod-shaped, nonmotile bacterium that is a member of the enteric bacteria. Shigella causes a gastrointestinal disease called "shigellosis." The genus *Shigella* is divided into four species: *Shigella dysenteriae* (*S. dysenteriae*), *S. flexneri*, *S. boydii*, and *S. sonnei*. Each of these species is divided into multiple serotypes. *S. dysenteriae* causes severe epidemic disease in less developed countries, and *S. flexneri* causes disease in developing countries. *S. boydii* is only found on the Indian subcontinent, and *S. sonnei* causes disease in developed and less developed (transitioning) countries.

Shigellosis is spread by fecal-oral contact. Transmission occurs when people ingest food or water contaminated with *Shigella*. Shigellosis can spread when food grows in a field with contaminated water. Flies can spread shigellosis by breeding in infected feces and landing on food or surfaces. Shigellosis can also spread when people drink, swim, or play in contaminated water. Transmission can be spread through sexual contact, particularly through anal and oral sex.

Shigellosis commonly occurs in developing countries with inadequate sanitation. It thrives in areas with overcrowding, poor handwashing techniques, and a lack of safe food and water protocols. The disease also spreads easily in close quarters, such as daycare centers, refugee camps, jails, and prisons.

Shigella can survive stomach acid and needs as few as ten microbes to cause disease. *Shigella*, therefore, is one of the most virulent organisms known to medicine.

RISK FACTORS

About eighteen thousand cases of shigellosis are reported in the United States alone each year. Many milder cases are not diagnosed or reported; public health officials estimate the number of cases could be as high as 360,000 annually. The infection is most common in children aged two to four years.

Shigellosis is the most common cause of diarrhea among visitors to developing countries. It infects hundreds of millions of people worldwide each year, resulting in an estimated one million deaths, mostly among children in countries with inadequate medical resources.

DISEASE PROCESS

After entering the gastrointestinal tract, *Shigella* passes through the stomach to the small intestine. After multiplying in the small intestine, it moves to the colon and targets microfold (M) cells. M cells take up the bacteria, but *Shigella* passes through the M cell to the underlying resident macrophage. The macrophage is part of a network of lymphoid tissue called "mucosal-associated lymphoid tissue" or MALT. MALTs extend into the submucosa and are loaded with macrophages and other immune cells.

Macrophages readily phagocytose *Shigella*, but it degrades the phagosome and escapes into the cytoplasm. Once in the cytoplasm, *Shigella* activates the macrophage's programmed cell death pathway, killing it. The dying macrophage releases several cytokines, including interleukin-1ß, that activate a robust inflammatory response. The inflammatory response damages and kills the colon's mucosal cells, resulting in ulcerations and abscesses. The released bacteria enter the mucosal cells from the bottom and spread throughout the mucosal epithelium, damaging it.

S. dysenteriae, serotype 1 produces Shiga toxin, which enters cells and turns off protein synthesis. The extensive damage to the colon wall causes bleeding and allows Shiga toxin to enter the bloodstream. If Shiga toxin travels to the kidney, it enters the epithelial cells of the delicate glomeruli and kills them. Dead glomerular endothelial cells make holes in the kidney's filtration system, and proteins start to leak into the urine (proteinuria). Endothelial cell death also triggers cytokine release, which evokes inflammation and initiates clot formation.

Shigella *seen in a stool sample. Photo via the CDC/Wikimedia Commons. [Public domain.]*

Blood clots within the glomeruli significantly reduce platelet numbers (thrombocytopenia) and form a network of tiny spaces through which red blood cells must pass. These clots act like cheese cutters as red blood cells pass through them, fragmenting them into schistocytes—a process known as microangiopathic hemolysis. Continuous red blood cell destruction causes anemia. The combination of blocked vessels and fewer red blood cells causes kidney ischemia. Since the ischemic kidney can no longer filter blood, metabolic wastes, like urea, accumulate in the blood, causing uremia. Uremia, hemolytic anemia, and thrombocytopenia characterize hemolytic uremic syndrome (HUS). HUS is a consequence of Shiga toxin entering the bloodstream.

SYMPTOMS
The symptoms of watery diarrhea, fever, vomiting, stomach and rectal cramps begin from one to three days after a person encounters the bacterium. In some cases, the incubation period is as short as twelve hours. Often, diarrhea contains blood and mucus, and the infected person may develop a fever. Some experience nausea, vomiting, anorexia, or cramping rectal pain. The symptoms usually resolve within five to seven days, even without treatment. However, the infected person may still be contagious for another week or two.

Some people do not experience symptoms, but they can pass *Shigella* to others while infected. Sometimes, dehydration occurs, leading to the death of a person who has severe shigellosis.

In developing countries, infected persons may experience prolonged, acute diarrhea, lasting seven to thirteen days, or persistent diarrhea, lasting fourteen days or more; this leads to malnutrition. These long-term conditions have the potential to be life-threatening.

About 3 percent of persons with shigellosis develop Reiter's syndrome, consisting of joint pain (usually the knee), irritation of the eyes, and painful urination. The syndrome can last for months or years, leading to chronic, treatment-resistant arthritis. Another rare complication is a hemolytic-uremic syndrome, a form of kidney failure that includes anemia and clotting problems.

Tonic-clonic seizures may occur in severe cases, especially in children. The person loses consciousness, followed by involuntary muscular contractions that cycle from a rigid (tonic) phase to a rhythmic contraction and relaxation (clonic) phase. Neonates and malnourished children have an increased risk of sepsis.

Persons with high fever, confusion, headache with a stiff neck, lethargy, or seizures should seek emergency care. These symptoms are most common in children.

SCREENING AND DIAGNOSIS
A stool culture identifies *Shigella* in the feces of an infected person. Because there are several different strains of *Shigella*, the stool culture will help determine the correct treatment. Fecal samples are usually cultured on MacConkey agar. On this medium, *Shigella* form white, non-lactose fermenting colonies. Staining stools with methylene blue show polymorphonuclear leukocytes. A blood test also may be done if symptoms are severe or to rule out other causes.

Polymerase chain reaction (PCR) directly identifies *Shigella* deoxyribonucleic (DNA).

TREATMENT AND THERAPY
Persons with mild cases of shigellosis usually recover quickly without treatment. However, antibiotics can shorten the course of the illness by a few days. Some *Shigella* bacteria have become resistant to antibiotics.

Severe cases require antibiotics, and the standard treatments include trimethoprim/sulfamethoxazole, fluoroquinolones, macrolides, and beta-lactams. However, third-generation cephalosporins like cefixime or ceftriaxone are the preferred treatment for drug-resistant strains.

Infected persons should drink water and electrolyte solutions (such as *Gatorade*) to replace fluids lost by diarrhea. They should follow their normal diet as much as possible to ensure nutrition. Doctors recommend that persons with shigellosis avoid foods that are high in fat and sugar, spicy foods, and alcohol and coffee until two days after all symptoms have disappeared.

Because shigellosis is particularly dangerous for children, research continues into *Shigella* vaccines. A person who has recovered from shigellosis is unlikely to be infected with the same strain for several years. Antidiarrheal medicines such as loperamide (Imodium) and atropine (*Lomotil*) should not be taken by persons with shigellosis, as they can make the illness worse.

PREVENTION AND OUTCOMES
Precautions for food and water safety will prevent shigellosis. Handwashing with soap can prevent the spread of shigellosis. Because of contagion, infected persons should be separated from those not infected.

People with shigellosis should not prepare food or pour water for others. Travelers should drink only treated or boiled water and eat cooked hot foods and self-peeled fruit. If a child in diapers is infected, all persons who change the diapers should observe strict sanitation and dispose of the diapers properly.

Government agencies in the United States are working to prevent outbreaks of shigellosis. *Shigella* infections are monitored by the Centers for Disease Control and Prevention and state and local health departments. These agencies investigate shigellosis, track how it is transmitted, and develop methods of controlling the disease. In addition, these agencies research ways to identify and treat *Shigella* infection. The US Food and Drug Administration checks imported foods and advocates for improved food-preparation techniques in restaurants and food-processing plants. The US Environmental Protection Agency checks the safety of drinking water.

—*Michael A. Buratovich, PhD*

For Further Information:

Aslam, Aysha, and Chika N. Okafor. "Shigella." *StatPearls*, 13 Feb. 2022, www.ncbi.nlm.nih.gov/books/NBK482337/. Accessed 5 Apr. 2022.

Graciaa, Daniel S., et al. "Outbreaks Associated with Untreated Recreational Water—United States, 2000-2014." *Morbidity and Mortality Weekly Report*, vol. 67, no. 25, 2018, pp. 701-6, doi:10.15585/mmwr.mm6725a1.

Roth, Erica. "Shigellosis." *Healthline*, 23 Jul. 2021, www.healthline.com/health/shigellosis. Accessed 5 Apr. 2022.

Shigella - Shigellosis. The Centers for Disease Control and Prevention, 7 Oct. 2020, www.cdc.gov/shigella/index.html. Accessed 5 Apr. 2022.

Shigella Infection (Shigellosis). San Francisco Department of Public Health, n.d., www.sfcdcp.org/infectious-diseases-a-to-z/shigella-infection-shigellosis/. Accessed 5 Apr. 2022.

Tack, Danielle M., et al. "Preliminary Incidence and Trends of Infections with Pathogens Transmitted Commonly Through Food—Foodborne Diseases Active Surveillance Network, 10 US-Sites, 2016-2019." *Morbidity and Mortality Weekly Report*, vol. 69, no. 17, 2020, pp. 509-14, doi:10.15585/mmwr.mm6917a1.

SHINGLES

Category: Disease/Disorder
Also known as: Herpes zoster
Anatomy or system affected: Nervous system, skin
Specialties and related fields: Dermatology, family medicine, gerontology, internal medicine, neurology, virology
Definition: Reactivation of the viral infection within a nerve cell that causes pain and a characteristic skin rash.

Key terms:
dermatome: a section of skin that is supplied by nerves that come from a single spinal nerve root
viremia: the presence of viruses in the blood

CAUSES AND SYMPTOMS

Shingles results from the same virus (*varicella zoster*) that causes chickenpox. All individuals who have had chickenpox are at risk for shingles. The disease most commonly affects those over age fifty but can develop at any age, especially in immunocompromised individuals. In the United States, over 1.2 million people suffer from shingles each year. Approximately 30 percent of the population will experience shingles in their lifetime.

Varicella-zoster virus (VZV) is transported through airborne droplets and infects the lymphoid tissue in the upper respiratory system (nasopharynx). The virus initially infects T lymphocytes, and these cells carry VZV throughout the body, resulting in a viremia. The long incubation period for chickenpox (a range of ten to twenty-one days, with an average of fourteen to sixteen days) results from the virus's ability to evade the immune system. The rash results from VZV infecting epidermal cells, and skin cell destruction produces virus-laden vesicles. The cell-free virus in the vesicles infects sensory nerve termini. It moves up (retrograde) to the sensory nerve cell bodies in the dorsal root ganglia. Cell-mediated immunity developed against VZV during chickenpox is required to end the infection.

After resolution of chickenpox, VZV remains dormant in dorsal sensory nerve roots or ganglia. During its latent phase, VZV expresses a few genes, and infectious virus is not detectable within the ganglia. Each dorsal root receives sensation from receptors in a strip of skin on only one side of the body that are arranged in a segmental distribution called "dermatomes" (map of the skin). Common sites for shingles outbreaks include the back along the distribution of a single dermatome wrapping around one side to the chest or abdomen. They may travel from the upper back to the arm or the lower back to the leg. Shingles can also occur on the face and rarely can involve the optic nerve of the eye.

Varicella zoster virus can stay inactive in the nerve root for decades. It appears to be reactivated by stress, illness, decreased immune function, or aging. Consequently, individuals with autoimmune diseases, compromised immune systems, active HIV infection, and transplant patients are at increased risk of VZV reactivation. Upon reactivation, VZV spreads within the ganglion and subsequently moves down the sensory nerve dendrites (anterograde) to infect the skin and cause the lesions characteristic of shingles. The first symptom is often a sensation of tingling, burning, or sharp

INFORMATION ON SHINGLES

Causes: Viral infection with *varicella zoster*; triggered by stress, illness, decrease in immune function, aging

Symptoms: Tingly, burning, or sharp pain; rash with blisters

Duration: Three days to several weeks

Treatments: Antiviral medications (acyclovir, famciclovir, valacyclovir); pain relief (cool compresses, anti-inflammatory drugs, mild narcotics)

pain over the skin area supplied by the affected nerve root. Damage to neurons is responsible for the neuropathic pain associated with shingles (also known as "herpes zoster"). Within several days, a rash appears, characterized by a cluster of blisters with surrounding redness spreading along the dermatomal pattern. The rash typically occurs only on one side of the body. Clinical diagnosis usually can be made by the characteristic rash. Alternately, fluid within the shingles blister may be sampled for viral culture to obtain a definitive diagnosis.

Shingles blisters scab over in about three days and clear within several weeks. Until the blisters are completely scabbed over, the fluid within the blisters can transmit chickenpox via contact. Unvaccinated individuals who have never had chickenpox can develop chickenpox following contact with the fluid in the shingles blisters (e.g., from a grandparent with shingles holding a young child). Even though the fluid from shingles blisters can transmit chickenpox, this same fluid cannot transmit shingles —individuals cannot acquire shingles from contact exposure. About 20 percent of people continue to have severe pain along the nerve course after the rash has cleared. This condition is called "postherpetic neuralgia" (PHN). It can last for weeks and be so severe as to interfere with activities of daily living.

TREATMENT AND THERAPY

If shingles is diagnosed within three days of the appearance of the rash, antiviral medications. Including acyclovir, famciclovir, and valacyclovir, are prescribed to stop viral replication and help shorten the duration of the illness and decrease the pain associated with it. Antiviral medications also encourage more rapid healing of skin lesions, prevent the formation of new lesions, decrease the risk of VZV transmission by reducing viral shedding, and prevent PHN. Acyclovir is poorly absorbed and requires dosing five times a day. Valacyclovir and famciclovir are dosed three times a day. All three medications are very well tolerated, but commonly, they may cause headaches, nausea, and diarrhea. Antiviral treatment usually lasts for seven days. The effectiveness of treating shingles over seventy-two hours after the onset of the rash has not been rigorously established. Pregnant women should be treated with acyclovir since this drug is the most heavily studied of the three. Intravenous acyclovir is used in patients with rare but severe VZV complications such as shingles infections of the eyes (herpes zoster ophthalmicus), retina (acute retinal necrosis), ears (Ramsay Hunt syndrome), or brain (VZV meningitis, encephalitis, or myelitis).

Treatment also involves pain control with local cool compresses, calamine lotion, anti-inflammatory medications, or even mild narcotics. Gabapentin, a drug similar in structure to an inhibitory neurotransmitter, gamma-aminobutyric acid (GABA), and its relative, pregabalin (Lyrica), are useful against pain experienced in PHN. Other nonopioid pain relievers effective against PHN pain include tricyclic antidepressants like amitriptyline, nortriptyline, imipramine, and glucocorticoids. Antiviral therapy does not affect PHN, but it can help prevent it.

In 2006, Zostavax (zoster vaccine live) was approved for use in the United States to reduce the risk of shingles in older adults. Zostavax is no longer sold in the United States as of July 2020 but is still used in other countries.

Shingrix is a recombinant zoster vaccine that contains VZV outer envelope glycoprotein E with adjuvant. Besides the United States, Shingrix is available in Canada, China, and several European countries. In clinical trials, Shingrix reduced the risk of shingles and PHN by over 90 percent. Shingrix is administered in two doses. Adverse effects of Shingrix include pain at the injection site, muscle aches, fatigue, headache, shivering, fever, and an upset stomach, all of which were of short duration. Hypersensitivity to Shingrix is rare but has been observed.

PERSPECTIVE AND PROSPECTS

In 1892, James von Bokay was the first to suggest a relationship between chickenpox and shingles. He hypothesized that the same virus causes both diseases. In 1888, he noted that homes with adults with shingles also usually had children with chickenpox. He also discovered that chickenpox and shingles caused skin lesions with similar macroscopic and microscopic appearances. The von Bokay hypothesis facilitated further research into shingles.

VZV belongs to a family of viruses called the "herpesviruses." "Herpes" is derived from the Greek word *herpein*, meaning "to creep."

Because more than 90 percent of adults in the United States harbor the varicella-zoster virus, shingles remains a significant clinical problem, particularly in the elderly and those with compromised immune systems.

—*Michael A. Buratovich, PhD*

See also: Blisters; Chickenpox; Herpes; Nervous system; Neuralgia, neuritis, and neuropathy; Neurology; Neurology, pediatric; Rashes; Viral infections.

For Further Information:

Davidson, Tish. "Shingles." *Vaccines: History, Issues, and Science*. Greenwood, 2017, pp. 116-18.

Doerr, Steven. "Shingles." *MedicineNet.com*, 5 July 2017.

Gagliardi, A. M., et al. "Vaccines for Preventing Herpes Zoster in Older Adults." *Cochrane Database Systemic Reviews*, vol. 3, 2016, CD008858.

Galetta, Kristin M., and Don Gilden. "Zeroing in on Zoster: A Tale of Many Disorders Produced by One Virus." *Journal of the Neurological Sciences*, vol. 358, no. 1-2, 2015, pp. 38-45, www.medicinenet.com/shingles_herpes_zoster/article.htm, doi:10.1016/j.jns.2015.10.004. Accessed 30 July 2017.

Janniger, Camilla K. "Herpes Zoster.." *Medscape.com*, 20 July 2017, emedicine.medscape.com/article/1132465-overview. Accessed 30 July 2017.

"Nonopioid Drugs for Pain." *Medical Letter on Drugs and Therapeutics*, vol. 64, no. 1645, 2022, pp. 33-40.

Oxman, M. N., et al. "A Vaccine to Prevent Herpes Zoster and Postherpetic Neuralgia in Older Adults." *New England Journal of Medicine*, vol. 352, 2005, pp. 2271-84.

"Shingles (Herpes Zoster)." US Centers for Disease Control and Prevention, 19 Aug. 2016, www.cdc.gov/shingles/index.html. Accessed 30 July 2017.

Watson, C. Peter, editor. *HerpesZosterand Postherpetic Neuralgia: Focus on Treatment and Prevention*. Springer Berlin Heidelberg, 2017.

Shock

Category: Disease/Disorder

Anatomy or system affected: All

Specialties and related fields: Critical care, emergency medicine, family medicine, internal medicine

Definition: Shock is a life-threatening condition that may occur in response to a variety of circumstances (allergic reaction, infection, injury, blood loss, heart attack, toxic substances in the blood) which causes the heart to be unable to pump enough blood to supply the vital organs, which are therefore deprived of oxygen and nutrients and lose normal function; symptoms include rapid and shallow breathing, clammy skin, low blood pressure, rapid and weak pulse, and dizziness and if untreated will progress to unconsciousness and death.

Key terms:

blood pressure: the amount of pressure on blood vessel walls when the heart contracts and relaxes

cardiovascular system: the organ system consisting of the heart and all blood vessels (vasculature)

vasculature: all the blood vessels, including the arteries (blood vessels carrying blood away from the heart), the capillaries (the smallest blood vessels, where fluid and nutrients are exchanged), and the veins (blood vessels that return blood to the heart)

vital organs: organs of the body essential to life; the brain, heart, lungs, and sometimes the kidneys

CAUSES AND SYMPTOMS

The primary goal of the cardiovascular system is to provide blood flow, carrying oxygen and other nutrients to all tissues to meet their requirements. The cardiovascular system performs this function by maintaining a blood pressure high enough to push sufficient blood flow throughout the body, especially the vital organs. To keep the blood pressure up, the heart must pump sufficient amounts of blood even when the demand for increased blood flow to some tissues occurs. The blood vessels also play an important role in maintaining blood pressure. The heart and the blood vessels work in a coordinated manner to maintain blood pressure and blood flow.

A healthy heart is capable of adjusting the strength of its beats and the rate of its beats (the heart rate) to produce enough flow to match the demands placed on it by the tissues of the body. For example, during exercise, the exercising muscles require greater blood flow. If the heart does not pump the increased amount of blood that is necessary, then the blood pressure will fall. Hormones such as adrenaline help the heart beat faster and harder to meet the increased demand for blood by the muscles.

The blood vessels (vasculature) have a special structure and function to help maintain blood pressure. The arteries and veins are elastic in nature and squeeze on the blood like an inflated balloon does to the air inside it. In addition, the walls of blood vessels have special muscle tissue, called smooth muscle, that can contract to make the vessels' internal diameter smaller, which helps keep pressure up. If the vessels' internal diameter becomes too small, however, then the blood flow through them will decrease. The concept of blood vessels getting narrow and making it more difficult to push blood through is termed resistance to flow or vascular resistance. The balance of blood flow produced by the heart (cardiac output) and vascular resistance keeps blood pressure at the proper level. When one or both of these components falter, cardiac output and blood pressure fall, which, if untreated, leads to shock.

When the cardiovascular system cannot supply blood flow to the essential organs that is adequate to sustain their function, the body is said to be in shock. A reduction in cardiac output is the primary problem in shock. There are two major ways in which cardiac output can decrease enough to cause shock. When the ability of the heart to pump falls to about 40 percent of its normal capacity, it is termed cardiogenic shock. Cardiogenic shock may occur after a heart attack, heart valve disease, lung collapse, and other disorders.

Cardiogenic shock may occur in several ways. The most common cause is a myocardial infarction (heart attack). During a heart attack, the heart is damaged, and like any other muscle when injured, does not have the strength to pump much blood. Thus, cardiac output goes down and a fall in blood pressure will follow. Cardiogenic shock will progress to death if medical treatment is not rapidly obtained. After a myocardial infarction, while the heart is still healing, it has a reduced ability to pump blood. Exercise, even light exercise such as walking, must be resumed gradually. If it is not, the heart may not be able to pump enough blood to supply muscles even though demand for more flow is only slightly increased. This inability to meet the oxygen demand of the heart will cause further damage to the heart.

In cardiac tamponade, a type of obstructive circulatory shock, the stiff but pliable sac surrounding the heart (pericardium) fills with fluid or swells. This takes up room in the sac, squeezing the heart and prohibiting it from filling adequately from beat to beat. Therefore, the amount of blood pumped decreases, and a drop in blood pressure occurs. Cardiac tamponade can occur for several reasons. It can occur rapidly after trauma or heart surgery if the heart is punctured and bleeds into the pericardial sac. Cardiac tamponade occurs much more slowly when excess fluid is produced by the pericardium or when the pericardium becomes swollen. Both of these conditions can be caused by an infection.

A less common form of cardiogenic shock is caused by an extremely high heart rate. Normally, the heart beats at a rate between sixty and one hundred beats per minute. When the heart rate exceeds one hundred, the resulting condition is called tachycardia. Occasionally, in some people, the heart rate can go rapidly up to near two hundred beats per minute. The time between beats becomes so short that the heart does not have enough time to refill and cardiac output falls. If this condition persists, the blood pressure may fall, causing shock. When this occurs, the combination of the rapid heart rate and low blood pressure may cause a myocardial infarction.

Shock caused by a problem in the vascular system, not by a primary decrease in heart function, is generally termed hypovolemic shock. It is characterized by a lack of sufficient blood volume returned to the heart by the vascular system. Hypovolemic shock can be caused by a decrease in the body's total blood volume.

Excessive bleeding (hemorrhage) is the most common form of hypovolemic shock. The blood vessels are

---

elastic in nature, and they must remain filled with blood for arterial pressure to be maintained. In addition, enough blood must be in the veins to push it back to the heart, to be pumped through the lungs and back out into the arteries. When blood loss is slight, the body attempts to compensate by contracting the veins and arteries, thereby maintaining enough pressure and sufficient cardiac output. When enough circulating blood volume is lost, approximately 15 percent to 20 percent, hypovolemic shock occurs.

There are other ways in which blood volume may decrease. When a person is burned severely, plasma (the fluid in which blood cells are suspended) is lost through the burn sites. Enough can be lost to cause hypovolemic shock. Different forms of dehydration can also result in shock. Prolonged diarrhea, vomiting, and sweating can ultimately result in shock if the person does not drink enough liquids to replace fluid lost. All these conditions lead to a loss in the circulating blood volume and subnormal return of blood to the heart, and thus reduced cardiac output.

A virtual loss in blood volume may also occur, resulting in neurogenic shock. Sometimes anesthesia, hypoxia (inadequate oxygen), low blood sugar, spinal cord injuries, or damage to the brain stem can cause the vascular smooth muscle around the arteries and veins to relax. This results in a loss of arterial and venous pressure. Blood tends to accumulate in the veins and is not returned to the heart, and cardiac output falls. A systemic (entire body) allergic reaction can cause a similar response, called anaphylactic shock. Severe infections, usually bacterial, can cause septic shock, which has a death rate of approximately 40 percent. In this type of shock, the immune system of the body responds to the infection. However, this response can cause damage to blood vessels or cause a release of chemicals that cause the vessels to dilate (expand). All types of shock can be deadly if they are not promptly treated.

APPLICATIONS

In spite of the different causes of circulatory shock, the symptoms are quite common in nearly all cases of shock. The pulse (heart rate) is usually rapid and feeble. Breathing is generally rapid and shallow. The skin is pale, cool, and sometimes moist. The mouth is dry, and thirst is intense. Blood pressure is decreased. Some of these signs are attributable to the body's attempt to alleviate the problem.

The body has several defense mechanisms to help avoid circulatory shock. Several reflex systems function to maintain cardiac output and blood pressure. The body has sensors in the cardiovascular system that tell the brain what the pressure is in the arteries and the veins. When the brain senses a change in either or both of these pressures, it calls on its defenses.

When the arterial pressure sensors tell the brain that blood pressure is falling, the brain produces several responses. Through the nerves, the brain can make the heart beat faster and with greater force. In addition, the nerves can cause vascular smooth muscle to contract, making the vessels squeeze against the blood and increasing pressure. When the smooth muscle contracts, the veins squeeze blood back to the heart to enable it to pump more. The brain can also cause the release of adrenaline into the blood. This hormone can also cause the heart to beat harder and faster. The combined actions of this reflex mechanism attempt to compensate for the decreased cardiac output and blood pressure; however, these responses are only temporary before the person progresses to decompensation and death.

The sensors in the large veins and atria of the heart can cause a different response. Since most (75 percent) of the blood in the body is in the veins at any point in time, a 10 percent to 15 percent decrease in volume triggers the release of a hormone called vasopressin into the blood, which constricts the blood vessels to increase both arterial and venous pressure. The increase in venous pressure squeezes more blood back to the heart to improve cardiac output. The squeeze on the arteries raises blood pressure. Vasopressin also causes the kidneys to retain water. This fluid retained by the kidney is returned to the blood to keep up the vascular volume.

Specialized blood vessels in the kidneys can also initiate a reflex response to a decrease in blood pressure. The kidneys release a hormone called renin into the blood. Renin activates another hormone, angiotensin, which is a powerful constrictor of blood vessels. Angiotensin increases the release of yet another hormone, aldosterone, which helps the kidneys to reabsorb more fluid. All the above reflexes work together to increase blood volume, cardiac output, and blood pressure, in an attempt to alleviate shock. Despite these mechanisms to prevent shock, however, the by-products of these reflexes actually produce negative effects in the body that eventually lead to more damage.

When average arterial blood pressure falls below 60 millimeters of mercury (mmHg), the blood flow to the blood vessels supplying the heart (coronary vessels) cannot be maintained. When this occurs in shock, it happens at a time when the heart needs its critical supply of oxygen. In fact, the heart is trying to beat harder and faster, which increases its need for oxygen. As a result, the heart can weaken. When weakened, it pumps less and thus cannot bring the pressure back to normal. The heart becomes weaker and weaker. This condition is termed cardiac failure. In addition to cardiac failure caused by reduced coronary blood flow, the body can produce a hormone called myocardial depressant factor (MDF). This hormone directly causes a weakening of the heart that is independent of coronary blood flow. MDF also causes the body's bacterial defense system to function poorly. The maintenance of heart function is important to defend against shock.

Because the blood vessels contract in most of the body during shock, blood flow to nonessential tissues such as skin, muscle, bone, and the intestines is reduced, depriving these tissues of oxygen. These tissues can tolerate short periods of low oxygen supply, but if shock persists for more than a few minutes, these tissues revert to other energy sources. The end products of these alternative energy sources are acids, which can begin a process of tissue damage. If this process is not controlled or reversed, tissues can die. If a critical amount of tissue in an organ dies, the organ cannot function and may fail. Acid produced by other tissues gets into the blood and can directly decrease the function of the heart and its ability to respond to beneficial reflex signals. Acid production makes it more difficult for the body to fight shock.

Derangements in blood clotting can occur during shock. Blood clots can form in the early stages of shock, blocking small vessels. This causes a loss of oxygen that results in acid production. Increased acid in the blood can increase the rate of formation of blood clots. Thus, the clotting system can start a vicious cycle that increases the severity of shock.

Even when shock is not bacterial in origin, the body needs its bacteria-fighting systems. During shock, the bacterial defenses are weakened. Normally, bacteria from the intestines constantly enter the blood and are rapidly neutralized. If this does not occur, endotoxic shock can intensify the already existing shock. Therefore, a capable bacteria-fighting system is important in defending against shock.

In shock, the blood vessels of the heart and brain are spared the constriction experienced by all other tissue blood vessels. In fact, arteries in these organs relax to permit as much blood flow as possible, maintaining oxygen supply to these vital organs. Even so, when very low blood pressure persists (less than 50 mmHg), the brain's function decreases. At this point, the brain sends fewer of the beneficial reflex signals to the heart and blood vessels. The final result is a continuous decline in blood pressure and death. Maintenance of brain blood flow is a very important factor in surviving shock.

TREATMENT AND THERAPY

Emergency procedures in response to circulatory shock entail contacting emergency service providers such as paramedics and keeping the victim warm and flat on his or her back, with slightly elevated legs. The victim must get medical attention immediately.

Treatment of shock can vary depending on the cause. In many cases, shock can be effectively treated with intravenous (IV) fluids and medication. Some cases require surgical intervention. In all cases, the status of body fluids must be monitored and treated. The body's blood volume is one of the most important things to maintain.

It is particularly important to optimize blood volume in forms of hypovolemic shock. With hemorrhagic shock, whole blood is given intravenously to replace lost blood. In other forms of hypovolemic shock, different intravenous fluids are usually given. In burn shock, when the blood's plasma weeps from the burn sites, blood plasma is the medicine of choice to restore lost volume. IV fluids are immediately started to restore lost volume until the needed blood products can be acquired. When hypovolemia is caused by excessive diarrhea, vomiting, or sweating, IV fluids are given to replenish lost volume.

In other cases of shock, special drugs are needed to alleviate the symptoms. Shock caused rapidly by a myocardial infarction, with cardiac arrest, can be immediately supported by cardiopulmonary resuscitation (CPR), provided by a trained individual. After resumption of the heartbeat, the heart can be helped with several types of drugs. In the case of sustained tachycardia, a drug such as amiodarone can lower the very rapid heart rate to normal, allowing the heart to fill properly and pump adequate blood. Cardiac tamponade must be corrected to allow the heart to pump usual amounts. If the onset is rapid, as when it is caused by chest trauma, then the fluid in the pericardial sac may need to be removed immediately. A needle is placed into the sac, and the excess fluid is removed to alleviate the pressure around the heart. If fluid accumulates slowly as with an infection and is recognized early, appropriate drug treatment for the infection (antibiotics) may resolve the problem. In cases of shock in which acidosis is a complication or even a potential complication, sodium bicarbonate, a chemical that can reduce the acidity of the blood, may be given. There is no universal treatment for the complex process of shock. For example, hemorrhage may become complicated by heart failure and/or septic shock. Each case must be treated in accordance with the patient's existing conditions.

PERSPECTIVE AND PROSPECTS

Chinese writings of more than three thousand years ago indicate that a connection existed between the heart and the blood. Until the second century, it was thought that arteries carried air, not blood. Through the Middle Ages, it was believed that "spirits" were the essence of life or "vitality." This belief encouraged "bloodletting" as a treatment for many ailments, including shock. Leeches were applied to remove the "evil spirit" causing the sickness. This was not a very successful mode of therapy.

It was not until the seventeenth century that blood transfusions were tried, with the first experiments conducted by Richard Lower. In the 1660s, Jean-Baptiste Denis administered lamb's blood to a sixteen-year-old boy who was very weak and who had a high fever. The condition of the boy, who had been bled several times, improved for a short period of time. Others continued to experiment with transfusion as the remedy for loss of blood, but until the discovery of blood typing at the turn of the twentieth century, most attempts were of limited success.

The practice of giving transfusions greatly increased after the discovery of blood types in 1901 by Karl Landsteiner, who won the 1930 Nobel Prize in Physiology or Medicine for his work. By 1920, blood could be transfused from a bottle, since Luis Agote had discovered that citrated blood would not clot after being removed from the body. Blood banking was established in the 1920s by Russian scientists who discovered that citrated blood could be stored at 40 degrees Fahrenheit.

All types of shock are treated by determining and correcting the underlying cause. Oxygen is given in shock to improve the amount of circulating oxygen to the tissues. In hypovolemic shock, the goal is to improve the amount of circulating volume. This volume is replaced by intravenous fluids until blood products are available. Potent intravenous cardiac drugs that improve the contractions of the heart, improve blood pressure, or cause vasoconstriction may be used in cardiogenic and other types of shock. Mechanical devices have been developed (an intra-aortic balloon pump and a ventricular assist device) to use in severe cardiogenic shock that has not responded to traditional therapy. Synthetic epinephrine (adrenalin) is the first-line treatment for anaphylactic (allergic reaction) shock. It causes the smooth muscle in the bronchioles (tubes into the lungs) to relax and constricts blood vessels. Other treatments may include oxygen, antihistamines and corticosteroids. Septic shock is treated with IV antibiotics and fluids. Shock is a dangerous process that can occur for a variety of reasons. Quick detection and medical treatment are required to prevent negative outcomes.

—*J. Timothy O'Neill, PhD;*
updated by Amy Webb Bull, DSN, APN

See also Allergies; Bites and stings; Bleeding; Blood and blood disorders; Blood pressure; Blood vessels; Burns and scalds; Cardiac arrest; Cardiopulmonary resuscitation (CPR); Critical care; Critical care, pediatric; Electrical shock; Emergency medicine; First aid; Heart attack; Heart failure; Hemophilia; Hemorrhage; Hypotension; Necrotizing fasciitis; Resuscitation; Septicemia; Transfusion; Unconsciousness; Vascular system.

For Further Information:

American College of Emergency Physicians. *Pocket First Aid.* New York: DK, 2003. An excellent reference guide illustrated with photographs and written in a clear, step-by-step format. Covers many first aid methods, from resuscitation of conscious and unconscious choking victims, to how to deal with bleeding, shock, spinal injuries, poisoning, seizures, fractures, and bandages.

Avraham, Regina. *The Circulatory System.* Philadelphia: Chelsea House, 2000. This text explains the function of the circulatory system in reasonably simple terms. Provides historical development of knowledge about the heart and blood vessels.

Holcomb, Susan Simmons. "Helping Your Patient Conquer Cardiogenic Shock." *Nursing* 32, no. 9 (September, 2002). 32cc1-32cc6. Reference for nurses who work in the intensive care unit.

Klein, Deborah G. "Shock and Sepsis." In *Introduction to Critical Care Nursing,* edited by Mary Lou Sole, Deborah G. Klein, and Marthe J. Moseley. 5th ed. St. Louis, Mo.: Saunders/Elsevier, 2009. A chapter in a critical-care nursing textbook.

Marx, John A., et al., eds. *Rosen's Emergency Medicine: Concepts and Clinical Practice.* 7th ed. Philadelphia: Mosby/Elsevier, 2010. A logical and straightforward presentation of current standards of emergency medicine. Intended to be a reference in busy emergency rooms. The writing is clear and to the point.

Porth, Carol M., and Glenn Matfin. "Heart Failure and Circulatory Shock." In *Essentials of Pathophysiology,* edited by Carol M. Porth. 2d ed. Philadelphia: Lippincott Williams & Wilkins, 2007. A chapter in a textbook on pathophysiology. Offers a detailed explanation of various types of shock.

SHUNTS

Category: Procedure
Anatomy or system affected: Abdomen, brain, circulatory system, gastrointestinal system, head, liver, nervous system
Specialties and related fields: General surgery, neonatology, perinatology, vascular medicine

Definition: Surgically inserted tubes that are used to bypass blocked vessels that normally allow fluid to move from one region of the body to another.
Key terms:
anesthesia: the use of drugs to inhibit pain and alter consciousness
catheter: a tube passed into the body for fluid transport
incision: a cut made with a scalpel
portacaval: referring to a type of shunt used to carry blood from the portal vein to the inferior vena cava, allowing blood to bypass the liver
ventriculoperitoneal: referring to a type of shunt used to carry cerebrospinal fluid from the brain to the abdominal cavity

INDICATIONS AND PROCEDURES

The surgical placement of shunts is performed to reduce fluid pressures when the vessel that normally carries the fluid is blocked. Two major types of shunts are ventriculoperitoneal and portacaval. Ventriculoperitoneal shunts are used to remove excess fluid from the brain in hydrocephalus. Shunts used to decrease blood pressure in the portal veins are known as portacaval shunts.

Hydrocephalus is a condition characterized by an excessive amount of cerebrospinal fluid in the brain caused either by too much cerebrospinal fluid production or by the blockage of its flow. Hydrocephalus can occur at birth or be caused by head trauma, infection, or brain hemorrhage. If it occurs at birth, the main signs are an enlarged head that continues to grow more rapidly than normal. An infant's skull bones have yet to fuse, and the fluid pressure causes them to expand. The infant may have seizures, vomiting, abnormal reflexes, and other neurological signs. If hydrocephalus occurs in an adult, when the skull bones cannot expand, the pressure on the brain causes headaches, mental deterioration, loss of consciousness, and, if not treated, death.

Physicians use computed tomography (CT) scanning or magnetic resonance imaging (MRI) to find the blockage. The patient is then prepared for surgery to have a shunt inserted to drain the accumulating fluid. After the individual is anesthetized, the head is prepared for the operation. An incision is made through the skin of the head and a hole drilled into the skull, a procedure called craniotomy. A catheter that is part of the ventriculoperitoneal shunt is inserted into the ventricles of the brain and passed under the skin into the abdominal cavity, which is lined by the peritoneum. The peritoneum is a large membrane capable of absorbing the excess cerebrospinal fluid.

Portacaval shunts are used to reduce the blood pressure in the veins carrying blood from the digestive tract to the liver. Patients with abnormally elevated blood pressure in these veins have portal hypertension. This pressure reduces blood flow from the esophagus, stomach, and intestines, which leads to a pooling of blood and an engorgement of these vessels that may lead to their rupturing. Fluid leaking from the portal vein accumulates in the abdominal cavity, a condition known as ascites.

The most common cause of portal hypertension is cirrhosis of the liver, in which the liver is diseased and scar tissue forms. This scar tissue can block blood entering the liver from the portal vein and lead to portal hypertension. Occasionally, a thrombus (blood clot) will form in the portal vein and cause portal hypertension when the liver is not diseased. The patient may have ruptured vessels that bleed into the digestive tract, causing the feces to appear black. If the physician suspects portal hypertension, he or she will perform an ultrasound and arteriography to view the vessels.

A portacaval shunt operation may be necessary to reduce the pressure in the portal vein if other treatments have failed. In this surgical procedure, the patient is anesthetized and prepared for a major abdominal surgery called a laparotomy. An incision is made into the abdominal cavity, and the portal vein is exposed. The surgeon must then carefully place a catheter between the portal vein and another large abdominal vein. The latter vein is the inferior vena cava, which helps return blood to the heart from the lower body and the abdominal cavity. Another surgical option is for the surgeon to connect part of the portal vein to the inferior vena cava directly without the use of a catheter. The portacaval shunt diverts some of the blood that normally goes to the liver directly into the inferior vena cava, thus reducing the pressure within the portal vein.

USES AND COMPLICATIONS

The major problem associated with the ventriculoperitoneal shunt is the fact that it will need to be replaced as the infant grows. It is also possible for this tube to become blocked or infected. If the shunt remains in place for a long period of time, it may spontaneously penetrate an abdominal organ.

Portacaval shunt operations reduce the high blood pressure in the portal vein and help prevent bleeding. Unfortunately, they do not significantly improve liver function in most patients and may even cause further liver damage.

PERSPECTIVE AND PROSPECTS

Early detection and treatment of increased intracranial pressure (pressure on the brain) in hydrocephalus and increased blood pressure in portal hypertension are important to the long-term health and survival of the patient.

Early treatment of hydrocephalus with shunt placement prevents further neurological damage and, if the increase in brain pressure is rapid, may even be necessary to prevent death. Drugs such as acetazolamide that inhibit the formation of cerebrospinal fluid may, in certain cases, prevent the need for shunt operations. These agents will likely prove most effective in patients with mild disease.

Physicians may try to stop bleeding from ruptured vessels that is caused by portal hypertension by injecting a solution into the veins to seal them (sclerotherapy). Dietary restriction of salt (sodium) and diuretic drugs may be tried to reduce blood pressure, vessel engorgement, and ascites fluid accumulation.

—*Matthew Berria, PhD and Douglas Reinhart, MD*

See also Abdomen; Blood vessels; Brain; Brain disorders; Bypass surgery; Catheterization; Cirrhosis; Craniotomy; Fluids and electrolytes; Hydrocephalus; Hypertension; Liver; Liver disorders; Vascular system.

For Further Information:
Brunicardi, F. Charles, et al., eds. *Schwartz's Principles of Surgery.* 9th ed. New York: McGraw-Hill, 2010. A standard textbook on the topic. Intended for practicing surgeons, but valuable to general readers for its details.
Leikin, Jerrold B., and Martin S. Lipsky, eds. *American Medical Association Complete Medical Encyclopedia.* New York: Random House Reference, 2003. A concise presentation of numerous medical terms and illnesses. A good general reference.
Parker, James N., and Philip M. Parker, eds. *The Official Parent's Sourcebook on Hydrocephalus.* San Diego, Calif.: Icon Health, 2002. Guides patients in using the Web to educate themselves about hydrocephalus and draws from public, academic, government, and peer-reviewed research to provide comprehensive information on a range of topics related to the condition.
Toporek, Chuck, and Kellie Robinson. *Hydrocephalus: A Guide for Patients, Families, and Friends.* Sebastopol, Calif.: O'Reilly, 1999. Covers a range of topics related to the condition, including detailed discussion of shunt revision surgery.

SICKLE CELL DISEASE

Category: Disease/Disorder
Anatomy or system affected: Blood, cells, kidneys, lungs, spleen
Specialties and related fields: Genetics, hematology
Definition: Genetic disorders of the hemoglobin molecule.
Key terms:
anemia: the pathologic state of decreased concentration of hemoglobin
aplastic crisis: a sudden decrease in the bone marrow release of red blood cells, associated with very severe anemia

hemoglobin: the substance within red blood cells that transports oxygen and carbon dioxide

infarction: death in a tissue or organ caused by the obstruction of blood flow

CAUSES AND SYMPTOMS

Sickle cell disease is a genetic disorder of hemoglobin, which gives the red color to blood. The hemoglobin molecule is made up of two pairs of globin polypeptide chains (two α chains and two β chains) and four heme molecules containing iron. Normal hemoglobin (hemoglobin A) is a remarkable protein that changes the biophysical configuration of its amino acid chains so that it can deliver oxygen safely to the tissues without oxidizing iron. Oxygen removal occurs during each cycle of blood flow from the lungs to the tissues. Sickle hemoglobin has a single amino acid substitution of valine for glutamic acid at the sixth position from the end of the β chain. Sickle hemoglobin has the unfortunate propensity to condense as rods in red blood cells when the oxygen is removed during the normal circulation of the blood. These rods distort the cells, making them stiff, rigid and unable to transverse the smaller blood vessels rapidly. The result is vasocclusion (obstruction) of the small and medium-sized blood vessels, damaging the endothelial inner lining of the blood vessel and thereby resulting in tissue necrosis (ischemia). Vaso-occlusive episodes are one of the hallmarks of sickle cell disease. Sickling of red blood cells can occur during deoxygenation and hemoglobin tetramers polymerize and become sickle shaped. Patients with only one mutated beta-globin chain can also observe sickling at a lower volume as compared to HbSS-genotype patients.

The incidence of sickle cell disease in the United States varies, with the highest population being African Americans, and about 1 in 360 newborn babies suffering from the disease. Globally, over 75 percent of Sickle Cell patients reside in Sub-Saharan Africa, with an estimated 230,000 individuals impacted. Sub-Saharan Africa also has the highest rate of disease burden, as over 50 percent of children affected die by five years of age. The most common genotypes of sickle cell disease are sickle cell anemia-homozygous sickle cell disease (SS disease), sickle cell hemoglobin C disease (SC disease), sickle cell β0 thalassemia (Sβ0 thalassemia), and sickle cell β+ thalassemia (Sβ+ thalassemia). Less common genotypes include sickle cell hemoglobin E disease (SE disease), sickle cell hemoglobin D Los Angeles (SD Los Angeles), and sickle cell hemoglobin O Arab (SO Arab). In addition to these conditions, more than four hundred other abnormal human hemoglobin's can combine with sickle hemoglobin. This genetic heterogeneity accounts for the wide spectrum of clinical severity in patients with sickle cell disease, with

---

> ### INFORMATION ON SICKLE CELL DISEASE
>
> **Causes:** Genetic disorder
> **Symptoms:** Severe anemia, episodes of acute pain; complications may include septicemia, meningitis, pneumonia, severe upper respiratory tract infections, bone infarctions, kidney infections
> **Duration:** Chronic with acute recurrent episodes
> **Treatments:** Prophylactic antibiotics, hospitalization, analgesics

---

some forms essentially asymptomatic, such as Hb SE or S deer lodge. HbS has reduced oxygen affinity when compared to HbA, the normal hemoglobin phenotype found in unaffected individuals. This reduced affinity worsens polymerization and sickling which further reduces oxygen-binding affinity. HbS polymerization and sickling has a direct relationship with the concentration of HbS within the erythrocyte. Red blood cells that undergo polymerization and sickling repeatedly will eventually become an irreversible sickle cell, which cannot return to a natural shape.

Sickle cell anemia (SS disease) is the most common and the most severe form of sickle cell disease. It results from the inheritance of the sickle cell gene from both parents. Its hallmark clinical manifestations are anemia and severe episodes of pain; similar but less frequent manifestations are seen with other forms of sickle cell disease. In sickle cell anemia, anemia is caused by the rapid destruction of the red blood cells as they circulate because of a shortened peripheral survival time of less than 30 days (normal is 120 days).

Acute painful episodes—particularly in the older child, adolescent, or adult—are characteristic of sickle cell anemia. Sickle cell crisis often begins with pain in the abdomen or extremities and joints. Painful sickle crisis in the young child is usually precipitated by an acute fever, with excruciatingly tender swelling of the hands and feet (dactylitis) caused by small infarctions of the small growing bones of the hands and feet. Approximately 25 percent of SS patients have endless and repeated painful episodes throughout life requiring frequent hospital care. The clinical course of sickle cell anemia involves intermittent episodes of acute painful illnesses interspersed with periods of clinical quiescence and relative well-being. Commonly occurring acute complications necessitating intensive medical care are septicemia and meningitis during childhood, recurrent sickle cell pain crises, cerebral infarction with stroke, acute chest syndrome (often termed "pneumonia"), severe upper respiratory tract infections, gallbladder disease with gallstones, aplastic crisis, hypersplenism with splenic sequestration crisis, bone infarctions, priapism (a painful erection of the penis not associated with sexual desire), and pyelonephritis (infection of the kidney).

Acute pain events usually affect the musculoskeletal (MSK) system: extremities, chest, and back being the most common. The treatment is guided by how bad the pain is and how much the patient can tolerate. When oral analgesics and hydration alone cannot decrease pain, opioids are recommended. Vaso-occlusive crises can also sometimes result in sudden unexpected death. Patients may also suffer from acute chest syndrome, the second most frequent reason for hospital visits behind MSK pain. The severity of these episodes increases with age, and patients often require hospitalization with antibiotics, bronchodilators and transfusions. Patients could also suffer from acute stroke or acute anemic events secondary to SCD. The risk of a child developing stroke increases by 300-fold if affected with SCA, and ischemic stroke can occur as a complication of an acute chest episode. Patients need to be monitored for risk of intracranial hemorrhage and bleeding. Acute anemic events such as splenic sequestration or aplastic crises happen in over half of patients diagnosed with SCD and are one of the early leading causes of infant mortality. Patients often require splenectomy and transfusion to correct the crisis. Finally, patients with SCD also may suffer from recurrent cholelithiasis secondary to hemolysis. Acute complications from gallstones such as cholecystitis and choledocholithiasis affect over 20 percent of patients by adulthood.

An increased incidence of invasive infections caused by the bacteria *Streptococcus pneumoniae* is found in children with SS disease who are between the ages of four months and five years; this is thirty to one hundred times that which would be expected in a healthy population of the same race and age. Blood infections in SS infants and young children are associated with a rapid elevation of temperature, often to 104 degrees Fahrenheit, and the patient becomes even more anemic. In the untreated patient, death occurs within eight to twelve hours. Prevention of infection with prophylactic penicillin has remained a safe practice, as well as vaccinations against pneumococcal disease.

Chronic major organ failure in SS disease is the direct consequence of irreversible and ongoing damage to the endothelial lining of the small blood vessels as a result of sickle cells (sickle vasculopathy). Vascular damage begins years before the overt clinical symptoms are apparent. The spleen is the first organ to be destroyed, usually by five years of age. During childhood (three to ten years of age), 10 percent of children with this disease will have strokes, with resulting severe brain damage. Strokes cause paralysis and weakness of the extremities and difficulties in learning. This devastating complication in young children often makes functioning in school or living as self-sustaining adults difficult. Brain

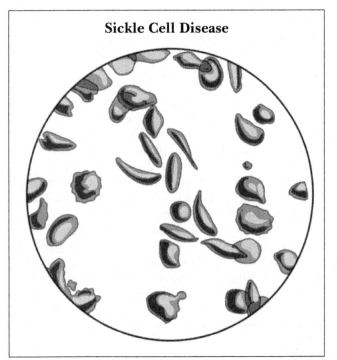

Sickle Cell Disease

The red blood cells are sickle-shaped rather than round, which causes blockage of capillaries. ©EBSCO

infarction can be accurately identified using computed tomography (CT) brain scans, magnetic resonance imaging (MRI), positron emission tomography (PET), and other diagnostic procedures. Sickle vasculopathy eventually culminates in young adulthood as end-stage kidney failure (glomerulosclerosis), sickle chronic restrictive lung disease, intracranial hemorrhages and brain damage, retinopathy with blindness, disabling leg ulcers, and painful generalized osteonecrosis of many of the bones of the body. Specialized medical care is required for the diagnosis and management of these permanent incurable complications. Patients may also suffer from pulmonary failure and myocardial injury due to chronic disease. SCA patients are recommended to undergo serial echocardiography every one to three years to screen for pulmonary hypertension.

TREATMENT AND THERAPY

Most acute complications of SS disease can be treated successfully so that the patient can attend school, be involved in social activities, and have a pleasant childhood and adolescence. Intensive care units with sophisticated monitoring equipment that are dedicated to infants and young children can manage and maintain the vital function of patients during severe illness episodes. The main stay of treatment for patients with SCD revolves around managing pain and monitoring for further sequelae of the illness. Patients who suffer from acute pain episodes are treated with analgesia and hydration as well as rest, until the pain becomes intolerable; at which point, opioids have proved helpful in treating the pain crises. Patients also need to be screened for and frequently follow up to detect for normal kidney, pulmonary and cardiovascular function. Prophylactic measures are recommended to those who are more susceptible to infection.

The institution of appropriate immunization programs for children with sickle cell anemia has substantially decreased their mortality and morbidity throughout the world. The importance of preventing the usual childhood infectious diseases such as hepatitis, whooping cough (pertussis), red measles (rubeola), rubella (German measles), diphtheria, tetanus, mumps, poliomyelitis, and *Hemophilus influenzae* septicemia allows 90 percent of these children to reach adulthood. The use of prophylactic antibiotics such as penicillin during young childhood (four months to five years) decreases the incidence of invasive pneumococcal blood infections. However, a recent ominous increase has been seen in penicillin resistance to pneumococcal serotype-specific strains, making prophylactic antibiotic prevention less effective. Salmonella contamination of chicken is still a major source of septicemia and salmonella osteomyelitis (bone infection).

Over time, children with sickle cell disease and their families begin to recognize the things that may precipitate a painful sickle cell crisis. Severe episodes require hospitalization and analgesic treatment, often with narcotic agents in addition to intravenous fluids.

PERSPECTIVE AND PROSPECTS

Sickle cell anemia is the prototypical molecular disease. The causative gene modifying the chemical structure of the hemoglobin β chain (βA to βS)—replacing the amino acid glutamic acid with valine—originated in Africa. The disorder was transmitted to the United States, Arabia, Europe, and South and Central America as part of the slave trade. At that time, healthy persons carrying the sickle gene, who are said to have sickle cell trait, survived the rigors of a slave ship. As persons carrying the sickle cell trait migrated throughout the North and South American continents and Europe, genetic drift occurred, accounting for the 15 percent of patients with the various forms of sickle cell disease who are not phenotypically African in appearance.

Improvements in acute medical care during childhood and in the social and environmental situation for patients, as factors taken together, have made it possible for most children with sickle cell anemia and other forms of sickle cell disease to survive childhood. In the United States, Great Britain, and most European countries, umbilical cord blood diagnosis or peripheral blood sampling of newborns can diagnose the disorder at birth. This allows early immunization for children and a responsive knowledgeable medical care.

The current focus of clinical investigations is prevention of the tissue destruction induced by the repeated endothelial damage caused when sickle cells obstruct blood vessels. Such prevention requires lifelong medical treatment. Drugs that can modify the rate of hemoglobin polymerization (precipitation) in the red blood cells include hydroxyurea, cytosine arabinoside, 5-azosididine, and other agents that increase the amount of fetal hemoglobin in red blood cells. By increasing the fetal hemoglobin, the rate of polymerization of hemoglobin S is modified so that there is less propensity for insoluble rods to be formed. The membranes of red blood cells become more flexible, allowing the cells to traverse the microvasculature and thereby decreasing the damage to blood vessels. Adhesion molecules (such as VCAM-1) act to provide the glue that binds the damaged sickle cell to the inner lining of the blood vessel, inducing permanent endothelial damage. Intensive search is underway to identify blocking agents for these adhesion molecules that can prevent the blood vessel occlusion.

Bone marrow transplantation with normal bone marrow (normal red blood cell precursors) from a donor with identical human leukocyte antigens (HLAs) is the only cure now available for sickle cell anemia. Bone marrow transplantation is limited by the paucity of HLA-compatible sibling donors who do not have sickle cell anemia. Erythrocyte transfusions have also been a helpful therapy which are associated with decreased endothelial injury and inflammatory damage. Chronic transfusion therapy, however, can have several adverse effects such as iron overload and hemolytic transfusion reactions. L-Glutamine has shown to have a positive impact in the treatment of SCD. L-Glutamine was approved in 2017 to reduce acute complications of SCA. Though the exact mechanism is unknown, it may involve prevention of oxidative damage of erythrocytes and prevent their hemolysis. Recent investigations target hemoglobin affinity for oxygen, inhibiting polymerization of HbS. Voxelotor, a treatment approved by the US Food and Drug Administration (FDA) in 2019, this increases the affinity of hemoglobin to oxygen and has shown improvement in the hemoglobin levels as well as decreases hemolysis. Although Voxelotor has shown a downward trend in vaso-occlusive crises in SCD patients, further investigation needs to be done to determine its efficacy in this respect.

Gene therapy holds the promise of a cure but has not been successfully developed for use in patients with sickle cell anemia. Gene editing utilizing CRISPR/CAS-9 focus on disrupting genes such as BCL11A, and are currently under phase I/II trials. The advantage of gene therapy is that no HLA-compatible donor is required.

—Fady Gendy, OMS-III

See also: African American health; Anemia; Blood and blood disorders; Bone marrow transplantation; Fatigue; Genetic diseases; Hematology; Hematology, pediatric; Pain management; Thalassemia.

For Further Information:

Ballas, S. K. "Sickle Cell Anemia: Progress in Pathogenesis and Treatment." *Drugs*, vol. 62, 2002, pp. 1143-72. A clearly presented review of sickle cell anemia, with available treatment options described.

Edelstein, Stuart J. *The Sickled Cell: From Myths to Molecules*. Harvard UP, 1986. A historical description of ancient African cultural beliefs and how they correlated to the modern molecular understanding of sickle hemoglobinopathies.

Embury, Stephen H., Robert P. Hebbel, Narla Mohandas, and Martin H. Steinberg, editors. *Sickle Cell Disease: Basic Principles and Clinical Practice*. Raven Press, 1994. Chapters 26, 30, 35, 38, and 40 offer an in-depth description of the molecular and biochemical nature of sickle hemoglobin and clinical correlations.

Kato, G. J., F. B. Piel, C. D. Reid, et al. "Sickle Cell Disease." *Nature Reviews Disease Primers*, vol. 4, 15 Mar. 2018, p. 18010, doi:10.1038/nrdp.2018.10, PMID: 29542687.

O'Malley, Paul D., editor. *New Developments in Sickle Cell Disease Research*. Nova Science, 2006. Covers a range of topics, from psychobiological reactivity to acute chest syndrome.

Osunkwo, I., D. Manwani, and J. Kanter. "Current and Novel Therapies for the Prevention of Vaso-Occlusive Crisis in Sickle Cell Disease." *Therapeutic Advances in Hematology*, vol. 11, 29 Sept. 2020, 2040620720955000, doi:10.1177/2040620720955000.

Pauling, Linus, H. Itano, S. J. Singer, and I. C. Wells. "Sickle Cell Anemia: A Molecular Disease." *Science*, vol. 110, 1949, pp. 543-48. The discovery of the electrophoretic mobility of sickle HbS as compared to normal HbA defines the first molecular disease to be identified.

Powars, Darleen R. "Management of Cerebral Vasculopathy in Children with Sickle Cell Anemia." *British Journal of Haematology*, vol. 108, 2000, pp. 666-78. Explains that brain infarction (stroke) is the most devastating complication of sickle cell anemia.

Serjeant, Graham R., and Beryl E. Serjeant. *Sickle Cell Disease*. 3rd ed., Oxford UP, 2001. Offers clinical observations of sickle cell disease based on long-term studies in Jamaica.

SIDS. SEE SUDDEN INFANT DEATH SYNDROME (SIDS).

SIGNS AND SYMPTOMS

Category: Procedure
Anatomy or system affected: All
Specialties and related fields: All
Definition: Characteristics of a disease state perceived either by the affected individual (symptom) or by someone other than the affected individual (sign).

Key terms:

asymptomatic disease: a disease that has no obvious symptoms

diagnosis: the act of identifying a specific disease using signs and symptoms as evidence

prognosis: the predicted outcome of a disease

symptomatic disease: a disease or disorder that displays overt symptoms

INTRODUCTION

It is common practice to use the words "sign" and "symptom" interchangeably. There is, however, a subtle difference between the two terms; it concerns who is making the observation. Symptoms are subjective qualities that indicate an abnormality or disease. In other words, they are perceived by the affected individual. Examples of symptoms that a patient may describe are an itchy sensation in the skin, headache, joint pain, or nausea.

Signs are objective. They can be noticed by persons other than the affected individual, such as physicians, nurses, and relatives. Examples of outward signs of disease include hyperactivity in a child, forgetfulness in an elderly person, fever, rash, a swollen ankle, or vomiting. Sometimes, signs may not be immediately apparent and further testing may be necessary in order to reveal them. For example, a physician or nurse may check a patient's blood pressure, blood may be drawn for analysis, or a colonoscopy may be ordered.

Health care professionals use a combination of the signs that they observe and the symptoms described by the patient in order to determine the presence of a particular disorder. This process is called diagnosis. Once a diagnosis has been made, an appropriate course of treatment is evaluated.

TYPES OF SIGNS AND SYMPTOMS

Signs and symptoms come in many different guises, and the way in which they present themselves gives health care professionals further clues as to the nature of the disorder-not only which disease is present but also how severe it is.

Blood pressure, pulse rate, body temperature, and breathing rate are known as vital signs. They are used as standard markers when monitoring an individual's state of health.

A sign or symptom is described as chronic if it is present for an extended period of time. For example, a chronic cough may be indicative of asthma, or a response to an environmental allergen. If a sign or symptom lessens in intensity or disappears, then it is a remitting symptom; conversely, if it worsens or reappears after a period of abatement, then it is relapsing. Some conditions are characterized by these types of signs. Relapsing-remitting multiple sclerosis is an example. In the relapse stage of this disease, the body's immune system attacks the sheath of myelin that surrounds nerves in the central nervous system. When the immune response has calmed down, special cells in the central nervous system, called glia, repair the myelin; the remission period is entered.

The presenting symptom is the symptom that first prompts the affected individual to consult a health care professional. If a symptom is general, involving the whole body-such as fatigue, weight loss, or fever-then it is called a constitutional symptom.

A condition that manifests in a tangible way is said to be a symptomatic disease or disorder. An asymptomatic condition, however, can be present without the affected individual being aware of it. Sometimes, routine screening methods such as a mammogram or prostate examination expose the presence of asymptomatic conditions before they become symptomatic, thereby increasing the chance for successful treatment. An asymptomatic infection is an infection by viruses or bacteria that does not result in obvious signs or symptoms. Often, sexually transmitted infections are asymptomatic: Examples include infection by the *Chlamydia trachomatis* bacterium (chlamydia) or the human papillomavirus (HPV). Some infections are asymptomatic while the bacteria or virus is incubating, which is the period of time between exposure to the infectious agent and the onset of symptoms. For example, the incubation period of the seasonal influenza virus is one to four days. Asymptomatic infections can be problematic because it is possible for the affected individual to transmit them to other people unknowingly.

Diseases can have primary and secondary symptoms. Alzheimer's disease is characterized primarily by symptoms such as memory loss and difficulty with concentration. As a result of the burden caused by these primary symptoms, an affected individual may develop depression. In the case of Alzheimer's disease, depression is a secondary symptom.

Prognostic signs or symptoms are those that give clues about the future course of the disease. The predicted outcome of the disease is called the prognosis. An example of a disease with an extremely poor prognosis is pancreatic cancer. Pancreatic cancer is rarely diagnosed in its early stages due to lack of symptoms; the chance of successful treatment becomes very low as the disease progresses. Less than 5 percent of pancreatic cancer patients survive for more than five years after diagnosis.

When an addictive substance is abruptly denied to an addicted body, withdrawal symptoms usually become apparent. In alcoholism, these symptoms range from headaches, nausea, and weakness to convulsions and delirium tremens (confusion and visual hallucination). Each addictive substance has a characteristic set of withdrawal symptoms.

Eponymous signs are named after the person who first described them. For example, Braxton Hicks' contractions (sometimes known as Hicks' sign), prelabor contractions occurring during pregnancy, were first described by John Braxton Hicks.

PERSPECTIVE AND PROSPECTS

Many years ago, physicians could use only their limited powers of observation, along with patients' description of their symptoms, to make a diagnosis. The development of progressively sophisticated equipment and new methods for clinical testing has made the diagnostic procedure faster and more accurate. As a consequence, treatment is becoming increasingly effective.

A vast amount of medical information is now available to the layperson. Online discussion groups and "symptom checker" Web sites encourage the practice of self-diagnosis. In fact, the act of researching a disease using the Internet as a resource, and subsequently worrying that one is suffering from symptoms of that particular disease, is termed cyberchondria.

—Claire L. Standen, PhD

See also Allied health; Alternative medicine; Biopsy; Blood pressure; Blood testing; Cancer; Cardiac rehabilitation; Death and dying; Diagnosis; Disease; Hospice; Imaging and radiology; Invasive tests; Laboratory tests; Noninvasive tests; Physical examination; Physical rehabilitation; Prognosis; Pulse rate; Screening; Syndrome.

For Further Information:

Kahan, Scott, Redona Miller, and Ellen Smith. *In a Page-Signs and Symptoms*. 2d ed. Philadelphia: Lippincott Williams & Wilkins, 2008.

Springhouse, ed. *Handbook of Signs and Symptoms*. 4th ed. Philadelphia: Lippincott Williams & Wilkins, 2009.

Tierney, Lawrence, and Mark Henderson. *The Patient History: Evidence-Based Approach*. New York: McGraw-Hill Medical, 2004.

SINGLE PHOTON EMISSION COMPUTED TOMOGRAPHY (SPECT)

Category: Procedure
Also known as: Single photon emission tomography (SPET)
Anatomy or system affected: Blood, blood vessels, brain, circulatory system, head, heart
Specialties and related fields: Cardiology, nuclear medicine, psychiatry, pulmonary medicine, radiology
Definition: A nuclear imaging test used to provide three-dimensional information about the flow of

blood through arteries and veins in order to diagnose a wide range of health conditions, including strokes, epilepsy, dementia, and tumors.

Key terms:

gamma rays: electromagnetic radiation emitted during radioactive decay with short wavelengths

ischemia: reduced blood flow

myocardial perfusion imaging (MPI): a type of cardiac stress test

neurotransmitter: a chemical that communicates nerve impulses from one nerve cell to another

photons: particles that travel at the speed of light

tracer: a substance that is injected into the body and releases energy which allows it to be followed along its path through the circulatory system and metabolism pathways

INDICATIONS AND PROCEDURES

Single photon emission computed tomography (SPECT) uses the radioisotopes xenon 133, technetium 99, and iodine 123 to acquire information about blood flow. A small amount of radioisotope is injected into a patient's vein to observe the flow of blood and metabolic pathways during the digestion of food. These radioisotopes are the radioactive forms of the naturally occurring elements of xenon, technetium, and iodine. These forms are referred to as radioactive because they emit gamma rays. These gamma rays can be measured directly by using a gamma ray detector containing a series of crystals that convert the gamma rays to photons of light. Photomultiplier tubes amplify the photons into electrical signals, which are then converted by a computer into detailed three-dimensional visual images on a screen.

SPECT is one of several nuclear imaging techniques used in medicine for diagnosis. Imaging is important as a noninvasive method of seeing inside the body, without requiring surgery. Other common techniques include X rays, magnetic resonance imaging (MRI) scans, computed tomography (CT) scans, and ultrasound. The other nuclear imaging techniques include cardiovascular imaging, bone scanning, and positron emission tomography (PET). All these techniques assist in the detection of inadequate blood flow to tissues, aneurysms (weak locations in the walls of blood vessels), various blood cell disorders, and tumors.

Of these techniques, SPECT is the most similar to PET, but SPECT is less expensive and more readily available. SPECT radioisotopes emit single gamma rays with longer decay times than in PET, and thus have the disadvantage of producing less detailed images than PET.

Tomography refers to the technique of using rotating X rays to record an image within the body. With today's computers, the terminology of computed tomography (CT) is used. The imaging process of SPECT combines CT with the use of radioisotopes. These radioisotopes are often referred to as tracers because they allow physicians to follow the pathway traveled by the blood through the body. Tracers emit gamma rays that are collected by a computer, which then translates the data into two-dimensional cross sections that are added together to form a three-dimensional image. These radioactive tracers decay within minutes to hours and are eliminated in the urine, thus posing negligible harm to the body.

USES AND COMPLICATIONS

The sharp images that can be obtained using SPECT enable it to be a useful diagnostic tool for a variety of cardiovascular, cerebrovascular, and neurological disorders. SPECT is more sensitive than an electrocardiogram (ECG) for detecting ischemia. In order to diagnose ischemic heart disease, SPECT scanning enhances myocardial perfusion imaging (MPI) after a patient exerts stress in order to compare images from before and after stress to assess blood flow. SPECT has become an extensively used tool to diagnose coronary artery disease (CAD). Because it is such a useful tool for detecting reduced blood flow, SPECT has also been widely used to detect tumors. For example, as part of the diagnosis of patients suspected of having aneurysms or tumors at the base of the skull, the internal carotid artery temporary balloon occlusion (TBO) test is enhanced by the use of SPECT to evaluate the cerebral blood flow. SPECT is also used to detect lymphoma tumors in the chest and abdomen, neuroendocrine tumors, stress fractures and stress

A SPECT brain study. Photo via Wikimedia Commons. [Public domain.]

reactions in the spine (known as spondylolysis), and liver lesions.

The high resolution of SPECT allows it to be a very useful tool for obtaining images of the striatum, a specific area of the brain containing the neurotransmitter dopamine. This dopamine activity can be monitored to help diagnose schizophrenia and various mood and movement disorders, including epilepsy, Alzheimer's disease, dementia, and obsessive-compulsive disorder.

PERSPECTIVE AND PROSPECTS

Although a SPECT scan exposes the body to less radiation than does a CT scan or a chest X ray, pregnant or nursing women should not receive a SPECT scan. A nuclear medicine technologist will inject a patient with a small amount of radioactive tracer. After enough time is allowed for the tracer to travel to the brain (usually ten to twenty minutes), a special camera called a gamma camera is used to acquire multiple images from multiple angles by rotating around the head. This gamma camera detects the gamma radiation emitted by the radioactive tracers. Thus, the patient needs to remain motionless during the scanning process so that clear images can be obtained. After the scanning process is finished, it is important for the patient to drink fluids to remove the radioactive tracers from the body.

—*Jeanne L. Kuhler, PhD*

See also Angiography; Angioplasty; Computed tomography (CT) scanning; Echocardiography; Imaging and radiology; Magnetic resonance imaging (MRI); Mammography; Neuroimaging; Noninvasive tests; Nuclear medicine; Nuclear radiology; Positron emission tomography (PET) scanning; Radiation sickness; Radiation therapy; Radiopharmaceuticals; Ultrasonography.

For Further Information:

American Academy of Neurology, Therapeutics, and Technology Assessment Subcommittee. *Assessment: Brain SPECT.* Minneapolis: American Academy of Neurology, 1995.

Frankle, W. G., et al. "Neuroreceptor Imaging in Psychiatry: Theory and Applications." *International Review of Neurobiology* 67 (2005): 385-440.

Masdeu, J. C., et al. "Special Review: Brain Single Photon Emission Tomography." *Neurology* 44 (October, 1994): 1970-1977.

Van Heertum, R. "Single Photon Emission, CT, and Positron Emission Tomography in the Evaluation of Neurologic Disease." *Radiologic Clinics of North America* 39 (May, 2001).

Single-port, four-arm surgery

Category: Procedure
Also known as: Robotic surgery, robot-assisted surgery, single-site robotic surgery

Anatomy or system affected: Skeletal system, muscular system, nervous system, endocrine system, cardiovascular system, lymphatic system, respiratory system, digestive system, urinary system, and reproductive system
Specialties and related fields: General surgery, bariatric surgery, breast surgery, colorectal surgery, endocrine surgery, gynecological surgery, neurosurgery, thoracic surgery, urological surgery
Definition: A surgical procedure performed through a small, strategically placed incision, with the aid of a four-armed robotic device.
Key terms:
da Vinci Surgical System: a popular robotic surgical system made by the American company Intuitive Surgical that was approved by the US Food and Drug Administration (FDA) in 2000
laparoscopic surgery: a technique in which short, narrow tubes are inserted into the abdomen through small incisions; surgeons may then insert instruments through the tubes to manipulate or cut tissue as needed
minimally invasive: refers to a surgical procedure requiring only a small incision or the insertion of an instrument into a body cavity; involving minimal damage to body tissue
patient cart: the portion of a robotic surgical system that holds the robotic arms and is placed alongside the patient
port: incision or cut through which the surgery is performed
surgeon console: the station at which the surgeon sits to operate the controls during robotic surgery
vision cart: a large viewing monitor through which the surgical team has broad perspective and visualization of the procedure

INDICATIONS AND PROCEDURES

In decades past, surgeons almost always made large incisions in skin and muscle, a technique that allowed them to readily see and work on the affected body part or system. While "open surgery," as it is called, is still commonly performed today, more minimally invasive procedures have also been developed. Many medical conditions can now be treated using single-port surgery—which requires only a small, strategically placed incision, or port and help from a robotic surgical system, most of which have four arms (three mounted with multiple small surgical instruments and a fourth with a high-definition, three-dimensional (3D) camera capable of magnifying the tissue and structures of the body by a magnitude of) 10.

Single-port, four-arm surgery is performed by a variety of general surgeons and surgical specialists, including those focused on airway, breathing, and lung conditions; surgical oncologists; cardiovascular surgeons; neurosurgeons; gastrointestinal experts; and those dealing with gynecological conditions.

Certain conditions lend themselves most readily to such procedures. Robotic systems are commonly used, for example, in bariatric surgery, and they have been deployed to treat conditions such as Crohn's disease, diverticulitis, hernias, and fistulas. In gynecology, robotic surgery is often used for procedures such as hysterectomy and fibroid removal, and cardiothoracic experts can turn to robotic instrumentation for endoscopic coronary artery bypass grafting, mitral valve repair, and atrial septal defect repair. Among the most common procedures performed using robotic systems is cholecystectomy (removal of the gallbladder).

USES AND COMPLICATIONS

Robotic surgical systems typically consist of a cart that is placed alongside the patient contained the robotic arms. These hinged arms hold a variety of instruments, such as scalpels, forceps, cautery, scissors, retractors, and suction irrigators. They are manipulated by a surgeon sitting at a separate console that serves as a control center, and other consoles allow the team to view the surgical field through a 3D endoscope or hold supporting components like pumps, fiber-optic devices, and light sources.

The benefits of most robotic surgery include increased precision by allowing the practitioner to operate near sensitive tissues, organs, and nerves without worrying about hand tremors or other mishaps. Surgeons also enjoy a better visual field, since high-definition cameras provide a magnified, detailed view of the affected area, and the ability to access hard-to-reach areas of the body. Patients are said to experience less pain, lower risk of infection or scarring, decreased blood loss, and shorter recovery times as compared to traditional surgery.

As robotic surgery increases in popularity, there has been some backlash, however, with critics suggesting that for routine procedures such as cholecystectomy, laparoscopic surgery is the accepted standard of care and can be performed by most general surgeons without the use of robotic systems.

Some studies have shown that while there may be benefits to robotic abdominal and pelvic surgery, any advantages over more conventional methods are virtually negligible. One 2021 survey found, for example, that while up to 9 percent of conventional laparoscopies required follow-up interventions, so did as much as 8 percent of robotic operations; similarly, while life-threatening complications occurred in up to 3 percent of all laparoscopic gastrointestinal surgeries, that figure decreased only to 2 percent in the case of

for robot-assisted surgery. (Additionally, the US Food and Drug Administration (FDA) has warned against the use of robotic surgery for the treatment of certain aggressive cancers, citing a lack of epidemiologic data on the practice.)

With long-term outcomes being similar no matter the surgical method used, and limited evidence to support its deployment, critics also point to the costs associated with robotic surgery—as much as 25 percent higher per incident compared with laparoscopic surgery. Pressure to purchase the systems also places undue burden on smaller or underfunded hospitals, with most systems costing upwards of $2 million to purchase and pricey service contracts required.

Furthermore, the specific modifications needed to decrease the number of ports used can mean poor ergonomics, loss of triangulation, and limited tissue retraction, thus compromising the unit's functionality, and experts urge regulators to continue to monitor the adoption of all types of robotic surgery across procedures and specialties to ensure that patient safety is protected and that hospitals carefully consider whether or not their patient volume warrants the acquisition of a system.

PERSPECTIVE AND PROSPECTS

It was National Aeronautics and Space Administration (NASA) that first began exploring the possibilities of remote surgery back in the 1970s; if a machine equipped with surgical instruments could be placed on a space station and controlled by a surgeon on Earth, it would be a boon for the space program. Similarly, the US Defense Advanced Research Projects Agency (DARPA) was interested in the potential for surgical procedures to be performed directly on the battlefield, by surgeons in a safe location.

In 1985, the first surgical robot, PUMA 560, extracted tissue from a patient for a brain biopsy, guided by computed tomography, and three years later a system developed at Imperial College London successfully performed transurethral prostate surgery. In 2000, the da Vinci Surgery System became the first robotic surgery system approved by the FDA for general laparoscopic surgery. By 2001 technology had advanced enough to allow surgeons in New York City to remove the gallbladder of a patient in Strasbourg, France.

Single-port robotic surgery was first used clinically in September 2018, and there are currently several new single-port systems in development. Although Intuitive Surgery's da Vinci platform has dominated in years past, newer technology companies are now entering the continually evolving field.

—*Mari Rich*

For Further Information:
Bakalar, Nicholas. "Are Robotic Surgeries Really Better?" *New York Times*, 16 Aug. 2021www.nytimes.com/2021/08/16/well/live/robotic-surgery-benefits.html?searchResultPosition=1. Accessed 7 Mar. 2021.
Brodie, Andrew, and Nikhil Vasdev. "The Future of Robotic Surgery." *Annals of the Royal College of Surgeons of England*, vol. 100, Suppl. 7, 2018, pp. 4-13, doi:10.1308/rcsann.supp2.4.
Childers, C. P., and M. Maggard-Gibbons. "Estimation of the Acquisition and Operating Costs for Robotic Surgery." *JAMA*, vol. 320, no. 8, 2018, pp. 835-36, doi:10.1001/jama.2018.9219.
Faust, Russell A. *Robotics in Surgery: History, Current and Future Applications*. Nova Science Publishers, 2007.
Novitsky, Yuri W. *Atlas of Robotic General Surgery*. Elsevier, 2021.
Sheetz, K. H., J. Claflin, and J. B. Dimick. "Trends in the Adoption of Robotic Surgery for Common Surgical Procedures." *JAMA Network Open*, vol. 3, no. 1, 2020, p. 1918911, doi:10.1001/jamanetworkopen.2019.18911.

SINGLE-PORT SURGERY

Category: Procedure
Also known as: Laparoendoscopic single-site (LESS) surgery, minimally invasive surgery, single-port robotic surgery, single-incision laparoscopic surgery (SILS), single-site surgery, "belly button" or "Band-Aid" surgery
Anatomy or system affected: Digestive system, reproductive system, respiratory system
Specialties and related fields: General surgery, gynecological surgery, bariatric surgery, oncology, otolaryngology
Definition: Single-port surgery refers to procedures that require only one small incision, most often in the abdomen, near the belly button.
Key terms:
bariatric surgery: procedures performed on the digestive system to induce weight loss
laparoscopic surgery: a surgical technique in which short, narrow tubes are inserted into the abdomen through multiple small incisions; long, narrow instruments are threaded through the tubes, allowing surgeons to cut and sew tissue
port: small incision or cut made in the body by surgeons
trocar: a device placed through the abdomen during laparoscopic surgery to serve as a portal for the placement of other needed surgical instruments

DIFFERENCES IN TECHNIQUE
There are several approaches that surgeons take when planning to operate on a patient. In traditional "open" surgery, a large incision is made, allowing the surgeon a wide visual field but resulting in greater pain levels and necessitating longer recuperation time.

In recent decades, minimally invasive techniques have been developed. These involve smaller incisions (typically three to five). Robotic surgery can be performed in this way: in those cases, robotic arms fitted with surgical instruments and a surgeon sitting at a remote console controls a tiny three-dimensional (3D) camera. The system allows the surgeon to make motions with a greater degree of precision and better range of motion than the human hand.

Laparoscopic surgery is another minimally invasive technique; in laparoscopic procedures, a needle or small tube called a "trocar" is inserted through a small incision in the abdomen, which is then inflated with carbon dioxide gas to allow surgeons to see the internal organs better. A small lighted camera called a "laparoscope" is inserted, and once surgeons determine the appropriate course of action to take, additional instruments can be threaded through other small incisions to complete the procedure.

By contrast, single-port surgery in conducted through a single port—or incision—in the abdomen, generally near the belly button. Although the exact position may vary depending on the patient, single-port surgery is sometimes referred to as "belly button surgery." The fact that it results in just a small, easily covered incision has also given rise to the nickname "Band-Aid surgery."

COMMON PROCEDURES
The single-port approach is used in many different types of procedures. Among the most common are cholecystectomy, or removal of the gallbladder, and numerous types of kidney surgery, including nephrectomy (in which surgeons remove all or part of the organ, often because of cancer), donor nephrectomy (the removal of the organ from a living person prepared to donate it to an ill recipient), pyeloplasty (blockage repair), and even transplantation. The first-ever robotic single-port kidney transplant was performed at the Cleveland Clinic's Glickman Urological & Kidney Institute in 2019, by the same team that had performed the world's first single-port radical prostatectomy the year before. Headlines at the time trumpeted the fact that the Institute was paving the way to make radical prostatectomy an outpatient procedure.

Prostatectomy—the partial or complete removal of the prostate in order to treat cancer or prostatic hyperplasia—is just one of the prostate procedures that can be performed with the single-port method. Others include transvesical enucleation of the prostate (removal of tissue blocking the flow of urine) and pelvic lymphadenectomy or lymph node resection (the removal of the nodes in the pelvic area. Urologists can also employ single-port techniques in cystectomies (bladder removal) or urinary tract reconstructions.

SLIS is now among the most commonly used method for the bariatric (weight-loss) procedure known as "sleeve gastrectomy," in which up to three-quarters of the stomach is removed, leaving a sleeve-shaped organ that can hold exponentially less food than before.

Single-port surgery is also increasing used by otolaryngologists to treat ear, nose, and throat (ENT) issues that may have previously involved painful and invasive procedures. In the 1990s, for example, removing tumors of the throat, palate, pharynx, tongue, and tonsils meant making a large incision in the neck and separating the jaw to gain access. The result was often such bad scarring and disfigurement, as well as permanent complications like inability to swallow, that many patients opted instead for radiation or chemotherapy—much less effective treatments that had their own set of debilitating side effects. By the early 2000s, however ENT surgeons began using robotic surgical that allowed them to remove tumors through the mouth, avoiding large incisions, and those methods have since continued to evolve.

THE BENEFITS

The benefits of single-port surgery for the patient include greatly reduced pain (and less need for opioid pain relief), as well as shorter hospital stays and subsequent cost savings. Cosmetically, the procedures leave either no scar or a barely noticeable one. Single-port methods have also been shown to reduce complications such as infection that can occur in traditional open surgery and some cases of laparoscopic surgery.

Additionally, even some patients who are not considered candidates for other robotic or laparoscopic surgeries—either because they have previously had multiple major abdominal surgeries or severe pulmonary or cardiac disease that puts them at heightened risk may be eligible for single-port procedures.

Another valuable advantage is that surgeons can perform more than one procedure using the same small incision, for example, removing the prostate and a cancerous portion of kidney—something that would have previously required two separate incisions or two surgeries.

RISKS

Some practitioners consider single-port approaches more challenging than traditional laparoscopy or robotic surgery because manipulating multiple instruments using one entry point limits freedom of motion. Additionally, some studies have shown that there is an increased risk of port-site hernias when only a single port is employed.

PERSPECTIVE AND PROSPECTS

Medical historians trace the dawning of single-port surgery to the development of multiport laparoscopic procedures. While there were scattered cases, including tubal ligation in 1969 and an appendectomy in the early 1990s, the use of single ports did not truly take off until robotic surgical systems were fully developed. These new systems allowed surgeons to better meet the general challenges of laparoscopy, and in 2009, the first successful series of single-port robotic surgeries was conducted, marking yet another milestone for the Cleveland Clinic, which performed eleven single-site robotic prostatectomies and eight single-site robotic nephrectomies.

As word of that clinical success spread, surgeons from all specialties began exploring the possibilities. Challenges remained: instruments were still difficult to maneuver and triangulating the trocars sometimes proved virtually impossible. Techniques evolved, however, and now single-port surgery is widely used around the world for a variety of procedures.

Some experts consider the field to still be in relative infancy, and research continues into better trocar design and systems that are more sophisticated.

—*Mari Rich*

For Further Information:
Barrera, Kaylene, David Wang, and Gainosuke Sugiyama. "Robotic Assisted Single Site Surgery: A Decade of Innovation." *Annals of Laparoscopic and Endoscopic Surgery*, Jan. 2020, ales.amegroups.com/article/view/5505/html#:~:text=The%20first%20single%20site%20surgery,way%20as%20an%20outpatient%20procedure. Accessed 28 Mar. 2021.
"Minimally Invasive Surgery." *Mayo Clinic*, 24 Sep. 2021, www.mayoclinic.org/tests-procedures/minimally-invasive-surgery/about/pac-20384771. Accessed 28 Mar. 2021.
Saidy, Maryam N., et al. "Single-Incision Laparoscopic Surgery—Hype or Reality: A Historical Control Study." *Permanente Journal*, vol. 16, no. 1, 2012, pp. 47-50, doi:10.7812/tpp/10-076. Accessed 28 Mar. 2021.
"Single Port Surgery." *Cleveland Clinic*, 21 Aug. 2021, my.clevelandclinic.org/health/treatments/17476-single-port-surgery. Accessed 28 Mar. 2021.
Spinoglio, Giuseppe, Alfredo Mellano, Domenico Conte, and Dario Ribero. "Single Site: Historical Perspectives and Current Application." Mar. 2021, doi:10.1007/978-3-030-53594-0_65. Accessed 28 Mar. 2021.

SINUSITIS

Category: Disease/Disorder
Anatomy or system affected: Nose, respiratory system
Specialties and related fields: Family medicine, internal medicine, otorhinolaryngology

Definition: Irritation and swelling of the sinuses.
Key terms:

deviated septum: a condition that causes a shift of the bones and cartilage from the middle of the nose to either side, making one side of the nasal passages much smaller than the other

nasal polyps: noncancerous growths inside the nose; usually associated with allergies or asthma, which can block the sinus drainage tract

orbit: the bones and other tissues that surround the eye, commonly known as the eye socket

CAUSES AND SYMPTOMS

The sinuses are airspaces in the skull's forehead just above the eyes, on either side of the nose below the eyes, and in the area just above the nose and in between the eyes. Mucus and tiny hairs, called "cilia," line the sinuses. Cilia trap inhaled particles and bacteria and move them back out through the nose, eliminating these potential irritants inhaled during normal breathing. The tracts through which the sinuses drain are relatively small and easily blocked by swelling of the area. Sinus blockage impairs drainage and causes the buildup of normal sinus secretions.

The term "sinusitis" refers to irritation or swelling of the sinuses and their membranes. Typical symptoms may include congestion or pressure in the nose or face and a runny nose with secretions that may vary in color from clear to yellowish-green to bloody. The facial pressure is often worse when bending forward.

Most often, sinusitis is precipitated by the common cold. Another frequent cause is allergies, with typical symptoms of sneezing, runny nose, and itchy, watery eyes. An allergic patient sensitive to a particular airborne substance (pollen, ragweed, dust, animal dander) has a particularly vigorous response when these particles land in the nose and enter the sinuses. Increased production of mucus and the body's natural

Illustration depicting Sinusitis. Image by BruceBlaus, via Wikimedia Commons.

INFORMATION ON SINUSITIS
Causes: Common cold; allergies; environmental exposure to smoke or air pollution; blockage from nasal polyps, deviated septum, or pregnancy
Symptoms: Irritation or swelling of sinuses, congestion or pressure in nose or face, runny nose with secretions varying from clear to yellowish green to bloody, decreased sense of smell, productive cough, fever, tooth pain, bad breath
Duration: Acute
Treatments: Increased fluid intake, antihistamines, anti-inflammatory drugs, decongestants, humidified air, nasal irrigation, oral or nasal allergy medications, antibiotics if needed

immune defenses combine to produce thick and copious nasal secretions that can fill the sinuses in an attempt to eliminate the offending agent.

Another factor predisposing a patient to sinusitis is environmental exposure to smoke or air pollution that irritates the sinuses. Problems that cause a blockage of the sinus drainage system, including nasal polyps, a deviated septum, or pregnancy (which leads to swelling of the nasal membranes due to hormonal changes), can interfere with mucus drainage from the sinuses. Finally, other genetic diseases like cystic fibrosis or immune system disorders can predispose patients to sinusitis.

Although viruses or allergies cause most cases of sinusitis, these can often lead to infection by bacteria if they do not resolve promptly. Bacterial sinusitis requires treatment with antibiotics to avoid the rare but severe complications of infection of the orbit or the brain and its surrounding tissues.

The distinction between bacterial and other causes of sinusitis depends on the patient's symptoms and a physical examination. A patient is more likely to have bacterial sinusitis if two or three of the following symptoms are present for at least seven days: facial pressure, nasal congestion, discolored nasal mucus, decreased sense of smell, productive or "wet" cough, fever, tooth pain on the upper jaw, or bad breath.

Sinus X-rays, done frequently in the past, are not considered a reliable diagnostic test for sinusitis. Though sinus computed tomography (CT) scans allow detailed visualization of sinus anatomy, they do not reliably distinguish bacterial sinusitis from other forms. They are helpful only in long-standing, refractory symptoms for which sinus surgery is considered.

TREATMENT AND THERAPY

The initial sinusitis treatment involves extra fluids, anti-inflammatory drugs such as ibuprofen, antihistamines, short-term use of nasal decongestant sprays (no longer than three days), and oral decongestants such as pseudoephedrine. Humidified air (e.g., steam from a hot shower) and nasal irrigation with water or saline can offer short-term symptom relief.

If allergies cause sinusitis, then oral or nasal allergy medications are appropriate. Examples are nonprescription antihistamines such as chlorpheniramine, brompheniramine, or diphenhydramine; they can cause drowsiness in some patients. Loratadine, fexofenadine and cetirizine, and other related, newer generation antihistamines are also available. They offer once-daily dosing and are significantly less sedating. Other nasal sprays such as topical steroids are available by prescription and provide significant relief.

Most sinusitis cases result from viral infections that do not require antibiotics. Symptomatic treatments include saline nasal washes, intranasal corticosteroids, and over-the-counter analgesics (e.g., acetaminophen, ibuprofen, aspirin, etc.). Nasal decongestants may help viral sinusitis cases, but there is no credible evidence that decongestants help with bacterial sinusitis infections.

If symptoms persist longer than ten days, antibiotic therapy may be necessary, and a healthcare provider evaluation is warranted. Other indications that antibiotics are warranted include pus-filled nasal discharge, facial pain for three to four days, or if symptoms improve after an upper respiratory viral infection and then become worse five to six days later. Many different antibiotics are effective for sinusitis, and prescription practices vary. Acute sinusitis treatment also differs from chronic sinusitis treatments. For mild to moderate acute sinusitis, *Augmentin* is the standard treatment twice a day for fourteen days. The alternative treatment is doxycycline, twice a day for seven days. If these initial treatments fail, then the patient is given one of three options: (1) high-dose *Augmentin* (2 grams) twice a day for fourteen days; (2) levofloxacin daily for seven days, or (3) moxifloxacin once daily for seven days. These treatment regimens are for outpatient cases. If the patient suffers from severe sinusitis that requires hospitalization, they are administered intravenous antibiotics.

PERSPECTIVE AND PROSPECTS
Before the antibiotic era, sinusitis treatment involved drainage of the sinuses by extracting a tooth, puncturing the roof of the mouth, or entering the nose and creating a drainage tract to drain the sinuses and subsequently irrigate them with fluid for cleansing. Given the invasiveness of these procedures, they have become uncommon with the development of effective antibiotic therapy.

The development of tiny, high-resolution cameras known as "endoscopes" in the 1950s created a revolution in understanding sinus disease. Direct visualization of the nasal passages and sinus drainage tracts allowed a better understanding of the sinus anatomy. It thus led to the use of this equipment to facilitate surgical treatment.

Occasionally, patients with recurrent symptoms require surgical removal of infected sinus tissue and en-

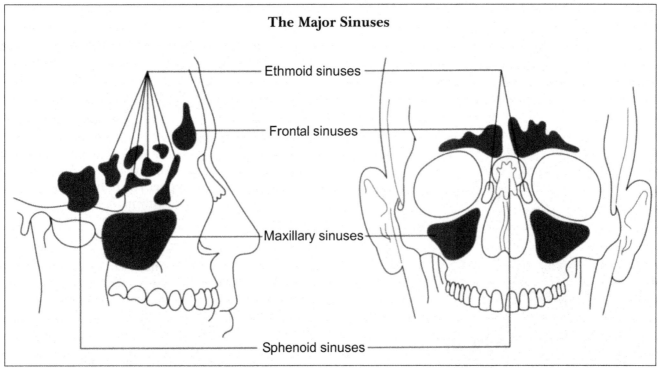

The Major Sinuses

Ethmoid sinuses

Frontal sinuses

Maxillary sinuses

Sphenoid sinuses

largement of the natural drainage tracts to minimize sinus obstruction. A specialist in otorhinolaryngology can perform such surgery using an endoscope without general anesthesia. Patients do not typically require hospitalization, and complications are rare.

—*Michael A. Buratovich, PhD*

For Further Information:

Acute Sinusitis. Mayo Clinic, 27 Aug. 2021, www.mayoclinic.org/diseases-conditions/acute-sinusitis/symptoms-causes/syc-20351671. Accessed 27 Aug. 2021.

Fried, Marvin P. "Sinusitis." *Merck Manual Consumer Version*, Dec. 2021, www.merckmanuals.com/home/ear,-nose,-and-throat-disorders/nose-and-sinus-disorders/sinusitis. Accessed 5 Apr. 2022.

Sinus Infection (Sinusitis). The Centers for Disease Control and Prevention, 27 Aug. 2019, www.cdc.gov/antibiotic-use/sinus-infection.html. Accessed 5 Apr. 2022.

Sinus Infection (Sinusitis). Cleveland Clinic, 6 Apr. 2020, my.clevelandclinic.org/health/diseases/17701-sinusitis. Accessed 28 Aug. 2021.

Sinusitis. American Academy of Otolaryngology-Head and Neck Surgery Foundation, Aug. 2018, www.enthealth.org/conditions/sinusitis/. Accessed 5 Apr. 2022.

"What are sinusitis, rhinosinusitis and sinus infections?" *YouTube*, uploaded by the American Academy of Allergy, Asthma, and Immunology, 10 Jul. 2019, www.youtube.com/watch?v=PRxGBrVufI0. Accessed 5 Apr. 2022.

"8 Hot Dog Gadgets put to the Test." *YouTube*, uploaded by Crazy Russian Hacker, 6 June 2016, www.youtube.com/watch?v=WBlpjSEtELs.

SJÖGREN'S SYNDROME

Category: Disease/Disorder
Also known as: Dry eye/dry mouth or sicca syndrome
Anatomy or system affected: Eyes, immune system, mouth
Specialties and related fields: Dentistry, family medicine, rheumatology
Definition: An autoimmune disorder resulting in the loss of tears and saliva.
Key terms:

Sicca syndrome: a condition characterized by dryness of the mouth and eyes
xerophthalmia: dry eyes
xerostomia: dry mouth

CAUSES AND SYMPTOMS

Sjögren's (pronounced SHOW-grins) syndrome is a chronic autoimmune disease. The body's immune cells attack and eliminate the glands that produce tears and saliva. This condition causes dryness of the eyes and mouth and is referred to as sicca syndrome. The causes of Sjögren's syndrome are unknown, although evidence suggests that viral infection, heredity, and

---

> **INFORMATION ON SJÖGREN'S SYNDROME**
>
> **Causes:** Unknown; possibly viral infection, heredity, hormones
> **Symptoms:** Dry eyes, dry mouth, blurred vision, eye discomfort, recurrent mouth infections, swollen salivary glands, hoarseness, difficulty swallowing and eating, extreme fatigue
> **Duration:** Chronic
> **Treatments:** Moisture replacement (eyedrops, saliva-stimulating drugs, salivary packets); immunosuppressive drugs or nonsteroidal anti-inflammatory drugs (NSAIDs)

hormones may be involved. Sjögren's syndrome is one of the more prevalent autoimmune disorders, affecting as many as four million Americans. Nine of ten patients with Sjögren's syndrome are female.

Sjögren's syndrome can be challenging to diagnose because the symptoms are similar to those caused by other diseases. The symptoms can also mimic the side effects of several medications and may vary from individual to individual. Even when the symptoms are reported to a physician, dentist, or eye specialist, the proper diagnosis can be overlooked.

The classic symptoms are dry eyes (xerophthalmia) and dry mouth (xerostomia). Individuals with Sjögren's syndrome often have blurred vision, constant eye discomfort, recurrent mouth infections, swollen parotid (salivary) glands, hoarseness, and difficulty swallowing and eating. Dryness of other mucous membranes of the body, such as the intestines, lungs, and reproductive system, may also occur. Extreme fatigue can also seriously alter the quality of life.

Sjögren's syndrome is most commonly diagnosed in people in their mid-forties. In some individuals, primary Sjögren's syndrome affects only the tear ducts and salivary glands. In other patients, it is present in conjunction with other diseases such as rheumatoid arthritis, systemic lupus erythematosus, systemic sclerosis (scleroderma), or polymyositis/dermatomyositis (secondary Sjögren's syndrome).

Sjögren's syndrome also adversely affects dental hygiene. Saliva contains many different compounds that discourage cavity formation in the teeth. Also, the constant washing of the teeth keeps them clean. The xerostomia experience by Sjögren's syndrome patients increases tooth sensitivity and the risk of dental caries and periodontal disease.

TREATMENT AND THERAPY

Once Sjögren's syndrome is suspected, a doctor will order blood tests for autoantibodies against nuclear or cytoplasmic proteins. Other tests for Sjögren's

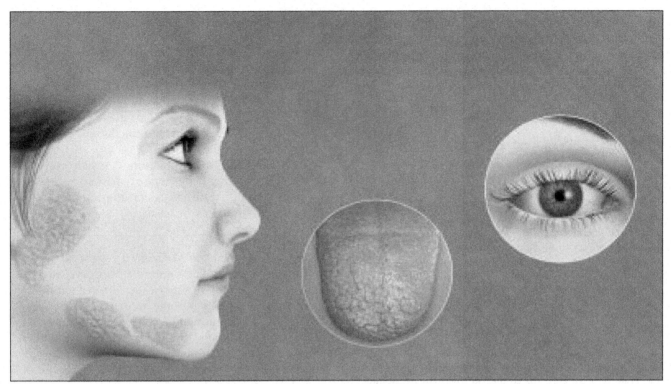

Characteristic dryness appears at multiple locations: the tongue, face, and eyes. Image by Scientific Animations, via Wikimedia Commons.

syndrome include the Schirmer's test, which measures tear production, and salivary scintigraphy, which determines salivary gland function, may also be performed. A lower lip biopsy to determine the extent of inflammation may also be needed.

Moisture replacement therapies are designed to ease the symptoms of dryness. Routine use of over-the-counter artificial tears effectively wets the eyes and temporarily relieves the pain of dry eyes. Many artificial tears preparations are available. They usually contain some form of cellulose as a lubricant and polyethylene glycol or polyvinyl alcohol to prevent evaporation. Some artificial tear formulations contain preservatives that may irritate the eyes, but other preparations are preservative-free. *Lacrisert*, a daily insert, gradually releases hydroxypropylcellulose, a lubricant, after placement.

Other ocular medications diminish eye inflammation. These include ocular cyclosporine preparations: 0.05 percent (*Restasis*) and 0.09 percent (*Cequa*) formulations. These drugs help tear formation and reduce inflammation at the eye surface. Another ocular anti-inflammatory is the 5 percent ophthalmic solution of lifitegrast (*Xiidra*).

The everyday use of eyedrops controls dryness of the eyes, and saliva-stimulating drugs and salivary packets help with difficulties in chewing and swallowing food. Their doctors may prescribe immunosuppressive or nonsteroidal anti-inflammatory drugs (NSAIDs).

Dentists and dental hygienists treat Sjögren's syndrome patients with local anesthetics to mitigate tooth sensitivity during dental cleanings. Additionally, dentists treat Sjögren's syndrome patients' teeth with fluoride applications to strengthen the tooth enamel and discourage tooth decay. Sjögren's syndrome patients have difficulty wearing dentures due to dry and sensitive gums. Consequently, tooth implants seem to be a better choice for these patients than dentures.

PERSPECTIVE AND PROSPECTS

Sjögren's syndrome is named after the Swedish eye doctor Henrik Sjögren, who first identified the syndrome in 1933. There is no known cure for Sjögren's syndrome or a current treatment to restore gland secretion. The outlook for individuals with this condition is usually good because Sjögren's syndrome is generally not life-threatening.

—*Michael A. Buratovich, PhD*

For Further Information:
Masterson, Susan. *You Mean It Isn't in My Head?: What Sjogren's Syndrome Is and What You Can Do About It.* Independently published, 2021.
Ng, Wan-Fai, editor. *Sjögren's Syndrome.* Oxford UP, 2016.
Sjögren Disease. Oral Health Topics, American Dental Association, 16 May 2019, www.ada.org/en/member-center/oral-health-topics/sjogren-disease. Accessed 28 Aug. 2021.
Sjögren Syndrome. American College of Rheumatology, Dec. 2021, www.rheumatology.org/I-Am-A/Patient-Caregiver/Diseases-Conditions/Sjogrens-Syndrome. Accessed 5 Apr. 2022.

Understanding Sjögren's. Sjögren's Foundation, n.d., www.sjogrens.org/understanding-sjogrens. Accessed 5 Apr. 2022.

Wallace, Daniel J., et al., eds. *The New Sjogren's Syndrome Handbook.* 3rd ed., Oxford UP, 2005.

SKELETAL DISORDERS AND DISEASES. SEE BONE DISORDERS.

SKELETON. SEE BONES AND THE SKELETON.

SKIN

Category: Anatomy

Anatomy or system affected: Nerves, nervous system

Specialties and related fields: Dermatology, neurology, oncology, plastic surgery

Definition: The largest organ of the body, which is vital to the survival of an organism for its protection against dehydration and abrasion, regulation of body temperature, and sensory reception.

Key terms:

basal cell carcinoma: the most common type of skin cancer; it grows slowly and seldom spreads beneath the skin

collagen: a fibrous protein found in the connective tissue, including skin, bone, ligaments, and cartilage

contact dermatitis: a common skin allergy characterized by inflamed skin; it occurs when skin comes in contact with substances such as poison ivy or allergenic cosmetics

dermatologist: a physician who treats the skin, including its structures, functions, and diseases

dermis: the layer of skin beneath the epidermis, consisting of dense connective tissue and blood vessels

epidermis: the outermost part of the skin, composed of four or five different layers called strata

keratin: an extremely tough protein that is the chief constituent of the epidermis, hair, nails, and tooth enamel

melanin: the dark pigment of the skin or hair that accounts for variations in skin color

melanoma: a cancer arising from a pigmented mole; it tends to spread to internal organs if left unchecked

psoriasis: a chronic skin disease characterized by red, scaly patches overlaid with thick, silvery gray scales

STRUCTURE AND FUNCTIONS

The anatomy of the skin consists of two major parts: the outer epidermis and the underlying dermis. The epidermis is composed of a particular kind of tissue called stratified squamous epithelium. Epithelium consists of cells that are packed together very tightly, a feature that is most important to an organ that must cover and protect the rest of the body. It is called squamous, which means "flat" in Latin, because its cells are flat and fit together like tiles. The word "stratified" describes the dozens of layers of cells that are piled up to create the epidermis. These cells form four or sometimes five strata, with their own characteristics and roles to perform.

The stratum basale, or basal layer, lies on a thin piece of tissue called the basement membrane, which is next to the dermis. The basal layer cells divide continuously throughout life, supplying new cells called keratinocytes for all the layers above the basal layer. About one-fourth of the stratum basale cells are called melanocytes because they produce the pigment melanin. As the keratinocytes are pushed up, they acquire a spiny shape; for this reason, the layer above the basal layer is called the stratum spinosum. While in the spiny layer, the upward-moving cells begin to produce the protein fibers that will eventually become waterproof keratin. As the spiny cells are moved further upward, they begin to flatten out. The layer that they form at this point is called the stratum granulosum because the keratin being formed is visible here, under the microscope, as large clumps or granules. Langerhans cells, which are very important in immunity and protection from disease, are also found in the granular layer. Only in thick skin, such as that found on the palms of the hands and the soles of the feet, do some of the migrating cells form a transparent layer of dead cells full of a shiny substance called eleidin. The shininess of this fourth layer earned it the name stratum lucidum.

The outermost part of the epidermis, the stratum corneum, is what most people think of as "the skin"-dead, dry cells that are completely waterproof because they are packed with keratin. The twenty-five layers of corneum cells form an efficient barrier to water loss and to the entrance of microorganisms. The epidermis has no blood vessels. The living, reproducing basal-layer cells must be nourished by nutrients passed from blood vessels in the dermis. Nerve endings that pick up the sensations of touch and pain extend upward into the epidermis, while those that sense pressure, heat, and cold extend only into the dermis.

Directly beneath the epidermis's basement membrane is the dermis. The dermis extends in a wavy or vertical tonguelike fashion into the epidermis to anchor it. The top of the dermis, which is called the papillary layer, thus forms ridges that account for one's fingerprints and toe prints. There are small blood vessels and fibers scattered throughout the papillary layer. The larger, lower part of the dermis is called the reticular layer. This thicker dermal layer has many more elastic and collagen fibers than does the papil-

The Structure of the Skin

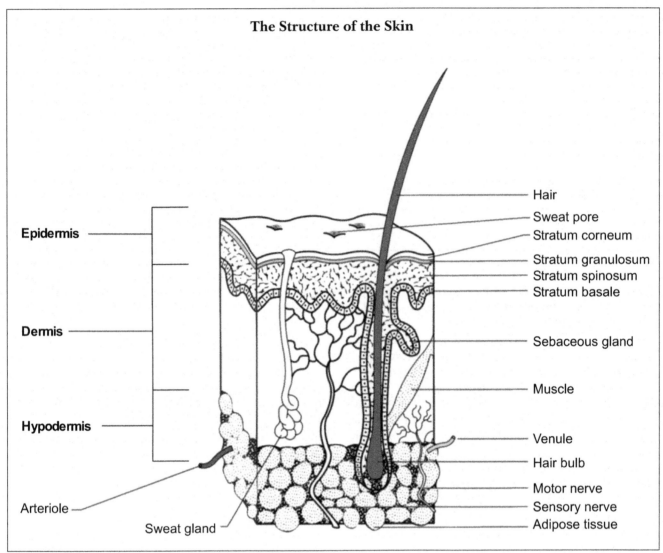

Epidermis

Dermis

Hypodermis

Arteriole

Sweat gland

Hair
Sweat pore
Stratum corneum
Stratum granulosum
Stratum spinosum
Stratum basale

Sebaceous gland

Muscle

Venule
Hair bulb
Motor nerve
Sensory nerve
Adipose tissue

©EBSCO

lary layer, and it is the location of oil glands, sweat glands, fat cells, hair follicles, and large blood vessels.

Directly under the skin, which is often called the cutis, is the jellylike, fat-filled subcutaneous layer. This packaging material provides heat insulation and energy storage, and it serves to attach the skin to the muscles and organs below.

The anatomy of the skin makes it able to perform a variety of functions. All these roles have one major purpose: to enable the skin to maintain homeostasis-that is, to keep the body relatively stable inside, in spite of constantly changing conditions outside.

The intact skin acts as a barrier to invasion by the multitude of microorganisms that come into contact with its surface. The waterproof keratin in the epidermis prevents all substances that are able to dissolve in water from entering the body through the skin. The presence of the pigment melanin enables the skin to absorb harmful radiation from the sun safely, up to a

point. Too much exposure to the sun causes sunburn, drying of the skin, a loss of elasticity, and wrinkling. More important, every sunburn increases the risk of skin cancer. Inheritance determines the amount of melanin possessed; although all races have the same number of melanocytes, people of different races differ greatly in the amount of melanin that their cells produce. The more melanin present, the darker the skin. The absence of a certain gene prevents melanin synthesis, causing those persons without the gene to be albinos. Skin color also varies because of the yellow pigment called carotene, which is found in the upper layers of the epidermis, and because of the red blood that is visible through the dermis of light-skinned people.

A very important function of skin is its role in temperature regulation. The body rids itself of excess heat by sweating. Excess heat passes from blood vessels into sweat glands, which conduct heat and perspiration to the surface. A large amount of heat can be lost as the sweat evaporates, thus maintaining normal body temperature. At other times, skin conserves heat by tightening blood vessels and reducing sweat secretion. Simultaneously, shivering, which is the involuntary contraction of skeletal muscles, releases internal heat to counteract excessive heat loss from the body. Only certain sweat glands-namely, those in the armpit and groin-produce the type of sweat that gives rise to an odor.

The waterproof quality of the skin prevents most substances from being absorbed through it into the body. Among the materials that can be absorbed are oxygen; vitamins A, D, E, and K; steroids such as cortisone cream; and, unfortunately, poisons such as insecticides.

The skin is able to produce a form of vitamin D that becomes active and useful to the body after passing through the kidneys. This synthesis requires a small amount of sunshine-far less than that necessary to cause a sunburn. If the skin does not produce enough vitamin D to enable the body to use calcium correctly, then vitamin D is needed in the diet.

Two very specialized accessory structures of the skin have their own particular functions. One of these skin derivatives is the pili, or hair. Except for the palms, soles, lips, and eyelids, the entire body contains hair. Each hair consists of a hair shaft that grows beyond the skin surface and a hair root lying inside a hair follicle. The follicle itself consists of epidermis that has grown downward into the dermis. Each hair follicle has an associated sebaceous gland that produces sebum, an oily substance, to lubricate the hair. Scalp hair protects the scalp from overexposure to the sun and from cold weather; eyelashes and tiny hairs inside the nose and ear canals help keep foreign material from entering.

The other important skin accessory is the nails. Each nail consists of a nail plate attached to a nail bed. Nails contain modified, highly keratinized cells from the stratum corneum. The basal cells that reproduce to make the nails grow lie under the cuticle at the base of the nail. Nails help to protect fingers and toes and enable humans to pick up tiny objects more efficiently.

DISORDERS AND DISEASES
The complex anatomy of the skin allows for the development of many possible defects and diseases. Three disorders that modern medical science attempts to understand and alleviate are psoriasis, cancer, and the many varieties of contact dermatitis.

Psoriasis, one of the most common of all skin conditions, is said to afflict about 3 percent of the American population. It commonly runs in families and affects both sexes equally. It may develop in childhood or old age but typically appears in the second or third decade of life. It most frequently occurs as scaly patches, or plaques, on the elbows, knees, and scalp but may appear on the back, belly, buttocks, and legs. Many people with psoriasis experience itching; surprisingly, some do not.

Human epidermis cells usually take about twenty-eight days to move from the stratum basale, where they are produced, to the top of the stratum corneum, where bathing removes them. This means that the cycle of normal epidermal cells in transit through the skin is accomplished in a month or more, allowing the cells time to mature. In psoriasis patients, this transit period is as short as four days. The reproducing basal cells divide five to ten times too rapidly, and the epidermis thickens enormously, but in patches. The skin cells of psoriasis patients are so abnormal that the patients' immune systems form antibodies that attack and destroy them, further damaging the ruptured, scaly surface. There is a notable tendency for psoriatic lesions or sores to form at sites of childhood injuries such as sunburns, scratches, scrapes, and areas where chickenpox was particularly widespread. These lesions often become pus-filled abscesses that contain enormous numbers of white blood cells. The epidermal cells no longer die at the stratum granulosum, and even the granules themselves are lost. The outermost corneum layer, which is usually dead, dry, and protective, is full of living but abnormally functioning cells. In the dermis below, large, dilated, thin-walled blood vessels appear, and the epidermis directly above them is disproportionately thin. Scratching or picking at the plaques causes bleeding.

The exact cause of psoriasis is not yet known. Genetic factors play a role in its development, since one-third of all patients have a family member who is also afflicted. In addition to the physical discomfort and damage to self-esteem caused by this very obvious skin condition, it can lead to heat loss, fever, severe arthritis, heart failure, and even death.

The many forms of skin cancer can also cause great disfigurement and even death. Two frequently observed types are basal cell carcinoma and malignant melanoma. Basal cell cancers, which may begin in the hair follicle epithelium, are the most common skin cancers, accounting for almost 70 percent of all cases. Fortunately, they are also the most easily treated. They are most often found where sunlight strikes the hardest, on the neck, scalp, face, and shoulders. Basal cell cancers often start as small bumps but grow wider and more elevated, usually with a cavity in the center. Although their surface is shiny and filled with tiny blood vessels, their color may still be like that of normal skin. If left untreated, basal cell carcinomas may develop a crust or an ulcer that cannot heal. Although they seldom metastasize, shifting or spreading through the bloodstream to another part of the body, they often do great damage to the tissues and structures directly under them. Those that grow near ears and eyes can cause loss of function of those organs.

In almost all cases, the appearance of basal cell carcinomas is directly related to sun exposure. A few seem to be related to previous scars, burns, tattoos, or exposure to arsenic. It is important to be aware of the warning signs of basal cell carcinomas. Some can be felt as well as seen as reddish or dotted lumps; others look like open sores caused by scratches or insect bites that do not heal. Because these cancers, which often grow for two years before detection, have such varied appearances, they can be diagnosed accurately only by biopsy.

The most dangerous skin cancers are the malignant melanomas. They begin in the pigmented cells called melanocytes but usually and quite rapidly invade deeper tissue. Severe sunburns early in life seem to be their usual cause. Many start as small dark brown growths similar to moles, although they may become white, blue, or reddish and irregular in shape as they grow. Often they will bleed if rubbed. People who have acquired one hundred or more moles by young adulthood are considered genetically predisposed toward these dangerous melanomas; such people should use sunscreens every day all year long. It should be noted that half of all melanomas arise from apparently normal skin that has no moles. The malignant melanomas are much more dangerous than the basal cell carcinomas because they tend to release cancerous cells into the bloodstream that latch on to and grow into numerous internal organs.

Seldom life-threatening, contact dermatitis can still be very uncomfortable for a patient. Dermatitis is an inflammation of the skin that usually is a result of an allergic reaction and may include redness, swelling, blistering, crusting, and scaling among its symptoms. In all its many varieties, it probably forms the bulk of a dermatologist's practice. Contact dermatitis results from coming into contact with a causing substance, such as poison ivy, poison oak, or poison sumac. The sap from these plants contains urushiol, a substance to which 70 percent of all people are allergic.

Large numbers of persons are allergic to the metal nickel and can develop inflammations from wearing nickel rings, watches, earrings, or other jewelry. Nickel zippers and clothing snaps, eyeglass frames and sewing needles, and even coins can cause a reaction.

The chemicals in permanent hair dyes cause terrible swelling and itching of the face and neck in some people. Oddly, the scalp under the dyed hair is often unaffected. When dermatitis seems to result from hair dyes, it is often because the affected person has simultaneously been using certain sunscreens, the pain reliever benzocaine, or one of many other common medicines.

The chemical potassium dichromate is found in many detergents. People who experience dermatitis caused by detergent use should avoid other chromate-containing products as well. These include inks, paints, bleaches, and spackling, to name only a few.

Other people contract dermatitis caused by a formaldehyde allergy. Permanent-press clothing and sheets are made wrinkle-proof by the use of a formaldehyde-based substance. Individuals with a formaldehyde allergy must also avoid many paper products, cosmetics, and disinfectants that contain formaldehyde derivatives.

Susceptibility to contact dermatitis from rubber products is widespread. Surprisingly, it often appears long after the exposure and is most common in manufacturing workers.

In modern society, with its heavy reliance on over-the-counter drugs, cleaning products of all kinds, deodorants and cosmetics, insecticides and weed-killers, and innumerable other chemical products, the potential causes of contact dermatitis have been and will continue to be multiplied.

PERSPECTIVE AND PROSPECTS

Research in dermatology both borrows from and sheds light upon many other branches of medical science. Immunology, endocrinology, biochemistry, surgery, and oncology are just a few of many.

Diseases of the skin can reveal the presence of many otherwise unseen internal disease conditions. Shiny, thin, reddish-yellow patches on the shins may be a sign of diabetes. Prediabetics are also susceptible to repeated yeast and fungal infections of the skin and have poor wound-healing ability.

Too little thyroid hormone causes coarse hair; thickened, dry, cool skin; and rough plaques on the shins. Too much thyroid hormone causes thin hair, excessive sweating, and, surprisingly, identical rough plaques on the shins.

Abnormally dark skin can be a sign of drug side effects, the presence of heavy metals, poor adrenal gland output, or pituitary tumors. Skin may also darken from excess iron intake or, very noticeably, from a widespread malignant melanoma.

Various bowel diseases may also cause skin conditions. The small intestine defect involving a flattened, malfunctioning lining can produce severely itchy blisters on the limbs and the back. Ulcers in the large intestine often produce deep, dirty-looking skin ulcers.

The presence of cancer in the breast, bowel, or lungs may precipitate thousands of external wartlike growths or flat, waxy-surfaced growths. Similarly, the gradual appearance, usually on the legs of the elderly, of fishlike skin may reveal the early presence of cancer of the lymph glands.

Alcoholism reveals itself in spider telangiectasia, webs of dilated capillaries on the skin surface. The presence of hepatitis, a serious viral infection of the liver, is indicated by the yellowing of the skin known as jaundice.

Two other links among dermatology, immunology, and oncology are the search for a vaccine against skin cancer and a new treatment called photopheresis. Since the late 1960s, there has been an ongoing attempt to develop a vaccine to prevent a recurrence of malignant melanoma. This is a particularly important pursuit because those who have survived one case of melanoma have a high risk of developing future ones.

Photopheresis patients take a drug called psoralen. Two hours later, their blood is drawn and exposed to ultraviolet light. The interaction between the psoralen and the light destroys abnormal white blood cells, after which the blood is returned to the body. Since 1987, photopheresis has been used to treat a cancer of the immune system that begins in the skin. Researchers hope eventually to use psoralen to treat arthritis and lupus, and to prevent the rejection of organ transplants.

For many years, drugs for internal conditions could be administered only orally or by injection. In both methods, the circulating amount may be too high to be safe immediately after it is given and too low to be effective as the hours go by. Dermatologists have greatly advanced medical science by developing transdermal patches. These patches enable a steady supply of a drug to enter the bloodstream by absorption through the skin. By the end of the twentieth century, patches had been developed to treat angina, high blood pressure, motion sickness, menopausal symptoms, and nicotine addiction.

One of the greatest traumas skin can suffer is a widespread burn. Although surgeons have had great success in transplanting many internal organs, they are unable to permanently transplant skin from another person. In 1981, they developed a marvelous technique to produce artificial skin. It uses animal skin protein seeded with a few skin cells taken from the patient. From this small patch, a large enough piece of skin can be grown to cover the wounds until the gradually healing skin replaces it.

From the earliest simple salves for skin rashes to the great discoveries of transdermal patches and artificial skin, dermatologists have done and continue to do their share in advancing medical science.

—*Grace D. Matzen*

See also Abscess drainage; Abscesses; Acne; Acupressure; Acupuncture; Age spots; Albinos; Allergies; Athlete's foot; Bedsores; Biopsy; Birthmarks; Bites and stings; Blisters; Boils; Bruises; Burns and scalds; Candidiasis; Canker sores; Cells; Chickenpox; Cold sores; Collagen; Corns and calluses; Cradle cap; Cryosurgery; Cyst removal; Cysts; Dermatitis; Dermatology; Dermatology, pediatric; Dermatopathology; Diaper rash; Eczema; Edema; Electrical shock; Electrocauterization; Face lift and blepharoplasty; Fifth disease; Frostbite; Fungal infections; Glands; Grafts and grafting; Hair; Hair loss and baldness; Hair transplantation; Hand-foot-and-mouth disease; Heat exhaustion and heatstroke; Hives; Host-defense mechanisms; Human papillomavirus (HPV); Hyperhidrosis; Impetigo; Insect-borne diseases; Itching; Jaundice; Kawasaki disease; Laceration repair; Laser use in surgery; Leishmaniasis; Leprosy; Lesions; Lice, mites, and ticks; Lower extremities; Measles; Melanoma; Moles; Morgellons disease; Nails; Necrotizing fasciitis; Numbness and tingling; Pigmentation; Pityriasis alba; Pityriasis rosea; Plastic surgery; Poisonous plants; Porphyria; Psoriasis; Radiation sickness; Rashes; Ringworm; Rocky Mountain spotted fever; Rosacea; Roseola; Rubella; Scabies; Scarlet fever; Scleroderma; Sense organs; Shingles; Skin cancer; Skin disorders; Skin lesion removal; Smallpox; Stevens-Johnson syndrome; Stretch marks; Styes; Sunburn; Sweating; Systemic lupus erythematosus (SLE); Tattoos and body piercing; Touch; Upper extremities; Vitiligo; Warts; Wrinkles.

For Further Information:
Goodman, Thomas, and Stephanie Young. *Smart Face*. Englewood Cliffs, N.J.: Prentice Hall, 1988. An easy-to-read explanation of skin structure, problems, and care, with special emphasis on delicate facial skin. Contains an extensive appendix of consumer product information.

Jacknin, Jeanette. *Smart Medicine for Your Skin*. New York: Putnam, 2001. An accessible and comprehensive guide to skin problems and solutions that include traditional therapies and alternative medicine choices.

Lamberg, Lynne. *Skin Disorders*. Philadelphia: Chelsea House, 2001. This brief volume is an introduction to the study of skin problems. Contains a very helpful glossary, a bibliography, and a list of organizations to contact for more information.

Lees, Mark. *Skin Care: Beyond the Basics*. 3d ed. Clifton Park, N.Y.: Thomson/Delmar Learning, 2007. A text for estheticians and students in the field that provides practical information on treating many kinds of skin problems and discusses topics such as rosacea, sensitive skin, hormones and menopause, and postlaser skin care.

Mackie, Rona M. *Clinical Dermatology*. 5th ed. New York: Oxford University Press, 2003. A text written for dermatology students but useful to the general public for more precise and detailed information than that contained in popular works. Illustrated in color.

Siegel, Mary-Ellen. *Safe in the Sun*. New York: Walker, 1995. Presents information from research of leading dermatologists and ophthalmologists showing the relationship between sun exposure and damage to skin and eyes. Easily understood by the general public. Contains an extensive glossary and many pages of helpful further sources of information.

Turkington, Carol, and Jeffrey S. Dover. *The Encyclopedia of Skin and Skin Disorders*. 3d ed. New York: Facts On File, 2007. More than one thousand entries on skin-related topics, including diseases, treatments, resources and organizations, skin cancer, acne treatment, FDA approvals of new treatments, and remedies for wrinkled skin.

Weedon, David. *Skin Pathology*. 3d ed. New York: Churchill Livingstone/Elsevier, 2010. Text with extensive photographs, covering tissue reaction patterns; the epidermis, dermis, and subcutis; the skin in systemic and miscellaneous diseases; infections and infestations; and tumors, among other topics.

SKIN CANCER

Category: Disease/Disorder
Anatomy or system affected: Lymphatic system, skin
Specialties and related fields: Dermatology, environmental health, immunology, oncology
Definition: Malignancies of the skin (that sometimes spread to the internal organs) caused by ultraviolet radiation in sunlight.

Cancer is the common term used to describe the large class of diseases called "malignant neoplasms." Neoplasms, which occur only in multicellular organisms, develop and function in an autonomous way that does not abide by the biological mechanisms that govern the growth and metabolism of the individual cells and the reactions that take place in a living organism. When such neoplasms grow at a rate faster than the tissues from which they arise, while at the same time invading those tissues, they are called "malignant" and are commonly described as cancerous. Benign neoplasms, which do not invade surrounding tissues, generally are not as dangerous as malignant ones.

Sun radiation is life-sustaining, but the higher-energy part of the sunlight spectrum brings the danger of skin cancer. When living tissue is irradiated, its molecular structure is disrupted, thus initiating a chain of reactions, many of which are not the usual ones associated with the living organism. Therefore, a change in the chromosomal composition and the development of unwanted cells is likely to occur. Such changes take place because of the formation of free radicals in the deoxyribonucleic acid (DNA) molecules that constitute the genetic code. The result is skin cancer, the most common form of cancer in both men and women in the United States.

TYPES OF SKIN CANCER

Skin neoplasms may be benign or malignant, acquired or congenital. The majority are benign and acquired. The common mole (the medical term for which is melanocytic nevus) is a neoplasm of benign

> **INFORMATION ON SKIN CANCER**
>
> **Causes:** Genetic factors, ultraviolet radiation from sun exposure
> **Symptoms:** Lesion that increases in size and turns several colors (black, blue, white, brown); in later stages, itching, bleeding, and pain
> **Duration:** Short-term to recurrent
> **Treatments:** Surgical removal, chemotherapy, radiation therapy

melanocytes that is often present at birth, and which is known as a "birthmark." Such moles are generally harmless unless they are large in which case, they may have up to a 10 percent chance of becoming malignant. Other benign skin lesions include strawberry hemangiomas and port wine stains, which are of vascular origin.

The two most common forms of skin cancer—basal cell carcinoma and squamous cell carcinoma—arise from the corresponding part of the keratinocytes of the epidermis and are caused by the cumulative effect of ultraviolet radiation on the skin. They are generally localized and rarely metastasize. These cancers are easily identified as persisting sores or crusting patches that grow mostly on sun-exposed parts of the body such as the hands, neck, arms, and nose. These usually can be treated with routine surgical procedures. A malignant melanoma is formed from the pigment-forming melanocyte and with enough time will almost certainly metastasize. Melanomas, therefore, should be removed surgically at the earliest possible stage. If a melanoma is detected at a later stage, chemotherapy and radiation are the techniques usually applied.

A malignant melanoma appears as an asymmetric lesion that increases in size over time, usually has a scalloped border, and is typically multicolored to include black, blue, white, and brown. Typically asymptomatic at first, symptoms such as itching, bleeding, and pain are may be encountered at later stages of development.

There are several other skin malignancies that are not as common. Two that have the potential for fatal outcome are mycosis fungoides and Kaposi's Sarcoma (KS). Mycosis fungoides is a skin lymphoma that may be confined to one location for ten or more years before it metastasizes to internal organs, which entails a high mortality. As a result, it is difficult to track this skin cancer, both clinically and histologically, and several biopsies (skin histological examinations) may be required to ascertain its presence. KS occurs as skin lesions commonly either among older Mediterranean men or in human immunodeficiency virus (HIV)-infected people. The sarcoma is derived from skin blood vessels and appears as violet patches or lesions. As long as it is contained only in the skin, KS typically is not fatal. Once the internal organs are affected, however, the prognosis is much worse even though the lesions may be treated with irradiation and chemotherapy.

THE EFFECTS OF SUNLIGHT ON SKIN
Extensive skin exposure to sunlight, such as at the beach, leads to the polymerization of skin chemicals (known as catecholamines) and the subsequent formation of different types of epidermal pigmentation (melanin), which are responsible for tanning. Tanning occurs only if there is gradual exposure to sunlight, while sudden and/or prolonged sun exposure often leads to a sunburn, particularly in fairer-skinned individuals. Photoprotection is believed to be one of the major biological functions of the melanin pigment. It appears that melanin formation can participate effectively in reducing the harmful effects of sunlight by an array of photoinduced chemical reactions, which result in the consumption of scavenging active oxygen species such as the superoxide anion and hydrogen peroxide. It has been determined that in biological systems, superoxide and hydrogen peroxide are formed in small quantities during normal processes. Both species are known to produce several biological effects, most of which are harmful to tissues. It should be pointed out, however, that although melanin may act as a free radical scavenger, it may also become energetically overloaded and may change to a toxic state. Evidence exists that melanin increases the radiative damage to cells which leads to sunlight induced skin cancer. In other words, melanin formation is good only when moderate exposure to sunlight occurs.

In the atmosphere 12 to 48 km above the earth's surface lies a small layer of ozone. Although this layer does not contain much ozone—it is estimated to be about 3 millimeters thick under normal conditions of temperature and pressure—it has a profound effect on life. The ozone layer absorbs the harmful ultraviolet radiation from the sun, thus providing the mechanism for the heating of the stratosphere. A reduction in the ozone layer would lead to a large increase of ultraviolet rays intruding into the atmosphere, thus increasing the incidence of skin cancer. F. S. Rowland and M. J. Molina declared in 1974 that the presence of the volatile chlorofluorocarbons would eventually reduce the ozone layer. Some measurements done by scientists in 1979 showed a decrease in the layer, which led to the action taken by several governments to decrease and replace the chlorofluorocarbons commonly used in aerosols. As the average life span steadily increases, the incidence of skin cancer will likely increase as well. The use of effective sunscreens and sunglasses to block

ultraviolet light is recommended for people who are exposed to large amounts of sunlight.

—*Darin Kennedy, MD and Rebecca Hayes, MD*

See also: Cancer; Carcinogens; Carcinoma; Chemotherapy; Dermatology; Dermatopathology; Kaposi's Sarcoma; Lesions; Lymphadenopathy and lymphoma; Malignancy and metastasis; Melanoma; Moles; Radiation therapy; Skin; Skin disorders; Skin lesion removal; Sunburn; Warts.

For Further Information:
Dollinger, Malin, et al. *Everyone's Guide to Cancer Therapy*. 5th ed., Andrews McMeel, 2008. An excellent source of medical information about cancer, written for the general public. Describes various cancer sites in the body. Includes a helpful glossary of medical terminology.
Firnhaber, Jonathon M. "Diagnosis and Treatment of Basal Cell and Squamous Cell Carcinoma." *American Family Physician*, vol. 86, no. 2, 15 July 2012, pp. 161-68. Medical article on basal and squamous cell skin cancers.
James, William D., Timothy G. Berger, and Dirk M. Elston. *Andrew's Diseases of the Skin: Clinical Dermatology*. 10th ed., Saunders/Elsevier, 2006. Includes discussions of skin cancer.
McClay, Edward F., and Jodie Smith. *One Hundred Questions and Answers About Melanoma and Other Skin Cancers*. Jones and Bartlett, 2004. Uses a reader-friendly format to survey a range of topics related to skin cancer.
Siegel, Mary-Ellen. *Safe in the Sun*. Walker, 1995. This comprehensive book describes the benefits of sunlight, the risks of exposure and how to protect the skin, and how damage that has already occurred can be treated.
Skin Cancer Foundation, www.skincancer.org. Promotes public education about skin cancer through campaigns against sun exposure and in support of early detection and research into new diagnostic techniques and therapies.
US Preventive Services Task Force. "Screening for Skin Cancer: Recommendation Statement." *American Family Physician*, vol. 94, no. 6, 15 Sept. 2016, pp. 479-81.
Weedon, David. *Skin Pathology*. 3rd ed., Churchill Livingstone/Elsevier, 2010. Text with extensive photographs, covering tissue reaction patterns; the epidermis, dermis, and subcutis; the skin in systemic and miscellaneous diseases; infections and infestations; and tumors, among other topics.

SKIN DISORDERS

Category: Disease/Disorder
Anatomy or system affected: Skin
Specialties and related fields: Dermatology, family medicine, occupational health
Definition: Diseases and conditions that affect the skin, ranging from harmless to life-threatening.
Key terms:
benign: in reference to a neoplasm, having a nonmalignant character
dermatology: the study of the skin, its chemistry, physiology, histopathology, cutaneous lesions, and the relationships of these lesions to systemic disease

malignant: in reference to a neoplasm, having the property of uncontrollable growth and dissemination, recurrence after removal, or both

melanin: dark brown or black molecules of pigment that normally occur in the skin, hair, pigmented coat of the retina, and pupil of the eye and in selected cells of the brain

metastasis: the shifting of a disease, or its local manifestations, from one portion of the body to another; in cancer, the appearance of neoplasms in parts of the body remote from the primary tumor

ANATOMY OF THE SKIN

The skin is the largest organ of the body. It provides a barrier between the external world and the internal world: It protects against external contamination and helps to maintain the sterility of the internal body. The skin also assists in temperature regulation; humans can survive only within a narrow temperature range. The skin has nerve receptors that supply the brain with information, providing an interface with the world. There are specialized receptors for touch, temperature, vibration, and position in space (proprioception).

Appendages to the skin are fingernails, toenails, and hair. They are mainly of psychological importance. Nails protect the tips of fingers and toes in humans but are not needed for protection as claws are in lower animals. Hair is analogous to feathers. In birds, tiny muscles attached to the base of each feather cause them to be ruffled; this creates air pockets and allows birds to conserve heat and keep warm. The same muscles persist in humans, causing "goose flesh," but they do not serve any other function. The main importance of these appendages is cosmetic. For example, people spend billions of dollars on hair care products each year. The motivation for this activity is psychological.

The two main layers in skin are the epidermis and dermis. The epidermis is the upper or outermost layer, and cells are continually formed at its base. As new cells are formed, existing cells are pushed toward the surface of the skin. These cells gradually lose their watery central contents, causing them to dry out (desiccate) and become flattened. This process normally spans approximately a month. Thus, the surface of the body is largely composed of dead cells that have become flattened. These cells are normally lost on a continual basis and create dandruff when shed from the scalp. On other parts of the body, sloughed cells provide excellent conditions for bacterial growth, accounting for the unpleasant odors that accompany poor hygiene habits.

Two other important types of cells are found in the epidermis: melanocytes and Langerhans cells.

INFORMATION ON SKIN DISORDERS

Causes: Infection, disease, allergies, environmental factors (e.g., ultraviolet radiation), hormonal changes, irritation, clogged sweat glands, eczema

Symptoms: May include inflammation, infection, flaking, pain, itching, redness, rashes, lesions, bleeding

Duration: Acute to chronic

Treatments: Topical ointments, antibiotics, corticosteroids, surgery, chemotherapy, radiation therapy

---

Melanocytes contain melanin and provide all the variations of pigmentation found in the human species. They multiply when stimulated by the ultraviolet radiation in sunlight. This causes the skin to become darker, a protective mechanism against damage from ultraviolet radiation. Langerhans cells contain surface receptors for immunoglobulins. They play a central role in allergic reactions of the skin, such as contact dermatitis or delayed hypersensitivity reaction.

The dermis is an inner layer of skin located beneath the epidermis. Its main function is protection. Within the dermis are highly specialized cells containing microscopic filaments. These cells impart tensile strength to the skin in much the same way that fibers strengthen fiberglass or reinforcing steel mesh strengthens concrete. Because they are so dense, they also serve as a barrier to the entry of most pathogens and many chemicals. Eccrine sweat glands are found in the dermis throughout the entire body. These produce a salty secretion (essentially salt water) that assists in thermoregulation through evaporative cooling. They are also sensitive to emotional stress. Apocrine sweat glands are primarily in the armpits (axilla) and groin and produce a milky secretion. When these secretions are broken down by bacteria on the surface of the skin, a characteristic odor is produced. The bases of hair follicles are also found in the dermis. The small sebaceous, or oil-secreting, gland associated with most hair follicles has the function of softening and moisturizing the hair.

Hair is found on most surfaces of the body; exceptions are the palms of the hands, the soles of the feet, and the glans penis in men. The texture and length of the hair vary with location on the body, gender, genetic heritage, and age. Dramatic increases in the growth and distribution of hair occur at puberty. With increasing age, hair is typically lost from the scalp and other body parts. It also changes color, assuming a gray or white color because of the loss of melanin at the base of the hair follicle.

COMPLICATIONS AND DISORDERS

When normal skin anatomy and physiology are upset, several common diseases or disorders result. When the barrier provided by the skin is broken, bacteria, viruses, fungi, and other pathogens can invade the body, leading to infections. Locally, these infections can cause inflammation (redness and pain) of the skin; if widespread, they can lead to systemic infections. When the cells and other substances found in the skin become irregular or are abnormal, skin disorders or conditions result.

Skin disorders and conditions. Pigmentation of the skin results from the presence of melanocytes, cells that manufacture and contain melanin. Most humans have pigmentation over their entire bodies; the degree of pigmentation varies with different racial and ethnic groups. Local areas of increased color have a range of names depending on the size of the pigmented area. A freckle is small and discrete. A nevus is a larger area of hyperpigmentation. These conditions are attributable to underlying variations in the distribution of melanocytes. They are genetic in origin and permanent; they are also accentuated by exposure to sunlight. Melasmas are irregular, flat, light brown areas on the neck, cheeks, or forehead. They are caused by hormonal changes associated with pregnancy or contraceptive pills and by exposure to sunlight. Melasmas fade with the reduction of excess hormones. There are also color changes in the labia of females during pregnancy; these changes are both harmless and permanent.

Generalized increases in skin coloration can occur with some metabolic diseases. Addison's disease involves an increase in melanocyte-stimulating hormone. This leads to an overall bronzing of the body, with accentuation in creases of the palms and soles. The condition subsides with treatment of the underlying cause of the disease. Similar pigment increases are associated with some forms of lung cancer, hemochromatosis, and chronic arsenic exposure. The latter two conditions are caused by the deposition of iron (hemochromatosis) and arsenic in the skin.

Generalized decreases in skin coloration can also occur. If melanocytes fail to migrate to the skin during embryologic development, hair follicles will lack color, resulting in a condition called piebaldism. Characteristically, this is a white patch in the hair of the forehead. Vitiligo is caused by an immunologically mediated loss of melanocytes. Individuals with phenylketonuria (PKU) experience a generalized depigmentation of hair and eye color, in addition to intellectual disabilities, if the condition is not adequately and promptly treated. An individual totally lacking melanocytes is called an albino; because melanin is also responsible for eye color, albinos have red eyes. The loss of hair is called alopecia. It can occur because of aging, sustained pulling on the hair with some hairstyles, and genetics. Women do not usually experience much alopecia until after the menopause. Conversely, some men start to lose their hair during their twenties.

Skin diseases. Eczema or dermatitis is a general term that describes a skin disease involving vesicles that ooze fluid. These conditions are usually characterized by a rash; they are inflammatory reactions, commonly caused by contact with a chemical or plant material. They can be caused by an adverse reaction to a drug or by sunlight. Bacteria, yeasts, or other fungi on the skin can cause eczema. Most rashes itch or burn; they can be spread by scratching. Athlete's foot is a common example of an eczematous dermatitis.

Maculopapular diseases encompass several common skin conditions, such as red measles (rubeola), German measles (rubella), and scarlet fever. Viruses that land on the skin cause these diseases. They are characterized by relatively large, localized areas of changed skin color (macules) that are also raised (papules) but not fluid-filled. After their clinical course is run, they disappear without leaving a scar. The more dangerous toxic shock syndrome also belongs to this group of diseases; it is caused by toxin from the bacteria *Staphylococcus aureus*.

Thickening of the skin and the formation of red to purple areas having sharply defined borders characterize papulosquamous skin diseases. The most common example is psoriasis. Other examples are pityriasis and ichthyosis. The pathology responsible for psoriasis is an alteration in the normal development of skin cells. In individuals with psoriasis, new skin cells develop and migrate to the surface in only five days instead of the usual thirty. This fact alone explains the flaking (rapid cell turnover), redness (thinner skin and a rich blood supply for new skin), and pain and itching (less protection for sensory nerve endings) experienced. Pityriasis includes a group of different conditions caused by different viruses. Patches or large spots develop on the skin. They usually resolve within a few weeks. Aside from being locally photosensitive, they usually are not serious. Ichthyosis describes a group of genetic conditions characterized by extreme scaling of the skin.

Vesiculobullous diseases have fluid-filled blisters that can vary in size from relatively small (vesicles) to relatively large (bullae). Insect bites, herpes, and some bacterial infections lead to the formation of vesicles or bullae. Such conditions are attributable to an immune reaction that leads to the formation of blisters at the junction between epidermis and dermis. They can be accompanied by intense pruritus (itching); scratching often leads to scarring.

Pustular diseases of the skin include acne, folliculitis, and candidiasis. They are characterized by the inflammation of hair follicles caused by surface bacteria or yeasts. Adequate personal hygiene is the most effective method of prevention. These diseases are usually not serious, but prolonged or repeated attacks can result in scarring and disfigurement. The sebaceous glands, which secrete oil at the base of hair follicles, can increase in size. The subsequent increase in oil output worsens the condition.

Clogged sweat glands can lead to acne. While this is primarily a problem for teenagers, it can affect individuals of any age. Exposure to cutting oils and other hydrocarbons such as gasoline and paint thinners can cause a similar condition called chloracne, which is inflammation in the base of hair follicles found on exposed skin in areas such as the nape of the neck, forearms, and face. The inability to sense temperature and regulate body heat through sweating is called anhidrosis, a condition that can cause shock and potentially death.

Other diseases that can affect the skin. Five such diseases are worthy of mention: leprosy, scleroderma, lupus, atherosclerosis, and diabetes mellitus. Leprosy, or Hansen's disease, is caused by infection by *Mycobacterium leprae*, a relative of the bacteria that cause tuberculosis. In leprosy, the causative organism accumulates in the skin and peripheral nerves. This causes disfigurement and loss of sensation, the latter being similar to that experienced by an uncontrolled diabetic. Disfigurement is responsible for the stigma associated with leprosy since ancient times: loss of fingers and toes, as well as mutilation of the nose and ears. Leprosy is caused by long-term association with the organism and can be adequately treated with appropriate antibiotics.

Scleroderma (literally, "hard skin") is an uncommon disease characterized by fibrosis of the skin and involvement of visceral organs. The skin involvement can range from an isolated, hardened patch to a life-threatening, generalized condition described as an ever-tightening case of steel. The skin becomes stretched tightly over the underlying skeleton. Skin tone is lost with restriction of movement.

Systemic lupus erythematosus is a disease of unknown etiology that is characterized by inflammation in many different organ systems. The skin is usually involved, as nearly all individuals with lupus develop a characteristic butterfly-shaped rash on their faces. This red coloration covers the cheeks and nose. Persons with lupus are also sensitive to sunlight, and many develop alopecia. Most of those affected are female. The disease waxes and wanes; treatment depends on the particular organs involved.

Atherosclerosis and diabetes can block the arteries supplying the nerves of the skin, leading to a loss of sensory input. When the patient is unable to experience pain, cuts and other abrasions on the skin are not noticed. Untreated, these lesions can lead to gangrene, sometimes requiring amputation of a body part.

Skin cancer. The most commonly diagnosed form of cancer is that involving the skin. It is not the most fatal form, but millions of cases are discovered annually. The origin of most skin cancers can be traced to excessive exposure to radiation from the sun. They can occur on any surface of the body, although they are more common on areas that are usually exposed to the sun, such as the face, the backs of the hand, and the neck. Skin cancers can arise in the epidermis or dermis. The majority are noncancerous, or benign. Epidermal nodules are characterized by local thickening of the epidermis, often accompanied by scaling of the skin in the affected area. Nodules in the dermis may appear as lumps with no alteration of the epidermis above them.

There are three malignant forms of skin cancer. Basal cell carcinoma arises from cells deep in the epidermis. This form of tumor rarely spreads (metastasizes), but it can be extensive and destructive locally. Squamous cell carcinoma is less common but can be invasive (involving adjacent tissues) and can metastasize. Melanoma is relatively uncommon but can grow extremely rapidly; it has the potential to be fatal in a matter of months. It involves the uncontrolled growth of melanocytes. Melanomas have irregular borders and color or pigmentation. Any pigmented lesion or suspicious change in the skin should be evaluated by a medical professional in a timely manner.

Prevention is the preferred method of dealing with skin cancer. When outside, loose-fitting clothing can provide protection from the sun, and a hat can protect the head. When exposure is unavoidable, a product with a sun-blocking agent will reduce exposure. Limiting the time of exposure to the sun until the body has reacted by producing additional melanocytes (tanned) is recommended.

Prolonged exposure to the sun also accelerates changes in the skin associated with aging. Collagen fibers provide the characteristic firm feel to the skin of a young person. With aging the skin becomes less firm, losing some of its tone, and begins to sag. Inadequate moisture also contributes to the loss of skin tone. Excessive exposure to the sun hastens both of these processes.

—*L. Fleming Fallon, Jr., MD, PhD, MPH*

See also Abscess drainage; Abscesses; Acne; Age spots; Aging; Albinos; Allergies; Bedsores; Birthmarks; Bites and stings; Blisters; Boils; Bruises; Canker sores; Carcinoma; Chickenpox; Cold sores; Corns and calluses; Cradle cap; Cyst removal; Cysts; Dermatitis; Dermatology; Dermatology, pediatric; Dermatopathlogy; Diaper rash; Eczema; Fifth disease; Grafts and grafting; Hair; Hair loss and baldness; Hand-foot-and-mouth disease; Herpes; Hives; Human papillomavirus (HPV); Hyperhidrosis; Impetigo; Inflammation; Insect-borne diseases; Itching; Kawasaki disease; Leprosy; Lesions; Measles; Melanoma; Moles; Morgellons disease; Necrotizing fasciitis; Neurofibromatosis; Pigmentation; Pityriasis alba; Pityriasis rosea; Poisonous plants; Psoriasis; Rashes; Ringworm; Rocky Mountain spotted fever; Rosacea; Scabies; Scleroderma; Skin; Skin cancer; Skin lesion removal; Stevens-Johnson syndrome; Stretch marks; Styes; Sunburn; Sweating; Systemic lupus erythematosus (SLE); Tattoo removal; Tattoos and body piercing; Vitiligo; Warts; Wrinkles.

For Further Information:

Burns, Tony, et al., eds. *Rook's Textbook of Dermatology.* 7th ed. Malden, Mass.: Blackwell Science, 2004. This is a core text in dermatology that will appeal to professionals and members of the general public who want a concise introduction to the subject. The aim of the book is to integrate basic science with clinical practice.

Frankel, David H., ed. *Field Guide to Clinical Dermatology.* 2d ed. Philadelphia: Lippincott Williams & Wilkins, 2006. Frankel, a noted internist and dermatologist, has enlisted widely respected and talented colleagues to help in the production of this book. It is a uniquely organized and easily readable field guide complete with 220 pages of excellent color illustrations.

Freinkel, Ruth K., and David T. Woodley, eds. *Biology of the Skin.* New York: Parthenon, 2001. Covers the basic biology of the skin, how the skin functions, effects of the environment, the molecules that direct cutaneous function, genetic influences, and methods in cutaneous research.

Goldsmith, Lowell A., Gerald S. Lazarus, and Michael D. Tharp. *Adult and Pediatric Dermatology: A Color Guide to Diagnosis and Treatment.* Philadelphia: F. A. Davis, 1997. This book provides excellent pictures to accompany good descriptions of dermatologic diseases.

Grob, J. J., et al., eds. *Epidemiology, Causes, and Prevention of Skin Diseases.* Cambridge, Mass.: Blackwell Science, 1997. This well-written book presents data on large groups of people. The sections on skin cancer are especially noteworthy.

Kenet, Barney, and Patricia Lawler. *Saving Your Skin: Prevention, Early Detection, and Treatment of Melanoma and Other Skin Cancers.* 2d ed. Chicago: Four Walls Eight Windows, 1998. Skin cancer is the focus of this title, which reviews the early symptoms of melanoma, its causes, and its treatment. Very few skin care titles do more than offer a chapter on the problem.

Sams, W. Mitchell, Jr., and Peter J. Lynch, eds. *Principles and Practice of Dermatology.* 2d ed. London: Churchill Livingstone, 1996. This is a new edition of a dermatology reference guide and text emphasizing accurate diagnosis by succinct discussions in eighty-five presentations featuring color photographs.

Weedon, David. *Skin Pathology.* 3d ed. New York: Churchill Livingstone/Elsevier, 2010. Text with extensive photographs, covering tissue reaction patterns; the epidermis, dermis, and subcutis; the skin in systemic and miscellaneous diseases; infections and infestations; and tumors, among other topics.

SKIN GRAFTING. SEE GRAFTS AND GRAFTING.

SKIN LESION REMOVAL

Category: Procedure
Anatomy or system affected: Skin
Specialties and related fields: Dermatology, general surgery, oncology, plastic surgery
Definition: The removal of cancerous and precancerous skin lesions under local anesthesia with a curette or scalpel, an electric needle, or liquid nitrogen.
Key terms:

anesthesia: the use of drugs to numb the pain and other unpleasant sensations during procedure

benign: having noncancerous characteristics

fusiform: spindle-shaped; wide in the middle and tapering at both ends

hemostasis: the cessation of bleeding

incision: a cut made with a scalpel

malignant: having cancerous characteristics, including uncontrollable growth and spread, recurrence after removal, or both

premalignant: precancerous

skin lesion: a growth or patch of skin that appears different from the surrounding area

suture: a thread used to stitch and hold together the edges of a wound or surgical incision

INDICATIONS AND PROCEDURES

Actinic (or solar) keratosis and skin cancers affect more than a half million Americans each year. Actinic keratosis, which are rough, scaly lesions considered to be premalignant, are often removed as a precaution. Among skin cancers, basal cell carcinoma is the least harmful. The lesion may appear on the skin surface as a small, flesh-colored or pale pink spot, usually with a raised edge that has a translucent, pearly appearance. It grows slowly and will rarely spread (metastasize) to other parts of the body. Squamous cell carcinoma is more dangerous. It appears on the surface as a small, firm, scaly tumor with an indistinct margin. Untreated squamous cell malignancies may metastasize. Melanoma, which literally means "black tumor," is the most dangerous of the three types of skin cancer. Melanoma lesions may resemble a mole with an irregular shape and can be red, blue, black, brown, gray, or even white. Melanoma rapidly invades nearby tissue and can metastasize readily to other parts of the body.

Most abnormal-appearing skin lesions are treated in the dermatologist or family physician's office under local anesthesia. More widespread lesions may need to be removed in the hospital under general anesthesia. Four primary ways to remove skin lesions are the shave, punch, elliptical, and snip excision methods. The site is first cleaned with a germicidal swab, and a local anesthetic (such as Lidocaine) is injected under the skin to numb the area. The shave technique utilizes a thin flexible blade (resembling a razor blade) to slice the lesion along the skin surface. The resultant wound is superficial and does not require closure with sutures. In contrast, punch and elliptical excisions result in deeper wounds that require suturing. The punch technique utilizes a circular cutting device (resembling a tiny cookie cutter) to enclose the lesion and remove it in a full-thickness cylindrical core of tissue. The elliptical excision technique utilizes a scalpel to cut a fusiform shape around the skin lesion and remove it completely, full-thickness, down to the fat layer under the growth. If there is concern for skin cancer, a small amount of normal tissue around the lesion (about 3 to 4 millimeters) may be removed to ensure that margins are clear of any possible cancerous cells. Finally, snip excision is performed using small, curved scissors to cut around and under the lesion, so is best for removing superficial growths that have a stalk.

Other methods of removing abnormal skin lesions are electrocautery, curettage, or cryosurgery. In electrocautery, an electric needle is used to burn the surface of any atypical growth and seal off small blood vessels. In curettage, the lesion is scraped away using an instrument with a small, scoop-shaped cutting head called a "dermal curette." In cryosurgery, cold liquid nitrogen is sprayed from a metal canister directly onto the lesion for a few seconds to freeze and destroy abnormal tissue.

Choosing the ideal method for skin lesion removal will depend on the type of growth, its location, size, spatial characteristics, and malignant potential. Skin lesions that appear benign can be treated with cryosurgery, destroyed with electrocautery or curettage, or removed with any of the excisional techniques above. The treatment of choice for precancerous lesions such as actinic keratoses is cryotherapy. In contrast, skin lesions that are suspicious for malignancy, particularly melanoma, should be fully removed with a scalpel by the elliptical excision technique. Skin lesions that are raised or protruding are best removed with the shave technique or snip excision, as long as there are no concerns for pathology in the deeper tissue layers.

For full-thickness excisions and larger lesions that are removed with a scalpel, sutures will be needed to close the wound and achieve hemostasis. Cancers on the eyelids, on the tip of the nose, or near facial nerves may be removed with radiation (using X-rays or another source). If the area treated is large, cosmetic or reconstructive surgery (such as Mohs procedure, a skin-sparing technique) is performed to restore the patient's physical appearance.

USES AND COMPLICATIONS

There is about a 95 percent cure rate for treated basal cell carcinomas. The cure rate for squamous cell carcinomas is only slightly less, especially if the lesion has been treated at an early stage. The cure rate for malignant melanomas is low unless they are diagnosed and treated early before metastasis occurs.

The possible risks and common complications of skin lesion removal procedures (punch, shave, elliptical excision, electrocautery and curettage) are pain, bleeding, infection, scarring, changes in skin color, recurrence of the growth, and local nerve damage or numbness. The risks and complications of cryosurgery are similar, but also include possible blister formation, as well as increased or decreased skin pigmentation at the treatment site. Prior to any surgery, informed consent should be obtained after clear discussion of these risks and complications, as well as benefits and alternatives of the procedure.

—*Cindy Yang, MD*

See also: Biopsy; Cancer; Carcinoma; Cryosurgery; Dermatology; Dermatopathology; Electrocauterization; Grafts and grafting; Laser use in surgery; Lesions; Melanoma; Oncology; Pigmentation; Plastic surgery; Skin; Skin cancer; Skin disorders; Warts.

For Further Information:
Fowler, Grant C. *Pfenninger and Fowler's Procedures for Primary Care*. 4th ed., Elsevier, 2019.
Hall, John C., and Brian J. Hall. *Sauer's Manual of Skin Diseases*. 11th ed., Lippincott Williams & Wilkins, 2017.
James, William D., et al. *Andrews' Diseases of the Skin: Clinical Dermatology*. 13th ed., Elsevier, 2019.
Mayeaux Jr, E. J. *The Essential Guide to Primary Care Procedures*. 2nd ed., Lippincott Williams & Wilkins, 2015.
Patterson, James W. *Weedon's Skin Pathology*. 5th ed., Churchill Livingstone/ Elsevier, 2010.
Russell, John J, and Edward F. Ryan. *Common Dermatologic Conditions in Primary Care*. Springer, 2019.
Turkington, Carol, and Jeffrey S. Dover. *The Encyclopedia of Skin and Skin Disorders*. 3rd ed., Facts on File, 2007.
Usatine, Richard P., et al. *Dermatologic and Cosmetic Procedures in Office Practice*. Saunders, 2011.
———. *Skin Surgery: A Practical Guide*. Mosby, 1998.
Wolff, Klaus, et al. *Fitzpatrick's Color Atlas and Synopsis of Clinical Dermatology*. 8th ed., McGraw Hill Medical, 2017.

SLEEP

Category: Biology
Anatomy or system affected: Brain, cells, glands, nervous system, psychic-emotional system

Specialties and related fields: Biochemistry, endocrinology, family medicine, internal medicine, neurology, pharmacology, preventive medicine, psychiatry, psychology

Definition: A quiescent period of rest characterized by decreased motor activity and diminished voluntary thought.

Key terms:

electroencephalograph (EEG): a device that records the electrical activity of the brain through electrodes attached to the scalp

insomnia: long-term deprivation of adequate sleep

neurotransmitter: a chemical that is stored in a neuron (nerve cell) and crosses the synaptic cleft (gap between neurons) to cause a change in another neuron

rapid eye movement (REM) sleep: a type of sleep characterized by heightened brain activity, vigorous eye movements, and relaxed postural muscles

sleep stage: the type of sleep based primarily on the EEG record; additional recordings of eye movements and muscle tension are used to determine the presence of REM sleep

STRUCTURE AND FUNCTIONS

All multicellular animals cycle through daily fluctuations in biological activity known as "circadian rhythms," with the alternation of sleep and wakefulness being the most obvious example. In humans, a polycyclic sleep/wake cycle—several periods of sleep and arousal during a twenty-four-hour period—becomes evident in the fetus during the latter stages of pregnancy. As children progress from infancy through childhood, they gradually settle into a mainly diurnal pattern, with one long period of sleep during the day. A complex interaction of several external and internal events determines the timing and duration of sleep.

The key exogenous factor that influences sleep is light. In the absence of the alternation of day and night, people will usually develop a sleep/wake cycle that is a little longer (from a few minutes to an hour) than a twenty-four-hour day. Two neurological structures detect light and synchronize the body's sleep/wake cycle with the presence or absence of light. The pineal gland is a photosensitive endocrine gland centrally located in the brain that secretes the hormone melatonin, which causes drowsiness. When darkness increases, the pineal gland steps up production of melatonin; levels of melatonin decline as light increases. Melatonin levels also affect the structure of the brain that plays the key role in regulating circadian rhythms, the suprachiasmatic nucleus (SCN) of the hypothalamus. The SCN serves as the body's primary biological clock, containing cells that will pulse in rhythmic activity in the absence of light. The activity of these cells, however, is influenced by output from the pineal gland and from the eye's retinal cells, providing two avenues by which light can affect the SCN. Light causes the SCN to alter levels of Tim, a protein which, when it interacts with two other proteins known as "Per" and "Clock," will induce sleepiness at high levels. Levels of "Tim," in turn, will increase activity in certain cells of the SCN. Thus, light serves as the *zeitgeber* (time-giver) for the sleep/wake cycle by changing the activity of the pineal gland and SCN, thereby altering levels of sleep-inducing chemicals.

Although damage to the pineal gland and SCN will significantly disrupt the quality and quantity of sleep, periods of sleep will still occur. That observation, in addition to the fact that animals will develop sleep/wake cycles in the absence of light changes, points to other, internal mechanisms that control sleep and arousal. One of these mechanisms is body temper-

Over an eight-hour sleep period, depth of sleep fluctuates, punctuated by periods of "rapid eye movement" (REM), which appear necessary for restful sleep. ©EBSCO

ature. Body temperature fluctuates from approximately 98° Fahrenheit (36.7° Celsius) to 99° Fahrenheit (37.2° Celsius) during the day. Rising body temperature is associated with arousal; declining body temperature is correlated with drowsiness. Vigorously rubbing the hands together can increase blood flow to the hands, dropping the blood supply to the brain, thereby decreasing the temperature of the brain and making it easier to fall asleep. While blood flow has an impact on the level of alertness, it is the flow of several neurotransmitters—chemicals that bridge the synaptic gap between one neuron (nerve cell) and another—that play the crucial role in regulating sleep and arousal.

Neurotransmitters generally have excitatory or inhibitory effects on arousal, but their impact on sleep is dependent on the neurological structures that they affect. Overall, more neurotransmitters appear to facilitate arousal rather than sleepiness. Acetylcholine and glutamate are the primary neurotransmitters for learning, so it is not surprising that they mediate the brain's alertness to external stimuli. The pontomesencephalon portion of the reticular formation—the brain's major arousal system—releases these two neurotransmitters, which activate regions of the brain from top (the cortex) to bottom (the medulla). Acetylcholine is also released by excitatory basal forebrain cells that have direct connections with the thalamus, the brain's center for the integration and processing of sensory information. Close to the bottom of the brain in the pons is the locus coeruleus, which promotes wakefulness and helps to consolidate memories.

Norepinephrine, the neurotransmitter involved in the display of active emotions such as fear or anger, is released from this structure and arouses many areas of the brain. Between the locus coeruleus and the basal forebrain is the hypothalamus, which influences many aspects of motivation and emotion, particularly through its regulation of the pituitary gland, the master gland of the endocrine system. Anterior cells of the hypothalamus release histamine, which, like acetylcholine, has widespread arousing effects on the brain. Taking antihistamine drugs to subdue the symptoms of allergies and colds will militate against those arousing effects. Lateral cells of the hypothalamus produce orexin, a neurotransmitter that is necessary for staying awake, especially as the day transpires.

Three neurotransmitters promote the induction and maintenance of sleep; two of them exert their effects via the basal forebrain. Gamma-aminobutyric acid (GABA), the brain's primary inhibitory neurotransmitter, is released by inhibitory cells in the basal forebrain and dampens arousal in the cortex and thalamus. Adenosine decreases activity in the acetylcholine-pro-

ducing cells of the basal forebrain, thereby inhibiting arousal. Caffeine derives its stimulating effects by blocking adenosine receptors. Moderate levels of serotonin have a calming effect and can facilitate the induction of sleep. However, serotonin (and norepinephrine) can decrease the quantity of REM sleep. Other chemicals, such as prostaglandins, work in conjunction with these three neurotransmitters to promote the induction and maintenance of sleep.

The interplay of various levels of neurotransmitters and hormones effect changes in the electrical activity of the brain. Recordings of the electrical potentials of brain cells made with an electroencephalograph (EEG) have resulted in the identification of four succeeding distinct patterns of brain wave activity that occur in approximately ninety-minute cycles. Prior to falling asleep, a person manifests mostly alpha EEG readings—high amplitude (top-to-bottom distance), medium wavelength (peak-to-peak distance) brain wave activity—characteristic of an alert, relaxed state. When a person slips into the first stage of sleep, a theta EEG pattern—low amplitude, short wavelengths—predominates. As sleep progresses, brief periods of very short wavelengths (sleep spindles) and bursts of high amplitude waves (K-complexes) punctuate the theta EEG pattern, marking the appearance of stage 2 sleep. Eventually, high amplitude and long wavelength brain activity—a delta EEG record—becomes more prevalent and stage 3 sleep is evident. Finally, delta EEG waves predominate as the person settles into stage 4 sleep. The individual will then cycle back through the third and second stages before reaching stage 1 sleep again, completing the ninety-minute biorhythm. The second period of stage 1 sleep is usually accompanied by the first appearance of rapid eye movement (REM) sleep in humans (many species lack the eye movements), a phenomenon in which brain activity is high but many signs of physiological arousal, such as muscle tension, are low. The time spent in each stage varies, depending on how long the person has been sleeping: stages 3 and 4 predominate during the first half of a sleep period, while stages 1 and 2 predominate (stage 4 sleep is often absent) during the second half.

Differences in sleep stage characteristics and their associated phenomena have led some researchers to distinguish between two basic types of sleep: S-sleep (more neural synchrony, similar activity in diverse brain regions), which combines stages 3 and 4, and D-sleep (more neural desynchrony, diverse brain regions active at different times), which combines stages 1 and 2. S-sleep is characterized by many signs of a deeper physical rest: lower body temperature, generally lower autonomic arousal, difficult arousal. Moreover, sleep loss and physical injuries or deprivations tend to increase the percentage of S-sleep over

D-sleep. In contrast, more signs of psychological restoration are associated with D-sleep: increased cortical blood flow and more vivid and prevalent dreams, especially during REM sleep. Additionally, deprivation of REM sleep tends to impair memory and increase irritability more so than deprivation of S-sleep. Because the distinctions between S-sleep and D-sleep are not always clear-cut—for example, S-sleep is essential for some types of memory formation—some researchers prefer to distinguish between REM sleep and non-REM (NREM) sleep.

DISORDERS AND DISEASES
Species vary in the amount of sleep that they require during a day, ranging from approximately two hours for a horse to twenty hours for a bat. Humans begin life averaging around sixteen hours of sleep a day as babies, progress to needing about half that much through most of adolescence and adulthood, and then typically get six to seven hours of sleep a day in later adulthood (partially due to age-related decreases in melatonin). No matter what the species or the age of the individual, problems with both the quantity and quality of sleep impair physical and psychological well-being.

Poor quantity of sleep, resulting in feeling tired during waking hours, is the primary characteristic of the most common class of sleep disorders known as "insomnia." Insomnia may be characterized by difficulty initially falling asleep (onset), problems in staying asleep (maintenance), or inability to fall back asleep when waking up early (termination). Termination and maintenance insomnia become more likely as people leave early adulthood. Rising body temperature is a factor in both onset and termination insomnia; breathing problems often induce maintenance insomnia.

Trouble breathing, leading to a drop of oxygen in the blood and frequent awakenings, is the main symptom of sleep apnea. Apnea can be caused by many factors, including obstructions of airway passages (often the result of obesity), the use of drugs (such as alcohol and tranquilizers, which relax breathing muscles), or deterioration of areas in the brain that control breathing (the pre-Botzinger complex of the medulla). Left untreated by surgery or breathing aids, apnea can result in numerous health problems, such as loss of cells in multiple areas of the brain, memory deficiencies, heart problems, and diabetes.

Insomnias and apnea, as well as numerous other sleep disorders, can also lead to poor quality of sleep. In particular, depressed amount of REM sleep is a common problem associated with sleep dysfunctions. Neurological depressants, such as alcohol and tranquilizers, have commonly been used to treat insomnia.

Unfortunately, such drugs can lead to iatrogenic (caused by medical treatment) insomnia in which a drug initially facilitates sleep but then tolerance develops, in which an increasing amount of the drug is needed to induce its primary effects, and insomnia recurs. Moreover, neurological depressants typically suppress REM sleep, further exacerbating the insomniac's condition.

In stress-induced insomnia, EEG records reveal that brain activity drifts in a twilight zone between sleep and wakefulness, with minimal REM sleep. People suffering from significant reactions to trauma, such as in posttraumatic stress disorder (PTSD), frequently reexperience their traumatic encounters in nightmares that are so vivid and horrifying that they are unable to stay asleep during REM periods. In contrast, it is the sleep partners of individuals with REM behavior disorder who have problems staying asleep, as the person with the dysfunction thrashes wildly about, perhaps acting out her or his dreams.

Overactive motor activity is also the primary symptom of two NREM disorders: restless leg syndrome(which is characterized by twitching and high muscle tension of the legs) and myoclonus(which involves body twitching, particularly of the arms and legs, while asleep). The extreme overactive muscle sleep disorder, however, is sleepwalking. Sleepwalking normally occurs in stage 4 sleep and is more common in children and adolescents. What sleepwalking is to motor activity, night terrors (extremely terrifying dreams) are to psychological activity. As with sleepwalking, night terrors are more common in children and adolescents and occur during stage 4 sleep. Sleep talking is not restricted to any particular age group or sleep stage.

Narcolepsy is a sleep dysfunction in which the main problem is evident during waking hours rather than during the sleep period. The four primary symptoms of narcolepsy are intense periods of sleepiness, cataplexy (muscle weakness), hypnogogic imagery (dreamlike hallucinations while slipping into sleep), and sleep paralysis (muscle immobility while moving into and out of sleep periods). Because most of the symptoms are associated with REM sleep, narcolepsy has been interpreted as a wakeful experience of REM-like sleep. Low levels of orexin have been implicated as a cause of this disorder.

PERSPECTIVE AND PROSPECTS
In his book *The Promise of Sleep* (1999), William C. Dement, one of the foremost researchers of sleep, describes the breakthrough research in the early 1950s that gave birth to the modern era of sleep understanding. Dement, working with Nathaniel Kleitman and Eugene Aserinsky, conducted the first research to measure simultaneously the electrical activity of the eyes

and brain while people were sleeping. The results of their work led to the identification of four distinct stages of sleep, the discovery of a ninety-minute sleep cycle, and the detection of REM sleep. REM sleep was later found to correspond with a discovery by Michel Jouvet called "paradoxical sleep," so named because animals in this type of sleep manifest high brain activity but relaxed postural muscles. Dement and Kleitman also discovered that people awakened from REM sleep were usually dreaming. These discoveries of the 1950s opened up new avenues of research, from empirical studies of dreaming to the interrelationship between sleep and health, and led to the development of better methods to diagnosis and treat sleep disorders.

By the mid-twentieth century, benzodiazepines (tranquilizers, such as Halcion, Valium, and Xanax), which facilitate the action of GABA and adenosine, became the primary treatment for diverse kinds of sleep disorders. Side effects such as REM suppression, increased likelihood of apnea, and drowsiness during waking hours, however, prompted researchers to search for alternatives to these highly addictive drugs. Safer alternatives for insomnia were developed in the late twentieth century as nonbenzodiazepines, GABA-facilitating sleep aids (such as Ambien, Lunesta, and Sonata). Rozerem, a melatonin receptor stimulant, offered physicians a new approach to treating insomnia in the twenty-first century. While medications, such as dopaminergic agents (Sinemet) for restless leg disorder and stimulants (Ritalin) for narcolepsy, can be useful in treating various sleep disorders, for the person suffering from insomnia, the best advice is often to avoid the substances—such as alcohol, caffeine, and nicotine—that will interfere with the natural mechanisms designed to promote sleep.

—Kendi Tang, DO

See also: Apnea; Caffeine; Chronobiology; Hallucinations; Narcolepsy; Nightmares; Paralysis; Physiology; Sleep apnea; Sleep disorders; Sleepwalking; Stress.

For Further Information:
Dement, William C., and Christopher Vaughan. *The Promise of Sleep: A Pioneer in Sleep Medicine Explores the Vital Connection between Health, Happiness, and a Good Night's Sleep.* Delacorte Press, 1999. Renowned sleep expert Dement presents an authoritative, yet accessible overview of sleep research and sets forth principles for healthy sleeping. An extensive list of sleep centers in the United States of America is included.
Hirshkowitz, Max, Patricia B. Smith, and William C. Dement. *Sleep Disorders for Dummies.* For Dummies, 2004. This easy-to-understand guide covers the causes, symptoms, and treatment options for numerous sleep disorders. Practical advice, humor, and numerous visual aids make this book a good reference for the person with little knowledge of sleep disorders.
Jacobs, Gregg D. *Say Goodnight to Insomnia.* Rodale, 2009. Jacobs outlines a drug-free program, developed at Harvard Medical School, for overcoming insomnia. Six basic strategies for conquering insomnia form the core of the program.
Kryger, Meir H., Thomas Roth, and William C. Dement, editors. *Principles and Practice of Sleep Medicine.* 4th ed., Saunders/Elsevier, 2005. A comprehensive textbook (1,517 pages) that is the standard reference for the field of sleep medicine. Written with the scholarly audience in mind.

SLEEP APNEA

Category: Disease/Disorder
Also known as: Obstructive sleep apnea
Anatomy or system affected: Respiratory system
Specialties and related fields: Otorhinolaryngology, pulmonary medicine
Definition: A sleep disorder characterized by intermittent cessation of airflow through the upper airway.
Key terms:
apnea: lack of airflow for more than ten seconds
hypopnea: a decrease in airflow greater than 50 percent
oxygenation: the process of getting oxygen into the bloodstream

CAUSES AND SYMPTOMS

Obstructive sleep apnea (OSA) is caused by repetitive upper airway obstruction. Soft tissue in the back of the mouth collapses during sleep and temporarily obstructs airflow into the lungs. Generally, OSA is due to obstruction or collapse of the nasopharynx, oropharynx and/or the hypopharynx. People with sleep apnea experience many periods of apnea and hypopnea. During such periods, the oxygen level in the bloodstream can decline significantly. Since these episodes occur throughout the night, the sleep cycle is interrupted, resulting in the person feeling sleepy during the day. Symptoms of OSA can be divided based on the time of day. Daytime symptoms can include morning headaches, fatigue, poor concentration, and daytime sleepiness (somnolence). The person might doze off while watching television, reading, or, more dangerously, driving. Nighttime symptoms include dry mouth, choking during sleep, and snoring. While the person may not be aware of apnea or the resultant snoring, a sleeping partner will frequently notice these symptoms. It should be noted, however, that snoring alone, without apnea, is very common and does not indicate sleep apnea.

Risk factors for the development of OSA include older age, obesity, a small jaw, a deviated septum of the nose, a big tongue, or enlarged tonsils. Smokers are also at higher risk of developing sleep apnea.

If OSA is left untreated, significant medical complications may result, including increased risks of hypertension, heart failure, strokes, and pulmonary hypertension. In pulmonary hypertension, the lungs become stiff and fail to provide normal oxygenation. OSA can also increase the risk of perioperative complications, especially respiratory failure. Therefore, it is extremely important to recognize and treat sleep apnea.

While the clinical triad of snoring, apneic episodes, and daytime somnolence suggests OSA, testing must be performed for a definitive diagnosis to be made. This diagnosis can be made at home by using Home Sleep Apnea testing (HSAT) or an overnight oximeter. An oximeter is a noninvasive device worn over a finger that measures the oxygen level in the bloodstream. It can be worn overnight at home and is useful for detecting any drop in oxygen level caused by apneic or hypopneic episodes. It must be noted however, that overnight desaturations using overnight pulse oximetry alone is not enough to diagnose OSA. The gold standard for OSA diagnosis is a formal sleep study known as "polysomnography."

Polysomnography requires an overnight observation in a sleep center where multiple monitors record brain waves, heart rate, breathing rate, abdominal muscle movement, and oxygen level. Based on these measurements, an apnea-hypopnea index (AHI), the average number of apneic and hypopneic episodes in one hour, is reported. An AHI of respiratory events per hour of sleep is normal, five to fourteen is considered mild sleep apnea, fifteen to thirty is moderate, and an AHI of greater than greater is considered severe.

An illustration depicting a sleep apnea monitor. Image by BruceBlaus, via Wikimedia Commons.

INFORMATION ON SLEEP APNEA

Causes: Upper airway obstruction; risk factors include obesity, small jaw, deviated septum, big tongue, enlarged tonsils, smoking

Symptoms: Periods of apnea and hypopnea during sleep, interrupting sleep pattern and resulting in snoring, daytime sleepiness, morning headaches, fatigue, difficulty with concentration; complications may include hypertension, heart failure, strokes, pulmonary hypertension

Duration: Chronic with acute episodes

Treatments: Lifestyle changes (weight loss, smoking cessation, avoidance of sedating medications and alcohol); continuous positive airflow pressure machine; in severe cases, surgery (removal of excess soft tissue, moving of tongue and jaw forward, tracheostomy)

TREATMENT AND THERAPY

Obese individuals with OSA should lose weight, quit smoking, and avoid sedating medications and alcohol as they may impair breathing even further.

Initial OSA treatment consists of a nasal continuous positive airflow pressure (CPAP) machine. A triangular mask fits over the nose and is hooked up to a machine that pushes pressured air into the upper airway to keep it open. A repeat sleep study using a CPAP machine can determine the level of pressure necessary to prevent apneic and hypopneic episodes. Such a device can be very effective in treating OSA. Side effects may include anxiety from using the mask, nasal congestion, nosebleeds, dry mouth, and irritation of the skin from the mask.

Some individuals require surgical treatment, especially those who cannot tolerate the use of a CPAP machine. The most common surgery performed for OSA is a procedure called "uvulopalatoplasty," which involves surgical removal of excess soft tissue including the tonsils in the back of the mouth. Laser-assisted uvulopalatoplasty, in which a laser is used to remove the soft tissue, can be performed in the office. Other surgeries, including maxillary and mandibular advancement can move the tongue and jaw forward to open up the airway in the back of the mouth. For very severe cases of sleep apnea, an opening can be made in the trachea (the windpipe in the upper neck) to bypass the obstruction in the mouth and nose; this procedure is known as a "tracheostomy." Since there is not a single "cure all" treatment for OSA, a complete surgical evaluation should include a proper physical exam, nasopharyngeal endoscopy and radiographic imaging to develop an individualized plan based on the severity and classification of an individual's OSA.

PERSPECTIVE AND PROSPECTS

Accounts of what may have been sleep apnea date back to 305 to 30 BCE and involve eleven members from seven generations of the Egyptian royal family. These individuals were obese and were reported by contemporary philosophers and historians to have a tendency toward falling asleep during social and political events.

Sleep apnea has sometimes made an appearance in literature. In the late sixteenth century, symptoms of OSA are suggested in characters created by William Shakespeare for this plays *Richard II* and *Henry IV.* In *Richard II*, the obese Sir John Falstaff snores and sleeps much of the day, interrupted by an apneic breathing pattern. In *Henry IV*, King Henry IV has trouble sleeping, with periods of not breathing in his sleep. Lewis Carroll described a character with sleep apnea in his book *Alice's Adventures in Wonderland* (1865). At the Mad Hatter's tea party, the Dormouse suffers from daytime sleepiness. The other characters try to help the Dormouse by putting him into a tight teapot, which would serve as a positive pressure to assist his breathing.

The famous composer Johannes Brahms (1833-97) was thought to have developed sleep apnea in his later years when he gained weight. He was known to his friends to snore loudly at night. He also fell asleep during a performance by another famous composer, Franz Liszt.

—*Zuha Anwar, OMS-III*

See also: Apnea; Asphyxiation; Cyanosis; Hypoxia; Lungs; Obesity; Pulmonary diseases; Pulmonary medicine; Pulmonary medicine, pediatric; Respiration; Resuscitation; Sleep; Sleep disorders.

For Further Information:
Goldman, Lee, and Dennis Ausiello, editors. *Cecil Textbook of Medicine*. 23rd ed., Saunders/Elsevier, 2007.
Lavie, Peretz. *Restless Nights: Understanding Snoring and Sleep Apnea*. Translated by Anthony Berris. Yale UP, 2003.
Mason, Robert J., et al., editors. *Murray and Nadel's Textbook of Respiratory Medicine*. 5th ed., Saunders/Elsevier, 2010.
Randerath, Winfried J., Bernd M. Sanner, and Virend K. Somers, editors. *Sleep Apnea: Current Diagnosis and Treatment*. S. Karger, 2006.
Rock, Peter, editor. *Obesity and Sleep Apnea*. Saunders/Elsevier, 2005.
Terris, David J., and Richard L. Goode, editors. *Surgical Management of Sleep Apnea and Snoring*. Taylor & Francis, 2005.
Salman, Salam O., editor. *Modern Management of Obstructive Sleep Apnea*. Springer Nature, 2019.

SLEEP DISORDERS

Category: Disease/Disorder
Anatomy or system affected: Brain, nervous system, psychic-emotional system
Specialties and related fields: Geriatrics and gerontology, neurology, psychiatry, psychology
Definition: Any abnormal pattern of sleep that threatens normal function, including conditions that cause too much as well as too little sleep, which may be both organic and nonorganic in origin.
Key terms:
circadian rhythm: a physiological process that occurs in twenty-four-hour cycles; examples include the sleep-wake cycle and the maintenance of body temperature
hypersomnia: a group of disorders in which the patient complains of excessive daytime sleepiness or of an inability to stay awake during the day
insomnia: the complaint of poor-quality sleep, which can be caused by a difficulty in falling asleep or a difficulty in maintaining sleep; the most common sleep disorder
narcolepsy: a disorder in which sufferers experience an overwhelming need to sleep during the day; other characteristics include sudden muscle weakness, hallucinations, or sleep paralysis
parasomnias: disorders, occurring primarily in children, in which the patient exhibits abnormal behavior during sleep; examples are sleepwalking and night terrors
periodic leg movements: a disorder in which muscle spasms in the legs partially awaken the sleeper, preventing the proper staging of the sleep cycle
polysomnogram: a collection of physiological information regarding brain waves, breathing, muscle movements, and blood oxygen levels used to diagnose sleep disorders
rapid eye movement (REM) sleep: the period of sleep in which intense brain activity can be measured; the stage of sleep in which dreaming occurs
sleep apnea: a cessation of breathing during sleep, which interrupts the normal sleep cycle; the patient must partially awaken in order to resume breathing

CAUSES AND SYMPTOMS

Sleep is more than the absence of wakefulness. While a person sleeps, the brain continues to be quite active—indeed, this activity is essential for human survival. Brain activity can be measured in sleeping subjects and has been used to classify sleep into stages 1 through 4, where stage 1 is the lightest sleep and stage 4 is the deepest. A sleeper moves from stage 1, through stages 2 and 3, and to stage 4, and then back through stages 2 and 3 to stage 1. This cycle occurs every ninety to one hundred minutes throughout the night. During the latter part of the sleep period, stage 1 sleep is associated with brain activity that is as intense as that seen in waking subjects. During these periods of intense brain activity, rapid eye movements (REMs) are observed, and as a result these periods are referred to as REM sleep, and the other sleep stages are referred to as non-REM sleep. Although the precise function of sleep is still hotly debated in scientific circles, most people can verify from experience that adequate sleep has a major impact on their ability to function effectively and on their emotional stability. For those who suffer from a sleep disorder, life can become a daily struggle; sleep disorders often have severe physical, financial, and social consequences.

Patients who are having difficulty with sleeping usually complain of insomnia, feeling sleepy during the day, or abnormal behaviors during sleep. Sleep disorders have been divided into four broad categories by the Association of Sleep Disorders Centers: the insomnias, or disorders of initiating or maintaining sleep; the hypersomnia's, or disorders of excessive sleep; disorders of the sleep-wake cycle; and the parasomnias, or disorders of partial arousal such as sleepwalking and night terrors. Of these, the most common complaint are the insomnias.

Insomnia is a subjective complaint of non-refreshing sleep. Patients believe that their ability to function during the day is impeded by short or poor-quality sleep. Since most people experience transient insomnia at various times in their lives, chronic insomnia is defined as insomnia lasting longer than three months. Individuals with insomnia have a variety of sleep patterns: Some may require a long period to fall asleep, some wake up after a few hours and cannot fall asleep again, and some may not know that they have awakened briefly hundreds of times during the night. The sleep patterns of the insomniac can vary from night to night, which increases the anxiety of the patient. Electrical monitoring of brain activity shows that most insomniacs have only a slightly reduced total sleep time, with few changes in sleep stages. Physiologically, poor sleepers have been shown to maintain a higher body temperature during sleep than normal sleepers, which may reflect a higher level of arousal. Insomnia is not a disorder in itself; instead, it can be a symptom of a large number of underlying disorders. These can be physiological, psychological, behavioral, or simply a normal part of the aging process.

Insomnia can be caused by medical problems that interfere with breathing, such as sleep apnea, in which patients have multiple episodes each night when they stop breathing. A single episode can last ten seconds to two minutes, and in some severe cases, up to 50 per-

---

INFORMATION ON SLEEP DISORDERS

Causes: May include sleep apnea, obesity, restless leg syndrome, stress, anxiety, caffeine use, aging process, jet lag, shift work, medications, psychiatric or medical problems

Symptoms: Varies widely; may include irregular snoring, daytime sleepiness, sudden muscle weakness, sleepwalking, night terrors

Duration: Acute to chronic

Treatments: Sleep clinic monitoring, drugs, technical aids, behavior modification

---

cent of sleep time can be spent without breathing. Sleep apnea is often seen in obese men and women because of obstruction of the air passage. Clinical signs include irregular snoring and daytime sleepiness. Insomnia can also be caused by neurological problems, muscular problems, or conditions that cause pain. Periodic leg movement can (but does not always) cause multiple awakenings during the night, as can a related disorder called "restless leg syndrome," which is characterized by a creeping sensation in the legs. Psychiatric research has demonstrated that insomnia can be a symptom of clinical depression. Surveys have shown that insomniacs have a higher level of stress, tension, and anxiety than normal sleepers. In addition, insomnia can occur when behavioral patterns do not encourage sleep. The use of caffeine or engaging in arousing activities, such as exercise, using social media or answering work emails prior to bedtime can contribute to poor sleep. The normal aging process usually causes a decrease in total sleep time and in stage 1 sleep and an increase in fragmented sleep, resulting in drowsiness and sometimes depression in the elderly.

In addition to all these causes, there are some individuals who complain of insomnia in which no abnormalities can be found. When comparing subjective reports from the patient to sleep recordings in the laboratory, there is a tendency for such insomniacs to report wakefulness even though the sleep recording indicates that the patient is sleeping normally. It appears that there are other sleep abnormalities that contribute to the quality of sleep which remain unknown.

Hypersomnia is defined as excessive daytime sleepiness (EDS) and include the group of patients who are unable to stay awake during the day. Several external circumstances can contribute to EDS, such as jet lag, shift work, medications, or some of the disorders underlying insomnia listed above. In addition, narcolepsy, a central nervous system disorder, is characterized by the overwhelming need to sleep several times a day. These sleep attacks often occur without warning. Narcoleptics can also experience cataplexy, or sudden muscle weakness when in emotionally charged situations that cause anger, laughter, or fear. They may also experience hallucinations when sleep begins or sleep paralysis upon waking that can last for several minutes. Narcolepsy affects 0.05 percent of the population and causes significant hardship to those afflicted. It can pose a danger if the person falls asleep while operating a car or when in a dangerous environment.

The daily cycle of wakefulness followed by a prolonged sleep period is controlled by circadian rhythms. People who travel across time zones or who work rotating shifts are often forced to sleep at a time when their circadian rhythm supports wakefulness and work when their circadian rhythm supports sleep. Other individuals have defects in the mechanisms that regulate circadian rhythms and may experience delayed or advanced sleep phase syndrome in which there is a shift of the normal twenty-four-hour cycle. If they follow their circadian rhythm, these patients will sleep for a normal amount of time; however, the social consequences of retiring at 7:00 P.M. or awakening at noon are prohibitive. Internal desynchronization between the sleep-wake cycle and the closely related circadian temperature cycle can also contribute to poor-quality sleep.

The parasomnias, or disorders of arousal, include sleepwalking and night terrors. Both of these disorders occur predominantly in childhood, although they can be experienced by adults. When brain activity is characterized by an electroencephalograph (EEG), there are elements of both wakefulness and REM sleep, often in the deepest stages (3 and 4). This finding dispels the myth that sleepwalkers are acting out dreams, since dreaming occurs during REM sleep. Sleepwalking activity can vary in length. The person usually has his or her eyes open, can respond verbally, and can move about normally. Sleepwalkers are usually aware of the environment at some level, although their judgment is impaired and they can sometimes injure themselves. Night terrors involve signs of panic such as shrieking, sweats, and frenzied movements and can be distinguished from nightmares, which involve little movement and more extensive memory. Both sleepwalking and night terrors are usually not recalled, and there is little connection between these syndromes and psychiatric disease. Both may be exacerbated by sleep deprivation, stress, fever, or medications.

TREATMENT AND THERAPY
One of the difficulties in diagnosing insomnia or one of the other sleep disorders is that there is much individual variability among normal sleepers in sleep needs and amount of sleep logged each night. Therefore, what may be adequate sleep for one person might cause another to report poor sleep. To

determine the causes of poor sleep, a person is usually referred to a sleep clinic. There, a detailed history of the problem as well as a description of the patient's sleep habits, lifestyle, and psychological state is recorded. Often, a description of behavior during sleep from someone who shares the bedroom can provide additional important information. Next, a polysomnogram, in which the sleeping patient is monitored with electrodes, is performed so that information on brain waves, breathing, muscle movements, and blood oxygen levels can be obtained. Sometimes this test is administered in the sleep center, and sometimes it is done in the more natural sleep environment of the person's home using ambulatory monitoring devices. From this information, a diagnosis usually can be made and the appropriate therapy determined.

When insomnia is associated with an underlying psychiatric or medical problem, treatment usually begins with the primary problem rather than with the symptom of poor sleep. When the primary problem is solved, the sleep pattern usually returns to normal. Symptomatic treatment of the insomnia itself is provided only when the cause of the sleep disturbance cannot be treated. There are two major approaches: treatments that emphasize the use of drugs or technical aids and treatments that emphasize a change in behavior.

Although over-the-counter aids cannot improve sleep, large numbers of prescription drugs can affect sleep patterns and influence alertness during waking hours. Historically, barbiturates were administered for insomnia, but in 1970, benzodiazepines were introduced; they are now the most commonly prescribed drugs for sleeplessness. These drugs are usually taken about thirty minutes before bedtime, causing drowsiness and thus decreasing the amount of time it takes to fall asleep. Benzodiazepines alter the stages of sleep, decreasing the amount of stage 1 and REM sleep and increasing the amount of stage 2 sleep. The significance of these changes is not understood. When used alone, benzodiazepines are safe and have few side effects; if they are combined with other drugs, however, there can be a toxic interaction. Although most people can tolerate these drugs and report no daytime grogginess, some impairment of function may exist upon waking. There is strong evidence to suggest that benzodiazepines be used for only a short period of time. With continued use (longer than thirty days), patients usually find that the drug becomes less effective unless the dosage is increased to an unsafe level. When the drug is discontinued, the original symptoms of insomnia usually recur and often a "rebound insomnia," which is even more severe than before the drug treatment began, may be present for a brief period. Because of these limitations, these "sleeping pills" are usually given when an acute but temporary situation exists. To treat insomnia that is caused by periodic leg movements, a muscle relaxant is sometimes used. For patients whose sleep apnea is not resolved by weight reduction, mechanical devices that hold the air passage open during sleep are usually employed. Orthodontic aids or tongue retainers may provide relief, and other patients wear masks that hold the air passage open, providing a continuous airflow during sleep.

Since insomnia is often caused by poor habits that condition the sleeper to remain awake, the problem can sometimes be solved by educating the patient about proper sleep hygiene. This involves a simple commitment to avoid naps, reduce caffeine and alcohol intake, eat light meals in the evening, reduce noise in the sleep environment, and establish a regular bedtime. Many insomnia sufferers are so preoccupied with the fear that they will not sleep well that they become tense as bedtime approaches. These fears may sometimes be put to rest by the knowledge that sleep needs vary greatly from individual to individual. In some cases, people may not physiologically require a "normal" amount of sleep but have been convinced that they have a sleep disorder by spouses who do. Another commonly held misperception that contributes to tension is the notion that, once sleep is lost, it can never be recovered. Studies have shown that sleep-deprived humans are able to return quickly to normal sleep patterns, and therefore a few nights of poor sleep is no cause for alarm.

For those whose anxiety about sleep persists, techniques that teach people to relax their muscles such as mindfulness or meditation to decrease mental activity may reduce this anxiety and promote sleep. Patients who experience better sleep when away from their normal sleeping location may have "learned" to associate the bedroom environment with wakefulness. To overcome this problem, stimulus control is used to try to strengthen the bedroom as a cue for sleep. This method requires that patients use the bedroom only for sleep and sex and go to bed only when sleepy. Most importantly, if they do not fall asleep within ten minutes of lying down, they should get up, go into another room, and engage in a mundane activity, coming back to the bedroom only when sleepy. This may be done several times, but the main goal is to associate the bedroom with falling asleep quickly. Regardless of the length of sleep, patients should always get up and go to bed at the same time and not nap during the day. This regimen may need to be continued for several weeks in order to overcome the previous habit and requires perseverance from the patient; however, the advantage of behavioral therapy lies in the absence of the side effects caused by medication.

Excessive daytime sleepiness is usually diagnosed by a polysomnogram followed by a Multiple Sleep Latency Test. In this test, patients are allowed to fall asleep several times a day, and if sleep occurs within five minutes multiple times during the day, the diagnosis is positive. EDS is treated in different ways depending on its cause. If the cause is sleep apnea or periodic leg movements, the disorder is handled as described above. In other cases of sleep fragmentation, medication is used to prevent arousal during the night. The excessive daytime sleepiness found in narcoleptics is usually treated with drugs that act as central nervous system stimulants. Other symptoms of narcolepsy are usually treated with antidepressant drugs that suppress REM sleep. Of these, gamma hydroxybutyrate has been shown to be effective and to cause limited side effects. Short naps taken throughout the day seem to prevent many of the symptoms associated with sleep attacks.

Problems with the circadian rhythms of the sleep-wake cycle are usually not helped by medication. Instead, chronotherapy may be effective in resetting the biological clock. Over the course of two weeks, the patient's bedtime is gradually moved forward or backward around the clock until the desired bedtime is reached. Similar effects may be seen using strong light to shift the sleep period.

PERSPECTIVE AND PROSPECTS

The field of sleep research is still in its infancy. For most of history, sleep was not studied at all because it was difficult to characterize the process without interrupting it. Early scientists such as Lucretius, however, made observations and suggested that the motions of sleeping animals might reflect their dreams. In the early nineteenth century, sleep was viewed simply as the absence of waking, and the treatment of lethargic patients with damage to the brain stem led doctors to postulate that this area of the brain had two centers—a waking center and a sleeping center. These two centers were thought to function and communicate with each other using chemical signals. As the field of neurobiology advanced, it became possible to measure the electrical properties of the brain using an electroencephalograph. By the 1930s, numerous studies had shown that the brain remains active during sleep and that the different stages of sleep have different patterns of electrical activity. REM sleep was first observed in 1953 and was linked to dreaming. Additional brain structures in the midbrain and pons were identified that controlled REM and non-REM sleep. An understanding of the neurotransmitters, or chemical substances involved in sleeping and waking, began in the 1960s when it was discovered that neurons in the pons contained serotonin and norepinephrine. Another neurotransmitter, acetylcholine, was found in neurons that were active during REM sleep.

It is only recently that the study of sleep disorders has been recognized as a legitimate pursuit. Most of the sleep disorders mentioned here were discovered in the 1960s and 1970s, and public opinion regarding those who complain of tiredness and fatigue is only gradually shifting from disdain to understanding that there might be a real physiological cause.

This greater acceptance might be due to a growing awareness of the toll of sleep deprivation. The 2000 Omnibus Sleep in America Poll completed by the National Sleep Foundation found that 43 percent of Americans reported that they are sleepy during the day and that the sleepiness was enough to interfere with daily activities. The National Sleep Foundation concluded that the consequences of sleep deprivation are more severe than most people realize and affect metabolism, endocrine functions, immune system function, memory, mood, and reaction time. The average adult sleeps about an hour less than the eight hours per night recommended by sleep experts. During the workweek, only 33 percent of adults get the necessary eight hours of sleep. Forty-three percent of the adults in the survey reported that they often stay up later than they should because of watching television or surfing the web. Also, 58 percent of adults experienced the symptoms of insomnia, and 15 percent experienced restless leg syndrome. The factors most often identified for disrupting sleep were stress and pain. Fifty-one percent of Americans reported driving while drowsy, and one in five said they have actually fallen asleep at the wheel. Sleep deprivation has also negatively impacted work performance for 27 percent of adults. The list of work-related problems included being late for work, making errors, reductions in quality of work, lower productivity, diminished concentration, and suffering injuries.

Perhaps because of such statistics and a growing public recognition of the dangers of sleep problems, the number of sleep centers and laboratories that are studying sleep and its accompanying disorders has grown tremendously. These sleep centers have been instrumental in elucidating the primary disorders of sleep and in educating the general public concerning sleep management and the safety risks that result from abnormal sleep. Research laboratories are investigating the anatomical, chemical, and physiological mechanisms of sleep and sleep abnormalities. Some of the most interesting areas of current research include genetic studies that determine whether sleep disorders are inherited. There appears to be a significant genetic component to several sleep characteristics, including bedtime, sleep duration, insomnia, narcolepsy, snoring, and sleep apnea. It is expected that, as scientists come to understand more about the nature and mechanisms of the brain and normal sleep, further understanding of the causes and treatments for sleep disorders will be forthcoming.

—*Trevor Prashad, DO*

See also: Aging; Anxiety; Apnea; Caffeine; Chronobiology; Depression; Hallucinations; Memory loss; Narcolepsy; Nightmares; Paralysis; Phobias; Sleep; Sleep apnea; Sleepwalking; Stress.

For Further Information:
Caldwell, J. Paul. *Sleep: The Complete Guide to Sleep Disorders and a Better Night's Sleep*. Rev. ed., Firefly Books, 2003. A thorough examination of sleep disorders constitutes a good portion of this book, including such topics as what causes sleep apnea, sleep disorders in children and seniors, what drugs interfere and help with sleep, and treatment guidelines.

Dement, William C., and Christopher Vaughan. *The Promise of Sleep*. Delacorte Press, 1999. Over this book's four sections, the authors cover the basics, such as "Daily Sleep Need," "Alternative Therapies," and "Sleeping Pills." Gives sleep, one of human beings' greatest basic needs, the attention it deserves.

Dotto, Lydia. *Losing Sleep: How Your Sleeping Habits Affect Your Life*. William Morrow, 1990. Discusses the physical and social consequences of sleep disorders, with an emphasis on sleep loss. In an easy-to-read style, the author reports on the effects that a modern, frenetic lifestyle has on sleep and its ramifications for waking hours as well.

Hobson, J. Allan. *Sleep*. Scientific American Library, 1995. This beautifully illustrated volume provides an overview of past and contemporary sleep research. The author draws upon neurology and psychology to provide an interdisciplinary approach to his topic.

Jameson, J. L., A. S. Fauci, D. L. Kasper, et al., editors. *Harrison's Principles of Internal Medicine*. 20th ed., McGraw Hill, 2018.

Montplaisir, Jacques, and Roger Godbout, editors. *Sleep and Biological Rhythms*. Oxford UP, 1990. This collection of articles highlights the role biological rhythms play in sleep, wakefulness, and psychological well-being. One chapter is devoted to explaining a possible mechanism for insomnia and another discusses drugs that are used in the treatments for restless leg syndrome and narcolepsy.

National Sleep Foundation, www.sleepfoundation.org. Along with good information about the range of sleep disorders, the site also gives information on sleep tips, children and sleep, and sleep services, among other features.

Reite, Martin, John Ruddy, and Kim E. Nagel, editors. *Concise Guide to Evaluation and Management of Sleep Disorders*. 3rd ed., American Psychiatric Press, 2002. Gives an overview of the symptoms and treatments available for different types of sleep disorders.

Walsleben, Joyce A., and Rita Baron-Faust. *A Woman's Guide to Sleep: Guaranteed Solutions for a Good Night's Rest*. Crown, 2001. Writing in an informal, easily comprehensible style, Walsleben, director of the Sleep Disorders Center at New York University School of Medicine, and freelancer Baron-Faust cover nearly every sleep disorder suffered by women.

SLEEPING SICKNESS

Category: Disease/Disorder
Also known as: West African trypanosomiasis, Gambian sleeping sickness, East African trypanosomiasis
Anatomy or system affected: Brain, heart, lymphatic system, nervous system, psychic-emotional system
Specialties and related fields: Environmental health, epidemiology, internal medicine, microbiology, neurology, public health
Definition: A parasitic disease caused by protozoa and transmitted to humans by the bites of infected tsetse flies.
Key terms:
acute: having a sudden, severe onset
blood-brain barrier: an anatomical barrier created by the modification of brain capillaries that prevents certain chemicals in the blood from crossing the capillary walls into the brain tissues
chronic: having a slow onset with progressively more serious symptoms
edema: water retention
parasite: an organism that lives off or in another organism without benefit to the host organism
protozoa: a phylum or subkingdom of mostly unicellular, mobile organisms that includes disease-causing parasites
vector: an organism that transmits a pathogen to another organism

CAUSES AND SYMPTOMS

Sleeping sickness is a vector-transmitted parasitic disease caused by *Trypanosoma*. These protozoa are transmitted to humans by the tsetse fly, genus *Glossina*, which is found only in moist savannas and forests in parts of sub-Saharan Africa. Rarely, transmission can occur from a mother to her unborn child or through blood transfusion or organ transplantation. There are two types of sleeping sickness. West African trypanosomiasis is found in both Central and West Africa. Also called Gambian sleeping sickness, it is caused by *Trypanosoma brucei gambiense*. East African trypanosomiasis is caused by *T. brucei rhodesiense*. Another human form of trypanosomiasis, Chagas' disease, is found in the Western Hemisphere.

Symptoms of the East African type emerge in three stages. Untreated victims of this acute form of the illness may die within weeks or one year later. The first stage begins with the reaction to the tsetse fly's bite. A painful sore, called a chancre, appears about forty-eight hours after the bite and lasts from two to four weeks. It is accompanied by swollen lymph nodes. The second or early stage includes high fever, severe headache, joint pain, and fatigue; symptoms appear in

---

INFORMATION ON SLEEPING SICKNESS

Causes: Parasitic infection transmitted by tsetse flies
Symptoms: Painful sore at bite, swollen lymph nodes, high fever, severe headache, joint pain, fatigue, rashes, liver and spleen enlargement, edema, weight loss, debilitation, heart failure; in late stage, appetite loss, listlessness, personality changes, insomnia, tremors, slurred speech, unsteady gait, uncontrollable drowsiness, coma, and death
Duration: A few weeks to months; progressive and fatal if untreated
Treatments: Toxic drugs (suramin, melarsoprol) for both types; nontoxic drug (eflornithine) for West African type

---

waves, with symptom-free periods that can last up to two weeks. Rashes, swollen lymph nodes, enlargement of the liver and spleen, and edema may also occur. As the disease progresses, weight loss and debilitation increase. Heart involvement may appear early; some patients succumb to heart failure before the parasites invade the central nervous system. In the late stage, which appears within a few weeks to months of the infection, loss of appetite, personality changes, headache, listlessness, and insomnia are seen, along with tremors, slurred speech, and unsteady gait. Uncontrollable drowsiness occurs late in the course of the disease, progressing to coma and finally death, often from secondary infections.

West African sleeping sickness is a chronic illness, though just as deadly as the East African variety if left untreated. Instead of three distinct stages, there is usually a long symptom-free period. Often, no chancre appears, and the early stage may be so mild as to be overlooked, although swollen lymph nodes on the back of the neck, called Winterbottom's sign, may be visible. Symptoms gradually appear weeks or years later but are often so subtle that they continue to be ignored. Ironically, the lack of symptoms can be very dangerous for the patient because early treatment of sleeping sickness is critical in avoiding disability or death.

TREATMENT AND THERAPY

All but one of the drugs used to treat sleeping sickness are highly toxic. Mortality from drug toxicity can reach 5 to 10 percent. In addition, some of the drugs cannot cross the blood-brain barrier, so they are useless in late-stage illness. The one nontoxic drug, eflornithine, not only crosses the barrier but also is highly effective in treating both early-stage and late-stage West African infection. It is not used for East African illness, however, because it is not consistently effective for that type. In addition, it is expensive and difficult to administer correctly. Thus, for both types of early-stage infection, intravenous suramin (or suramine) is often used after giving a test dose to see how patients will tolerate the drug, with intravenous melarsoprol given for late-stage disease of both types. With treatment, most patients recover. However, irreversible brain damage or death is common when therapy is attempted at the later stage.

PERSPECTIVE AND PROSPECTS
Sleeping sickness is endemic in about one-third of Africa's total land area and threatens more than sixty million people in thirty-six countries. The World Health Organization (WHO) estimates that between 300,000 and 500,000 people are infected annually, despite much smaller numbers of cases reported. In some areas of Angola, the Democratic Republic of Congo, and southern Sudan, sleeping sickness has become the first or second greatest cause of mortality, ahead of human immunodeficiency virus (HIV) or AIDS. Its worst effects are felt in remote, rural areas where health infrastructure is often nonexistent. War, poverty, and lack of education hamper efforts at controlling the disease by shrinking tsetse fly populations through insect abatement programs, treating livestock harboring the parasites, and testing and treating asymptomatic human carriers.

Suramin was discovered in 1921. Pentamidine, sometimes used in treating the early stage of West African sleeping sickness, was discovered in 1941. Melarsoprol, the last arsenic-based medicine still in use, was discovered in 1949. Eflornithine was registered for use in sleeping sickness in 1990 and is approved in the United States for topical use in removing facial hair. None is an ideal drug, and most are difficult to administer under less-than-ideal conditions. Early diagnosis is likewise not easy or inexpensive.

The tragedy is that sleeping sickness had almost disappeared by the early 1960s, but strict screening and control efforts were allowed to lapse, allowing the disease to reestablish itself and become endemic in many areas. In an effort to once again reverse the spread of the disease, WHO has created the Program for Surveillance and Control of African Trypanosomiasis (PSCAT), which unites national programs, nongovernmental organizations, private foundations, universities, regional centers, and donor countries in an effort to reach the common goal of permanent eradication.

—*Sue Tarjan*

See also Bites and stings; Insect-borne diseases; Parasitic diseases; Protozoan diseases; Tropical medicine.

For Further Information:
Dumas, Michel, Bernard Bouteille, and Alain Buguet, eds. *Progress in Human African Trypanosomiasis, Sleeping Sickness*. New York: Springer, 1999.
Hoppe, Kirk Arden. *Lords of the Fly: Sleeping Sickness Control in British East Africa, 1900-1960*. Westport, Conn.: Praeger, 2003.
Lyons, Maryinez. *The Colonial Disease: A Social History of Sleeping Sickness in Northern Zaire, 1900-1940*. New York: Cambridge University Press, 1992.
Ramen, Fred. *Sleeping Sickness and Other Parasitic Tropical Diseases*. New York: Rosen, 2002.
World Health Organization. *Control and Surveillance of African Trypanosomiasis: Report of a WHO Expert Committee*. Geneva: Author, 1998.

SLEEPWALKING

Category: Disease/Disorder
Also known as: Somnambulism
Anatomy or system affected: Brain, musculoskeletal system, nervous system, psychic-emotional system
Specialties and related fields: Neurology, psychology
Definition: Repeated episodes of arising from bed during sleep and walking about, without being conscious of the episodes or remembering them.
Key terms:
electroencephalogram (EEG): a report of brain wave activity, achieved through attaching conductors to the scalp
parasomnia: normal waking behavior appearing within sleep (including sleepwalking) that is not caused by psychiatric illness
sleep stages: the division of sleep into rapid eye movement (REM) sleep, in which dreaming occurs, and non-REM sleep divided into four progressive levels, the first two being drowsiness and light sleeping and the last two involving deep sleep

CAUSES AND SYMPTOMS
Sleepwalking occurs during stages 3 and 4 of non-REM sleep and most frequently between one to four hours after falling asleep. Electroencephalograms (EEGs) indicate that children usually make a sudden transition into lighter sleep at the end of the first period of deep sleep. Some children do not make the transition rapidly and engage in parasomnia, or a simultaneous functioning of deep sleep and waking known as sleepwalking. An episode lasts from a few minutes to about an hour.

An estimated 40 percent of children ranging from six to sixteen years have reported sleepwalking, with twelve being the age of prevalence. While sleepwalking before the age of four is rare, partial wakings can affect toddlers and infants. Although sleepwalking usually ends around the age of seventeen, it can continue on into the early twenties. It is slightly more common in boys. Although most children sleepwalk infrequently, some sleepwalk frequently and for a period of five years or longer.

Sleepwalkers may have blank, staring faces and remain unresponsive to the attempt of others to communicate with them. They can be awakened only through great effort. Although sometimes sleepwalking children possibly see and walk around objects during their episodes, their behavior may involve leaving the bed violently and running without regard for obstacles. Partial awareness of their environment may be evident in their ability to negotiate hallway turns or objects on the floor. Some children stumble on stairs, crash into glass windows or doors, or walk out of the house into traffic. Serious injuries have occurred. While memory of these episodes is often absent, there may be a dim recall of the need to escape.

During sleepwalking, aggression toward others or toward objects in the vicinity is rare. The activity may be accompanied by sleeptalking that is characterized by poor articulation. Sleepwalkers also have increased incidence of other sleep disorders associated with non-REM sleep, such as night terrors.

Hormones or other biological factors may affect the character of these nighttime arousals. Statistics show that as many as 50 percent of sleepwalking children have close relatives with a history of similar phenomena. Although sleepwalking in very young children is developmental, many older children exhibit both a biological and an emotional predisposition for frequent sleepwalking. Some children who struggle to avoid expressing their feelings develop sleep problems.

TREATMENT AND THERAPY

Ensuring adequate sleep and providing a normal schedule are the best ways to treat partial wakings in young children. Although these remedies can help, some parents may have to learn to live with their children's sleepwalking. Understanding what is happening will prevent the parents from intervening by attempting to awaken or question children or returning them to bed immediately. Instead, parents should talk quietly and calmly to sleepwalking children. If the children spontaneously awake after the episode, parents should avoid negative comments and treat the event matter-of-factly. In the case of agitated sleepwalking, restraint merely intensifies and increases the length of time of the episode. One should approach the child only to prevent injury, thus allowing the sleepwalking to run its course.

The child's environment should be made as safe as possible to prevent accidental injury. Floors and stairs

---

INFORMATION ON SLEEPWALKING

Causes: Developmental disorder, hormones, hereditary factors
Symptoms: Blank, staring face; unresponsiveness; running without regard for obstacles; poor articulation
Duration: Acute to chronic
Treatments: Monitoring in sleep clinic, drugs, technical aids, behavior modification

---

should be cleared, and hallways should be lit. For young children, gates may be installed at their bedroom doors or at the stairs, and should they attempt to leave the house, chain locks above their reach should be affixed to the doors.

Richard Ferber, director of the Center for Pediatric Sleep Disorders in Boston and author of *Solve Your Child's Sleep Problems* (1985), believes that older children whose sleepwalking may involve both psychological and inherited factors will benefit from psychotherapy. They may find it very difficult to express their feelings, especially if they are involved in situations in which things are happening outside their control. In the event of changes, losses, or an absence of warmth or love within a family, Ferber believes that children are often quite angry about the circumstances but do not express it outwardly. Psychotherapy or counseling will encourage children to believe that their feelings are not dangerous and will help them express these feelings. Medication is prescribed reluctantly-only to prevent self-injury-and is decreased as the benefits from psychotherapy increase.

PERSPECTIVE AND PROSPECTS

As late as the 1960s, sleepwalking was believed to be a neurotic or hysterical manifestation or an acting out of a dream. Contemporary studies have confirmed that sleepwalking is a sleep disorder that is not caused by psychiatric illness and is not a walking dream state.

Fortunately, sleepwalking can be outgrown by adulthood. Meanwhile, investigations into the nature of sleep, sleep and waking patterns, and biological rhythms continue to provide the best insight into this distressing family problem.

—*Mary Hurd*

See also Nightmares; Psychiatry, child and adolescent; Sleep; Sleep disorders.

For Further Information:
Ferber, Richard. *Solve Your Child's Sleep Problems*. Rev. ed. New York: Simon & Schuster, 2006. This concise volume is illustrated and includes an index.
McMillan, Julia A., et al., eds. *Oski's Pediatrics: Principles and Practice*. 4th ed. Philadelphia: Lippincott Williams & Wilkins, 2006. A text that offers clear descriptions of diseases and illustrations.

Parkes, J. David. *Sleep and Its Disorders*. London: W. B. Saunders, 1985. This volume is aimed at the medical professional and includes illustrations, bibliographical references, and an index.

Reite, Martin, John Ruddy, and Kim E. Nagel, eds. *Concise Guide to Evaluation and Management of Sleep Disorders*. 3d ed. Washington, DC: American Psychiatric Press, 2002. Gives an overview of the symptoms and treatments available for different types of sleep disorders.

Sutton, Amy L., ed. *Sleep Disorders Sourcebook: Basic Consumer Health Information About Sleep and Sleep Disorders*. 2d ed. Detroit, Mich.: Omnigraphics, 2005. Covers topics such as insomnia, sleepwalking, sleep apnea, restless leg syndrome, narcolepsy, and their treatment options.

SLIPPED DISK

Category: Disease/Disorder

Also known as: Herniated disk, ruptured disk, prolapsed disk, intervertebral disk displacement

Anatomy or system affected: Arms, back, legs, musculoskeletal system, neck, nerves, nervous system, spine

Specialties and related fields: Exercise physiology, family medicine, occupational health, orthopedics, osteopathic medicine, physical therapy, preventive medicine, sports medicine

Definition: A condition in which the soft, gelatinous center part of an intervertebral disk pushes out through a weakened portion of the disk, often placing pressure on a spinal nerve.

CAUSES AND SYMPTOMS

The spinal column has small bones called vertebrae that connect the skull to the pelvis. It is divided into regions: cervical (neck), thoracic (chest), and lumbar

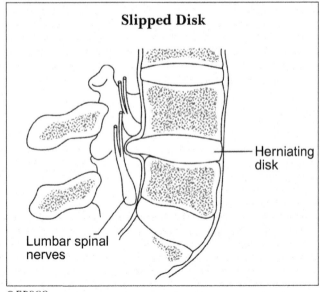

Slipped Disk

Herniating disk

Lumbar spinal nerves

©EBSCO

> ### INFORMATION ON SLIPPED DISK
>
> **Causes:** Aging process (degeneration and loss of water in disks); trauma (improper lifting, excessive weight, vertical pressure on spine, twisting)
>
> **Symptoms:** Varies with region affected and with degree of protrusion and nerve compression; may include low back pain (dull ache or sharp, burning sensation), neck pain, numbness, tingling, weakness, loss of bladder or bowel control, muscle spasms
>
> **Duration:** Chronic
>
> **Treatments:** Initially bed rest, then activity and physical therapy; medications (pain relievers, anti-inflammatory drugs, muscle relaxants, steroid injections); surgery (diskectomy, microdiskectomy, spinal fusion); chemonucleolysis

(lower back). Separating the vertebrae are intervertebral disks that provide cushioning and shock absorption during movement. The spinal column also has a hollow center portion called the spinal canal, which contains the spinal cord and nerves.

A slipped disk occurs when the outer portion of the intervertebral disk, called the annulus fibrosus, becomes weakened and allows the center portion, called the nucleus pulposus, to push out or leak through. There are various reasons that such bulging may occur. The process of aging is associated with degeneration and loss of water content in the disk material, which causes it to weaken over time, becoming less elastic. Improper lifting, excessive weight or vertical pressure on the spine, twisting, or forceful trauma can also cause a disk to rupture. Slipped disks are most common in the lumbar region, occur less frequently in the cervical region, and occur rarely in the thoracic region.

Symptoms vary with the degree of disk protrusion and nerve compression. In the lumbar region, the main symptom is low back pain, which may be a dull ache or a sharp and burning sensation radiating to the buttocks, legs, and feet (sciatica). Other symptoms include weakness or tingling in one leg and loss of bladder or bowel control. In the cervical region, symptoms include neck pain, often radiating to the shoulder, arm, or hand, and numbness, tingling, or weakness in any of these areas. All cases may include muscle spasms, and pain may be worsened upon movement, coughing, or straining.

TREATMENT AND THERAPY

Conservative treatment with initial bed rest, over-the-counter pain relievers, and anti-inflammatory medications is standard for a slipped disk. Muscle relaxants may be prescribed for muscle spasms. After forty-eight hours, activity and physical therapy is recommended. Most patients recover with this regimen. In cases of acute pain, steroid injections in the back may be used to reduce inflammation. Various surgical approaches, involving diskectomy, microdiskectomy, and spinal fusion, exist for patients who do not improve with conservative treatment.

An often effective alternative to surgery is chemonucleoylsis, wherein the orthopedist injects an enzyme that dissolves the ruptured portion of the disk. In 2007, the Food and Drug Administration approved lumbar disc replacement as a treatment option for some types of low back pain. Some clinical researchers believe that as new materials and placement techniques are developed, spinal disc-replacement surgery may become a standard treatment for some types of low back pain.

—*Barbara C. Beattie*

See also Anti-inflammatory drugs; Back pain; Laminectomy and spinal fusion; Numbness and tingling; Orthopedic surgery; Orthopedics; Sciatica; Spinal cord disorders; Spine, vertebrae, and disks.

For Further Information:

Gunzburg, Robert, and Marek Szpalski, eds. *Lumbar Disc Herniation.* Philadelphia: Lippincott Williams & Wilkins, 2002.

Icon Health. *Herniated Disk: A Medical Dictionary, Bibliography, and Annotated Research Guide to Internet References.* San Diego, Calif.: Author, 2004.

"Information from Your Family Doctor: When You Have a Herniated Disk." *American Family Physician* 67, no. 10 (May 15, 2003): 2195-2197.

Porter, Robert S., et al., eds. *The Merck Manual Home Health Handbook.* Whitehouse Station, N.J.: Merck Research Laboratories, 2009.

SMALL INTESTINE

Category: Anatomy

Also known as: Small bowel, small gut

Anatomy or system affected: Abdomen, endocrine system, gastrointestinal system, immune system, intestines, lymphatic system, nervous system

Specialties and related fields: Alternative medicine, biochemistry, endocrinology, gastroenterology, general surgery, histology, immunology, internal medicine, nutrition, oncology, osteopathic medicine, pathology, pediatrics, pharmacology

Definition: The section of the alimentary canal where the digestion of nutrients is completed and nutrients, vitamins, minerals, and fluids are absorbed. It is connected proximally to the stomach and distally to the large intestine and divided into the duodenum, jejunum, and ileum.

Key terms:

absorption: the passage of simple nutrients from the food compartment of the small intestine to the blood

chyme: food in a semifluid state that reaches the small intestine after partial digestion in the stomach

epithelium: tissue made up of tightly adherent cells, usually lining the surfaces of the body and organs

intestinal lumen: the inner cavity of the intestine; represents the food (chyme) compartment

STRUCTURE AND FUNCTIONS

In the average adult man, the small intestine is about 6 to 7 meters long, with a diameter of 2.5 to 3.0 centimeters. Its wall contains layers of smooth muscle and nervous tissue, which allow contraction movements and their control; its inner layer consists of absorptive mucosa, rich in blood and lymph vessels that drain into the portal vein. The mucosa is lined with absorptive epithelium.

Chyme from the stomach is mixed in the duodenum with bile and pancreatic enzymes, which neutralize its acidity and digest nutrients to simpler molecules. Proteins are degraded to smaller peptides, fats to fatty acids and glycerol, and carbohydrates to oligosaccharides. Enzymes linked to mucosal cells complete the breakdown, so nutrients can cross the epithelium and reach the bloodstream (absorption).

The mucosa is lined with millions of fingerlike projections (villi), 0.5 to 1.5 millimeters long, surrounded by moatlike invaginations (crypts), and each absorptive cell has microvilli protruding into the lumen. This yields an enormous absorptive area: about 250 meters^2 (the size of a tennis court). The mucosa includes absorptive, secretory, endocrine, and antimicrobial cells and is constantly renewed. Absorptive cells originate in the crypts and migrate up the villus, where they become mature and fully functional. Here they live for about three days, then are shed into the lumen. Nutrients enter the absorptive cells either via specialized cellular transport mechanisms (simple sugars and amino acids) or by simple diffusion (lipids), exit the cell through the basolateral membrane, and diffuse into the villus capillary vessels. Chyme is then moved down the intestinal lumen.

Three layers of smooth muscle allow segmentation contractions that mix the chyme and peristaltic movements that propel it distally. Between meals, periodic contractions called "migrating motor complex" propagate caudally along the small intestine and remove residual debris and bacteria. Intestinal movements are controlled locally by the enteric nervous system (a network of nerve fibers in the intestinal wall) and are modulated by the central nervous system. Hormones secreted by the small intestine regulate gastrointestinal secretion and motility and interact with the nervous system in modulating hunger and satiety.

DISORDERS AND DISEASES

Absorption-related disorders are linked to defects of mucosal enzymes or transporters and are usually genetic: In lactose intolerance (not to be confused with milk allergy), the enzyme lactase is lacking or insufficient; in glucose-galactose malabsorption, the mucosal transporter for glucose and galactose is defective. Unabsorbed sugars in the lumen cause gastrointestinal symptoms, which are reversed by avoiding the offending sugars.

Celiac disease is caused by an immunological response to gluten (a protein present in wheat, barley, and rye) and causes chronic intestinal inflammation with flattening of the villi. Mucosal surface and function are restored by a gluten-free diet.

Tropical sprue is a disorder of unknown cause (possibly an infection) in tropical areas, which causes abnormalities in the lining of the small intestine and anemia. It is treated with tetracycline.

In intestinal lymphangiectasia (idiopathic hypoproteinemia) the mucosal lymph vessels are enlarged and obstructed, so that fat and proteins cannot be absorbed. A low-fat, high-protein diet with supplements can help manage the resulting diarrhea. Short bowel syndrome occurs after surgical removal of a large portion of the small intestine. It causes diarrhea and malabsorption and often requires long-term total parenteral nutrition.

Whipple's disease (intestinal lipodystrophy) is a rare bacterial infection that damages the mucosa. It is successfully treated with antibiotics but can recur. Bacterial overgrowth syndrome is the result of slow peristalsis, which allows intestinal bacteria to grow excessively, causing diarrhea and malabsorption. It is treated with antibiotics.

Cancerous tumors in the small intestine are rare. Adenocarcinoma develops in the glandular cells of the mucosa. It requires surgical removal. Noncancerous (benign) tumors can affect different kinds of intestinal cells. Small noncancerous growths may be destroyed by endoscopic surgery.

Parasitic infestations include giardiasis (caused by a unicellular organism, mainly treated with metronidazole) and ascariasis (treated with mebendazole) and tapeworm infections (treatments vary widely), both caused by worms.

PERSPECTIVE AND PROSPECTS

Intestinal ailments and remedies are documented in ancient civilizations. Medieval anatomists maintained the gut could influence the humoral balance of the body. In the seventeenth century, intestines were described as being "made up of tunics, and these from fibers, flesh, parenchyma, veins, arterie, mesenterics, mucous crust, and fat." It was not until the mid-twentieth century that the complexity and importance of the small intestine became apparent. The glucose-transport mechanism was discovered in the 1960s, and molecular mechanisms of absorption have been studied throughout the late century. Recent techniques now allow investigation of their regulation through transporter gene expression. Also, the discovery of a host of intestinal hormones has opened the exploration of the endocrine and neural pathways that regulate nutrient intake, particularly in connection with the problem of obesity control.

—*Donatella M. Casirola, PhD*

See also Abdomen; Abdominal disorders; Appendicitis; Colitis; Colon; Colonoscopy and sigmoidoscopy; Colorectal cancer; Colorectal polyp removal; Colorectal surgery; Constipation; Crohn's disease; Diarrhea; Digestion; Diverticulitis and diverticulosis; Endoscopy; Gastroenterology; Gastroenterology, pediatric; Gastrointestinal disorders; Gastrointestinal system; Internal medicine; Intestinal disorders; Intestines; Irritable bowel syndrome (IBS); Laparoscopy; Nutrition; Obstruction; Peristalsis.

For Further Information:

Badman, Michael K., and Jeffrey S. Flier. "The Gut and Energy Balance: Visceral Allies in the Obesity Wars." *Science* 307 (March 25, 2005): 1909-1914. An article about intestinal hormones and nervous signaling, within a special section about the gut in a scientific magazine.

Levin, Roy J. "Digestion and Absorption of Carbohydrates: From Molecules and Membranes to Humans." *American Journal of Clinical Nutrition* 59, 3d suppl. (March, 1994): 690S-698S. A scholarly article discussing intestinal sugar absorption in detail.

Sherwood, Lauralee. "The Digestive System." In *Human Physiology: From Cells to Systems*. 7th ed. Belmont, Calif.: Brooks/Cole Cengage Learning, 2010. A chapter in a textbook for undergraduate students, easily accessible to the nonspecialist.

SMALLPOX

Category: Disease/Disorder

Also known as: Variola

Anatomy or system affected: Gastrointestinal system, muscles, skin

Specialties and related fields: Dermatology, environmental health, epidemiology, histology, immunology, pathology, preventive medicine, public health, virology

Definition: An acute, systemic, highly contagious disease caused by a viral infection; there are two forms, the more deadly and feared "classic" smallpox and a milder variety known as alastrim, which has a fatality rate of about 1 percent.

Key terms:

Centers for Disease Control and Prevention (CDC): a government facility, located in Atlanta, that coordinates investigations of disease occurrence in the United States; the CDC stockpiles smallpox vaccine for distribution if and when needed

incubation period: after initial infection, the period of time before any symptoms appear

quarantine: the sequestering of individuals who have been exposed to the infectious phase of a disease until any threat of contagion has passed; with smallpox, this period is seventeen days following last contact with a known case

vaccination: a process whereby live or attentuated virus is introduced into the skin tissue of healthy people in an effort to provide immunity

CAUSES AND SYMPTOMS

The variola virus that causes smallpox is spread through physical contact with infected victims, sometimes through droplets from nasal or oral secretions and sometimes through contact with scabs carried on bedding, towels, clothing, or other fabrics. After exposure to the variola virus, the incubation period ranges from seven to seventeen days. Early symptoms resemble influenza and include headache, muscle ache, and sometimes vomiting. When the characteristic rash appears, the infected person is already very ill. In unvaccinated persons not treated with antiviral medications, between 20 and 40 percent of persons infected with classic smallpox (variola major) would be expected to die. Death most often occurs between the fifth and seventh day of illness.

The initial deep-seated rash characteristic of smallpox develops into lesions, which then follow a progressive sequence of fluid-filled vesicles, then pustules, and finally scabs. Lesions often appear first on the face. In contrast to chickenpox, in which "crops" of lesions appear, all smallpox lesions are at the same phase in development. Smallpox cases become contagious when the first lesions appear and remain so until the last scab separates from the skin. After the scabs are completely shed, the recovered smallpox victim is left with characteristic pitted scars over large portions of the body. Some victims are rendered permanently blind as a result of contracting smallpox; males may be left sterile. Survival is generally accompanied by lifetime immunity to further infections.

TREATMENT AND THERAPY

Smallpox may be prevented through vaccination. Live vaccinia virus is introduced into the skin tissue of healthy people in an effort to provide immunity against smallpox. The vaccinia virus is very similar to the variola virus that causes smallpox. Live vaccinia virus has been used for smallpox vaccinations since the time of Edward Jenner, the Englishman who pioneered vaccination in the late eighteenth century.

There is no treatment known to cure smallpox, although vaccination may be effective in lessening disease severity when administered within four days of exposure. In the 1970s, methisazone (N-methylisatin beta-thiosemicarbazone), trade name Marboran, was believed to afford some protection when administered early in the incubation period. Isolation of victims, burning of all contaminated discharges, concurrent disinfection of the isolation environment, and sterilization of bedclothes and fabrics, combined with quarantine and vaccination of all persons susceptible to smallpox, has been used to contain epidemics in the historical past.

One of the last outbreaks of smallpox in the United States occurred in New York in 1947. To prevent a nationwide outbreak that year, the New York City Board of Health vaccinated about six million people (80 percent of the city's population) within a four-week period.

This young girl in Bangladesh was infected with smallpox in 1973. Freedom from smallpox was declared in Bangladesh in December, 1977 when a WHO International Commission officially certified that smallpox had been eradicated from that country. Photo via CDC/Wikimedia Commons. [Public domain.]

The final smallpox outbreak in the United States occurred in the Rio Grande Valley of Texas in 1949. The last case reported in the Western Hemisphere was in Brazil in 1971. Prior to the official "last case" of smallpox observed in human populations in October, 1977, international travelers were responsible for introducing the disease into areas where people had not received vaccinations to prevent smallpox. A laboratory accident in England in 1978 caused several cases of smallpox. In 1980, the World Health Organization (WHO) officially declared that smallpox had been eradicated. Major world powers, including the United States and the Soviet Union, maintained stocks of viable smallpox virus for further study.

PERSPECTIVE AND PROSPECTS

There are no natural carriers of smallpox virus; prior to its eradication, it was an endemic urban disease found only in humans, spread as healthy people came into contact with smallpox cases or with fabrics containing scabs shed by smallpox patients.

Following the terrorist attacks on the United States on September 11, 2001, a series of letters containing anthrax spores were sent through the U.S. mail. These letters caused inhalation anthrax, resulting in severe illnesses and several fatalities. Governments became concerned that terrorists would attempt to cause smallpox epidemics. Within the United States, a program was initiated in 2002 to vaccinate "first responder" health professionals in the event of a bioterrorist attack using smallpox. Few people volunteered for vaccination, but among the outwardly healthy people who were vaccinated, two died unexpectedly from cardiovascular disease. News reports of these deaths made people who were offered vaccination less willing to participate, although subsequent study seemed to indicate that these deaths were not directly attributable to receiving the vaccine.

Few Americans, even those now involved in research on the smallpox virus, have ever seen an active case. If a bioterrorist attack using the smallpox virus were to occur, then medical personnel might have some initial difficulty identifying the disease. The general public would need to be informed about the disease in a manner that would avoid widespread panic and ensure that those exposed were immediately vaccinated and quarantined.

By 2004, no medication had been approved to treat smallpox within the United States. Various antiviral agents had been investigated; the drug cidofovir (Vistide), at that time approved only to treat cytomegalovirus retinitis, was identified by several authorities as a potential agent to treat smallpox. Supportive measures that may be used include fever reducers, pain control medication, intravenous rehydration, and antibiotics to control secondary infections.

INFORMATION ON SMALLPOX

Causes: Infection with variola virus

Symptoms: Rash (progressing from lesions to fluid-filled vesicles to pustules to scabs); flulike symptoms (headache, muscle ache, sometimes vomiting); complications may include blindness and sterility

Duration: About one week

Treatments: Prevention through vaccination, antiviral drugs

A single case of smallpox occurring anywhere in the world at any time in the future would constitute an immediate epidemiological emergency. Smallpox is a "Class 1" internationally quarantinable disease; any cases must be reported immediately to local, state, national, and international health authorities.

The resurgence of interest in smallpox at the start of the twenty-first century brought forth many new ideas about all aspects of the disease and its prevention. In 2003, several researchers noted that the increase in numbers of people infected by human immunodeficiency virus (HIV) corresponded with the decline in smallpox vaccinations worldwide. Laboratory research has since determined that prior infection with the vaccinia virus (through vaccination) may confer some immunity to HIV.

—Anita Baker-Blocker, MPH, PhD

See also Biological and chemical weapons; Childhood infectious diseases; Epidemics and pandemics; Immunization and vaccination; Monkeypox; Rashes; Viral infections.

For Further Information:

Baciu, Alina, et al., eds. *The Smallpox Vaccination Program: Public Health in an Age of Terrorism.* Washington, DC: National Academies Press, 2005. A report from the Committee on Smallpox Vaccination Program Implementation from the Board on Health Promotion and Disease Prevention.

Benenson, Abram S., ed. *Control of Communicable Diseases in Man.* 16th ed. New York: American Public Health Association, 1995. This handbook, written after the last reported case of smallpox in the Western Hemisphere but before smallpox was declared eradicated, contains a complete description of methods of control, including preventive measures; the control of patients, contacts, and immediate environment; epidemic measures; and international measures.

Frieden, T., et al. "Cardiac Deaths After a Mass Smallpox Vaccination Campaign-New York City, 1947." *Morbidity and Mortality Weekly Report* 52, no. 39 (October 3, 2003): 933-936. Briefly reviews the history of the New York City 1947 epidemiological emergency and the Board of Health response. According to the New York City data, no unexpected increase in cardiovascular mortality occurred as a result of mass vaccination.

Glynn, Ian, and Jenifer Glynn. *The Life and Death of Smallpox*. New York: Cambridge University Press, 2004. Takes a historical view of the disease.

Heymann, David L., ed. *Control of Communicable Diseases Manual*. 19th ed. Washington, DC: American Public Health Association, 2008. An official report of the American Public Health Association. Includes an index.

SMELL

Category: Biology
Anatomy or system affected: Nervous system, nose
Specialties and related fields: Neurology, otorhinolaryngology
Definition: One of the five special senses; chemicals interact with receptor sites in specialized structures of the nasal cavity, and the resulting nerve impulses are classified as certain kinds of odor.

Key terms:

anosmia: a loss of the ability to detect aromas; general anosmia describes a lost ability to detect or identify any odors, while specific anosmia describes a lost ability to detect or identify a specific class of odors

Bowman's glands: one of three sources of the olfactory mucus that moistens the membranes of the olfactory center, thereby allowing odoriferous molecules to adhere to the olfactory hairs; glands that are located between olfactory supporting cells

chemoreceptors: in olfaction, specific structures in the nasal cavity upon which odoriferous, gaseous molecules adhere; this attachment induces a neural response that the brain interprets as smell

olfaction: the sense of smell; a process in which nerve impulses caused by chemicals interacting with chemoreceptors in the nose arrive in the olfactory center of the brain and are classified as certain kinds of odor

olfactory adaptation: the relatively quick response to and subsequent fatigue of the sense of smell that allows the presence of odoriferous chemicals to be recognized quickly and then become less and less noticed until they are soon ignored

olfactory bulb: an extension of the brain located below the frontal lobes of the cerebrum and above the ethmoid bone (extending back from the nose); one of a pair of gray masses into which the olfactory nerves terminate, thus serving as the first synaptic sites in olfactory neural pathways

olfactory epithelium: the surface covering of the olfactory region of the nasal cavity from which tiny, hairlike projections monitor the external world; a mucus-coated layer made of olfactory cells, supporting cells, and basal cells

olfactory hairs: the small, cilia-like projections extending from olfactory knobs into the conchae of the nasal cavity; at these projection sites, odoriferous molecules may interact chemically with the hairs to cause a nervous impulse to be sent to the brain

olfactory knobs: unmyelinated, tiny, rounded nerve endings of the sensory cells found at the mucus-coated olfactory membrane; each knob has five to eight extensions, called olfactory hairs, that branch out into the nasal cavity and monitor the environment

olfactory receptor cells: bipolar nerve cells surrounded by supporting cells in the olfactory epithelium; each cell body has one dendrite that terminates as an olfactory knob with hairlike projections

olfactory tract: the canal running posteriorly from the nose into the primary olfactory area of the cerebral cortex of the brain; the tract that houses large, myelinated olfactory nerves

STRUCTURE AND FUNCTIONS

Smell, one of the five special senses, plays an important role in both conscious and subconscious thought. While the loss of smell (anosmia) is troublesome, in isolation it is not a life-threatening problem. Nevertheless, anosmia is frequently an indication of an underlying pathology in either the olfactory or related organs; some of these pathologies may be life-threatening.

Of the special senses-gustation (taste), sight, olfaction (smell), audition (hearing), and equilibrium (balance and direction)-smell is the most primitive. As such, the organs that compose the olfactory system in humans are essentially identical to those found in other animals, including lampreys, cats, or dogs. The olfactory region of the nose is a very discriminating organ. Humans are able to classify smells according to at least seven agreed upon, although vague, classifications of primary odors: camphorlike, musky, floral, minty, ethereal, pungent, and putrid. Other categories that have been suggested are woody, spicy, and burned.

Within each odor category, the olfactory nerves and the brain are able to identify specific aromas with precision. For example, within the category of pungent, smells of onion, garlic, or skunk spray are easily discerned as similar, yet different, odors. Within the floral category, the human mind can readily distinguish among rose, lavender, and gardenia. The human olfactory sense can even distinguish between "left-handed" or "right-handed" molecules. In other words, the olfactory system can identify mirror-image molecules, in which one molecule is the spatial reverse of the other. An example is the substance carvone: When a person sniffs one form of carvone, the smell is spearmint; a sniff of the other form of carvone smells of caraway seed.

While studies of the anatomy and physiology of olfaction have not been finalized, the most accepted model of olfaction depends on the concept of odoriferous molecules attaching to olfactory receptor sites; the size and shape of both the odor molecules and the receptor sites are essential elements in currently adopted theories and descriptions of the mechanics of olfaction. Molecules of an odor-emitting substance chemically interact at receptor sites within specialized structures of the nasal cavity. The olfactory dendrites that are in contact with the external environment are directly linked to the neural centers of the brain. The olfactory tract connects these nerves directly to the hypothalamus region of the brain, which is associated with basic instinctual responses including fight-or-flight cues, food intake, or sexual curiosity and drive. This direct link to the brain causes a rapid and powerful response in animals to odor stimuli.

Because there is no physical barrier to protect olfactory receptors from the outside world, these nerve endings have a certain vulnerability to harm or damage. Olfactory nerves constantly regenerate in about a twenty-eight-day cycle; they are the only nerves that are capable of readily regenerating themselves and returning to full function. Nevertheless, it is estimated that about 1 percent of all olfactory receptors in an in-dividual die each year because of externally induced damage and general wear. Therefore, the sense of smell becomes less sensitive in older adults, which can minimize or repress the desire to eat and result in malnutrition.

The nasal cavity has two roles, one associated with respiration and the other with the sense of smell. The region that is dedicated to olfaction is small and evenly divided between the two septa of the nose. Within each nostril are folds called conchae. Humans have three conchae pairs-lower, middle, and upper. The specialized sensing structures for olfaction are found inside the middle and upper conchae. It is currently believed that olfactory receptors are regions of specialized molecular architecture located on cilia-like fibers called olfactory hairs. Olfactory hairs are extensions, or branches, of the olfactory sensing cells. The hairs, which are actually made of microfilaments, are dispersed over the surface of the olfactory sensing region of the nasal cavity.

While the size of the olfactory region of the nasal cavity is small (about the size of a dime), its surface area is comparatively large because of the many olfactory hairs coating the surface, or epithelium, of the olfactory cleft. It is estimated that humans have between 10 and 40 million olfactory receptors. The number of

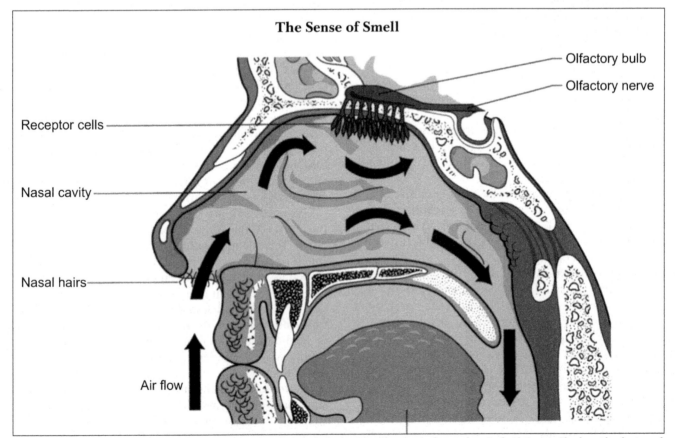

The Sense of Smell

Olfactory bulb

Olfactory nerve

Receptor cells

Nasal cavity

Nasal hairs

Air flow

Humans detect odors by a complex series of interactions—some only theoretical—involving receptors in the nasal cavity that interact with odor molecules to send nerve impulses to the brain through the olfactory nerve. ©EBSCO receptor hairs varies among species; dogs have about 1 million receptors on their olfactory cleft alone and are far more sensitive to specific odors than are humans. This feature explains why dogs can be trained for hunting game, finding missing persons, and locating drugs or explosives. A person can smell a pot of soup cooking and know it is soup, but a dog smelling the same pot of soup smells each ingredient of the soup, not the scent of the mixture. Nevertheless, among the senses, the sense of smell in humans is second only to vision in terms of number of receptors per unit of surface area.

The olfactory hairs are surrounded by a thick, brown-colored mucus and are partially covered and partially exposed. Thus, the mucosal lining on the epithelium of the olfactory region is a thin and poor protective barrier for the specialized structures that it coats. The mucus on the olfactory epithelium has three structures of origin: Bowman's glands, the goblet cells of the respiratory regions of the nose, and the supporting cells of the olfactory epithelium. Most of the mucus around the olfactory hairs is secreted from Bowman's glands, and only the Bowman's secretions contain the brown pigment that colors the mucus. It is known that, in other species, pigment is connected to olfactory ability; for example, albino pigs, which are lacking all pigments, are unable to smell toxic plants and often die from ingesting native plants that are poisonous to their species. The true significance of the brown pigment in humans, however, remains unclear.

The significance of the olfactory mucus itself is not in question. Odoriferous molecules must be trapped by the mucus so that they can travel to chemoreceptor sites on the olfactory hairs. The interaction between the odor molecules and the chemoreceptors of the olfactory hairs requires a mutual attraction, originating from small electrostatic forces. The shape, size, and polarity or nonpolarity of molecules causing odor are important factors in the creation of a smell stimulus.

From the olfactory hairs in the membrane structure, the odor molecules travel through the cribriform plate and into the olfactory tract, which leads directly to the hypothalamus in the brain. The olfactory hairs extend from the olfactory knobs, unexposed sensory cell endings completely covered by brown mucus. Five to eight hairs extend from each knob; electron micrographs show that the hairs are actually dendrites extending from the cell body into the external environment, while the axons of the cells carry nerve impulses toward the brain.

The sensory cells are found about midway in the olfactory epithelium. Other cells in the epithelium are the supporting cells and the basal cells. The supporting cells provide a scaffolding for the sensory cells and

also contribute fluids to the mucus layer. Basal cells are able to assist in the replenishment of receptor cells.

The cribriform plate, often described as a wafer-thin structure, is an important separation point between unmyelinated sensory nerves, which are in touch with the environment, and the myelinated nerves that direct the tiny electrical impulses of smell to the brain. Myelinated olfactory nerves are large and function with great speed and efficiency in comparison to the unmyelinated sensory cells. Thus, the original nerve signal prompted by an odoriferous molecule is slow, but this time is more than recovered in the myelinated nerve fibers. Working together, the unmyelinated and myelinated nerve bundles detect, transmit, and deliver nerve impulses of smell in fractions of a second, aided by the relatively short path between the nasal cavity and the hypothalamus.

The hypothalamus is located under the thalamus in the brain. It is the center into which nerve impulses originating at the sensory organs of sound, taste, smell, and the somatic senses are delivered. The activity of this portion of the brain is closely linked to the activity of the pituitary gland. This association is important in the sense of smell and sexual maturation, which is triggered by hormones released by the hypothalamus. In addition to these attributes, the hypothalamus is essential to regulating the autonomic nervous system, body temperature, and food intake.

DISORDERS AND DISEASES

Loss of the ability to sense all smells is called anosmia. Hyposmia (a decrease of smell function), dysosmia (an altered sense of smell), and anosmia can manifest themselves in numerous ways.

Most people are well acquainted with the inability to smell during a heavy cold. This condition is a temporary one caused by the presence of excessive mucus. The presence of a cold virus causes the respiratory region of the nose to respond by producing excessive volumes of cleansing mucus from goblet cells. Unfortunately, there tends to be so much mucus that the olfactory region becomes flooded; instead of swimming in mucus, the olfactory hairs are drowning. A thick coating over the hairs prevents odoriferous molecules from reaching the chemoreceptors. The sense of smell is lost until partial recovery decreases the mucus levels and once again allows the olfactory hairs to be partially exposed to the exterior world. The ability to sense odors fully returns once recovery from the head cold is complete.

Because it is uncommon to lose the ability to smell all odors, true anosmia is a rare condition. Furthermore, anosmia is seldom a problem found in isolation. Often there are simultaneously occurring symptoms such as a loss of taste (gustatory) function, undeveloped ovaries and testes, or head injury. In diagnosing possible causes of anosmia or dysosmia, a physician must obtain a complete medical history and perform a thorough physical exam. Special attention is given to the nasal cavity, the head and neck area, and, perhaps surprisingly, to genital maturation and function. Smell function is measured by passing vials containing increasing concentrations of an odoriferous chemical under a patient's nose until a scent can be detected. It is also important to assess whether the patient can properly identify the smell; if not, further studies must be done.

Olfactory problems can originate in one of the three structures that are involved in olfaction: in the sensory receptors, which convert chemical signals arising from odor molecules into electrical impulses; in the sensory nerve cells, which transmit these electrical impulses to the brain; and in the brain, which interprets the incoming electrical signals.

Abnormalities in the nasal cavity that can modify or destroy olfaction may include nasal polyps, a tumor located in an olfactory bulb, or allergic rhinitis (irritated and swollen membranes of the nose). Other olfactory maladies may be of an indirect origin, such as nutritional abnormalities or the presence of a toxic trace metal. Endocrine imbalances can be particularly pertinent in olfaction function.

An example of an endocrine imbalance that can influence the olfactory sense is seen in the cooperative workings of the hypothalamus and the pituitary gland. The hypothalamus receives impulses from olfactory nerves. It also lies just above the major endocrine gland, the pituitary gland. The pituitary gland receives regulating chemicals from the hypothalamus that either stimulate or inhibit the anterior portion of the gland. The anterior region of the pituitary gland monitors the levels of steroid hormones circulating in the body. Steroid hormones are essential to complete sexual maturation in both males and females. A congenital defect that affects both the nose and sexual maturation is Demorsier's olfactogenital dysplasia. Individuals with this malady are anosmic as a result of underdeveloped olfactory lobes. Low levels of gonadotropic hormones are also found in afflicted persons, resulting in undeveloped ovaries or testes. A somewhat similar (but not congenital) problem can be seen in Kohn's syndrome. In this syndrome, the ovaries or testes are underdeveloped and the olfactory nerves are abnormally formed, halting the sense of smell.

Olfaction is believed to play a role in the timely onset of sexual maturation in puberty. It seems that both male and female pheromones, oily scents that subconsciously cause sexual excitement in a species, can assist in or accelerate the events of sexual maturation. Although researchers are still exploring the role of pheromones in the human species, it appears that smell is relevant to the onset of menstruation in pubescent girls. Scents also contribute to sexual arousal in males.

An altered sense of smell can occur with pregnancy because of the resulting changes in hormone levels. For some pregnant women, formerly pleasant aromas may become repugnant, sometimes contributing to the feeling of nausea that some pregnant women experience. In addition, the increased mucus production that occurs with pregnancy works to block full smell function.

Brain tumors or lesions can sometimes account for anosmia, hyposmia, or dysosmia. Head injury is another possible cause because nerves or the hypothalamus itself can be crushed or otherwise damaged. Tumors, lesions, and neural damage can be detected using positron emission tomography (PET) scanning or magnetic resonance imaging (MRI). Some neurological diseases may be considered when diagnosing these olfactory disorders since the sense of smell requires only organs found in the nervous system.

Treatment of olfactory malfunctions varies greatly depending on the origin of the problem. Surgery may be needed to remove tumors. Allergies may be treated by shots; corticosteroids may be used to prevent the inflammation of nasal mucous membranes. Drugs may be administered to either inhibit or activate nerve conduction. Treatment often results in the recovery of olfaction, but not in all cases.

PERSPECTIVE AND PROSPECTS

The sense of smell has been recognized as one of the most primitive attributes of the human species, and it once held a high position in the hierarchy of skills required for species survival. Olfaction has long been a topic of intrigue in intellectual circles. The Greek philosopher Democritus of Abdera (384-322 BCE) proposed his theory of the atom in a time when modern science and scientific methods did not exist. Democritus incorporated his description of atoms into an explanation of olfaction. He presumed that the sense of smell in humans resulted from some kind of connection that formed when atoms of odor-emitting substances entered the nose. Different odor sensations, he proposed, would result from differences in the texture and shape of these atoms. The anatomy of the nose and brain was not considered in his philosophy. Democritus's idea of atoms was largely rejected in Greek circles of thought, however, and the concept of atoms combining to form molecules would not appear for hundreds of centuries. Modern understanding of the sense of smell is largely a more advanced, more informed, and more technical description of the very ideas imagined by this great Greek philosopher.

Another Greek contemplating the subject of smell was the physician Galen of Pergamum (129-c. 199 CE), who proposed an insightful description of the neuroanatomy of olfaction which also proved to be validated, with some alterations, centuries later. Whether he accepted the notion of atoms or not, Galen believed that particles actually tunneled into what are now called olfactory bulbs, thereby causing an odor to be detected. Galen also believed that these olfactory bulbs were extensions connected directly to the brain. Living in an era when microscopes and the scientific method did not exist, Galen could only describe what he saw with the unaided eye and reason intuitively. It is fascinating, therefore, to learn that his belief that the olfactory bulbs were extensions of the brain has been proven correct.

As the most primitive, and thus less evolved, of the five special senses, smell is associated with basic instincts, reactions or responses to external stimuli that aid an individual organism. Smell influences instincts of aggression when odors are released in fighting or battle through sweat and perhaps blood. These odors may inspire fight-or-flight responses in the brain and body. Social groups, such as a street gang, a group of soldiers, or a den of lions, can learn to recognize the scent (or the absence of scent) of its members in training or other group activities, helping to identify safe and unsafe groups in darkness or battle when other cues may be masked. Thus, while it is a subtle form of recognition often registered in the subconscious, smell apparently plays a role in modern survival tactics as well.

Another basic instinct that utilizes the sense of smell is the so-called mothering instinct. For example, new mothers are better able to identify their newborns by scent than by sight only hours after delivery. This sense seems adaptively helpful to the exhausted mother-who may have been in labor for days and is likely to be suffering from general exhaustion and diminished energy-in locating and feeding her baby. In a primitive human culture, this ability would help mothers identify babies if a flight from danger or a search for food or water caused a temporary separation of the mother-child pair. In addition, a nursing baby is guided to the mother's nipple by the scent released from the sweat glands surrounding the nipples.

Mate selection is believed to be linked to scents and olfactory appeal. There is some evidence that even the most heavily perfumed person of modern society emits pheromones that are sexually alluring to some and repulsive to others. This allure or repulsion seems to occur in the subconscious mind, or the limbic region of the brain.

On a more conscious level, the sense of smell is sometimes useful as a warning of a health problem; thus odors can be helpful in either describing or diagnosing a disease. For example, some people with epilepsy, days or only minutes before the onset of an epileptic seizure, have olfactory hallucinations-they smell odors in the absence of any stimulating molecules. The odor is usually described as either a scent of decay, as at a fish market, or a chemical, such as ether or petroleum. The sweet smell of acetone on a person's breath can indicate a diabetic who is in danger of coma, or who is already in a coma and cannot ask for help. Vincent's angina can be suspected if a foul breath odor is present, while diphtheria causes a sweet scent.

Because of the unique regenerative capacity of the olfactory neurons, neurologists and other researchers are actively attempting to understand the mechanisms that allow these nerves to be so efficient and effective in nerve regeneration. Such research may have an impact upon the understanding and treatment of a variety of neurological disorders that are not directly affiliated with olfaction.

—*Mary C. Fields, MD*

See also Allergies; Anosmia; Antihistamines; Aromatherapy; Common cold; Decongestants; Nasal polyp removal; Nasopharyngeal disorders; Otorhinolaryngology; Polyps; Respiration; Rhinoplasty and submucous resection; Sense organs; Sinusitis; Taste.

For Further Information:

Engen, Trygg. *The Perception of Odors*. New York: Academic Press, 1982. Designed for the beginner, this text describes the anatomy, physiology, and psychology behind olfaction. Provides detailed explanations of the classification of odors, odor theories, and the tests that are used to assess olfactory function.

Finger, Thomas E., Wayne L. Silver, and Diego Restrepo, eds. *Neurobiology of Taste and Smell*. 2d ed. New York: Wiley-Liss, 2000. Introduces the study of taste and smell, focusing on the way chemical senses work, with coverage ranging from microorganisms to humans and from genetics to behavior.

Møller, Aage R. *Sensory Systems: Anatomy, Physiology, and Pathophysiology*. Boston: Academic Press, 2003. An excellent text that describes how human sensory systems function, with comparisons of the five senses and detailed descriptions of the functions of each of them. Also covers how sensory information is processed in the brain to provide the basis for communication and for the perception of one's surroundings.

Schmidt, Robert F., ed. *Fundamentals of Sensory Physiology*. Translated by Marguerite A. Biedermann-Thorson. Rev. 3d ed. Berlin: Springer, 1986. Chapter 9, "Physiology of Olfaction," addresses the organization of the olfactory system and its relevant connections in the brain.

Shier, David N., Jackie L. Butler, and Ricki Lewis. *Hole's Essentials of Human Anatomy and Physiology*. 10th ed. Boston: McGraw-Hill, 2009. Covers the sense of smell and related topics, such as the anatomy and organization of the brain and nervous system. Although this academic textbook is more advanced than an introductory biology book, its definitions and excellent diagrams and drawings assists readers at all levels.

Tortora, Gerard J., and Bryan Derrickson. *Principles of Anatomy and Physiology*. 12th ed. Hoboken, N.J.: John Wiley & Sons, 2009. This text offers a brief treatment of the topic of smell, but perusal of the book will allow the reader to place this special sense within the context of the whole human anatomy.

Wolfe, Jeremy M., et al. *Sensation and Perception*. 2d ed. Sunderland, Mass.: Sinauer, 2009. Addresses all five senses. Includes a detailed section on olfaction.

SMOKING

Category: Disease/Disorder
Anatomy or system affected: Circulatory system, respiratory, throat, gastrointestinal, bladder
Specialties and related fields: Oncology, pulmonary medicine, vascular medicine, addiction medicine
Definition: The inhalation of tobacco in the form of cigarettes or cigars, which poses important health risks; those risks can be significantly decreased by smoking cessation, even in older age.

CAUSES AND EFFECTS

Cigarette smoking has long been known to have adverse effects. Smokers get more wrinkles than nonsmokers and brown/black discoloration of teeth so they tend to look older than their chronological age. They also are more likely to develop worsening of age-related problems such as gum disease, loss of teeth, and alteration in sense of smell and taste. Loss of teeth leads to difficulty chewing, which in turn leads to difficulties with digestion. Most people who lose teeth eventually develop loss of the bone that should support their teeth, making it increasingly difficult to fit dentures.

Smokers are ten times more likely to get lung cancer than nonsmokers. Lung cancer is now the number one cause of cancer deaths in women, as well as in men. In addition to lung cancer, smokers have a higher incidence of cancers of the head and neck, esophagus, colon, rectum, kidney, bladder, and cervix. Smokers are three to six times more likely to have a heart attack than are nonsmokers. In older people, the major risk factor for disease of the coronary arteries is hypertension, but smoking is still significant, especially when combined with other risk factors for heart disease, such as diabetes or high cholesterol. Smoking and diabetes are also the two most important risk factors for diseases of the veins and arteries of the lower leg. Those who continue to smoke once these diseases develop are much more likely to require limb amputation than those who quit. Smokers may develop chronic obstructive pulmonary disease (COPD), which includes emphysema and chronic bronchitis, and are eighteen

---

INFORMATION ON SMOKING

Causes: Addictive properties of drug

Symptoms: Increased incidence of lung cancer, pancreatic cancer, oral cancer, esophageal cancer, bladder cancer, emphysema, and chronic bronchitis; increased risk of gum disease; impaired sense of smell and taste; tooth loss; difficulty with digestion including acid reflux; decreased muscle strength, agility, coordination, gait, and balance; wrinkles

Duration: Often chronic

Treatments: Support groups, hypnosis, increased exercise; use of nicotine replacement systems (patches, gum), medications, electronic cigarettes

---

times more likely than nonsmokers to die of diseases of the lungs other than cancer. Older smokers also show a decrease in muscle strength, agility, coordination, gait, and balance. The changes in these areas make them seem older than their actual age.

Smoking has long been thought to be associated with peptic ulcer disease. In addition, smoking makes the symptoms of many diseases worsen or increases the risk of complications in patients with allergies, diabetes, hypertension, and vascular disease. Male smokers are at greater risk of experiencing sexual impotence. Female smokers tend to experience an earlier menopause, bone loss called "osteoporosis" and are therefore at increased risk for hip fracture than nonsmokers. Smokers are more likely to develop glaucoma than nonsmokers. (Studies completed in 1996 indicated an increased risk with smoking for macular degeneration, the leading cause of blindness in older adults. The evidence is mixed on smoking and Alzheimer's disease, but a 1998 study contradicted earlier work and found that the risk is greater in smokers than in nonsmokers.) Finally, smokers are at greater risk of death or injury caused by cigarette-related fires.

Cigarette smoking tends to speed up the processes in the liver for breaking down, using, and eliminating medications, both nonprescription and prescription. This means that medications may not perform as expected in the body. Smokers may need to take medications more frequently or in greater doses than nonsmokers, so it is important for health care providers to know that a person smokes. The drugs known to be affected by smoking include sedatives, narcotic and synthetic narcotic painkillers, certain antidepressants, anticoagulant medications, asthma medications, and certain blood pressure medications. These changes are of particular concern in the older population for a number of reasons. First, older people (whether smok-

Smoking is known to cause a variety of health problems. Photo via iStock/skynesher. [Used under license.]

ers or nonsmokers) tend to need more medications than younger people. With each additional drug, the risk of serious drug interaction and other adverse effects increases. Second, changes in body composition and function that alter the metabolism of drugs come with age, making medication use somewhat riskier in older persons, in terms of adverse effects and complications. The additional changes associated with smoking increase these risks significantly.

The dangers of passive smoking are well-documented. More than fifty compounds in secondhand smoke are identified as carcinogens in humans. The effects seem to be more harmful in children than in adults, but adults who are affected are at increased risk for cancer, heart disease, cancerous lung diseases, and allergies.

TREATMENT AND THERAPY

Numerous studies have shown that smoking cessation has health benefits in as little as one year, such as reducing the risk of heart attack and coronary artery disease. Within two years of smoking cessation, the risks of stroke and diseases of the blood vessels in the lower leg are reduced as well. Even though chronic lung disease is not reversible, those who quit smoking slow the decline in lung function considerably. Risks for cancers also decrease significantly with smoking cessation and are similar to the cancer risk for nonsmokers in ten to thirteen years. These findings indicate that it is worthwhile even for older people to give up smoking. An average forty-year-old gains approximately nine additional years of life by quitting smoking, and a sixty-year-old gains approximately three additional years.

Because smoking is an addiction, it may be difficult to quit, particularly after years of cigarette use. Most smokers have to stop several times before quitting permanently. Setting a quit date, attending support group meetings, taking it one day at a time, undergoing hypnosis, making a contract with a friend or a health care provider, substituting carrot sticks for cigarettes, increasing exercise (particularly swimming), and breathing deeply all seem to be helpful techniques. Nicotine replacement systems are available in the United States on a nonprescription basis, but it is important for older people, particularly those with health problems or who are taking multiple medications, to consult a health care professional prior to using them. Some forms of nicotine replacement include lozenges, patches, gum. It is also important that anyone using these aids stop smoking completely. Continuing to smoke while using nicotine replacement could potentially cause toxicity, and it decreases the success of cessation attempts, since the behavior of smoking is still present. Two non-nicotine-containing medications are available by prescription for smoking cessation: the antidepressant bupropion SR (Wellbutrin, Zyban) and varenicline (Chantix). Both medications significantly increase the success rates at the end of treatment and one year later. The mechanism of action is by stimulating chemical messengers in the brain that are affected by nicotine. The use of nicotine replacement in conjunction with these two non-nicotine-containing medications may increase the likelihood of smoking cessation. Wellbutrin may work better in patients who have depression-like symptoms.

Electronic cigarettes are used as a tool for smoking cessation. A battery-powered device that can deliver nicotine without the combustion or smoke. Use and awareness of e-cigarettes has dramatically increased over the past few years. Studies have suggested that physical and behavioral stimuli, such as holding a cigarette, can reduce the craving to smoke. Recent findings suggest that individuals who used e-cigarettes reduced the number of tobacco cigarettes they smoked. These findings suggest that e-cigarettes may be an important tool for reducing the harm that tobacco cigarettes can cause. Unfortunately, the benefits and risks of electronic cigarettes as of 2013 are still uncertain. More studies are needed for further investigation of their safety and efficacy.

PERSPECTIVE AND PROSPECTS
Smoking is the main avoidable cause of death in the United States and many other developed nations. More than 10 percent of North Americans over the age of sixty-five smoke cigarettes. This put them, and those with whom they live, at risk for significant health problems. These risks appear to increase both with age and with the number of years of smoking. After World War II, more women began smoking. Because the diseases related to smoking usually take years to develop, it was only in the last part of the twentieth century that rates of smoking-related disease among women began to approach those of men. Research indicates that smoking cessation appears to be beneficial, even in a person who has smoked for many years.

—Trevor Prashad, DO

See also: Addiction; Amputation; Bronchitis; Caffeine; Cancer; Carcinogens; Chronic obstructive pulmonary disease (COPD); Dental diseases; Diabetes mellitus; Emphysema; Eyes; Fracture and dislocation; Gingivitis; Glaucoma; Heart attack; Lung cancer; Lungs; Macular degeneration; Nicotine; Osteoporosis; Pulmonary diseases; Pulmonary medicine; Respiration; Sexual dysfunction; Skin disorders; Strokes; Substance abuse; Teeth; Vision disorders; Wrinkles.

For Further Information:
Britton, John. *ABC of Smoking Cessation*. Blackwell, 2004. This guide provides practical information for smoking cessation and discusses the public health and individual health problems associated with smoking.
Hales, Dianne. *An Invitation to Health Brief*. Updated editor. Wadsworth/Cengage Learning, 2010. This updated, helpful resource covers many aspects of health, including mental health, physical fitness, stress management, and preventive medicine.
Jameson, J. L., A. S. Fauci, D. L. Kasper, et al., editors. *Harrison's Principles of Internal Medicine*. 20th ed., McGraw Hill, 2018. Accessed 19 Apr. 2020.
Jorenby, Douglas E., et al. "Efficacy of Varenicline, an a4ß2 Nicotinic Acetylcholine Receptor Partial Agonist, versus Placebo or Sustained-Release Bupropion for Smoking Cessation." *Journal of the American Medical Association*, vol. 296, no. 1, 5 July 2006, pp. 56-63. This article compares two non-nicotine smoking-cessation products to a placebo in a smoking-cessation study with evaluation at the end of treatment and at fifty-two weeks. Varenicline was found to be significantly more effective than bupropion. Both agents were more effective than a placebo.
Marcus, Bess H., Jeffrey S. Hampl, and Edwin B. Fisher. *How to Quit Smoking without Gaining Weight*. Simon & Schuster, 2004. This paperback book from the American Lung Association provides expert advice on quitting smoking without gaining substantial weight. It provides motivation and discusses physical activity and many strategies to help with cravings. Includes recipes and meal plans.
Parles, Karen, and J. H. Schiller. *One Hundred Questions and Answers about Lung Cancer*. 2nd ed., Jones and Bartlett, 2010. A patient-oriented guide that covers a range of topics related to lung cancer, including risk factors and causes; methods of prevention, screening, and diagnosis; available treatments and how to choose among them; and ways of coping with common emotional and physical difficulties associated with the diagnosis and treatment.
Pirozynski, Michael. "One Hundred Years of Lung Cancer." *Respiratory Medicine*, vol. 100, no. 12, Dec. 2006, pp. 2073-84. Lung cancer is the most common cause of cancer death in the world, and cigarette smoking remains the major risk factor. Discusses treatment and prognosis.
Sloan, Frank A., et al. *The Price of Smoking*. MIT Press, 2006. This book contains a thorough analysis of the costs of smoking, which have often been ignored. These costs are carefully and comprehensively discussed by a group of economists.

SNAKEBITES

Category: Disease/Disorder
Anatomy or system affected: Blood, circulatory system, nervous system
Specialties and related fields: Emergency medicine, hematology, serology
Definition: The penetration of skin or flesh by the fangs of a snake. Although a snakebite often involves a poisonous snake, not all bites include venom injection into the bloodstream.

antivenin: an antidote given to snakebite victims to combat the effects of venom that has been injected into the bloodstream

venom: the substance that is often injected into the affected part of the flesh during a snakebite

CAUSES AND SYMPTOMS

A snakebite is a wound that results from the flesh penetration created by the hollow teeth, or fangs, of a snake and sometimes the injection of venom into the bloodstream. Venom is usually encountered in snakes, although other animals and insects use it, often as part of their defense system. In Australia, for example, several creatures are classified as venomous, such as twenty-two types of spiders, four types of ants, two types of beetles, two types of caterpillars, all platypus variations, two types of blue-ringed octopi, seven types of jellyfish, and eleven types of rays.

Venomous snakebites have a different effect based on the size of the victim, the location of the bite, the quantity of venom injected, and the time elapsed between the snakebite and the administration of antivenin therapy. Any part of the body is subject to this injury, but statistically legs, feet, and arms are by far the most commonly affected areas.

The symptoms of a snakebite include swelling or discoloration of the skin, a racing pulse, weakness, shortness of breath, nausea, and vomiting. Other symptoms include dilation of the pupils, shock, convulsions, twitching, and slurred speech. In extreme cases, severe pain and swelling and sometimes paralysis, unconsciousness, and even death may occur.

Snake venom contains an array of substances that are usually proteins in nature and that create tissue damage in several ways. The most important kinds of damage are nerve destruction, in which case the venom is called neurotoxic, and blood and tissue destruction, in which case the venom is hemotoxic. Neurotoxins have the tendency to paralyze the nervous system and lead to heart and respiratory failure. Hemotoxins destroy arteries, veins, and blood corpus-

Common North American Poisonous Snakes

Western diamondback rattlesnake
Location: West, Southwest, esp. arid zones
Color: Brown to reddish
Features: Diamond pattern on skin, rattle on tail

Eastern diamondback rattlesnake
Location: Southeast
Color: Brown
Features: To 8 feet long, diamond pattern on skin, rattle on tail

Prairie rattlesnake
Location: Great Plains
Color: Greenish-gray to brown
Features: To 4 feet long, rattle on tail

Timber rattlesnake
Location: Forests, swamps, hillsides in Midwest, Northeast
Color: Pale brown with black bands
Features: Rattle on tail

Sidewinder rattlesnake
Location: West, Southwest deserts, arid zones
Color: Pale brown
Features: Hornlike eyelash scales above eyes, rattle on tail

Water moccasin (cottonmouth)
Location: South, Southeast in or near water
Color: Brown with dark crossbands or black
Features: To 5 feet long, opens mouth to show white interior, no tail rattle

Copperhead
Location: East (north to south), South
Color: Russet with dark bands, yellowish head
Features: Vibrates tail when angry

Eastern coral snake
Location: Southeast
Color: Yellow-black or yellow-red recurring ring pattern
Features: To 4 feet long, slender

cles and lead to internal hemorrhaging. Different snakes have various degrees of toxins. Cobra venom is usually neurotoxic, while rattlesnake venom is hemotoxic. The development of gangrene in the location of the snakebite is possible unless the victim is treated promptly.

TREATMENT AND THERAPY

The victim of a snakebite may exhibit mild to severe symptoms. Although the strength of venom of different snakes differs widely, snakebite treatment should be imposed as soon as possible in order to reduce the possibility of a fatality. This treatment should address two points: how to restrict the venom to the smallest body area possible and how to remove as much venom as possible. Thus, all contractions of the body and limb movement should be reduced immediately to a minimum to avoid spreading the venom. This is accomplished by immobilizing the affected area, preferably in a horizontal position and definitely lower than the heart. Any exertion and/or excitement by the bitten person increases the pulse rate and blood circulation, which leads to easier spreading of the venom. This is the same reason that stimulants should be avoided.

Statistically, more than three-quarters of snakebites occur on the lower leg or forearm. Current first aid recommendations do not include ice, any incision, the application of oxidizers such as potassium permanganate, or the administration of aspirin, ibuprofen, acetaminophen, or alcohol. Instead, the bitten part should be wiped, and a relatively tight tourniquet that reduces the lymphatic flow without cutting off the blood supply to the affected area should be applied. A nurse or other emergency medical service employee should check the pulse at the bitten area to ensure adequate blood flow. It is also recommended that the bandage be released every half hour for half a minute. It is also helpful to take the snake, whether alive or dead, to the hospital for proper identification.

If the swelling extends more than 5 inches within the first twelve hours after the bite, antivenin is given through intravenous transfusion in a hospital. Antivenin preparations are created through the immunization of animals such as horses, and their efficiency is dependent on the purification and concentration of the substance. Antivenins are usually specific, but some, such as that for tiger snake venom, appear to protect against the venom of more than one snake. If there is no swelling and increasing pain around the bite within thirty minutes, then the wound is one of the approximately one-third of bites by poisonous snakes in which venom is not injected. A notable exception is the bite of the coral snake, in which swelling takes place regardless of the venom infusion.

INFORMATION ON SNAKEBITES

Causes: Penetration of skin or flesh by fangs of snake

Symptoms: Swelling or discoloration of skin, racing pulse, weakness, shortness of breath, nausea, vomiting, dilation of pupils, shock, convulsions, twitching, slurred speech

Duration: Acute

Treatments: Tight tourniquet to reduce lymphatic flow without cutting off blood supply, antivenin

---

After the patient sees a doctor, several nutrients can be taken that appear to relieve pain and symptoms. They include vitamin C (approximately 10,000 milligrams every hour), which serves as a detoxifier and lessens infection; calcium gluconate (500 milligrams every four to six hours), which relieves pain; and pantothenic acid (500 milligrams every four hours for two days), which serves as an antistress vitamin.

PERSPECTIVE AND PROSPECTS

Snakebites have been recorded in history for thousands of years, including such well-known examples as during Moses and the Israelites' flight from Egypt and Cleopatra's suicide with an asp. Traditionally, American Indians have had snakebite victims use echinacea, either by chewing the leaves and roots of the plant or drinking it in a tea form. They have also used its pulp placed on the affected area after making an incision and sucking the venom out until blood flows freely.

Approximately one-third of the three thousand snake species are poisonous, and only about three hundred can kill humans. The efficiency of emergency services and the wide availability of antivenins have reduced the death rates from snakebites dramatically. As a result, the number of people killed because of bee, wasp, and scorpion stings in the United States is higher than the deaths attributed to snakebites.

—*Soraya Ghayourmanesh, PhD*

See also Bites and stings; Emergency medicine; Emergency medicine, pediatric; Nervous system; Neurology; Neurology, pediatric; Numbness and tingling; Poisoning; Seizures; Toxicology; Zoonoses.

For Further Information:
Altimari, William. *Venomous Snakes: A Safety Guide for Reptile Keepers*. St. Louis, Mo.: Society for the Study of Amphibians and Reptiles, 1998. This concise volume covers the handling of poisonous snakes, offering information on snakebites and venom. Includes bibliographical references and an index.

Campbell, Jonathan A., and William W. Lamar. *The Venomous Reptiles of the Western Hemisphere*. Ithaca, N.Y.: Cornell University Press, 2004. Provides valuable information about the medical aspects of snakebite.

Julivert, Maria Angels. *The Fascinating World of Snakes.* New York: Barron's Educational Series, 1993. Vivid, full-color illustrations provide much detail, especially of predatory activities. Includes a glossary and an index.

Mattison, Christopher. *The Encyclopedia of Snakes.* New York: Facts On File, 1995. This volume discusses aspects of the life cycle of snakes-their biology, history, and taxonomy. Chapter topics include origin and evolution, morphology and function, feeding, defense, and reproduction.

"Squamata." In *McGraw-Hill Concise Encyclopedia of Science and Technology.* 6th ed. New York: McGraw-Hill, 2009. A section in a reference for the nonspecialist that offers articles written by world-renowned scientists and engineers.

Thorpe, Roger S., Wolfgang Wüster, and Anita Malhotra, eds. *Venomous Snakes: Ecology, Evolution, and Snakebite.* New York: Oxford University Press, 2002. Offers a multidisciplinary approach to research into venomous snakes, focusing on the medical aspects of snake venoms and the effects of snakebites.

Tilton, Buck. *Backcountry First Aid and Extended Care.* 5th ed. Guilford, Conn.: Falcon, 2007. A small, portable guide to the myriad emergencies and medical problems encountered in the wilderness.

Tu, Anthony T., ed. *Reptile Venoms and Toxins.* New York: Marcel Dekker, 1991. In twenty-four contributed chapters, thirty-seven international specialists describe the latest developments in research on snake venom and summarize what is known to date on Gila monster and frog toxins.

SODIUM

Category: Biology

Anatomy or system affected: All

Specialties and related fields: Multiple health related fields

Definition: Sodium is a chemical element with symbol Na (from Latin natrium) and atomic number. It is a soft, silvery-white, highly reactive metal.

Key terms:

diuretic: a drug that removes water from the body by increasing urine production, colloquially called "water pills."

ion: an atom or molecule that has an electric charge.

BACKGROUND

Sodium is one of about one hundred chemical elements, the mineral substances that make up everything in the universe. Sodium is one of the most vital chemical characteristics of animal life, which could not exist without it. Because of sodium's high reactivity—its ability to combine with other elements to form compounds-people have used sodium for a variety of purposes, including to make rock salt, baking soda, and table salt. Though nearly all foods in human diets contain some amount of sodium, consuming too much of it over long periods can cause a range of health problems such as hypertension and kidney disease.

THE CHEMISTRY OF SODIUM

Pure sodium is a semisolid silver metal with a softness and composition like butter. Because it lacks much density-solidity or compactness-sodium is extremely light and can float on water. As with many metals, it conducts, or transmits, electricity and heat extremely well.

The periodic table of the elements, a scientific chart containing chemical information for all known elements, reveals more facts about sodium. Its chemical symbol, the lettered representation of an element's name, is "Na," which is derived from the ancient Latin word for sodium, natrium. The name "sodium" itself descends from the Latin sodanum, a word that past civilizations gave to a form of sodium that alleviated headaches. English-speaking people later referred to this chemical as "soda."

The periodic table also provides information about sodium's atomic state. An atom is the most basic chemical unit of everything that exists. One atom of sodium has an atomic number of 11. An element's atomic number is determined by the number of protons and electrons, two types of subatomic particles, contained within one of its atoms. An atom of sodium therefore has eleven of each of these particles.

One of sodium's defining traits is its reactivity. The element is so versatile and so easily combines with other elements that it cannot be found in pure form in nature. Rather, sodium must be chemically extracted from compound substances such as sodium chloride, the rock salt that forms naturally in oceans. Over many years, people around the world have discovered myriad uses for sodium and the range of compounds it can help create.

HUMAN USES OF SODIUM

Sodium compounds have been used to create now-commonplace household products such as baking soda (sodium bicarbonate), soda (sodium carbonate), paper and photographs (sodium sulfate), and borax (sodium borate), the chemical used in laundry detergents. Sodium also can be combined with small amounts of the element neon to create sodium vapor lamps. These lights are bright and inexpensive to maintain, which is why they commonly are used in stadiums and on highways.

The most common natural compound of sodium is sodium chloride, composed of sodium and chlorine, the same substance that forms oceanic rock salt. People have used this naturally occurring chemical to manufacture road salt, which is used in winter to melt snow and ice on roads. Sodium chloride also can be mixed with water and applied to pottery and ceramics as a salt glaze finish. A related process involves making substances called *frits*. Essential components in glassmaking, frits are made from sodium carbonate created from a sodium chloride base.

A highly popular domestic use of sodium chloride is table salt. Salt is used for many culinary purposes, including cooking, baking, preserving perishable foods, and adding extra flavor to prepared meals. Edible salt was an especially valuable commodity in less industrialized times when countries around the world sometimes raided foreign salt mines to build up their own supplies. Although the human body requires a certain daily amount of sodium, too much can instigate a range of health problems, including increased risk of heart attack and stroke.

SODIUM AND HEALTH
Sodium exists in the body in the form of an ion Na+ with a positive charge. As an ion, it is active in controlling the distribution of fluids, maintaining blood pressure, creating an electrical gradient that allows nerve transmission and muscle contraction to occur, maintaining the mechanisms that allow wastes to leave cells, and regulating the acidity (pH) of the blood. Healthy foods that contain natural quantities of sodium include milk, celery, beets, and a variety of other vegetables and fruits. Most of the processed foods available in grocery stores and restaurants, however, contain added sodium, which has been cooked or baked into the items and is impossible to separate. Foods generally high in added sodium include snack foods such as potato chips, canned foods, and frozen meats such as sausage and bacon.

People can remain healthy while consuming as little as 500 milligrams (mg) of sodium daily. This amount is in slightly less than 1/4 teaspoon of table salt, which is 40 percent sodium by weight. The United States Centers for Disease Control and Prevention (CDC) suggests that healthy adults younger than age 51 consume no more than 2,300 milligrams of sodium daily. The CDC also urges adults older than fifty-one, especially those with histories of diabetes or heart, liver, or kidney disease, to limit their daily sodium intake to 1,500 milligrams because consuming too much sodium over an extended period can lead to hypertension (high blood pressure). Hypertension strains the body's blood vessels; over time, this strain can increase a person's risk of suffering a heart attack or stroke.

Certain drugs, most commonly diuretics and non-steroidal anti-inflammatory drugs (e.g. Aleve, Motrin, Advil) and some anti-depressant drugs cause large amounts of sodium to be excreted in urine and may result in low sodium levels. This becomes a health issue most often if the individual has other complex health problems.

—Michael Ruth;
updated by Tish Davidson

For Further Information:
"Health Risks and Disease Related to Salt and Sodium." Harvard University School of Public Health. www.hsph.harvard.edu/nutritionsource/salt-and-sodium/sodium-health- risks-and-disease (accessed August 1, 2017). An easy-to-read summary of the diseases and disorders that are associated with salt and sodium consumption.
"Salt." U. S. Centers for Disease Control and Prevention June 27, 2017 www.cdc.gov/salt (accessed August 1, 2017). A comprehensive set of recommendations for decreasing sodium in the diet of both children and adults.
"Sodium & Salt." American Heart Association 2017. www.heart.org/HEARTORG/HealthyLiving/HealthyEating/Nutrition/Sodium-and-Salt_UCM_303290_Article.jsp#.WYAsyFFlCic (accessed August 1, 2017). A gateway site with links to multiple articles about almost every health issue concerning salt and dietary guidance on salt consumption.
U.S. National Library of Medicine. "Sodium in Diet." Medline Plus July 5, 2017. www.nlm.nih.gov/medlineplus/ency/article /002415.htm (accessed August 1, 2017). A summary of the health issues surrounding sodium in easy-to understand form.

SOILING

Category: Disease/Disorder
Also known as: Encopresis
Anatomy or system affected: Anus, gastrointestinal system, intestines, psychological or emotional system
Specialties and related fields: Gastroenterology, pediatrics
Definition: The passage of fecal material into inappropriate places, usually underclothes.
Key terms:
functional megacolon: the rectal dilatation characteristic of fecal soiling
psychogenicmegacolon: fecal soiling as part of a constellation of behavioral disorders

CAUSES AND SYMPTOMS
Some authors use the term "encopresis" to mean the passage of an entire bowel movement into the underwear and reserve the term "soiling" for the seepage of small amounts of semisolid feces. The term "encopresis" was derived by combining the Greek terms *enourein* (meaning "to pass urine") and *kopros* (meaning "feces") to form a term that is analogous to enuresis, which describes bed-wetting.

The term "functional megacolon" is used to describe the rectal dilatation characteristic of this disorder and distinguishes it from congenital aganglionic megacolon (Hirschsprung's disease). In this much less common and far more serious disorder, the failure of development of part of the autonomic nervous system in the intestines results in a failure of propagation of colonic contractions (peristalsis), which in turn results in distention of the colon. As a general statement, children with Hirschsprung's disease rarely, if ever, have fecal soiling.

The term "psychogenic megacolon" implies fecal soiling as part of a constellation of behavioral disorders. Although behavioral abnormalities occur in children with soiling, most recent studies indicate that they are no more common in soiling children than in normal children and that they tend to be a response to the soiling.

Soiling is caused by chronic constipation in school-aged children. About 1.5 percent of second-graders experience fecal soiling, which is six times more common in boys than in girls. Constipation and its associated complications are common symptoms in young children, accounting for 25 percent of visits to pediatric gastroenterologists. Constipation becomes less frequent with age and usually resolves as puberty approaches. The basis of constipation is slow motility of the colon, usually present in several family members, which allows excessive water absorption from the stool, causing hard stools that are difficult to expel.

Typically, the child will begin having frequent episodes of fecal soiling at ages five to seven. Parents are mystified by this symptom and bring the child to the physician because of the impending forced socialization of beginning school. Upon questioning, a history of infrequent, large-caliber bowel movements, sometimes too large to be accommodated by the plumbing, is often obtained. The size of these bowel movements is evidence of distention of the rectum as a result of long-standing constipation, which is the basis of this disorder.

The rectum normally functions as a sensory organ, responding to rectal distention by alerting the brain that a bowel movement is imminent and that appropriate arrangements should be made. Persistent rectal distention (megacolon) as a result of chronic constipation results in decreased sensitivity of the rectum to acute rectal distention. These children frequently admit that they do not sense an impending bowel movement before or during episodes of soiling, and studies with distention of balloons passed into the rectum bear out this lack of sensitivity to acute rectal distention. Much more air has to be pumped into a rectal balloon before a soiling child can sense it than for a normal child.

In soiling children, the rectum functions as a storage organ, and does so rather poorly. Storage of fecal material in the rectum bypasses the normal mechanisms of continence and leaves the external anal sphincter, a circular muscle holding the anus closed, as the sole mechanism of continence. The external anal sphincter is under voluntary control. To keep it closed, the child

---

INFORMATION ON SOILING

Causes: Behavioral disorders, chronic constipation, gastrointestinal disorders, disease
Symptoms: Loss of control of bowel movements
Duration: Acute to chronic
Treatments: Oral cathartic agents (citrate of magnesia, sodium phosphate, colonic lavage solutions), stool softeners, biofeedback training

---

must keep all the muscles of the pelvic floor contracted. Any distraction or relaxation of the pelvic floor muscles to urinate can lead to leakage of semisolid stool.

TREATMENT AND THERAPY

Since soiling results from rectal distention (megacolon), effective therapy should empty the rectum (catharsis) and keep it empty (maintenance), allowing reversal of the rectal distention and return of normal rectal sensitivity. Several regimens are available, with most using a saline cathartic agent-that is, one that works by pulling water out of the circulation and into the colon, thus flushing out the contents of the colon. Hypertonic sodium phosphate enemas are frequently recommended but carry the risk of dehydration and electrolyte disturbances. In addition, these children are very sensitive to anorectal manipulation. For these reasons, using an oral cathartic is preferable. Such agents include citrate of magnesia, sodium phosphate, and colonic lavage solutions designed for cleaning the colon before an endoscopic examination. Stool softeners are usually prescribed as maintenance therapy to keep the water content of the stool high. Preparations such as mineral oil, milk of magnesia, lactulose, and sorbitol are generally safe and effective. Stool softeners are safe for long-term use and, unlike stimulant laxatives such as senna and phenolphtha- lein, do not cause dependence. The goal of therapy is resolution of the fecal soiling, since this is the only symptom that causes the child to suffer. Constipation is usually benign and self-limiting, and regularity of bowel movements should be seen not as a goal but rather as an indication that the rectal distention is reversing. Even with no treatment, soiling resolves spontaneously around the time of puberty as the underlying constipation resolves. This therapy is usually very successful if applied consistently, and no child should have to suffer the humiliation of fecal soiling. Many studies indicate that an effort by the child and his or her family to keep track of the episodes of soiling, passage of bowel movements, and dosage of medicine is required for the best outcome. Even if the soiling is resolved, however, the tendency toward constipation remains until puberty, and if the problem falls on the family's list of priorities as it resolves, the chance of recurrence is high.

PERSPECTIVE AND PROSPECTS

The earlier treatment is started for encopresis, the better the outcome. Clearing the colon of retained stool is the first step, followed by encouraging healthy bowel movements. In those children who are thought to have emotional disorders, psychotherapy is also helpful. Mental health professionals trained in behavior modification can be especially helpful in establishing techniques for teaching children to have regular bowel movements. If the encopresis is thought to be related to emotional issues a psychotherapist may be helpful, particularly if the child experiences shame, guilt, depression, or low self-esteem related to the encopresis. (Mayo Clinic, Encopresis, 2017)

—Wallace A. Gleason, Jr., MD;
updated by Mary Dietmann, EdD, APRN, CNS

See also: Anus; Bed-wetting; Colon; Constipation; Gastroenterology; Gastroenterology, pediatric; Gastrointestinal disorders; Gastrointestinal system; Hirschsprung's disease; Peristalsis; Psychiatry, child and adolescent; Rectum; Toilet training.

For Further Information:

Cooper, Candy J., Heidi Murkoff, and Teresa Martinez. "Bye-bye, Diapers." Parenting 14, no. 5 (June/July, 2000): 98-105. The authors highlight eight potty predicaments and how to solve them. Somesuggestions for picking the perfect potty are offered as well.

Kuhn, Brett R., Bethany A. Marcus, and Sheryl L. Pitner. "Treatment Guidelines for Primary Nonretentive Encopresis and Stool Toileting Refusal." American Family Physician 59, no. 8 (April 15, 1999): 2171-2178. Six guidelines for managing children with primary nonretentive encopresis, or stool toileting refusal, are outlined. Acase study demonstrates the efficacy and simplicity of these guidelines.

Loening-Baucke, Vera. "Clinical Approach to Fecal Soiling in Children." Clinical Pediatrics 39, no. 10 (October, 2000): 603. Fecal soiling is common in childhood and can be caused by stool toileting refusal, fecal incontinence due to organic disease, or encopresis due to functional constipation.

Wicks-Nelson, Rita, and Allen C. Israel. Behavior Disorders of Childhood. 6th ed. Upper Saddle River, N.J.: Pearson/Prentice Hall, 2008. An accessible text that details childhood behavior disorders, related clinical and research data, and updated coverage of treatment.

Woolf, Alan D., et al., eds. The Children's Hospital Guide to Your Child's Health and Development. Cambridge, Mass.: Perseus, 2002. An authoritative and comprehensive guide to children's health, providing a guide to every common illness or condition that affects children and a carefully designed emergency section.

SOLUTION-FOCUSED BRIEF THERAPY

Category: Treatment
Definition: Solution-Focused Brief Therapy is goal-orientated, solution-focused therapy that focuses on patients present and future.
Specialties and related fields: Brief Therapy, Psychotherapy, Psychology

Key terms:

miracle questions: questions that focus on identifying behaviors that would change if a patients problem miraculously resolved overnight

scalingquestions: questions that help patients quantify their situation, their objectives and overall prognosis for their own recover as a tool to track progress and make clear distinctions

exception questions: questions that focus on the 'exception to the rule' and help patients identify times where they could manage their problems and what behaviors were different in that time

coping questions: questions used to compliment the patient for managing with their problems thus far and identify the strengths they already possess that have helped them do so

E.A.R.S. (Elicit, Amplify, Reflect and Start): A process in which therapists elicit examples of what has changed for a patient, amplify those changes by identifying what specifically happened, reinforcing those changes by positive responses and having patients identify how they were able to accomplish them, and lastly, starting over with a new scenario

OVERVIEW

Solution-Focused Brief Therapy (SFBT) is a therapy practice that focuses on patients present and future over delving into their past. It is goal-orientated to help patients identify first what they want their future to look like and how they can create that future. Rather than problem-solving, SFBT's approach is to solution-build. Typically, SFBT only takes around 3-5 sessions which are spent creating an image of what the 'solution' is and discovering the tools needed to attain it. SFBT is based of the idea that focusing on solutions and positive aspects increases the brevity of therapy. The first session is spent helping patients clearly identify what their goals are and what are skills they have that can achieve the goals.

SBFT believes that patients can be effective in solving their problems and this capacity can be reached if they change their own negative ideas of the situation and focus on the exceptions to their problems. SBFT breaks the barrier of singular, permanent view a patient has on their problem and encourages them to see things in a different way. They can see big results by taking small steps. Based on the fact the patients are there to change, they can and will do their best to create a better world for themselves.

FIRST SESSION

The first session can use a number of techniques and lines of questioning to help identify the solution to a patient's problem.

The therapist would like to know, initially who the patient is and what he/she is hoping to gain from the sessions. The patient identifies his/her problem, how often and how intensely it happens. The idea is that the knowledge of and change for the problem comes from the patient, not the professional. Identifying a clear baseline helps track the progress of the patient and shows what the patient would like their life to be like once the knowledge and change needed is identified.

Another activity is to have the patient identify pre-session changes. This exercise uncovers what the patient has tried on their own to manage the problem prior to making the appointment and to make note of what changes they have noticed since beginning their journey.

The next element of the first session is the miracle question. Professionals ask if the patient goes to bed that night and wakes up to the problem resolved, what would be different in the patient's life tomorrow. This question separates patient from problem and results in the patient identifying what their own behaviors would look like if their world was miraculously changed. What would they do differently? Thus, miracle questions begin forming concrete ideas of what a resolved situation could look like and begin gaining a sense that this miracle outcome is attainable.

Another important factor is identified through exception questions. Exception questions can vary but primarily ask patients to identify the last time they didn't experience the problem, the last time they successfully managed the problem, and determine what was the exception with those times. Therapists want to learn what makes those times different as a way to identify the beneficial tools their patients already possess. These questions have the patient think of times when the problem was managed appropriately, escapable, or all together non-existent. Therapists also ask what are the times like where the 'miracle' is already happening. Patients are able to see their problems as temporary and can realize the skills they have at managing them.

Scaling questions usually use a scale of 1-10 to give patients a quantifiable way to describe their situation and potential outcomes. This gives patients a way to measure their progress. They are asked where on the scale was the problem at its worst, where the patient feels they are now on the scale and talk about the last time they were a 10. They also rank how much they feel change is possible. Scaling is also used to identify how long patients believe it will take to see results. What life would be like and how they would interact and behave in the world if they were up by one point.

Another line of questions is about coping. These questions ask patients how they have been dealing with their problems so far and how they keep going despite the hardship. It is a compliment to the person and gives them a feeling of power over their situation. This acclamation encourages patients to see the strengths they already have as a means to see themselves more positively. Rather than trying to reassure, or disvaluing a patient's view of the problem, coping questions help show patients their capabilities.

SECOND AND SUBSEQUENT SESSIONS

The second session seeks to identify what positive changes have happened for the patient thus far and takes a progress-focused approach. To identify this, therapists follow a process called E.A.R.S. This stands for Elicit, Amplify, Reflect and Start over.

Eliciting questions are used to explore what positive changes are already happening for the patient. Therapists ask the patient questions that promote reflection to consider what is better, however slightly the change may be. If a patient can not identify a positive change, the therapist instead asks how they have managed, what they have learned, what was the best part so far. Once a patient can recognize some positive difference, however small, the therapist's goal is to amplify those differences.

Amplifying questions help the patient focus on what made that situation different. It expands on the particulars of each situation. They ask patients when and how something happen, and how patients knew to do something. Exploring each situation can help patients see the importance and value of the changes. Once they can notice it, the therapist does their best to reinforce the change.

Reinforcing the change encourages patients to continue their path to positive change. It can be from complimenting them on their success to even non-verbal messages like leaning in, seeming impressed, raising eyebrows etc. Asking questions like how a patient did something can help reinforce their own internal tools to change.

Lastly, start over. Once a situation has been thoroughly examined for all the positive things patients have done to improve, the therapist then starts over. This plans for more change, identifies more situations they improved on and finds out what else is better.

—Briana Moglia

For Further Information:

Dolan, Yvonne. "What is Solution-Focused Therapy?" *Institute for Solution-Focused Therapy,* solutionfocused.net/what-is-solution- focused-therapy/. Overview of SFBT, it's key concepts, techniques, types of questions and a brief summary of a research studying supporting the effectiveness of SFBT.

Iveson, Chris. "Solution-Focused Brief Therapy." *Advances in Psychiatric Treatment,* The Royal College of Psychiatrists, 8 Mar. 2002, apt.rcpsych.org/content/8/2/149. History of SFBT and the basis behind the therapeutic process.

Northfield, John. "Solution-Focused Brief Therapy shows goal attainment gains in people with mild learning disabilities." *National Elf Service,* 26 Jan. 2016, www.nationalelfservice.net/learning-disabilities/challenging-behaviour/solution-focused-brief-therapy-shows-goal-attainment-gains-in-people-with-mild-learning-disabilities/. Summary of a study done in the Netherlands that compared using SFBT's to help people with mild learning disabilities to reach treatment goals versus people who received 'care as usual.'

"Solution Focused Therapy." *Solution Focused Therapy,* www.psychpage.com/family/library/sft.htm. Gives the steps of the process with examples of possible conversations between client and therapist.

SORE THROAT

Category: Disease/Disorder
Anatomy or system affected: Nose, respiratory system, throat
Specialties and related fields: Family medicine, otorhinolaryngology, pediatrics
Definition: Discomfort and/or pain experienced in the throat, which sometimes indicates the presence of a more serious disorder.

CAUSES AND SYMPTOMS

Sore throat, termed pharyngitis by medical practitioners, is a common cause of patient discomfort and visits to the doctor's office. Though many people equate sore throat with strep throat, in reality there are many infectious and noninfectious causes of this symptom. Sore throat can even be a sign of disease in another part of the body. The sensation, which may be described by sufferers as scratchy, raw, tight, burning, or achy, may last from minutes to months, depending on the underlying cause, and may be accompanied by related complaints such as fever, runny nose, hoarseness, or difficulty swallowing.

Most sore throats are caused by infection in the upper respiratory tract, including the ears, nose, and sinuses as well as the throat and tonsils. Research has demonstrated that more than half of these infections are caused by common viruses. Epstein-Barr virus, which causes mononucleosis, accounts for less than 10 percent. Most of the remainder are caused by various

INFORMATION ON SORE THROAT

Causes: Allergies, bacterial or viral infections, ingestion of foreign objects, thermal injury from hot beverage, chemical injury, external force from blow to neck, environmental irritants, lymph node inflammation
Symptoms: Scratchy, raw, tight, burning, or achy throat; may be accompanied by fever, runny nose, hoarseness, difficulty swallowing
Duration: Acute to several months
Treatments: Rest, increased fluid intake, analgesics, antibiotics if needed

bacteria. Of the bacterial causes, strep, more specifically group A beta-hemolytic *Streptococcus pyogenes*, is the most common pathogen (disease-causing organism). Additional bacterial causes include species of *Staphylococcus, Hemophilus, Mycoplasma,* non-group A streptococcus, and others. More rarely, fungi may account for a larger portion of throat infections in patients with weakened immune defenses.

Noninfectious causes of sore throat are quite varied. Although most are self-limited (resolving over time without treatment), some represent serious illness. These come into consideration especially if the duration of symptoms is longer than usual and if other aspects of the patient's health history suggest the likelihood of secondary causes.

Traumatic causes of throat discomfort include swallowing foreign objects, such as fish bones; thermal injury from a hot beverage; chemical injury from an ingestion, such as bleach; and external force from a blow to the neck. Environmental irritants, such as smoke and solvent fumes or allergies to dusts and pollens, cause symptoms in susceptible, exposed persons. Regurgitated stomach acid causes discomfort, which may be more pronounced when the patient is lying down. Enlargement of the thyroid gland or the salivary glands, cysts arising from embryonic structures such as the thyroglossal duct, or inflammation of lymph nodes can exert local pressure on the throat itself or on adjacent nerves, thereby eliciting symptoms. Cancer is the most ominous cause of sore throat symptoms, and it needs to be considered in patients with risk factors such as smoking and alcohol consumption.

Considering this expansive list of possibilities, which does not include every possible cause of sore throat, it is evident that the expedient diagnosis of sore throat is challenging. Though most sore throats resolve without treatment or complication, the practitioner must consider the possibility of rarer but potentially life-threatening diseases. The initial history and physical examination are sufficient in most cases to separate those patients who are likely to have an infectious cause from those who are unlikely to have one. Since most patients are initially concerned about the possibility of strep throat and the need for antibiotics, clinical algorithms, such as the Centor score, have been developed to assist this process. By tallying associated signs, symptoms, and patient characteristics, the practitioner may increase diagnostic accuracy. In some cases, additional testing, such as a rapid streptococcal antigen throat swab or a culture, is needed.

The search for noninfectious causes often begins when the patient returns with persisting symptoms. Since most throat infections resolve within a week or two, lingering discomfort suggests the need for further evaluation. In many cases, additional historical information from the patient and a follow-up physical examination will significantly narrow the list of possibilities. Clues such as weight loss, hoarseness, and a history of cigarette smoking and alcohol consumption increase the probability of cancer. Occupational information may uncover exposure to noxious dust or vapors. In difficult cases, diagnosis may require examination and biopsy of the throat during a procedure called laryngoscopy.

TREATMENT AND THERAPY

The treatments of noninfectious sore throat are as varied as the diagnoses themselves. The treatment of infectious sore throat depends on the underlying cause, ranging from rest, fluids, and analgesics (painkillers) for viruses to antibiotics for certain bacteria and fungi. Penicillin has been the mainstay of strep throat treatment since the mid-twentieth century. Before the discovery of penicillin, throat infection sometimes resulted in serious complications, such as rheumatic fever (which damages the heart valves) and glomerulonephritis (which damages the kidneys). Although group A *Streptococcus pyogenes* has remained remarkably sensitive to penicillin, reports have suggested that the treatment of strep throat is becoming more complex. The presence of other bacteria in the throat, some of which have developed the ability to inactivate penicillin, may actually protect the strep bacteria from the antibiotic. Interestingly, some research suggests that antibiotic treatment very early in the course of disease may even increase the likelihood of subsequent recurrence. Infections by bacteria other than strep or by fungi are treated with other antibiotic and antifungal drugs.

Given this scenario, one may wonder why doctors do not treat everyone with antibiotics, rather than going to the trouble and expense of diagnosing strep throat. Antibiotic treatment is complicated by many

factors, including cost, drug interactions, and the potential for fatal allergic reactions. Widespread use has led to the development of antibiotic-resistant strains of "super bacteria," which are very difficult if not impossible to treat.

—*Louis B. Jacques, MD*

See also Acid reflux disease; Antibiotics; Common cold; Epiglottitis; Influenza; Mouth and throat cancer; Multiple chemical sensitivity syndrome; Nasopharyngeal disorders; Otorhinolaryngology; Pharyngitis; Pharynx; Quinsy; Strep throat; Streptococcal infections; Tonsillectomy and adenoid removal; Tonsillitis; Tonsils; Voice and vocal cord disorders.

For Further Information:
Coutts, Cherylann. "A New Way to Treat Tonsil Trouble." *Parenting* 14, no. 10 (December, 2000/January, 2001): 33. If a child's physician determines that a tonsillectomy is required, a promising new procedure may be used. It uses radio-frequency energy to shrink tonsils, allowing for less pain and a much speedier recovery.
Evans, Julie A. "Thirteen Old-Fashioned Cold Remedies That Really Work!" *Prevention* 52, no. 11 (November, 2000): 106-113. Argues that good science is behind homemade elixirs for sniffles, sneezes, and other woes. Old-fashioned cold remedies, like honey and lemon for sore throats and chicken soup for a stuffy head, are discussed.
Ferrari, Mario. *PDxMD Ear, Nose, and Throat Disorders.* Philadelphia: PDxMD, 2003. A clinical yet accessible reference text that provides a comprehensive list of disorders, with a summary of the condition, background, diagnosis, treatment, outcomes, prevention, and resources.
Kemper, Kathi J. *The Holistic Pediatrician: A Pediatrician's Comprehensive Guide to Safe and Effective Therapies for the Twenty-five Most Common Ailments of Infants, Children, and Adolescents.* Rev. ed. New York: Quill, 2002. Integrates mainstream and alternative medicine to aid parents in dealing with the most common childhood health problems, such as fever, diaper rash, sore throats, ear infections, and allergies.
Kimball, Chad T. *Colds, Flu, and Other Common Ailments Sourcebook.* Detroit, Mich.: Omnigraphics, 2001. A comprehensive guide for general readers covering treatment issues and controversies surrounding common ailments and injuries. Includes discussions on ailments of the nose, throat, lungs, ears, eyes, and head; common injuries; alternative therapies; choosing a doctor; and buying drugs and finding health information online.
Litin, Scott C., ed. *Mayo Clinic Family Health Book.* 4th ed. New York: HarperResource, 2009. Perhaps the best general medical text for the layperson, this book covers the entire medical field. While the information is derived from a wide variety of highly technical sources, the articles are written to be easily understood by a general audience.
McIsaac, Warren J., Vivel Goel, Teresa To, and Donald E. Low. "The Validity of a Sore Throat Score in Family Practice." *Canadian Medical Association Journal* 163, no. 7 (October 3, 2000): 811. This study assessed the validity of a previously published clinical score for the management of infections of the upper respiratory tract accompanied by sore throat.

SPEECH DISORDERS

Category: Disease/Disorder
Anatomy or system affected: Ears, muscles, musculoskeletal system, psychic-emotional system
Specialties and related fields: Audiology, psychiatry, psychology, speech pathology
Definition: Dysfunction in the brain-coordinated use of speech organs, such as problems with language, vocal quality, articulation, fluency, and dementia.
Key terms:

aphasia: a partial or total loss of the ability to articulate ideas; often results from brain damage

articulation: the act or process of speaking correctly, as a result of appropriate movement and coordination of the speech organs

connective tissue: tissues possessing a highly vascular structure that form support and connecting structures of the body (for example, cartilage, ligaments, and tendons)

dysfluency: another term for stuttering

dysfunction: the disordered or impaired function of a body system or organ

organic: pertaining to, arising from, or affecting a body organ

psychogenic: originating in the mind or in mental conditions and activities

stuttering: a disorder involving speaking with spasmodic hesitation, prolongation, and/or repetition of sounds

CAUSES AND SYMPTOMS

Learning to speak correctly is of great importance to all people. It involves the brain-coordinated use of the mouth, jaws, lips, and tongue, as well as of the vocal cords, lungs, and diaphragm. On average, children learn to talk during their second year by imitating the speech of those persons, mostly family members, with whom frequent and close contact is maintained. Hence, it is important that young children hear correct speech.

The development of speech is viewed as occurring in several distinct stages. First, babies make involuntary noises in response to physical stimuli. Then, they begin to enjoy making these noises at about two months of age. Next, about nine months after birth, they start to imitate the sounds and inflections of the speech of others around them. Beginning at twelve to eighteen months of age, children start to vocalize in a meaningful way, and in due time, they learn to speak.

In many cases, however, a child is quickly found to have some difficulties with the use of speech or with its development to levels viewed as appropriate within expected time spans. Such children suffer from speech

---

INFORMATION ON SPEECH DISORDERS

Causes: Dementia, brain injury, neurologic disorders, birth defects, cleft palate
Symptoms: Inappropriate pitch or sound quality (e.g., hoarseness), lack of audibility, inappropriate loudness, stuttering, speech rate and speech rhythm problems, aphasias
Duration: Temporary to chronic
Treatments: Surgical and dental treatment, behavior and speech modification

---

disorders including stuttering, lisping, and lack of speech comprehension. They should receive appropriate professional help as soon as possible. Others are born with physical problems, such as cleft palate, which make appropriate speech impossible without medical intervention. Smaller numbers of people develop speech disorders later in life for various reasons, including accidents that damage the brain or the mechanical organs of speech, as well as the physical and mental ravages of advanced age.

Speech disorders fall into three main categories: problems associated with speech production, difficulties of articulation, and dysfunction in the ability to utilize language. These disorders have been known since antiquity and although they are frequently hereditary, the genetic cause is often unclear. In fact, there is often a psychogenic aspect to their origin as well.

Another broad means of categorizing speech disorders is by dividing them into causative organic and nonorganic groups. The term "organic speech disorder" is used to indicate birth defects or later injuries to the brain or the structures, muscles, and connective tissues that are required to produce speech. The disorders for which no such origin can be clearly identified with existing techniques fall into the nonorganic group. Usually, they are attributed solely to psychogenic factors. It is probable, however, that they have subtle organic causes that are beyond present methods of identification.

Speech disorders may be associated with articulation, voice, fluency, language, and dementia. The cures for all these types of speech disorders vary; they include the interactive participation of teachers in school systems and the attention of speech professionals such as audiologists, surgeons, psychiatrists, and physical therapists. Each case must be analyzed carefully and then treated individually. Even so, varied success is obtained from patient to patient, regardless of the disorder, the nature of the therapeutic procedures utilized, and the therapists who are involved.

Articulation disorders are attributable to the inappropriate sequential movement of the jaw, tongue, and related speech structures. Minor, nonpathological differences result in regional differences (accents) in the spoken language within a country. Pathological problems that cause speech that cannot be understood are most often organic in nature. Examples include cleft palate and neurologic dysfunction. Voice disorders include inappropriate pitch, sound quality (for example, hoarseness), lack of audibility, or inappropriate loudness. Fluency disorders are most often identified with stuttering, speech rate problems, and speech rhythm problems. The best-known language disorders are the aphasias, which are characterized by poor language comprehension and childhood language impairment (often resulting from developmental problems). Dementia can impair speech at any age, but it is most common in the elderly, for whom memory, language, and cognitive ability may be greatly impaired.

TREATMENT AND THERAPY

Many viewpoints exist concerning the treatment of speech disorders. All agree, however, that interaction between family, patient, teachers, and various clinicians is essential. Disorders of articulation are quite common and range from mild problems (for example, a lisp) to those which are so extreme that the speech of afflicted individuals becomes unintelligible. Many of the most severe of these speech disorders arise from the organic impairment of motor control in the speech musculature, which may be attributable to stroke, cleft palate, or even the loss of lips or other speech system components.

Frequently, efforts at remediating such problems must include surgical and dental treatment. After any necessary corrective surgery and/or dentistry, many treatment regimens focus on behavior modification. Affected individuals receive instruction regarding the physical basis of their problems and are then trained to overcome them as effectively as possible.

In many cases, the use of psychological and psychiatric counseling is considered to be of great value. Some experts suggest, however, that the main effect of such therapy is to enable afflicted individuals to live comfortably with the imperfections in articulation that remain after all treatments are tried.

Voice disorders occur when the phonatory mechanism is dysfunctional. They range from the consequences of laryngeal, oral, or respiratory disease to the misuse of the phonatory system, which may reflect psychological state. Such functional disorders, if left untreated for too long, may lead to organic damage. In the case of pitch abnormalities, causative factors may include psychological tension, an undersized larynx, misformed vocal cords, and hearing problems, either individually or in various combinations.

Disorders of voice quality likewise have many physical sources, including larynx and vocal cord abnormalities, and ones of psychogenic origin. The disorders associated with loudness range from overly loud voices caused by workplace noise or hearing loss to extremely soft ones that are generally psychogenic. Treatment of all such disorders begins with the disqualification of treatable organic problems. In the case of psychogenic disorders, psychiatric counseling can be extremely helpful. Psychological and medical treatments must be followed, however, by very thorough interaction with speech-language pathologists if optimum results are to be obtained.

Disorders of fluency most often involve stuttering, also called dysfluency, which features spasmodic hesitation and the prolongation or repetition of sounds. In addition, stuttering is often accompanied by tics and other uncontrolled body movements. The basis for the problem is unclear, and different experts point to learned behavior, psychogenic origins, or organic roots. There is no cure for dysfluency, but it (and the accompanying nonspeech problems) can be greatly diminished. Treatment usually involves both psychiatric counseling and behavior and/or speech modification by speech-language pathologists as well as by other related speech professionals. Such therapy varies widely from individual to individual and with the age of the patient.

Language disorders are characterized by the diminished ability to use or to understand spoken language. In children, these disorders are often identified as language delay or development aphasias. They are most often thought to be attributable to intellectual disabilities, hearing loss, or autism. When lost hearing is not the main problem, the treatments for such language problems often involve behavior modification techniques. In all cases in which hearing loss is an important component, its correction is the first effort; such efforts may work wonders. When hearing problems cannot be remediated entirely, however, the overall treatment will be much less successful because hearing the speech of others is so important to speech development.

True aphasia is very often viewed as speech impairment; it occurs in adults as a result of stroke, accidents that produce severe head trauma, or dementia. It is desirable to begin treatment of afflicted persons as soon as possible after aphasia is observed. Some rapid and spontaneous healing of lost language ability occurs, and this healing can be maximized by the efforts of speech-language pathologists. The continued treatment of aphasias is very important and usually follows careful evaluation of its causes. It is often possible to make progressive, long-term advances in healing aphasias. Complete recovery is rare, however, and the use of sign language or personal computers for interpersonal communication may be necessary.

PERSPECTIVE AND PROSPECTS

For many years, it was thought that speech disorders were caused only by insoluble psychological problems in the very young or by severe head, facial, and brain trauma later in life. It is now clear that they have other causes, ranging from hearing loss to dementia. Furthermore, it is currently understood that speech problems of every type can attack anyone-young children, adolescents, and adults of all ages.

These problems often have disastrous psychological and economic effects on the afflicted person. Young children may be traumatized if speech disorders are not treated early; in severe cases, they may later be unable to enter the workforce in meaningful positions or to receive anything above the most rudimentary education. This is unfortunate because many such problems of childhood, adolescence, and even young adulthood can be almost completely solved by careful medical examination, followed quickly by appropriate corrective action.

There is also help available for older people who develop speech problems because of aging, dementia, or harmful workplace conditions. In all cases, once a sound treatment plan is developed, it is essential that the afflicted person follow it rigorously. Miracles should not be expected; rather, sustained interaction between the treatment team-especially the patient and a speech-language pathologist-must be undertaken. Furthermore, the psychological support of the patient's family and friends has been recognized as a crucial factor in many successful treatment plans.

In the case of the young child, the diagnosis of speech problems by schoolteachers can be another important means to treatment. Once a problem is observed, the child's family can be advised concerning special education available through the school system or local programs. Teachers should be cautioned, however, against attempts to treat the child in question unless they have adequate training. The job of unspecialized teachers should be diagnosis and the recommendation of an appropriate treatment group. When speech disorder therapy results in less-than-adequate treatment of extremely serious problems, the use of sign language, special typewriters, and computer-assisted communication, as well as psychotherapy, should be considered.

Overall, the treatment of speech problems has improved, and its sensible application can enable patients to enter into or return to the workforce at levels commensurate with their abilities, can prevent them from becoming maladjusted, and can enrich society as a whole. Dealing with such problems in the young is particularly important because it may help to prevent neuroses and psychoses from developing. It is hoped that ongoing research will continue to increase the avenues available for the prevention and cure of speech disorders, to identify additional methods for treating them, and to result in their eradication.

—*Sanford S. Singer, PhD*

See also Alzheimer's disease; Aphasia and dysphasia; Audiology; Autism; Birth defects; Brain damage; Cerebral palsy; Cleft lip and palate; Cleft lip and palate repair; Deafness; Dementias; Developmental disorders; Dyslexia; Ear surgery; Ears; Electroencephalography (EEG); Jaw wiring; Laryngitis; Learning disabilities; Lisping; Paralysis; Strokes; Stuttering; Tics; Tonsillitis; Tourette's syndrome; Transient ischemic attacks (TIAs); Voice and vocal cord disorders.

For Further Information:

American Psychiatric Association. *Diagnostic and Statistical Manual of Mental Disorders: DSM-IV-TR*. 4th ed. Arlington, Va.: Author, 2000. This classic text contains diagnostic criteria and other useful facts about a variety of mental disorders, including those associated with speech dysfunction.

Beers, Mark H., et al., eds. *The Merck Manual of Diagnosis and Therapy*. 18th ed. Whitehouse Station, N.J.: Merck Research Laboratories, 2006. Contains useful data on the characteristics, etiology, diagnosis, and treatment of speech disorders and related processes. Although the text is designed for physicians, the material should be useful to general readers as well.

Cole, Patricia R. *Language Disorders in Preschool Children*. Englewood Cliffs, N.J.: Prentice Hall, 1982. This book by an expert speech-language pathologist explains the modalities associated with solving speech-language disorders. Solid and well referenced, it covers language development, disorders, diagnosis, and treatment. Much useful information concerning learning semantics and syntax.

Gelfand, Stanley A. *Essentials of Audiology*. 2d ed. New York: Thieme, 2009. Undergraduate text covering a wide range of relevant topics, including acoustics, anatomy and physiology, sound perception, auditory disorders and their related speech disorders, and the nature of hearing impairment.

Lubinski, Rosemary, and Carol M. Frattali, eds. *Professional Issues in Speech-Language Pathology and Audiology*. San Diego, Calif.: Thomson/Delmar Learning, 2007. For those interested in entering the field of audiology. Covers the practicalities of a career path, ethical-legal considerations, professional organizations, and ongoing issues in health care, among other topics.

Paul, Rhea. *Language Disorders from Infancy Through Adolescence: Assessment and Interventions*. 3d ed. St. Louis, Mo.: Mosby/Elsevier, 2007. An introductory text that covers pediatric language disorders across various ages, assessment and treatment of those disorders, public policy, and special pediatric populations.

Winitz, Harris, ed. *Human Communication and Its Disorders: A Review*. Vol. 4. Timonium, Md.: York Press, 1995. This authoritative text covers in detail the prominent disorders of human communications: their occurrence, symptoms, and treatment. Both organic and nonorganic aspects of these communication problems are carefully explored and referenced.

SPERM BANKS

Category: Organization
Anatomy or system affected: Genitals, psychic-emotional system, reproductive system, uterus
Specialties and related fields: Biotechnology, ethics, genetics, infertility, obstetrics, urology
Definition: The identification of suitable sperm donors and the evaluation, processing, storage and distribution of their semen for use in assisted reproductive technology.
Key terms:
insemination: the process of placing semen in the female reproductive tract; natural insemination occurs during sexual intercourse, while artificial (or donor) insemination is performed with medical instruments in a clinic
semen: the male reproductive fluid consisting of two parts, a liquid called seminal plasma and living reproductive cells called sperm

INDICATIONS AND PROCEDURES

Sperm banks exist primarily to help women with normal adult premenopausal reproductive function to become pregnant. A woman seeking pregnancy may need the services of a sperm bank if her male partner is infertile, if she is in a lesbian relationship, or if she chooses to be a single mother. When a man in a heterosexual relationship produces too few sperm for his female partner's pregnancy, sperm from a sperm bank can help the couple become pregnant through artificial (or donor) insemination. An additional purpose of sperm banking is to allow men who have cancer to preserve their sperm before undergoing chemotherapy or radiation, which might render them infertile or compromise the quality of their sperm.

A sperm bank makes available the sperm from a number of qualified donors. The primary task of a clinical sperm bank is to preserve sperm and identify suitable donors, based upon medical and biological criteria. The sperm bank does a medical physical examination of donor candidates and obtains an extensive medical and family history from them. Special attention is given to semen quality and to the risk of transmitting infectious or genetic diseases.

Semen quality has two major components. The first component is whether the semen has enough fertile sperm with appropriate motility and morphology to create a pregnancy. The second component is whether enough sperm in the semen survive freezing. Freezing in a special way (cryopreservation) to keep sperm alive is the only way a sperm bank can store its semen inventory. Another important reason for cryopreservation is related to infectious disease testing. For example, a donor is tested for acquired immunodeficiency

syndrome (AIDS) at the time he produces the semen, but the test is repeated six months later to increase its certainty. The cryopreservation allows the semen to be stored during this "quarantine" period. Donors are tested for a variety of diseases that can be transmitted through semen: AIDS, gonorrhea, chlamydia, syphilis, trichomonas, and well-known sexually transmitted infections (STIs); and viral hepatitis, cytomegalovirus, and human T-lymphotropic virus (HTLV).

The genetics of a donor is very important. Genes are responsible for each person's positive attributes and negative ones (genetic diseases). There are no genetically perfect persons; there are no perfect donors. There are only a few hundred genetic tests for more than five thousand genetic conditions; therefore comprehensive testing for genetic disease is impractical. Sperm banks usually screen donors routinely for a few very common diseases with a genetic component, such as diabetes, gout, and high cholesterol. Additional tests may be done on donors of certain ethnic backgrounds for diseases linked to specific ethnicities: cystic fibrosis, Canavan disease, Gaucher disease, sickle cell disease, Tay-Sachs disease. Each sperm bank will have its own list.

Fortunately, both parents determine a child's genetics. The genetic attributes of one often will compensate for the liabilities of the other. A person choosing a donor would be wise to seek the help of a certified genetics counselor. A genetics counselor will help match the genetics of the woman with the genetics of possible donors.

Considering all that is involved in identifying each suitable donor, a sperm bank requires donors to provide many "samples," not only of semen but also of blood. Additionally, there are annual physical exams, perhaps a psychological exam, and other tests. It is understandable that the bank compensates donors for their time and effort in participating; this is different from "buying sperm." Similarly, sperm banks receive a fee for their efforts in recruiting and evaluating donors plus their work in evaluating, processing, and providing semen to physicians and their patients.

Semen is normally available to a patient through a physician or other medical clinician trained in artificial insemination. Sometimes a patient will request self-inseminating at her home. This is possible with physician authorization, meaning that the physician retains responsibility for mistakes that might occur. The requested semen is delivered frozen by the sperm bank in a shipping container similar to a thermos. The semen is thawed immediately before insemination.

USES AND COMPLICATIONS

There are many personal decisions to be made regarding artificial insemination. Often there are psychological effects on the woman to be inseminated and her partner. Usually artificial insemination is done with semen from an anonymous donor, thus preventing any social contact between donor and recipient. The use of an anonymous donor usually conveys full parental rights and responsibilities on the partner of the recipient, relieving the donor of any responsibility. Sometimes the recipient or her partner want to use a donor known to them, a directed donor. Although this is possible, it raises legal and psychological issues that are not fully known. These issues about the kind of donor also have implications for the psychology of the offspring. There are many medical decisions to be made regarding artificial insemination. The procedure must be done at the time of ovulation, an event occurring between menstrual periods. The occurrence of ovulation can be determined in several ways, often by hormonal tests. The physician must decide whether to do one or more inseminations at ovulation. If the timing is off, the patient will not become pregnant. Another attempt can be made on the next monthly cycle.

Although many women will become pregnant with semen placed in the vagina at the entrance to the uterus, many physicians and other clinicians will increase the success of insemination by placing the se-men into the woman's uterus. Intrauterine insemination (IUI) requires removing the semen from the seminal plasma, administering substances that cause the uterus to contract strongly, and discharging the sperm into the uterus through a catheter.

Other complications include the possibility of infection or genetic problems. Although the sperm has been properly tested, tests are not perfect. The patient must remember that even when all aspects of insemination are technically perfect, the complex biology of making a baby from a fertilized egg can go wrong.

PERSPECTIVE AND PROSPECTS

Horse breeders may have successfully used artificial insemination as early as the fourteenth century. In 1776, John Hunter, an English surgeon, may have been the first person to successfully artificially inseminate a woman. Cryopreservation of bull semen was developed in England in the early 1950s. An American urologist, Raymond H. Bunge, was the first physician to successfully use cryopreserved human semen. Many sperm banks were established in the early 1980s so that semen could be quarantined to prevent the transmission of AIDS. Today, sperm banks are being used to guarantee male fertility for men with medical problems as well as to allow women to reproduce. Sperm banks

Example of a liquid nitrogen cryogenic tank at life sciences laboratory Photo via iStock/anamejia18 {Used under license.]

have expanded to become embryo banks. Future technology will permit cryopreservation of human eggs. These banks will be contributing components of genetic medicine.

*—Armand M. Karow, PhD;
updated by Robin Kamienny Montvilo, RN, PhD*

See also Assisted reproductive technologies; Childbirth; Cloning; Conception; Gynecology; Infertility, female; Infertility, male; Men's health; Obstetrics; Pregnancy and gestation; Reproductive system; Screening; Semen; Uterus.

For Further Information:
Bahadur, G., et al. "Factors Affecting Sperm Banking for Adolescent Cancer Patients." *Archives of Diseases in Children* 91, no. 8 (2006): 715-716.
Berger, Gary S., Mark Fuerst, and Marc Goldstein. *The Couple's Guide to Fertility.* 3d ed. New York: Broadway Books, 2001.
Critser, J. K. "Current Status of Semen Banking in the USA." *Human Reproduction* 13, supp. 2 (1998): 55-65.
Doherty, C. Maud, and Melanie M. Clark. *Fertility Handbook: A Guide to Getting Pregnant.* Omaha, Nebr.: Addicus Books, 2002.
Mohler, Marie, and Lacy Frazer. *A Donor Insemination Guide: Written by and for Lesbian Women.* New York: Alice Street Editions/Harrington Park Press, 2002.
Pence, Gregory E. *Re-creating Medicine: Ethical Issues at the Frontiers of Medicine.* Lanham, Md.: Rowman & Littlefield, 2007.
Schover, Leslie R., and Anthony J. Thomas. *Overcoming Male Infertility: Understanding Its Causes and Treatments.* New York: John Wiley & Sons, 2000.
Vercollone, Carol Frost, Heidi Moss, and Robert Moss. *Helping the Stork: The Choices and Challenges of Donor Insemination.* New York: John Wiley & Sons, 1997.
Zouves, Christo. *Expecting Miracles: On the Path of Hope from Infertility to Parenthood.* New York: Berkley, 2003.

SPHINCTERECTOMY

Category: Procedure
Anatomy or system affected: Anus, bladder, eyes, intestines, muscles, musculoskeletal system
Specialties and related fields: General surgery, ophthalmology
Definition: The surgical removal of all or a portion of a sphincter, a ring of muscle that closes or constricts an opening or passage in the body when the muscles contract.

INDICATIONS AND PROCEDURES

In the human body, sphincters can be found in the internal and external region of the anus, in the area that joins the large and small intestine, between the urinary bladder and the urethra, at the lower end of the esophagus, and in the pupil of the eye. While located in a variety of areas of the body, each has in common the ability to allow or prevent the passage of something (solid, liquid, or light) through it when relaxed or constricted, respectively. A variety of conditions may lead to the need for surgical intervention to restore proper functioning of a sphincter or an associated organ.

Spinal cord injuries may lead to the need for bladder management intervention, especially in men. An option for those who do not prefer intermittent catheterization for bladder control is to slit the urethral sphincter to create a low-pressure bladder system that allows evacuation without need for muscular control of the sphincter.

Splits in the lining of the rectum called anal fissures can be caused by hard bowel movements. For chronic conditions that do not heal because of anal spasms, cutting the outermost portion of the anal sphincter may relieve the spasms and speed healing.

In patients afflicted with both cataracts and glaucoma, excision of a portion of the pupillary band of the iris can aid in removing the cataract while dealing with potential pressure buildup caused by glaucoma.

USES AND COMPLICATIONS

Although surgery to correct tears or defects in sphincters is more common than their removal, in cases of extreme damage or disease, useless sphincters must be surgically excised. For the removal of internal sphincters, the patient is opened surgically and the appropriate organs are moved to expose the sphincter in question; external sphincterectomies are performed without incisions in the body cavity. A scalpel is used to dissect the sphincter away from the surrounding tissue. Bleeding vessels are repaired, and the incisions are closed.

After removal, an individual will lack the control provided by the sphincter, such as control of defecation or urination, and alternative means of compensating for this loss will be presented to the patient. As in all surgeries, patients must be aware of any potential indications of infection such as fever, redness at the area of incision, and bleeding.

—Karen E. Kalumuck, PhD

See also Anus; Cataract surgery; Cataracts; Colon; Esophagus; Eye infections and disorders; Eye surgery, Eyes; Gastroenterology; Gastroenterology, pediatric; Gastrointestinal disorders; Gastrointestinal system; Glaucoma; Intestinal disorders; Intestines; Muscle sprains, spasms, and disorders; Muscles; Peristalsis; Rectum; Small intestine; Urinary disorders; Urinary system; Urology; Urology, pediatric.

For Further Information:
Daniel, Edwin E., et al., eds. *Sphincters: Normal Function-Changes in Disease.* Boca Raton, Fla.: CRC Press, 1992.
Friedman, Scott L., Kenneth R. McQuaid, and James H. Grendell, eds. *Current Diagnosis and Treatment in Gastroenterology.* 2d ed. New York: Lang Medical Books/McGraw-Hill, 2003.

Griffith, H. Winter. *Complete Guide to Symptoms, Illness, and Surgery.* Revised and updated by Stephen Moore and Kenneth Yoder. 5th ed. New York: Perigee, 2006.

Holschneider, Alexander M., and Prem Puri, eds. *Hirschsprung's Disease and Allied Disorders.* 3d ed. New York: Springer, 2008.

Janowitz, Henry D. *Your Gut Feelings: A Complete Guide to Living Better with Intestinal Problems.* Rev. ed. New York: Oxford University Press, 1995.

SPIDER BITES. SEE BITES AND STINGS.

SPINA BIFIDA

Category: Disease/Disorder
Also known as: Myelocele, meningomyelocele, lipomeningocele
Anatomy or system affected: Bones, brain, nervous system, spine
Specialties and related fields: Embryology, neonatology, perinatology, plastic surgery
Definition: A birth defect that results from a mistake early in the development of the spinal cord.
Key terms:
central nervous system: the brain and spinal cord
hydrocephalus: the abnormal accumulation of fluid within the developing brain
neural plate: a layer of tissue in the early embryo from which the brain and spinal cord will develop
neuropore: a small opening into the interior of the brain or spinal cord of the embryo
vertebra: an individual bone in the spine

CAUSES AND SYMPTOMS

The development of the fetal nervous system is the most complicated process during pregnancy. It starts a few weeks after conception and continues until well after birth. The earliest steps are the most crucial, because the basic plan of the nervous system must be established accurately if it is to work properly later.

The central nervous system begins with the formation of a thickened layer of tissue, called the neural plate, along the back of the embryo. The edges of this plate curl up to form ridges, and the whole plate rolls up into a slender tube running from the head to the rump. This cylinder is then covered over by tissues that will form the surface of the back. The front end of this tube will soon expand to become the brain, and the rest of the tube will form the spinal cord. In order for these processes to proceed properly, the tube must seal itself along its entire length. If there are any gaps where the tube does not close, it will leak and will not be able to expand and develop properly. Without such expansion,

> ### INFORMATION ON SPINA BIFIDA
> **Causes:** Birth defect
> **Symptoms:** Bulging spinal cord, hydrocephalus, paralysis in lower back and legs, bladder and bowel malfunction, loss of sensation, mental impairment
> **Duration:** Chronic
> **Treatments:** Surgery, catheterization, prostheses, physical therapy, sometimes fetal surgery

all the later stages of nervous system development will also be prevented from occurring properly.

If the neural tube fails to seal, a small opening called a neuropore will remain at some point along its length. Depending on where the opening is, a variety of abnormalities can result. When the posterior region of the neural tube fails to close, the result is spina bifida. This flaw in the neural tube in turn affects the assembly of the muscle, bone, and skin in this region. In spina bifida, which means "divided spine," the vertebrae of the backbone do not join together properly.

The severity of spina bifida depends on how much damage has been done to the lower spinal cord region. In its mildest form, the only evidence of a problem may be that two of the bones in the spine fail to form quite right. If several vertebrae are involved, the membranes that protect the surface of the spinal cord can bulge outward, forming a ball-like mass in this region. The problems that result depend on how much of the spinal membrane is involved in this bulge. In the most severe cases, the vertebrae fail to protect the spinal cord, so that the nervous tissue itself is also involved and an opening to the outside remains at the base of the spinal cord. Additional problems with nervous system development may result, including improper fluid balances in the brain (hydrocephalus).

Because the brain and spinal column fail to develop properly in spina bifida, a variety of mental, behavioral, and physical symptoms can result. The nerve connections at the base of the spine are likely to be affected, resulting in paralysis in the lower back and legs, problems with bladder and bowel function, and loss of sensation. Because the development of the brain can also be affected, mental abilities may be impaired.

TREATMENT AND THERAPY

Effective measures have been developed to minimize the effects of spina bifida. Often, surgery is performed within twenty-four to forty-eight hours of birth to close any opening in the child's lower back and to reconstruct the spine and other tissues in this area. Problems with feet and legs may also be dealt with surgically. If the

Types of Spina Bifida

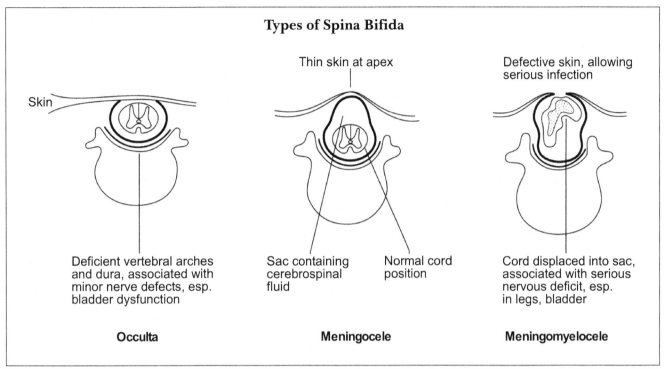

Occulta — Skin; Deficient vertebral arches and dura, associated with minor nerve defects, esp. bladder dysfunction

Meningocele — Thin skin at apex; Sac containing cerebrospinal fluid; Normal cord position

Meningomyelocele — Defective skin, allowing serious infection; Cord displaced into sac, associated with serious nervous deficit, esp. in legs, bladder

©EBSCO

child has symptoms of hydrocephalus, the excess fluid will be drained. Bladder and bowel function will be regulated, such as by catheterization. Eventually, prosthetic devices may be fitted to assist the child's movement. Mental health and physical therapy experts will also be involved to assist in overcoming learning hurdles, monitoring physical development and training, and making emotional adjustments.

PERSPECTIVE AND PROSPECTS
Spina bifida has been known since ancient times, but little could be done then to ease the mental and physical damage that it causes. By the 1960s, surgical procedures were being developed that could repair the damage to the spinal cord and other parts of the lower back. Improvements in physical therapy methods, as well as improved prosthetic devices, also began to make physical activity a realistic prospect for these children.

Late in the twentieth century, new insights were gained into the causes of spina bifida. The mutated genes involved were identified, and it was learned why they do not work properly. Studies of neural tube defects in mice revealed how these defects occur and how best to prevent them.

It is now known that the diet of a pregnant woman can influence neural tube development. One of the most effective measures for preventing spina bifida has been shown to be the daily intake of folic acid. Recommended doses vary from 0.4 to 4.0 mg per day based on risk status, such as prior delivery of a baby with

neural tube defects. Preconceptual counseling includes recommendations for prenatal vitamins (which contain significantly more folic acid than other multivitamins) to be taken even before pregnancy. In 2000, it was reported that a folic acid supplement program for pregnant women that took place over a six-year period in South Carolina cut in half the rate of neural tube defects, including spina bifida. Doctors now know that folic acid supplements starting at the point of conception can decrease the risk of spina bifida by as much as 75 percent.

For fetuses that develop spina bifida, fetal surgery, which occurs while the fetus is in the womb, has become an option for parents. Fetal surgery can improve brain malformations, making it unnecessary for many babies to need lifelong shunts-devices that allow drainage of fluid that has accumulated around the brain. Even with the demonstrated benefits of the surgery, however, there is no guarantee that the surgery can correct all neurological functions or that it will be successful for all babies. In fact, it has been shown that fetal surgery increases the risk of a baby being born prematurely, which poses a whole new set of problems.

Support organizations for families can help them cope with the challenges of caring for children with spina bifida. Physical therapy, counseling, and various group activities are available. Thanks to improved treatment and support, it is now possible for children with this condition to lead long and healthy lives.

—*Howard L. Hosick, PhD*

See also Amniocentesis; Birth defects; Brain damage; Chiari malformations; Congenital disorders; Embryology; Fetal surgery; Genetic diseases; Hydrocephalus; Intellectual disability; Neonatology; Nervous system; Neurology; Neurology, pediatric; Neurosurgery; Perinatology; Plastic surgery; Spinal cord disorders; Spine, vertebrae, and disks; Stillbirth.

For Further Information:

Bloom, Beth-Ann, and Edward L. Seljeskog. *A Parent's Guide to Spina Bifida*. Minneapolis: University of Minnesota Press, 1988. Designed to assist the parents of children with spina bifida. The book includes chapters on the nature of the disorder and how it is treated, the medical problems associated with spina bifida, and how to help the afflicted child while he or she is growing up.

Kimball, Chad T. *Childhood Diseases and Disorders Sourcebook: Basic Consumer Health Information About Medical Problems Often Encountered in Pre-adolescent Children*. Detroit, Mich.: Omnigraphics, 2003. Offers basic facts about cancer, sickle cell disease, diabetes, and other chronic conditions in children and discusses frequently used diagnostic tests, surgeries, and medications. Long-term care for seriously ill children is also presented.

McLone, David. *An Introduction to Spina Bifida*. Reprint. Washington, DC: Spina Bifida Association of America, 1998. A concise report on spinal dysraphism and related disorders. Illustrations illuminate the text.

Martin, Richard J., Avroy A. Fanaroff, and Michele C. Walsh, eds. *Fanaroff and Martin's Neonatal-Perinatal Medicine: Diseases of the Fetus and Infant*. 2 vols. 8th ed. Philadelphia: Mosby/Elsevier, 2006. This classic reference work is one of the most comprehensive to date and features discussions on the diverse practice of neonatal-perinatal medicine, pregnancy disorders and their impact on the fetus, delivery room care, provisions for neonatal care, and the development and disorder of organ systems.

Moore, Keith L., and T. V. N. Persaud. *The Developing Human*. 8th ed. Philadelphia: Saunders/Elsevier, 2008. An outstanding textbook on human embryonic development, with specific information about the causes of congenital malformations and common defects occurring in each of the body's systems.

Nightingale, Elena O., and Melissa Goodman. *Before Birth: Prenatal Testing for Genetic Disease*. Cambridge, Mass.: Harvard University Press, 1990. Offering practical guidance to prospective parents, this volume addresses the question of whether or not to undergo testing, and if elected, how best to use the results.

Spina Bifida Association. www.sbaa.org. Promotes the prevention of spina bifida and strives to enhance the lives of all affected. Offers newsletter, physician referrals, and scholarship funds, among other services.

Spinal cord disorders

Category: Disease/Disorder
Anatomy or system affected: Bones, musculoskeletal system, nerves, nervous system, spine
Specialties and related fields: Emergency medicine, neurology, physical therapy

Definition: Conditions that adversely affect the spinal cord, which normally carries sensory information from the skin and muscles to the brain and returns with information to control movement.

Key terms:

congenital malformation: an abnormal condition that exists at birth

lesion: damage to cells, tissues, or organs that results in lost or impaired function; spinal cord lesion usually involves motor and/or sensory nerve fiber tracts

neuroglia: nonneuronal support cells of the central nervous system; oligodendrocytes are one type of neuroglia that myelinate nerve fibers

neuron: a nerve cell, the functional unit of the nervous system, containing dendrite and axon processes specialized for carrying information toward and away from the cell body, respectively

neurotrophic factor: a chemical signal that is required for the normal differentiation and function of neurons; this signal is often produced by neuroglia or by the cells with which neurons form synapses

plasticity: the ability of the nervous system to change its function over time by experience; includes changes in nerve fiber networks

teratogen: a chemical that causes abnormal embryonic development; often an environmental pollutant or something to which the mother is exposed during pregnancy, such as alcohol or other drugs

CAUSES AND SYMPTOMS

Most people take certain basic tasks for granted, such as walking up a flight of stairs, brushing their teeth, or using a personal computer. Motor neurons in the spinal cord control the hundreds of muscle fibers that are involved in each of these activities. At the same time, other neurons of the spinal cord serve as part of the sensory pathways that provide information regarding body position and motion that contributes to the coordination of these activities. In amyotrophic lateral sclerosis (ALS), also known as Lou Gehrig's disease, the motor neurons in the spinal cord die, leaving patients without control of their muscles. This example of a spinal disorder serves to emphasize the important role that the spinal cord plays as it serves as an interface (input-output system) between the brain and the body.

Similarly, most people have experienced pain in the hand, which is followed by an instantaneous, automatic movement of the hand away from the object causing that pain. Such reflexes represent the simplest of movements, yet they still require the integrative and relay action of neurons of the spinal cord to cause immediate hand withdrawal without requiring the individual to think about the act consciously. Only after the reflex has occurred does the spinal cord activity "inform" the brain that something happened. Therefore, in addition to sensory and motor interface functions for the brain, the spinal cord performs basic integration tasks as it controls reflexes, contributes to the coordination of movement between the left and right sides of the body and prevents opposing muscle groups from trying to move a joint in opposite directions at the same time. As with any other vital organ of the body, spinal cord damage or defects have serious consequences for the health and well-being of humans.

In the medical research laboratory, paralysis results from complete or partial transection of the spinal cord. In the real world, a fracture or dislocation of vertebrae or damage done by a bullet can cause paralysis in the same fashion. Acute transection of the spinal cord can also result from an inflammatory condition or from any situation in which the spinal cord is compressed, such as by a tumor. The spinal cord is contained within the vertebral column, which is divided into the cervical, thoracic, lumbar, and sacral regions, each of which is associated with a specific set of functions. Transection typically results in the loss of sensory and motor functions below the level of the lesion.

Spinal cord injuries and defects are the result of three basic types of pathological conditions. The first of these conditions is traumatic physical injury to spinal cord tissue, such as the severing of the spinal cord during a car accident. The second condition is a congenital or inherited genetic problem with spinal cord development and function, as illustrated by spina bifida. The third is an acquired condition such as damage caused by a viral or bacterial infection. In each case, the severity of the pathological condition is dependent upon the location and extent of the resultant spinal cord lesion. In the clinical setting, physicians utilize information regarding all aspects of spinal cord function (such as sensory, motor, reflex, and coordination functions), as well as information from a variety of imaging techniques to diagnose pathological conditions and to select appropriate treatments.

Trauma. The neurons of the spinal cord carry out their functions by way of their long nerve processes (axons), which extend to form synapses with, and control, target cells (muscles and other neurons). Some of these nerve processes extend out of the spinal cord to the body, others extend either up to or down from higher-brain regions, and yet others extend from one side of the spinal cord to another. Trauma mainly damages the nerve process of cells and in this fashion disrupts their function in controlling target neurons and muscles. Often, after nerve processes have been damaged, the neuron itself will die because of loss of neurotrophic influences from their target cells. It has been estimated that every year between ten thousand and twelve thousand people in the United States are disabled by some degree of paralysis resulting from

INFORMATION ON SPINAL CORD DISORDERS

Causes: Injury, congenital or hereditary defects, disease, infection, tumors or cysts
Symptoms: Varies; may include impaired movement, pain, tingling or numbness, loss of sensation
Duration: Acute to chronic
Treatments: Depends on cause; may include surgery, antiviral drugs, antibiotics

traumatic injury to the spinal cord. The spinal cord can be also damaged by blocked blood flow to the cord, blood accumulation (hematoma) in or near the cord, or the presence of a ruptured or herniated disk, all of which can be caused by trauma.

Congenital defects. Spinal cord defects are not the result of trauma but rather are generally attributed to abnormal events during embryonic development. In particular, most major spinal cord defects arise around the third week of development. During this time, the flattened neural plate is beginning to fold upward as its lateral edges come together and fuse to form the top margin (dorsal aspect) of the neural tube. If this process is incomplete, then the spinal cord remains open and exposed along the embryo's back, accompanied by the failure of the vertebral bones to surround the spinal cord tissue completely. This condition is referred to as spina bifida. Often, rather than simply being exposed, some normal contents of the vertebral canal, including spinal cord tissue, protrude out of the back as a bulge. Spina bifida is most common in the lower lumbar and upper sacral regions of the spine, but more severe cases may involve the cervical and thoracic regions. Depending on the level and extent of the defect, the clinical symptoms of spinal abnormalities range from mild impairment to fatality. This type of neural tube defect often causes some degree of motor and sensory handicap. The cerebrospinal fluid is continuous from the ventricles of the brain to the central canal of the spinal cord. If the spinal defect impairs the normal flow of cerebrospinal fluid, other problems may occur, such as intellectual disability resulting from hydrocephalus (fluid on the brain). Although there is still much to learn about the causes of spinal cord defects, in many cases scientific evidence points the finger at genetic problems (mutations) and the disruptive action of teratogens such as environmental pollutants and drugs.

Infections. Acquired spinal cord lesions are not the result of trauma or developmental problems but rather are related to such conditions as tumor development or viral and bacterial infections. In general, invasion of the spinal cord by viruses or bacteria can produce inflammation known as myelitis. Multiple sclerosis (MS) and ALS are the two most common nontraumatic disorders of the spinal cord. Many of the nerve fibers of the central nervous system are covered by a myelin sheath produced by neuroglia cells, known as oligodendrocytes. This sheath contributes to the speed and efficiency of the nerve cells as they carry electrical information. MS involves the destruction of this important myelin sheath, leading to the disruption of motor and sensory nerve pathway functions manifested by such symptoms as abnormal sensations, paralysis, and exaggerated reflexes. Although its cause is not clearly understood, researchers believe that viral infections are involved in some cases, while in others the individual's own immune system might be mistakenly destroying normal myelin tissue (an autoimmune disorder). ALS is a fatal condition that is restricted to the loss of motor neurons. As with MS, there is much speculation regarding the causes of ALS. Acquired immunodeficiency syndrome (AIDS) is a viral infection that can involve the disruption of spinal cord neuron function.

Other infections that can cause spinal cord lesions include tabes dorsalis, poliomyelitis, meningitis, and syringomyelia. Tabes dorsalis involves the degeneration of sensory neurons from the dorsal region of the spinal cord as a result of the invasion of the syphilis spirochete bacterium. The polio virus infects and kills spinal motor neurons in a disease called poliomyelitis; if the disease destroys the brain-stem neurons that control respiration and heart rate, then this condition is fatal. Meningitis is a bacterial inflammation of the layers of cells that cover the spinal cord (collectively referred to as meninges), producing high fever and sometimes inducing a comatose state that can lead to death.

Tumors and cysts. Growths within the spinal cord can also disrupt normal spinal cord function. Syringomyelia is such a condition, in which fluid-filled cysts develop among the neurons of the spinal cord. Cancerous tumors are often the result of uncontrolled growth of the neuroglia cells, which can damage neurons and nerve fiber pathways.

TREATMENT AND THERAPY

Spinal cord defects, either congenital or hereditary, pose serious challenges for the medical community. Surgical intervention is the only option in mild cases of spina bifida, but in severe cases there is no effective treatment. The advent of intrauterine surgery (prior to the birth of the baby) for the correction of minor cases of spina bifida is a major step toward alleviating

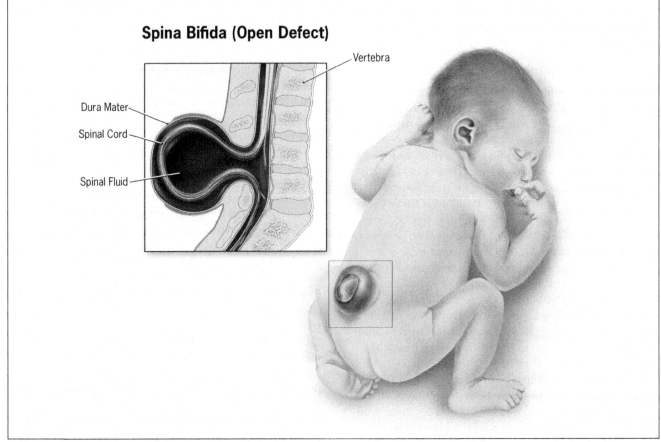

An illustration of an infant with Spina Bifida. Image via CDC/Wikimedia Commons [Public domain.]

serious problems. It is believed that better prenatal care may reduce the risk of spinal cord defects. For example, consumption of the vitamin folic acid in pregnancy greatly reduces the incidence of spina bifida. Numerous other causative factors have been implicated in spinal cord defects, including alcoholism, drug use, and even environmental pollution. In some cases, genetic screening may provide a method to reduce certain types of defects, while in other cases reduced exposure to risk elements is the most effective preventive action.

Treatments for acquired spinal cord injury involve antiviral and antibacterial drugs that combat infection and in so doing reduce inflammation and cell damage. It is clear that early detection and intervention is an important factor in being able to save as many neurons as possible and to limit the extent of the lesion. Neurotrophic factors are likely to be important therapeutic agents as doctors try to stimulate the maximum recovery of neuronal function. In cases in which the immune system itself may be damaging healthy neurons, as is suspected in some cases of MS, drugs are used to suppress immune function.

PERSPECTIVE AND PROSPECTS

Medical researchers are taking numerous approaches to understand spinal cord development and function, in the hope of utilizing that information to develop new therapies to prevent or treat these clinical conditions. An interesting aspect of the problem is that, unlike most other organ systems, the adult nervous system appears to retain only a few selected stem cell populations after embryonic development. Stem cell populations are groups of cells that divide to produce cells for the growth and regeneration of tissues and organs.

It was believed that human babies were born with all the neurons in their central nervous system that they would ever have, meaning that no new neurons would be produced. Recent work in rodents and nonhuman primates, however, has unequivocally demonstrated that neural stem cells exist in the adult mammalian brain and give rise to millions of new neurons during an individual's life span. This process generates new neurons predominantly in two areas of the brain-in the olfactory bulb, which controls the sense of smell, and in the hippocampus, a memory center-but not to any appreciable extent in other brain areas. Scientists are beginning to identify stem cells in other brain regions, but there appear to be only a few, and those lack the ability to repair spinal cord injuries. Many laboratories are working on harnessing the potential of stem cells for cell replacement therapies, which hold significant promise for brain repair. As the individual ages, the nervous system becomes more efficient in processing

information as neural networks are modified. This modification involves changes in nerve cell connections, a process referred to as plasticity, and new neuron generation (neurogenesis), but only in a few areas of the adult brain. Researchers hope to utilize information about the biological basis of normal plasticity to help repair damaged or impaired nervous systems.

Modern neuroscience research quickly vanquished the long-held belief that it is impossible to repair neurons damaged by trauma or disease. Experiments with animals and in tissue culture have demonstrated that damaged neurons can survive, regrow nerve processes, and once again carry electrical impulses. In fact, neurons from human spinal cords have been grown in tissue culture under conditions that stimulated them to regrow their axonal process. One of the most important aspects of understanding nervous system development is the fact that the cells communicate with one another not only with neurotransmitters but also with neurotrophic factors. Basic research and clinical trials are being done on neurotrophic factors with the expectation that they will become important parts of therapeutic treatments to stimulate the repair and regeneration of damaged neurons. These neurotrophic factors hold such promise because they are important in stimulating normal cell differentiation during embryonic development and for the subsequent survival of neurons after birth into adulthood. Therefore, clinical treatments are being designed to recreate the embryonic conditions that contributed to normal development. In addition, it is believed that one of the major factors in the lack of a regeneration response in damaged spinal cords is that the neuroglia cells, known as astrocytes, form scar tissue that is not conducive to nerve fiber regeneration. Therefore, medical researchers are looking at treatments that, in addition to prolonging the life of neurons, reduce the formation of scar tissue.

—*William L. Muhlach, PhD;* *updated by W. Michael Zawada, PhD*

See also Amyotrophic lateral sclerosis; Anesthesia; Anesthesiology; Back pain; Bone cancer; Bone disorders; Bones and the skeleton; Brain damage; Cerebral palsy; Chiari malformations; Chiropractic; Congenital disorders; Disk removal; Fracture and dislocation; Head and neck disorders; Kinesiology; Kyphosis; Laminectomy and spinal fusion; Lumbar puncture; Meningitis; Motor neuron diseases; Multiple sclerosis; Muscle sprains, spasms, and disorders; Muscular dystrophy; Nervous system; Neuralgia, neuritis, and neuropathy; Neurology; Neurology, pediatric; Neurosurgery; Numbness and tingling; Osteoarthritis; Osteoporosis; Paget's disease; Paralysis; Paraplegia; Physical rehabilitation; Poliomyelitis; Quadriplegia; Radiculopathy; Sciatica; Scoliosis; Slipped disk; Spina bifida; Spine, vertebrae, and disks; Spondylitis; Sports medicine; Sympathectomy.

For Further Information:

Carey, Joseph, ed. *Brain Facts: A Primer on the Brain and Nervous System.* 5th ed. Washington, DC: Society for Neuroscience, 2006. A publication by the Society of Neuroscience directed at educating the general public about the value of neuroscience research.

Carlson, Bruce M. *Human Embryology and Developmental Biology.* 4th ed. Philadelphia: Mosby/Elsevier, 2009. This textbook presents human development in the context of modern scientific and medical research. Includes a consideration of basic normal spinal cord development, as well as a detailed look at developmental defects.

Kandel, Eric R., James H. Schwartz, and Thomas M. Jessell, eds. *Principles of Neural Science.* 5th ed. Norwalk, Conn.: Appleton and Lange, 2006. This massive, comprehensive book serves as the bible for the field of neuroscience. In spite of its tremendous breadth and depth, this book contains excellent basic explanations and illustrations, and thus serves as a valuable reference for people of all academic backgrounds.

Larsen, William J. *Human Embryology.* Edited by Lawrence S. Sherman, S. Steven Potter, and William J. Scott. 3d ed. New York: Churchill Livingstone, 2001. Basic coverage of human embryonic development, including both normal and abnormal spinal cord development.

Litin, Scott C., ed. *Mayo Clinic Family Health Book.* 4th ed. New York: HarperResource, 2009. Discusses both muscles and bones, underscoring the intimate relationship between disorders in the two systems. The text and illustrations are complete and easy to understand.

National Institute of Neurological Disorders and Stroke (NINDS). *Disorder Index.* www.ninds.nih.gov/disorders/disorder_index.htm. The site provides information about various spinal cord diseases and injury, current research, and support organizations.

Nicholls, John G., A. Robert Martin, and Bruce G. Wallace. *From Neuron to Brain.* 4th ed. Sunderland, Mass.: Sinauer, 2007. An excellent and detailed undergraduate neurobiology text that describes how nerve cells transmit signals, how signals are put together, and how higher functions emerge from this integration.

Palmer, Sara, Kay Harris Kriegsman, and Jeffrey B. Palmer. *Spinal Cord Injury: A Guide for Living.* Baltimore: Johns Hopkins University Press, 2000. Sets expectations for recovery from and life after a spinal cord injury. Covers initial hospitalization, rehabilitation therapy, readjusting to home, the effects of spinal cord injury on other family members, dating and sexuality, independent living choices, and current research.

Salter, Robert Bruce. *Textbook of Disorders and Injuries of the Musculoskeletal System.* 3d ed. Baltimore: Williams & Wilkins, 1999. Four sections of the book-"Basic Musculoskeletal Science and Its Applications," "Musculoskeletal Disorders: General and Specific," "Musculoskeletal Injuries," and "Research"-examine the diagnosis and treatment principles of disorders and trauma of the musculoskeletal system.

SPINAL FUSION. SEE LAMINECTOMY AND SPINAL FUSION.

SPINAL TAP. SEE LUMBAR PUNCTURE.

SPINE, VERTEBRAE, AND DISKS

Category: Anatomy

Anatomy or system affected: Back, bones, musculoskeletal system, nerves, nervous system

Specialties and related fields: Alternative medicine, geriatrics and gerontology, neurology, orthopedics, physical therapy, preventive medicine, sports medicine

Definition: The supporting structures of the trunk, from the base of the skull to the end of the tailbone; the vertebrae form a small, central canal for the sensory and motor nerves that constitute the spinal cord.

Key terms:

disk: a soft, cushionlike structure that lies between bony vertebrae from the base of the skull to the sacrum of the pelvis; it has a soft liquid in the center (the nucleus pulposus) and is surrounded by a thickened ligament (the annulus fibrosis)

intervertebral foramina: openings between two adjacent vertebrae to permit the exit of nerve structures from the spinal cord

spinal cord: a cord in the trunk containing nerve cells that transmit impulses to and from the brain

spinous processes: bony projections from vertebrae (horizontally in the neck, tilting downward in the thoracic area, and horizontally in the lumbar area) that are connected to one another by the interspinous and supraspinous ligaments and that control extremes of trunk motion

transverse processes: projections from the sides of vertebrae, to which are attached muscles and ligaments, that assist in motor function by enhancing leverage and limiting extremes of motion

vertebra: a bony structure in the back with a central spinal canal surrounded by an arch; the back part of the arch (the lamina) and the front part of the arch (the pedicle) are joined together by muscles, ligaments, and cartilage for motion, stability, and posture

STRUCTURE AND FUNCTIONS

The spinal column undergoes developmental changes from infancy to the adult state and then degenerative changes with aging. The alignment of the spinal column at birth is in the shape of a C curve, the fetus having been curled up. This forward-tilted curve is retained except in the neck and lower back. As the infant raises its head and attempts to see things, head control and vision gradually require the head to tilt back, resulting in a posterior curve at the neck. As children progress to standing and walking, the lower spine also develops a posterior curve (a normal lumbar lordosis).

As individuals increasingly use the predominant upper extremities, these muscles become stronger and increase the pull on that side of the spine, resulting in a lateral curve (a normal scoliosis).

Humans generally have thirty-three vertebrae, but abnormalities can occur in their numbers, shape, alignment, density, and maturation. There are seven vertebrae in the neck or cervical area, twelve in the chest or thoracic area, five in the lower back or lumbar area, five usually joined together in the pelvic region to form the sacrum, and three or four rudimentary vertebrae partially fused to form the coccyx. The typical vertebra develops embryologically from two bone growth centers. The front of one bone growth center becomes the body and part of the arch, while the other bone growth center evolves into the spinous processes, the transverse processes, the articular processes, and the back portion of the arch.

The thirty-three vertebrae of the spine have various defined parts and characteristics. The oval or round vertebral body has a spongy center surrounded by a dense bone. Above and below it are layers of cartilage. Lack of the mineral calcium reduces the density of the bone, resulting in osteoporosis. This condition may occur in postmenopausal women, causing pain, fractures, and kyphosis (a thoracic humpback). The pedicle portions of this anterior arch have an upper and lower notch called the intervertebral foramina, through which the spinal nerves exit from the spinal canal. At the junction of pedicle and lamina are projections upward and downward that form the articular processes, or joints. The alignment and direction of these joints vary with the spinal region and serve to control spinal motion. The transverse processes assist in the movement of muscles and at the chest level act as links between the ribs. There are generally twelve thoracic vertebrae and twelve ribs. On occasion, an extra cervical rib may be present; this extra rib narrows the exit space at the neck and can pinch the cervical nerves and blood vessels.

The upper two cervical processes are different from all other vertebrae. The first cervical vertebra supports the head and is called the atlas. Instead of a body, it has an enlarged anterior arch and a groove on which the head rests. Its transverse processes are long, but its spinous process is a little knob. The second cervical vertebra is also unique, with an upward projection called the dens that is like a pole fitting into the ring of the first cervical vertebral arch. It represents the body of the first cervical vertebra. This pole and ring permit the head to rotate.

The cervical transverse processes or lateral projections have holes, the transverse foramina, through which the vertebral arteries send blood to the brain. As one progresses downward, the vertebrae become larger

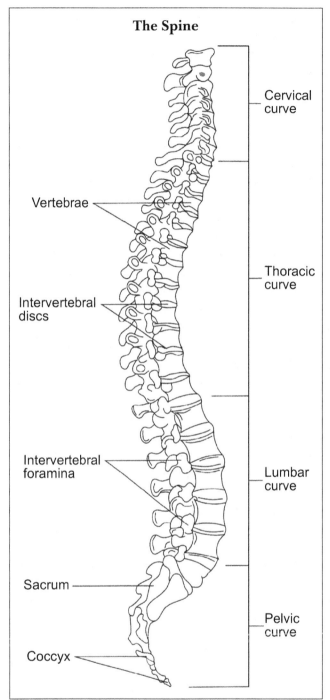

The Spine

Vertebrae

Intervertebral discs

Intervertebral foramina

Sacrum

Coccyx

Cervical curve

Thoracic curve

Lumbar curve

Pelvic curve

©EBSCO

and bear more weight. The thoracic vertebrae have their joint surfaces in the frontal plane, and the transverse processes are solid. The ribs share half of the joint surfaces with the adjoining vertebrae, except for the first, tenth, eleventh, and twelfth vertebrae; these vertebrae join only their corresponding ribs. As one continues down the spine, the spinous processes become more slender and project downward, almost touching one another. The lower thoracic vertebrae are closer to the lumbar vertebrae in appearance.

The lumbar vertebrae are more massive, carry more stress, and support the weight of the body. The transverse processes in this region are thinner but longer, increasing the leverage action for muscles. The joint surfaces tilt upward, backward, and toward the center, opening the joint space when one bends forward. This action permits side bending, increasing the side pressures on the disks. The five sacral vertebrae are fused, with small ridges representing the sites of fusion. Small openings allow the upper four sacral nerves to exit the spine. The sacrum contributes the back portion of the pelvis. The coccyx, or tailbone, is composed of three or four rudimentary vertebrae, with the first distinct and separate from the other two or three, which are fused. The back of the spine is layered with muscles going to the upper extremities, with long vertical muscles underneath, intermediate-length muscles under these, and the deepest muscle groups closest to the spine and only two or three vertebrae in length.

Vertebrae are separated by washers called disks. The central portion of a disk is a gel-like substance, the nucleus pulposus, which offers hydraulic cushioning and allows some movement. This substance is enclosed in a ligamentous covering called the annulus fibrosis. Disks contribute approximately one-fourth of body length, can add about eight degrees in motion per vertebra, and can alter their shape to accommodate the solid vertebrae when the body is bent. The nucleus pulposus is 70 to 80 percent water, and about 14 kilograms (30 pounds) of pressure must be exerted constantly by ligaments to maintain the shape of the disk. Dehydration, aging, compressive forces, and simply a day of normal activity can temporarily reduce the amount of the watery nucleus pulposus, increase the bulging of the disks, and shorten one's stature.

The spinal cord connects the peripheral structures of the body to the brain and the nerve cells in the spinal cord itself. Until about the third month of life, the spinal cord occupies the entire length of the spinal canal. The vertebrae grow faster than the spinal cord, however, and later in life it occupies two-thirds of the length of the spinal canal (approximately 42 to 45 centimeters) and ends at about the second lumbar vertebra. The coverings on the cord continue as the filum terminale, which is attached to the sacral vertebrae.

There are three coverings of the spinal cord within the spinal canal. The outermost, toughest, and fibrous covering, called the dura, is separated from the bony

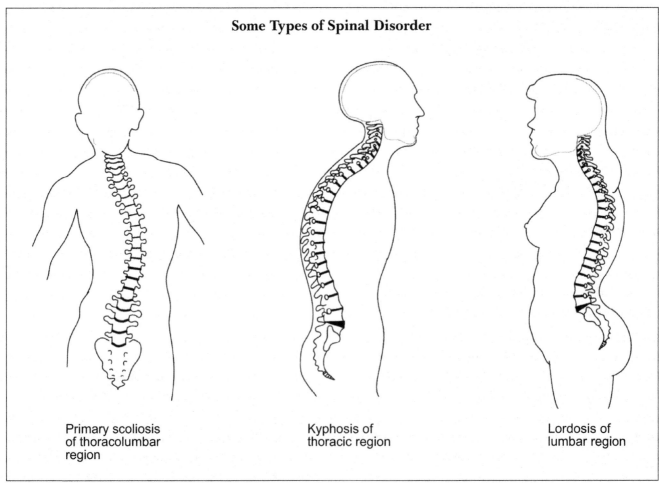

Some Types of Spinal Disorder

Primary scoliosis
of thoracolumbar
region

Kyphosis of
thoracic region

Lordosis of
lumbar region

surfaces by fat and blood vessels. The spinal cord is covered by a thin layer called the pia that enters into the spinal cord and separates various portions of the cord. Surrounding the pia is a protective fluid, the spinal fluid, which is held in place by the arachnoid layer; this fluid can be aspirated for analysis, as in a lumbar puncture, or spinal tap. The nerves exiting from the spinal cord are also segmental. There are only seven cervical vertebrae but eight cervical nerves. The eighth cervical nerve exits below the seventh cervical vertebra, and thereafter all roots from the vertebrae leave below the corresponding vertebra. These segmental nerves then join, divide, send messages to the brain and other organs, and control bodily functions and motion.

Ligaments run vertically in front of the vertebral bodies (the anterior longitudinal ligament) and in back of the vertebral bodies and within the spinal canal (the posterior longitudinal ligament). These ligaments support the vertebrae and disks and limit excessive motion forward and backward. The posterior longitudinal ligament ceases at about the fourth lumbar vertebra, and thus farther down the spine the fibrous rings about the disks are weaker, permitting herniations. Such leakages from the disks may press on nerve roots exiting at these levels and cause pain. These ruptures of the disks occur mostly when lifting with the trunk bent forward and sideways. There are additional ligaments between the spinous processes at the tips (the supraspinous ligament) and along the length of the spinous processes (the interspinous ligament). The portion of the arch between the spinous processes and the transverse processes is the lamina. Between the laminae are the ligamentum flavum. The interspinous ligament, ligamentum flavum, and nucleus pulposus have no pain fibers. The laminae and disks may be removed when disk surgery is performed, and pieces of bone from the hip may be used to fuse and reduce motion at this level.

Motion between each vertebra is about eight degrees. Motion is enhanced by the facets, vertical bony projections with joint surfaces. They are structured like the other joints of the body, and thus are subject to irritation and arthritic changes. Flexion of the trunk opens the spaces in the lumbar joints and allows side bending and rotation in the same direction. Extension of the trunk compresses and limits motion in these facets.

The blood supply to the spinal cord and the surrounding tissues diminishes progressively downward. Excessive activity can lead to insufficient circulating blood to these nerves and give rise to symptoms in the lower extremity called intermittent claudication. The front portion of the spinal cord contains motor nerve cells, leading to the trunk and the muscles of the extremities, that can be inhibited or activated by im-

pulses. The lateral areas of the spinal region contain messenger tracts and the autonomic nervous system. The back portion of the spinal cord has sensory structures that carry messages of pain, temperature, position, and touch to the brain. The different levels within the spinal cord connect to different segmental structures of the body. The fifth cervical nerve down to the first thoracic nerve connect to the upper extremities, and the second lumbar to second sacral roots connect to the lower extremities. Compression of these nerve roots at the spine may cause symptoms in areas distant from the spine.

DISORDERS AND DISEASES

The anatomy of the trunk regulates the erect, or standing, posture. It is influenced by the structure of the vertebrae and extremities and even by the tilt of the head. It is also influenced by cultural factors, emotion, habits, and occupation. Good posture involves standing straight with the head up, the shoulders back and up, the stomach in, and the hips and knees straight. This position also is most efficient in energy expenditure, since it requires the least amount of muscle activity in order to balance the weights in the front and back of the trunk, as well as the weights on the left and right sides of the body. Looking at the front of the body, the central gravitational, or weight-bearing, line falls in line with the nose and between the pelvis, knees, and ankles. From the back, the gravitational line follows the center of the head, the spinous processes, the gluteal fold between the buttocks, and between the knees and ankles. The weight stresses should be balanced between the right side and the left side of the body and between the front and the back. The head should be maintained so that the eyes and the labyrinth in the inner ear are level. Any deviations cause imbalance in the trunk, resulting in muscle strain, ligament sprains, pain, and possibly deformities. Abnormalities in posture and gait may be attributable to muscle imbalance, deformities at birth, problems in development, disease, or surgical procedures.

There are several birth defects that affect the spine. Occasionally, during embryonic development, the two bone growth regions that form a vertebra do not fuse together, causing an opening in the arch in the back called spina bifida. Spondylolysis occurs when the articular process remains unattached. Ligaments, muscles, and tendons are unable to attach to these areas securely, and the result is weakness in the vertebra and a reduction in stability. Occasionally, this weakness permits the upper vertebra to slide forward, a condition called spondylolisthesis. The misalignment and narrowing of the spinal canal can compress the nerve structures within it, a condition known as spinal stenosis. The lower cervical and lower lumbar regions, which need more nerve tissue to supply the extremities, are especially vulnerable to pressure symptoms.

Inequality in leg lengths or pain in the lower extremities, upper extremities, abdomen, chest, or neck can lead to compensatory reactions in the trunk. These may then cause misalignment in the spine with side deviations (scoliosis), backward deviations (kyphosis, or humpback, in the thoracic area), and forward deviations (lordosis in the low back). Other contributing factors are overuse, muscle spasm or weakness, birth defects, developmental abnormalities, diseases, aging, and trauma. Some misalignments occur after surgery on the chest, back, or abdomen. Idiopathic scoliosis (scoliosis of unknown cause) may occur in adolescent girls; when it is severe, lung and heart functions can be impaired. Temporarily increased lordosis can occur in pregnancy, to compensate for the extra weight in the abdomen. Lordosis may be permanent because of structural changes in the spine, pendulous abdomen and/or breasts, or poor muscle balance. Therefore, back problems may be caused by poor posture, behavior, occupation, and structural, neurologic, or muscular factors. Pain located only in the back is generally attributable to poor posture, trauma, or inflammation. If pain extends below the knees, the cause may be nerve pressure at the fifth lumbar or first sacral nerve roots. Bladder and rectal sphincter disturbances may indicate sacral nerve or cord involvement and may require immediate surgical care.

The body's center of gravity is in the front portion of the second lumbar vertebra. Thus, the compressive force of body weight is increased when one lifts an object with the arms in front of the trunk. The greater the distance of the object from the center of the body, the greater the need for the back muscles to contract. Lifting a 45-kilogram (100-pound) object may require a 545-kilogram (1,200-pound) muscle pull and compressive force. The posterior longitudinal support for the disks that is provided by ligaments narrows in the sides at the level of the fourth and fifth lumbar vertebrae. Herniations through the fibrous disk ring at these levels are more likely, and a ruptured disk can pinch the nerves exiting at these levels.

Stresses that bear on the spine are categorized as compressive, shearing, elongating, or rotational. Compressive forces may involve the muscles, disks (possible ruptures), vertebrae (fractures), and the facet joints. Shearing stress may lead to forward slippage of the fourth or fifth vertebra from the segment below. This is most common in individuals with incomplete bony union of vertebrae. Rotatory stress may affect the joints, the facets of the spine, the short spine muscles, or the ligaments. On rare occasions, an elongating stretch or traction may strain muscles and sprain or tear ligaments.

PERSPECTIVE AND PROSPECTS

Examinations of the spine usually include the history of the problem: whether it is sudden or gradual and whether it is influenced by certain activities or climates. The physician checks the patient's posture for abnormal curvatures and determines whether they are fixed or functional. Functional curves disappear when the patient is lying down. The gait should be evaluated for symmetry, balance, and deviations. The physician will measure leg lengths for inequalities, the circumference of the chest for rib flare, and the circumferences of extremities for swelling or shrinkage. Next, the trunk's range of motion will be evaluated, followed by palpation to discover tender spots and muscle spasms.

With spinal problems, a full examination of the entire body is indicated since pain can be referred to the back from other organs. Changes in function, sensation, and motor strength can indicate spinal cord or nerve involvement. Simple X rays of the spine will indicate alignment of the vertebrae, bone density, fracture lines, extraneous bone growth, cartilage thickness, and unusual soft tissue densities caused by hemorrhage or calcification. For problems other than bone and cartilage tissue involvement, a computed tomography (CT) scan or magnetic resonance imaging (MRI) may be needed; these techniques provide images of the area to be examined that are at different levels or depths.

—*Eugene J. Rogers, MD*

See also Anesthesia; Anesthesiology; Back pain; Bone cancer; Bone disorders; Bones and the skeleton; Braces, orthopedic; Cerebral palsy; Chiari malformations; Chiropractic; Disk removal; Fracture and dislocation; Head and neck disorders; Kinesiology; Kyphosis; Laminectomy and spinal fusion; Lumbar puncture; Meningitis; Motor neuron diseases; Multiple sclerosis; Muscle sprains, spasms, and disorders; Muscular dystrophy; Nervous system; Neuralgia, neuritis, and neuropathy; Neurology; Neurology, pediatric; Neurosurgery; Numbness and tingling; Orthopedic surgery; Orthopedics; Orthopedics, pediatric; Osteoarthritis; Osteoporosis; Paget's disease; Paralysis; Paraplegia; Physical rehabilitation; Poliomyelitis; Quadriplegia; Radiculopathy; Sciatica; Scoliosis; Slipped disk; Spina bifida; Spinal cord disorders; Spondylitis; Sports medicine; Stenosis; Sympathectomy; Whiplash.

For Further Information:
Fine, Judylaine. *Conquering Back Pain: A Comprehensive Guide.* Rev. ed. Englewood Cliffs, N.J.: Prentice Hall, 1987. This softcover book summarizes the anatomy of the back, discussing its various structures, types of pain, and areas where pain may be distributed. Also enumerates the treatments, both conservative and surgical, of back pain.

Jenkins, David B. *Hollinshead's Functional Anatomy of the Limbs and Back*. 9th ed. Philadelphia: Saunders/Elsevier, 2009. An easy-to-understand and well-illustrated book designed for physical therapy students. It can be useful for those individuals wishing more information about the muscles of the back and extremities, their nerve and blood supplies, and the function of these structures.

Palastanga, Nigel, Derek Field, and Roger Soames. *Anatomy and Human Movement: Structure and Function*. 5th ed. New York: Butterworth Heinemann/Elsevier, 2007. This large volume contains excellent illustrations, definitions, and indexes and is written to simplify the more complex aspects of anatomy using understandable terms.

Scott, Judith. *Good-bye to Bad Backs: Stretching and Strengthening Exercises for Alignment and Freedom from Lower Back Pain*. 3d ed. New York: Princeton Book, 2002. Provides visualizing techniques, gentle exercises, and specific workouts for alleviating back pain. Medical line drawings illustrate and teach about muscles and their relationship to posture and lower back pain.

Tortora, Gerard J., and Bryan Derrickson. *Principles of Anatomy and Physiology*. 12th ed. Hoboken, N.J.: John Wiley & Sons, 2009. This introductory college textbook offers an excellent survey of human anatomy and physiology. Several chapters are devoted to the musculoskeletal system. In addition to normal structure and function, each chapter includes sections on abnormalities (including both injuries and diseases) and their treatment.

SPINOCEREBELLAR ATAXIA

Category: Disease/Disorder
Also known as: Olivopontocerebellar atrophy, Maria's ataxia, Cerebellar degeneration
Anatomy or system affected: Arms, brain, eyes, feet, hands, head, legs, muscles, musculoskeletal system, nerves, nervous system
Specialties and related fields: Genetics, occupational health, ophthalmology, optometry, physical therapy, speech pathology
Definition: A group of inherited diseases that cause degeneration in the brain and spinal cord, resulting in progressive loss of coordination.
Key terms:
ataxia: poor coordination and unsteadiness that result from damage to the brain
dysarthria: speech disorder as a result of nerve damage
macular degeneration: damage to the photoreceptors in the retina that causes loss of vision in the center of the visual field

CAUSES AND SYMPTOMS

Located at the base of the brain, the cerebellum receives neural input from the overlying cerebral hemispheres, spinal cord, and sensory receptors, and integrates these inputs in order to precisely coordinate

INFORMATION ON SPINOCEREBELLAR ATAXIA

Causes: Inherited mutations in various genes that cause the death of brain cells
Symptoms: Symptoms vary but they have in common progressive loss of coordination and tremors
Duration: Onset of symptoms varies; disease lasts a lifetime
Treatments: Physical and occupational therapy, speech pathology, supportive devices to help with movement

movement. Damage to the cerebellum causes dizziness, nausea, poor balance, and coordination problems.

Spinocerebellar ataxia (SCA) is a group of hereditary diseases of the nervous system characterized by the progressive onset of ataxia or inability to coordinate muscle movements. The symptoms of SCA are a consequence of gradual, progressive damage to the cerebellum.

Over 30 different types of SCA have been described, and they are named SCA1, SCA2, and so on. Mutations in distinct genes cause the different types of SCAs, and their inheritance patterns also vary.

The specific symptoms of each type of SCA vary as do the age when symptoms first appear, but virtually all of them cause ataxia and tremors. For example, people with SCA1 begin with an abnormal gait and gradually progress into ataxia of all four limbs and speech problems (dysarthria). Within 15-20 years, the disease confines most patients to a wheelchair. SCA2 has similar symptoms except that the fast, jerky movements the eyes make when changing their focus from one object to another (saccades) significantly slow. In addition to ataxia, SCA7 causes macular degeneration and blindness, and SCA10 and 17 cause seizures.

TREATMENT AND THERAPY

Diagnosis of SCA requires brain imaging, which can detect atrophy of the cerebellum, the symptoms of the patient, and, since these diseases are inherited, their family history. However, because the symptoms of these diseases show so many similarities, molecular genetic tests remain the only way to definitively determine which type of SCA ails a patient.

No cure exists for SCA, and treatments consist of addressing symptoms. Balance and mobility problems may require a cane, walker, or wheelchair. Physical therapy has been shown to improve mobility for patients, and occupational therapy can also assist patients with independent living. Speech pathology can also help with speech problems. Sleep disorders afflict some SCA patients, and prescribed sleep aids may provide relief.

Experimental treatments with stem cell transplantations have shown promise in laboratory animals, and a small clinical trial in China with umbilical cord stem cells showed definite promise, but such treatments remain in the experimental stages.

—*Michael A. Buratovich, PhD*

See also Genetic counseling; Neurology; Occupational health; Quadriplegia; Terminally ill: extended care

For Further Information:
Hong, Sunghoi, ed. *Ataxia: Causes, Symptoms and Treatment.* Hauppauge, NY: Nova Science Publishers, 2012.
McArthur, Sara. *Ataxia: How I Had to Cope with an Untreatable, Incurable Neurodegenerative Cerebellum Disease.* Frederick, MD: PublishAmerica, 2010.
Schuman, Tammy L. *Scooter Sagas: Coping With Ataxia.* Bloomington, IN: iUniverse, 2013.

SPLENECTOMY

Category: Procedure
Anatomy or system affected: Abdomen, lymphatic system, spleen
Specialties and related fields: Emergency medicine, general surgery
Definition: The surgical removal of the spleen.

INDICATIONS AND PROCEDURES
Splenectomy is often performed after trauma to the upper left abdominal cavity that results in injury to the spleen. When the spleen is damaged in such cases, life-threatening intra-abdominal hemorrhage may occur. Surgical repair of the damaged spleen is sometimes difficult, but the lack of a spleen has relatively few ill effects, as other organs such as the liver and tissues of the lymphatic system compensate for its absence. Therefore, splenectomy is usually the indicated treatment for damage to the spleen.

Patients undergoing splenectomy are first anesthetized by an anesthesiologist. Surgical assistants then prepare the patient by scrubbing the upper abdomen to rid the skin of pathogens. The surgeon than makes an incision in the upper left abdomen or along the midline of the abdomen. He or she will then expose the spleen and tie off blood vessels to the spleen with sutures. The surgeon then cuts the attachments that anchor the spleen in the abdomen and removes the organ. This procedure takes approximately one hour to complete, provided that there are no complications. Most patients are allowed to leave the hospital after about one week or less. Although surgical infections

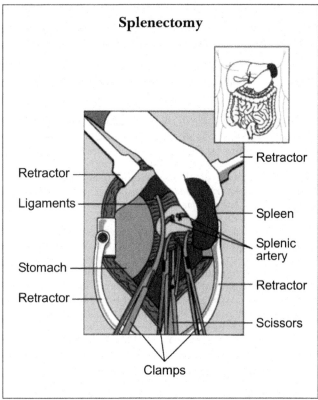

Splenectomy

The removal of the spleen is required when the organ has sustained damage from injury or disease; the inset shows the location of the spleen. ©EBSCO

are rare, they may require the patient to remain hospitalized for a few more days.

USES AND COMPLICATIONS
Splenectomy is also performed to treat patients with certain types of anemia and hypersplenism. Since the normal function of the spleen is to destroy aged or nonfunctional red blood cells and platelets, overactivity of the spleen in hypersplenism results in excessive destruction of these blood cells and leads to anemia and blood-clotting disorders.

Even though splenectomy has few long-term adverse effects, some adult patients have a slightly increased risk of contracting infections. Splenectomy in children, however, results in greater susceptibility, particularly to pneumococcal pneumonia. Physicians often recommend that children who have undergone splenectomy be immunized against this bacterial pneumonia, and many of these patients even receive long-term prophylactic antibiotic therapy to prevent the disease.

—*Matthew Berria, PhD,*
and Douglas Reinhart, MD

See also Abdomen; Abdominal disorders; Anemia; Bleeding; Hematology; Hematology, pediatric; Immune system; Immunology; Internal medicine; Lymphatic system; Metabolism; Pneumonia; Wounds.

For Further Information:
Griffith, H. Winter. *Complete Guide to Symptoms, Illness, and Surgery*. Revised and updated by Stephen Moore and Kenneth Yoder. 5th ed. New York: Perigee, 2006.
Hiatt, J. R., E. H. Phillips, L. Morgenstern, eds. *Surgical Diseases of the Spleen*. New York: Springer, 1997.
Kasper, Dennis L., et al., eds. *Harrison's Principles of Internal Medicine*. 16th ed. New York: McGraw-Hill, 2005.
Schwartz, Seymour I., James T. Adams, and Arthur W. Bauman. *Splenectomy for Hematologic Disorders*. Chicago: Year Book Medical, 1971.
Wilkins, Bridget, and Dennis H. Wright. *Illustrated Pathology of the Spleen*. New York: Cambridge University Press, 2000.
Zollinger, Robert M., Jr., and Robert M. Zollinger, Sr. *Zollinger's Atlas of Surgical Operations*. 8th ed. New York: McGraw-Hill, 2003.

SPLIT-BRAIN

Category: Disease/Disorder
Anatomy or system affected: Brain
Specialties and related fields: Neurology, neuroscience, psychiatry, psychology
Definition: A condition that results from cutting the corpus callosum, which is the major connection between the two cerebral hemispheres of the brain.

Key terms:
cerebral hemispheres: refers to the two halves of the cerebrum that includes the cerebral cortex, containing both white and gray matter of the brain
commissure: a connection or link between two structures such as the two cerebral hemispheres
contralateral: referring to the opposite side
epilepsy: a neurological condition that results in seizure activity
epileptic focus: the point in the brain where a seizure originates
glia: the most numerous cells within the brain; in contrast to neurons, they do not conduct impulses but provide various supportive functions such as cleaning up waste products
laterality: refers to unique functions that occur within only one cerebral hemisphere
myelin: glia cells that wrap themselves around nerve axons

CAUSES AND SYMPTOMS
Split-brain is a condition that develops when the two cerebral hemispheres in the brain cannot easily and efficiently communicate with each other. In early usage, it was referred to as the bisected brain. The corpus callosum (CC) is the largest of several connections between the two hemispheres. The CC is made up of mostly nerve axons (approximately 350 million in the human brain), which are covered with glia cells that form a myelin sheath. The density of the myelinated

axons is such that it alters the color of the CC giving it a whitish appearance-hence, the name "white matter" as opposed to "gray matter" found in the brain. The central purpose of the CC is to allow for the transference of massive amounts of information to flow across the two hemispheres. When this connection is severed, the brain receives information but becomes limited in how it can process it.

Immediately after the CC is surgically cut, a patient will typically experience trouble coordinating their behavior. Investigators have described the split-brain condition as though two people are in control of a single body. For example, a split-brain person who removes an item from a closet with one hand could find that the opposite hand attempts to put it back. Fortunately, the internal competition that results from two independent hemispheres dissipates after a few weeks. The brain, through the process of neuroplasticity, begins to alter itself in ways that allow the two hemispheres to cooperate better. One way it does this is by allowing additional commissures (e.g., anterior commissure) to transfer information that had been previously sent across by the CC. It is also believed that the left hemisphere suppresses the right hemisphere's ability to interfere with coordination by taking control.

Although severing the CC is an intrusive surgical procedure, it usually does not lead to a permanent debilitating outcome. Most patients lead a normal life postsurgery. For physicians and neuroscientists, one unexpected windfall from the procedure was that it created an opportunity to learn more about the independent nature and functionality of the two hemispheres. Although it was previously known that each hemisphere controlled the sensory and motor information on the contralateral side of the body, the split-brain condition revealed the laterality for different language functions, memory processes, and different types of attentional processes. Experimental testing performed by Michael Gazzaniga and his colleagues found that visual information could be presented in such a way that only one hemisphere could learn it. If a word such as "spoon" was presented to the right hemisphere, the split-brain person showed signs of knowing the word yet could not verbalize it. The inability to say "spoon" was due to the lack of language centers in the left hemisphere for the vast majority of people. However, when the person is asked to point to the object from a group of objects, he has no difficulty identifying the spoon. This apparent lack of "knowing" how to verbalize the object is due to the fact that information was placed into the nonspeaking hemisphere, which could not transfer the information into the left hemisphere via the CC.

TREATMENT AND THERAPY

The split-brain procedure is most often performed on patients who suffer from epilepsy. Epilepsy occurs in one to two percent of the population. In the majority of cases, epileptic seizures can be controlled using antiseizure medication such as tegretol. When medicines do not adequately control seizure activity, surgical procedures are considered to remove the epileptic focus with the goal of eliminating the seizures. In rare instances, a patient might have multiple focus points within the same hemisphere whereby surgically removing all of them would be too dangerous. An alternative surgical procedure is a corpus callostomy. This is a procedure that severs the CC, resulting in the split-brain condition. Surgeons will consider cutting about two-thirds of the CC and then evaluating the results as a means to avoid some of the split-brain symptoms. This procedure does not prevent seizures from occurring; instead, it isolates the seizures in one hemisphere by preventing the malevolent electrical signals to propagate through the CC to the opposite hemisphere, thus minimizing its disrupting influence on the brain. A corpus callostomy is a last resort treatment to stop the hemispheres from sharing seizure activity, but it can come at a cost.

Different degrees of split-brain conditions can occur as a result of abnormal neural development. A rare genetic disorder, callosal agenesis, occurs when the CC forms improperly or not at all. This condition can lead to developmental delays and difficulties in language as well as spatial reasoning. Whether the split-brain condition arises from corpus callostomy or from callosal agenesis, cognitive rehabilitation can be prescribed as a means to improve overall cognitive functioning.

PERSPECTIVE AND PROSPECTS

While William P. van Wagenen and R. Yorke Herren, in 1940, were the first to create the split-brain condition by surgically cutting the CC as a means to control epileptic seizures, it was Michael Gazzaniga, Joseph Bogen, and Roger Sperry who adapted more modern techniques, which were initially performed on animals, to human patients in the early 1960s. Today, while corpus callostomy surgeries are still being performed to help patients suffering from epileptic seizures, most neuroscientists have turned to functional brain imaging technologies such as fMRI and PET as a means to investigate the unique processing capabilities of the two cerebral hemispheres.

—*Bryan C. Auday, PhD, and Daruenie Andujar*

See also Epilepsy; Neurology; Neuroscience

For Further Information:
Epilepsy Foundation of America.
  www.epilepsyfoundation.org.

Gazzaniga, Michael. "Forty-Five Years of Split-Brain Research and Still Going Strong." *Nature Reviews Neuroscience* (August, 2005): 653-659.
Gazzaniga, Michael. "The Split Brain Revisited." *Scientific American: The Hidden Mind; Special Editions* (May, 2002): 27-31.
Reuter-Lorenz, Patricia Ann, and Michael S. Gazzaniga. *The Cognitive Neuroscience of Mind: A Tribute to Michael S. Gazzaniga.* Cambridge, MA: MIT Press, 2010.
Springer, Sally, and Georg Deutsch. *Left Brain Right Brain Perspectives from Cognitive Neuroscience.* New York: W.H. Freeman and Company, 2003.
Stirling, John D. *Cortical Functions.* London: Routledge, 2000.

SPONDYLITIS

Category: Disease/Disorder
Also known as: Ankylosing spondylitis
Anatomy or system affected: Joints, spine
Specialties and related fields: Cardiology, ophthalmology, orthopedics
Definition: A form of arthritis that affects the spine.

CAUSES AND SYMPTOMS

Spondylitis, also known as ankylosing spondylitis, is a form of arthritis that is chronic and affects the spine. It is a specific disease within a family of diseases called spondyloarthropathies. Examples include psoriatic arthritis, Reiter's syndrome, and arthritis associated with inflammatory bowel disease (IBD). Spondylitis has unique features differentiating it from the other spondyloarthropathies and its own prognosis. The cause of spondylitis is unknown, but the condition may be genetic. Most people with this condition or other spondyloarthropathies are born with a particular gene, HLA-B27. However, having the gene does not mean that a person will develop spondylitis.

Symptoms include mild to severe back and buttock pain that is often worse in the early morning hours. This pain usually decreases with activity. The condition may begin in the teens or twenties and appears gradually over time. Continued inflammation of the ligaments and joints of the spine can cause the spine to fuse together, leading to deformity and disability. The inflammation of ankylosing spondylitis can affect other parts of the body, most commonly other joints and the eyes, but sometimes the lungs and heart valves. Other complications include arthritis of the hip joints and the joints between the ribs and sternum, bone spurs and inflammation in the feet, inflammation of the eyes, scarring of the lungs, inflammation of the prostate, and inflammation of the aorta and aortic valve. Severe disease may lead to poor posture and deformities.

It is reported that men are more likely than women to develop spondylitis; however, females may develop milder cases that sometimes go undiagnosed. Most symptoms of spondylitis appear in early adulthood, prior to age forty, although young males may have symptoms in early adolescence, or even in childhood.

The hallmark signs and symptoms are stiffness and pain in the lower back, buttocks, and hips upon waking in the morning or after a period of inactivity; back pain relieved by movement and exercise; difficulty bending the spine; pain in the hips and difficulty walking; pain in the heels and soles of the feet; bent posture; straightening of the normal curvature of the spine; fever; loss of appetite and weight loss; fatigue and decreased energy; eye swelling, redness, and pain; sensitivity to light; difficulty with chest expansion for deep breathing; heart failure; and heart block.

No definitive test can diagnose ankylosing spondylitis. Most doctors expect to see X-ray evidence of inflammation of the joint between the sacrum and the ilium, as well as any one of the following: inflammatory back pain, reduced mobility of the spine, and reduced ability to expand the chest. Blood tests results that can suggest spondylitis include an elevated erythrocyte sedimentation rate and anemia. The aspiration of synovial fluid from the joint will confirm inflammation.

TREATMENT AND THERAPY

Treatment includes exercise and physical therapy to help reduce stiffness and to maintain good posture and mobility. Medications for pain and inflammation, such as nonsteroidal anti-inflammatory drugs (NSAIDs), are prescribed. Treatment of iritis involves regular eye examinations. Assistive devices, such as a cane or walker, are used to help reduce joint stress and inflammation. Surgery is rarely performed. Patients should choose chairs that help them avoid slumped or stooped postures. Other treatments include hip replacement surgery, treatment for iritis with steroid and dilating drops, and a pacemaker for severe heart block.

—*Jane C. Norman, PhD, RN, CNE*

See also Arthritis; Back pain; Joints; Paralysis; Rheumatoid arthritis; Rheumatology; Spine, vertebrae, and disks.

For Further Information:
Klippel, John H., Paul A. Dieppe, Fred F. Ferri. *Primary Care Rheumatology*. Philadelphia: W. B. Saunders, 2002.
Koopman, William J., and Larry W. Moreland, eds. *Arthritis and Allied Conditions: A Textbook of Rheumatology*. 15th ed. Philadelphia: Lippincott Williams & Wilkins, 2005.
Royen, Barend J. van, and Ben A. C. Dijkmans, eds. *Ankylosing Spondylitis: Diagnosis and Management*. New York: Taylor & Francis, 2006.
Van der Linden, S., and D. van der Heijde. "Ankylosing Spondylitis: Clinical Features." *Rheumatic Disease Clinics of North America* 24, no. 4 (1998): 663-676.
Weisman, Michael H., Désirée van der Heijde, and John D. Reveille, eds. *Ankylosing Spondylitis and the Spondyloarthropathies*. St. Louis, Mo.: Mosby/Elsevier, 2006.

SPORTS MEDICINE

Category: Specialty
Anatomy or system affected: Bones, circulatory system, feet, hands, head, heart, joints, knees, legs, ligaments, muscles, musculoskeletal system, nervous system, spine, tendons
Specialties and related fields: Cardiology, emergency medicine, exercise physiology, family medicine, internal medicine, nutrition, orthopedics, pharmacology, physical therapy, preventive medicine, psychology, rheumatology
Definition: A medical subspecialty concerned with the care and prevention of athletic injuries, primarily those related to the musculoskeletal system.
Key terms:
joint: a specialized structure in the body where bones come together and motion occurs
ligament: a tough, rubber-band-like structure that connects one bone to another and prevents the abnormal motion of these bones in relationship to each other
musculoskeletal: a term used to describe the relationship between bones and muscles within the framework of the body and the way in which they provide stability and locomotion
musculotendinous unit: a structure that consists of a muscle that provides motion of a bone and its attachment to the bone, the tendon, which is a tough, inelastic fibrous structure

orthopedic surgery: the field of surgery that deals with the musculoskeletal system

SCIENCE AND PROFESSION

Sports medicine is a field that has become popular as the number of people who exercise has increased. More than 50 percent of people in the United States exercise on a daily basis. People all over the country are participating in sports, from recreational sports to professional competitive sports. There has been a growing trend of participation in exercise as more and more studies have proved that exercise is beneficial to health; however, exercise places people at risk for injuries that a sedentary person would not have. This fact has led to the emergence of sports medicine, with its specially trained health care professionals. These professionals include physical therapists, athletic trainers, nutritionists, exercise physiologists, cardiologists, sports psychologists, family practitioners, internists, and orthopedic surgeons. They all contribute by bringing special knowledge and understanding to the care of athletes and athletic injuries. Such knowledge can relate to nutrition, strength training, cardiovascular conditioning, psychosocial issues, musculoskeletal care, or one or more of many other areas related to the health of athletes. Therefore, sports medicine is a very broad and diverse field that requires a team approach.

Athletic injuries occur with regularity, but very few injuries are unique to sports. Yet treating an injured athlete does not necessarily require the same process as that used to treat an injured sedentary person. The athlete tends to have greater expectations than does the average sedentary person. These expectations usually increase proportionately with the competitive level of the athlete. For example, the athlete with an ankle sprain will spend ten to twelve hours per day performing treatment and rehabilitation supervised by a physical therapist or athletic trainer. The sedentary person, however, might go to physical therapy three times per week. Although the philosophy of the treatment is the same, the number of treatments and the desired outcomes are completely different. Athletes also require an extensive amount of information regarding their injuries, treatment, and rehabilitation. Athletes are not afraid to ask questions regarding their injuries because they want to know when they will be able to return to competition.

Sports medicine is a challenging and rewarding profession. It is enjoyable working with patients who have a high level of compliance and motivation. The reward of watching an athlete recover from an injury and compete is exceptional. The sports medicine physician must realize, however, that he or she will also be called upon by the athlete and the athlete's coach and parents to communicate the severity of the injury and its

significance—a process that can be difficult at times, especially when what the physician has to say is not what anyone wants to hear. Nevertheless, it is the role of the physician to act in the best interest of the athlete. In order for the physician to be prepared to handle this, he or she must fully understand the demands of each sport. Attendance at games is usually not enough to achieve this level of knowledge and experience. Observing practice sessions and workouts is often useful. With the exception of high-impact collision sports, such as hockey and football, most injuries occur during practice and workout sessions. Furthermore, such observation gives the physician an opportunity to be involved in education and injury prevention. Many athletic injuries are witnessed by an athletic trainer or physician who may be called upon to administer first aid in the field or provide treatment for injuries.

By attending practices or competitions, the physician may also have the opportunity to observe the actual mechanism of injury, which can be useful in evaluating the type and severity of the injury. Many physicians call the first twenty minutes after an injury has occurred, prior to the onset of swelling and spasm, the "golden period." It is at this time that an accurate and meaningful physical examination can be performed on the injured athlete. The recreational athlete, however, usually will arrive at the physician's office one to two days after the injury, when swelling and spasm are maximal. At this time, examining the injured body part is quite difficult and may not be meaningful. This may result in delays in diagnosis and definitive treatment. For the sedentary person and the occasional athlete, such delays will probably not be significant. However, the highly competitive athlete would be dissatisfied if an injury delayed his or her return to competition. Although most athletic injuries differ very little from other cases of musculoskeletal trauma, the finer points of managing them are unique.

Most athletic injuries affect one of three structures in the body: bones, ligaments, or musculotendinous units. These injuries may be acute or chronic in onset. Most acute injuries occur as a result of trauma, with presentation being soon after the incident. Chronic injuries, which are often insidious in onset, usually result from a change in the athlete or the athletic environment. Chronic injuries tend to be difficult to recognize and treat effectively. The best approach to chronic injuries is prevention. Most acute injuries can be classified as sprains, strains, or fractures and most chronic injuries can be classified as strains or stress fractures.

Sprains are injuries to ligaments; strains are injuries to the musculotendinous unit. Sprains occur when there is excessive abnormal motion at a joint. This results in overstretching of the ligaments and produces local pain, swelling, limitation of motion, and a sense of instability. Such overstretching can result in partial tears (mild) or complete tears (severe) of the ligament. Strains are usually the result of an abrupt increase in the tension of the musculotendinous unit. For example, they may occur when one lifts weights that are too heavy. This increase may result in partial or complete tears of the muscle, the tendon, or the bone to which the tendon is attached. The most important principle is to realize that strains are not the result of overstretching but occur well within the normal limits of motion. Strains are also graded from mild to severe. Often, there is an obvious deformity at the site of injury because the muscle rolls up into a ball. Fractures are breaks in the bones of the body. Stress fractures occur when excessive demands are placed on the bone. Eventually, the bone fails to accommodate these demands, and microscopic breaks result.

DIAGNOSTIC AND TREATMENT TECHNIQUES
The initial management of acute injuries is the same in athletics as it is in other musculoskeletal trauma. Treatment should be directed at prevention of bleeding and edema. These conditions usually lead to pain and decreased function of the injured body part, which requires the application of ice, compression, elevation, and rest. Other methods of treatment used in the professional setting are also useful in preventing or reducing bleeding and edema. These include electric stimulation, contrast baths, ultrasound, and compression stockings. After the initial phase of bleeding and edema, therapy should be directed at restoring range of motion, strength, and, finally, functional tasks that will ultimately result in the athlete's return to competition. Chronic injuries, however, usually require elimination of the precipitating factors as well as increased rest while the injured body part is allowed to heal. This may require a special taping procedure, a brace, a change in footwear, the alteration of practice sessions or simply refraining from that activity for a short period.

Chronic injuries and overuse injuries are usually caused by change. Change can occur in the athlete, the environment, or the activity. Identifying these changes can be helpful in injury prevention, since the majority of injuries in athletics are chronic. In addition, the treatment requires elimination of the offending change and restoration of the proper condition. Strains to the musculotendinous unit can also occur chronically. They tend to result from muscle fatigue, too much training too fast, or poor training conditions. Many of these injuries are called "tendinitis," which means inflammation of the tendon. The most prominent aspect of such an injury is pain, which is almost always located in the region of the injured structure. Management is directed at avoidance of painful

activity, elimination of the offending factor, and symptomatic relief of pain with ice, ultrasound, injections, electric stimulation, and medications. Rehabilitation is aimed at restoring strength and flexibility as well as avoiding the initial cause.

Most sprains can be treated with routine physical therapy and rehabilitation, but many severe sprains will require surgery. Average time lost from athletics ranges from seven days (for example, for a mild ankle sprain) to one year (for example, for a severe knee sprain with reconstruction of ligaments). With strains, complete tears of the tendon usually require surgery, while injury to the muscle itself does not. Treatment is similar to that for sprains; rehabilitation should be directed at regaining strength and flexibility. The diagnosis of a fracture can be made through X-ray imaging. Treatment of fractures requires immobilization either in a cast, special splint, or brace. Some fractures will require the placement of plates or screws by an orthopedic surgeon. Rehabilitation of fractures involves restoration of motion, strength, flexibility, and proprioception. Proprioception is the unconscious awareness of where a body part is in space (for example, a person can tie his or her shoes with eyes closed because the brain knows where the hands are in space). The treatment of stress fractures is different from treatments of other fractures in that immobilization is almost never necessary. Adaptation of activity and relative rest are usually all that is required. Return to competition averages three to six weeks but may be longer.

Sports medicine personnel also provide education and guidance to coaches, athletes, and parents. They make themselves available to provide the best and most efficient care possible. It is the responsibility of the sports medicine physician to coordinate this care. This all begins with the preseason screening history and physical exam.

The preseason screening also identifies athletes who are at risk for developing strains and sprains because their flexibility is lower than normal. Identifying these athletes allows the athletic trainer to work with them on a stretching program intended to reduce the number and severity of such injuries. It is during the preseason that the athletes are at greatest risk for injury, since the workouts are long and numerous and most athletes are not yet in shape. Injuries may occur at any time during practice or a game. However, most injuries occur during practice, and especially at the end of the session, because athletes are tired and their concentration level is low.

Prior to the commencement of each athletic season, athletes are usually required to provide a medical history and undergo a physical examination. The requirements of such examinations vary from state to state, college to college, and professional league to professional league. The purpose of these examinations is to identify athletes who may have potential problems in the sport in which they have chosen to compete. Below are some example patient cases that show the role of preparticipation sports evaluations in keeping individuals healthy and safe.

Julian is a fifteen-year-old high school student who would like to try out for the football team. During his preparticipation sports evaluation, the doctor listens to his heart and hears a heart murmur. Julian's murmur intensity is worse with the Valsalva maneuver, which is a diagnostic technique that may be used to evaluate for a cardiac condition. The Valsalva maneuver decreases the cardiac preload, which is the force that stretches the heart prior to its contraction. Maneuvers that increase the amount of blood in the ventricles of the heart, such as squatting and passive leg elevation, decrease the intensity of his heart murmur. Julian notes that both his father and paternal uncle died suddenly during intense exercise at age thirty. The physician refers Julian to a cardiologist for further workup. Evaluation by the cardiologist reveals that Julian has hypertrophic cardiomyopathy. Hypertrophic cardiomyopathy is a genetic condition that results in enlargement and thickening of the walls of the left ventricle. The left ventricle is the part of the heart that is responsible for pumping blood into the circulation for the rest of the body. Hypertrophic cardiomyopathy may lead to ventricular stiffness and decreased outflow of blood into the systemic circulation. Patients with hypertrophic cardiomyopathy are at an increased risk for sudden death, especially while in a state of high myocardial oxygen demand such as during physical exertion. The cardiologist strongly advises Julian to avoid heavy lifting or doing any strenuous exercise. Hypertrophic cardiomyopathy is an important cause of sudden cardiac death in young patient populations, thus supporting the value of preparticipation sports evaluation.

An incoming freshman college student went to a family medicine physician to establish care and request a preparticipation physical examination for volleyball. On review of her medical history, she tells the physician that she has been healthy but has visited the hospital twice previously. The first time she went to the hospital was at age ten when she had retinal detachment after her head was hit by a ball. Two years ago, she was evaluated at an emergency room after a left shoulder dislocation. When asked about medical conditions that run in her family, she states that she has one brother who is healthy and plays basketball in high school. However, her mother passed away from a ruptured cerebral aneurysm when she was forty-nine. On physical exam, the patient is six feet one, has long

extremities, and slender fingers. The doctor asks the patient to place her thumbs in the palms of the same hand and form a fist. When the patient does this, in both hands, the tips of her thumbs protrude beyond the fifth digit. This is called a "positive thumb sign." After considering the information obtained from the medical history and the physical exam findings, the family medicine physician refers this patient for an ultrasound imaging of the heart called "echocardiography." The results of this test showed mild dilation of the aortic root. The patient is referred for genetic testing, which confirmed the family medicine physician's clinical suspicion for Marfan syndrome. Marfan syndrome is an inherited medical condition that causes a defect in the connective tissue of the body. This disease results in various clinical manifestations, such as cardiovascular disorders, joint hypermobility, tall stature, and retinal detachment. Early diagnosis of this medical condition is especially important in athletes because sports activities that involve high levels of dynamic exercise can increase aortic wall stress, which could put an athlete with Marfan syndrome at a higher risk for aortic dissection. Aortic dissection is a condition where the blood enters between blood vessel layers to create a false lumen, which could then lead to fatal consequences like cardiac tamponade. Cardiac tamponade is a compression of the heart by fluid, which impairs the heart's ability to circulate blood throughout the body. This is another scenario that demonstrates the importance of preparticipation sports history and physical exam. In this case, example, confirming this patient's diagnosis may also prove beneficial for her brother. If Marfan syndrome is diagnosed early and treated prior to development of fatal complications, athletes may be counseled appropriately about sports activities.

Dean is a twenty-year-old college soccer player who went to an urgent care center for one week of fever, malaise, and sore throat. He is diagnosed with infectious mononucleosis, an infection caused by the Epstein-Barr virus. His trainer advises him to follow up with the team physician for return to sport evaluation. During his evaluation by the team physician, Dean is informed that he is at high risk for splenic rupture due to infectious mononucleosis. In infectious mononucleosis, the spleen, a small organ that filters the blood, enlarges due to the proliferation of immune cells in response to the viral infection. Splenic rupture from infectious mononucleosis is rare, but it is the most common cause of death in individuals with this infection. Splenic rupture is considered a medical emergency since it may cause massive intra-abdominal bleeding which can lead to rapid clinical deterioration. Strenuous contact sports like soccer is associated with an increased risk of splenic rupture after infectious mononucleosis; thus, the team physician advises Dean to refrain from his sports activities for a minimum of four weeks. Dean recovers and returns gradually to his sports activities after six weeks. With the aid of the trainer and prompt attention by the team physician, a potentially fatal medical emergency was prevented.

Mary is a fifteen-year-old high school all-state cross-country runner. She is now entering her junior year and is expected to compete on the national level. Six weeks into the fall season, Mary's times begin to decrease slightly. When asked about her performance, she states that she has been experiencing pain in both her shins, particularly the one on the right, for two weeks. Her coach asks Mary to see her family doctor since the school does not have an athletic trainer or team physician. Mary's doctor tells her that she has shin splints and that she should rest. Mary does not accept this, and continues to run against her doctor's advice. In the next race, Mary finishes last. The pain has become unbearable. Mary is then referred to a sports medicine physician, who discovers several relevant facts. Mary is underweight and has not been eating well. She has been forcing herself to vomit for a number of days prior to each race. She has also not experienced her first menses. X-rays of Mary's right leg reveal severe stress fractures. Mary is referred to several specialists, including an orthopedic surgeon who places her in a cast, a nutritionist, a psychologist who evaluates and treats her eating disorder, and a gynecologist who proceeds with a workup for her late development. Mary is diagnosed with functional hypothalamic amenorrhea, which is a menstrual dysfunction in the setting of restrictive eating and excessive exercise. This condition is also referred to as the female athlete triad of functional hypothalamic amenorrhea, and is characterized by strenuous physical activity or low intake of calories, low bone mineral density, and amenorrhea, which is a lack of menses. The pathophysiology of functional hypothalamic amenorrhea involves low energy availability (due to caloric restriction and/or excessive exercise) and elevated cortisol levels (secondary to stress or excessive exercise), which results in decreased hypothalamic gonadotropin-releasing hormone (GnRH) pulsatile secretion. Normally, GnRH from the hypothalamus stimulates the release of luteinizing hormone (LH) and follicle-stimulating hormone (FSH) from the anterior pituitary. In functional hypothalamic amenorrhea, the decreased GnRH pulsatile secretion results in decreased secretion of both LH and FSH, which consequently decreases estrogen levels. The reduced estrogen levels in individuals with functional hypothalamic amenorrhea leads to anovulation and amenorrhea. After several months of collaborative treatment by several health care professionals, Mary begins retraining on a bicycle

under the direction of an athletic trainer and a physical therapist. She moves on to compete in the spring season of track and field and becomes a national champion. Without the collaborative care of the sports medicine team, Mary's condition could have progressed to serious complications or even death. This is a common scenario among adolescent athletes. The pressures placed upon them by friends, coaches, and parents can become detrimental to their emotional and physical well-being.

Henry is a fifty-five-year-old businessman who spends five days a week playing tennis at the local health club to stay in shape. After buying a new racket, he begins to experience pain in his right elbow. An orthopedic surgeon who specializes in sports medicine evaluates him. After speaking with Henry and examining his elbow, the doctor recommends anti-inflammatory medication, a special forearm strap, and use of the old racket. Henry's condition, which is called "tennis elbow" or lateral epicondylitis, is quite common. Lateral epicondylitis is a condition caused by excessive pronation, supination, and extension motions of the wrist, resulting in inflammation of the wrist extensor muscles. After several weeks of the initial treatment, Henry does not feel any better. His doctor, therefore, injects him with a medication to ease the pain and calm the inflammation. Henry is instructed to rest his arm for a week prior to starting tennis again. Henry follows the doctor's instructions carefully. He begins to play tennis again and feels fine for about a month, after which he begins to experience the same discomfort. This time, the doctor recommends surgery for Henry's elbow. Three months after the surgery, Henry is free of pain.

These examples have demonstrated how sports medicine can be beneficial to athletes. Each scenario differs in type of athlete, location, diagnosis, and treatment.

PERSPECTIVE AND PROSPECTS
Sports medicine is assuming a significant role in the medical profession today. Sports medicine was first recognized in the days of the early Olympics. It was not until the final decades of the twentieth century, however, that it emerged into a field of its own. Sports medicine training programs have been developing at an exponential rate. Interest in sports medicine can be pursued in various ways. Most sports medicine physicians undergo a one-year fellowship either after either a five-year orthopedic residency training program or after completion of either a family medicine residency, internal medicine, pediatrics, emergency medicine or physical medicine and rehabilitation training program.

Athletic trainers must pass a national examination for certification. Most have master's degrees, and all have some form of bachelor's degree. Their expertise is in the prevention, treatment, and rehabilitation of athletic injuries. These are the primary caregivers of the sports medicine world. Certified athletic trainers are being hired at all major universities, many high schools, and many health clubs across the country. Various types of sports medicine centers are continually being developed. These centers offer a wide range of services to both professional and amateur athletes. As more and more people begin to exercise, the need for sports medicine professionals will increase.

Athletes' needs and goals are different from those of most other people. Although the injuries that they experience are not unique to sports, the rapidity with which they recover is of utmost importance. This identifies them as a distinct group of people with special demands for medical care. It is because of this and because of the growing number of people who exercise on a daily basis, that sports medicine has evolved into a viable medical field. Sports medicine will continue to grow and will play an important role in preventing many of the injuries that afflict people in the United States.

—Jason Pyon, MD and Marichelle Pita, OMS-III

See also: Acupressure; Anorexia nervosa; Arthroplasty; Arthroscopy; Athlete's foot; Biofeedback; Bones and the skeleton; Braces, orthopedic; Bruises; Cardiology; Concussion; Critical care; Eating disorders; Emergency medicine; Ergogenic aids; Exercise physiology; First aid; Fracture and dislocation; Fracture repair; Glycolysis; Head and neck disorders; Heat exhaustion and heatstroke; Hydrotherapy; Joints; Kinesiology; Muscle sprains, spasms, and disorders; Ligaments; Muscles; Nutrition; Orthopedic surgery; Orthopedics; Orthopedics, pediatric; Oxygen therapy; Over-the-counter medications; Overtraining syndrome; Physical examination; Physical rehabilitation; Physiology; Preventive medicine; Psychiatry; Psychiatry, child and adolescent; Rotator cuff surgery; Spine, vertebrae, and disks; Steroid abuse; Steroids; Tendinitis; Tendon disorders; Tendon repair; Whiplash.

For Further Information:
Ahmad, Z., N. Siddiqui, S. S. Malik, et al. "Lateral Epicondylitis: A Review of Pathology and Management." *Bone Joint Journal*, vol. 95-B, no. 9, Sept. 2013, pp. 1158-64, doi:10.1302/0301-620X.95B9.29285. PMID:23997125.
Auwaerter, P. G. "Infectious Mononucleosis: Return to Play." *Clinical Sports Medicine*, vol. 23, no. 3, July 2004, pp. xi, 485-97, doi:10.1016/j.csm.2004.02.005. PMID:15262384.
Blumenstein, Boris, Michael Bar-Eli, and Gershon Tenenbaum, editors. *Brain and Body in Sport and Exercise: Biofeedback Applications in Performance Enhancement.* John Wiley & Sons, 2002. Notes that technical advances in biofeedback have made it a vital method of training athletes in order to increase individual awareness and control over the body and reduce habitual physiological tensions. Brings together current research and applications and shows how different biofeedback approaches can be used in various sports.
De Souza, M. J., A. Nattiv, E. Joy, et al. "Expert Panel: 2014 Female Athlete Triad Coalition Consensus Statement on Treatment and Return to Play of the Female Athlete Triad: 1st International Conference held in San Francisco, California, May 2012 and 2nd International Conference held in Indianapolis, Indiana, May 2013." *British Journal of Sports Medicine*, vol. 48, no. 4, Feb. 2014, p. 289, doi:10.1136/bjsports-2013-093218. PMID: 24463911.
Delforge, Gary. *Musculoskeletal Trauma: Implications for Sport Injury Management.* Human Kinetics, 2002. Covers the therapeutic management of sport-related soft tissue injuries, fractures, and proprioceptive/sensorimotor impairments. Reviews the major categories of intervention and presents fifty illustrations to accompany the text.
Gordon, C. M., K. E. Ackerman, S. L. Berga, et al. "Functional Hypothalamic Amenorrhea: An Endocrine Society Clinical Practice Guideline." *The Journal of Clinical Endocrinology & Metabolism*, vol. 102, no. 5, 1 May 2017, pp. 1413-39, doi:10.1210/jc.2017-00131. PMID: 28368518.
Landry, Gregory L., and David T. Bernhardt. *Essentials of Primary Care Sports Medicine.* Human Kinetics, 2003. This book explains general health issues for athletes.
Loeys, B. L., H. C. Dietz, A. C. Braverman, et al. "The Revised Ghent Nosology for the Marfan Syndrome." *Journal of Medical Genetics*, vol. 47, no. 7, pp. 476-85, doi:10.1136/jmg.2009.072785.
McArdle, William, Frank I. Katch, and Victor L. Katch. *Exercise Physiology: Energy, Nutrition, and Human Performance.* 7th ed., Lippincott Williams & Wilkins, 2010. A wide-ranging text on exercise and the human body, covering topics such as nutrition, energy transfer, exercise training, systems of energy delivery and utilization, enhancement of energy capacity, the effect of environmental stress, and the effect of exercise on successful aging and disease prevention.
Nishimura, R. A., H. Seggewiss, and H. V. Schaff. "Hypertrophic Obstructive Cardiomyopathy." *Circulation Research*, vol. 121, no. 7, 2017, pp. 771-83, doi:10.1161/circresaha.116.309348.
O'Connor, T. E., L. J. Skinner, P. Kiely, and J. E. Fenton. "Return to Contact Sports Following Infectious Mononucleosis: The Role of Serial Ultrasonography." *Ear, Nose & Throat Journal*, vol. 90, no. 8, Aug. 2011, pp. E21-24, doi:10.1177/014556131109000819. PMID: 21853428.
Pelliccia, A., F. M. Di Paolo, E. De Blasiis, et al. "Prevalence and Clinical Significance of Aortic Dilatation in Highly Trained Competitive Athletes." *Circulation*, vol. 122, 2010, pp. 698-706.
Scuderi, Giles R., and Peter D. McCann, editors. *Sports Medicine: A Comprehensive Approach.* 2nd ed., Mosby/Elsevier, 2005. This text covers all types of athletic injuries and offers useful illustrations. Includes a bibliography and an index.
Small, Eric, et al. *Kids and Sports: Everything You and Your Child Need to Know About Sports, Physical Activity, and Good Health.* Newmarket Press, 2002. Reminds parents that children are physiologically and psychologically different from adults and thus experience sports and their injuries in different ways. Covers which sports are suitable for which age, how to prevent and treat injuries, how to plan sports programs for children with chronic conditions such as asthma or diabetes, and the importance of good nutrition and exercise.

Warren, M. P., and N. E. Perlroth. "The Effects of Intense Exercise on the Female Reproductive System." *Journal of Endocrinology*, vol. 170, July 2001, pp. 3-11, doi:10.1677/joe.0.1700003. PMID:11431132.

Won, A. C., and A. Ethell. "Spontaneous Splenic Rupture Resulted from Infectious Mononucleosis." *International Journal of Surgery Case Reports*, vol. 3, no. 3, 2012, pp. 97-99, doi.org/10.1016/j.ijscr.2011.08.012.

SPRAINS. SEE MUSCLE SPRAINS, SPASMS, AND DISORDERS.

SQUAMOUS CELL CARCINOMA. SEE SKIN CANCER.

STAPHYLOCOCCAL INFECTIONS

Category: Disease/Disorder
Also known as: Staph infections
Anatomy or system affected: Blood, circulatory system, gastrointestinal system, musculoskeletal system, nervous system, respiratory system, urinary system
Specialties and related fields: Bacteriology, cardiology, dermatology, epidemiology, general surgery, internal medicine, microbiology, orthopedics, urology
Definition: infections caused by bacteria from the genus *Staphylococcus*
Key terms:
antistaphylococcal penicillins: a group of penicillin antibiotics that kill methicillin-sensitive *Staphylococcus aureus* strains and other staphylococci
beta-lactam antibiotics: antibacterial drugs that inhibit cell wall synthesis in bacteria and contain a beta-lactam ring in their structure
methicillin-resistant Staphylococcus aureus: also known as MRSA; is an S. aureus strain that has acquired antibiotic resistance genes and causes several community- and hospital-acquired infections
Panton-Valentine leucocidin: a toxin produced by some strains of *Staphylococcus aureus* that destroys white blood cells and damaged tissues
superantigens: a class of antigens that result in excessive activation of the immune system
toxic shock syndrome toxin: a superantigen produced by some *Staphylococcus aureus* and *Streptococcus pyogenes* isolates that causes toxic shock syndrome

CAUSES AND SYMPTOMS

Under the microscope, staphylococci bacteria grow in irregular, grapelike clusters from which they derive their name. Individually, the organisms are spherical and appear purple (positive) when stained with the Gram technique. Staphylococci are found predominantly on mammals' and birds' skin and mucous

> **INFORMATION ON STAPHYLOCOCCAL INFECTIONS**
>
> **Causes:** Bacterial infection with staphylococci; often from food poisoning, contamination of catheter or shunt
> **Symptoms:** Depends on type; may include vomiting, fever, rashes, pus-producing lesions
> **Duration:** Acute
> **Treatments:** Depends on type; may include alleviation of symptoms, drainage or cleansing of site, antibiotics (vancomycin, methicillin, oxacillin)

membranes. Usually, they exist in a benignly symbiotic relationship with their hosts. When the barrier imposed by either the skin or mucous membranes is breached, however, staphylococci may cause disease, assisted by various enzymes and toxins they can manufacture. Many strains of staphylococci, such as *Staphylococcus aureus*, produce coagulase, which catalyzes the formation of a clot from fibrinogen proteins in the blood. Hyaluronidases, lipases, and other proteolytic enzymes carve out a cavity within the clot, covered by a coagulase-generated fibrin coat, and an abscess is formed. Abscess formation is one of the hallmarks of staphylococcal infection and can be found in virtually any organ in the body because of local invasion or spread to the site via the bloodstream. Staphylococcal strains can produce a variety of proteins called "exotoxins" that have significant roles in determining the type of illness that results. Superantigens, such as toxic shock syndrome toxin-1 (TSST-1), target the circulatory system and can markedly lower blood pressure. TSST-1 producing strains have caused disease by growing in vaginal tampons and simultaneously causing postsurgical wound infections. Food poisoning results after ingesting food contaminated with staphylococcal strains that produce enterotoxins. The toxins are produced in the food after contamination from the colonized noses or infected skin of food handlers through sneezing or direct contact. The enterotoxins are relatively heat-stable and do not result in any unusual taste, odor, or appearance of the food. Abdominal cramps, nausea, vomiting, and diarrhea occur one to six hours after ingesting the food containing the toxin. Toxic shock syndrome is not an actual infection, as it is the pre-formed toxin that produces the illness. The exfoliative toxin is produced by the strains causing scalded skin syndrome. The illness is manifested by fever and reddened skin that subsequently peels off.

Staphylococci can form a variety of cytotoxins that damage the membranes of bodily tissues. These toxins can destroy red and white blood cells and organ cells. White blood cell-killing toxins from staphylococci were

SEM micrograph of S. aureus *colonies; the grape-like clustering is common to Staphylococcus species. Photo via Wikimedia Commons. [Public domain.]*

first reported in 1932, and the Panton-Valentine leukocidin (PVL) was named in honor of these scientists. PVL is produced by strains of *S. aureus* that cause skin and soft tissue infection and pneumonia in the community (outside the hospital). *S. aureus* is the preeminent pathogen causing infection in hospitalized patients. It is the most common cause of surgical wound infections. It is joined by another species, *S. epidermidis*, which can produce slime, enabling the bacteria to adhere to the surfaces of medical devices such as vascular catheters, central nervous system shunts, artificial heart valves, and prosthetic joints. Together, these two species account for many hospital-acquired infections. Skeletal muscle and adjacent tissue infections are called "pyomyositis" or "necrotizing fasciitis." This type of infection has been common in developing countries with tropical climates. However, since the 1970s, it has been seen more frequently in modern countries with temperate climates. The pathogenesis of pyomyositis is not entirely understood. Some cases follow trauma, and there are several risk factors, such

as intravenous drug abuse, human immunodeficiency virus (HIV) infection, and skin diseases. Other cases occur in healthy individuals without any apparent risk factor. Recently, virulent strains of community-acquired methicillin-resistant *S. aureus* (MRSA) have caused pyomyositis in the United States. *S. saprophyticus* is an important cause of urinary tract infections in sexually active young women. Bladder infections caused by this organism usually produce painful urination (dysuria), urinary urgency, pain in the lower abdomen below the navel, and, occasionally, blood in the urine.

TREATMENT AND THERAPY

Specific treatment of staphylococcal infection hinges on administering an effective antibiotic. Staphylococci are resistant to a host of regularly prescribed antibiotics. Therefore, drug developers discovered a group of antistaphylococcal penicillins to treat staphylococcal infections specifically. These drugs include methicillin (which was removed from human use because it causes kidney damage), nafcillin, oxacillin, and dicloxacillin. Unfortunately, some *Staphylococcus aureus* strains acquired a gene called *mecA* from nonpathogenic staphylococci. The *mecA* gene encodes an abnormally low-affinity cell wall-synthesizing enzyme, PBP2a, that helps the organism grow and divide in the presence of antistaphylococcal penicillins and other antibiotics like them. *Staphylococcus aureus* strains with the *mecA* gene are called "methicillin-resistant *Staphylococcus aureus*" or "MRSA."

MRSA is resistant to beta-lactam antibiotics, including penicillin, amoxicillin, oxacillin, and other related antibiotics. Vancomycin, a glycopeptide antibiotic developed in the 1950s, has remained effective for nearly all strains. Still, it must be given intravenously and has some serious potential side effects. Some newer antibiotics, daptomycin, dalfopristin/quinupristin, ceftaroline, linezolid, and tedizolid, are effective against MRSA and successfully treat infections.

Antibiotics are not the only measure necessary to cure these infections. Surgical or percutaneous catheter drainage of abscesses, surgical debridement of dead tissue, and the removal of medical devices or prostheses are often necessary. Other medical supportive modalities, such as fluid replacement, vasopressors, or mechanical ventilation, may be required.

PERSPECTIVE AND PROSPECTS
The Centers for Disease Control and Prevention (CDC) collaborates with other medical organizations to develop and promote strategies to reduce the transmission of staphylococci, primarily MRSA, in both health care and community settings. The CDC has also launched a campaign to prevent antimicrobial resistance by educating the public and healthcare providers about unnecessary and inappropriate antibiotic usage. Legislative efforts have been directed at eliminating the use of antibiotics in animal feed to prevent resistance.

Newer antimicrobial agents continue to be developed, but the stream has slowed. Molecular-based treatments directed toward toxins and other virulence factors are being actively pursued.

—*Michael A. Buratovich, PhD*

For Further Information:
Bush, Larry M. "*Staphylococcus aureus* Infections." *Merck Manual Consumer Version.* Mar. 2021, www.merckmanuals.com/home/infections/bacterial-infections-gram-positive-bacteria/staphylococcus-aureus-infections. Accessed 5 Apr. 2022.
Koneman, Elmer W. *The Other End of the Microscope: The Bacteria Tell Their Own Story.* ASM Press, 2002.
McCarthy, Matt. *Superbugs: The Race to Stop an Epidemic.* Avery, 2019.
Staph Infections. Mayo Clinic, 6 May 2020, www.mayoclinic.org/diseases-conditions/staph-infections/symptoms-causes/syc-20356221. Accessed 5 Apr. 2022.
Staph Infections: What You Should Know. Penn Medicine, 7 May 2018, www.pennmedicine.org/updates/blogs/health-and-wellness/2018/may/staph-infections. Accessed 5 Apr. 2022.
Staphylococcal Skin Infection. DermNet NZ, Dec. 2015, dermnetnz.org/topics/staphylococcal-skin-infection. Accessed 5 Apr. 2022.

STATINS

Category: Biology
Anatomy or system affected: Cardiovascular, endocrinology
Specialties and related fields: Biochemistry, metabolism
Key terms:
3-hydroxy-3-methylglutaryl CoA (HMG CoA): the substrate from which cholesterol is synthesized
3-hydroxy-3-methylglutaryl CoA (HMG CoA) reductase: the main controlling enzyme of cholesterol biosynthesis
atherosclerosis: a condition where fatty plaques are deposited in the inner arterial walls
dyslipidemia: the imbalance of cholesterol, triglycerides and lipoproteins
hypercholesterolemia: high serum cholesterol levels
lipoproteins: protein/lipid complexes that transport cholesterol and glycerides in the blood and lymph
myocardial infarction: a heart attack

STRUCTURE AND FUNCTIONS
Statins are a group of drugs that inhibit the enzyme 3-hydroxy-3-methylglutaryl CoA (HMG CoA) reductase, a liver enzyme that functions in the biosynthesis of cholesterol. The enzyme converts acetyl CoA and acetoacetyl CoA to mevalonate. Since statins resemble the structure of HMG CoA and easily fits into the active site of HMG CoA reductase, they are competitive inhibitors of the enzyme. Statins reduce total serum cholesterol by at least 20 percent. Statins are preferably taken in the evening, since cholesterol is produced by the liver during the night. Statins are one of the best-selling drugs in history. Many statins are on the market and include atorvastatin and rosuvastatin among many others. In terms of clinical efficacy, some statins are more potent in lowering the "bad cholesterol" levels, and some have fewer side effects than the others. However, statin intolerance is far less common than previously reported.

DISORDERS AND DISEASES
According to the World Health Organization (WHO), ischemic heart disease and stroke are the two major causes of death. Apart from age, gender, and family history, the majority of these cardiovascular events are caused by modifiable risk factors: high blood

pressure, tobacco use, overweight/obesity, lack of physical activity, diabetes, and high blood cholesterol levels. Reducing cholesterol levels is one of the therapeutic targets in reducing the prevalence of cardiovascular mortality. Furthermore, statins reduce the risk of thrombosis and stenosis. Statins are therefore the first choice of therapeutic cholesterol-lowering agents in the prevention of cardiovascular events.

Hypercholesterolemia is an elevated level of serum cholesterol. Low-density lipoproteins (LDLs), as part of total serum cholesterol, can provoke or intensify the process of atherosclerosis. LDLs are particles that transport cholesterol and other lipids in the blood. Because of an excess of cholesterol in the blood, LDLs accumulate in the arterial walls. This accumulation of cholesterol is followed by a gradual process of chronic inflammation in the walls. This creates plaques that compromise blood flow and ultimately can lead to thrombosis or stenosis. In sum, the amount of LDL in the blood is a strong predictor of cardiovascular events.

Statins can reduce the cardiovascular risk by the inhibition of the biosynthesis of endogenous cholesterol and additionally, by the retardation and stabilization of the plaque development in arterial walls. Statins have demonstrated their therapeutic benefits both in patients with no history of cardiovascular diseases (primary prevention), and in patients who have already experienced a cardiovascular event (secondary prevention). Despite underreporting of side effects, it is believed that the potential benefits of statins may outweigh their potential risks.

When statins were used for primary prevention, a significant reduction was observed in the prevalence of cardiovascular events and mortality rates in patients with a high cardiovascular risk profile. This finding was confirmed by a systematic literature review conducted in 2013 by the Cochrane Collaboration, led by Huffman Taylor, et al. Patients with a high initial cardiovascular risk show greater cardiovascular absolute risk reductions caused by statins than those with lesser initial risk. This was demonstrated by the Cholesterol Treatment Trialists in 2012 which stated that for each reduction of 40mg/dl LDL caused by statins, a relative risk reduction of 21 percent in major vascular events was documented in patients. A relative risk reduction in vascular mortality of 12 percent was documented. In terms of age, there is little evidence supporting that the use of statins in elderly patients in primary prevention has net benefits. A meta-analysis conducted by Gotto Savarese, et al. in 2013 stated that in the case of the elderly who have a high cardiovascular risk yet no established cardiovascular diseases, statins did not seem to prolong life in the short term, even though the incidence of

myocardial infarction (MI) and stroke was reduced. Based on these and other studies, in 2021 the United States Preventive Services Task Force recommended that statins be used as a primary preventative for everyone between the ages of forty and seventy-five years of age who have at least one risk factor for developing heart disease and at least a 10 percent risk of heart disease. Many other organizations including the National Institute for Health and Clinical Excellence (NICE), the European Society of Cardiology, the American College of Cardiology and the American Heart Association also recommend statins as a primary preventative of cardiovascular disease.

In secondary prevention, statins are effective in the prevention of major coronary events for almost all patients. In patients with a history of ischemic stroke or patients with coronary artery diseases (heart attack, angina), statin therapy showed a significant reduction in the incidence of vascular events.

Despite all the documented benefits, statins do have some side effects including muscle and liver problems and diabetes mellitus. Muscle effects are the most reported and documented adverse effect (AE), and are dose-dependent. Severe muscle damage can lead to renal dysfunction and renal failure (rhabdomyolysis), sometimes causing death. It is possible that muscle damage and diabetes mellitus may result from the inhibition of HMG CoA reductase, which is also used to synthesize CoQ10, a compound necessary for muscle integrity and blood sugar regulation. Although cognitive problems have been reported there seems to be little evidence for a link to statins. Elevated transaminase levels, an indicator of liver damage, has also been reported. Observational and limited data, though conflicting, suggest that dietary supplementation with CoQ10 may improve statin-induced AEs.

PERSPECTIVE AND PROSPECTS

Cholesterol is an essential structural component of cell membranes where it functions in nerve conduction, an intracellular transport and signaling molecule. It is also a precursor molecule for steroid hormones, vitamin D and bile. Cholesterol can be synthesized by the liver (endogenous) or can be obtained from food such as animal fats (exogenous). Dietary cholesterol is transported to the liver by chylomicrons. These are a type of lipoproteins, molecules that can carry cholesterol through the blood. Lipoproteins vary in density from very-low- (VLDL) to high-density lipoproteins (HDL). The liver can regulate its endogenous cholesterol production according to the amount of dietary cholesterol intake. It can also remove cholesterol to extrahepatic tissues in the form of VLDL particles. After removing triglycerides from VLDL-particles by hydrolysis, low-density lipoproteins (LDL particles) remain in the blood plasma where they bind to LDL receptors in the liver and are taken up by the liver thereby removing cholesterol from circulation. Cholesterol, packed in LDL particles, accounts for 70 percent of the plasma cholesterol in most people and is considered "bad cholesterol." High-density lipoprotein particles (HDL particles) remove cholesterol from cells and transport it to the liver. HDL particles are considered to be "good cholesterol." The sum of LDL and HDL in blood plasma is referred to as the total cholesterol (TC). TC is expressed in mg/dl and is recommended to be lower than 200 mg/dl.

—*Marija Petrovic, MD*

For Further Information:

Bytyçi, Penson, et al. "Prevalence of Statin Intolerance: A Meta-Analysis." *European Heart Journal*, 2022 Feb. 16, ehac015, doi: 10.1093/eurheartj/ehac015. PMID: 35169843.

Cholesterol Treatment Trialists, et al. "The Effects of Lowering LDL Cholesterol with Statin Therapy in People at Low Risk of Vascular Disease: Meta-Analysis of Individual Data from 27 Randomized Trials." *The Lancet*, vol. 380, 2012, pp. 581-90.

Golomb, Beatrice, and Marcella Evans. "Statin Adverse Effects: A Review of the Literature and Evidence for Mitochondrial Mechanism." *American Journal of Cardiovascular Drugs*, vol. 8, no. 6, 2008, pp. 373-418.

Insull, William. "The Pathology of Atherosclerosis: Plaque Development and Plaque Responses to Medical Treatment." *The American Journal of Medicine*, vol. 122, no. 1, 2009, pp. 3-14.

Manktelow, Bradley, and J. F. Potter. "Interventions in the Management of Serum Lipids for Preventing Stroke Recurrence." *The Cochrane Library*, vol. 3, 2009.

Mills, O'Regan, et al. "Intensive Statin Therapy Compared with Moderate Dosing for Prevention of Cardiovascular Events: A Meta-Analysis of 40000 Patients." *European Heart Journal*, vol. 32, no. 11, 2011, pp. 1409-15.

Pagano, Irwin S., and Nathan B. Strait. *HDL and LDL Cholesterol: Physiologyand Clinical Significance*. Nova, 2009.

Savarese, Gotto, et al. "Benefits of Statins in Elderly Subjects without Established Cardiovascular Disease: A Meta-Analysis." *Journal of the American College of Cardiology*, vol. 62, no. 22, 2013, pp. 2090-99.

Taylor, Huffman, et al. "Statins for the Primary Prevention of Cardiovascular Disease." *The Cochrane Library*, vol. 1, 2013.

US Preventive Services Task Force. "Statin Use for the Primary Prevention of Cardiovascular Disease in Adults: Preventive Medication." Nov. 2016.

Visseren, F. L.J., F. Mach, et al. "2021 ESC Guidelines on Cardiovascular Disease Prevention in Clinical Practice." *European Heart Journal*, vol. 42, 2021, pp. 3227-337.

Ward, Lloyd Jones, et al. "A Systematic Review and Economic Evaluation of Statins for the Prevention of Coronary Events." *Health Technology Assessment*, vol. 11, no. 14, 2007, pp. 1-160.

STEM CELLS

Category: Biology
Anatomy or system affected: All
Specialties and related fields: All
Definition: Cells that are not terminally differentiated that have the ability to self-renew and differentiate into more mature cell types, and have the potential to replace dead or damaged cells and regenerate diseased tissues and organs.

Key terms:

differentiation: The process by which less specialized cells develop or mature into more specialized cells that are distinct in function and form.

multipotency: The ability of some stem cells to differentiate into subsets of various types of adult cell types.

pluripotency: The ability of certain stem cells to differentiate into any adult cell type.

stem cells: Undifferentiated cells that can self-renew and differentiate into specialized cells with diverse functions.

totipotency: The ability of specific types of stem cells to differentiate into any adult or embryonic cell type.

STRUCTURE AND FUNCTIONS

Highly touted for future applications in regenerative medicine, stem cells have gained notoriety over the past decades due to their ability to extensively multiply and potential to differentiate into specific cell types. In their 1961 paper, scientists Ernest McCulloch and James Till observed that mouse bone marrow tissue contained cells that could grow, or generate colonies, in the spleen. Two years later, another paper from their lab showed these colonies' ability to self-renew and make several different cell types—a balance between proliferation and differentiation.

Since then, research has focused on understanding these cells both in early stages of human development and later in life. Different stem cell types have been discovered or generated in the laboratory. The cells formed from an egg fertilized by a sperm were considered to have totipotency, meaning that these early cells from the first days after conception could turn into any cell type in the human body. In 1981, embryonic stem cells (ESCs) were isolated from early mouse embryos, and in 1998, a laboratory technique was established by which human ESCs can be made in the laboratory from donated embryos left over from in vitro fertilization. Human ESCs are isolated from 4-5-day-old human embryos that have grown into a hollow sphere called a blastocyst. The inner cells of the blastocyst, the cells of the *inner cell mass*, are isolated and cultured in a special medium. If these blastocyst-derived cells grow and establish a cell line, they have formed an

ESC line. ESCs are *pluripotent*, which means that they can differentiate into or give rise to most cell types found in the human body. Both *totipotent* and pluripotent cells have the capability to self-renew, which is highly important for human development.

As embryos mature, the cells of the inner cell mass divide and differentiate into hematopoietic stem cells (HSCs) and other stem cell types that lead to the production of blood, nerves, bones, muscles, and other tissues important for survival. HSCs are an example of cells in the *multipotent* stage, a stage where a cell can self-renew but cannot turn into as many different cell types. Multipotent HSCs can generate either the myeloid (creates red blood cells and white blood cells) or lymphoid cells (white blood cells that are specific to different pathogens and can create immunologic memory). Stem cells' ability to self-renew also decreases with maturity until they eventually reach their final developmental stage, where they differentiate into parts of a functional organ system.

Adults harbor stem cells to regenerate organ systems, though these cells are rare and not fully understood. In the early 60s, there was a suspicion that stem cells might exist in the brain to replace old cells (neurogenesis) due to the findings of Leblond and others. This led to another experiment in 1965 by Altman and Das which found evidence of new brain cells, or neurons, forming in the olfactory bulb, which conveys smells to the brain. The proliferative cells were from a specific part of the brain called the subventricular zone (SVZ). Other organ systems have also demonstrated some ability to harbor stem cells, though none can provide complete self-renewal if disease or trauma does severe damage to an organ.

Recently, excitement around stem cells picked up again when, in 2006, scientist Shinya Yamanaka showed that human differentiated cells can be reverted or "reprogrammed" back to pluripotent stem cells by inserting specific genes that encode proteins involved with cell replication and self-renewal. Yamanaka and his colleagues used four transcription factors: Sox2, cMyc, Oct4, and Klf4. When the expression of these four genes is forced in adult cells, they dedifferentiate into ESC-like cells called induced pluripotent stem cells (iPSCs). iPSCs offer the potential of creating limitless batches of proliferating stem cells with a specific patient's genetic code that could be differentiated into most cell types throughout the body. This technology would circumvent the ethical questions that surround ESCs since the derivation of ESC lines destroys embryos. Also iPSC technology would provide scientists with a novel way to study diseases and open the door

A technician cultures stem cells. Photo via iStock/Andrei Tchernov. [Used under license.]

to medical treatment personalized to a patient's specific genetic code. iPSC generation is still being perfected, but it aims to one day use iPSC-derived cells for transplantation or accurately predict disease or reactions to new medications. This iPSC technology earned Yamanaka the Nobel Prize in 2012, along with Sir John Gurdon, who in the '60s reprogrammed frog cells into non-specialized cells.

DISORDERS AND DISEASES

Stem cells have the promise of treating diseases or disorders, but there is one condition that is considered a stem cell disorder: myelodysplastic syndrome (MDS). It is characterized by irregular hematopoiesis that could eventually lead to acute myeloid leukemia, a cancer of white blood cells. In 2014, Woll and others found that stem cells had mutations that caused MDS. They isolated stem cells by looking for cell surface markers from general MDS cells and saw that the cancerous properties, also known as driver mutations, originated in these stem cells and were key to the progression of the syndrome. If scientists are able to target these stem cells, it could serve as a potential cure for the disorder, since their elimination would cause the cancer to cease. Since other types of cancers also seem to stem from *cancer stem cells*, research into these rogue stem cells could potentially revolutionize cancer diagnosis and treatment.

PERSPECTIVE AND PROSPECTS

Politically, stem cells have been a controversial topic in the United States, with Congress going back and forth on the ethical questions that surrounds stem cells derived from an embryo. In 1996, the Dickey-Wicker Amendment put an end to the use of government money for research that created ESCs, and President George W. Bush signed an executive order in 2001 prohibiting any US funds from being used for research relating to ESCs. However, the private sector was still allowed to use these stem cell lines. In 2009, President Barack Obama overturned his predecessor's policy, and in 2016, he signed the 21st Century Cures Act to help regulate ESC-based technologies.

Despite the increased funding for embryonic stem cell research in recent years, stem-cell-based treatments have been slow to roll out due to continued efforts to understand stem cell biology. The best stem cell therapy to-date is bone marrow transplantation, which has saved countless lives due to its ability to replace irregular bone marrow cells with new, healthy ones. Today, not many therapies exist using ESCs or IPSCs, though there are several clinical trials using this technology that are ready to recruit human subjects. In the past five years, several stem cell clinical trials on macular degeneration (a condition of the eye which ul-

Embryonic stem cells under a microscope. Photo via iStock/Andrei Tchernov. [Used under license.]

timately results in loss of central vision) were carried out around the world, but they achieved mixed results: few patients enrolled in these studies experienced even limited success while several were blinded. A wide range of stem cells was used in the study, from ESCs and iPSCs to "autologous" (stem cells from the patients' own body) stem cells derived from body fat, and the level of differentiation in these studies varied.

Mesenchymal stem cells (MSCs), first isolated in 1974, have been recently publicized in the media, especially for athletes, to aid in healing. Simple to obtain from bone marrow, body fat, and other tissues, MSCs can differentiate into bone, cartilage, fat, and smooth muscle, and they can easily be grown in the laboratory. Some of these treatments remain highly experimental without proper data to support claims that MSCs can fully regenerate tissues.

The theoretical potential for stem cells as regenerative therapies is widely acknowledged, but the technology has not yet been properly harnessed for safe treatments in humans. The main concern comes from a stem cell's potential to cause cancers and tumors. Despite this fear, some clinics around the world offer expensive stem cell treatments without proper testing or proof of efficacy. The FDA has recently taken a stronger stance against these types of clinics that offer stem cell treatments, as major infractions by some clinics have been found. Until these treatments are deemed safe, stem cell therapy remains in its early experimental stages.

—*Brian Campos*

For Further Information:
Berman, Mark and Elliot Lander. *The Stem Cell Revolution.* Bloomington, IN: AuthorHouse, 2015.

Buratovich, Michael A. *The Stem Cell Epistles*. Cascade Books, 2013.

Burgess, Rob. *Stem Cells: A Short Course*. Hoboken, NJ: Wiley-Blackwell, 2016

Knoepfler, Paul. *Stem Cells: An Insider's Guide*. Singapore: World Scientific Publishing Company, 2013.

Pereira, Lygia V. *Stem Cells: Promise and Reality*. Singapore: World Scientific Publishing Company, 2016.

STENOSIS

Category: Disease/Disorder

Also known as: Stricture, arctation, coarctation

Anatomy or system affected: Blood vessels, circulatory system, gastrointestinal system, heart, spine

Specialties and related fields: Cardiology, exercise physiology, gastroenterology, nephrology, neurology, oncology, orthopedics

Definition: An abnormal narrowing or constriction of a canal or passageway in the body that is caused by the buildup of cholesterol, fats, or other substances (called plaque); the swelling or overgrowth of cells, tissue, or an organ; or a deformity.

CAUSES AND SYMPTOMS

Stenosis can occur in many areas of the body, such as an artery, heart valve, or vertebral (spine) canal. It may stem from many causes, depending on the area affected. In an artery, stenosis occurs with the buildup of cholesterol, fats, or other substances (called plaque). A stenotic heart valve can be a congenital (birth) defect or result from an infection (endocarditis), rheumatic fever, or aging. The septum (dividing wall in the heart) can enlarge and lead to an abnormally small ventricle (heart chamber). Spinal stenosis is caused by a deteriorating or herniated disk, arthritis, tissue enlargement inside the spinal canal, deformities of the spinal column (Paget's disease), or an injury.

Symptoms of this disorder relative to an artery, heart valve, or ventricle include high blood pressure, pain or tightness in the chest (angina pectoris), shortness of breath, dizziness or fainting with exertion, fatigue, palpitations (rapid heartbeat), or a heart murmur. In more severe cases, it can develop into a heart attack or stroke. The symptoms of spinal stenosis include back, neck, leg, or buttocks pain or numbness that worsens with standing or exercising.

TREATMENT AND THERAPY

Medication is commonly used to treat or relieve the symptoms caused by a stenosis. Blood thinners (aspirin, Coumadin) allow easy passage of blood through a stenosed area to lower the risk of high pressure. Cholesterol-lowering medications slow the buildup of

---

INFORMATION ON STENOSIS

Causes: Buildup of plaque; swelling of tissue, cells, or organ; deformity

Symptoms: Varies by area affected

Duration: Temporary or permanent

Treatment: Various medications, invasive interventions, surgery

---

plaque in the artery. Antibiotics help repair damaged heart valves, with a long course and high dosage used if the cause is infectious endocarditis. Finally, anti-inflammatory medications or steroid injections are the first line of treatment for spinal stenosis.

A number of interventions can be used to correct this disorder. Balloon angioplasty flattens plaque buildup, while valvuloplasty widens the valve opening. Stent placement (wire mesh tube) often follows an angioplasty to hold the artery open. An alternative is atherectomy, in which a laser or rotary shaver breaks up the plaque. If a patient has multiple severely stenosed arteries, then coronary artery bypass surgery may be recommended. Finally, artificial heart valve replacement surgery or corrective surgery for spinal stenosis may be warranted.

—*Christine G. Holzmueller*

See also Angiography; Angioplasty; Arteriosclerosis; Bypass surgery; Cholesterol; Circulation; Claudication; Endocarditis; Heart; Heart attack; Heart disease; Hypercholesterolemia; Hypertension; Plaque, arterial; Spine, vertebrae, and disks; Stents; Strokes; Vascular medicine; Vascular system; Venous insufficiency.

For Further Information:

American Heart Association. www.american heart.org.

Dorland's Illustrated Medical Dictionary. 30th ed. Philadelphia: Saunders, 2003.

North American Spine Society. www.spine.org.

STENTS

Category: Procedure

Anatomy or system affected: Abdomen, blood vessels, circulatory system, heart

Specialties and related fields: Cardiology, radiology, vascular medicine

Definition: Wire mesh tubes permanently implanted to prop open arteries or veins.

Key terms:

angioplasty: insertion of a long, flexible tube into a narrowed or blocked blood vessel in order to repair it; in balloon angioplasty, a small balloon is inflated at the end of the tube to compress fatty blockage in the blood vessel so blood flow increases

atherosclerosis: a blood vessel disease characterized by plaques of fat-like substances accumulated on the inner walls of the blood vessel

coronary artery disease: also called, CAD, it occurs when the arteries bringing blood to the heart are impeded from supplying enough blood, nutrients, and oxygen; it is the most common heart disease in the United States

plaque: arterial plaque is the name given to fatty material deposited on the inside of blood vessels

restenosis: one of the two reasons coronary stents fail to maintain blood vessel patency; restenosis occurs when there has been a gradual re-narrowing of the stent, so blood flow again becomes impeded; if it is going to happen, it usually does so between three and twelve months after stent placement and repeating a percutaneous revascularization is the management of choice; the other reason stents fail is stent thrombosis, an abrupt thrombotic occlusion of a stent that had been successfully widened previously

stenosis: stenosis occurs when cholesterol, fats, or plague cause an abnormal narrowing or constriction of blood vessels; it can also apply to any canal or passageway in the body that is blocked or constricted; types of stenosis discussed elsewhere in *Magill's* include aortic, mitral, pulmonary, spinal, and urethral

INTRODUCTION

A stent is a wire mesh tube inserted into a blood vessel to keep it open, in the setting of a stenosis (narrowing) or occlusion (blockage). While the location of where the stent is placed will determine its material composition, most are made of stainless steel or platinum-chromium, cobalt-chromium, or nickel-titanium alloys. Using stents to keep blood vessels open is possible because of endovascular surgery and its use of minimally invasive percutaneous techniques. Percutaneous access of the vessel is usually some distance away from the diseased area.

A wire is inserted through a hollow needle into the cavity (lumen) of the blood vessel. The needle is then removed, and a catheter and/or sheath is placed over the wire for stability. This is known as the Seldinger technique. The wire can then traverse across the plaque and the intervention can proceed over the wire.

Different endovascular techniques treat vascular disease. The most common technique uses an over-the-wire balloon. First described by two researchers, Charles Dotter and Melvin Judkins in 1964, Andreas Grüntzig first performed the procedure in 1977. The surgeon inflates the balloon intentionally creating a vessel with the goal of increasing the size of

the lumen cavity and thus, blood flow. This is percutaneous transluminal angioplasty. If the procedure involves the coronary arteries supplying the muscle of the heart, it is called "percutaneous transluminal coronary angioplasty."

There are complications of balloon angioplasty. The first involves the artery snapping back to near its original lumen prior to ballooning, "recoiling." The second involves the linings of the arteries separating from each other, leading to more than one channel of blood flow to the target organ, "artery dissection." Dissections can lead to the vessel clotting off, "thrombosing," and results in poor perfusion of the issue, "ischemia." The final complication, "rupture," occurs in mismatched balloon-vessel sizes or in calcified vessels. Despite these challenges, these percutaneous techniques make it possible to treat patients who otherwise might not receive treatment because of the risk in undergoing open surgery.

Stents are placed commonly in the coronary arteries, but by no means are they limited to that territory. Stents can be placed in any vascular bed including the arteries supplying the lower extremities, kidneys, intestines, and brain as well as the aorta. They can also be placed in veins draining blood from those same structures. They are used the treatment of coronary artery disease, which can present with stable angina (chest pain), unstable angina, or a heart attack. They are also indicated in the treatment of atherosclerosis in other vascular beds as previously mentioned.

The first stent was placed in a human coronary artery in 1986 in France. In general, stents are placed either primarily if the vessel will have a higher likelihood of staying open, or secondarily if there is a complication as mentioned previously (recoil, dissection, rupture). Apart from the material from which they are made, stents can be either self-expanding or balloon-expandable in nature. A self-expanding stent (SES) is deployed by unsheathing the catheter, which is constraining them on the wire, whereas a balloon-expandable stent (BES) is deployed by inflating the balloon, which is inside the stent. The choice of which stent to use depends on several factors, including the pathology of the lesion as well as its location in the body. An SES tends to be elastic but applies low radial force, whereas a BES is often rigid with high radial outward force, thus allowing the BES to be deployed with greater precision.

In 1999, the first drug-eluting stent (DES) was placed in a human coronary artery, continuing the development of stent technology. This strategy was developed to combat restenosis, which can occur even after placement of a bare metal stent (BMS). The science behind restenosis involves the proliferation and migration of vascular smooth muscle cells as well as a cascade of other cell types and chemical messengers. Therefore, drugs were identified that would be able to inhibit this process and subsequently were implanted onto the stent to release onto the inner lining of the vessel wall. A polymer coating is also necessary to adhere the stent to the drug. The most common drugs used in this setting are sirolimus (or one of its chemical analogues) and paclitaxel. Due to instances of late stent thrombosis with a first-generation DES, a second-generation DES was developed with more biological polymers and thinner platforms.

Despite the advancements that have been made with stent technology, there are still limitations and modes of failure that lead to complications and deaths each year. Medications have been developed and refined to help tackle these challenges. These medications fall into the category of "antiplatelet" therapy; however, the exact mechanisms vary. The most prescribed medication is aspirin. Aspirin inhibits an enzyme producing a chemical called thromboxane A2. Its production by platelets results in a greater degree of platelet accumulation and vasoconstriction (circumferential tightening of the vessel). If a stent is placed, though, patients will be put on dual antiplatelet therapy (DAPT). The most common second medication is clopidogrel, which has a mechanism distinct from that of aspirin. Clopidogrel belongs to a class called P2Y12 inhibitors. P2Y12 is a platelet cellular receptor that binds to ADP (adenosine diphosphate), leading to more production and release of chemicals from the platelet inner core and prolonged accumulation of the platelets to each other. Newer P2Y12 inhibitors have been developed (prasugrel and ticagrelor) as well. The length of time that DAPT therapy is continued after coronary stents are placed depends on the initial clinical presentation of the patient as well as the stent type used. The more severe the clinical entity and the use of DES typically lead to a greater duration of DAPT therapy.

The future direction for stents is twofold. One, there is a push to develop adjunctive methods to assist with stenting to make the lesion more amenable to it and hopefully lead to less likelihood of stenosis or thrombosis in the future. Two, stents reduce the inflammatory response and as they leave the smallest footprint possible it promises the greatest possible results. Creating stents with thin struts and a maximally biocompatible structure is of utmost importance.

—*Paul Moglia, PhD and Anubhav Agarwal, MD*

For Further Information:
Iqbal, Javaid, Julian Gunn, and Patrick W. Serruys. "Coronary Stents: Historical Development, Current Status, and Future Directions." *British Medical Bulletin*, vol. 106, 2013, pp. 193-211, doi.org/10.1093/bmb/ldt009.

Khan, Safdar A. "Analgesics (Toxicity)." *Merck Manual (Vet Manual)*. June, 2016, www.merckvetmanual.com/toxicology/toxicities-from-human-drugs/analgesics-toxicity#:~:text=Aspirin%20reduces%20prostaglandin%20and%20thromboxane,an%20effect%20on%20platelet%20aggregation.

Safi, U., Maninder Singh, Shahul Valavoor, et al. "Dual Antiplatelet Therapy After Percutaneous Coronary Intervention and Drug-Eluting Stents: A Systematic Review and Network Meta-Analysis." *Circulation*, vol. 142, 2020, pp. 1425-36, doi:10.1161/circulationaha.120.046308. This article was a large investigation and analysis of research on almost 80,000 patients. While its conclusion is straightforward, its discussion and analysis of data is for the specialist.

STERILIZATION

Category: Procedure
Anatomy or system affected: Abdomen, genitals, reproductive system, uterus
Specialties and related fields: Family medicine, general surgery, gynecology, urology
Definition: The surgical prevention of pregnancy, as performed on males through the cutting of the vas deferens (vasectomy) or on females through the blockage or cutting of the Fallopian tubes, the removal of the ovaries, or the removal of the uterus (hysterectomy).
Key terms:
contraception: the prevention of pregnancy
corpus luteum: a yellow cell mass produced from a graafian follicle after the release of an egg
endometriosis: a disease of the female reproductive system that occurs when cells of the uterine lining (endometrium) grow outside the uterus and cause severe pain
Fallopian tubes: the two tubes that connect the ovaries to the uterus and through which an egg travels during ovulation
graafian follicle: any of the ovarian follicles that produce eggs
hormone: a substance made by a body organ and carried through the blood to a second (or target) organ in order to optimize the operation of that target organ
hysterectomy: a surgery that removes part or all of the uterus
laparoscopy: a surgical procedure in which a small incision is made near the navel and the organs of the abdominal cavity, including the uterus and Fallopian tubes, are viewed with a lighted tube called a laparoscope
ovariectomy: the removal of the ovaries

peritoneal cavity: the abdominal cavity that contains the visceral organs

INDICATIONS AND PROCEDURES

Sterilization, of either a woman or a man, is a permanent method of surgical contraception that is used to render a couple incapable of conceiving children. Female sterilization involves the blockage or removal of the Fallopian tubes, the ovaries, or the uterus. Male sterilization involves the interruption of the vas deferens, the pathway of sperm from the testicles. The vas deferens may be reconnected, while many of the sterilization procedures performed on women are considered irreversible. Although the most frequently utilized types of female sterilization possess the potential for reversal at a later date, attempted reversals are often unsuccessful. Therefore, a woman choosing this type of contraception should be quite sure that she does not want another child. By the beginning of the twenty-first century, sterilization was the most prevalent form of contraception worldwide, with an estimated one hundred million women choosing the procedure. In the United States, approximately 700,000 women are sterilized each year. One reason that female sterilization is a popular form of contraception with women is because it represents a onetime effort that is usually both simple and the cause of only mild side effects. Another advantage of sterilization over the use of birth control pills is its high success rate: Less than a tenth as many sterilized women will become pregnant (as a result of improperly performed or incomplete procedures) as will women who rely on birth control pills for their contraception. The use of condoms, diaphragms, and all the other barrier pregnancy prevention devices are even less effective than birth control pills.

Before considering the various aspects of sterilization, it is useful to describe the female reproductive system and its biological operation. This organ system consists of two ovaries connected to paired Fallopian tubes that open up into the uterus. The entire system passes through a monthly menstrual cycle that is controlled by the female hormones progesterone and the estrogens. During each menstrual cycle, an ovary produces one egg (sometimes more) in a graafian follicle. The egg then enters one of the Fallopian tubes, which carries it to the uterus. If an egg is fertilized, it then implants in the endometrial tissue that lines the interior of the uterus and subsequently develops into an embryo.

Egg formation and uterus preparation for implantation are controlled by the female hormones. Once an egg implants, the uterus is kept in a state that optimizes pregnancy with the production of progesterone and related hormones, first by the corpus luteum

(originally the graafian follicle that yielded the egg) and then by the placenta that forms from commingled uterine and fetal tissue. In the absence of fertilization, the menstrual cycle continues, most of the endometrium breaks down into the monthly menstrual flow, and the process begins over again.

Menstruation stops between forty-five and fifty-five years of age in most women, causing them to undergo a process called the menopause. After hundreds of repeated menstrual cycles since puberty, the graafian follicles stop producing eggs. Cessation of the menstrual cycle means that female hormone production stops almost entirely. Therefore, the menopause is accompanied by gradual atrophy of the sex organs and possible related symptoms, including hot flashes, depression, and irritability. When ovariectomy or hysterectomy is performed to achieve sterilization, these symptoms of the menopause may be induced prematurely.

For pregnancy to occur, then, a woman must have at least one functional ovary that produces eggs, an intact and operational Fallopian tube to transport the egg, and a functional uterus. The surgical methods that are used for sterilization must, therefore, make one of these reproductive organs nonfunctional. Most often, sterilization cuts and then blocks or removes the Fallopian tubes. Such interruption of the Fallopian tubes is the preferred form of female sterilization surgery for three reasons. First, these operations are relatively minor surgical procedures and are unlikely to be very risky. In addition, premature menopausal symptoms are not produced because the menstrual cycle continues. Finally, when carried out appropriately, interruption of the Fallopian tubes can sometimes be reversed if the patient changes her mind as a result of altered marital arrangements, lifestyle, or financial circumstances.

In many cases, a 1-centimeter to 1.5-centimeter section in the middle of each Fallopian tube is removed surgically or burned away via electrocoagulation. Alternatively, plastic or metal clips are used to close off each tube, or similar tube closure is effected by making a loop in each Fallopian tube and closing it off with a tight plastic ring or band.

Very frequently, the method that is used to damage the Fallopian tubes is a form of surgery called a laparoscopic procedure. The patient is given a general anesthetic, a very small incision is made close to the navel, and a flexible lighted tube-a laparoscope-is inserted into the incision. The laparoscope is equipped with fiber optics and enables an examining physician to see into the abdominal (peritoneal) cavity. Visibility of the Fallopian tubes and the other abdominal organs with laparoscopic examination is enhanced by pumping harmless carbon dioxide gas or nitrous oxide gas into the abdomen, to distend it. This process is called pneumoperitoneum.

After laparoscopic examination identifies the operation site in the peritoneal cavity, the surgical tools for cauterization, cutting, banding, and other aspects of interrupting the Fallopian tubes are passed through the laparoscope, and the chosen surgical interruption procedure is carried out. An entire laparoscopic procedure often takes less than thirty minutes, which is one of the reasons for its great popularity. In addition, women who choose to undergo such surgery can usually go home in a few hours and are fully recovered after only one to two days of postoperative bed rest, followed by a week or so of curtailed physical and sexual activity.

Despite the popularity of the laparoscopic procedure for sterilization, some physicians prefer to carry out sterilization by use of a larger surgical incision through which the tubes are altered directly. Despite the larger size of the incision, the physicians who use this method believe that it is safer and more sure of success and that it has a greater potential for reversibility.

Other methods for sterilization through Fallopian tube surgery are culdoscopy and chemical means. Culdoscopy, in which an optical instrument and surgical tools reach the Fallopian tubes through the uterus, has a somewhat lower success rate than do the laparoscopic procedure and the direct method. Chemical methods for tubal closure have also been attempted and are not viewed as viable because of a low success rate and frequent, serious postoperative complications.

The other avenues available for sterilization are ovariectomy (removal of the ovaries) and hysterectomy (removal of the uterus). Both of these types of sterilization surgery are much more serious and risky. In addition, ovariectomy and hysterectomy are totally irreversible. Ovariectomy, a more complicated procedure than the one inactivating the Fallopian tubes, is usually utilized only when both ovaries are diseased. This procedure produces an early menopause because most of a woman's female hormones are made by the ovaries' graafian follicles.

Hysterectomy is the most uncommon form of female sterilization because it requires even more extensive surgery and can have fatal complications. While the operation is sometimes carried out when a woman has completed her desired family, most hysterectomies are curative. They are performed in cases of very severe and widespread endometriosis and in the presence of other serious gynecological problems.

An alternative available to couples is sterilization of the male partner. This type of surgery, a vasectomy, is quite simple, brief, and relatively painless and only rarely results in physical or psychological complications. In addition, after vasectomy only one-tenth of a

percent of involved couples experience undesired pregnancies. Vasectomy has no effect on sexual desire or male hormone production. It is also relatively easy to reverse such surgery, if so desired later in life. Consequently, the method has become quite popular. In the United States, for example, it was estimated in the early twenty-first century that approximately 500,000 men undergo this sterilization surgery each year.

Vasectomy involves the surgical interruption of the tube-the vas deferens-through which sperm leave the testicle. Vasectomy is carried out after identifying the position of each tube and injecting it with a local anesthetic. A 1-inch-long incision is made in the scrotum, each tube is cut near its middle, a small piece of the tube is removed to keep the cut ends apart, and all the ends are closed with sutures, by cauterization, or with metal or plastic clips.

Vasectomy has a short recovery period and does not stop ejaculation during postoperative intercourse. It is important to note, however, that azoospermia (a lack of sperm in the ejaculate) is achieved only after six to fifteen postoperative ejaculations. Therefore, to ensure sterility, it is critical that the condition of azoospermia has been achieved before the patient carries out intercourse without using condoms or other protective measures. After two consecutive sperm counts indicate azoospermia, unprotected intercourse is deemed safe.

USES AND COMPLICATIONS

The most popular method of female sterilization is to block or damage both Fallopian tubes so that eggs cannot pass through them to the uterus. In some cases, the tubes are removed completely. While removal ensures successful sterilization, it is irreversible and considered too drastic by women who might someday wish to reverse the operation. Several popular alternatives to removal are the methods that interrupt the tubes, retaining the potential for reversal at a later date. Women undergoing this type of surgery are warned, however, that such reversal may be impossible.

When the Fallopian tubes are damaged but not entirely closed off, they may reconnect and cause an ectopic pregnancy, in which a fertilized egg implants in one of the tubes and begins to grow into a fetus. Ectopic pregnancy can be fatal to the pregnant woman, and when identified, it is corrected by surgical removal of the fetus. Although the cause of this problem is not clear, there is some thought that alteration of the interior wall of the tube or slowed passage of an egg through the tube may be the causative agent. Fortunately, ectopic pregnancy is relatively uncommon.

Whether the laparoscopic method or the direct approach is utilized, the best time to carry out female sterilization is at the end of a menstrual cycle; at this time, early pregnancies cannot be compromised. It is advised that the patient discontinue intercourse and the use of birth control pills for at least a month prior to the surgery. The cessation of intercourse eliminates the chance of unexpected pregnancy at the time of surgery, while stopping the use of birth control pills decreases the possibility of blood-clotting problems.

The complications of all types of Fallopian tube surgery can include internal bleeding, blood-clotting problems, injury to the intestines and the other abdominal organs, and abnormal postoperative menstrual cycles. It is estimated, however, that these complications occur in less than 1 percent of patients. A more frequent problem is the difficulty of restoring fertility by reconnecting the Fallopian tubes (with only a 20 to 40 percent success rate).

Hysterectomy is never a highly recommended female sterilization operation. Rather, it is used mostly in those cases where other uterine health problems are sufficiently severe to make the process sensible. These problems may include recurrent and heavy vaginal bleeding, severe endometriosis, and chronic pelvic inflammatory disease (PID). This extensive surgery results in a high rate of complications and a significant number of deaths.

A woman may seek sterilization when she is having an abortion or soon after giving birth to an undesired child. Such a decision, perhaps made hastily at a time of intense emotional stress, is not advisable. It is essential that a sterilization operation be performed only after careful reflection. Divorce or the death of a spouse and subsequent remarriage may cause a sterilized woman regret should she desire more children.

Severe psychological problems for both the patient and her family may accompany female sterilization. Therefore, it is highly recommended that these women, their families, and both partners in married couples consult a gynecologist and a psychological counselor before proceeding with female sterilization surgery.

In contrast to the complications associated with female sterilization, with vasectomy a day of bed rest and a week of avoidance of all strenuous physical activity usually produce complete recovery. Health complications occur in less than 5 percent of vasectomy patients. In addition, these problems are usually minor and almost never lead to fatalities. Skin discoloration, swelling, and oozing of clear fluid from the scrotum incision are common symptoms immediately following the surgery, but they spontaneously disappear as the healing process continues. Less frequently, inflammation and a condition called sperm granuloma can occur when sperm leak out of the cut portion of the vas deferens closest to the testicle. A granuloma produces severe inflammation, pain, and swelling. When this condition does not subside spontaneously, the granuloma must be removed surgically.

PERSPECTIVE AND PROSPECTS

While surgical sterilization was first described in the nineteenth century, it was not widely available for contraception until the 1920's, nor did it become popular immediately. Though voluntary sterilization began slowly in the 1950s, its use accelerated until it became a popular form of fertility control in the industrial and developing nations of the 1970s.

A source of discontent with the sterilization techniques that are available is their total or poor reversibility when fertility reinitiation is desired later in life. This discontent has occurred because, with passing time, an unexpectedly large segment of sterilized men and women have come to regret their decisions regarding sterilization. All hysterectomies and Fallopian tube removals are forever irreversible, and a low reversibility rate is seen even in the two most popular-and potentially reversible-sterilization methodologies: Fallopian tube interruption and vasectomy.

Consequently, the development of sterilization surgery has been directed toward devising methods that will enable much larger incidences of reversibility, where desired. One direction has been to expand the understanding of Fallopian tube and vas deferens anatomy and functionality. Particularly useful results obtained include the realization that destruction of the nerves that control the operation of these organs can make the recovery of fertility incomplete or impossible even when excellent corrective surgery reverses the original interruption of continuity. This discovery has led to the development of more sophisticated interruption surgery that is less likely to damage the vas deferens or Fallopian tube nerve integrity. Some improvement of the reversibility of these operations has been obtained in this manner, but the overall results are still far from satisfactory.

Consequently, many other surgical techniques have been attempted, including the placement of removable plugs in the Fallopian tubes or of tiny, faucetlike valves in the vas deferens that allow or stop the ejaculation of sperm. Other useful methods to ensure reversible sterilization may include hormones, vaccines against eggs and sperm, and chemical treatments. It is hoped that improved antifertility methodologies will be developed that combine more reversible surgical sterilization, vaccines, chemicals, and various contraceptives.

—*Sanford S. Singer, PhD*

See also Conception; Contraception; Gynecology; Hysterectomy; Laparoscopy; Menopause; Men's health; Menstruation; Ovaries; Pregnancy and gestation; Reproductive system; Tubal ligation; Uterus; Vas deferens; Vasectomy; Women's health.

For Further Information:

Ammer, Christine. *The New A to Z of Women's Health: A Concise Encyclopedia.* 6th ed. New York: Checkmark Books, 2009. A respected classic that covers the full spectrum of women's health issues, including reproduction and methods of contraception.

Connell, Elizabeth B. *The Contraception Sourcebook.* Chicago: Contemporary Books, 2002. A straightforward guide that provides comprehensive coverage of each contraceptive method, including a clear and understandable analysis of its advantages and disadvantages as well as a lively discussion of its origins.

Denniston, George C. *Vasectomy.* Victoria, BC: Trafford, 2002. Provides a range of information for men who are considering a vasectomy.

Mastroianni, Luigi, Jr., Peter J. Donaldson, and Thomas T. Kane. *Developing New Contraceptives: Obstacles and Opportunities.* Washington, DC: National Academy Press, 1990. This book on contraceptive measures other than sterilization by surgery also contains considerable useful information on sterilization practices and legalities. Provides useful insights and allows the reader to consider other effective, long-term methods of contraception, excluding surgery.

Parker, James N., and Philip M. Parker, eds. *The Official Patient's Sourcebook on Vasectomy.* San Diego, Calif.: Icon Health, 2002. Draws from public, academic, government, and peer-reviewed research to provide a wide-ranging handbook for patients considering a vasectomy.

Sherwood, Lauralee. *Human Physiology: From Cells to Systems.* 7th ed. Pacific Grove, Calif.: Brooks/Cole/Cengage Learning, 2010. This college text provides details about the menstrual cycle, hormones, and the endometrium. Many useful definitions, diagrams, and glossary terms are included.

Wigfall-Williams, Wanda. *Hysterectomy: Learning the Facts, Coping with the Feelings, and Facing the Future.* New York: Michael Kesend, 1986. Discusses sterilization as a motive for hysterectomy, in addition to severe endometriosis. Offers guidelines for the choice of a physician or surgical procedure and explores possible aftereffects, such as depression and changes in sexual function.

STEROID ABUSE

Category: Disease/Disorder

Anatomy or system affected: Circulatory system, endocrine system, heart, muscles, psychic-emotional system, reproductive system

Specialties and related fields: Exercise physiology, psychiatry, psychology, sports medicine

Definition: The use of illegal anabolic steroids to increase athletic performance, with negative side effects on physical and psychological health.

CAUSES AND SYMPTOMS

Steroids provide many valuable medical benefits for various conditions ranging from asthma, infections, and delayed puberty to spastic colon. Unfortunately, steroid abuse has become an increasingly prevalent issue. Steroid abuse has gained attention in the past few years mainly due to its relation to professional sports. Numerous well-known athletes have admitted to using steroids in order to increase their athletic edge. A lack of social acceptability around steroid use has resulted from the more than seventy side effects associated with steroid use, including such immediate problems as rage, depression, and highly aggressive behavior. Reports have included findings of teenagers committing acts as brutal as murder, without any prior history of criminal or aggressive behavior, while under the influence of steroids. While such acts are rare, the connection between steroids and out-of-control rage is well known. In addition, steroid abuse has been linked with such long-term problems as heart attacks, strokes, and changes in the reproductive system. It is likely that increasing attention will be focused on these kinds of long-term effects, both in research and in terms of problem reporting. Increases in the access to anabolic steroids are also partly responsible for an increase in the visibility of and attention to such problems.

Social research also has demonstrated important findings related to steroid use in college students and in athletes. One study, for example, demonstrated that college students consistently rated anabolic steroid-using athletes more negatively than drug-free athletes. In fact, students tended to evaluate anabolic steroid-using athletes just as negatively as they would an athlete who was using cocaine. In another study, researchers demonstrated that steroid use is not only physically reinforcing but also psychologically reinforcing. Specifically, in interviews with thirty-five male self-reported anabolic steroid users, lower levels of anxiety related to the perception of one's physique and higher levels of satisfaction with one's upper body were demonstrated, relative to the control subjects. There was a psychological gain associated with the steroid use that was directly related to the shorter-term physical benefits of their use.

PERSPECTIVE AND PROSPECTS

Recent estimates suggest that about 1.4 percent of college athletes are using anabolic steroids. A 2001 report by the National Collegiate Athletic Association (NCAA) demonstrated that this was a decrease from the 4.9 percent of student athletes who reported using steroids in 1985. Nationwide, according to the NCAA, collegiate football players were reported to have the highest rate of use, at 3.0 percent. The survey suggested, however, that this lowered rate may reflect underreporting. Factors such as the illegality of drug use or a lack of social acceptability in acknowledging such personal behavior may be responsible.

Such assertions of underreporting also are based on other reports that 2.6 percent of male high school students and 0.4 percent of female high school students have used anabolic steroids. Furthermore, among athletes not in college, reported rates are much higher. The highest reported usage rates were found in weight lifters, power lifters, track-and-field athletes, football players, and sprinters. Major League Baseball banned steroids in 2002 and instituted a testing program after several top players admitted to steroid use. Future work in this area will likely explore these psychological factors and focus on how to intervene effectively. Additionally, it is likely that social interventions will be explored. Athletics remain competitive and financially lucrative, so special attention will need to be paid to the social context in which steroid abuse occurs. There is little research or studies on the treatment of steroid abuse. Most knowledge on treatment comes from the experience of a small number of physicians who have treated steroid withdrawal themselves. The most effective treatment is prevention.

—*Roman J. Miller, PhD and Nancy A. Piotrowski, PhD; updated by Samar Aslam, MD*

See also Addiction; Ergogenic aids; Ethics; Exercise physiology; Hormones; Hypertrophy; Muscles; Psychiatry, child and adolescent; Puberty and adolescence; Sports medicine; Steroids

For Further Information:
www.drugabuse.gov/publications/drugfacts/anabolic-steroids
Craig, Charles R., and Robert E. Stitzel, eds. *Modern Pharmacology with Clinical Applications.* 6th ed. Philadelphia: Lippincott, 2004.
Kronenberg, Henry M., et al., eds. *Williams Textbook of Endocrinology.* 11th ed. Philadelphia: Saunders/Elsevier, 2008.
Taylor, William N. *Anabolic Steroids and the Athlete.* 2nd ed. Jefferson, NC: McFarland, 2002.
Yesalis, Charles E., ed. *Anabolic Steroids in Sport and Exercise.* 2nd ed. Champaign, IL: Human Kinetics, 2000.
Yesalis, Charles E., and Michael S. Bahrke. "Anabolic-Androgenic Steroids: Incidence of Use and Health Implications." *President's Council on Physical Fitness and Sports Research Digest* 5, no. 5 (2005): 1-8.

STEROIDS

Category: Biology
Anatomy or system affected: Endocrine system, glands
Specialties and related fields: Biochemistry, endocrinology, pediatrics, pharmacology, sports medicine
Definition: Organic compounds, both natural and synthetic, that enhance specific activities of the body and that can be used as therapeutic agents in the treatment of many clinical disorders.

Key terms:
anabolic steroids: a class of steroids that stimulate body reactions to build up more complex molecules and structures from simpler molecules; most are synthetic derivatives of testosterone
cholesterol: a fatlike steroid alcohol that is found in animal fats, oils, and tissues; most of the body's supply is manufactured in the liver, while some is absorbed from the diet
corticosteroids: the group of steroid hormones produced by the adrenal cortex, which includes the classes of mineralocorticoids, glucocorticoids, and sex steroids
glucocorticoids: steroid hormones that regulate the metabolism of glucose and other organic molecules
mineralocorticoids: steroid hormones that regulate the body levels of sodium and potassium
sex steroids: steroid hormones such as androgens and estrogens that influence the activity of reproductive organs and development
steroid nucleus: the molecular arrangement of four carbon rings that makes up the backbone of all steroids
sterol: a steroid that has long side chains of carbon compounds attached to it and contains at least one hydroxyl group; cholesterol is one type of sterol

STRUCTURE AND FUNCTIONS

Steroids are a group of organic compounds that are distinguished by a unique molecular arrangement of seventeen carbon atoms situated in four adjacent rings. This set of four rings is referred to as the steroid nucleus and is common to all steroid compounds. Three of these rings are hexagonal six-carbon rings arranged in a bent-line fashion to form what is called a "phenanthrene group." The fourth group or ring contains only five carbon atoms. Steroids vary with the nature of the attached groups, the position of a given attached group, or some alteration to the configuration of the steroid nucleus. Small chemical differences in the structure of steroids can reflect very great differences in specific biological effects. Steroids are included in the lipid category of biological molecules because they are nonpolar and insoluble in water.

Any steroid that contains a hydroxyl group (-OH) is called a *sterol*. This term comes from a Greek word meaning "solid"; sterols were so named because they were among the earliest compounds that were found to be solid at room temperature. Once chemical structures were determined, then other compounds with similar structures were given the name steroid, which means "sterol-like." The suffix *-oid* comes from the Greek and means "similar to."

Chemists have isolated hundreds of different steroids from plants and animals; additionally, thousands have been made by chemically modifying natural steroids or by synthesizing the entire molecule. The parent compound for steroids is acetic acid. Assisted by a variety of enzymes, acetic acid is altered and transformed into several other compounds before cholesterol is formed. Cholesterol serves as the parent, or precursor compound, for bile acids and for the steroids that are biologically important to the body.

Cholesterol is the most common steroid in the human body, as it is a structural component of cellular membranes. The prefix *chole-* comes from the Greek word for liver bile, which is a digestive fluid manufactured by the liver and secreted into the intestines. The name is appropriate since the bile contains a considerable amount of cholesterol. Bile is stored in the gallbladder and becomes concentrated there. Cholesterol is not very soluble, and if it accumulates in great enough quantities, it will form small crystals in the bile. These crystals may join to form larger particles that can block the narrow duct that leads from the gallbladder to the intestines. These aggregations of particles are called "gallstones" and are composed of almost pure cholesterol. The blockage can result in a buildup of pressure and cause much pain. Often, a surgical operation is required to remove the obstruction.

Cholesterol is also an important molecule because it is the precursor or parent molecule for the steroid hormones produced by the gonads and the adrenal cortex. The gonads, a collective term referring to the testes and ovaries, secrete the sex steroids. These sex steroids include estradiol and progesterone from the ovaries and testosterone from the testes. The adrenal cortex secretes the corticosteroids, which include cortisol and aldosterone as well as other steroid compounds. Most of the steroid hormones are specialized in their function and do not produce general effects on metabolism. The sex hormones influence reproduction by acting on sexual organs to stimulate their development and function, by influencing sexual behavior, and by stimulating the development of secondary sex characteristics. Some of the steroids secreted by the adrenal cortex have more general effects on the metabolism of carbohydrates and proteins in many tissues.

Steroid hormones combine with specific receptors that are in the cytoplasm of the responsive tissues. Since these hormones are lipid-soluble, they pass readily through cell membranes, which are largely composed of lipids. Inside the cytoplasm, a steroid-specific protein receptor will bind to the hormone. Upon binding, the hormone-receptor complex becomes activated or transformed and is then translocated to the nucleus. In the nucleus, the activated steroid receptor complex binds to the chromatin, or genetic material, causing an activation of a certain set of genes. Gene activation results in the production of messenger molecules that induce the production of specific proteins that are either used by the cell or secreted elsewhere.

The steroid hormones of the adrenal cortex fall into three categories, each having separate actions and sites of actions. Aldosterone is the principal mineralocorticoid and plays an important role in regulating body levels of sodium and potassium. Cortisol, the major glucocorticoid, regulates carbohydrate metabolism. Adrenal androgens are also produced, but they have only weak activity and play a minor physiological role under most conditions. All adrenal steroids are derived from cholesterol.

Mineralocorticoids are the adrenal steroids that regulate levels of potassium and sodium in the body. Aldosterone, the most potent mineralocorticoid, is secreted by the adrenal cortex at the rate of about 0.1 milligram (mg) per day. Mineralocorticoids affect the distal tubules of the kidney by stimulating the excretion of potassium and the reabsorption of sodium. The net effect of these actions is to increase the volume of body fluids.

Glucocorticoids are the adrenal steroids that regulate glucose metabolism. In humans, cortisol is responsible for most of the glucocorticoid activity. It is secreted by the adrenal cortex in a pulsatile fashion following a circadian rhythm. The release is greatest in the morning hours and declines throughout the day. Cortisol is regulated by the central nervous system and by permissive or stimulatory messenger molecules of the body. Generally, glucocorticoids stimulate the production of glucose and enhance the use of fat and protein as energy sources.

Androgens are steroid hormones that are secreted primarily by the testes but also by the adrenal glands and ovaries. Testosterone is the principal androgen that is secreted by the testes; it regulates the development and function of male sex accessory organs. Increased testosterone secretion during puberty is required for the growth of the seminal vesicles and prostate. Removal of androgens by castration results in these organs undergoing atrophy.

Androgens stimulate growth of the larynx and cause lowering of the voice. They increase hemoglobin synthesis, which is higher in males than females, and affect bone growth by causing the conversion of cartilage to bone. Androgens also promote protein synthesis or anabolic activity in skeletal muscle, bone, and kidneys. As a class of compounds, androgens are reasonably safe drugs, since they have a limited and relatively predictable set of side effects. In human males, testosterone is synthesized by the testes at the rate of about 8 mg per day.

Estrogens and progesterones are primarily produced in the ovaries of nonpregnant adult women. In pregnancy, the placenta is the major site of estrogen and progesterone production. Smaller amounts of estrogen synthesis involve the liver, kidney, skeletal muscle, and testes. Estrogens cause the growth of the female reproductive organs and are responsible for the expression of female secondary sex characteristics, such as breast enlargement, female body contours, skin texture, and distribution of body hair. Estrogens are thought to protect against atherosclerosis and heart attacks since occurrence of these health problems in mature women is much lower than in males of similar ages.

USES AND COMPLICATIONS

When cortisone was initially discovered, it was labeled a "wonder drug" and was thought to possess widespread effectiveness in many areas of medicine. Although these expectations have not been realized, a variety of steroids are found to be effective in medical practice and treatment. Steroids are commonly prescribed to serve as replacements for those persons whose bodies are unable to produce specific steroid hormones in adequate quantities. Steroids are effective as anti-inflammatory agents, reducing inflammatory reactions in a variety of body tissues. They are also prescribed for patients who have undergone an organ transplantation or have highly sensitive allergies because they inhibit the responsiveness of the immune system.

The primary therapeutic use of androgens is for testicular deficiency in which the induction and maintenance of male secondary sex characteristics are desired. In these cases, supplemental doses of androgens are given to stimulate and enhance the development of secondary sex characteristics. Historically, androgens were used in the therapy of some anemias when persons have reduced levels of red blood cells.

Steroids also have anabolic activities that are manifested by stimulating increases in protein production, by enhancing the uptake of amino acids into cells, and by inhibiting the glucocorticoids from breaking down proteins. They influence embryonic development, especially the differentiation of the central nervous system and the male reproductive tract. The excitatory function of androgens occurs at puberty, during which

the reproductive organs are activated to produce sex cells. Androgens also maintain the body's sexual characteristics in the adult. Thus, in cases of androgen deficiency there is a regression of male sexual behavior, libido, and reproductive function; depending on the cause this regression maybe reversible with treatment.

It should be noted that anabolic steroids are frequently abused because of these kinds of effects. Athletes and body builders in search of accelerated muscle building or physical definition are two groups in which such abuse has been seen. A complication has been that stimulatory effects of the anabolic steroids make drug administration reinforcing and therefore loaded with addiction potential. As such, frequent users of anabolic steroids should be aware of conditions such as dependence, as well as withdrawal and other problematic side effects of heavy steroid use. Such effects may include increased periods of sleep disturbance, paranoia, anger and agitation, mood swings or instability of mood, violence or other impulsive behavior, and concentration and memory disturbance. Physical problems may include severe acne, jaundice, excess water retention, decreased sperm count, high cholesterol, liver disease, and difficulty with blood sugar control.

Addison's disease is caused by a failure of the adrenal gland to secrete adequate amounts of both glucocorticoids and mineralocorticoids. The symptoms of this disease are imbalances of body levels of sodium and potassium, dehydration, reduced blood pressure, rapid weight loss, and generalized weakness. A person with Addison's disease will die if not treated with corticosteroids because of the severe electrolyte imbalance and dehydration.

Cushing's syndrome is the manifestation of corticosteroid excess. Symptoms include high blood pressure, alterations in protein and carbohydrate metabolism, high blood sugar concentrations, weight gain, and muscular weakness. This syndrome is often caused by a tumor in the adrenal gland that promotes the secretion of corticosteroids. Surgical intervention is often used to remove the portion of the gland that is malfunctioning. Symptoms like those seen in Cushing's syndrome are found in people with inflammatory diseases who receive lengthy treatments with corticosteroids in order to reduce the inflammation.

Congenital adrenal hyperplasia is a collection of disorders that result from alterations in the synthesis of adrenal steroid hormones. The severity of these disorders can range from death in utero to not life threatening. In these conditions excess in androgens can present as a newborn with ambiguous genitalia, premature puberty in a child, or increased amounts of body hair. Mineralocorticoids can also be synthesized in excess resulting in high blood pressure and low potassium levels.

The greatest use of estrogens as therapeutic agents is in oral contraception, or "the pill." This method is convenient, reversible, and relatively inexpensive; its use is worldwide and includes up to 25 percent of American women of childbearing age. Most oral contraceptives are active combinations of estrogen and progesterone. Users take a daily pill containing both steroids for twenty or twenty-one days of the menstrual cycle and then a placebo for seven or eight days. Withdrawal bleeding occurs two to three days after discontinuing the pill. The mechanism for the effectiveness of these steroids involves inhibiting the release of hormones that would normally stimulate ovulation. Hormone therapy was the primary treatment for menopausal symptoms. However, the Women's Health Initiative Study showed that while hormone therapy had some benefits, it also increased the risk for blood clots, breast cancer, heart attacks, and strokes.

Breast cancer tumor growth is stimulated by estrogen in up to 80 percent of cases. This is the basis of hormone therapy including tamoxifen, a selective estrogen receptor modulator or SERM, and anastrozole, an aromatase inhibitor, which is an enzyme the body uses in estrogen synthesis. Possible side effects of these drugs include those associated with decreasing estrogen, hot flashes, bone fracture, and strokes.

Antiandrogens are substances that prevent or depress the action of androgens, or testosterone, on the body. They are of value in the management of patients whose bodies are producing abnormally high levels of androgens, who are undergoing a premature puberty, or who are affected with acne, hirsutism (excessive hairiness, especially in women), and certain tumors or neoplasms. Potentially, these drugs can be utilized to cause sterility in males.

Natural body androgens stimulate the growth of the prostate gland in males and enhance the proliferation of many prostate cancers. Treatment of abnormal growths, malignant cancers, or benign tumors in the male prostate gland has frequently used either natural or synthetic steroids. Estradiol, a form of the female sex steroid estrogen, has been used to control the advancement of prostate carcinoma but this has largely been replaced with other hormone-based therapies due to the risk of cardiovascular events. Androgen-deprivation therapy is currently the mainstay of most prostate cancer treatments. Benign prostatic hypertrophy or hyperplasia is a benign enlargement of the prostate gland and is sensitive to the highly potent androgen dihydrotestosterone. Finasteride is a medication that inhibits the enzyme that is necessary for dihydrotestosterone synthesis and thus is used in the treatment of benign prostatic enlargement.

PERSPECTIVE AND PROSPECTS

The use of steroids as therapeutic agents began in the early 1930s. At that time, Philip Showalter Hench, who was working in the Mayo Clinic, noticed that the symptoms of arthritic women were alleviated when they became pregnant. He suggested that increased secretions from the adrenal cortex might be the responsible agents. Later, clinical trials were conducted to test the role of corticosteroids in treating acute arthritis. With the use of adequate dosages, the clinical response was impressive. The 1950 Nobel Prize in Physiology or Medicine was awarded to Hench and his coworkers for their finding that cortisone was effective in treating arthritis.

Pharmaceutical firms have manufactured numerous steroid derivatives, all of which have different effectiveness levels as glucocorticoids, mineralocorticoids, or sex steroids. Organic chemists synthesize analogues of adrenal steroids in order to create compounds that produce heightened biological effects with a minimum or lack of side effects. Consequently, hundreds of different steroids are available. Most of these are characterized according to their biological effectiveness, such as their ability to reduce inflammation or to inhibit the immune system. When determining a course of treatment, a physician chooses a particular steroid that enhances the effects that are desired and has minimal effects in related areas. Some pharmaceutical derivatives of adrenal steroids are very poorly absorbed by the skin. These derivatives are especially useful to apply to the skin when a maximal local effect is desired without a generalized effect on other body regions.

Steroids, however, can also have negative, and sometimes dangerous, effects on the body, whether they are ingested (cholesterol) or injected (anabolic steroids). Evidence indicates that high blood cholesterol levels, specifically LDL-cholesterol or "bad" cholesterol levels, are associated with an increased risk of atherosclerosis, a clinical condition in which localized plaques (or atheromas) build up in the walls of arteries, reducing blood flow. Atheromas serve as locations for blood clot formation, which can further block the blood supply to a vital organ such as the heart, brain, or lung. High blood cholesterol may result from a diet rich in cholesterol and saturated fat, or it may result from an inherited condition in which affected individuals have extremely high cholesterol concentrations, regardless of their diet. These persons may suffer heart attacks during their childhood.

Cholesterol is found in foods that are based on animal products. Cholesterol-rich foods include most meats, eggs, and dairy products such as cheese, cream, and butter. Humans readily absorb cholesterol from dietary sources. Most Western diets contain 400 to 600 milligrams of cholesterol per day, of which about 75 percent is readily absorbed into the bloodstream from the dietary tract. Cholesterol is carried to the arteries by proteins in the blood plasma called "low-density lipoproteins," or LDLs. A given cell may engulf the LDLs and use the cholesterol for different purposes. The LDLs in a given location may stimulate other cells to secrete growth factors that either begin or contribute to the development of an atheroma. Thus, the risk of atherosclerosis is greatly increased. Most people can significantly lower their blood cholesterol levels through controlled exercise and diet. Since saturated fat raises blood cholesterol levels, foods such as fatty meat, egg yolk, and liver should be eaten sparingly so that fat contributes less than 30 percent to the total calories of a diet.

The use and abuse of anabolic steroids to increase muscle mass and strength are widespread in both amateur and professional sports. Although those promoting steroid use claim increases in muscle mass, strength, and endurance, controlled clinical trials show minimal, if any, enhancement of muscle mass and strength. Testosterone may also enhance training efforts by promoting aggressive behavior. Use of these compounds poses ethical questions and increases the risk of serious toxicity because of the extremely high doses that are administered, often as much as one hundred times the usual therapeutic dosages.

—*Joshua Kingman, MS-III*

See also: Addison's disease; Adrenal glands; Cholesterol; Contraception; Cushing's syndrome; Endocrine disorders; Endocrine glands; Endocrinology; Endocrinology, pediatric; Ergogenic aids; Glands; Growth; Gynecology; Hormone therapy; Hormones; Hypercholesterolemia; Metabolism; Muscles; Ovaries; Pain management; Pharmacology; Prostate cancer; Prostate gland; Puberty and adolescence; Reproductive system; Sports medicine; Steroid abuse.

For Further Information:

Craig, Charles R., and Robert E. Stitzel, editors. *Modern Pharmacology with Clinical Applications*. 6th ed., Lippincott, 2004. This college-level pharmacology text contains easy-to-comprehend sections on steroids, including their chemistry, synthesis, physiological activity, and pharmacological activity.

Guyton, Arthur C., and John E. Hall. *Human Physiology and Mechanisms of Disease*. 6th ed., W. B. Saunders, 1997. Guyton is a nationally recognized authority on medical physiology, having written and edited numerous college-level and medical school textbooks on the subject. His writing style is flowing and understandable to the nonmedical specialist and student.

Henry, Helen L., and Anthony W. Norman, editors. *Encyclopedia of Hormones*. 3 vols. Academic Press, 2003. A comprehensive overview of the role of hormones, the major physiological systems in which they operate, and the biological consequences of an excess or deficiency of a particular hormone.

Kronenberg, Henry M., et al., editors. *Williams Textbook of Endocrinology*. 11th ed., Saunders/Elsevier, 2008. Comprehensive information regarding endocrine diseases, pathophysiology, diagnoses, treatment, and prognoses.

Montgomery, Rex, et al. *Biochemistry: A Case-Oriented Approach*. 6th ed., Mosby Year Book, 1996. Surveys the field of biochemistry, examining steroids and steroid hormones in that context. A major section describes the essential role of cholesterol in the body, as well as in the synthesis of other steroids.

Tortora, Gerard J., and Bryan Derrickson. *Principles of Anatomy and Physiology*. 12th ed., John Wiley & Sons, 2009. This popular college-level undergraduate anatomy and physiology text contains well-written sections on major biological molecules such as steroids, as well as longer sections on steroid hormones and their specific effects.

Zelman, Mark, et al. *Human Diseases: A Systemic Approach*. 7th ed., Pearson, 2010. This well-written and interesting book uses a case-oriented approach to explore the essential concepts of physiology and health. Numerous examples of pathologies relating to steroids or steroid hormones are illustrated.

STEVENS-JOHNSON SYNDROME

Category: Disease/Disorder

Also known as: Toxic epidermal necrolysis

Anatomy or system affected: Abdomen, back, breasts, eyes, feet, gastrointestinal system, genitals, hands, head, immune system, knees, legs, lungs, neck, nose, reproductive system, respiratory system, urinary system

Specialties and related fields: Critical care, dermatology, emergency medicine, family medicine, gastroenterology, immunology, internal medicine, ophthalmology, pediatrics, pulmonary medicine, urology

Definition: A severe immune response-mediated hypersensitivity reaction to particular drugs or infections that causes a rash, sloughing of the skin, and the disruption of mucous membranes.

Key terms:

dermis: the middle layer of the skin, which lies below the epidermis and above the subcutaneous layer

epidermis: the outermost layer of the skin

erythema multiforme: a skin disorder that produces multiple skin lesions and results from an allergic reaction or infection

Fas ligand: a membrane protein that is a member of the tumor necrosis factor family of signaling proteins; it binds to a Fas receptor and induces programmed cell death

CAUSES AND SYMPTOMS

Stevens-Johnson syndrome begins with a nonspecific upper respiratory tract infection or after the

2748 • Stevens-Johnson syndrome

> ### INFORMATION ON
> ### STEVENS-JOHNSON SYNDROME
>
> **Causes:** Hypersensitivity to infections and drugs
> **Symptoms:** Fever, headache, cough, rash, blistering
> **Duration:** Lasts minimum of two to three weeks; convalescence can be very long
> **Treatments:** Discontinuation of offending drug, intravenous fluids and salts, symptom management, treatment of secondary infections

consumption of a particular drug. The early symptoms last for one to fourteen days and consist of fever, sore throat, headache, cough, body aches, and sometimes vomiting and diarrhea. Subsequently, a flat, red rash (erythema multiforme) breaks out over the face and trunk that later spreads to the rest of the body. Painful blisters form in the center of the rash, and the skin around the blisters is quite loose and rubs off easily. Patients have a headache, fever, weakness (malaise), and a cough that produces thick, pus-filled material.

Blisters can form on the mucous membranes that line the mouth (preventing the patient from eating or drinking), throat, genitals, eyes, and anus. If the urinary tract is involved, then the patient will not be able to urinate. Eye involvement causes the eyes to swell and fill with pus so that they seal shut. Blisters on the surface of the eyes (corneas) can scar them. Lesions in the respiratory tract restrict breathing, and tissue sloughing can cause respiratory collapse. Sores in the digestive tract can cause diarrhea and narrowing of the esophagus. The open, skinless sores are also susceptible to infections.

Stevens-Johnson syndrome is classified according to the percentage of the skin affected. If 10 percent or less of the body surface area detaches, then the patient has Stevens-Johnson syndrome. If 10 to 30 percent of the skin detaches, then the patient has overlapping Stevens-Johnson syndrome/toxic epidermal necrolysis (TEN). If more than 30 percent of the skin is detached, then the patient has TEN.

Drug reactions cause most cases of Stevens-Johnson syndrome. The drugs that may trigger it include antibiotics, such as penicillin, ciprofloxacin, and sulfa drugs; anticonvulsant drugs, such as phenytoin, carbamazepine, and barbiturates; nonsteroidal anti-inflammatory drugs (NSAIDs); the antigout drug allopurinol; the narcolepsy treatment modafinil (Provigil); anti-human immunodeficiency virus (HIV) drugs; diuretics; and topical ocular medications. Viral, bacterial, fungal, and protozoan infections can also cause the disease, as can various types of cancers. Between one-quarter and one-half of all cases of

Stevens-Johnson syndrome are idiopathic, which means that there is no discernable cause. There is also a genetic basis for this disorder.

Diagnosis requires a skin biopsy, which shows extensive cell death, detachment of the upper layer of the skin (epidermis) from the middle layer of the skin (dermis), and infiltration of the skin with particular white blood cells called lymphocytes.

The large amount of skin loss in TEN is similar to a severe burn and is life threatening. Water and salts leak through the denuded areas and can produce organ failure. Infection at the damaged areas is also a major cause of death in TEN patients.

TREATMENT AND THERAPY
The most important therapeutic step is to discontinue all drugs suspected of triggering the disease. Management of symptoms is also essential. Mouthwashes can treat oral lesions and allow fluid intake, which, when coupled with the intravenous replacement of fluid and salts, can prevent dehydration and electrolyte imbalance. Skin lesions are treated as burns. Topical anesthetics can reduce pain, and denuded skin areas are covered with saline compresses. Any secondary infection that develops must be rapidly identified and treated.

There is no universally accepted drug treatment for Stevens-Johnson syndrome. Oral corticosteroids appear to help during the first few days, but not after that. In advanced cases of TEN, corticosteroids increase the incidence of complications. Intravenous delivery of antibodies (immunoglobulins) against the Fas ligand that mediates cell death has helped small groups of TEN patients, but this treatment has not been systematically evaluated. Also, drugs that down-regulate the immune system have been used, but too little data exist to evaluate their efficacy properly.

PERSPECTIVE AND PROSPECTS
Stevens-Johnson syndrome was first described in 1922 by Albert Mason Stevens and Frank Chambliss Johnson. They encountered two young boys who showed inflammation of the mucous lining of the cheeks, pus-filled eyes, and the generalized skin blisters that are now commonly associated with the disease. Stevens and Johnson originally thought that the boys suffered from a type of unknown infectious disease. Bernard Thomas named the condition in 1950. The condition gained public attention in 2010 when it contributed to the death of former professional basketball player Manute Bol.

No treatment for Stevens-Johnson syndrome provides consistent benefits to patients in systematic studies. Nevertheless, several treatments have shown promise in small studies. For example, intravenous immunoglobulin treatments, skin grafts, the antitransplant rejection drug cyclosporine, and a blood filtration procedure called plasmapheresis have successfully treated small groups of patients with few complications and little mortality. However, until larger, double-blind, placebo-based studies establish the efficacy of these treatments, they will remain experimental.

—*Michael A. Buratovich, PhD*

See also Allergies; Antibiotics; Blisters; Eye infections and disorders; Eyes; Human immunodeficiency virus (HIV); Immune system; Lesions; Necrosis; Pus; Rashes; Skin; Skin disorders; Ulcers.

For Further Information:
Boyer, Woodrow Allen. *Understanding Stevens-Johnson Syndrome and Toxic Epidermal Necrolysis*. Raleigh, N.C.: Lulu Press, 2008.
Koh, Mark-Jean-Aan, and Kwang-Yong Tay. "An Update on Stevens-Johnson Syndrome and Toxic Epidermal Necrolysis in Children." *Current Opinion in Pediatrics* 21, no. 4 (August, 2009): 505-510.
Parrillo, Steven J. "Stevens-Johnson Syndrome and Toxic Epidermal Necrolysis." *Current Allergy and Asthma Reports* 7, no. 4 (July, 2007): 243-247.
Warn, Dana, and Nancy Matharu. *Stevens-Johnson Syndrome: A Booklet for Children and Their Families*. Vancouver, BC: Provincial Health Services Authority, 2006.

STILLBIRTH

Category: Disease/Disorder
Anatomy or system affected: Fetus
Specialties and related fields: Obstetrics and gynecology, perinatology, women's health
Definition: The death or loss of a baby before or during delivery.
Key terms:
antiphospholipid syndrome: also known as Hughes syndrome, is a disorder of the immune system that causes an increased risk of blood clots
cholestasis: any condition in which substances normally excreted into bile are retained; bile flow is decreased due to impaired secretion by hepatocytes or by obstruction of bile flow through intra- or extrahepatic bile ducts
fetoscopy: an endoscopic procedure during pregnancy to allow surgical access to the fetus
isoimmunization: the development of antibodies against antigens from the same species
karyotyping: test to determine the presence of chromosomal abnormalities
placenta abruptio: the premature separation of the placenta from the uterus

preeclampsia: a pregnancy complication characterized by high blood pressure and signs of damage to another organ system, most often the liver or kidneys
thrombophilias: an abnormality of blood coagulation that increases the risk of blood clots in blood vessels
ultrasonography: a technique using echoes of ultrasound pulses to delineate objects of different densities in the body

CAUSES AND SYMPTOMS

There are many causes of stillbirth, but the precise cause of fetal death is not known in many cases. The causes of stillbirth can be grouped into general categories such as fetal asphyxia; hematologic, chromosomal, or developmental problems with the *fetus*; and maternal illness. Fetal asphyxia occurs when the blood supply to the fetus is reduced or cut off, such as in cases of umbilical cord entanglement or placenta abruptio (abnormal detachment of the placenta from the uterus caused by such factors as maternal high blood pressure or preeclampsia, trauma, or certain drugs). Hematologic causes of stillbirth include isoimmunization (maternal antibodies attack fetal blood cells) or thrombophilias (abnormalities in blood clotting). Maternal illnesses such as *diabetes*, infections (such as listeria), cholestasis, and antiphospholipid syndrome are also associated with an increased risk of stillbirth.

The primary symptom of fetal demise is the absence of fetal movement. The death can be confirmed on ultrasonography or fetoscopy, which reveals the absence of a fetal heartbeat. Stillbirth may be associated with other symptoms, depending on its cause. For instance, if it results from placenta abruptio, the woman may experience bleeding and contractions.

TREATMENT AND THERAPY

Once a stillbirth has been confirmed, treatment is directed at helping the woman and her family cope with the loss. Grief counseling is an important component of therapy. If the patient is already in labor, minimizing obstetric trauma to the mother is of prime concern. If the patient is not in labor, then plans regarding labor induction are made since prolonged retention of the dead fetus and placenta may result in disseminated intravascular coagulation (DIC), a dangerous blood condition. The patient also receives treatment to control any maternal illnesses, such as diabetes or preeclampsia. Suppose no obvious conditions contributed to the stillbirth. In that case, the patient may be offered an investigation into the causes of the demise. This investigation may involve tests on maternal blood for blood clotting abnormalities, infections, abruption, diabetes, and liver abnormalities. With appropriate consent, witnessed sampling, and

INFORMATION ON STILLBIRTH

Causes: Often unknown but may include lack of oxygen to fetus (umbilical cord entanglement, placenta abruptio); hematologic factors (iso-immunization, thrombophilias); chromosomal or developmental problems with fetus; maternal illnesses (diabetes, infections)

Symptoms: Absence of fetal movement or heartbeat, sometimes bleeding and contractions in mother

Duration: Acute

Treatments: Grief counseling, induction of labor, minimization of trauma to mother during labor, control of any maternal illnesses, investigation into cause (fetal autopsy, karyotyping)

chain of custody handling, a urine specimen may be evaluated for the maternal ingestion of toxic substances. The stillborn fetus may be sent for autopsy and karyotyping.

No effective means exist for preventing stillbirth. With advances in medical care, by 2003, the stillbirth rate in the United States had fallen to about 7.5 per 1,000 births, about half of what it was in the mid-1940s. If a pregnant woman has conditions putting her at increased risk of fetal demise or a history of stillbirth, then increased surveillance using ultrasonography and fetal heart tone monitoring may be indicated.

—*Anne Lynn S. Chang, MD.*

For Further Information:

Other FAQs About Pregnancy Loss (Before 20 Weeks of Pregnancy). National Institute of Health: Eunice Kennedy Shriver National Institute of Child Health and Human Development, 1 Sept. 2017, www.nichd.nih.gov/health/topics/pregnancyloss/more_information/faqs. Accessed 3 Apr. 2022.

Pregnancy Loss. US Department of Health and Services, Womenshealth.gov, 30, Jan. 2019, www.womenshealth.gov/pregnancy/youre-pregnant-now-what/pregnancy-loss. Accessed 3 Apr. 2022.

Stillbirth. March of Dimes, Oct. 2020, www.marchofdimes.org/complications/stillbirth.aspx. Accessed 3 Apr. 2022.

Stillbirth. National Health Service, 16 Mar. 2021, www.nhs.uk/conditions/stillbirth/. Accessed 3 Apr. 2022.

Stillbirth: Trying to Understand. American Pregnancy Association, n.d., americanpregnancy.org/getting-pregnant/pregnancy-loss/stillborn-trying-to-understand/. Accessed 3 Apr. 2022.

What is a Stillbirth? Pregnancy, Birth & Baby, Jul. 2020, www.pregnancybirthbaby.org.au/what-is-a-stillbirth. Accessed 3 Apr. 2022.

What is Stillbirth? The Centers for Disease Control and Prevention, 16 Nov. 2020, www.cdc.gov/ncbddd/stillbirth/facts.html. Accessed 3 Apr. 2022.

STINGS. SEE BITES AND STINGS.

STOMACH, INTESTINAL, AND PANCREATIC CANCERS

Category: Disease/Disorder
Anatomy or system affected: Abdomen, gastrointestinal system, intestines, pancreas, stomach
Specialties and related fields: Gastroenterology, immunology, oncology
Definition: Malignant tumors of the small intestine, stomach, or pancreas, the latter two types being difficult to detect and treat.

Key terms:

carcinogen: anything that initiates cancer

endoscope: a long, flexible fiber-optic tube used to examine the gastrointestinal tract; the tube's accessories can also remove tissue or stones

gastric: pertaining to the stomach

jaundice: a yellowing of the skin and eyes from an excess of bile pigment caused by a blocked duct or injured liver

metastasis: the dispersal of cancer cells from a tumor to other parts of the body, where they begin secondary tumors

pancreas: a secretory organ behind the stomach and connected to the duodenum; it produces enzymes to digest food and insulin to metabolize sugar

small intestine: the region of gut between the stomach and the colon that comprises the duodenum, jejunum, and ileum; also called the small bowel

tumor: a mass of new cells growing independent of surrounding tissues; either benign (noncancerous) or malignant (cancerous)

CAUSES AND SYMPTOMS

The section of the gut from the esophageal sphincter in the upper stomach to the ileocecal valve at the end of the small intestine digests food taken into the body and absorbs its nutrients. This vital function also exposes the gut and its organs, the liver and pancreas, to ingested toxins that can initiate cancer and to materials that damage the gut lining, also potentially leading to cancer. Because diet greatly influences the chances for contracting these cancers, it is understandable that stomach cancer is the world's most common type. Surprisingly, however, cancers of the small bowel are rare. Pancreatic cancer is the most lethal of these cancers and one of the most difficult to detect before irreversible damage has been done: Few patients live long after diagnosis. These facts and the large number of suspected carcinogens make the stomach and pancreatic cancers a pressing challenge for physicians and public health.

Broad similarities characterize the types of cancers throughout the upper gastrointestinal (GI) tract. The majority, adenocarcinomas, grow in and mimic gland tissue, but possible as well are cancers of the lymph tissue (lymphoma), hormone-secreting cells (carcinoid tumors), and the muscle wall of the bowel (sarcoma). Early symptoms tend to be vague and do not necessarily point specifically to cancer: abdominal pain, loss of appetite, weight loss, and perhaps diarrhea or vomiting.

While diet is a major factor in stomach cancer, its role in pancreatic and intestinal cancers is not as clear. A diet consisting mainly of pickled, smoked, or salted food with few fruits and vegetables, especially those containing vitamins A and C, is thought to be risky. In fact, countries with the highest rates of gastric cancer, such as Japan, are those that have long relied on such chemical preservation techniques rather than on refrigeration. It is probably no coincidence that the stomach cancer rate in the United States declined sharply after refrigeration became widespread in the 1930s; moreover, Japanese immigrants to the United States have sharply fewer gastric cancers than do their relatives in the homeland.

The presence of nitrites in the diet, alcohol consumption, radiation exposure, chronic gastritis (inflammation of the stomach lining), and cigarette smoking have also been suspected as gastric carcinogens. Hereditary susceptibility may sometimes play a role, although it is also possible that family members, living under the same conditions, are simply exposed to the same carcinogens and that no genetic susceptibility is involved. Finally, chronic stomach infection with the bacterium *Helicobacter pylori* has been linked to gastric cancer development.

Risk factors for the pancreas and small intestine are much less clear. Chronic pancreatitis, gallstones, and cirrhosis (scarring) of the liver pose some danger of initiating pancreatic cancer, and smokers and diabetics are twice as likely to develop it than are others. Chemists and others who work with organic solvents and petrochemicals also run a slightly higher risk. Intestinal cancer becomes more likely after the immune system has been damaged or late in the course of chronic intestinal diseases, such as Crohn's disease and sprue.

Risky foods, diseases, or occupations do not inevitably lead to cancers. Tumor growth requires at least three factors: some agent that initiates a change in a cell's genetic structure so that a new type of cell is created, called a mutation; an agent that enhances the cell's response to the initiator, encouraging it to reproduce; and the failure of the immune system to destroy the abnormal cells. Most small bowel and gastric can-

---

INFORMATION ON
STOMACH, INTESTINAL, AND
PANCREATIC CANCERS

Causes: Gastric carcinogens (high-nitrate diet, alcohol consumption, radiation exposure, cigarette smoking); chronic gastritis; genetic predisposition; chronic stomach infection; gallstones; chronic pancreatitis; cirrhosis; exposure to chemicals

Symptoms: May include abdominal pain, appetite loss, weight loss, diarrhea, black blood in stool, general weakness, vomiting blood, swollen abdomen, noticeable mass in stomach, iron-deficiency anemia

Duration: Chronic, possibly recurrent

Treatments: Surgery, chemotherapy, radiation therapy

---

cers probably result from long-term overstimulation of the glands or mucosa. This overstimulation occurs when the body fights chemical irritants that have been ingested with food, drink, or air; the body's defense mechanisms lead to inflammation in the damaged area. Chronic inflammation and continually stimulated cell division to repair damage eventually is likely to produce a mutated cell. If adapted to the harsh environment that produced it, the cell can multiply unchecked, overwhelm the immune system, and invade normal tissue; eventually, it may metastasize. A potentially lethal cancer can grow for months or years before its victim notices any definite changes in particular body functions or general health.

Eventually, however, danger signs begin. After initially complaining of abdominal pain, loss of appetite, and difficulty keeping food down, stomach cancer patients may have black, digested blood in the stool, weight loss, general weakness, bouts of vomiting blood, a swollen abdomen, a noticeable mass in the stomach, and iron-deficiency anemia. When the disease is well advanced, metastases become increasingly common, invading the lymph nodes, bile ducts, and liver and eventually spreading to the lungs, bones, and brain. The cancer becomes symptomatic relatively quickly. On average, patients go to their doctors about six months after noticing symptoms.

Pancreatic cancer is much less likely to cause early symptoms, and by the time patients seek medical help, the cancer is usually too far advanced to cure. Physicians suspect pancreatic adenocarcinoma when a patient complains of food aversion, progressive weight loss, and abdominal and back pain, especially when accompanied by vomiting, diarrhea, and jaundice. A rare form of pancreatic cancer (less than 5 percent of cancers in the pancreas) develops from the insulin-producing cells of the organ and makes abnormally high amounts of insulin; in this case, the symptoms are attributable to low blood sugar (hypoglycemia) and include weakness, loss of energy, dizziness, chills, muscle spasms, double vision, and, in extreme cases, coma.

Adenocarcinomas, lymphomas, carcinoid tumors, and sarcomas may form in the small bowel, and most of these grow slowly. Intestinal adenocarcinomas show up primarily in the jejunum or duodenum of elderly patients. Often, they first become apparent when they clog the bowel or bleed. Usually appearing in the stomach, lower jejunum, or ileum, lymphomas are sus-

pected when the patient has fever, night sweats, weight loss, and abdominal pain. Intestinal carcinoid tumors may actively secrete hormones. If they metastasize, release of the hormones sometimes causes a bizarre group of symptoms that are collectively known as carcinoid syndrome: diarrhea, flushing, itching, low blood pressure, and heart disease. Intestinal sarcomas can occur anywhere in the small bowel and reveal themselves by bleeding.

TREATMENT AND THERAPY
Since other diseases also cause the weight loss, abdominal pain, and nausea common to these cancers-for

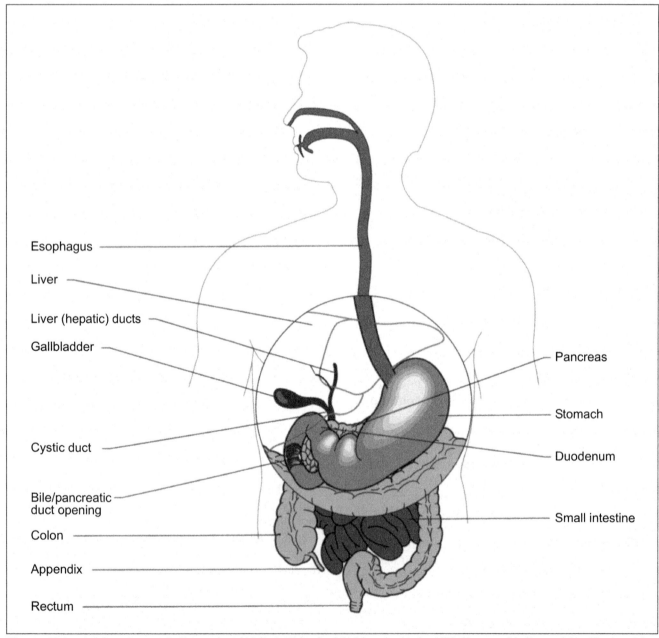

The magnified section shows the stomach, the pancreas (which lies behind and to left of the stomach), the gallbladder, part of the liver, and the midsection of the large colon. ©EBSCO

example, pancreatitis, malabsorption, inflammatory bowel disease, and gastritis-the diagnosis of cancer requires specific evidence from chemical tests, imaging, endoscopic procedures, or surgery. Suspecting stomach cancer, the physician may send the patient for an upper GI barium study. For this procedure, the patient drinks a mixture containing barium sulfate; the radio-opaque barium coats the stomach and under X-ray photography can be seen to outline a tumor if one is present. Tests to check for anemia and blood in the stool may also be ordered. If imaging and tests support a diagnosis of cancer, a gastroenterologist, inserting an endoscope through the patient's mouth, will obtain biopsies of the tumor so that a pathologist can determine if the tumor is malignant. Since biopsies remove such small samples and can miss a cancerous portion of a tumor (especially a lymphoma or sarcoma), surgical biopsy may be necessary to settle the diagnosis beyond doubt.

Similarly, initial tests for pancreatic and intestinal cancer rely on imaging and chemical assays. A barium X-ray study of the small bowel, a computed tomography (CT) scan, or ultrasonography may locate the tumor. Again, endoscopic or surgical biopsy alone can verify the diagnosis of malignancy. Tumors in the small bowel usually lie beyond the reach of endoscopy, so when a barium study reveals a tumor, surgical biopsy is most often necessary to obtain tissue samples; at the same time, the tumor is usually removed to relieve or prevent obstruction of the bowel.

If a tumor has not spread and is well defined, cutting it out provides the best chance of a cure for cancers throughout the stomach, pancreas, and small bowel. Such surgeries are often technically difficult, however, because the patients are typically malnourished and weak and have difficulty enduring the rigors of surgery. When a stomach tumor is single and small, surgeons remove it and a small margin of tissue around its edges. Larger or multiple tumors force the removal of larger portions of the stomach and adjacent lymph nodes. For pancreatic cancer, if more than a single area of the pancreas is involved, the surgeon may remove the entire organ and, depending on the size and location of the tumor, parts of the duodenum and stomach as well. Cancers of the intestines are cut away along with a section of bowel, whose ends are then reconnected by suturing. Chemotherapy and radiation on their own have not proved reliable for shrinking stomach, pancreatic, and intestinal cancers (except lymphomas) and are usually used in conjunction with surgery, especially when a primary tumor has metastasized.

Sometimes endoscopic maneuvers can stop bleeding or relieve pain by clearing out obstructions or, in the case of an obstructed bile duct, by inserting a small perforated tube called a stent to ensure that bile and pancreatic juices flow freely. Pain management, whether with manipulative procedures or with drugs, becomes the primary focus of treatment when surgical cure for a cancer is unlikely. Surgeons do not attempt curative operations if the cancer has metastasized. At this point, surgery, if possible at all, is for relieving pain, preventing blockage, or minimizing blood loss.

PERSPECTIVE AND PROSPECTS

The frequency of these cancers and their distribution in the world vary considerably. Intestinal cancers make up less than 1 percent of all cancers and less than 5 percent of gastrointestinal cancers; pancreatic cancer accounts for only about 3 percent of all cancers. Yet the incidence of both cancers has been rising. In the United States, for example, pancreatic cancer increased about 25 percent from the 1950s to the 1990s. By 2002, it was the fourth leading cause of cancer death, and more than 30,000 Americans were diagnosed with the disease annually. At the same time, stomach cancer decreased dramatically, dropping from the United States' most common cancer in the 1930s to about 2 percent of all cancers in the 1990s. Yet in Japan, Iceland, and parts of Central and South America and of Eastern Europe, the stomach cancer rate is very high, accounting for most of the nearly 700,000 new cases yearly. In some countries, such as Japan, it is higher than all other cancer types combined. Until the 1990s, men contracted and died from stomach, pancreatic, and intestinal cancers more often than women; thereafter, however, women and men began to die from pancreatic cancer in nearly equal numbers. In the United States, African Americans get these cancers more often than Caucasians. Probably because of their diet, poor people develop them more often than middle-class or upper-class people. The peak age group is fifty to fifty-nine years for stomach cancer and seventy to seventy-nine years for pancreatic and intestinal cancer.

The chances for successfully treating or drastically curtailing small bowel cancer are reasonably good; 20 percent of patients with adenocarcinomas in the small intestine survive for at least five years following diagnosis, and patients with carcinoid tumors have lived ten and even fifteen years after surgery. Treatment of small bowel or stomach lymphomas can result in a cure or prolonged survival in a significant percentage of cases. The prospects for pancreatic and stomach adenocarcinomas, however, are another story entirely. Overall, in the United States about 10 percent of gastric cancer patients are alive five years later. Pancreatic cancer is even deadlier, with 90 percent of patients dying in the first year after diagnosis, regardless of treatment. Of those with cancer of the pancreatic duct, only about 4 percent survive three years. Those with cancer in the insulin-producing cells fare better-a 30 percent survival rate-but this is a very rare type of cancer.

Japan has higher survival rates of stomach cancer than does the United States; 50 percent of Japanese patients survive at least five years. The reason is simple. Because gastric cancer is common in Japan, doctors routinely screen patients for it by endoscopy or photofluorography (a type of X ray). Many more cancers are caught early, while they are still surgically treatable. Endoscopic and chemical screenings for pancreatic cancer are also possible, but since the disease is so much less common, doctors do not perform the tests unless they already have good reason to suspect cancer. Avoidance of carcinogens, especially alcohol, remains the most promising way to escape gut cancers.

—Roger Smith, PhD

See also Alcoholism; Bladder cancer; Cancer; Carcinoma; Chemotherapy; Colorectal cancer; Gallbladder cancer; Gastrectomy; Gastroenterology; Gastroenterology, pediatric; Gastrointestinal disorders; Gastrointestinal system; Gastrostomy; Ileostomy and colostomy; Intestinal disorders; Intestines; Jaundice; Kidney cancer; Liver cancer; Malignancy and metastasis; National Cancer Institute (NCI); Oncology; Pancreas; Pancreatitis; Radiation therapy; Small intestine; Tumor removal; Tumors.

For Further Information:

American Cancer Society (ACS). www.cancer.org. Web site is divided into sections for patients, family, and friends; survivors; health information seekers; ACS supporters; and professionals. Information on all cancers is wide ranging.

Daly, John M., Thomas P. J. Hennessy, and John V. Reynolds, eds. *Management of Upper Gastrointestinal Cancer.* New York: W. B. Saunders, 1999. This book addresses such topics as surgical management of gastric cancer, gastric lymphoma, esophageal cancer, and the various treatments associated with these and other ailments.

Eyre, Harmon J., Dianne Partie Lange, and Lois B. Morris. *Informed Decisions: The Complete Book of Cancer Diagnosis, Treatment, and Recovery.* 2d ed. Atlanta: American Cancer Society, 2002. This text from the American Cancer Society is intended for the layperson. It is exemplary in its discussion of cancer.

Kapadia, Cyrus R., James M. Crawford, and Caroline Taylor. *An Atlas of Gastroenterology: A Guide to Diagnosis and Differential Diagnosis.* Boca Raton, Fla.: Parthenon, 2003. Provides a fully illustrated, nonspecialist understanding of myriad gastrointestinal diseases, including gastrointestinal cancers. Includes bibliographic references and an index.

Levine, Joel S., ed. *Decision Making in Gastroenterology.* 2d ed. Philadelphia: B. C. Decker, 1992. This text for physicians contains detailed information about the symptoms and development of cancers. Accompanying charts explain the sequence of examination, testing, and treatment, and dedicated laypersons can glean much of value from them.

O'Reilly, Eileen, and Joanne Frankel Kelvin. *One Hundred Questions and Answers About Pancreatic Cancer.* 2d ed. Sudbury, Mass.: Jones and Bartlett, 2010. Gives both a doctor's and patients' points of view and covers treatment options, post-treatment quality of life, and sources of support.

Parker, James N., and Philip M. Parker, eds. *The Official Patient's Sourcebook on Gastric Cancer.* San Diego, Calif.: Icon Health, 2002. Guides patients in using the Web to educate themselves about the disease and draws from public, academic, government, and peer-reviewed research to provide information on virtually all topics related to gastric cancer, from the essentials to the most advanced areas of research.

Rustgi, Anil K., and James M. Crawford, eds. *Gastrointestinal Cancers.* New York: W. B. Saunders, 2003. This book discusses cancer of the digestive organs, as well as the growth and development of the gastrointestinal system. Includes a bibliography and an index.

Sachar, David B., Jerome D. Waye, and Blair S. Lewis, eds. *Pocket Guide to Gastroenterology.* Rev. ed. Baltimore: Williams & Wilkins, 1991. Contains outlines of the medical subspecialty's basics. An invaluable reference for symptoms, tests, and treatments.

Steen, R. Grant. *A Conspiracy of Cells: The Basic Science of Cancer.* New York: Plenum Press, 1993. Thorough, lucid explanations of all physiological aspects of cancer make this book instructive for readers willing to slog through the subject's complexity and terminology.

STOMACH REMOVAL. SEE GASTRECTOMY.

STONE REMOVAL

Category: Procedure

Anatomy or system affected: Abdomen, bladder, gallbladder, kidneys, urinary system

Specialties and related fields: Gastroenterology, general surgery, nephrology, urology

Definition: An operation that extracts solidified substances (stones) from an organ; typically, these stones block the organ's ability to release fluid.

Key terms:

calculus: an abnormal crystalline formation of a mineral salt; also called a stone

cholecystectomy: the removal of a diseased gallbladder or one that contains many gallstones

cholelithiasis: the formation of gallstones in the gallbladder or the ducts that connect the gallbladder to the liver or small intestine

ureterolithotomy: the surgical removal of a stone in the ureter

ureters: the two muscular tubes that connect the kidneys to the urinary bladder and that serve as conduits for urine

urolithiasis: the formation of stones in the urinary tract

The Removal of Stones

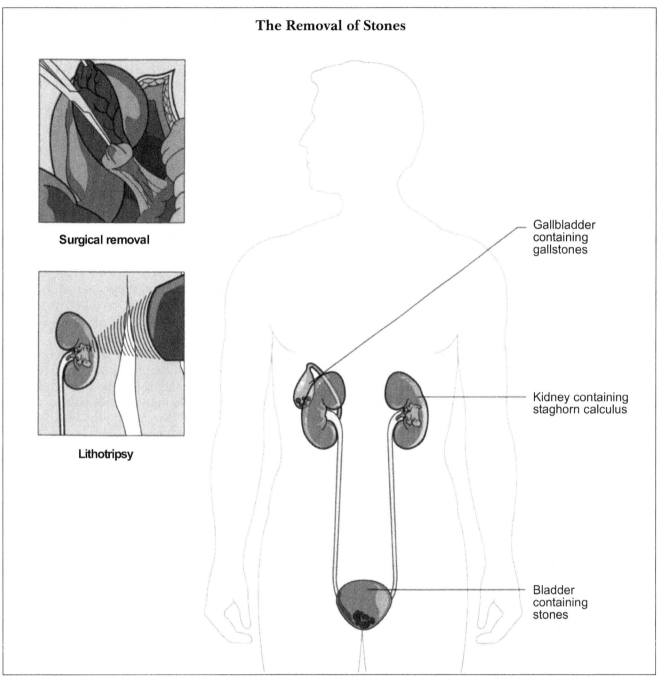

Surgical removal

Lithotripsy

Gallbladder containing gallstones

Kidney containing staghorn calculus

Bladder containing stones

The formation of large calcium deposits in the gallbladder and parts of the urinary system such as the kidneys and bladder can cause pain and obstruction of the ureters or bile ducts. In the case of gallstones, treatment may involve the removal of the entire organ, while kidney or bladder stones can be destroyed using lithotripsy, in which shock waves are used to break up the stones. ©EBSCO

INDICATIONS AND PROCEDURES

Urinary tract stones can occur in the kidneys, ureters, or urinary bladder. These stones, or calculi, are caused by substances that precipitated in the urine. The most common substance that solidifies in the urine is calcium oxalate. Stones referred to as infective, however, are present in about 20 percent of patients with urinary tract stones. These stones typically occur in patients with chronic urinary tract infections. Bacteria in the urinary tract produce ammonia, which combines with calcium or magnesium. Infective stones have the potential to block large areas of the urinary tract.

Patients with urinary tract calculi may experience a variety of symptoms depending on where the stones are located. If a stone is in the ureter, then a sharp pain that extends from the middle of the back to the groin is felt; this pain is called renal colic. Bladder stones are usually not as painful, but they may obstruct the flow of urine from the urinary bladder.

The patient's physician will have the urine examined for the presence of blood (hematuria) and crystals. X rays and/or ultrasound will show the location of the stone. Blood tests may or may not be ordered depending on whether a metabolic disorder is suspected. Hypercalcemia and hyperparathyroidism can be detected by a blood test; both indicate a problem of excess calcium.

If the urinary tract stone is relatively small, the renal colic is treated with bed rest and an analgesic, along with adequate fluid intake to promote passing of the stone. Larger stones, infective stones, or severe obstruction of urinary flow requires surgery to remove the stone. The patient is usually under general anesthesia and has a small surgical scope (a cystoscope for the bladder or a ureterorenoscope for the ureter) passed up the urethra. These scopes give the surgeon the ability to visualize and crush the stones with attachments on the instruments.

The gallbladder, which stores and concentrates bile, also has the potential for stone formation. Gallstones are usually composed of cholesterol and may be found in the ducts that connect the gallbladder to the small intestine or liver. If a stone has obstructed one of these ducts, the resulting symptoms can include intense pain known as biliary colic. This pain is usually felt in the upper right side of the abdomen or between the shoulder blades.

Ultrasound scanning of the upper abdomen can almost always detect the presence of gallstones. If the gallstones do not cause symptoms, they may be left alone, or drugs such as chenodiol and ursodeoxycholic acid may be tried to dissolve them. When symptoms are severe, removal of the gallbladder (cholecystectomy) is indicated. This surgery involves an incision under the ribcage on the right side. A laparoscope may be used or a larger incision made for an open procedure. In either case, the liver is gently lifted to expose the gallbladder, and the blood vessels and cystic duct are tied off so that blood and bile do not leak from the excised organ. The wound is then closed, and the patient may return home within a week.

USES AND COMPLICATIONS
Complications from removing urinary tract stones include infections, scarring, bleeding, and anesthesia risks. These complications are rare when the operation is performed by a competent surgical team. An uncommon but significant adverse result from obstruction relief is an excessive amount of urine loss, sometimes greater than 10 liters per day, which places the patient at risk for dehydration. Reducing fluid intake helps the kidney return to normal function slowly. Occasionally, this complication does not resolve. If the obstruction is not removed, however, the patient is at

risk for developing chronic urinary tract infections and even renal failure.

The major risk in performing cholecystectomy is damage to the bile duct that leads to the small intestine. If scarring or inflammation occurs in this duct, it may lead to obstruction of the flow of bile from the liver. This in turn may lead to obstructive jaundice, in which pigments normally released into the intestines accumulate in the liver and blood. The patient may have a yellowish tinge to the skin and eyes until the obstruction is corrected.

If there are no complications during the cholecystectomy, then the outcome of the surgery is usually good. Approximately 90 percent of the patients have no further symptoms and recover completely in about three weeks.

PERSPECTIVE AND PROSPECTS
Advances in medical technology have aided physicians in the removal of stones. Kidney and urethral stones now can be broken up using a technique called lithotripsy. An ultrasonic lithotripsy probe can break the stones using externally applied sound waves that penetrate the skin and other soft tissues. For some patients, a noninvasive technique takes advantage of sound waves transmitted through the abdominal cavity and directed at the stones. This procedure is known as extracorporeal shock-wave lithotripsy. The latter technique is also used to treat some patients with gallstones.

—*Matthew Berria, PhD and Douglas Reinhart, MD*

See also Bile; Cholecystectomy; Cholecystitis; Cystoscopy; Gallbladder; Gallbladder diseases; Hematuria; Kidney disorders; Kidneys; Laparoscopy; Lithotripsy; Nephrology; Stones; Ultrasonography; Urinary disorders; Urinary system; Urology.

For Further Information:
Alexander, Ivy L., ed. *Urinary Tract and Kidney Diseases and Disorders Sourcebook: Basic Consumer Health Information About the Urinary System.* 2d ed. Detroit, Mich.: Omnigraphics, 2005. Covers diagnosis and treatment of a range of disorders, including kidney and bladder stones.
Blumgart, L. H., and Y. Fong, eds. *Surgery of the Liver and Biliary Tract.* 3d ed. 2 vols. New York: W. B. Saunders, 2000. This authoritative text offers a comprehensive, detailed description of the subject.
Leikin, Jerrold B., and Martin S. Lipsky, eds. *American Medical Association Complete Medical Encyclopedia.* New York: Random House Reference, 2003. A concise presentation of numerous medical terms and illnesses. A good general reference.
Parker, James N., and Philip M. Parker, eds. *The 2002 Official Patient's Sourcebook on Kidney Stones.* San Diego, Calif.: Icon Health, 2002. Draws from public, academic, government, and peer-reviewed research to provide a wide-ranging reference about the causes, treatments, and risk factors of kidney stones.

Tierney, Lawrence M., Stephen J. McPhee, and Maxine A. Papadakis, eds. *Current Medical Diagnosis and Treatment 2007*. New York: McGraw-Hill Medical, 2006. This book is revised annually. Contains several chapters that address stones. An excellent and concise text, but written for professionals.

Walsh, Patrick C., et al., eds. *Campbell-Walsh Urology*. 4 vols. 9th ed. Philadelphia: Saunders/Elsevier, 2007. A classic urology text.

STONES

Category: Disease/Disorder
Also known as: Calculi
Anatomy or system affected: Abdomen, bladder, gallbladder, kidneys, urinary system
Specialties and related fields: Gastroenterology, internal medicine, nephrology, urology
Definition: Hard deposits of material in the body associated with urine and bile.

CAUSES AND SYMPTOMS

Stones may form in the kidneys, ureters, bladder, and gallbladder. Kidney and ureter stones are typically calcium-based, while bladder stones are most frequently composed of uric acid (a by-product of protein metabolism) or struvite (a result of chronic urinary infection). Gallstones contain very little calcium; they are primarily composed of cholesterol.

The symptoms that accompany urinary stone disease are dependent on the location of the stone, the size of the stone, how long the stone has been present, whether infection is associated with the stone, and the degree of obstruction to urinary flow caused by the stone. Urine, which is produced by the kidneys, located beneath the ribs of the back, is collected into a structure just outside the kidney known as the renal pelvis. From the renal pelvis, urine passes into a thin narrow tube called the ureter and travels a relatively long distance to the urinary bladder. It is easy to envision how a stone traveling along such a narrow, long tube can get stuck and dam the further flow of urine.

Stones caught in the renal pelvis, prior to entry into the ureter, generally cause an intermittent, sharp pain in the back or side. Stones that pass into the ureter can cause pain in the back as well as points distant from the urinary system (the groin, the lower abdomen, and the testicles and penis in men); this phenomenon is known as referred pain. Occasionally, stones in the lowest portion of the ureters will cause pain only with urination or produce the desire to urinate frequently but only in small amounts. Often, blood not visible to the naked eye can be found in the urine with a simple chemical dipstick or by looking at the urine under a

INFORMATION ON STONES

Causes: Metabolic disorders, chronic urinary infection, high levels of cholesterol, prostate enlargement, narrowed urethra, abnormal pouching of bladder, neurologic dysfunction leading to poor bladder emptying
Symptoms: Sharp and sudden pain in lower abdomen that worsens with movement, intermittent blockage of urine stream, weak urine stream, increased frequency of urination, urgency, recurrent urinary tract infections, blood in urine
Duration: Acute
Treatments: Extracorporeal shock-wave lithotripsy, surgery (laser and conventional), endoscopy

microscope, both easily accomplished in most doctors' offices.

Several radiological tests can be performed to pinpoint the location of a stone lodged in the urinary tract. An intravenous pyelogram (IVP) is a series of X rays performed following the administration of a dye into the patient's vein. This dye is concentrated in the urine and can be visualized as it travels through the urinary tract. High-frequency sound waves, or ultrasound, can determine if obstruction is present in the kidneys but will frequently miss stones lodged in the ureters. A computed tomography (CT) scan is similar to an IVP but uses advanced computer technology to visualize better all contents of the body. While the CT scan is the most sensitive test for the detection of urinary stones, certain situations may necessitate the use of different tests. Frequently, people with poor renal function cannot receive the X-ray dye because of its potential harmful effects on the kidneys. A CT scan without contrast or ultrasound will frequently be performed in this situation.

Bladder stones are found much less frequently than stones in the kidney and ureter. Perhaps the most famous person to have suffered from bladder stones is Benjamin Franklin, who reportedly stood on his head to urinate. Throughout the world, bladder stones are almost exclusively a disease of the older, male population. They are most frequently found in association with enlargement of the prostate that obstructs the bladder's ability to empty and allows these stones to crystallize in the urine. Other causes of bladder stone formation should be excluded, such as a narrowed urethra, an abnormal pouching of the bladder, a chronic urinary infection, or a neurologic dysfunction leading to poor bladder emptying.

Symptoms of a bladder stone are pain in the lower abdomen that worsens with movement, intermittent blockage of the urinary stream, a weak urine stream, increased frequency of urination often associated with a strong and urgent need to void, recurrent urinary tract infections, or blood in the urine. Definitive diagnosis of a stone can be made with a simple X ray of the abdomen alone; however, the physician will often need to perform additional tests, including a direct look into the bladder.

Diseases affecting the gallbladder and bile ducts occur commonly in the elderly. By the age of seventy, stones in the gallbladder and bile duct represent the most frequently occurring disorder affecting this organ system. In the late 1990s, it was estimated that 33 percent of the U.S. population over seventy would be diagnosed with gallstones at some point in their lives.

The symptoms associated with stones in the gallbladder or bile duct are numerous and depend on the location and size of the stone and whether there is an associated infection. Frequently, patients complain of pain in the right upper part of the abdomen. This pain often occurs after the consumption of a fatty meal, which causes the gallbladder to contract and release its bile. Fever, sweats, and chills may accompany the pain if there is infection present. Jaundice, a yellowish discoloring of the skin, may occur if the common bile duct or hepatic duct becomes obstructed with a gallstone. As with stones in the urinary tract, it is the blockage of flow of bile from the gallbladder that leads to the symptoms. Elderly patients who appear jaundiced may not always be suffering from gallstones, especially if there is no associated pain. Other diseases

of the liver and biliary system, such as cirrhosis of the liver or hepatitis, will also cause jaundice and are frequently found in the elderly.

The biliary system stores bile formed in the liver and delivers it to the intestines following a meal, aiding in the digestion of fat and the absorption of certain vitamins. The gallbladder is a blind-ending pouch that comes off of the bile duct as it courses from the liver to the small intestine. After consumption of a fatty meal, its muscle-lined wall contracts to release bile into the intestine. Stones can form in the gallbladder and can cause pain or infection when lodged in the bile duct or common hepatic (liver) duct. If a stone causes blockage and infection, the patient can become very sick and require emergency medical care.

Unlike kidney stones, gallstones are frequently not visible upon plain X-ray examination of the abdomen. Despite their hard nature, gallstones contain very little calcium. They are primarily composed of cholesterol, which, unlike calcium, is not dense enough to be visible on an X ray. Ultrasound examination of the liver and gallbladder is almost always the first test ordered by a physician who is suspicious that a patient may have a gallstone. To determine if obstruction of the bile duct is present, a physician can also use nuclear medicine studies, which use a radioactive material concentrated by the gallbladder, similar to the concentration of X-ray dye used in the diagnosis of kidney stones. On occasion, the diagnosis of a gallstone lodged in the bile duct requires the placement of a telescope into the patient's stomach and intestine and direct visualization of the common bile duct's entry into the intestine.

TREATMENT AND THERAPY

Treatment of any stone depends on the location of the stone, its size, the time it has been in place, and any complicating issues such as infection. The methods for treatment are broad, and the specific means by which a stone should be removed are often debated among the experts in this field. Some stones-especially if they are small, cause no pain, and are not significantly obstructing-are given a chance to pass on their own, a treatment termed watchful waiting. The most frequent noninvasive means to treat a small stone located in the urinary tract above the pelvic bone is extracorporeal shock-wave lithotripsy (ESWL). This procedure involves the use of high-energy sound waves created by a machine outside the body and focused through the skin onto the stone. These sound waves break the stone into fine sand, which passes in the urine without symptoms. This is frequently the best method to deal with stones in elderly patients who have other medical problems that can make surgical means of removing a stone risky. Endoscopic removal of a stone involves the use of small telescopes passed into the urinary

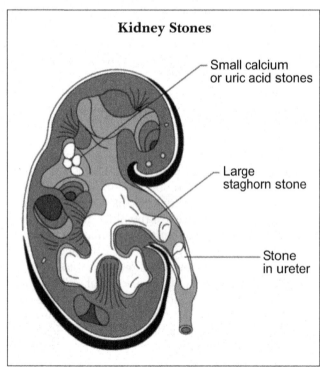

Kidney Stones

Small calcium or uric acid stones

Large staghorn stone

Stone in ureter

©EBSCO

tract either through the urethra or through the back directly into the kidney. Different means of fragmenting the stone into smaller pieces for direct removal are then employed through the telescopes. This method is highly successful and often used for larger stones. Like ESWL, this low-invasive, endoscopic means of removing the stone places minimal stress on the elderly patient with other medical problems.

The development of these minimally invasive procedures for stone removal has led to a significant decrease in the need for open surgery. Nevertheless, there are special situations when an open surgical procedure may be the first reasonable option for the elderly patient with a urinary stone. These situations include abnormal urinary tract anatomy, concurrent urinary tract pathology other than the stone, or the failure of less invasive means to remove the stone.

Treatment of bladder stones is very successful and appropriate for the elderly. As with stones of the kidney and ureter, endoscopic removal of a bladder stone using small telescopes frequently can be performed. Most bladder stones, however, are removed with open surgery. Paramount to the successful treatment of a bladder stone is the treatment of the underlying cause for its formation, which frequently dictates the method of removal. Whether endoscopic or open surgery is chosen, both are generally well tolerated by elderly patients even if significant other medical problems exist.

Treatment of symptomatic gallstones almost always involves surgery using lighted telescopes passed either directly into the abdomen (laparoscopes) or through the stomach and intestine (endoscopes), or open surgery. Unlike the removal of kidney and bladder stones, which most often merely involves the removal of the actual stone and not the kidney, ureter, or bladder, treatment of gallstones usually also involves the removal of the gallbladder itself. The loss of this unpaired organ often does not lead to significant digestive problems, though in the elderly loose, foul-smelling bowel movements may result from the altered digestion of fats.

The choice of surgical approach again depends on whether an infection is associated with the stone, how severe the symptoms are, whether any liver dysfunction is associated with the stone, and the overall health of the patient. Gallstones not causing symptoms are generally not removed. Patients with diabetes mellitus and other complicating medical conditions are dealt with in a more cautious manner and frequently undergo surgery to remove the gallstone and gallbladder even if symptoms do not exist.

PERSPECTIVE AND PROSPECTS

While there is no evidence of increased incidence of urinary stones with increasing age, stones of the biliary tract (cholelithiasis) do increase with age, affecting approximately 33 percent of the U.S. population over seventy years old.

Kidney stones or stones in the urinary tract affect 5 to 10 percent of the general population of the United States. The likelihood of a person to form a stone for the first time in their life decreases with advancing age. In people who have a prior history of urinary stone formation, however, the incidence, recurrence, and severity of urinary stone disease is similar between the geriatric and younger populations. The composition of urinary stones in the older population is no different from that of those found in younger patients; however, the underlying urinary abnormality leading to the stone formation is different. More frequently, urinary stones in the elderly are caused by high uric acid levels and low citrate levels in the urine. Similar difficulties in the disposal of protein metabolites can lead to gouty arthritis.

—*John F. Ward, MD and Prodromos G. Borboroglu, MD*

See also Bile; Cholecystectomy; Cholecystitis; Endoscopy; Gallbladder; Gallbladder diseases; Gout; Jaundice; Kidney disorders; Kidneys; Laparoscopy; Lithotripsy; Nephritis; Nephrology; Nutrition; Stone removal; Urethritis; Urinary disorders; Urinary system; Urology.

For Further Information:
Gillenwater, Jay Y., et al., eds. *Adult and Pediatric Urology.* 4th ed. Philadelphia: Lippincott Williams & Wilkins, 2002. A three-volume clinical set that covers a range of urologic diseases and disorders in adults and children.
Moran, M. E. "Uric Acid Stone Disease." *Frontiers in Bioscience* 8 (September, 2003): 1339-1355. Details the rise of uric stone formation throughout the world, examining its history, diagnosis, treatments, and risk factors.
Saunders, Carol S. "Urolithiasis: New Tools for Diagnosis and Treatment." *Patient Care* 33, no. 15 (September 30, 1999): 28-44. Noncontrast helical CT has replaced IV pyelography as first-line imaging for suspected acute renal colic, and treatment decisions have been simplified with new guidelines. This and other advances in prevention are discussed.
Walsh, Patrick C., et al., eds. *Campbell-Walsh Urology.* 4 vols. 9th ed. Philadelphia: Saunders/Elsevier, 2007. This edition of a classic urology text maintains its encyclopedic approach while following a new organ systems orientation. Halftone illustrations and contributions by multiple authors. Includes a CD-ROM.

STRABISMUS

Category: Disease/Disorder
Also known as: Crossed eyes
Anatomy or system affected: Eyes, muscles
Specialties and related fields: Ophthalmology
Definition: The improper alignment or crossing of the eyes.

CAUSES AND SYMPTOMS

Strabismus affects approximately 5 percent of the population. It may be caused by a problem with the nerve supply to the muscles that move the eye or by poor vision or obstruction of vision in one or both eyes.

The most common type of strabismus is an esotropia (inward deviation) of the eye, which accounts for 75 percent of the cases of crossed eyes. There is also exotropia (outward deviation), hypertropia (upward deviation), and hypotropia (downward deviation) of the eye. When a child with strabismus has a penlight shone in the eye, the light reflected back does not fall on the pupil in the same place. This is referred to as the corneal light reflex test. When the eyes are aligned, the corneal light reflex will be placed symmetrically on the pupil. It is important to identify strabismus and to have it evaluated to prevent amblyopia (dimness of vision) or blindness in the eye that is deviated. It is also important because without input from both eyes, it is difficult to perceive depth.

A condition called pseudostrabismus gives the appearance of having crossed eyes. It occurs because there is a flat bridge of the nose or extra skin near the nose. In this situation, the corneal light reflex will be symmetrical in the pupil.

TREATMENT AND THERAPY

Treatment of strabismus is aimed at avoiding amblyopia and realigning the eyes to restore depth perception. This realignment frequently requires surgery. Some cases can be treated with glasses and bifocals. An ophthalmologist should be consulted for the treatment of strabismus.

—*Sheila J. Mosee, MD*

See also Blindness; Botox; Eye infections and disorders; Eyes; Optometry; Optometry, pediatric; Sense organs; Vision; Vision disorders.

For Further Information:
Buettner, Helmut, ed. *Mayo Clinic on Vision and Eye Health: Practical Answers on Glaucoma, Cataracts, Macular Degeneration, and Other Conditions.* Rochester, Minn.: Mayo Foundation for Medical Education and Research, 2002.
Eden, John. *The Physician's Guide to Cataracts, Glaucoma, and Other Eye Problems.* Yonkers, N.Y.: Consumer Reports Books, 1992.
Flynn, John T. *Strabismus: A Neurodevelopmental Approach.* New York: Springer, 1991.
Riordan-Eva, Paul, and John P. Whitcher. *Vaughan and Asbury's General Ophthalmology.* 17th ed. New York: Lange Medical Books/McGraw-Hill, 2007.
Sutton, Amy L., ed. *Eye Care Sourcebook: Basic Consumer Health Information About Eye Care and Eye Disorders.* 3d ed. Detroit, Mich.: Omnigraphics, 2008.
Van Noorden, Gunter K., and Emilio C. Campos. *Binocular Vision and Ocular Motility: Theory and Management of Strabismus.* 6th ed. St. Louis, Mo.: Mosby, 2002.

STRENGTH TRAINING

Category: Procedure
Anatomy or system affected: Musculoskeletal
Specialties and related fields: Physiology, fitness, gerontology
Definition: Strength training is a type of physical exercise specializing in the use of resistance to induce muscular contraction which builds the strength, anaerobic endurance, and size of skeletal muscles

Key terms:

anabolism: the repair/growth stage of muscle development
body weight: the use of the person's natural weight as the form of resistance while exercising
catabolism: damage to muscles
free weight: a freestanding object whose weight is used as resistance while exercising
stretchable tubing: elastic workout object with little to no weight that uses tension to create resistance for exercise
spotter: a person who assists with a person exercising to ensure proper technique and injury prevention; this can hands-on, by being in a physical position to prevent accidents, or hands-off by watching the exercising person and being ready to assist as needed
weight machine: a stationary machine used for exercise that uses attached weights and gravity to offer resistance

INTRODUCTION

Strength training, also called "resistance training" or weight lifting, is a type of exercise that uses resistance to build strength, muscle mass, and endurance. Resistance may be in the form of weights, weight machines, stretchable tubing, or body weight. Using resistance causes muscles to contract, or shorten, which strengthens them.

When a person creates resistance on a muscle, tiny tears damage the muscle cells. After strength training, hormones, nutrients, and proteins in the body repair and replenish muscles, helping them to grow. The damage to the muscles is called "catabolism," and the repair/growth stage is called "anabolism." Building muscle has many positive health effects. It has been shown to help people manage their weight, strengthen their bones, and build up their stamina.

TYPES OF STRENGTH-TRAINING EXERCISES

Fitness experts group strength-training exercises by the type of resistance used. These exercises can be performed by using free weights or items found in the home, specialized machines found at gyms, resistance tubing, or even one's own body weight. People can use a combination of different strength-training exercises along with cardiovascular exercise to achieve maximum health and performance.

Free Weights. Free weights, such as barbells and dumbbells, can be used to provide resistance. Lifting free weights has many advantages. People do not need expensive equipment or even a gym membership to lift free weights. At home, they can use heavy objects—such as canned goods, bricks, or bottles of water—to exercise their muscles.

Moving and controlling free weights takes great focus and helps people improve their coordination skills. People who have injuries or limited movement can adjust the way they lift free weights to accommodate their needs. In addition, lifting free weights exercises many muscles at once, even ones that are not being specifically targeted. For example, if people stand and raise weights in front of them, the muscles in the abdomen and back will work to help keep the body steady.

Nevertheless, there are some disadvantages to lifting free weights. If people do not use proper form while lifting weights, they may risk serious injury. To prevent injury, people should not lift weights that are too heavy. Furthermore, they should always lift weights—especially heavy weights—with another person, known as a "spotter," to ensure they are using correct form. Other disadvantages involve the storage and cost of free weights. Storing free weights and designating an area to lift can be an issue in homes with little free space. Free weights can also be costly if people purchase multiple pieces of equipment, such as weight benches, bars, and weight plates.

Weight Machines. Weight machines are relatively easy to use. People position themselves on the machines, move a pin in the weight stack to the desired weight, and then move the machine by either pushing or pulling on handles or bars. They are safer to use than free weights and do not require as much coordination. Still, people must use good form on the machines so they do not injure themselves, and they should avoid lifting weights that are too heavy.

Using weight machines has several disadvantages. They are large and expensive, so most people must join a gym to use them. Machines usually target only one set of muscles, which means a person must use multiple machines to work different muscle groups. People who are not of average size may have difficulty using the machines correctly, and most machines cannot be adjusted to accommodate people who have limited movement or injuries.

Stretchable Tubing. Stretchable or resistance tubing is made of elastic tubes that stretch to provide resistance. They come in different sizes and thicknesses, which create more or less tension. To use them, people put them around a body part and pull on them to create tension. This causes the muscle to contract. Stretchable tubes are inexpensive, portable, easy to use, and take up little space. They can also target a variety of muscle groups. However, these tubes lose elasticity over time and may need to be replaced. Additionally, they can snap and cause injury.

Body Weight. People do not need free weights, machines, or stretchable tubing to strength train. They can use their own body weight as resistance to perform exercises such as abdominal crunches, leg squats, lunges, pull-ups, push-ups, and more. These types of exercises use the weight of a person's body as resistance. The major advantage to using one's body weight is that it is free. No special equipment is needed. Also, exercises that rely on body weight can be performed anywhere. A disadvantage to this form of strength training is that the resistance cannot be decreased. Yet, resistance may be increase by altering the way some exercises are performed.

BENEFITS OF STRENGTH TRAINING

Strength training has many benefits. These benefits include improved athletic performance, injury rehabilitation, weight loss and stress, and to combat effects of ageing. According to the American College of Sports Medicine, a person should work out all the muscle groups to fatigue at least two to three days a week with rest days in between active workout days to achieve maximum results. The major muscle groups include the abdominals, arms, back, chest, legs, and shoulders. Working out a muscle to fatigue means people should perform an exercise with weights that are heavy enough so that they can only perform eight to twelve repetitions. This is just an average number and can change depending on several factors, such as the age, health, goals, and strength of a person.

Strength training is one of the primary methods used by persons to improve athletic performance. Strength training programs can improve an athlete's muscle power and economy. An improvement in economy allows an athlete's body to burn through less energy at lower levels of intensity, as well as slowing down the draining of carbohydrate stores. An improvement in muscle power allows an athlete to increase the amount of force produced which can improve performance.

Injury rehabilitation, facilitated by a physical therapist, often utilizes body weight, resistance bands, and at latter stages weight machines, to regain muscle strength and function. Regaining muscle strength is accomplished through a focus on stabilizing muscles. Increased function is accomplished through a program designed to increase the muscles range of motion.

Research has indicated that the average American does not move enough and leads a sedentary lifestyle. Many people have jobs that keep them inactive during the day. In addition, many people spend much of their free time doing sedentary activities, such as watching television or playing on computers, instead of engaging in physical exercise. These conditions can lead to weight gain and stress. Strength training releases the brain neurotransmitters dopamine and serotonin, which when released help combat depression. Muscles during strength training also burn through carbohydrates, which when combined with a healthy diet, results in weight loss.

Research has shown that specific effects of aging on the brain, muscle strength and muscle density, can be slowed down through the incorporation of strength training. Strength training increases neurogenesis, neuroplasticity, and cognition performance, slowing down the deterioration of brain function. After the age of thirty, people lose five pounds of muscle every decade. In addition, people lose bone density as they age. Research has proven that performing resistance exercises can help slow or even reverse age-related muscle and bone loss. Strength training also helps to reduce the loss of motor function.

RISKS OF STRENGTH TRAINING

Strength training can also have harmful effects on the body. These effects usually occur due to overtraining or improper technique. Through proper research and consulting with strength and conditioning professionals, the risks of strength training can be greatly reduced.

Overtraining occurs when the intensity and frequency of strength training routines over an extended period of time doesn't allow the body significant time to recover. This has a variety of negative consequences, including muscle weakness, decreased athletic performance, reduction in quality of sleep, and increased resting heart rate. Overtraining is easily preventable by recognizing body fatigue and allowing ample time for the body to recover following strength training.

Improper technique occurs when a strength training exercise is done incorrectly. This can have immediate and long-term effects on the body. Improper technique adds additional pressure on joints and muscles, stretching of soft-tissue muscle, and can make preexisting injuries worse. Ways to avoid improper technique involve the use of a spotter to monitor exercise, proper research on exercises, and avoiding continuing exercise when muscle fatigue occurs.

—*Bradley R. A. Wilson, PhD*

For Further Information:
Collins, A. *Strength Training Over 40: A 6-Week Program to Build Muscle and Agility.* Rockridge Press, 2020.
Haff, G. Gregory, and N. Travis Triplett. *Essentials of Strength Training and Conditioning.* 4th ed., Human Kinetics, 2016.
Hunt, K. *Beginner's Guide to Weight Lifting: Simple Exercises and Workouts to Get Strong.* Rockridge Press, 2020.
———. *Bodybuilding for Beginners: A 12-Week Program to Build Muscle and Burn Fat.* Rockridge Press, 2019.
———. *Strength Training for Beginners: A 12-Week Program to Get Lean and Healthy at Home.* Rockridge Press, 2020.
Noelle, B. *Weight Training for Women: Exercises and Workout Programs for Building Strength with Free Weights* 2020.
"Strength Training: Get Stronger, Leaner, Healthier." *Mayo Clinic.* Mayo Foundation for Medical Education and Research, www.mayoclinic.org/healthy-living/fitness/in-depth/strength-training/art-20046670.
Derived from "Strength Training." *Salem Press Encyclopedia of Health*, Salem Press. Accessed 15 May 2021.

STREPTOCOCCAL INFECTIONS

Category: Disease/Disorder
Also known as: Strep infections
Anatomy or system affected: Arms, back, chest, circulatory system, ears, feet, genitals, hands, heart, joints, legs, muscles, neck, skin, throat
Specialties and related fields: Bacteriology, critical care, dermatology, emergency medicine, family medicine, general surgery, internal medicine, microbiology, obstetrics, pediatrics
Definition: Infections caused by bacteria belonging to the genus *Streptococcus*, such as strep throat, scarlet fever, impetigo, cellulitis, rheumatic fever, and necrotizing fasciitis.
Key terms:
cephalosporins: a class of antibiotics that attack the synthesis of the bacterial cell wall and were originally derived from the fungus *Acremonium*, previously called *Cephalosporium*
macrolides: a class of antibiotics that inhibit bacterial protein synthesis *erythromycin* : was the first macrolide antibiotic discovered

meningitis: infection of the meningeal coverings of the brain and/or spinal cord

pharyngitis: sore throat caused by inflammation of the pharynx

puerperal infection: infection of the female reproductive system after she has given birth or suffered a miscarriage

CAUSES AND SYMPTOMS

Among the bacteria that belong to the genus *Streptococcus*, the two major pathogens are group A streptococci, represented by *Streptococcus pyogenes*, and group B streptococci, which consist of *Streptococcus agalactiae*. Group A streptococci, common pathogens found in the throat and skin, cause various diseases listed in Table 1.

Group B streptococci cause severe disease and mainly affect newborns and pregnant women. These bacteria, found in the genital and intestinal tracts of 20 to 35 percent of healthy adults, can infect a newborn during the birth process and cause early-onset neonatal disease, which occurs within seven days of birth, or late-onset neonatal disease, which occurs more than one week after birth. Infected newborns develop the signs and symptoms of meningitis, pneumonia, and sepsis. *Streptococcus agalactiae* is the most common cause of neonatal meningitis and sepsis and can cause of neonatal death. This microorganism can also infect pregnant women and cause postpartum endometriosis, urinary tract and wound infections. Bacteremia (colonization of the blood by bacteria) and disseminated complications can also occur, resulting in stillbirth. In adult patients, particularly the elderly, *S. agalactiae* can cause bacteremia, pneumonia, bone, and joint infections, and skin and soft tissue infections.

Other pathogenic streptococci include group C streptococci, which includes *S. dysgalactiae*, group D streptococci, represented by *S. gallolyticus*, group F and G streptococci, which includes *S. anginosus*, and a member of the *S. mitis* group, *S. pneumoniae*. *S. dysgalactiae* can cause pharyngitis, and acute glomerulonephritis. *S. anginosus* causes deep tissue abscesses, and *S. gallolyticus* tends to be associated with gastrointestinal cancer and causes meningitis, endocarditis, and bacteremia. *S.*

INFORMATION ON STREPTOCOCCAL INFECTIONS

Causes: Bacterial infection with streptococci

Symptoms: Depends on type; may include sore throat, otitis media, sinusitis, tonsillitis, impetigo, cellulitis, necrotizing fasciitis, toxic shock syndrome

Duration: Acute

Treatments: Depends on type; may include antibiotics (penicillin, cephalosporins), prevention through good hygiene and wound cleansing, emergency care if severe

Table 1. Diseases Caused by Group A Streptococci

Disease	Clinical summary
Pharyngitis	Reddened throat with exudate (a mass of fluid and cells that has seeped from blood vessels during inflammation)
Scarlet fever	Diffuse rash that begins at the chest and spreads to the extremities
Pyoderma	A skin infection that begins with blisters that evolve into pustules
Erysipelas	Skin infection with pain, inflammation, lymph node enlargement, and systemic symptoms
Cellulitis	Infection of the skin that includes the deeper tissues
Necrotizing fasciitis	A deep skin infection that includes the destruction of underlying fat and muscle
Streptococcal toxic shock syndrome	Multiorgan systemic infection that resembles staphylococcal toxic shock syndrome, but with bacteremia and fasciitis
Puerperal sepsis	Bacterial infection of the female reproductive tract after childbirth or a miscarriage
Lymphangitis	Infection of the lymphatic system
Pneumonia	Lung infection
Rheumatic fever	Nonsupperative infection that does not involve actual infection of the tissues but includes inflammation of the heart, joints, blood vessels, and subcutaneous tissues
Acute glomerulonephritis	Acute inflammation of the kidney

pneumoniae is a common cause of pneumonia, meningitis, and bacteremia, particularly in elderly patients.

TREATMENT AND THERAPY

Streptococcal pharyngitis or Strep throat is diagnosed readily in the clinic by a rapid strep test. It can be treated easily with common antibiotics, such as oral penicillin V or amoxicillin, but cephalosporins or a macrolide should be used for patients who are allergic to penicillin. Antibiotic treatment of pharyngitis speeds recovery and, if initiated within ten days of the initial appearance of symptoms, will prevent rheumatic fever. Patients with rheumatic fever require long-term antibiotic prophylaxis to prevent the disease from returning, and during all dental procedures to prevent the colonization of the heart valves by bacteria. Prevention is the key to avoiding complications of the disease. Maintenance of hygiene (such as washing hands after sneezing or coughing), visiting a doctor to rule out streptococcal disease in case of severe sore throat, and taking any antibiotics prescribed should keep complications at bay. Keeping all wounds clean should prevent the occurrence of skin infections.

Table 2. Conditions for which *Pneumovax23* vaccination is recommended in adults aged nineteen to sixty-four years

Normally functioning immune system	Subfunctional immune system
Chronic conditions	Missing a spleen (anatomically or functionally)
Chronic heart disease	Sickle cell disease or other hemoglobin-based disorder (hemoglobinopathy)
Chronic lung disease (e.g., asthma and chronic obstructive pulmonary disease)	Human immunodeficiency virus (HIV) infection
Chronic liver disease	Chronic kidney diseases
Poorly controlled diabetes mellitus	Blood-based cancer (leukemia or lymphoma)
Cigarette smoking	Cancer in general
Alcohol abuse	Solid-organ transplantation
Those at high risk for meningitis	Bone marrow transplantation
Cochlear implant placement	Long-term glucocorticoid steroid or radiation treatment (also known as iatrogenic immunosuppression)
Cerebrospinal fluid leak	Genetically determined immune system disabilities
History of pneumococcal meningitis	
Prior head injury or head, neck, or spinal surgery	

Streptococcal toxic shock syndrome is a medical emergency and requires hospitalized care.

Group B streptococci are typically susceptible to penicillins, and high-dose penicillin G and ampicillin are the drugs of choice. In penicillin-allergic patients, ceftriaxone, vancomycin, linezolid, and daptomycin are viable alternatives. Resistance to macrolides, tetracyclines, and clindamycin has steadily increased in group B streptococci. To prevent neonatal disease, pregnant women should be screened for group B streptococci, and antibiotics are administered during labor to women who are carriers of these bacteria. This practice effectively prevents neonatal meningitis and sepsis. Babies affected by the disease can be treated effectively with antibiotics and management of symptoms. A vaccine against group B streptococcal infection is under development.

Ceftriaxone or vancomycin effectively treat *S. anginosus* infections. For *S. gallolyticus* infections, ceftriaxone, vancomycin, daptomycin, linezolid, and tigecycline are highly effective. *S. dysgalactiae* is quite susceptible to penicillin, and penicillin G remains the drug of choice, but cefotaxime and ceftriaxone are suitable alternatives.

Treatment of *S. pneumoniae* (or pneumococcal) infections presents a challenge because of extensive drug resistance. Historically, this organism was susceptible to penicillin, but in 1977, penicillin-resistant strains were isolated in South Africa. Since then, multidrug resistant *S. pneumoniae* strains have proliferated. For penicillin-resistant strains, ceftriaxone or cefotaxime are the preferred treatments for pneumococcal pneumonia. Alternative treatments include cefpodoxime, cefprozil, cefuroxime, levofloxacin, and clindamycin. For severely ill patients, combination treatments are used, such as vancomycin plus ceftriaxone, followed by an additional drug. *Prevnar13* (PVC13) is a vaccine for children six weeks to seventeen years. It protects against thirteen different *S. pneumoniae* strains. PCV13

is normally given to children at two, four, six, and twelve to fifteen months. Between four to six years, children receive a booster immunization with a different vaccination called *Pneumovax23* (PPSV23). PPSV23 contains purified carbohydrates from twenty-three different *S. pneumoniae* strains. It is also recommended for adults over sixty-five to immunize them against *S. pneumoniae* infections and protect them from infections that routinely plague older patients. Pneumococcal vaccination is not recommended for healthy adults younger than sixty-five years. However, the Centers for Disease Control and Prevention (CDC) recommends that all adults aged nineteen to sixty-four years with preexisting health conditions (see Table 2 above) that increase their risk of pneumococcal infections should receive *Pneumovax23*.

—*Michael A. Buratovich, PhD*

See also: Antibiotics; Bacterial infections; Ear infections and disorders; Impetigo; Infection; Necrotizing fasciitis; Peritonitis; Pharyngitis; Pneumonia; Quinsy; Rheumatic fever; Scarlet fever; Sinusitis; Sore throat; Strep throat; Tonsillitis; Toxic shock syndrome.

For Further Information:
Efstratiou A., and T. Lamagni. "Epidemiology of *Streptococcus pyogenes*." *Streptococcus pyogenes: Basic Biology to Clinical Manifestations*, edited by J. J. Ferretti, D. L. Stevens, and V. A. Fischetti, University of Oklahoma Health Sciences Center, 2016.
Frazier, Margaret Schell, and Tracie Fuque. *Essentials of Human Diseases and Conditions*. 7th ed., Saunders, 2020.
Loscalzo, Joseph, et al., editors. *Harrison's Principles of Internal Medicine*. 21st ed., McGraw-Hill, 2022.
Murray, Patrick R., Ken S. Rosenthal, and Michael A. Pfaller. *Medical Microbiology*. 9th ed., Elsevier, 2020.
"Pneumococcal Vaccine: What Everyone Should Know." *Center for Disease Control and Prevention*, 24 Jan. 2022, www.cdc.gov/vaccines/vpd/pneumo/public/. Accessed 6 Mar. 2022.
Ryan, Kenneth J., et al., editors. *Ryan & Sherris Medical Microbiology*. 8th ed., McGraw-Hill, 2021.

Stearns, Jennifer, and Michael Surette. *Microbiology for Dummies*. For Dummies, 2019.

STRESS

Category: Disease/Disorder
Anatomy or system affected: All
Specialties and related fields: Dermatology, environmental health, epidemiology, family medicine, immunology, internal medicine, oncology, psychiatry, psychology
Definition: A psychophysiological response to perceived pressures in the environment, including danger; prolonged stress contributes to hormonal imbalances, immune system collapse, susceptibility to disease, cancer, and death.

Key terms:

alarmone: a type of intracellular hormone which alerts the cell to various chemical imbalances in the cellular environment

anxiety: a type of stressful condition in which heightened neural activity accentuates an individual's anticipation of a stress-producing event

cellular transformation: carcinogenesis; the biochemical conversion of a cell from a normal state to a cancerous one of uncontrollable proliferation

chaos: a disorderly shift from predictable, linear behavior to nonlinear randomness, a situation which often occurs in stress and homeostatic breakdown

fight-or-flight response: a stressful biochemical reaction in animals, usually involving the adrenal hormone epinephrine, that prepares the animal for confrontation with predators or competitors

homeostasis: the maintenance of constant, linear conditions within a system, such as the maintenance of human body temperature, pH, and hormonal levels at stable states

hormone: a gene regulatory molecule which is produced in one body tissue region and which targets or controls cells in another region

nonlinear system: a process which is unstable and unpredictable in nature; such a process often results from a disturbance to a linear, predictable system

tend-and-befriend response: a neuroendocrine-linked stress response observed in females characterized by a tendency to respond to stressful situations by protecting self and young through nurturing behaviors and forming alliances with a larger social group

type A behavior: a psychological behavior classification for individuals who exhibit stressful, time-conscious lifestyles

type B behavior: a psychological behavior classification for individuals who exhibit unstressed, relaxed lifestyles

CAUSES AND SYMPTOMS

Stress is a psychophysiological response, within an individual animal, to a perceived danger. Stress involves a complex interplay of nervous and hormonal reactions to internal and external stimuli. All living organisms respond to stimuli, usually by means of gene-regulating chemical messengers called hormones.

Chemistry of stress. Hormones are produced in certain cells within the individual and then target tissues elsewhere in the body; these hormones control by controlling the gene regulation within their target cells. Hormones will activate certain genes within target tissue cells while inactivating other genes. If a hormone activates the control region of a gene so that the gene is "on," then it can be "read" by an enzyme (RNA polymerase), thereby leading to RNA and protein production. The produced protein may affect cellular chemical processes or may affect the expression (the on/off status) of other genes. In the latter case, the protein would be a type of intracellular hormone called an alarmone.

If a hormone inactivates the control region of a gene so that the gene is "off," then RNA polymerase will be unable to read the DNA nucleotide sequence of the gene. Therefore, no RNA and no protein will be produced. In this fashion, a hormone may activate certain genes while inactivating others. Consequently, a hormone controls what happens within the cell.

Such control is critical within complex multicellular organisms such as animals. Different cells specialize to become different tissues and organs (such as eyes, ears, hair, intestines, the heart, and so on) under the specific influence of hormones. Additionally, changes in the development of an organism over time involve changes in gene expression caused by hormones. Critical developmental changes in an individual must occur at precise times when a hormone is produced and acts correctly upon the proper array of genes in target cell tissues. When a hormone does not act correctly or issues incorrect instructions to genes, the homeostatic stability of the organism becomes disrupted. Incorrect proteins are produced in the wrong cells at the wrong times, thereby disturbing development and possibly threatening the organism's survival.

In higher animals, including humans, the body is regulated by hormones and by complex nervous systems that evolved from hormones. Most hormones are produced and secreted from the glands of the endocrine system, including the pituitary, thyroid, and adrenal glands as well as numerous organs, tissues, and cells throughout the body. The nervous system is an array of several trillion nerves concentrated in the brain and spinal cord and extending peripherally to virtually every cellular region of the body. The two systems are tightly interconnected. Both the endocrine and nervous systems at some point involve the secretion of hormones. Nerve tissue secretes hormones called neurotransmitters between electrically conducting cells called neurons.

Physiological responses to stress. Stress is therefore a biochemical response to danger that occurs within animals. The nervous system detects danger from internal or external stimuli, usually external stimuli such as predators, competitors, or life-threatening events. Increased electrical conductivity along millions of nerve cells targets various tissues to prepare the body for maximum physical activity. Among the tissues affected will be the skeletal muscles, the heart muscle, the hormone-secreting glands of the endocrine system, the immune system, the stomach, and blood vessels. Under nerve-activated stress, skeletal muscles will be poised for contraction. The heart will beat faster, thereby distributing more blood and nutrients to body cells, in the process accelerating the breathing rate to distribute more oxygen. Blood vessels will constrict. The stomach and other intestinal organs will decrease their activity, including a decreased production of mucus that protects against acid.

Heightened nerve activity also will trigger the production of various hormones from the immune system, specifically hormones that influence bodily metabolism such as thyroxine and epinephrine (adrenaline). These hormones target body tissue cells to prepare the body for increased output in the face of danger. Massive production of epinephrine will trigger maximum physical readiness and extraordinary muscular output, a phenomenon often referred to as the fight-or-flight response.

These physiological changes within an animal facing danger are important survival adaptations that evolved very early in the history of animal life on earth. Stress is a fact of life for animals because they must eat to survive. Competition for available food resources and avoidance of predators must be faced by all animals, including humans. While predation by larger animals is of little worry to current-day modern humans, the struggle for available resources remains. Furthermore, human technology has created stresses of an entirely different character.

The fight-or-flight stress response and other evolutionary stress adaptations endure within the individual for only seconds or minutes. Such natural stresses are to an individual's advantage, ensuring survival. The stresses that humans face are based on these behavioral adaptations. Much human stress is artificial, however, and lasts not for minutes but for hours, days, weeks, months, and years. Such stresses involve the same nervous and endocrine system responses, but they are usually brought about by perceived danger, not true danger.

INFORMATION ON STRESS

Causes: Nervous system and hormonal reactions to internal and external stimuli

Symptoms: Hormonal imbalances; immune system collapse; increased susceptibility to disease, cancer, ulcers, high blood pressure, and heart disease

Duration: Temporary to chronic

Treatments: Lifestyle modification, relaxation, time management, peer counseling and support, strengthening family bonds, improving self-esteem, exercise

---

Human societies impose norms and rules for the behavior of the individuals who compose the society. People must adhere to the societal norms or face punishment. In fast-paced technological societies, increasing bureaucratization and organization place less emphasis on the individual and more emphasis on process and productivity. People must face deadlines, be on time, produce quotas, generate company profit, and meet the demands of family, colleagues, and administration simultaneously. The result is a continuous fight-or-flight response in which individuals fear losing their jobs and thus the means of supporting themselves and their families.

The physiological manifestations of prolonged stress are devastating. Continued hyperactivity of nerve impulses and overproduction of hormones at incorrect developmental stages lead to the abnormal functioning of internal organs. The stomach undersecretes mucus, thereby leading to ulcers. The heart muscle contracts too rapidly, leading to higher pulse and respiration rates. The blood vessels constrict for lengthy periods of time, thereby causing the heart to pump harder and leading to high blood pressure and heart disease. Hormone overproduction leads to incorrect cell instructions and gene activation/inactivation, causing abnormal tissue functioning and cellular transformation leading to cancer. The immune system weakens under abnormal signaling by hormones, thereby decreasing the body's ability to defend itself from disease.

Newer research on stress response in women has uncovered a mechanism of stress response that is of interest given this upswelling of constant stress. Work by Shelley E. Taylor has documented an alternative to "fight or flight" known as "tend and befriend." Potentially linked to oxytocin, such tend-and-befriend behavior may help to facilitate relaxation and interpersonal bonding in response to stress. The potential stress response promises longer-lasting benefits, adaptively connecting humans to their social groups.

Stress and disease. A wide variety of human illnesses and disorders have been associated with stress. Heart disease, cancer, stroke, mental illness, allergies, accidents, asthma, chronic fatigue, depression, suicide, and deviant behavior are among the many illnesses and disorders that are considered by scientists to be stress-related illnesses. These stress-related diseases and disorders are responsible for the majority of deaths, hospitalizations, and visits to physicians by people in highly technological societies such as the United States, Japan, and Western Europe. In the United States alone, several billion dollars are spent each year for medications to treat stress-related illnesses that otherwise could be prevented by antistress methodologies.

Before the advent of industrialization in Europe and North America, the leading killers of humans were bacterial and viral diseases, which continue to be the principal killers of humans in the pretechnological and emerging technological countries of the Middle East, Asia, Africa, Latin America, and Oceania. European and North American industrialization has been accompanied by prodigious advances in medical science and the eradication or control of many microorganismal diseases. The psychological demands of fast-paced living and the dehumanized expectations of technological societies, however, have produced a plethora of stress-generated diseases and disorders, some of which had been masked by microorganismal diseases.

There still is some debate concerning the causal relationship between stress and illness, despite overwhelming scientific evidence demonstrating bodily responses to stressful situations. Abnormal nerve hyperactivity and prolonged, abnormal secretions of gene regulatory hormones from various endocrine glands disrupt the balanced homeostasis of many different body systems. Immune system reduction often occurs during stress, thereby making a stressed individual more susceptible to contracting infectious bacterial and viral diseases.

A clear linkage exists between the occurrence of stress in people and their subsequent susceptibility to infectious disease. Furthermore, there is a tendency for strokes, heart attacks, cancer, and sudden death to occur in individuals who recently have experienced major traumatic events in their lives. Too little attention has been given to the effects of everyday living upon the physical well-being of people. Environmental stimuli, nervous and endocrine systems, and physiological rhythms within the body are intricately connected.

Most bodily processes follow a self-regulatory, homeostatic pattern that is rhythmic, linear, stable, and predictable. For example, the beta cells of the islets of Langerhans in the pancreas secrete the hormone insulin in response to elevated blood glucose levels, whereas the alpha cells in these same islets secrete the hormone glucagon in response to low blood glucose levels. Likewise, the body chemically maintains a constant blood temperature (37 degrees Celsius), pH (7.35 to 7.45), calcium levels, and so on. The heart muscle requires an electrical stimulus approximately once per second to trigger a wave of muscular contractions throughout the myocardium via the sinoatrial and atrioventricular nodes.

Linear, balanced physiological rhythms are sensitive to subtle chemical changes in the cellular and organismal environment. An orderly, homeostatic process in the body can collapse into disorderly, nonlinear, and unpredictable chaos because of the slightest disturbance. Stress is a disturbance that imbalances the nervous and endocrine systems, which subsequently imbalance cells and organ systems throughout the human body. Physiological systems become unstable, and disease or cancer may ensue.

TREATMENT AND THERAPY

Psychologists, psychiatrists, physicians, and other medical professionals are becoming more aware of the physiological effects of stress. Through this awareness, professionals have sought to examine whether there are any characteristic styles of stress response. In response, psychologists have identified two principal behavioral types when it comes to stress among humans: type A behavior pattern and type B behavior pattern. Type A individuals are highly anxious, task-oriented, time-conscious, constantly in a rush to accomplish their jobs and other objectives, and somewhat prone to hostility. Research indicates that type A individuals may have a higher incidence of heart disease. Increasingly, the hostility component of type A behavior is seen as a very important contributing factor. On the other hand, type B individuals are more relaxed and experience less stress. Nevertheless, it should be emphasized that behavior is a continuum: Different people may exhibit varying degrees of type A and B behavior patterns. Given this discovery, it is not uncommon for professionals to recommend to their stressed clients to monitor their participation in type A behavior and to try behaving more in kind with type B behavior patterns.

Another important focus for health care has become the prevention, management, and treatment of stress itself. Health education programs emphasize the importance of physical fitness and stress reduction in everyday living. Stress-reducing methodologies for the individual include time management, peer counseling and support, spending longer amounts of time relaxing, strengthening family bonds, improving self-esteem, exercise, and learning to reframe how daily life events are interpreted, such as may be done through cognitive behavior therapy. These approaches greatly enhance an individual's quality of life and help the individual to cope positively with stressful events. All these stress reduction techniques emphasize an individual's personality and the more efficient use of an individual's free time. Relaxation, social interaction, and physical activity help the body to return to normal physiological rhythms following the numerous stressful events that every person faces daily. Individuals in American and Western societies are coming to realize that a slower, more relaxed living pace is essential for reducing stress and the millions of cases of stress-related disease that occur each year.

PERSPECTIVE AND PROSPECTS

Because stress is a major contributor to illness and disease in American and Western societies, a major objective of health care professionals in these countries is the identification of stress initiators and the reduction of stress in the general population. Stress cannot be eliminated entirely in any individual. Humans always will experience stress as a result of their continuous interactions with one another and with the environment. Stress is an important survival adaptation for animal life on earth. Nevertheless, stressful events in an individual's life serve as negative environmental stimuli that hyperactivate the human nervous and endocrine systems to create a fight-or-flight response. When this fight-or-flight response is maintained for abnormally long periods of times, prolonged elevations in nervous and hormonal activity modify body tissues and the developmental gene expression within cells to produce abnormal growths (such as cancers) and abnormal system functioning (such as diabetes mellitus). Breakdown of the human immune system under stress makes the body less capable of fighting spontaneous tumors, cancers, and infectious disease. The net result from physiological stress is illness, disease, rapid aging, and death.

Stress reduction should be a prime focus of medical research and education. The simplicity of educating the public with respect to stress can yield incredible savings in terms of lives saved, quality of lives improved, length of human life spans increased, and money saved. Some researchers propose that stress reduction not only can yield enormous health benefits but also can produce greater industrial productivity, happier people, and considerably less crime. It is expected that additional research into oxytocin, the tend-and-befriend response, and yet undiscovered mechanisms of stress response will contribute meaningfully to decreased stress and increased mental and physical well-being.

—*David Wason Hollar, Jr., PhD;*
updated by Nancy A. Piotrowski, PhD

See also Addiction; Alcoholism; Alternative medicine; Antianxiety drugs; Antidepressants; Anxiety; Appetite loss; Bipolar disorders; Caffeine; Cancer; Canker sores; Death and dying; Depression; Domestic violence; Eating disorders; Factitious disorders; Grief and guilt; Hallucinations; Hormones; Hypochondriasis; Midlife crisis; Neurosis; Obsessive-compulsive disorder; Panic attacks; Phobias; Postpartum depression; Post-traumatic stress disorder; Psychiatric disorders; Psychiatry; Psychiatry, child and adolescent; Psychiatry, geriatric; Psychoanalysis; Psychosis; Psychosomatic disorders; Schizophrenia; Sexual dysfunction; Sibling rivalry; Sleep; Sleep disorders; Stress reduction; Suicide.

For Further Information:
Bremner, Douglas J. *Does Stress Damage the Brain? Understanding Trauma-Related Disorders from a Neurological Perspective*. New York: W. W. Norton, 2002. Questions whether what one sees, hears, feels, and in other ways experiences, especially during times of stress, can result in permanent changes to the brain and argues that extreme stress may result in lasting damage to the brain, especially a part of the brain involved in memory.
Day, Stacey B., ed. *Cancer, Stress, and Death*. 2d ed. New York: Plenum Press, 1986. This informative work is a collection of scientific survey papers that demonstrate the relationship between stress and disease. The papers are clearly written for both scientific and general audiences.
Goodman, H. Maurice. *Basic Medical Endocrinology*. 4th ed. Boston: Academic Press/Elsevier, 2009. Focuses on research advances in the understanding of hormones involved in regulating most aspects of bodily functions. Includes in-depth coverage of individual glands and regulatory principles.
Henry, Helen L., and Anthony W. Norman, eds. *Encyclopedia of Hormones*. 3 vols. San Diego, Calif.: Academic Press, 2003. A comprehensive overview of the role of hormones, the major physiological systems in which they operate, and the biological consequences of an excess or deficiency of a particular hormone.
Kronenberg, Henry M., et al., eds. *Williams Textbook of Endocrinology*. 11th ed. Philadelphia: Saunders/Elsevier, 2008. Text that covers the spectrum of information related to the endocrine system, including hormones and their relation to stress.
Monroe, Judy. *Coping with Ulcers, Heartburn, and Stress-Related Stomach Disorders*. New York: Rosen, 2000. Designed for students in grades seven and up, this book discusses different types of ulcers, irritable bowel syndrome, food intolerances and allergies of all types, and heartburn and acid reflux.
Newton, Tim, with Jocelyn Handy and Stephen Fineman. *Managing Stress: Emotion and Power at Work*. Newbury Park, Calif.: Sage, 1996. This book addresses job stress and offers stress management techniques for coping with it. Includes a bibliography and an index.
Orth-Gomér, Kristina, Margaret A. Chesney, and Nanette K. Wenger, eds. *Women, Stress, and Heart Disease*. Mahwah, N.J.: Lawrence Erlbaum, 1998. This is a comprehensive and ground-breaking book on women's heart health.
Taylor, Shelley E. *The Tending Instinct: How Nurturing Is Essential to Who We Are and How We Live*. New York: Times Books, 2002. Presents a discussion of stress response in women and explores a strategy of tend and befriend instead of fight or flight.

STRESS REDUCTION

Category: Treatment
Anatomy or system affected: All
Specialties and related fields: Alternative medicine, environmental health, immunology, occupational health, preventive medicine, psychiatry, psychology
Definition: A set of procedures with the goal of decreasing bodily and mental tension by increasing rest and coping skills.
Key terms:
palliative treatments: therapies that reduce symptoms without completely eradicating a disorder
psychotherapy: treatment using the mind to remedy problems related to disordered behavior or thinking, emotional problems, or disease
stress: physical, environmental, or psychological strain experienced by an individual that requires adjustment

INDICATIONS AND PROCEDURES

Stress can exacerbate difficulties in daily functioning, slow recovery from mental or physical problems, and impede immunological functioning. Stress reduction techniques represent a cluster of procedures that share the goal of reducing bodily and emotional tension: drug and physical therapies, exercise, biofeedback training, meditation, hypnosis, psychotherapy, relaxation training, and stress inoculation therapy.

The drugs used in stress reduction are designed to provide overall bodily relaxation, to induce rest, or to decrease the anxious thinking that exacerbates stressful experiences. Sedatives, tranquilizers, benzodiazepines, antihistamines, beta-blockers, and barbiturates are examples of such drugs. Similarly, physical therapies and exercise are recommended for these purposes. Baths (hydrotherapy), massages, and moderate exercise can also be part of a stress reduction program.

Psychotherapy is a common treatment for stress implemented by psychiatrists, psychologists, social workers, psychiatric nurses, and counselors. Not only does it help individuals to sort out their problems mentally but it is also an effective stress management strategy. When individuals analyze their lifestyles and life events, stress-inducing behaviors and life patterns can be explored and targeted for modification.

Biofeedback training, meditation, hypnosis, and relaxation training all focus on inducing relaxation or altered consciousness by shifting a person's attention. Biofeedback uses monitoring devices attached to the body to provide visual or aural feedback to the trainee. Such devices include the electromyograph (EMG), which measures muscle tension, and the

psychogalvanometer, which measures galvanic skin response (GSR). An EMG involves placing sensors on various muscle groups to record muscular electrical potentials. GSR also relies on sensors, but these sensors record bodily responses caused by sweat gland activity and emotional arousal. The feedback from such devices allows a trainee to learn to control certain bodily processes (for example, muscle tension, brain waves, heart rate, temperature, and blood pressure). Biofeedback training is used to treat headaches, temporomandibular joint (TMJ) syndrome, high blood pressure, and tics, and it can also facilitate neuromuscular responses in stroke patients.

Meditation is a focused thinking exercise involving a quiet setting and the repetition of a word or phrase called a mantra. By blocking distracting thoughts and refocusing attention, meditation reduces anxious thinking. It is useful for mild anxiety, minor concentration difficulties, and daily relaxation.

Hypnosis involves the use of suggestion, concentrated attention, and/or drugs to induce a sleeplike state, or trance. Hypnosis can be induced by a hypnotist or via self-hypnosis. Hypnotic states are characterized by increased suggestibility, ability to recall forgotten events, decreased pain sensitivity, and increased vasomotor control. The ability to be hypnotized varies from person to person based on susceptibility to suggestion and psychological needs. Hypnosis is used as a brief therapy targeting such problems as insomnia, pain, panic, and sexual dysfunction. In addition, hypnosis is sometimes used when drugs are contraindicated for anesthetic use, particularly for dental procedures.

Relaxation training involves three primary methods: autogenic training, which involves such techniques as head, heart, and abdominal exercises; progressive relaxation, which involves becoming aware of tension in the various muscle groups by relaxing one group at a time in a specific order; and breathing exercises. Relaxation training is best learned when a therapist trains an individual in person and then the exercises are practiced independently. Relaxation can be practiced several times daily, as well as in response to stressful events. High blood pressure, ulcers, insomnia, asthma, drug and alcohol problems, spastic colitis, tachycardia (rapid heartbeat), pain management, and moderate-to-severe anxiety disorders are treated with relaxation training.

Stress inoculation therapy is a specific type of psychotherapy involving techniques that alter patterns of thinking and acting. It comprises three steps: education about stress and fear reactions, rehearsal of coping behaviors, and application of coping behaviors in stress-provoking situations. It is useful for treating anxiety disorders related to stress.

USES AND COMPLICATIONS

Individuals should not apply stress reduction procedures without proper consultation; medical conditions that might be causing symptoms should be assessed or ruled out first. Biofeedback training for headaches, for example, would be unwarranted until other, more serious causes of headaches had been eliminated from consideration. Similarly, exercise, drug, and physical therapies could actually worsen conditions such as high blood pressure, alcohol and drug problems, and chronic pain if applied incorrectly. For example, where stress or pain is chronic, drug therapies might encourage the development of drug dependence.

Instead, skilled providers should administer these procedures. Training via self-help materials alone or by an unskilled provider may provide no benefit or create difficulties. Poor training could result in frustration, hypervigilance, heightened anxiety, depression, or pain caused by overattention to symptoms or conflicts. In fact, some individuals are prone to these effects even with good training. Therefore, ongoing assessment is necessary. Finally, interpretation of any memories provoked by hypnosis should be done with caution because of the suggestibility that is characteristic of hypnotic states.

PERSPECTIVE AND PROSPECTS

Stress reduction techniques evolved from ancient meditation practices and simpler methods of pain management predating the development of modern anesthetics. The palliative and preventive effects of these techniques have given these procedures a sure hold in future medical practice, while benefits such as decreased absenteeism and increased feelings of wellness in employees have secured these strategies in the workplace. The expanded use of stress reduction procedures in prenatal care and with the elderly is likely.

—*Nancy A. Piotrowski, PhD*

See also Acupressure; Acupuncture; Alternative medicine; Antianxiety drugs; Antidepressants; Anxiety; Aromatherapy; Biofeedback; Caffeine; Cardiac rehabilitation; Chiropractic; Electrocardiography (ECG or EKG); Environmental health; Headaches; Hypertension; Hypnosis; Meditation; Occupational health; Palliative medicine; Stress; Temporomandibular joint (TMJ) syndrome; Tics; Yoga.

For Further Information:
Davis, Martha, Elizabeth Robbins Eshelman, and Matthew McKay. *The Relaxation and Stress Reduction Workbook*. 5th ed. Oakland, Calif.: New Harbinger, 2000. Provides guidance for different stress management techniques.
Humphrey, James H. *Stress Among Older Adults: Understanding and Coping*. Springfield, Ill.: Charles C Thomas, 1992. A rich overview of general and geriatric stress management issues and techniques.
Manning, George, Kent Curtis, and Steve McMillen. *Stress: Living and Working in a Changing World*. Duluth, Minn.: Whole Person Associates, 1999. Road rage and workplace violence are but two of the more obvious symptoms of increasingly stressful times. Manning and his partners have put together this comprehensive manual to show individuals how to manage stress and help managers, counselors, and teachers develop programs that reduce stress.
Newton, Tim, with Jocelyn Handy and Stephen Fineman. *Managing Stress: Emotion and Power at Work*. Newbury Park, Calif.: Sage, 1996. This book addresses job stress and offers stress management techniques for coping with it. Includes a bibliography and an index.
Pelletier, Kenneth. *The Best Alternative Medicine*. New York: Fireside, 2002. Explains mind/body medicine, herbal and homeopathic remedies, spiritual healing, and traditional Chinese systems, and discusses their effectiveness, the ailments each is most appropriate for, and how they can help prevent illness.
Schafer, Walt, and Sharrie A. Herbold. *Stress Management for Wellness*. 4th ed. Belmont, Calif.: Thomson/Wadsworth, 2000. Describes how stress affects the body and how it may contribute to illness and death. Includes tests for identifying high personal stress levels and discusses stress reduction measures.
Seaward, Brian Luke. *Managing Stress: Principles and Strategies for Health and Well-Being*. 6th ed. Sudbury, Mass.: Jones and Bartlett, 2009. Blends techniques from stress management with health psychology to offer a holistic approach to a healthy, relaxed lifestyle.

STROKES

Category: Disease/Disorder
Also known as: Cerebrovascular accidents (CVAs)
Anatomy or system affected: Blood vessels, brain, circulatory system, head, heart, nervous system, psychic-emotional system
Specialties and related fields: Emergency medicine, neurology, speech pathology, vascular medicine
Definition: Stroke, or a cerebrovascular accident (CVA), is the severe reduction or cessation of blood flow to the brain, resulting in a variety of serious and often permanent impairments depending on the area of the brain affected. A transient ischemic attack (TIA) is a temporary, brief loss of blood to the brain, accompanied by temporary impairment of vision, numbness, or other symptoms; it may herald a stroke.

Key terms:
amaurosis fugax: temporary blindness in one eye
angiography: radiological modality to visualize the arteries in the body; involves the placement of a catheter in an artery and the injection of dye
embolus: a small piece of atherosclerotic plaque, thrombus, or other debris that breaks off and lodges in a blood vessel

endarterectomy: a surgical technique in which an atherosclerotic plaque is excised

hemorrhagic: weakened blood vessel ruptures, as a result of aneurysm or arteriovenous malformation

infarct: tissue death resulting from lack of blood flow

ischemia: lack of blood in a particular tissue

revascularization: procedures to reestablish the circulation to a diseased portion of the body

thrombosis: the aggregation of platelets and other blood cells to form a clot

transient ischemic attacks(TIAs): commonly known as mini strokes; associated neurological deficits last less than twenty-four hours and usually only minutes

CAUSES AND SYMPTOMS

Strokes produce damage to portions of the brain as a result of decreased blood supply due to occlusion or hemorrhage. Strokes are commonly known as cerebrovascular accidents (CVAs). Symptoms of strokes will vary depending on the part of the brain that is affected. Rapid intervention is critical to management of stroke. The American Stroke Association has developed a guide to recognizing stroke symptoms to encourage the public to seek immediate emergency care. Using the word "FAST" to represent facial drooping, arm weakness, speech difficulty and time to call 911, allows individuals to recognize the symptoms of stroke and seek immediate treatment. Other symptoms of stroke may include trouble speaking, confusion, difficulty understanding simple commands such as "raise your right arm", trouble walking and severe headache.

Resulting speech disorders may include aphasia (loss of the ability to speak) or dysarthria (difficulty in speaking). A sudden weakness or numbness of one side of the body is known as hemiparesis or hemiplegia. The eyes can also be involved. A dimness or transient loss of vision, particularly in one eye, is called amaurosis fugax. Occasionally, it can involve the same portion of the visual field in both eyes. Other symptoms of stroke may include dizziness, unsteadiness, sudden falls, headaches, confusion, or stupor. Coma is less commonly involved in a stroke.

Predisposing factors to strokes include hypertension (high blood pressure), diabetes, high cholesterol, smoking, atherosclerotic disease in other portions of the body (such as the heart or legs), and a previous or family history of strokes or transient ischemic attacks. Gender and age are also associated with the incidence of strokes.

In cerebrovascular disease, atherosclerosis affects the arteries that circulate blood to the brain. The brain receives blood from two major sets of arteries. The carotid arteries, in the front of the neck, supply the anterior (front) portions of the brain. The vertebral arteries travel through the transverse processes of the

---

INFORMATION ON STROKES

Causes: Hypertension, diabetes, cerebral aneurysm, high cholesterol levels, smoking, atherosclerosis, personal or family history of strokes or TIAs

Symptoms: Vision impairment, numbness, aphasia, slurred speech, relaxed facial muscles, general muscle weakness, dizziness, unsteadiness, sudden falls, headaches, confusion, stupor

Duration: Acute

Treatments: Surgical revascularization (endarterectomy), balloon angioplasty, drugs, physical therapy

---

spine and join the basilar artery to provide blood to the posterior (back) portion of the brain. Both circulatory systems are joined within the brain in a structure known as the circle of Willis, a composite of arteries that join to form an anatomical circle. The various arteries supply the necessary blood flow to different areas of the brain. Only 25 to 50 percent of people have a complete circle of Willis; this anatomical variance may be a factor in the severity of the stroke.

In atherosclerotic disease, fat, cholesterol, and calcium deposits are laid down along the walls of the arteries, primarily at sites where arteries divide and natural turbulence tends to occur. These components build up to form plaques, which may cause stenosis (narrowing) and occlusion (closure) of the arterial lumen. Accumulation of platelets and other blood cells can form a thrombus (blood clot) along with plaque buildup, which also may obstruct the arteries. Pieces of plaque or thrombotic material may break off and cause emboli to lodge acutely in the main vessels or their more distant branches.

The most common components of cerebrovascular disease are transient ischemic attacks (TIAs), also referred to as ministrokes. By definition, TIA s last less than twenty-four hours; usually, they last only a few minutes or hours. Most TIAs are produced by emboli. An embolus occurs when a piece of plaque from the lining of a major artery breaks off and temporarily blocks the blood flow to a particular area of the brain. If the symptoms last for more than twenty-four hours, a cerebrovascular accident, cerebral infarct, or stroke has occurred. A reversible ischemic neurological deficit (RIND) is similar to a stroke in that it is an event that lasts for more than twenty-four hours but resolves in about seventy-two hours.

The majority of strokes in the United States (85 percent) are the result of impaired blood flow (ischemia) to the brain. Atherosclerosis in the cerebrovascular system will cause similar symptoms of ischemia in other portions of the body. There is increasing narrowing, or stenosis, of blood vessels. Eventually, they will close off completely and become occluded. The development of new, small vessels that bypass a diseased artery is called collateralization. This process requires weeks or months to occur. Collateralization seems to be especially prominent in the cerebrovascular system, since the brain is an organ that requires constant blood flow at all times. Eventual occlusion or thrombosis of a major vessel causes the majority of CVAs, producing significant ischemia in a portion of the brain. In certain cases, the blockage is acute, having resulted from an embolus or thrombus that blocks an artery. If collateralization has not developed, the damage to an affected structure is more severe. A thrombus or embolus can also arise from the heart. This is most common in individuals who have had a recent heart attack, who have disease that involves the mitral valve, or who have atrial fibrillation, a variety of irregular heartbeat.

Another cause of stroke is cerebral hemorrhage, or bleeding into the brain, resulting in loss of consciousness or incapacity. An older term rarely used now for cerebral hemorrhage is apoplexy. Hypertension is the most common cause of intracranial bleeding and accounts for 10 to 15 percent of cases. Other causes of strokes are cerebral aneurysms (5 to 7 percent), tumors that have developed blood supplies (3 to 5 percent), and genetic bleeding tendencies (1 to 2 percent). A cerebral aneurysm occurs when the wall of an artery becomes weak and enlarges like a balloon. These aneurysms often rupture. With a ruptured cerebral aneurysmand subsequent hemorrhage, by-products of red blood cell degeneration may produce a condition called vasospasm, wherein the arteries will constrict. This often leads to ischemia. One or more thrombi are often formed in an aneurysm. If they break loose, they can become emboli, float until they become lodged in a small blood vessel, block the flow of blood, and cause ischemia. This can ultimately lead to a stroke.

Stroke refers to the disease process that is mainly produced by atherosclerotic changes in the arteries to the brain. Contributing or significant risk factors in the development of atherosclerosis include hypertension (high blood pressure), hyperlipidemia (high levels of cholesterol in the blood), smoking, diabetes mellitus, and a family history of similar incidents. Evidence of atherosclerotic disease in other portions of the body, such as the heart or legs, increases the risk of stroke. Atherosclerosis is a generalized disease process that affects arterial beds throughout the body.

Symptoms of TIAs in structures near the front of the brain, the area supplied by the carotid arteries, include hemiparesis, a numbness or loss of function in half of the body. Hemiplegia, a weakness of an arm or leg (or both), can be attributable to disease in the carotid ar-

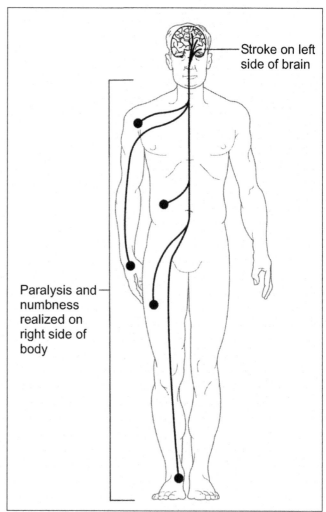

A major stroke to one hemisphere of the brain generally results in impairment of motor functions on the opposite side of the body. In addition, because the two brain hemispheres control different mental and autonomic functions, impairments will vary; for example, left-brain stroke is usually associated with some degree of speech impairment, because the speech centers are located in the left brain. ©EBSCO

tery on the side of the body opposite to the affected body part. Another relatively common problem usually caused by disease in the left carotid artery is aphasia, a speech disorder. Disease in either carotid artery can cause amaurosis fugax, or blindness in one eye. Victims often describe this condition as a shade being drawn over the eye.

Other, more generalized symptoms are the result of problems in the vertebral arteries or the blood vessels at the base of the brain, which supply the back portions of the brain. Associated symptoms include dizziness, a loss of orientation often produced by decreased blood flow to the brain. Dizziness is frequently caused by abrupt positional changes, in which blood pressure will suddenly fall with rapid standing or sitting, or by cardiac arrhythmias (irregular heartbeats), which prevent adequate amounts of blood flow from being delivered during certain cardiac cycles.

Vertigo is different from dizziness. Individuals suffering from vertigo experience a spinning sensation that may be accompanied by nausea. A common cause for vertigo is a condition known as subclavian steal, in which atherosclerotic disease affects the arteries of the arms just prior to the point where the vertebral arteries branch off. As an arm is used, or with abrupt changes in head position, blood will flow out of the vertebral arteries in a reverse manner (the so-called steal) to aid circulation in the arm (via the subclavian arteries) and vertigo will ensue. In addition, imbalance and other visual disturbances may be associated with problems in the vertebral arteries. These symptoms may also result from cerebrovascular disease in which inadequate blood supply to multiple areas of the brain can produce diverse symptoms. In the majority of strokes, symptoms last twenty-four to seventy-two hours. Approximately 25 percent of patients will develop permanent deficits that will affect them for the rest of their lives. Approximately 20 percent of individuals who have strokes will experience no symptoms (be asymptomatic) and not know that they have had a stroke. They are unlikely to even develop TIAs. Such unheralded events result from occlusion or thrombosis of the blood vessels in the brain. This causes ischemia that leads to infarction or cell death in a particular section of the brain.

Asymptomatic cerebrovascular disease, however, can often be detected by the presence of a bruit, a French word meaning "noise." Stenosis in arteries can be compared to rapids in a river. Blood will flow very quickly through the narrow area and create turbulence, producing a bruit that can be heard with a stethoscope. Patients with narrowing in the carotid arteries ranging from 20 to 80 percent may possess a bruit. The absence of a bruit does not mean that the carotid arteries are disease-free. Once the stenosis reaches critical proportions, the flow is diminished and turbulence may be negligible, indicating a severe stenosis or an occluded artery. Often, doctors will recommend elective surgery to patients with coronary artery stenosis between 60 and 80 percent in an effort to reestablish blood flow and prevent eventual occlusion and possible stroke. About 75 percent of strokes are caused by ischemia that results from the above process. Crescendo TIAs, in which multiple TIAs occur in a brief period of time, and evolving strokes require immediate medical treatment. Appropriate diagnosis and treatment may prevent a stroke or decrease its severity.

Although disease caused by an aneurysm is a separate entity, it may be associated with atherosclerotic disease in certain cases. Most aneurysms within the brain produce no symptoms. As aneurysms increase in size, the probability of rupture increases; therefore, elective surgery may be recommended. Occasionally, diagnoses of cerebral aneurysms are made during investigations of other cerebral events, such as headaches. Acute onset of severe headaches or stiff neck should mandate immediate medical attention, since rupture of a cerebral aneurysm often manifests itself in this manner.

TREATMENT AND THERAPY
Strokes and TIAs often occur quickly and without warning. The best treatment for them is preventive behavior to avoid the atherosclerotic disease leading to such events.

Immediate medical care is critical to managing stroke and minimizing the long-term effects of the event, including the potential to prevent death. Medical advances in radiological imaging and stroke treatments have improved survival rates over the past decade. When a stroke is caused by a clot, Alteplase IV r-tPA may be administered in an attempt to dissolve the clot. As the only FDA-approved treatment for ischemic stroke, Alteplase IV r-tPA is a tissue plasminogen activator that works to improve blood flow by dissolving the clot and restoring blood flow to the brain. It must be administered within three hours of initial stroke symptoms, although certain patients may benefit up to 4 1/2 hours post symptoms. Often patients delay seeking hospital care resulting in permanent disability reflected by the tissues in the brain deprived of oxygen. If a patient experiences a stroke during the night or has no recollection of when symptoms began, the use of r-tPA is limited. Continued research may allow longer periods of time from onset to drug delivery. An endovascular procedure may be used to send a catheter to the site of blockage in an attempt to remove the clot and r-tPA may be injected intra-arterially into the clot in some instances. The best clinical protocols for endovascular procedures are still being researched.

When a stroke or TIA is suspected upon arrival to the Emergency Room, it is imperative to determine the time of onset of symptoms. A brief history and physical examination followed by a CT scan follows to determine the type of stroke and the patient's eligibility for r-tPA. Because of the three-hour time window for administration, determining symptoms and noting significant risk factors and findings upon physical examination will help a physician determine the primary area of the brain affected, schedule the appropriate tests for further diagnosis, and choose the best course of therapy. If the patient is documented to be well outside the three to 4 1/2 hour accepted window, a more comprehensive work-up may be acceptable. The National Institutes of Health Stroke Scale (NIHSS) was developed by national and international panels to provide a quantitative measure of stroke-related neurologic deficit. It provides baseline data for a comprehensive clinical assessment of stroke patients and may be a predictor of outcomes in stroke patients.

Stroke care has evolved over time and continues to be the focus of research due to the debilitating and costly impacts on the patient. Because of the high incidence of death and disability associated with strokes, a variety of diagnostic tests have been developed since the 1950s. One of the oldest noninvasive methods is the directional Doppler test. A Doppler device employs a probe with one or two piezoelectric crystals. An ultrasonic signal using a frequency of 2 to 5 megahertz (MHz) is sent into the body. Movement of red blood cells causes a shift in the frequency of the signal that is transmitted back. The amount of shift is proportional to the speed of blood flow. This device can also be used to determine the direction of blood flow. By listening with a continuous-wave Doppler over a branch of the ophthalmic artery at the corner of the eye and performing certain compression maneuvers on the arteries that supply the face, information regarding possible collateral pathways can be obtained concerning internal carotid artery blockages of greater than 75 percent.

The vascular surgeon William Gee developed another device, called an ocular pneumoplethysmograph (OPG). The OPG utilizes cups placed in the eye to measure the ocular pressure. A vacuum is applied to the eyes, effectively blocking the ophthalmic arteries, which are the first major branches of the internal carotid artery. As the vacuum is released, the blood flow is reestablished and the appearance of arterial pulsations is noted on a strip chart. These pulsations denote systolic blood pressure in the ophthalmic arteries. A pressure difference of 5 millimeters of mercury (mm Hg) between the two eyes or an index of less than 0.66 (comparing the systolic blood pressure in the ophthalmic artery with that in the brachial artery) is consistent with carotid artery blockage of more than 50 to 75 percent.

Both of these methods are indirect tests, in which significant internal carotid artery disease is implied if the test is positive. Deficiencies in the test procedures include quantification of the percentage of carotid artery disease or differentiation of significant stenosis from occlusions. They also may be wrong if the vertebral or basal arteries contribute significant collateral blood flow. The OPG is still used in certain situations as a quick screening tool, but the directional Doppler has lost favor as an accurate diagnostic test. Duplex ultrasound machines, first employed in the early 1980s, utilize B-mode (brightness-mode) ultrasound to visualize the vessels and type of plaque. In comparison,

Doppler ultrasound can audibly evaluate the blood flow in the vessels. Using real-time spectrum analyzers, the Doppler signals are then analyzed in terms of velocity (speed of the blood flow) and waveform characteristics. The greater the velocity, the greater the amount of stenosis. Absence of blood flow will denote occlusions.

Much research has been done in evaluating plaque morphology and its association with the incidence of TIAs, but results have been controversial using the standard gray-scale duplex devices. The use of color duplex ultrasound, in which the Doppler signals are color-coded in terms of flow direction and speed to denote the various flow patterns in normal and diseased vessels, has enhanced the diagnostic accuracies of the examinations. The use of color Doppler in many ultrasound machines is allowing more rapid detection of arterial lesions in blood vessels both inside and outside the skull. Transcranial Doppler uses a MHz pulsed Doppler probe through various normal anatomic windows (holes) in the skull. Measurements can be made through the side of the head (transtemporal), from the back of the head (transoccipital), and through the eye (transocular). The purpose of the examination is to assess the blood circulation in the circle of Willis. The transcranial Doppler gives information concerning various collateral pathways established when significant disease is present in blood vessels outside the skull. It is also useful when there is stenosis of arteries inside the skull. It is extremely accurate in detecting and monitoring early vasospasm in individuals with bleeding inside the skull. Additional research with this device is ongoing in other areas, such as in the detection of cerebral aneurysms and arteriovenous malformations in which there is an abnormal connection between the arteries and the veins.

Computed tomography (CT) scanning is a radiological technique that provides a three-dimensional picture of the brain and its structures. Occasionally, a contrast medium is also used in this examination. CT scanning is especially useful in the diagnosis of cerebral aneurysms and areas of infarct. Magnetic resonance imaging (MRI) is a nonradiological technique that also provides exceptional three-dimensional images of the soft tissue structures of the brain. MRI can detect cerebral infarcts at an earlier stage than can CT scanning. Arteriography or angiography is an invasive procedure that is performed in a hospital setting. A catheter is placed in one of the arteries, and dye containing iodine is injected. Multiple X rays are then taken to visualize the circulation. Arteriograms are considered to be standard in diagnosis. The delineation of the blockages and collateral pathways is then used primarily to plan surgical procedures.

Aspirin is often prescribed to alleviate symptoms of TIAs and to help protect patients from strokes or heart attacks. Although it is a powerful drug in decreasing the incidence of embolus formation, a national study has demonstrated that patients with a history of TIAs and carotid artery stenosis of greater than 60 percent should undergo surgical revascularization to protect against major strokes. The chances of having a stroke after suffering a TIA are approximately 40 percent greater.

Endarterectomy is a surgical technique in which the inner wall and part of the middle wall of the carotid artery are excised, effectively scraping out atherosclerotic plaques. Although used in other arterial segments, endarterectomy is the most common surgical procedure used to revascularize the carotid arteries. Occasionally, procedures are performed to bypass diseased segments of the cerebral vessels. Long-term research has shown that they have limited effectiveness. Consequently, many have been abandoned.

Other techniques for intervention have been developed. Percutaneous balloon angioplasty involves placing a balloon catheter in the diseased segment during an angiogram. When the balloon catheter is inflated, it opens up the area of stenosis or small segment of occlusion. This method has been employed in the coronary arteries as well as in the vessels leaving the aorta, the iliac arteries, and arteries in the lower extremities. It is not used often in the treatment of atherosclerotic plaques in the cerebral circulation because of the possibility of emboli traveling to the more distant blood vessels of the brain or eye. Some success in the use of balloon angioplasty has been reported in the treatment of vasospasm.

PERSPECTIVE AND PROSPECTS

Stroke is the third-leading cause of death in the United States, with approximately 158,000 deaths annually. There are 700,000 strokes annually, and about one-fourth of all nursing home patients are permanently impaired from strokes. These statistics have a great impact on the amount of money spent annually on care for victims of strokes.

Since the 1960s, the death rate from strokes in the United States has decreased significantly, by about 60 percent. Control of blood pressure and diet, the development of new drugs and diagnostic techniques, and the advent of cardiovascular surgery in the early 1950s have contributed to these results. Unfortunately, strokes are still prevalent given the extent of atherosclerotic disease in the American population, which is largely attributed to a high-fat diet. Autopsies of U.S. soldiers killed in the Korean and Vietnam Wars demonstrated evidence that atherosclerosis begins at a

very early age, often by age eighteen. Atherosclerosis is more prevalent in males. Females have more protection until the onset of the menopause. Within five years of the menopause, however, the stroke and death rates of men and women tend to equalize.

High-salt diets, which contribute to hypertension, also contribute to the development and progression of atherosclerosis, as well as hemorrhagic strokes. Ethnic African and Asian populations appear to be at greater risk in this respect. Since the 1960s, however, extensive education of the American public concerning diet and the control of blood pressure has had a favorable impact. More recently, the increase in individuals who have stopped smoking and who have undertaken regular exercise has helped to lower stroke rates further.

Since the 1950s, a number of both noninvasive and invasive procedures have been developed to diagnose atherosclerotic disease. Cardiovascular surgical techniques were developed in the 1950s. The first bypass surgery (arterial autograft) probably occurred during the Korean War. The development of ultrasound devices in the 1950s initiated the research into using these noninvasive devices to diagnose cerebrovascular disease. The duplex devices introduced commercially in the late 1970s and early 1980s have spurred the development of new diagnostic devices for detecting atherosclerotic disease. These devices allow for visualization of plaque morphology (composition of the plaque, such as thrombus, calcium, hemorrhage, and other particulate matters) and blood flow characteristics for a better understanding of the disease process. Future developments in the field of ultrasound include holographic imaging for the three-dimensional visualization of plaques. These noninvasive technologies will also allow physicians to monitor the effects of new drugs and techniques in the treatment of atherosclerosis. Advances in digital subtraction and computer enhancement of angiographic techniques, along with new contrast media, have made arteriograms safer and more accurate.

Color duplex devices are utilizing low-frequency probes to visualize and produce color scans of blood vessels that lie inside the skull. By analyzing the blood flow direction and velocity in the circle of Willis and within the blood vessels of the skull, physicians will come to a better understanding of the formation of collateral pathways and will learn how to detect other pathological conditions that lead to cerebrovascular disease. Magnetic resonance imaging (MRI) is also being utilized to measure actual flow in individual arterial segments of the body.

Carotid endarterectomies, which lost favor for a period of time, have become the preferred therapeutic treatment for individuals with episodes of TIAs and severe atherosclerotic plaques in the carotid arteries. Additional studies will further delineate which other patient populations may benefit from this surgery. Aspirin still remains a potent drug in the treatment of TIAs in patients with lesser degrees of disease and in post surgery patients. Recognition and prompt treatment of symptomatic cerebrovascular symptoms remain the key to better survival rates.

—Silvia M. Berry, MSc, RVT, and L. Fleming Fallon, Jr., MD, PhD, MPH; updated by Bradley R.A. Wilson, PhD, and Patricia Stanfill Edens, PhD, RN, LFACHE

See also: Angiography; Angioplasty; Aphasiaand dysphasia; Arteriosclerosis; Blood vessels; Brain; Brain disorders; Bypass surgery; Carotid arteries; Cholesterol; Circulation; Congenitalheart disease; Edema; Embolism; Endarterectomy; Heart attack; Heart disease; Heart failure; Hyperlipidemia; Hypertension; Ischemia; Numbnessand tingling; Paralysis; Physical rehabilitation; Plaque, arterial; Speech disorders; Thrombolytictherapyand TPA; Thrombosisand thrombus; Vascularmedicine; Vascularsystem.

For Further Information:

American Medical Association. *American Medical Association Family Medical Guide*. 4th rev. ed. Hoboken, N.J.: JohnWiley & Sons, 2004. Provides updated, understandable medical information about various diseases including stroke.

American Stroke Association. www.stroke association.org. Gives information on current treatments, warning signs, stroke care, and stroke programs. Offers newsletters and scientific and professional research links, among other features.

Marler, John R. *Stroke for Dummies*. Indianapolis, Ind.: John Wiley & Sons, 2005. Offers general information about strokes for nonscientists.

National Institutes of Health Stroke Scale. www.nihstroke scale.org/ A systematic assessment tool that provides a quantitative measure of stroke-related neurologic deficit.

Rao, Paul R., Mark N. Ozer, and John E. Toerge, eds. *Managing Stroke: A Guide to Living Well After Stroke*. Washington, DC: ABI Professional, 2000. The staff of the National Rehabilitation Hospital in Washington, DC, has created an instructional guide for those who have suffered a stroke.

Senelick, Richard C., and Karla Dougherty. *Living with Stroke: A Guide for Families*. 3d ed. Albany, N.Y.: Delmar, 2001. Provides a range of information for stroke patients and their families, including data on strokes, current theories on neural plasticity, and the process of rehabilitation, especially the emotional component of recovery.

Wiebers, David O., Valery L. Feigin, and Robert D. Brown, Jr. *Handbook of Stroke*. Philadelphia: Lippincott Williams & Wilkins, 2006. Based on extensive experience at the Mayo Clinic, this book provides a concise and easy-to-read guide for the evaluation and management of stroke. It is filled with algorithms that put pertinent information at the reader's fingertips.

Zamanlu M, Farhoudi M, Eskandani M, et al. Recent advances in targeted delivery of tissue plasminogen activator for enhance thrombolysis in ischemic stroke. *J Drug Target*. 2017 Aug 10:1-42. Doi 1.1080/1061186X.2017.1365874.

STURGE-WEBER SYNDROME

Category: Disease/Disorder
Also known as: Sturge-Weber-Dimitri syndrome, encephe-lotrigeminal angiomatosis
Anatomy or system affected: Blood, blood vessels, brain, circulatory system, eyes, head, nerves, nervous system, skin
Specialties and related fields: Dermatology, neurology, ophthalmology, pediatrics, plastic surgery, psychology, vascular medicine
Definition: A disorder associated with partial facial disfigurement which involves vascular accumulations that affect the central nervous system.

CAUSES AND SYMPTOMS

Although the precise causation of Sturge-Weber syndrome has not been established, medical researchers have found a relationship to excess circulatory vessels remaining from embryonic development. Professionals estimate that approximately 15 percent of newborns with port-wine stains have this syndrome. Patients usually exhibit a facial port-wine stain along the trigeminal nerve on one side. The size of the birthmark and the area covered depend on which, and how many, of the three branches of this nerve-found in the brow, cheek, and jaw-are affected by excessive capillaries delivering blood to the skin. Sometimes, the birthmark appears on other parts of the body or the entire head. Infrequently, patients with this syndrome do not have a port-wine stain.

Neurological activity is often disrupted and slowed in these patients because of the massing of circulatory vessels on the brain adjacent to the port-wine stain. As a result, patients sometimes experience calcium buildup in brain tissues and epileptic seizures on the side without the birthmark. Approximately half of patients suffer developmental problems, including intellectual disabilities. Because circulation to the eyes is altered, fluid drainage is sometimes disrupted and pressure intensifies, resulting in swelling, glaucoma, and possible blindness. Partial paralysis occasionally accompanies this syndrome.

TREATMENT AND THERAPY

Many patients with Sturge-Weber syndrome suffer only facial birthmarks and mild neurological symptoms that do not affect their life span. Lasers can erase port-wine stains, and cosmetics are a less expensive but temporary solution. Psychological counseling can help patients cope with societal reaction to their birthmarks, including bullying and rejection.

Patients whose brains are significantly affected have higher risks. Medications can treat convulsions. In ex-

Guttman, Cheryl. "Location of Port-Wine Stains May Signal Syndromal Associations." *Dermatology Times* 19, no. 7 (July, 1998): 25.
Sturge-Weber Foundation. www.sturge-weber.org.

STUTTERING

Category: Disease/Disorder
Anatomy or system affected: Nervous system
Specialties and related fields: Family medicine, neurology, pediatrics, speech pathology
Definition: Breaks in the smooth flow of speech.

CAUSES AND SYMPTOMS

Stuttering is usually recognized as a child develops enough language skill to speak in complete sentences, beginning around three years of age. Typically, the child repeats the beginning sounds of a word, or whole words, before continuing with the sentence, as in, "I l-l-l-like to p-p-p-pet my ca-ca-cat." True stuttering must be differentiated from developmental dysfluency and dysfluency caused by unusually severe environmental or social pressures. Developmental dysfluency is normal, occurring in the three- or four-year-old child whose brain works faster than his or her mouth. This child may repeat parts of words, words, or parts of phrases, especially when excited. When a child feels significantly anxious, language may become dysfluent, or broken up and difficult to understand. This is not true stuttering, and treatment should be aimed at alleviating the anxiety or stress.

True stuttering is less common than the two dysfluencies just described, and it occurs more often in boys. Frequently, the true stutterer is consistently dysfluent on the same sounds or words. There is consistency in repetitions, prolongations, pauses, grammatical forms, and rate of emission of dysfluency. Often, the child will overcome a verbal hurdle by using certain actions such as eye blinking, finger snapping, or foot tapping.

INFORMATION ON STURGE-WEBER SYNDROME

Causes: Unknown; possibly excess blood vessels remaining from embryonic development
Symptoms: Port-wine stain, seizures, intellectual disabilities, eye disorders (swelling, glaucoma, possible blindness), sometimes partial paralysis
Duration: Chronic
Treatments: Depends on severity; may include cosmetic correction, including laser removal), psychological counseling, anticonvulsive medications, surgery to remove damaged tissues

---

treme cases, surgery may be required to remove damaged tissues. Medical professionals X-ray patients to assess brain calcification and to locate any tumors. The eyes are examined regularly to detect problems and are treated with medication or surgery as applicable. Physical therapy can strengthen weakened muscles in cases of partial paralysis.

PERSPECTIVE AND PROSPECTS

William Allen Sturge hypothesized in 1879 that a six-year-old patient suffering from seizures had a brain lesion on the same side as her port-wine stain. His peers rejected his theory. By 1901, Siegfried Kalischer verified Sturge's hypothesis through pathological studies. In 1922, Frederick Parkes Weber used radiography to document calcification inside the craniums of patients with port-wine stains. The next year, Vincente Dimitri added his insights; he is sometimes incorporated into the name of this syndrome. E. Steve Roach described three types of Sturge-Weber syndrome in 1992. His categories are based on trait occurrence and extent.

Established in 1987, the Sturge-Weber Foundation has created a registry of individuals with this syndrome. In the early twenty-first century, researchers continued their investigations of possible genetic factors in this syndrome.

—Elizabeth D. Schafer, PhD

See also Birthmarks; Blood vessels; Brain damage; Circulation; Congenital disorders; Dermatology; Dermatology, pediatric; Eyes; Glaucoma; Nervous system; Neuralgia, neuritis, and neuropathy; Neurology; Neurology, pediatric; Paralysis; Plastic surgery; Seizures; Skin; Skin disorders; Vascular medicine; Vascular system.

For Further Information:
Ball, Karen Fisher, ed. *Sturge-Weber Syndrome: The Resource Guide for a Reason, a Season, and a Lifetime.* Mt. Freedom, N.J.: Sturge-Weber Foundation, 2003.
Bodensteiner, John B., and E. Steve Roach, eds. *Sturge-Weber Syndrome.* Mt. Freedom, N.J.: Sturge-Weber Foundation, 1999.

INFORMATION ON STUTTERING

Causes: Developmental and physical defects, emotional stress, anxiety
Symptoms: Repeating beginning sounds of word or whole words; concomitant eye blinking, finger snapping, or foot tapping
Duration: Often short-term, may be chronic
Treatments: Speech therapy, reading aloud, singing

TREATMENT AND THERAPY

Treatment of true stuttering by a competent speech pathologist is imperative, and the prognosis, although variable, can be good. Parents and teachers should be alerted to alleviate any emotional stress that is unusual or severe. Absolutely essential is the ability of all adults to deal with the stuttering child without calling attention to the speech patterns or mannerisms. Practicing reading aloud, especially poetry, and singing-all in the privacy of the company of a caring adult-may help.

PERSPECTIVE AND PROSPECTS

The great ancient Greek orator Demosthenes was dysfluent and allegedly practiced talking with pebbles in his mouth until he could speak clearly. Stuttering does not preclude a person becoming successful in any endeavor. Modern speech therapy and understanding adults can be of great benefit to a child who stutters.

—*Robert W. Block, MD*

See also Antianxiety drugs; Anxiety; Lisping; Phobias; Psychiatry, child and adolescent; Speech disorders.

For Further Information:
Cole, Patricia R. *Language Disorders in Preschool Children.* Englewood Cliffs, N.J.: Prentice Hall, 1982.
Hamaguchi, Patricia McAleer. *Childhood Speech, Language, and Listening Problems: What Every Parent Should Know.* 2d ed. New York: Wiley, 2001.
Martin, Katherine L. *Does My Child Have a Speech Problem?* Chicago: Chicago Review Press, 1997.
Pinker, Steven. *The Language Instinct: How the Mind Creates Language.* New York: HarperCollins, 2007.
Plante, Elena, and Pelagie M. Beeson. *Communication and Communication Disorders: A Clinical Introduction.* 3d ed. Boston: Pearson/Allyn & Bacon, 2008.
Stuttering Foundation. www.stuttersfa.org.

STYES

Category: Disease/Disorder
Also known as: External hordeolum
Anatomy or system affected: Eyes, skin
Specialties and related fields: Bacteriology, dermatology, family medicine
Definition: Inflammations of hair follicles or glands of the eyelids that become infected by bacteria, usually *Staphylococcus aureus.*

CAUSES AND SYMPTOMS

The most common symptoms that accompany styes are swelling, redness, and pain to an area of the eyelid. A pimple often appears in the area of the swelling. There may also be excessive watering of the infected eye and an increased sensitivity to light. A chalazion can sometimes be mistaken for a stye because it too is marked by swelling. A chalazion is a lump on the edge of the eyelid that is caused not by bacteria but rather by a blocked mucous gland under the eye. Unlike a stye, a chalazion is a painless swelling.

While styes have no specific causes, they often develop when staphylococci bacteria are transferred from nose to eye by excessive rubbing. Stress has also been named as an influence on the frequency of recurring styes. Styes are not harmful to vision and can occur at any age.

> **INFORMATION ON STYES**
>
> **Causes:** Bacterial infection with staphylococci; may be triggered by rubbing or stress
> **Symptoms:** Swelling, redness, and pain in eyelid; excessive eye watering; increased sensitivity to light
> **Duration:** Usually a few days; sometimes recurrent
> **Treatments:** Warm compresses, antibiotic creams or ointments if infection persists

TREATMENT AND THERAPY

Some styes heal on their own within a few days. Healing may be encouraged by applying localized warm compresses (with a clean cloth) to the infected area for ten minutes, four to eight times throughout the day. The warmth of the compress assists in speeding the white blood cells to the infected area, which in turn accelerates the crowning of the stye and subsequent drainage of the abscess through the opening at the margin or underside of the eyelid. Once drainage of the pus begins, the swelling and pain associated with most styes begin to subside. Though the temptation may be great, styes should never be ruptured or "popped," as is often done with a pimple. This may spread the infection to other follicles of the eyelid, or it may spread the infection to the tissue of the eye, causing eyelid cellulitis.

Antibiotic creams and ointments are sometimes prescribed in cases of persistent and recurrent styes. Rarely do styes require lancing by a doctor. However, a health care provider should be consulted if the swelling on the eyelid continues to enlarge or if it does not cease on its own within a two-week period.

To prevent stye recurrence, it is important to keep the eyelid and lashes clean. Careful attention should be placed on cleaning excessive oil from the edges of the lids. Hands should be washed regularly, especially if they have touched the nose. Separate washcloths and towels should be used among members of a shared household. Styes pose no danger to the eye, and therefore the prognosis is usually quite positive.

—*Nicholas Lanzieri*

See also Abscess drainage; Abscesses; Bacterial infections; Boils; Dermatology; Dermatology, pediatric; Eye infections and disorders; Eyes; Ophthalmology; Skin; Skin disorders; Staphylococcal infections.

For Further Information:

Anshel, Jeffrey. *Smart Medicine for Your Eyes: A Guide to Safe and Effective Relief of Common Eye Disorders*. Garden City Park, N.Y.: Avery, 1999.

Porter, Robert S., et al., eds. *The Merck Manual Home Health Handbook*. Whitehouse Station, N.J.: Merck Research Laboratories, 2009.

Riordan-Eva, Paul, and John P. Whitcher. *Vaughan and Asbury's General Ophthalmology*. 17th ed. New York: Lange Medical Books/McGraw-Hill, 2007.

SUBDURAL HEMATOMA

Category: Disease/Disorder
Anatomy or system affected: Blood, brain
Specialties and related fields: Hematology, neurology, ophthalmology, speech pathology
Definition: Collection of blood (clotted and partially clotted) in the subdural space.

Key terms:

dura mater: tissue layer between the brain and the skull

hypoxia: lack of oxygen

subdural space: space between the brain tissue and the dura mater

tonic-clonic seizure (grand mal seizure): two-phase seizure common in epilepsy attacks that consists of a tonic phase, in which the body becomes rigid, and a clonic phase, which involves uncontrolled jerky movements

CAUSES AND SYMPTOMS

Subdural hematomas are caused by either a major head injury (acute subdural hematomas) or by a relatively minor head injury (chronic subdural hematomas). Acute subdural hematomas usually occur after a major head injury in which the rotational or linear forces cause veins in the subdural space to break. These types of subdural hematomas are the most common form of sports-related brain injury, especially in professional boxers because of the multiple head blows that they receive. Chronic subdural hematomas, on the other hand, typically develop days to weeks after relatively minor head injuries. This type of hematoma mainly afflicts the elderly, who are more likely to have brain shrinkage, which causes the subdural veins to stretch in order to cover the greater distance created between the brain and the dura mater. These stretched veins are more vulnerable to breakage, even from a minor head injury. Some cases of subdural hematomas occur without

INFORMATION ON SUBDURAL HEMATOMA

Causes: Usually major or minor head injuries; some cases arise without apparent head injury

Symptoms: In adults and older children, persistent headache, drowsiness, loss of consciousness, paralysis, seizures, memory problems, confusion, nausea, numbness, visual abnormalities, slurred or confused speech and language, weakness; in infants, focal seizures, generalized tonic-clonic seizures, increased sleepiness, irritability, vomiting

Duration: May occur immediately or develop in days to weeks

Treatments: For smaller hematomas, hole drilled in skull for drainage; for larger hematomas, craniotomy

apparent head injury, which may be due to the fact that many minor head injuries go unnoticed. Blood-thinning drugs such as Coumadin, alcohol abuse, seizures, repeated falls, shunts draining excess cerebrospinal fluid (CSF) from the brain, and very young or very old age increase the risk of developing a subdural hematoma.

A subdural hematoma can compress the brain, frequently leading to brain injury. Symptoms in adults and older children include a persistent headache, drowsiness, loss of consciousness, paralysis on the opposite side of the body, seizures, memory problems, confusion, nausea, numbness, visual abnormalities, slurred or confused speech and language, and weakness. An elderly person with memory loss or drowsiness may be mistakenly thought to have dementia when he or she actually has a subdural hematoma. In professional boxers, symptoms include neurological abnormalities, deteriorating dementia, and death.

In infants, subdural hematomas occur as part of shaken baby syndrome. Symptoms of a subdural hematoma in infants include swollen fontanelles ("soft spots" in a baby's skull), focal seizures, generalized tonic-clonic seizures, increased sleepiness, irritability, and vomiting. In all cases, acute subdural hematomas carry a high risk of death and are considered medical emergencies. The cause of shaken baby syndrome remains controversial. Initially, shaking was thought to induce shear forces that cause breakage of the bridging veins in the subdural space, resulting in the subdural hematomas, retinal hematomas, and encephalopathy characteristic of shaken baby syndrome. However, more recent research suggests that these symptoms are more likely caused by vein damage due to impact and hypoxia. Subdural hematomas may also be caused by the birth process.

TREATMENT AND THERAPY

Computed tomography (CT) scanning and magnetic resonance imaging (MRI) can detect most subdural hematomas. MRI is more sensitive and may be able to detect hematomas that may not show up on CT scans.

Treatment is based on the type and size of hematoma and the amount of pressure that has accumulated in the brain. Small subdural hematomas may resolve when head injuries heal. For small subdural hematomas that do not resolve, a hole may be drilled in the skull and the blood mass drained from the subdural space via a catheter. This procedure can be performed at the patient's bedside. Large hematomas, however, may require a surgical procedure known as a craniotomy, in which the skull is surgically opened and the blood mass removed. Surgical removal of acute subdural hematomas is associated with a significant risk of death. On the other hand, treatment of chronic subdural hematomas has a relatively good prognosis.

PERSPECTIVE AND PROSPECTS

In 1946, pediatrician John Caffey described the relationship between long bone injuries and subdural hematomas. Since then, subdural hematomas have been reported in the elderly, professional athletes such as boxers and hockey players, and in abused children.

There is considerable uncertainty about the long-term effects of subdural hematomas. Although it is not known if suffering a subdural hematoma puts someone at greater risk of experiencing subdural hematomas in the future, boxing commissions in several states have banned boxers with a history of subdural hematomas from competing. Boxers diagnosed with subdural hematomas risk being banned from boxing, a fact that prevents some professional boxers from seeking a diagnosis. A well-known case involves a thirty-one-year-old boxer, Joe Mesi, who was suspended by the Nevada Athletic Commission after he developed subdural hematomas as a result of head injuries sustained in a March, 2004, fight. Mesi lost an appeal to lift his medical suspension in 2005. Another athlete, a professional hockey player, suffered a subdural hematoma after receiving a hit to the head during a game. However, his wounds healed and his doctors allowed him to return to professional hockey, believing that there would be no negative consequences. Until more is known about the long-term effects of subdural hematomas, there will continue to be controversy over whether athletes with a history of hematomas should be allowed to compete.

—*Ing-Wei Khor, PhD*

See also Accidents; Bleeding; Blood and blood disorders; Brain; Brain damage; Circulation; Emergency medicine; First aid; Hematology; Hematology, pediatric; Hematomas; Hemorrhage; Intraventricular hemorrhage; Sports medicine; Vascular medicine.

For Further Information:
Heller, J. L. "Subdural Hematoma." www.nlm.nih.gov/medlineplus/ency/article/000713.htm. This MedLine Plus page (a service of the National Library of Medicine and the National Institutes of Health) provides an overview of the topic that is appropriate for a lay audience. Brief descriptions of symptoms, tests, treatment, and prognosis are included.
Miele, V. J., et al. *Subdural Hematomas in Boxing: The Spectrum of Consequences*. Medscape Today. www.medscape.com/viewarticle/553965_3. The causes and effects of subdural hematomas in professional boxers are presented, along with a discussion of the conflict between the need for diagnosis and treatment and the risk of being barred from boxing.
Squier, W. "Shaken Baby Syndrome: The Quest for Evidence." *Developmental Medicine & Child Neurology* 50, no. 1 (January, 2008): 10-14. Discusses the causes of shaken baby syndrome.
Squier, W., and J. Mack. "The Neuropathology of Infant Subdural Hemorrhage." *Forensic Science International* 187, nos. 1-3 (May 30, 2009): 6-23. Describes the neurological symptoms of subdural hematomas in infants.

SUBSTANCE ABUSE

Category: Disease/Disorder
Also known as: Substance-related disorders
Anatomy or system affected: All
Specialties and related fields: All
Definition: A pattern of social, psychological, and/or biological problems caused by the way in which a person uses drugs such as alcohol, nicotine, and prescription or illegal drugs.
Key terms:
abuse: a pattern of substance use observed in a twelve-month period resulting in occupational, safety-related, legal, and/or social problems as a consequence of the substance use
addiction: a condition in which an individual is compelled to use a drug, such as alcohol, despite the fact that it is causing significant problems
co-occurring disorders: a situation in which a person has more than one diagnosable problem
dependence: a pattern of substance use problems in a twelve-month period that demonstrates physiological or psychological reliance on a specific substance that results in conditions such as tolerance, withdrawal, inability to regulate one's use, and desire to control or reduce one's use
psychotropic drugs: substances that affect the mind through their influence on the central nervous system

substance of abuse: a drug that affects the mind and body in a reinforcing manner, causing a person to want to repeat use of the drug for its positive effects

tolerance: using a drug and getting less and less effect from the same amount of the drug, or needing more of the drug to get the same effect

withdrawal: symptoms that result when a person ceases or abstains from using a drug; vary from substance to substance and may range from mild irritability to hallucinations, seizures and death

OVERVIEW, CAUSES AND SYMPTOMS

There are many substances of abuse, including ubiquitous drugs such as caffeine, alcohol and nicotine, and the misuse of the latter two cause the greatest harm psychologically, medically, and economically. Substances of abuse also include illegal and regulated drugs such as marijuana, cocaine, amphetamines, heroin, and hallucinogens. Often overlooked, however, are medicinal drugs, such as one might get via a prescription from a doctor, and even common household substances ingested as inhalants, including glue and paint.

According to the *Diagnostic and Statistical Manual of Mental Disorders, Fifth Edition (DSM-V)*, the diagnostic handbook for mental health professionals, in order to be diagnosed with a substance abuse problem a person must have significant difficulty in fulfilling social and work-related obligations. These persons have frequent encounters with the law due to their drug problem and put themselves in danger physically either through the use of the substance itself or by driving under the influence, for example, over a twelve-month period. Substance dependence differs by definition in that those who have a substance abuse problem may require more of the drug to achieve the same effect, develop withdrawal symptoms when they do not have the drug, have difficulty quitting, and/or use the drug despite the negative social, legal, psychological, or physical effects.

Environmental and genetic factors also play a strong role in substance use disorder. Individual differences in genetics have been demonstrated to influence stress response and predispose some individuals to develop a substance use disorder.

The Adverse Childhood Experience Study (ACES) demonstrated that exposure to a range of traumatic events during childhood is associated with an increased risk of substance use later in life. This risk association was demonstrated to follow a pattern where increased trauma exposure was directly correlated with an increased risk of developing a substance use disorder.

Substance use disorders involve both psychological and physical dependence on the substance(s) of use.

Dependence is characterized by an inability to regulate use. Substance use disorders and addiction stem in part from adaptive changes in the brain as it seeks to regain homeostasis. Chronic and/or prolonged stress plays a strong role in developing drug-seeking behavior; it alters the corticotropin-releasing factor and hypothalamic-pituitary-adrenal axis (CRF/HPA).

Stimulants, such as cocaine and amphetamines, exert their effect by preventing the recycling of dopamine, norepinephrine, and serotonin. This results in increased concentrations of these neurotransmitters within the synaptic cleft. The influx of these neurotransmitters gives the user a euphoric effect.

Nicotine influx in the central nervous system (CNS) leads to neurotransmitters' release, specifically dopamine, which stimulates the brain's reward region. Chronic nicotine use results in tolerance. Chronic and excessive stimulation of nicotine acetylcholine receptors results in desensitization of the receptors; these neuroadaptations produce a state where the brain requires nicotine to function in homeostasis. This is known as "physiological dependence."

Alcohol produces euphoric effects through the dopamine neurons of the mesolimbic system. Alcohol inhibits N-methyl-D-aspartate receptor (NMDA) receptors and results in the upregulation of gamma-aminobutyric acid (GABA) receptors. Chronic consumption of alcohol leads to GABA receptor desen-

---

INFORMATION ON SUBSTANCE ABUSE

Causes: Exposure to addictive substances, repetitive use, genetic risks, other biological risk factors such as other diseases and disorders, social risk factors such as peer and family use, stress, poverty

Symptoms: For abuse, impaired occupational functioning, using in unsafe situations, legal problems, social problems; for dependence, sometimes tolerance, withdrawal, loss of control of use, desire to control use, excessive time spent related to use, reduction of other activities, use despite psychological or physical problems caused or made worse

Duration: Repeated pattern of problems established within any twelve-month period and time-limited, intermittently repeating, or continuing lifelong

Treatments: Medications, psychotropic drugs, cognitive and behavioral treatments, motivational treatments, family-based treatment, harm reduction treatments, self-help treatments, group-based support, integrated treatments with co-occurring disorders sitization and tolerance, potentiating the loss of drinking control.

Opioids include codeine, heroin, hydrocodone, hydromorphone, methadone, meperidine, morphine, and oxycodone. Opioids bind to delta, kappa, and mu receptors, which provide analgesia for severe pain and produce euphoria feelings. Higher doses may lead to respiratory suppression and death. Individuals with chronic exposure to opioids can experience profound withdrawal symptoms if opioid use is stopped abruptly. The withdrawal symptoms include but are not limited to diarrhea, excess sweating, excess lacrimation, nausea, vomiting, and insomnia.

Sedatives, hypnotics, and anxiolytics are a class of medications that can cause CNS depression, and if taken inappropriately, the effects can be fatal. They include benzodiazepines (alprazolam, clonazepam, lorazepam, diazepam) and barbiturates (phenobarbital, pentobarbital, butabarbital) and other hypnotics and sedatives.

Problems with substance use may result from many different causes. For conditions such as substance dependence, there can sometimes be a biological component related to genetics. Individuals who have a family history of these problems may carry a genetic risk. It is not a guarantee that they will have a problem, but they can have increased risk of developing one. In the same way, even if a person does not have a family history of a problem, it does not mean that they are risk-free. Using substances repetitively, particularly in large doses or very frequently, can also cause problems such as dependence. Patterns of use and frequent use can develop because an individual regularly has access to the drugs through family and/or friends. Also, people may learn how to use the drugs in ways that are not adaptive through these same individuals. Peers who use are a risk factor for their teenage friends.

Family history of other problems or characteristics can also contribute to having a greater risk for substance use problems. For instance, a family history of other mental health problems, such as depression, can be a risk factor for developing a substance use problem. Even social characteristics, such as a high amount of family stress, can be a risk factor because individuals may use substances to cope with stress and other life difficulties. Additionally, some individuals may never learn of the risks and consequences associated with substance use because of lack of education or prior exposure to the problems, and so they may use unwittingly and develop problems.

TREATMENT AND THERAPY

Treatments for substance-related disorders vary by the substance involved and the specific type of problem. For instance, if one is experiencing withdrawal from alcohol as compared to another drug such as heroin, different medications are given for treatment. This is the case because the different drugs affect different neurotransmitters in the brain. Also, depending on the severity of the problems or presence of other problems, more than one drug treatment may be used. If a person withdrawing from alcohol was also showing signs of depression, that individual might be given an additional psychotropic drug to address the depression. In fact, many patients have co-occurring problems, so integrating treatment of the varied problems is important.

It is also important to note that while some treatments focus on reducing symptoms such as withdrawal or sleep problems that are biological in nature, others focus on the more social and behavioral aspects of the problem. Treatments may also vary in their goal. Some treatments may focus on having an individual achieve abstinence from the problem drug(s), while other treatments may focus on reducing the amount or frequency of drug use, or even reducing other harm from the substance use. Approaches focusing on reducing frequency and amount of use are often focused on moderation as a goal. Approaches focusing on reducing harm are usually known as "harm reduction treatments" and may focus on reducing associated problems. An example of harm reduction is having individuals who use drugs avoid doing dangerous things such as driving after they have used (thereby reducing risks related to driving while under the influence) or having individuals who inject drugs not share needles (thereby reducing risks related to blood-borne problems such as hepatitis or human immunodeficiency virus, or HIV).

Nonpharmacological treatments include therapies that focus on changing specific behaviors or thoughts related to the problem use. They may also include treatments focusing on helping address the motivation of the individual to change. More specifically, not all people with substance use problems are ready to change immediately. Therefore, sometimes the first treatment needed may be to work on the motivation to change. In fact, sometimes individuals work on their problem on their own, using self-help materials before seeking out treatment professionals. Additionally, it is not uncommon for individuals to seek help for substance use problems through support groups, such as twelve-step groups (e.g., Alcoholics Anonymous).

PERSPECTIVE AND PROSPECTS

Problems related to substances of abuse have been affecting human behavior for all of human existence. Exposure to substances initially tried as foods or medicines that may have had psychotropic effects, such as fermented berries or mushrooms and plants, are probably some of the first experiences leading to both positive and negative consequences related to substance use. In fact, addictive substances have been an integral part of human society, used in religious and medicinal ceremonies from our beginnings as hunter-gatherers to Ancient Greece and beyond. As such, it is a long-standing problem that is likely to stay with human society and require management as time goes on.

While the formal diagnosis known as "substance abuse" is likely to change in terms of how it is recognized, the problems related to the condition as currently defined will remain a target of intervention and concern. For example, the parameters defining legal consequences may adjust with new laws as legislation evolves and even new substances of abuse are identified. In 2012, Washington and Colorado became the first states in the United States to legalize the recreational use of marijuana, and as a result, several other states are now showing increased pressure from voters and advocates alike to follow suit. The long-term legal and social effects of these measures are yet to be determined. Similarly, the type and scope of social and safety problems may increase as substances are used in new contexts and with new behaviors. Problems related to role functioning, legal issues, use in unsafe situations, and use resulting in consequences that disturb social relationships remain significant problems and will need continued attention by treatment providers and prevention specialists to address the problem of substance use whether it stands as a condition on its own or as part of a larger spectrum of substance dependence problems and formally diagnosable conditions.

The future is likely to bring continued fine-tuning of diagnoses to isolate and identify genetic and physiological aspects of these problems so as to refine prevention and treatment of drug problems involving more biological causes. The balance of the work to refine prevention and treatment will focus on the behavioral and social causes of these conditions which, on their own, may cause problems and also may interact with biological risk factors. Continued understanding of how substance-related conditions interact with other mental health problems, physical conditions, and even cultural differences are also efforts that will improve treatment and prevention.

—*Shuba Samuel, PhD*

See also: Addiction; Alcoholism; Antidepressants; Caffeine; Club drugs; Geriatrics and gerontology; Herbal medicine; Homeopathy; Metabolism; Narcotics; Nicotine; Over-the-counter medications; Pain; Pain management; Pharmacology; Pharmacy; Polypharmacy; Prescription drug abuse; Psychiatry; Psychiatry, child and adolescent; Psychiatry, geriatric; Self-medication; Smoking; Toxicology.

For Further Information:
Advokat, C. *Julien's Primer of Drug Action.* 14th ed., Worth, 2018. This is a more technical work that presents a more academic description of what different drugs are, how drugs are processed by the body, their safety issues, and their other effects on the body and brain.
DiClemente, Carlo C. *Addiction and Change: How Addictions Develop and How People Change.* 2nd ed., Guilford Press, 2018. Provides an easy-to-understand description of problems with addictions, along with useful concepts for thinking about how these problems develop for many people, as well as practical strategies for thinking about how to change.
Jahan, A. R., and D. M. Burgess. "Substance Use Disorder." *StatPearls,* 18 Aug. 2021, www.ncbi.nlm.nih.gov/books/NBK570642.
McNeece, C. Aaron, and Diana M. DiNitto. *Chemical Dependency: A Systems Approach.* 4th ed., Pearson, 2011. This textbook provides an integrated way of thinking about substance use problems and their treatment, starting with definitions, epidemiology, etiology, and the biological aspects and other consequences of these problems, while also addressing more advanced topics related to treatment of different types of individuals, such as adolescents, adults, elders, and whole families.
Rosen, Winifred, and Andrew T. Weil. *From Chocolate to Morphine: Everything You Need to Know about Mind-Altering Drugs.* Rev. ed., Houghton Mifflin, 2004. Source for varying ages provides insight into the broad range of substances that affect the mind.
"Trends & Statistics: National Institute on Drug Abuse." *NIDA,* 2021, nida.nih.gov/drug-topics/trends-statistics. This website offers current statistical information on various substance abuse trends in America, ranging from prescription drugs to teenage substance abuse.
Williams, Angela, *Tobacco and e-Cigarette Information for Teens.* 4th ed., Omnigraphics, 2020. This resource focuses on one of the most abused drugs in society, nicotine, and provides basic descriptions of key health problems related to its use in varied forms.

SUCCESSFUL AGING

Category: Biology
Anatomy or system affected: Biopsychosocial
Specialties and related fields: Gerontology
Definition: Successful aging (American English) or successful ageing (British English) refers to physical, mental and social well-being in older age. The concept of successful aging can be traced back to the 1950s, and was popularized in the 1980s.

Seniors are living longer and becoming a greater percentage of the population in the twenty-first century. Advances in medicine enable people to live longer and healthier lives. Since the early twentieth century, the average life span worldwide has increased from forty-seven to sixty-eight years old; in developed countries the average is around eighty. The traditional retirement age of sixty-five is no longer considered old, since many live into their eighties and nineties.

The growing number of seniors is redefining aging. Concerns have surfaced about society's ability to cope with an aging population that puts greater demands on health care and community caregiving resources. However, many individuals entering their later years are healthy, active, and involved in their communities. They are willing and able to contribute to society. Seniors are at the forefront of the movement to discover strategies for successful aging.

BACKGROUND

The perception of aging has changed since the beginning of the twentieth century. Retirement was for the rich only until Social Security was introduced in the United States in 1935. Everyone could expect to live decently in old age. Retirement communities sprang up to cater to the aging with the funds and leisure time to enjoy retirement. Today, many older adults continue to work and volunteer after retirement. Culture and genetics influence how people age. Scientists have discovered places in the world where people live a long time with a high quality of life, including Sardinia in Italy, Okinawa in Japan, and Loma Linda in California. Genetics, healthy eating habits, and a culture promoting freedom and well-being are factors in the successful aging process in these locations. Researchers studying centenarians have found that both health and life span are determined by genetics; however, genes can be influenced by lifestyle, diet, and environmental factors. The mapping of the human genome promises new possibilities to extend life expectancy and promote healthy aging.

Healthy aging is a combination of physical, mental, and social well-being. In general, older individuals today are in better physical shape than their predecessors. In the United States, chronic diseases are affecting people later in life. According to a 2009 study conducted by Pew Research, older individuals do not feel "old." One-third of respondents between the ages of sixty-five and seventy-four felt ten to nineteen years younger than their chronological age. Seniors who continue to maintain an active social life with family, friends, and community feel free to remain independent as they age successfully.

OVERVIEW

Successful aging begins with intentional effort to continue participating in life. In *Living the Good Long Life* (2013), lifestyle specialist Martha Stewart says, "The quality of the rest of your life is more within your control than you think." Many chronic diseases can be prevented or managed by making positive lifestyle choices. Healthy habits such as staying physically

active, reducing stress, maintaining a healthy weight, not smoking, and drinking moderately have been proven to improve the quality of life and reduce the incidence of chronic diseases. Physical activity in the form of daily exercise totaling at least two and a half hours a week keeps both the brain and the body healthy.

In a longitudinal study conducted in the United Kingdom, the strongest predictor of successful aging was shown to be socioeconomic status at midlife. After adjustment for socioeconomics, not smoking, diet, exercise, moderate alcohol intake (only in women), and work support (only in men) predicted successful aging.

Another effective aging strategy is to challenge the brain by working on stimulating mental activities, such as solving puzzles, learning a language, or traveling. Giving the gift of time as a volunteer benefits others but also keeps older citizens engaged in their community. More wealthy individuals are reinventing themselves as they age. For example, Bill Gates left Microsoft to devote his time to combating malaria and solving the world's energy problems through the Bill and Melinda Gates Foundation.

Having an active social life reduces loneliness and being involved also alleviates symptoms of depression and other mental illnesses. Engaging with active social groups is essential to successful aging. Social interaction improves life at all ages but is particularly important for older individuals who need the support of a circle of friends to provide counsel, affection, and the freedom to interact with others. According to Pew Research, 70 percent of respondents over sixty-five enjoy spending time with family members.

Perhaps the most important strategy for successful aging is having a positive attitude about life. Staying curious about the world and finding one's passion promotes joy in life. Acceptance of life's challenges reduces stress. Sharing this positive attitude with others is an important aspect of aging. Passing on knowledge, compassion, and beliefs to the younger generation unites the generations and builds a better world. When older individuals engage in their community, they are leaving a valuable legacy to the world as well as creating a blueprint for successful aging.

—*Yuji Yamada, MD*

For Further Information:

Adams, K. B. "Mid-Life: What Crisis? Planning for 'Successful Aging' at Mid-life." *Psychology Today*, 2012, www.psychologytoday.com/blog/mid-life-what-crisis/201210/planning-successful-aging-mid-life.

Arrison, Sonia. *100 Plus: How the Coming Age of Longevity Will Change Everything, from Careers and Relationships to Family and Faith.* Basic, 2011.

Chappell, Neena L., and Marcus J. Hollander. *Aging in Canada.* Oxford UP, 2013.

Cravit, David. *The New Old: How the Boomers Are Changing Everything—Again*. ECW, 2008.

"Growing Old in America: Expectations vs. Reality." *Pew Research Center*, 29 June 2009, www.pewsocialtrends.org/2009/06/29/growing-old-in-america-expectations-vs-reality.

Gurian, Michael. *The Wonder of Aging: A New Approach to Embracing Life after Fifty*. Atria, 2013.

Horstman, Judith. *The Scientific American Healthy AgingBrain*. Jossey, 2012.

Novelli, Bill. *50+: Igniting a Revolution to Reinvent America*. St. Martin's, 2006.

Reichstadt, J., G. Sengupta, C. A. Depp, et al. "Older Adults' Perspectives on Successful Aging: Qualitative Interviews." *The American Journal of Geriatric Psychiatry: Official Journal of the American Association for Geriatric Psychiatry*, vol. 18, no. 7, 2010, pp. 567-75, ncbi.nlm.nih.gov/pmc/articles/PMC3593659.

Stewart, Martha. *Living the Good Long Life: A Practical Guide to Caring for Yourself and Others*. Clarkson Potter, 2013.

Taubes, Gary. "Live Long and Prosper." *Discover*, vol. 31, no. 8, 2010, p. 80. Accessed 19 May 2015.

Sudden infant death syndrome (SIDS)

Category: Disease/Disorder

Anatomy or system affected: All

Specialties and related fields: Neonatology, pediatrics, psychiatry, psychology

Definition: The abrupt and inexplicable death of any infant or young child, and the most common cause of infant death between the ages of two weeks and one year; postmortem examination fails to demonstrate a definitive cause of death.

Key terms:

apnea: absence of breathing

bradycardia: slowness of the heartbeat

hyperthermia: environmentally influenced elevated body temperature

hypothermia: environmentally influenced lower-than-normal body temperature

hypoxemia: subnormal oxygenation of arterial blood

neonatal: the period of time succeeding birth and continuing through the first twenty-eight days of life

prone: lying face-downward

supine: lying face-upward

tachycardia: rapid beating of the heart

thermolabile: unstable when heated

CAUSES AND SYMPTOMS

Sudden infant death syndrome (SIDS) is considered a subcategory of sudden unexpected infant deaths (SUID) which is a term used to describe the sudden and unexpected death of a baby less than one year of age in which the cause was not obvious prior to

---

> **INFORMATION ON**
> **SUDDEN INFANT DEATH SYNDROME (SIDS)**
>
> **Causes:** Unknown; may involve interrelated genetic, environmental, and social factors (sleep disorders, sleep position, cold weather, overheating, poor socioeconomic conditions, premature birth)
>
> **Symptoms:** Varies and often has no warning signs or symptoms; may include sleep apnea, slow heart rate, low body temperature
>
> **Duration:** Acute, with little warning
>
> **Treatments:** Parent education, placing infants to sleep on their backs

investigation. The term SUID encompasses SIDS, accidental suffocation and strangulation in bed (ASSB), and unknown causes. After investigation, 37 percent of SUIDs are attributed to SIDS. The cause of sudden infant death syndrome is unknown, but a variety of genetic, environmental, and social factors have been associated with an increased risk of SIDS. The current theory for the cause of SIDS is a combination of intrinsic vulnerability such as a baby with dysfunctional or immature cardiorespiratory system and some extrinsic stressor such as prone sleep position or airway obstruction that converges during a critical developmental period. This combination of factors and timing leads to the symptoms of asphyxia, low heart rate, low blood pressure, metabolic acidosis, ineffectual gasping, and death.

The distribution of sudden infant death syndrome is worldwide. Incidence rates vary from 0.12 to 3.0 for every thousand live births. In the United States, rates range from 1.6 to 2.3 for every thousand live births, with considerable ethnic variation: 0.5 among Asians, 1.3 among whites, 1.7 among Latinos, 2.9 among African Americans (5.0 for those of low socioeconomic status), and 5.9 among American Indians.

There are several factors associated with an increased risk of SIDS. Sleeping in the prone position, soft or loose bedding, feeding formula, infant sleeping in a separate room, lack of prenatal care in birth parent, smoking during pregnancy, alcohol or illicit substance use during pregnancy, and overheating are risk factors associated with SIDS. Of note, studies have shown that recent immunization is not a risk factor.

TREATMENT AND THERAPY

Since the causes and mechanisms of death from SIDS is not fully understood, strategies have been implemented that work to reduce the incidence of this syndrome. The American Academy of Pediatrics "Safe to Sleep" campaign is credited with the considerable decline in SIDS from 130.3 deaths per 100,000 live births in 1990 to 33.3 deaths per 100,000 live births in 2019. In 2016, they released updated, evidence-based recommendations for safe infant sleeping. Their recommendations were split into "A" recommendations for those that has solid epidemiological evidence of risk reduction, "B" for those with less evidence, and "C" recommendations based on expert opinion and consensus. "A" level recommendations include placing baby on back to sleep, using a firm sleep surface, breastfeeding, room sharing between caregiver and infant, keeping soft or loose objects away from sleep environment, avoiding overheating, receiving recommended immunizations, and pacifier use. They also recommend that pregnant individuals obtain routine pre-natal care, avoid alcohol and illicit drug use, and avoid smoking. They do not recommend home cardiorespiratory monitors as a strategy to reduce SIDS.

In New Zealand, the government initiated a program of education for parents recommending that the prone sleeping position be avoided, that mothers not smoke, and that breastfeeding be encouraged. A similar education program for parents in Avon, England, was initiated, but it omitted advice on breastfeeding and included suggestions to avoid overheating after a retrospective case-control study that suggested a nearly ninefold relative risk for SIDS from infants sleeping prone. New Zealand and Avon both reported fewer deaths from SIDS after their parental education programs were introduced. The Department of Health extended Avon's campaign nationally.

Focus on risk reduction has had great public health success in reducing SIDS rates, but it is worth mentioning that such a focus is detrimental for parents who have lost a child to SIDS as it can call into question their role in the child's death. Parents who have lost a child to SIDS are grief-stricken. They are not prepared for such a tragedy, and their grief is compounded by guilt, because no definitive cause for SIDS has been identified and, as a result, parental behavior seems to be implicated. Investigations conducted by police, social workers, or others who become involved only add to this guilt. Parents may be confronted by questions of whether they positioned their infant correctly or over-dressed the child. Regardless of these behaviors, however, the factors causing the death may not have been under the parents' control.

SIDS will continue to occur until the exact etiologies of the syndrome, its mechanisms, and its correct treatment are identified. Until that time, it is expected that incidence rates will continue to go down, based on what is now known of the risk factors and recommendations against prone sleeping positions and overwarming.

PERSPECTIVE AND PROSPECTS

The term "sudden infant death syndrome" was popularized by Abraham Berman's book on SIDS in 1969, which grew out of a conference on that subject. Since then, recognition of the syndrome has led to the creation of organizations dealing with it. The Sudden Infant Death Foundation merged, on January 1, 1991, with the National Center for the Prevention of SIDS to form one organization, the Sudden Infant Death Alliance.

In dealing with SIDS, one factor looms most important: Education of parents makes all the difference. In 1991, for example, England's Scarborough district reported a 50 percent fall in the SIDS death rate after parents were advised not to overwarm their small infants. That same year, four other districts in England reported a similar reduction after parents were advised not to let their infants sleep in a prone position. The Foundation for the Study of Infant Deaths and the Department of Health recommend both procedures: a supine sleeping position and prevention of overwarming. Similarly, the United States experienced a significant decrease in SIDS following a "Safe to Sleep" campaign that aimed to educate caregivers about safe sleep.

—*Rachelle G. Ford, MD*

See also: Apnea; Death and dying; Grief and guilt; Hyperthermia and hypothermia; Neonatology; Premature birth; Respiration.

For Further Information:
Beers, Mark H., et al., editors. *The Merck Manual of Diagnosis and Therapy.* 18th ed., Merck Research Laboratories, 2006. Published since 1899, this classic medical book covers SIDS thoroughly and is easy to read.
Behrman, Richard E., Robert M. Kliegman, and Hal B. Jenson, editors. *Nelson Textbook of Pediatrics.* 18th ed., Saunders/Elsevier, 2007. This standard pediatric textbook has been around for years and deservedly so. Its excellent chapter on sudden infant death syndrome is a thorough review of the disease.
Byard, R. W., and H. F. Krous. *"Sudden Infant Death Syndrome: Overview and Update."* Pediatric and Developmental Pathology 6, no. 2, Mar./Apr. 2003, pp. 112-27. Details the research advances in the understanding of SIDS since 1990 and discusses historical background, epidemiology, pathology, and pathogenesis.
Moon, R. Y., R. A. Darnall, L. Feldman-Winter, et al. "SIDS and Other Sleep-Related Infant Deaths: Evidence Base for 2016 Updated Recommendations for a Safe Infant Sleeping Environment." *Pediatrics*, vol. 138, no. 5, 2016, doi.org/10.1542/peds.2016-2940. Accessed 14 Mar. 2022.
Samuels, M. *"Viruses and Sudden Infant Death."* Pediatric Respiratory Reviews, vol. 4, no. 3, Sept. 2003, pp. 178-83. Examines the role of viral respiratory tract inflammation in SIDS, as well as a preceding history of symptoms of minor illness.

SIDS Network, sids-network.org. Provides news about current research, frequently asked questions about SIDS, and fact sheets on such topics as sleep, smoking, and apnea.

Southall, D. P., and M. P. Samuels. *"Reducing Risks in the Sudden Infant Death Syndrome." British Medical Journal*, vol. 304, 1 Feb. 1992, pp. 265-66. These acknowledged experts in SIDS have written a thoughtful, thorough review on reducing the risks of SIDS. They strongly suggest that current interventions and socioeconomic factors need monitoring.

SUFFOCATION. SEE ASPHYXIATION.

SUICIDE

Category: Disease/Disorder
Anatomy or system affected: Psychic-emotional system, all bodily systems
Specialties and related fields: Geriatrics and gerontology, psychiatry, psychology
Definition: The deliberate taking of one's own life, usually the result of a mental disorder although sometimes deliberated in the face of life-threatening physical illness, significant interpersonal stress, or when under the influence of one or more substances of abuse.
Key terms:
"no suicide" contract: an agreement, verbally or in writing, that a suicidal person will not act on his or her urges to commit suicide and instead will take other more adaptive action
psychosomatic: referring to physical symptoms interacting with psychological problems
rational suicide: suicide to avoid suffering when there is no underlying cognitive or psychiatric disorder
ritual suicide: a formal, ceremonial, and proscribed form of suicide performed for social reasons in Japanese history
serotonin: an abundant neurotransmitter in the brain that affects many emotional states
suicide cluster: the occurrence of several suicides immediately following a much-publicized suicide
suicide gesture: a superficial suicidal action in which the intention is not to die but to solicit help

CAUSES AND SYMPTOMS

Suicide is the deliberate taking of one's own life. Most often, suicidal individuals are trying to avoid emotional or physical pain that they believe they cannot bear; sometimes, they are very angry and take their lives to lash out at others. Suicide is seen as a solution to an otherwise insoluble problem. Each year, there are about 500,000 self-inflicted injuries and 30,000 completed suicides, with 200,000 family survivors in the

INFORMATION ON SUICIDE

Causes: Psychological and emotional factors, depression, mental disorders, substance abuse
Symptoms: Depressed and/or anxious mood, hopelessness, loss of normal pleasure in life activities, diminished problem-solving skills, borderline personality disorder, unstable relationships
Duration: Temporary or recurrent
Treatments: Psychotherapy, counseling, drug therapy

United States. In 2006, there were 33,000 suicides, and estimates suggest there were between twelve and twenty-five times as many attempted suicides the same year. Women attempt suicide more often than men, but men complete suicide more often than women because men tend to use more lethal means, such as a gun. It should also be noted that adolescents and the elderly are two high-risk groups.

When an individual contemplates suicide to avoid the physical pain of a terminal illness and does not have a mental disorder, that form of suicidal thought is often called "rational" suicide. This does not imply that this form of suicide is appropriate, moral, or legal but merely that the suicidal thoughts do not arise from a mental disorder (nonrational). Social views on rational suicide vary by culture. For example, many Dutch people consider rational suicide to be acceptable, whereas most Americans do not.

Most suicidal people encountered by physicians, psychologists, social workers, and other mental health professionals experience suicidal thoughts as a result of a mental disorder. The suicidal thoughts and impulses are seen as symptoms of the underlying disorder and require treatment just as any other symptom. The treatment may involve protecting the person against his or her suicidal actions, even to the point of involuntary commitment to a mental hospital.

The rationale behind society's willingness temporarily to deny suicidal individuals' usual civil rights by involuntary commitment is that they are considered to be not "acting in their right mind" by virtue of their mental illness. Thus, they deserve the protection of society until their illness is treated. In fact, suicidal thoughts usually do abate when suicidal patients are treated. The vast majority of these individuals are appreciative afterward; they are glad that they were prevented from killing themselves, as they no longer wish to do so.

The most common mental illness that causes suicidal thoughts is depression. In fact, suicidal thoughts are considered to be a symptom of clinical depression. Other mental disorders associated with suicidal ideation include anxiety disorders such as panic disorder, psychotic disorders such as schizophrenia, substance use disorders such as alcohol dependence, and certain personality disorders such as borderline personality disorder.

Although suicide may occur at any time of the year, there is a seasonal variation in its peak incidence. Suicides are most common in both men and women in May; women have a second peak around October and November. This seasonal variation may be attributable to seasonal differences in the incidence of depression.

Suicide appears to have multiple factors involved in its etiology. There are biological, psychological, social, and contextual factors that interact in a complex way to contribute to the causes of suicide in any given individual. The biological factors include genetic contributions to the development of mental disorders such as clinical depression. This may be attributable in part to problems in the neurotransmitter systems in the brain, such as those that control levels of serotonin and dopamine.

Alcohol and other substances of abuse may also cause suicidal ideation. Suicidal thoughts may occur while the individual is using, intoxicated, or in withdrawal. Paradoxically, suicidal thoughts may also arise while the patient is taking antidepressant medications. Fortunately, this side effect is uncommon. and most antidepressant medications do not have such effects. The fact that suicidal thoughts may occur even when on medication, however, underscores the need for individuals taking medications to stay in regular contact with the prescribing physician and to never discontinue their medication without medical consultation. If family members observe a depressed individual taking medication become more depressed, hostile or angry, or suddenly happy or relieved, or if the individual has no apparent response to the medication, then it would be wise to consult with the prescribing physician. This is especially true for family members of children or elders on antidepressant medication.

Psychological factors contributing to suicide include a depressed and/or anxious mood, hopelessness, and a loss of normal pleasure in life activities. Chronically depressed people often have diminished problem-solving skills during periods of depression and can see no way out of their difficulties; suicide is seen as the only solution. There are also personality characteristics that contribute to suicide. In women, borderline personality disorder is often associated with suicide attempts. This disorder is characterized by widely fluctuating moods, rages, feelings of emptiness or boredom, and unstable relationships.

The social factors involved in suicide include cultural acceptance or rejection of suicide. Historically, Japanese people have accepted ritual suicide within their culture and somewhat sanction suicide as a response to a severe loss of face or social esteem. This does not mean that they embrace it, but rather that the history contributes to cultural norms where this is thought of as an option for dealing with shame. Similarly, the Dutch government has legalized rational suicide as an option for dying. In contrast, most Americans have a more negative view of the suicide act. Other social factors that increase the likelihood of suicide include social instability, divorce, unemployment, immigration, and exposure to violence as a child. In the United States, European Americans commit suicide more often than African Americans. Native Americans have a high incidence of suicide. In general, good social support reduces the risk of suicide.

Some patients engage in suicidal gestures; that is, they say they want to kill themselves and take actions such as swallowing some pills or superficially cutting their wrists, but there is no real intention to die. They act this way as a cry for help. For some, this may be the only way to receive attention for what troubles them. Unfortunately, the suicide gesture may go awry and unintended death may occur. Anyone who speaks of suicide or engages in what may appear to be a gesture should be taken seriously.

Most people who are suicidal have ambivalent feelings: Part of them wants to die, part does not. This is one of the reasons that the majority of suicidal people tell others of their intention in advance of their attempts. Most have visited their personal physician in the months prior to the suicide. Adolescents sometimes hint at their wish to die by giving away their prized possessions just prior to an attempt.

Contextual factors, or the circumstances in which people find themselves, can also contribute to individuals attempting suicide. Access to means of self-harm, such as weapons or drugs, can increase the likelihood of a suicide attempt. Similarly, physical isolation from others can also increase the odds, as there is no one to readily intervene. Even painful emotional or physical states, such as exhaustion or those that might be brought on by substance use, can set the stage for impulsive behavior to increase the likelihood of suicide attempts. In contrast, simply talking to someone about suicidal thoughts will not cause someone to commit suicide and instead may be a way to get help from a professional.

Anyone experiencing suicidal thoughts should be thoroughly evaluated by a professional trained in the assessment of suicidal patients. If the risk of suicide is considered to be high enough, the patient will have to be protected. This may require hospitalization, either voluntary or involuntary. It may mean removing suicidal means from that person's environment, such as removing guns from the home. Having someone stay with the patient at all times may be required. These steps should be individualized, taking into account the patient's situation.

Treatment of the underlying cause of the suicidal ideation is very important. Depression and anxiety can be treated with medications and/or psychotherapy. There are treatment programs for alcoholism and drug abuse. Usually, successful treatment of the underlying mental disorder results in the suicidal thoughts going away.

While they await the resolution of the suicidal ideation, patients need to be offered support and hope. Sometimes, a "no suicide" contract is helpful. This is simply a commitment on the part of the patient not to act on any suicidal thoughts and to contact the health professional if the urges become worse. While this contract may be written down, it is usually verbal.

Suicide prevention includes the early detection and management of the mental disorders associated with suicide. Because social isolation increases the risk of suicide, patients should be encouraged to develop and actively maintain strong social supports such as family, friends, and other social groups (church, clubs, and sports teams).

It may also be helpful to provide counseling to teenagers after an acquaintance has committed suicide, as this may prevent social contagion and suicide clusters. A suicide cluster is when several individuals (often teenagers) commit suicide after learning of the suicide of an acquaintance or a person who is attractive to them, such as a music or film star. Suicide clusters have increased among the young.

Family members of a suicide victim often go through a grieving process which is more severe than that which occurs after death from other causes. The stigma of suicide and mental illness is strong, and surviving family members often have greater feelings of both guilt and abandonment. Family survivors also have increased psychosomatic complaints, behavioral and emotional problems, and risk of suicide themselves. Referral to a suicide survivor group may be helpful.

TREATMENT AND THERAPY

An understanding of the causes, detection, and treatment of suicide has led to the development of a number of suicide hotlines and suicide prevention centers. There is evidence that, after these support groups are introduced into a community, the suicide rate for young women decreases. It is not yet known if they have any effect on other groups, such as young men or the elderly.

Most people who contemplate suicide do not seek professional treatment even if they tell people around them of their suicidal ideas. Thus, it is important for physicians, clergy, teachers, parents, and mental health workers to remain alert to the possibility of suicidal thoughts in those in their care. Someone who is depressed or very anxious should be asked about suicidal thoughts. Such a question will not plant the idea in his or her head, and the person may feel relieved after being asked. Once someone with suicidal ideation is identified, evaluation and treatment should proceed quickly. The following sample composite cases illustrate the application of the concepts described in the overview.

Mary is a seventeen-year-old senior in high school. She is from a broken home and was severely abused by her father prior to her parents' divorce ten years ago. Her teachers think that she is a bright underachiever who has a rather dramatic personality. Her friends see her as moody and easily angered. Her relationships with boyfriends are intense and always end with deep feelings of hurt and abandonment. Her mother is best described as cold, aloof, and preoccupied with herself.

Mary is brought to the school counselor by one of her friends when Mary threatens to kill herself and superficially scratches her wrists with a safety pin. The counselor learns that Mary has just broken up with her boyfriend, a young man at a local junior college. She is devastated. When she tried to tell her mother about it, her mother seemed uninterested and said that Mary always makes too much of such little things. It was the next morning that she scratched herself in front of her friend.

While more information is needed, this case illustrates a suicide gesture. In this case, Mary does not want to die but instead wants someone to realize how distressed she is. She feels rejected by her boyfriend and then by her mother. One can suspect a gesture rather than a serious suicide attempt by the superficial, nonlethal means (scratching with a safety pin) and by the likelihood of discovery (done in front of a friend).

Here is a second case. Tom is a forty-eight-year-old accountant. He is separated from his wife and three children and lives alone in an apartment. He has no real friends, only drinking buddies. Like his father and two uncles, Tom is an alcoholic. Each day after work, he stops at his favorite bar and drinks between eight and twelve beers.

He is brought to the emergency room of the local hospital by the police, who found him sitting on the steps of a church sobbing. He threatened to kill himself if his wife did not take him back. The emergency room doctor noted the strong odor of alcohol on his breath and ordered a blood alcohol test, which showed that he was legally intoxicated. Tom insisted that he would kill himself by running in front of a moving bus if he could not be with his family. The emergency room doctor had Tom's belt, pocketknife, and other potentially dangerous items taken from him and arranged for a staff member to sit with him until he was sober. Six hours later, his blood alcohol had returned to near zero. Tom no longer felt despondent and had no more suicidal thoughts. He was embarrassed by his statements a few hours before. An alcoholism counselor was called, and outpatient treatment for his alcoholism was arranged.

This case illustrates suicidal ideation caused by alcohol intoxication. As often happens, the suicidal ideation resolves when the patient becomes sober. The primary treatment is for the underlying addictive disorder.

Here is a third case. Sally is a fifty-three-year-old married mother of two. She is a part-time hairdresser and normally a very active, happy person. For the past three weeks, however, she has gradually lost all interest in her job, her children, her home, and her hobbies. She feels irritable and sad most of the time. Although she is tired, she does not sleep well at night, waking up very early each morning, unable to return to sleep. She is worried by the fact that she is having intrusive thoughts of killing herself. Sally imagines she could end all this dreariness by overdosing on sleeping pills and never waking up. She is a strict Catholic and knows it is against her religion to commit suicide. She calls her parish priest.

After a brief conversation, her priest meets her at the office of a psychiatrist who acts as a consultant for the diocese. The psychiatrist diagnoses major depression as the cause of Sally's suicidal ideation. She has a good social support network, so the psychiatrist decides to treat her as an outpatient and has her agree to a "no suicide" contract. Sally is also started on antidepressant medication, which gradually lifts her depression over a period of two to three weeks. Simultaneously, her suicidal thoughts leave her.

This case illustrates suicidal thoughts caused by depression. If Sally had been more depressed or her suicidal urges stronger, she would probably have needed hospitalization. If she had required hospitalization and had refused to go voluntarily, the psychiatrist could have had her committed according to the laws of the state where he practiced. Most states require a signed statement by two physicians or one physician and a licensed clinical psychologist. They must attest that the patient is a danger to himself or herself and that no less restrictive form of treatment would suffice.

Finally, here is a fourth case. Harry is a sixty-seven-year-old resident of a hospital, where he has been for the past two years. He has a serious neurological disorder called amyotrophic lateral sclerosis (also called Lou Gehrig's disease). It has caused progressive weakness such that he cannot even breathe on his own. Harry is permanently connected to a respirator attached to a tracheotomy tube in his throat. He has few visitors and mostly stares off and thinks.

Harry tells his nurse that he is "sick of it all" and wants his doctors to disconnect him from the respirator and let him die. His neurologist requests a psychiatric evaluation. The psychiatrist confirms the patient's wish to die. There is no evidence of dementia or other cognitive disorder, nor is the patient showing any evidence of a mental illness. Subsequently, a meeting is called of the hospital ethics committee to make recommendations. Membership on the committee includes physicians, nurses, an ethicist, a local minister, and the hospital attorney.

This case illustrates a difficult example of rational suicide request. The patient has a desire to die and is not suffering from any mental disorder. In this case, he is requesting not to take his own life actively but to be allowed to die passively by removal of the respirator. Some people do not consider this to be suicide at all. They make a distinction between passively allowing a natural process of dying to occur and actively taking one's own life. If this patient requested a lethal overdose of potassium to be injected into his intravenous tubes, such action would be considered suicide and ethically different. In either event, these matters are more ethical, social, and legal than psychiatric.

PERSPECTIVE AND PROSPECTS

Throughout history, there have been numerous examples of suicide. In Western culture, early views on the subject were mainly from a moral perspective and suicide was viewed as a sin. Mental illness in general was poorly understood and often thought of as weakness of character, possession by evil spirits, or willful bad behavior. Thus, mental illness was stigmatized. Even though society now has a better medical understanding of mental illness, there is still a stigma attached to mental illness and to suicide. This stigma contributes to underdiagnosis and undertreatment of suicidal individuals, as many sufferers are reluctant to come forth with their symptoms.

Suicide remains an important public health problem. In 2006, it was the eleventh most common cause of death in the United States (although it was third for adolescents and second for young adults). Each year, there are about thirty thousand known suicides in the United States. The actual incidence may be higher because an unknown number of accidental deaths or untreated illnesses may actually be undiagnosed suicides. For every suicide death, between eight and twenty-five other individuals attempt suicide.

Unfortunately, most cases of suicidal ideation never come to the attention of health professionals. Therefore, when someone talks of suicide, a high index of suspicion should be maintained. Those people who express suicidal thoughts should be taken seriously and thoroughly evaluated. Increased levels of awareness of suicide may help to improve detection and treatment of this potentially preventable cause of death. Research in this area continues to focus on prevention and early identification and treatment for individuals who are distressed.

—*Peter M. Hartmann, MD;*
updated by Nancy A. Piotrowski, PhD

See also Addiction; Alcoholism; Antidepressants; Anxiety; Death and dying; Dementias; Depression; Euthanasia; Grief and guilt; Hypochondriasis; Midlife crisis; Neurosis; Panic attacks; Phobias; Postpartum depression; Post-traumatic stress disorder; Psychiatric disorders; Psychiatry; Psychiatry, child and adolescent; Psychiatry, geriatric; Psychoanalysis; Psychosomatic disorders; Puberty and adolescence; Schizophrenia; Stress; Terminally ill: Extended care.

For Further Information:

DePaulo, J. Raymond, Jr., and Leslie Alan Horvitz. *Understanding Depression: What We Know and What You Can Do About It.* New York: Wiley, 2003. A leading expert on depression examines the disease's nature, causes, effects, and treatments.

Hafen, Brent Q., and Kathryn J. Frandsen. *Youth Suicide: Depression and Loneliness.* 2d ed. Evergreen, Colo.: Cordillera Press, 1986. An excellent review of all aspects of teenage suicide, with practical suggestions for helping the suicidal young person.

Jamison, Kay Redfield. *Night Falls Fast: Understanding Suicide.* New York: Alfred A. Knopf, 2000. Jamison, a distinguished psychologist and academic, brings a rare combination of personal and academic experience to bear in this monumental work on suicide.

Kolf, June Cerza. *Standing in the Shadow: Help and Encouragement for Suicide Survivors.* New York: Baker Books, 2002. The author, a veteran of hospice work, addresses the impact of suicide on family members and friends, and explores such emotions as forgiveness and depression, as well as the search for answers.

Koplewicz, Harold S. *More than Moody: Recognizing and Treating Adolescent Depression.* New York: Penguin, 2003. A leading clinician and researcher helps parents distinguish between normal teenage angst and depression, examining the warning signs, risk factors, and key behaviors, as well as treatment options.

Lester, David. *Making Sense of Suicide: An In-Depth Look at Why People Kill Themselves.* Philadelphia: Charles Press, 1997. This book may be helpful for beginning counselors and family members or friends interested in learning more about suicidal behavior.

Peck, M. Scott. *Denial of the Soul: Spiritual and Medical Perspectives on Euthanasia and Mortality.* New York: Random House, 1998. This book discusses controversial issues related to euthanasia and suicide.

Roesch, Roberta. *The Encyclopedia of Depression.* 2d ed. New York: Facts On File, 2001. This volume was written for both laypersons and professionals. Covers all aspects of depression, including bereavement, grief, and mourning. The appendixes include references, self-help groups, national associations, and institutes.

Suicide Awareness Voices of Education. www.save.org. Offers resources for suicide prevention, suicide survivors, and for families coping with a suicide loss.

SUPPLEMENTS

Category: Treatment
Anatomy or system affected: All
Specialties and related fields: Alternative medicine, family medicine, internal medicine, nutrition
Definition: Chemical compounds, concentrated into pills, powders, and capsules, that are taken to prevent or treat diseases.

THE ROLE OF SUPPLEMENTS

Adequate nutrition is the foundation of good health. Everyone needs the four basic nutrients: water, carbohydrates, proteins, and fats. It is important to choose the proper foods to deliver these nutrients and, as necessary, to complement the diet with supplements.

Health-conscious adults have heard the message repeatedly that they can get the vitamins they need from the foods they eat, but surveys have shown that people in many countries fail to eat adequate amounts of fruit, vegetables, whole grains, and low-fat dairy foods. Should public health officials or registered dieticians recommend that people take supplements to compensate for poor eating habits? The answer to this question can be found in a discussion of vitamin supplements.

The 1990s brought to light much new information about human nutrition, its effects on the body, and the role that it plays in disease. The fuel for the body's engine comes directly from the food that one eats, which contains many vital nutrients. Nutrients come in the form of vitamins, minerals, enzymes, water, amino acids, carbohydrates, and lipids (fats). These nutrients provide people with the basic materials that human bodies need to sustain life.

One of the latest types of dietary supplements are nutraceuticals. These supplements are obtained from naturally derived chemicals in plants, called photonutrients, that make the plants biologically active. They are not nutrients in the classic sense. They are what determine a plant's color, ability to resist disease, and flavor.

Nutritionists have discovered that fruits and vegetables, grains, and legumes contain other healthful nutrients called phytochemicals. Researchers have identified thousands of phytochemicals and have the ability to remove these chemical compounds and concentrate them into pills, powders, and capsules. Phytochemicals are believed to be powerful ammunition in the war against cancer and other cellular mutations. In simple

Pharmacies and supermarkets in the U.S. sell a large variety of vitamin dietary supplements. Photo via Wikimedia Commons. [Public domain.]

terms, cancer is a mutation of body cells through a multistep process. Phytochemicals are hypothesized to fight that disease by stopping one or more of the steps that lead to cancer. For example, a cancer process can be kindled when a carcinogenic molecule invades a cell, possibly from foods eaten or from air breathed. Sulforaphane, a phytochemical commonly found in broccoli, is then hypothesized to activate an enzyme process that removes the carcinogen from the cell before harm is done.

Researchers and pharmaceutical companies sell concentrated forms of various phytochemicals found in such vegetables as broccoli, brussels sprouts, cauliflower, and cabbage. Because no single supplement can possibly compete with nature, some nutritionists recommend a shopping basket full of fruits and vegetables, as opposed to using expensive bottled supplements. Tomatoes, for example, are believed to contain an estimated ten thousand different phytochemicals.

Natural food supplements can be high in certain nutrients. Examples are aloe vera, bee pollen, fish oils, flaxseed, primrose oil, ginseng, ginkgo biloba, garlic, and oat bran. In general, natural food supplements are composed of by-products of foods that can provide a multitude of health benefits. One caution, however, is that supplements of this type may not have the same

kind of quality control or oversight as medications prescribed by a doctor and bought from a pharmacy. As such, the effects of supplements may vary from pill to pill and bottle to bottle.

THE PROMISE OF ANTIOXIDANTS

No discussion of supplements would be complete without mention of antioxidants. They are a group of vitamins, minerals, and enzymes that help to protect the body from the formation of free radicals. Free radicals are groups of atoms that can cause damage to cells and thus impair the immune system. This damage is also thought to be the basis for the aging process. Free radicals are believed to be formed through exposure to radiation and toxic chemicals such as cigarette smoke, as well as overexposure to the sun's rays.

Some common antioxidants are vitamin A and its precursor, beta carotene; vitamin C; and vitamin E. Zinc and the trace mineral selenium are thought to play an important role in neutralizing free radicals. Each vitamin or mineral has a recommended daily allowance (RDA).

Some in the field of nutrition have recommended higher supplementation doses of antioxidants and specific use of four antioxidant supplements-vitamins C and E, selenium, and mixed carotenes-to protect the immune system even further. Recommendations such as this are numerous and related to different kinds of supplement use, and they must be weighed carefully against data obtained from controlled clinical trials. While many of the substances touted as beneficial to health may have some benefits, supplements can be harmful in the wrong person; at the wrong dose; if taken in combination with the wrong medications or diet; or if taken in the presence of certain health conditions. For example, it is possible to overdose on vitamins such as A, B, and E, or on iron supplements. Some supplements, like St. John's wort, may create a side effect of light sensitivity, and discontinuing drugs such as valerian root can lead to heart problems. Also, it is easy to succumb to the temptation to seek "health in a bottle" instead of engaging in proven preventive practices. For these reasons, careful consideration and consultation with one's doctor should occur before embarking on any regimen of supplements.

PERSPECTIVE AND PROSPECTS

Use of supplements is based both on modern research and development and on discoveries by mainstream scientists about the benefits of various substances. Substances such as garlic and aloe vera are examples of home remedies that have shown some promise for different kinds of ailments. Natural supplements have been used for centuries in many parts of the world as alternative medicines.

Considered and careful examination of supplement regimens in controlled clinical trials will serve as the ultimate test on the utility of these substances for health purposes. Simultaneously, consumers must remain aware that personal use of these supplements may, at times, be somewhat experimental. Quality control concerns and interactions between supplements and prescribed medications are an important consideration. Additionally, knowledge of the supplements found in pills or popular beverages and how they may interact with street drugs of different types is also important in order to avoid unnecessary harm. This is especially true for children and elders.

—Lisa Levin Sobczak, RNC;
updated by Nancy A. Piotrowski, PhD

See also Aging; Alternative medicine; Antioxidants; Digestion; Ergogenic aids; Food biochemistry; Herbal medicine; Macronutrients; Malnutrition; Nutrition; Osteoporosis; Over-the-counter medications; Phytochemicals; Self-medication; Vitamins and minerals.

For Further Information:

Balch, James F., and Phyllis A. Balch. *Prescription for Nutritional Healing: A Practical A to Z Reference to Drug-Free Remedies Using Vitamins, Minerals, Herbs, and Food Supplements.* 4th rev. ed. Garden City Park, N.Y.: Avery, 2008.

Hendler, Sheldon Saul. *The Doctors' Vitamin and Mineral Encyclopedia.* New York: Simon & Schuster, 1990.

Murray, Michael. *The Pill Book Guide to Natural Medicines: Vitamins, Minerals, Nutritional Supplements, Herbs, and Other Natural Products.* New York: Bantam, 2002.

The PDR Family Guide to Nutritional Supplements: An Authoritative A-to-Z Resource on the One Hundred Most Popular Nutritional Therapies and Nutraceuticals. New York: Ballantine Books, 2001.

Weil, Andrew. *Eight Weeks to Optimum Health: A Proven Program for Taking Full Advantage of Your Body's Natural Healing Power.* Rev. ed. New York: Ballantine Books, 2007.

SURGERY, GENERAL

Category: Specialty
Anatomy or system affected: All
Specialties and related fields: Anesthesiology, radiology
Definition: A field of medicine that involves a wide range of surgical procedures, from the simple removal of warts and bunions in the doctor's office to complex organ transplantation requiring a large staff in the operating room.

Key terms:
aseptic techniques: procedures that allow surgeons to operate in a germ-free environment
excision: the surgical removal of an organ or tissue

SCIENCE AND PROFESSION

In all probability, surgery has been practiced as long as humans have had cutting tools. Ample reports of battlefield amputations exist almost from the beginning of reported time. Historians tell of rough field surgery, the hacking off of wounded limbs and the sealing of the wounds by searing the lacerated flesh. There are even suggestions that ancient civilizations, such as that of the Egyptians, practiced trepanning, cutting into the skull to operate on the brain.

Until the latter half of the nineteenth century, surgery was a brutal, dirty, and dangerous practice. About this time, the relationship between microorganisms and diseases was first enunciated, a relationship which explained why so many surgery patients sickened and died. It was also at this time that anesthetics were developed, which for the first time allowed the surgeon to deaden the patient's pain.

Surgery today is one of the most respected medical specialties, requiring full training in the disciplines of medicine, as well as years of extensive work in surgical procedures. After becoming physicians, candidates for surgery spend years working under established surgeons learning the techniques that they will use in practice. They are subjected to intensive examination and receive certification only when their peers are convinced that they can perform their duties capably.

The tools and techniques of surgery that the surgical candidate must master present multiple challenges. In their training phase, surgeons learn to become skilled in the manipulation of all the basic instruments used in surgery, such as the various designs of scalpels, scissors, retractors, forceps, and sutures. The training surgeon learns a wide variety of stitching techniques and the materials used in suturing. Most challenging perhaps is mastery of the many new techniques and instruments that modern surgeons use.

After training and certification, some surgeons elect to practice general surgery. As the term implies, this field covers such diverse areas of the body as the stomach, gallbladder, liver, intestines, appendix, breasts, thyroid gland, salivary glands, main arteries

and veins, lumps under the skin, hernias, and hemorrhoids. Other surgeons choose to specialize in disciplines that require still more training, such as heart surgery, bone (or orthopedic) surgery, and eye (or ophthalmic) surgery, to name some of the more prevalent specialties.

Modern surgery is a far-ranging practice involving all body structures and systems. It is also a practice that sees constant advancements and improvements in operating techniques, in instrumentation and tools, and in high-tech equipment. Microsurgery, in which the surgeon uses a microscope to view the operating field and manipulates tiny instruments to repair or excise tissue, was virtually unheard of at the middle of the twentieth century. It is now common practice in virtually every surgical facility in the United States. At one time, a severed limb could never be reconnected,

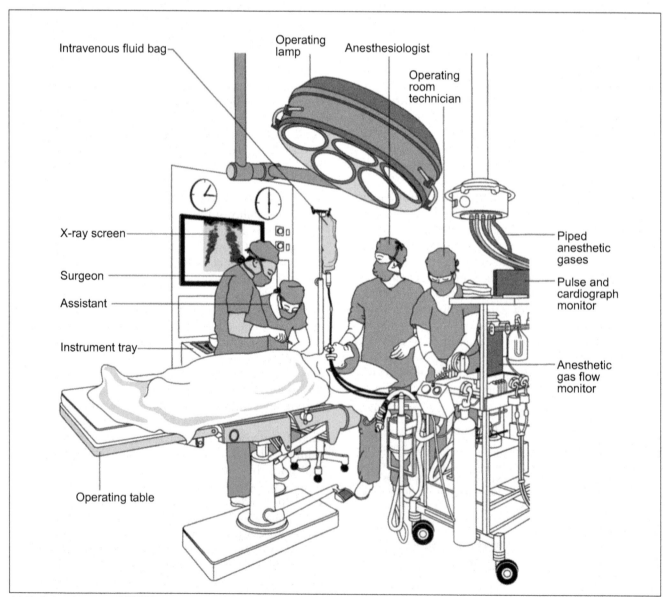

A typical operating room. ©*EBSCO*

largely because it was impossible to repair severed nerves. Now, because of microsurgery, arms, legs, hands, digits, and other severed body parts can be stitched back on to the body, often with much of their mobility restored.

Much minor surgery takes place in the physician's office or clinic. These procedures are generally simple, involving the excision of skin growths such as warts or cancers, hemorrhoids, and other surface conditions. Emergency surgery in the office, clinic, or emergency room may be necessary to open an airway for a patient whose breathing is impaired or to remove obstructions.

Major surgery usually requires a hospital stay, and its main characteristics are anesthesia and aseptic technique. Anesthesia may be local, regional, or general. For local anesthesia, anesthetic is injected into the site of the operation. The patient is usually fully awake during the surgery but feels no pain in the affected area. In regional anesthesia, a whole part of the body is anesthetized, such as a leg or an arm. As with local anesthesia, the patient is awake during the procedure but may be sedated for comfort. In general anesthesia, the patient is put to sleep and immobilized, usually by injections, and inhaled anesthetics are administered throughout the course of the operation.

To create an aseptic, germ-free environment, the operating room and everything in it are subjected to rigorous sterilization. Surgeons and all operating room staff scrub with antiseptic soaps. They don complete uniforms of sterilized cloth or paper: caps, masks, gowns, gloves, and foot coverings. Avoiding transmission of disease in the operating room can be said to be as important as the operation itself. It is vital that the patient be made safe from infection by the staff and from pathogenic organisms in the ambient atmosphere of the hospital.

It is equally important that staff be protected from infection by the patient. Operating room personnel are particularly vulnerable to blood-borne infections, such as hepatitis B and human immunodeficiency virus (HIV). Surgery can be a bloody procedure. In some operations, copious blood spurts are common, and the likelihood of staff being spattered is high, as is the possibility of disease transmission. It is possible that there will be a cut or tear in the staff's protective clothing and that the patient's blood or other body fluids can make contact with an abrasion on the body or even land on mucous membranes of the mouth, nose, and throat, where they can infect the caregiver. This has happened so often that the U.S. government has issued rigorous guidelines to high-risk health care personnel-particularly operating room staff-detailing specific procedures to follow to avoid disease transmission.

DIAGNOSTIC AND TREATMENT TECHNIQUES

The surgeon is rarely the first physician whom the patient sees. Usually, a primary care physician makes a diagnosis and may confer with or send the patient to a specialist for confirmation of the diagnosis. When surgery is recommended, the surgeon confers with the primary care physician and/or the consulting specialist and is fully apprised of the patient's condition. He or she reviews the patient's history and inspects all relevant documents and diagnostic reports, such as X rays, computed tomography (CT) scans, and other information that he or she needs to plan and perform the procedure.

For the most part, surgeons deal with their patients only in the immediate context of the operation. They meet before the operation, and surgeons look in on patients afterward to check their progress and recovery. In some cases, follow-up visits to the surgeon are required.

In the operating room, the surgeon assembles the staff needed for the particular procedure. There will be an anesthesiologist, perhaps other specialized surgeons, and various general and specialized operating room nurses. The surgeon or the staff will also order everything needed for the procedure. There is an enormous range of specialized equipment that surgeons can use in their procedures. Cardiac surgeons use heart-lung machines, which take over the task of circulating the patient's blood and allow the surgeon to open and enter the heart itself. The neurosurgeon may operate through specialized microscopic instruments.

A catalog of specialized endoscopes is now available to surgeons, many of which allow them to operate through a tiny hole in the patient's skin, rather than having to make massive cuts with a scalpel. Pulmonary surgeons use a bronchoscope to look down into the patient's bronchial tubes, where they can perform such surgical operations as removing obstructions and excising cancerous tissue. Gastrointestinal surgeons use a gastroscope both to investigate conditions in the stomach and to take small tissue samples for biopsy. Colon and rectal surgeons use a colonoscope to remove polyps from the colon and rectum, a major step in the prevention and treatment of colon cancer. Major surgery, however, still involves cutting the patient open to repair what has gone wrong inside the body. Fortunately, this procedure is now safer and more specialized than it has ever been before.

Management of disease in the United States has reached the point where there are surgical specialties to cover virtually all parts of the body individually. Some surgeons specialize in individual organs, such as the heart, lungs, brain, eyes, and ears. Some surgeons specialize in body systems such as bones or circulation.

Furthermore, many surgeons hone their skills in certain specialized surgical techniques and become so adept that they are recognized as experts in highly complex and critical procedures, such as repairing detached retinas, performing heart transplants, correcting slipped disks, or sealing brain aneurysms.

Surgeons are major inventors and designers. Much of the instrumentation and many of the surgical tools that are used in the operating room were invented by surgeons. They often direct the fabrication of specialized tools and instruments to help them in their work. Most of the metal and plastic prostheses implanted to replace damaged internal structures were designed by surgeons. Orthopedic surgeons design prosthetic hips, knees, and other implants. Ophthalmic surgeons design corneal implants. The specialized surgeon knows his or her area of the body better than anyone else does and can visualize what sort of equipment or device is needed to improve the patient's condition.

Surgeons are also at the forefront of major technical innovations that reach across the entire surgical field. They are adept at recognizing potential applications for new technology and adapting it to surgery. For example, fiber-optic science has been applied in surgical endoscopes. Cryosurgery, a technique of freezing tissue, is used in a wide range of procedures, from the removal of hemorrhoids to the reattachment of retinas.

Laser technology is employed in hundreds of surgical procedures. The laser is used for making incisions, for repairing tissue, and for excising diseased tissue, among other applications. One of the major areas that can benefit from the unique advantages of laser use is eye surgery. Ophthalmic surgeons use lasers to relieve diabetic retinopathy, glaucoma, macular degeneration, cataracts, and certain tumors, as well as to reattach torn retinas.

One of the critical qualities of the competent surgeon is judgment. No matter how thoroughly a surgeon may prepare for a procedure, there may be some surprises on the operating table. The surgeon learns the patient's history and status and also reviews all the appropriate diagnostic documents, X rays, and other visualizations, but unforeseen complications may arise during the operation. The surgeon must have the experience and competence to deal with the unexpected.

PERSPECTIVE AND PROSPECTS

Up to the mid-nineteenth century, surgical procedures were probably responsible for as many deaths as cures. Today, surgery extends the lives of millions: heart disease victims, cancer patients, and victims of infection and accidents. Surgery helps improve the quality of life for patients with arthritis and rheumatism, gastrointestinal problems, lung disorders, and circulation problems.

Furthermore, surgery is entering new areas of medicine. For example, operations can now be performed in the uterus to correct anomalies in unborn fetuses. Many more such procedures are predicted for the future.

New areas of surgical expertise are opening constantly; new techniques, instrumentation, and equipment are making many old procedures obsolete. Practicing surgeons face a constant challenge in keeping abreast of what is happening all over the world and deciding what avenues to explore for the benefit of their patients.

—*C. Richard Falcon*

See also Abscess drainage; Adrenalectomy; Amputation; Anesthesia; Anesthesiology; Aneurysmectomy; Appendectomy; Biopsy; Bladder removal; Bone marrow transplantation; Breast biopsy; Breast surgery; Bunions; Bypass surgery; Cardiac surgery; Cataract surgery; Catheterization; Cervical procedures; Cesarean section; Cholecystectomy; Cleft lip and palate repair; Colorectal polyp removal; Colorectal surgery; Corneal transplantation; Craniotomy; Cryosurgery; Cyst removal; Disk removal; Ear surgery; Electrocauterization; Endarterectomy; Endometrial biopsy; Eye surgery; Face lift and blepharoplasty; Facial transplantation; Fistula repair; Ganglion removal; Gender reassignment surgery; Gastrectomy; Grafts and grafting; Hair transplantation; Hammertoe correction; Heart transplantation; Heart valve replacement; Heel spur removal; Hemorrhoid banding and removal; Hernia repair; Hypospadias repair and urethroplasty; Hysterectomy; Kidney transplantation; Kneecap removal; Laceration repair; Laminectomy and spinal fusion; Laparoscopy; Laryngectomy; Laser use in surgery; Liposuction; Liver transplantation; Lung surgery; Mastectomy and lumpectomy; Myomectomy; Nail removal; Nasal polyp removal; Nephrectomy; Neurosurgery; Ophthalmology; Oral and maxillofacial surgery; Orthopedic surgery; Parathyroidectomy; Penile implant surgery; Periodontal surgery; Phlebitis; Plastic surgery; Prostate gland removal; Refractive eye surgery; Rhinoplasty and submucous resection; Shunts; Skin lesion removal; Sphincterectomy; Splenectomy; Sterilization; Stone removal; Surgery, pediatric; Surgical procedures; Surgical technologists; Sympathectomy; Tattoo removal; Tendon repair; Testicular surgery; Thoracic surgery; Thyroidectomy; Tonsillectomy and adenoid removal; Tracheostomy; Transfusion; Transplantation; Tumor removal; Ulcer surgery; Vagotomy; Varicose vein removal; Vasectomy.

For Further Information:
Brunicardi, F. Charles, et al., eds. *Schwartz's Principles of Surgery.* 9th ed. New York: McGraw-Hill, 2010. A standard textbook on the topic. Intended for practicing surgeons, but valuable to general readers for its details.
Griffith, H. Winter. *Complete Guide to Symptoms, Illness, and Surgery.* Revised and updated by Stephen Moore and Kenneth Yoder. 5th ed. New York: Perigee, 2006. Covers more than five hundred diseases and disorders and includes information about causes and risk factors, preventive techniques, diagnostic tests, and surgical treatment.

Litin, Scott C., ed. *Mayo Clinic Family Health Book*. 4th ed. New York: HarperResource, 2009. This book covers the surgical aspects of medicine admirably, with clear and concise descriptions of surgical procedures.

Mulholland, Michael W., et al., eds. *Greenfield's Surgery: Scientific Principles and Practice*. 4th ed. Philadelphia: Lippincott Williams & Wilkins, 2006. Covers scientific reviews of wound biology, inflammatory mediators, immunology, and the management of trauma and transplantation in the first part and an overview of surgical practice according to anatomic region and specialty in the second part.

Zollinger, Robert M., Jr., and Robert M. Zollinger, Sr. *Zollinger's Atlas of Surgical Operations*. 8th ed. New York: McGraw-Hill, 2003. A comprehensive examination of surgery. Covers basic surgical anatomy and vascular, gynecologic, gastrointestinal, and miscellaneous abdominal procedures.

SURGERY, PEDIATRIC

Category: Specialty
Anatomy or system affected: All
Specialties and related fields: Anesthesiology, general surgery, neonatology, pediatrics
Definition: The surgical correction of medical conditions of infants and children.
Key term:
congenital defect: an anatomic defect present at birth; it is not necessarily hereditary

SCIENCE AND PROFESSION

A pediatric surgeon is a general surgeon who has received additional training in operating on infants and children. The full course of training includes four years of medical school, followed by five years of general surgery residency and two years of pediatric surgery residency. Pediatric surgeons generally practice in large referral hospitals or children's hospitals.

Children experience some different surgical disorders than adults, especially congenital defects. Their ability to withstand the stress of surgery is less than that of an older person. Also, many of their surgical problems require years of follow-up care by a surgeon who understands child growth and development.

In the first half of the twentieth century, when pediatric surgery was developing as a specialty, the pediatric surgeon was trained to operate on all parts of the child's body. As the specialty matured, however, the pediatric surgeon was in charge of general surgical procedures on infants and children. This was possible due to development of pediatric subspecialties in the other surgical fields, such as neurosurgery and cardiac surgery. In addition, pediatric surgeons work closely with pediatricians, neonatologists, and family physi-

cians. As a team, they partake in the well-being of children from well childcare to preoperative and postoperative care.

The difference between a general surgeon and pediatric surgeon is due to the type of knowledge requirement. Pediatric surgeons have to manage their child patients and keep up their constantly changing body systems and the ability of a child's body to cope with disease along with surgery alters with age. It is therefore imperative for the pediatric surgeon to understand child growth and development.

Although a disorder may be surgically corrected in infancy, the child may continue to have postoperative difficulty for many years. An example is the removal of a large amount of intestines, which must sometimes be done with premature infants. It takes considerable patience and expertise to follow this sort of patient for years, adjusting the child's diet and treatment to achieve as nearly normal growth as possible. The pediatric surgeon's expertise comes in handy to provide this sort of care.

The organs and tissues of an infant or child are much smaller than those of an adult. The pediatric surgeon requires meticulous operative skills, great dexterity, and sharp intelligence to reduce the stress on pediatric patients.

Congenital defects are, fortunately, relatively uncommon. The pediatric surgeon treats relatively more of these conditions than a general surgeon would and therefore has greater experience in caring for them. Examples of congenital defects treated by pediatric surgeons include defects of the abdominal wall and diaphragm and the obstruction or absence of a part of the intestinal tract.

The pediatric surgeon should effectively communicate with all age groups as including parents in their child's care is important. This specialist is trained to build a supportive relationship with parents and to teach them about their child's disorder so that they can be informed participants in decisions regarding the patient's care. Especially with chronic diseases, the parents must be kept aware of their child's progress and changing needs so that they can participate fully in the child's recovery.

DIAGNOSTIC AND TREATMENT TECHNIQUES

The pediatric surgeon's day is split between the operating room and the clinic. This specialist spends relatively more time in the clinic than does a general surgeon. Surgical correction is only one-step in pediatric surgery. Careful evaluation, planning, and research must precede any procedure. Afterward, extended follow-up care is often necessary, sometimes for years. This type of care requires patience and an interest in long-range planning on the surgeon's part.

The pediatric surgeon relies heavily on history taking and physical examination of the patient. This information, plus knowledge of the incidence of specific disorders at different ages, leads the surgeon to the most likely diagnosis. Specific laboratory and radiographic tests are ordered to aid in the diagnostic process.

The pediatric surgeon works very closely with the anesthesiologist, the physician responsible for keeping the patient anesthetized and his or her vital functions stable during surgery. The needs of a child are different from those of an adult during surgery. Many hospitals with pediatric surgeons are also staffed with pediatric anesthesiologists. The pediatric surgeon can also further specialize in fetal surgery to treat complex prenatal disorders.

Like other surgeons, the pediatric surgeon also performs minor surgery on children, often in the clinic. Examples of minor procedures are the suturing of lacerations, the drainage of small abscesses, and the excision of small benign growths under the skin.

PERSPECTIVE AND PROSPECTS
Pediatric surgery began in the United States as an offshoot of general surgery in the first half of the twentieth century. The American Academy of Pediatrics was first to recognize the value of pediatric surgeons and, following a meeting by the academy in 1948, established a surgical section. C. Everett Koop, the surgeon general under President Ronald Reagan, was a vigorous advocate of pediatric surgical education and a developer of new surgical techniques for children from 1946 through the 1990s. He was an important proponent in the eventual recognition of pediatric surgery as a surgical specialty. It was not until 1973, however, that the Board of Pediatric Surgery certified the first specialists in the field. The Future Docs model that predicts the rapid growth of supply surgeons who treat pediatric patients have predicted that supply of pediatric surgeons will relatively grow rapidly through 2030 based upon the current demand. There are currently 59 pediatric surgery fellowships, a major growth from twenty-eight programs in the 1990s. Pediatric surgeons over all have increased to more than 1100+ in the last decade and continue to do so as the demand of pediatric surgeries have also been increasing over the years.

—*Vaidehi Patel, MS, MS-III*

See also: Abscess drainage; Adrenalectomy; Amputation; Anesthesia; Anesthesiology; Aneurysmectomy; Appendectomy; Biopsy; Bone marrow transplantation; Cardiac surgery; Cardiology, pediatric; Catheterization; Cleft lip and palate repair; Craniotomy; Cryosurgery; Ear surgery; Electrocauterization; Endocrinology, pediatric; Eye surgery; Fistula repair; Gastroenterology, pediatric; Genetic diseases; Genetics and inheritance; Grafts and grafting; Heart transplantation; Heart valve replacement; Hernia repair; Hypospadias repair and urethroplasty; Kidney transplantation; Laceration repair; Laparoscopy; Laser use in surgery; Lung surgery; Nasal polyp removal; Nephrectomy; Nephrology, pediatric; Neurology, pediatric; Neurosurgery; Ophthalmology; Oral and maxillofacial surgery; Orthopedic surgery; Orthopedics, pediatric; Parathyroidectomy; Pediatrics; Plastic surgery; Pulmonary medicine, pediatric; Shunts; Splenectomy; Surgery, general; Surgical procedures; Surgical technologists; Sympathectomy; Tattoo removal; Tendon repair; Thoracic surgery; Thyroidectomy; Tonsillectomy and adenoid removal; Tracheostomy; Transfusion; Transplantation; Urology, pediatric.

For Further Information:

Cockburn, Forrester, et al. *Children's Medicine and Surgery*. Oxford UP, 1996. This volume discusses the basics of pediatrics and features illustrations and an index.

Fraher, E. P., A. Knapton, G. F. Sheldon, et al. "Projecting Surgeon Supply Using a Dynamic Model." *Annals of Surgery*, vol. 257, 2013, pp. 867-72.

Glick, Philip L., et al. *Pediatric Surgery Secrets*. Hanley & Belfus, 2001. An accessible question-and-answer format addresses general and critical care, thoracic surgery, cardiovascular surgery, gastroenterology, hepatobiliary and spleen surgery, head and neck surgery, genitourinary surgery, trauma, tumors and oncology, and special topics.

Koop, C. Everett. "Pediatric Surgery: The Long Road to Recognition." *Pediatrics*, vol. 92, Oct. 1993, pp. 618-21. The history of pediatric surgery is discussed. Some believe that pediatric surgery would never have gotten off the ground without the development of pediatric anesthesiology.

Livingston, E. H., and J. Cao. "Procedure Volume as a Predictor of Surgical Outcomes." *JAMA*, vol. 304, 2010, pp. 95-97.

O'Neill, James A., Jr., et al., editors. *Principles of Pediatric Surgery*. 2nd ed., Mosby, 2004. This is a new edition of a classic textbook of pediatric surgery. It is the most comprehensive text available on the subject, a must for all practicing and aspiring pediatric surgeons. Perhaps a bit too comprehensive for nonpediatric surgeons looking for a simple reference book to keep on their shelf.

Ricketts, Thomas C. William T. Adamson, Erin P. Fraher, et al. "Future Supply of Pediatric Surgeons." *Annals of Surgery*, vol. 265, no. 3, Mar. 2017, pp. 609-15, doi: 10.1097/SLA.0000000000001810.

SURGICAL PROCEDURES

Category: Procedures
Anatomy or system affected: All
Specialties and related fields: Anesthesiology, general surgery, nursing, plastic surgery
Definition: The treatment of diseases or disorders by physical intervention, which usually involves cutting into the skin and other tissues.

Key terms:

anesthesia: the use of drugs to inhibit pain and other sensations

hemostasis: the control of bleeding

incision: a cut made with a scalpel

suture: a thread used to unite parts of the body

INDICATIONS AND PROCEDURES

Surgery has progressed as rapidly as other areas of medicine. Early surgeries consisted of gross excision (the cutting out of abnormal or diseased tissue). Today, surgery has been transformed by scientific advances so that surgeons commonly use microscopes, lasers, and endoscopes that allow the surgeon to make small incisions in order to gain access to the surgical site. Modern operations are much more precise and emphasize repair or replacement rather than excision.

When a patient requires surgery, several preoperative procedures are performed to increase the chances of a successful outcome. First, the patient is asked to abstain from eating for at least eight hours prior to surgery. This action reduces the chances of the individual vomiting during surgery and aspirating the gastric contents into the trachea (windpipe). After arriving at the hospital or clinic, the patient removes his or her clothes and puts on a gown. This provides the medical staff easy access to the patient for catheter insertion, intravenous line insertion, monitor placement, and preparation of the surgical site. Next, an intravenous (IV) line is placed in a vein of the hand or arm and connected to a bottle or bag of solution, which is suspended above the level of the patient's arm. The intravenous line gives the physician rapid vascular access for sampling blood and injecting drugs. Directly before the actual surgery, the patient is usually given a sedative by an anesthesiologist, and a blood pressure cuff and electrocardiogram (ECG or EKG) leads are applied to the patient to monitor blood pressure, heart rate and heart rhythm. The anesthesiologist will then anesthetize the patient further while the surgical team prepares the site for the operation. Preoperative antibiotics may be given if there is a significant risk of infection.

The surgery may require either general anesthesia, in which the patient is unconscious, or local anesthesia, in which a specific region of the body is anesthetized. For general anesthesia, the patient will be injected with an intravenous anesthetic and quickly intubated, a procedure in which a tube is inserted into the trachea and attached to a ventilator. This arrange-

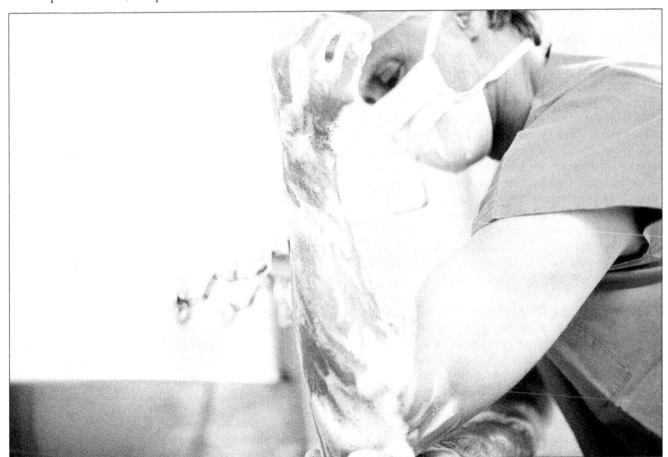

Surgeons scrub their hands and arms before performing an operation. Such procedures are essential to the maintenance of an antiseptic environment. Photo via iStock/kupicoo. [Used under license.]

ment gives the anesthesiologist the ability to administer gaseous drugs such as nitrous oxide and halothane as well as to control the patient's breathing. Surgical assistants prepare the operative site by cleansing the skin with a disinfectant. A sterile drape is used to cover all areas of the body except the surgical site. Surgeons and assistants must mask themselves and prepare for surgery by thoroughly washing their hands and arms. They then carefully put on a sterile gown and gloves. At this point, they must not come into contact with anything nonsterile.

The surgeon uses a scalpel to make an incision through the skin and any underlying structures in order to gain access to the area of the body needing attention. When blood vessels are cut, bleeding must be controlled by cauterizing, clamping, tying off with sutures, or applying direct pressure to the vessel; this process is known as "hemostasis."

After the surgery, the incision sites are closed with sutures, and the anesthetic is reversed. The patient is then taken to a recovery room to be monitored closely. Routine care of the patient recovering from anesthesia includes repeated evaluation of body temperature, pulse, blood pressure, and respiration. Postoperative pain medication (e.g., meperidine, morphine, or fentanyl) is given as needed.

USES AND COMPLICATIONS

Complications from surgery can result from surgical errors, infections, and abnormal patient reactions to the procedure or medications (idiosyncratic reactions). Occasionally, surgery involves damage to healthy tissues, including nerves and blood vessels. Significant intraoperative blood loss may also occur, requiring transfusion. An incision into any part of the body provides an opportunity for bacteria to enter and infect the surgical wound; prophylactic antibiotics help reduce the chance of surgical infection. Rarely, a patient may have an unexpected response to the procedure or drugs, which could result in permanent disability or death. These very infrequent reactions may include a blood clot causing a stroke or heart attack, an abnormal heart rhythm, or severe allergic reactions to medication.

PERSPECTIVE AND PROSPECTS

Modern surgery includes the use of surgical implants, microsurgery, laser surgery, endoscopic surgery, and transplant surgery. Surgery implants are used to replace a part of the body with an artificial implant. These implants include joints, heart valves, eye lenses, and sections of blood vessels or of the skull. During microsurgery, the surgeon uses specially designed instruments and a microscope to perform an operation on minute structures such as blood vessels, nerves, and parts of the eyes or ears. Microsurgery is also being

used to reattach severed fingers and toes. Laser surgery utilizes a high-energy, narrow beam that can cut through tissues like a scalpel but also cauterizes blood vessels during the incision. Lasers can be used on the retina, skin blemishes, and even tumors. Recovery from endoscopic surgery, in which a fiber-optic tube is inserted into the body to view the surgical site, is generally faster than from conventional operations because a smaller incision is made and less tissue damage results. Endoscopes are used to remove stones from the urinary tract and gallbladder and to remove or repair damaged cartilage in joints. With the availability of drugs that suppress tissue rejection, damaged organs can now be surgically replaced by donated organs. The most common examples are the heart, lungs, liver, kidneys, and bone marrow.

—*Chanel Rutledge, MS-III*

See also: Anesthesia; Anesthesiology; Biopsy; Bypass surgery; Catheterization; Cervical procedures; Colon and rectal surgery; Craniotomy; Cryosurgery; Cyst removal; Electrocauterization; Eye surgery; Fistula repair; Ganglion removal; Grafts and grafting; Hernia repair; Laparoscopy; Laser use in surgery; Lung surgery; Neurosurgery; Orthopedic surgery; Periodontal surgery; Plastic surgery; Shunts; Surgery, general; Surgery, pediatric; Surgical technologists; Thoracic surgery; Tracheostomy; Transfusion; Transplantation; Tumor removal.

For Further Information:
Brunicardi, F. Charles, et al., editors. *Schwartz's Principles of Surgery*. 11th ed., McGraw-Hill, 2019. A standard textbook on the topic. Intended for practicing surgeons, but valuable to general readers for its details.
Leikin, Jerrold B., and Martin S. Lipsky, editors. *American Medical Association Complete Medical Encyclopedia*. Random House Reference, 2003. A concise presentation of numerous medical terms and illnesses. A good general reference.
Mulholland, Michael W., et al., editors. *Greenfield's Surgery: Scientific Principles and Practice*. 7th ed., Lippincott Williams & Wilkins, 2006. Covers the scope and practice of surgery and includes reviews of wound biology, immunology, the management of trauma and transplantation, surgical practice according to anatomic region and specialty, and musculoskeletal, neurologic, genitourinary, and reconstructive surgery.
Zollinger, Robert M., Jr., and Robert M. Zollinger, Sr. *Zollinger's Atlas of Surgical Operations*. 8th ed., McGraw-Hill, 2003. A comprehensive examination of surgery. Covers basic surgical anatomy and vascular, gynecologic, gastrointestinal, and miscellaneous abdominal procedures.

SURGICAL TECHNOLOGISTS

Category: Specialty
Anatomy or system affected: All
Specialties and related fields: Anesthesiology, emergency medicine, general surgery, nursing

Definition: Surgical team members whose primary functions are to prepare surgical instruments and hand them to the surgeon as needed and to prevent infection by maintaining a sterile field in the operating room.

Key terms:

analgesia: the absence of pain

anesthesia: the absence of sensation; anesthesia may be achieved systemically (general anesthesia) or in a specific region of the body (regional or local anesthesia)

aseptic techniques: the standard procedures that help prevent wound contamination during the performance of surgical procedures; contamination may be followed by infection or death

circulator: the worker in the operating room whose responsibility is to keep records and to open sterile supplies for the team members wearing gowns and gloves

inpatient procedure: a surgical procedure performed on a patient who comes from a room in the hospital and who will return to a room in the hospital

operating room: a room in which surgical procedures are performed

outpatient procedure: a surgical procedure performed on a patient who comes from outside the hospital and who will most likely leave the hospital after a short stay in the recovery room

prep: a short form of the word "prepare"; to prep means to wash and shave the surgical area and to clean the skin surface immediately before a surgical procedure

recovery room: the room where a patient returns to full consciousness after a surgical procedure; in an outpatient facility, patients can change clothes in the recovery room, which may serve double duty as the preoperative waiting room

scrub: to wash one's hands and forearms in preparation for donning gown and gloves, which protect the patient from the surgical technologist and protect the surgical technologist from the patient

sterile field: an area where only sterile supplies may be placed and that only those wearing sterile gowns and gloves may touch; includes the surgical wound, the surgical drapes, and the extra tables

surgical team: the people working together in the operating room during a surgical procedure, including the surgeon, first assistant, surgical technologist, anesthesiologist and/or anesthetist, and circulator

SCIENCE AND PROFESSION

Surgical technologists work as part of the surgical team in an operating room, so they must be familiar with many aspects of patient care. The surgical team typically includes at least one of each of the following: a surgeon, a first assistant, a surgical technologist, an anesthesiologist and/or anesthetist, and a circulator. As a member of the surgical team, a surgical technologist anticipates the needs of the surgeon, prepares the instruments to be used for surgery, hands instruments to the surgeon, promotes efficiency, and at the same time helps prevent infection by maintaining the sterile field. A surgical technologist may also be referred to as a scrub nurse, a surgical assistant, a private scrub, or simply a scrub.

Surgical technologists work in many types of operating rooms, so their training must be fairly extensive. Courses may be taken at community colleges in one-year or two-year programs. Some of the two-year programs are accredited by the Association of Surgical Technologists. In 2001, the Commission on Accreditation of Allied Health Education Programs (CAAHEP) recognized 350 accredited programs. The courses taken include medical terminology, anatomy, and physiology. Classes specifically focused on surgical technology may include surgical conscience and ethics, the organization of an operating room, principles of microbiology, sterilization and disinfection, aseptic techniques, preoperative preparation and care of the patient, anesthesia, medications used during surgery, proper positioning of a surgical patient, preparation of the surgical site, methods of closing the surgical wound, surgical routines, the supplies found in the operating room, and the legal aspects of surgery.

A surgical technologist may work in one or all of many surgical services, so coursework must provide information about general surgery; obstetrical and gynecological surgery; plastic and reconstructive surgery; ear, nose, and throat procedures; surgery on the mouth and face; orthopedic surgery; neurosurgery; open-heart surgery; lung surgery; pediatric surgery; and surgery on blood vessels not located in the chest.

Students are required to gain experience in an operating room, which is usually done under supervision at a local teaching hospital. At such a hospital, a student gains experience in appropriate operating room procedures and learns the universal precautions against the transmission of infectious diseases.

Although the surgical technologist may work in any of the available medical services, some hospitals require their surgical technologists to specialize-that is, to rotate through different services so that they will gain familiarity with many operative procedures. At other facilities, the surgical technologist will work primarily in one area. For example, if the facility is a plastic surgeon's clinic, only these types of procedures will be performed.

A surgical technologist who has gained some experience may gain a specific area of interest within a broader field and decide to become a specialist. Common areas in which to specialize include eye surgery, neurosurgery, orthopedics, and plastic surgery. If this is the case, the technologist might be invited to work for a certain doctor or may find a number of (perhaps unaffiliated) doctors with whom to work. Working as a private scrub offers a different way to practice in the field. The surgical technologist works directly for the surgeon, instead of working for the hospital or surgical facility, and can usually expect to charge and earn more. There is also the possibility of greater camaraderie with the physician and more trust of the surgical technologist by the physician. Concentrating in a specific area may offer greater remuneration to the surgical technologist, greater rapport with a familiar surgeon, and a more regular schedule, with no requirement for working on the weekends.

DUTIES AND PROCEDURES

Surgical technologists typically work in many areas, both inside and outside the operating room. Within the operating room, they may be either scrubbed or not scrubbed. After washing his or her hands, the surgical technologist dons a gown and gloves, which provides a sterile surface to reduce the possibility of transmission of infection, either from the patient to the surgical technologist or from the surgical technologist to the patient. When scrubbed, surgical technologists perform many duties. They assist surgeons during surgical procedures by handing them instruments, following routine procedures. They promote efficiency by keeping the instrument tables neat and organized. They must anticipate the needs of surgeons, so it is necessary that they know the steps of a procedure and monitor its progress. A surgical technologist places instruments in the surgeon's hands so that the surgeon does not have to look away from the wound in search of an instrument. Surgical technologists also help prevent injuries to the patient.

When necessary, the scrubbed surgical technologist may be asked to act as a first assistant for a procedure. In this capacity, it may be necessary for the surgical technologist to hold tissue out of the way (retract it), so that the surgeon can reach deeper tissues. Surgical technologists may also be required to sponge blood out of the wound or to rinse the surgical site to promote visibility of the tissues. They may also cut sutures. Surgical technologists help count sponges, needles, and instruments when such counts are required; items must be counted so that none are left behind in the patient. These items are counted before, during, and after the surgical procedure, in a specified and orderly manner. It is also the responsibility of the scrubbed surgical technologist to keep track of surgical specimens, pieces of tissue removed from the patient that will be sent to the laboratory for analysis. Many speci-

mens may be taken from a particular procedure, so the surgical technologist must hand them off the sterile field to the circulator and make sure that the circulator labels the specimens properly. Specimens must also be handled and treated properly. Some are sent to the laboratory in preserving solutions, some are sent in salt water, and some are sent dry. It is important to keep track of specimens, to identify them, and to put them in the proper container for transportation to the laboratory.

When the surgical technologist is working in the operating room and is not scrubbed, a registered nurse must be immediately available in case there is an emergency. A registered nurse must also be present if medications are needed on the sterile field. A surgical technologist who is not scrubbed may function as a circulator. The circulator opens sterile supplies onto the operative field. Supplies are wrapped in many different ways, and the circulator must be able to pass the contents of a sterile package to the scrubbed surgical technologist without dropping them. Expiration dates must be checked on all supplies opened. Once the patient for a particular procedure is brought into the operating room, the circulator will help position the patient on the surgical table. The surgical technologist knows the position necessary for the particular procedure. Safe positioning methods prevent injury to patients. Once the patient is on the surgical table, the circulator washes the area with specified soaps and solutions and, if necessary, will shave the area around the surgical wound so that the area can be cleaned for the incision. The circulator ties the gowns of the scrubbed surgical technologist as well as the surgeon and other scrubbed assistants. If the anesthesiologist or anesthetist asks for help, the circulator provides that help, which may include holding, informing, or reassuring the patient.

It is the function of the circulator to connect tubings and electrical wires from instruments that may be needed on the sterile field, including power cords for cautery units, special lights, and drills, as well as fluid lines and suction cords. The circulator may need to focus or aim the surgical lights. With the scrubbed surgical technologist, the circulator performs the count of the items that need to be counted, including the sutures, sponges, and instruments. The circulator keeps the official legal record of the procedure, the operative report. On this document, the circulator records the particulars of the procedure, including the counts, what was done, and the medications that were given. It is the responsibility of the circulator to receive surgical specimens from the surgical technologist, and to record properly where they came from, before they are sent to the laboratory. It might be necessary for the circulator to wipe the brow of any of the scrubbed personnel, so that sweat will not fall onto the sterile field; however, this is a rare event. The circulator handles all the nonsterile equipment present in the operating room during the surgical procedure. This could involve moving or connecting equipment. In addition, the circulator helps to move the patient from the operating room to the recovery room after the procedure is over.

When not scrubbed for a procedure or functioning as a circulator, a surgical technologist may be asked to perform other duties in the surgery department. Surgical technologists need to be familiar with the protocols for receiving patients in the department. They may be asked to take patients to and from the surgical area or within the surgery department. Surgical technologists may help to order supplies for a department and, when they arrive, may help transport the supplies to the appropriate storage cupboard. Supplies need to be ordered from the central supply department or directly from manufacturers. In the operating room, not only must supplies be restocked but the expiration dates on sterile items must be inspected as well, to ensure that no outdated supplies are present in the operating room and given inadvertently to the patient. Surgical technologists may assist in cleaning instruments and supplies after a surgical procedure and preparing them for sterilization and subsequent reuse. They must be familiar with ways to sterilize instruments and supplies and must know which methods to use for which items. If equipment is working improperly, it is the responsibility of the surgical technologist to make sure that the equipment is repaired or replaced.

Working in an operating room is a very demanding occupation. It requires first of all personal integrity. As with any professional, the surgical technologist must be willing to admit mistakes. Often mistakes can be corrected if they are detected early. For example, the surgical technologist might have to say, "I forgot to sterilize the instruments, so we'll have to wait another fifteen minutes," rather than rush ahead to meet a particular deadline. In addition, a surgical technologist has to be able to handle stress-from providing fast and accurate care to a very sick patient, to having a patient die on the operating room table, to working with individuals with whom one does not get along on a personal level, to changing schedules for emergency procedures, to not being able to take a break to go to the restroom, to standing in one position for a whole day or a whole procedure.

No discussion of surgical technology would be complete without some mention of its legal aspects. As of the early twenty-first century in the United States, no state had licensed or defined the practice of surgical technology, although several states, including Texas, Oregon, and Georgia, were working on licensing initiatives. Therefore, the surgical technologist has only the common rights of a citizen on the street. Although no special license is required for surgical technologists, most hospitals prefer, and others require, certification. Surgical technologists can become certified surgical technologists by completing an approved program of at least one year and passing an examination given by the Association of Surgical Technologists (AST). One thing is certain: The surgical technologist is not allowed to practice medicine or nursing.

Since surgical technologists are not physicians, they may not diagnose or treat disease, inject medicine into the human body, or pronounce death. These actions are limited to physicians, and in some states, a physician may not delegate certain actions (such as suturing, cutting or penetrating the human body, and clamping) to a surgical technologist. Similarly, since the surgical technologists are not nurses, they may not administer medications, which is a practice relegated to the field of nursing. At one time, only registered nurses were permitted to act as circulators. Many hospitals now allow surgical technologists to circulate, with a registered nurse standing by for emergencies. When circulating, however, a surgical technologist must remember that only nurses may select and measure medications, a right that cannot be delegated to someone without a license.

Surgical technologists must obey the laws in the performance of their duties. They can be prosecuted for breaking a law or for failing to perform a proper job. Surgical technologists must pay attention to laws involving the respecting of property rights, both of patients and of hospitals. In addition to not exceeding the scope of practice, there is another area of concern for surgical technologists: negligence. Any act of carelessness is called negligence, which is legally defined as "the failure to exercise the care that a reasonably prudent person would exercise under similar circumstances." Although negligence itself is not a crime, surgical technologists must remember that carelessness could endanger the safety of the patient.

The most common areas of negligence (and subsequent malpractice lawsuits) that affect surgical technologists involve the following: proper positioning of side rails and patient supports, abandonment of the patient, surgical consent, patient identification, loss of items inside the patient, specimen collections, burns, and explosions. Carelessness involving side rails could result in an anesthetized patient falling on the floor. Abandonment refers to the careless act of leaving an incompetent patient alone. The patient must sign a consent, in which he or she agrees to the surgical procedure; this detailed legal document must be present before the procedure is begun, and the procedure may not wander from the permission given. Sponges, instruments, and needles are counted many times before, during, and after the surgical procedure, which helps to reduce the possibility of leaving anything inside the patient. Burns could be caused by the improper grounding of electrical devices used in the operating room, by the application of the wrong soap to the wrong area, or by the use of recently sterilized instruments, which may be too hot to be placed directly in contact with the patient. Explosions are less likely now than they used to be, because explosive medications are no longer used for general anesthesia. Nevertheless, the presence of oxygen in tanks and tubing increases the possibility of explosion and fire. In summary, there are many things about which the surgical technologist must be careful in order to avoid legal complications and injuries to patients.

PERSPECTIVE AND PROSPECTS

Historically, surgical technology began during World War II, when medical and nursing personnel in the armed forces trained men and women to assist in surgery in order to increase the availability of surgical procedures for the wounded. At that time, workers in this area were called operating room technicians. The name has gradually evolved to reflect the many areas where surgical procedures now take place-not only in hospitals but also in outpatient clinics, delivery rooms, and doctors' offices. In the beginning, surgical technologists had to work directly under the supervision of a registered nurse, who was legally required to be present in the operating room at all times.

The Association of Surgical Technologists began as a wing within the Association of Operating Room Nurses, but it later broke away to become the Association of Operating Room Technicians before later changing its name to the current one. Its headquarters are located in Littleton, Colorado. The AST provides many services for its members. It is a private organization that provides a certificate to those surgical technologists who pass a national examination. Certification, however, has little legal significance. States may not delegate their power to provide licenses to a private organization. The certified surgical technologist has demonstrated a level of skills and knowledge; however, one does not have to be certified in order to work as a surgical technologist. The AST also provides continuing education credits, insurance programs, and a magazine, as well as other services.

As the baby boom generation ages, the numbers of surgical procedures are expected to increase. Technological advances, such as fiber optics and laser technology, also allow new surgical procedures to be performed. For these reasons, the U.S. Bureau of Labor projects that employment opportunities for surgical technicians will grow by approximately 35 to 40 percent through the year 2010.

Working as a surgical technologist can be very demanding, but satisfaction, as in any profession, comes from working with a team in a complex situation in order to achieve a goal. There is satisfaction in a job well done, in being able to work well in stressful situations. There is great satisfaction in seeing the human body in all its complexity and in helping restore it to health. There is satisfaction in knowing in advance what the surgeon is going to use and having it ready at the moment it is needed. It is the excellent surgical technologist who can give the surgeon what is needed and not merely what is asked for.

—*William F. Taylor*

See also Allied health; Anesthesia; Anesthesiology; Education, medical; Malpractice; Nursing; Surgery, general; Surgery, pediatric; Surgical procedures.

For Further Information:
Caruthers, Bob, et al., eds. *Surgical Technology for the Surgical Technologist: A Positive Care Approach*. Florence, Ky.: Cengage Learning, 2009. Includes bibliographical references and an index.
Fuller, Joanna Kotcher. *Surgical Technology: Principles and Practice*. 4th ed. St. Louis, Mo.: Saunders/Elsevier, 2005. An accessible work that functions as a textbook for surgical technologists. Fuller has assembled a wealth of practical clinical information about caring for patients in surgery.
Miller, Benjamin F., Claire Brackman Keane, and Marie T. O'Toole. *Miller-Keane Encyclopedia and Dictionary of Medicine, Nursing, and Allied Health*. Rev. 7th ed. Philadelphia: Saunders/Elsevier, 2005. A comprehensive work which contains much information about the full spectrum of allied health.
Phillips, Nancymarie Fortunato. *Berry and Kohn's Operating Room Technique*. 11th ed. St. Louis, Mo.: Mosby/Elsevier, 2007. Another accessible textbook. This one contains much practical information about what goes on in the operating room.
Rothrock, Jane C., ed. *Alexander's Care of the Patient in Surgery*. 13th ed. St. Louis, Mo.: Mosby/Elsevier, 2007. The bible of surgical techniques and practices. A detailed reference work of the most common surgical procedures.

SWEATING

Category: Biology
Also known as: Perspiration
Anatomy or system affected: Glands, skin
Specialties and related fields: Dermatology, exercise physiology
Definition: The excretion of fluid from the sweat glands in order to cool the body.

STRUCTURE AND FUNCTIONS

Sweat glands are exocrine glands, which secrete products that are passed outside the body. There are two major types. Eccrine sweat glands excrete sweat that contains water and several salts. They are located in the skin throughout the body but are found in greater concentrations in the palms of the hands, soles of the feet, and forehead. Apocrine sweat glands excrete sweat that contains water and fatty substances. They are primarily found in the armpits and genital area. When bacteria break down the fatty materials, distinctive sweat odors develop.

The primary function of sweating in humans is to regulate body temperature. When the body temperature rises, the blood flow to the skin increases by opening more capillaries in the skin. Since blood can hold heat and circulates throughout the body, the blood can transport heat from the inner core of the body, where the temperatures are higher and the heat is more insulated, to the surface, where the heat is less insulated. In the skin, the warm blood will transfer the heat to the surface, where sweat glands release sweat. When the sweat evaporates, changing its physical state from a liquid to a gas, significant amounts of heat are removed from the body.

DISORDERS AND DISEASES

Sweating is a normal process that is important for the temperature regulation (thermoregulation) of the body, but complications can arise. The most critical result of excess sweating is dehydration. The biggest risk for dehydration occurs when people exercise in hot, humid environments. Therefore, it is important to drink plenty of water. Additionally, when sweating a lot for a period of days, additional salts may be beneficial. Most sports drinks supply adequate salts. In extreme conditions, the excess loss of water in sweat can lead to heatstroke and death. When the body loses too much water, the sweating mechanism shuts down. Without the advantage of sweat evaporation to cool the body, the temperature will continue to rise until death ensues. Anyone who has symptoms of heat stress-such as a body temperature over 105 degrees Fahrenheit, cessation of sweating, or altered mental state-should get immediate medical attention. The intravenous administration of fluids by medical personnel will rehydrate the body quickly.

A less concerning disorder of sweating is hyperhidrosis. People with this condition sweat frequently and in excess of what is required to regulate body temperature. About 1 percent of people have this condition; it is often linked to obesity. There are numerous treatments but no cure. Typical treatments include surgery, medications, biofeedback, relaxation, hypnosis, and weight loss.

—*Bradley R. A. Wilson, PhD*

See also Dehydration; Dermatology; Exercise physiology; Fever; Glands; Heat exhaustion and heatstroke; Host-defense mechanisms; Hyperhidrosis; Physiology; Signs and symptoms; Skin; Sympathectomy.

For Further Information:
Brooks, George A., Thomas D. Fahey, and Kenneth M. Baldwin. *Exercise Physiology: Human Bioenergetics and Its Applications*. 4th ed. Boston: McGraw-Hill, 2007.
McArdle, William, Frank I. Katch, and Victor L. Katch. *Exercise Physiology: Energy, Nutrition, and Human Performance*. 7th ed. Boston: Lippincott Williams & Wilkins, 2010.
Powers, Scott K., and Edward T. Howley. *Exercise Physiology: Theory and Application to Fitness and Performance*. 7th ed. New York: McGraw-Hill, 2009.

SYMPATHECTOMY

Category: Procedure
Anatomy or system affected: Back, neck, nerves, nervous system, spine
Specialties and related fields: General surgery, neurology
Definition: The surgical interruption of part of the sympathetic nerve pathway.

INDICATIONS AND PROCEDURES

The autonomic nervous system controls the involuntary internal environment of humans, and the sympathetic nerves increase energy expenditures by accelerating the heart rate, increasing the metabolic rate, and constricting and dilating blood vessels, among other actions. Occasionally, the proper regulation of vasoconstriction or vasodilation goes awry, and the sympathetic nervous system causes prolonged and inappropriate constriction of the blood vessels to a specific area. In Raynaud's phenomenon, there is intermittent constricting of blood vessels when the fingers, toes, ears, or nose is exposed to cold. The affected areas change color from white to blue to red, and the condition can be associated with numbness, tingling, burning, and pain. Symptoms of long-term blood vessel constriction associated with decreased blood flow include cold and clammy skin, areas of gangrene, and painful fibrous growths and infections. In other cases, excessive sweating and facial blushing may be candidates for correction with sympathectomy.

After the specific nerves are located, the patient is prepared for surgery and opened in the location of the nerves, typically the neck or back area. Organs are moved or adjusted as needed. The offending region of nerve is clipped from the remainder and removed. The organs are replaced or repaired, and the incisions are closed. Normal vascular dilation will return rapidly and with it warmth to the area and healing of the infections, fibrous tissue, and areas of gangrene.

In the treatment of excessive sweating, often sympathectomy can be performed as an outpatient procedure under local anesthesia. A small incision is made under the armpit and air is introduced into the chest cavity. The surgeon inserts a fiber-optic tube, or endoscope, which projects an image onto a screen. Lasers are used to destroy the ganglia involved in the excessive sweating.

USES AND COMPLICATIONS

To determine if sympathectomy is an appropriate treatment, the nerve in question is injected with a steroid and anesthetic to block the nerve function temporarily. If the condition in question is relieved, then the patient will likely benefit from sympathectomy. After surgery is completed, Doppler ultrasonography, which uses sound waves to measure blood flow, can be used to determine whether the procedure has succeeded in increasing circulation.

Potential complications include those common to all major surgeries. Depending on the type of sympathectomy performed, side effects may involve a decrease in blood pressure when standing, which can lead to fainting spells. About 30 percent of cases of sympathectomy for treatment of excessive sweating result in an increase in sweating of the chest, but the procedure is 90 percent effective in alleviating excessive sweating of the face, hands, and feet.

—*Karen E. Kalumuck, PhD*

See also Circulation; Nervous system; Neuralgia, neuritis, and neuropathy; Neuroimaging; Neurology; Neurosurgery; Sweating; Vascular medicine; Vascular system.

For Further Information:

Ernst, Calvin B., and James C. Stanley, eds. *Current Therapy in Vascular Surgery*. 4th ed. St. Louis, Mo.: Mosby, 2001.
Ganong, William F. *Review of Medical Physiology*. 23d ed. New York: Lange Medical Books/McGraw-Hill Medical, 2009.
Griffith, H. Winter. *Complete Guide to Symptoms, Illness, and Surgery*. Revised and updated by Stephen Moore and Kenneth Yoder. 5th ed. New York: Perigee, 2006.
Rutherford, Robert B., ed. *Vascular Surgery*. 6th ed. Philadelphia: Saunders/Elsevier, 2005.

SYNDROME

Category: Disease/Disorder
Also known as: Condition, disease, disorder
Anatomy or system affected: All
Specialties and related fields: All
Definition: A group or pattern of recognizable symptoms or conditions that occur together and indicate a specific disease, psychological disorder, or other abnormal condition.
Key terms:
disorder: abnormal physical or mental condition
symptom: indication of a disorder

CAUSES AND SYMPTOMS

A syndrome is a collection of symptoms that characterize a disorder. For example, metabolic syndrome is the name given to a group of symptoms that warn of potential heart disease, stroke, or diabetes. The symptoms of metabolic syndrome are obesity, high blood pressure, low levels of insulin, and high cholesterol.

Syndromes can be grouped into roughly fourteen categories: environmental (caused by the environment); congenital (existing at birth); gastrointestinal (affecting the stomach and intestines); cardiovascular (involving the heart and blood vessels); iatrogenic (induced by a treatment or procedure); neoplastic (caused by a malignant or benign tumor); endocrine (affecting glands, including sex glands); pulmonary (involving the lung); infectious (caused by a virus, bacterium, or fungus); renal (involving the kidneys); reticuloendothelial (affecting cells, including blood cells); neurological (affecting the nervous system); psychopathological (affecting the mind and behavior); and medically unexplained (cause uncertain).

The causes of syndromes vary. Some come from a single, clear source. For example, toxic shock syndrome is caused by the bacterium *Staphylococcus aureus*. The bacterium enters the body through wounds from injuries or surgery incisions. It also breeds in superabsorbent tampons and contraceptive sponges. Symptoms of this syndrome include fever, headache, vomiting, diarrhea, and muscle aches.

Chinese restaurant syndrome is caused by monosodium glutamate (MSG), a chemical compound widely used to enhance the flavor of foods. MSG can induce headache, dizziness, giddiness, a feeling of facial pressure, tingling sensations over parts of the body, and chest pain.

Some syndromes result from any one of an array of causes. Fanconi syndrome, for instance, activates the release of certain substances from the kidney into the urine instead of the bloodstream. It can be caused by genetic defects, inherited diseases, exposure to heavy metals, a kidney transplant, or any number of medicines or diseases that damage the kidneys.

Other syndromes, such as carpal tunnel syndrome, arise from a combination of causes. This syndrome stems from increased pressure on certain nerves and tendons in the carpal tunnel in the wrist. Most people prone to carpal tunnel syndrome are born with a comparatively small carpal tunnel. This condition is complicated by injury to the wrist, an overactive pituitary gland, an underactive thyroid, rheumatoid arthritis, or repeated use of vibrating hand tools.

The causes of some syndromes remain uncertain. For example, Reye's syndrome is a rapidly appearing, deadly disorder that affects all body organs, most seriously the brain and liver. It attacks adults but is primarily a children's disease. Symptoms include personality changes, seizures, and loss of consciousness. There is no cure. The cause is unknown, but there seems to be a link to the use of aspirin taken for a previous viral disease.

Restless legs syndrome is the nighttime twitching of the legs that often leads to insomnia. The cause is unknown, but there seems to be some connection to a family history of the disorder. Also associated with this syndrome are anemia, diabetes, kidney failure, and certain prescription and nonprescription medicines.

Just as the causes vary, so too do the number and severity of symptoms, depending on the syndrome. Barrett's esophagus, for example, is a condition in which the esophagus (the tube that carries food to the stomach) develops new cells similar to those found in the intestines. Symptoms are nonexistent, and the cause is unknown. It can, however, lead to a deadly type of esophageal cancer.

The symptoms of premenstrual syndrome (PMS) vary widely in number and severity from woman to woman. Some women experience few symptoms; others need several days of bed rest. Symptoms include irritability, headache, backache, weight gain, swelling or tenderness of the breasts, depression, fatigue, and loss of sex drive.

Some fifty different symptoms, or characteristics, are associated with Down syndrome. Characteristics include intellectual disability; short stature; slow physical growth; weak muscles; short, stocky arms and legs; a wide space between the big toe and second toe; small, low-set ears; a narrow roof of the mouth; crooked teeth and other dental problems; heart defects; an underactive thyroid; and hearing problems. So many symptoms require a lifetime of care.

Asperger's syndrome produces no symptoms that require medical attention, but people with this disorder display abnormal behaviors and have limited social skills that can bring on unwanted consequences, such as being shunned by others. Some people with this disorder seem "normal" most of the time. Others just seem odd or different from other people, quieter and disinterested. Still others exhibit somewhat bizarre, or at least socially unacceptable, behaviors, such as inflexible routines, a narrow but intense focus of interests, an inability to empathize with other people, and difficulty understanding some types of humor, especially teasing and sarcasm. Yet they are often above average in intelligence and do no more harm than so-called

normal people. The odd behaviors lead people to think that Asperger's syndrome is a mental disorder. In fact, it is a type of autism, a developmental disorder that affects how the brain processes information. The cause is unknown.

TREATMENT AND THERAPY

Treatment of a syndrome depends on the underlying causes and the severity and number of symptoms. Because syndromes run the full range of medical problems, treatments run the full range as well. Drugs, surgery, physical therapy, diet and lifestyle changes, alternative medicine, and psychotherapy are all used to treat syndromes.

PERSPECTIVE AND PROSPECTS

Both Western and Eastern medical practitioners have long recognized that a set of symptoms can describe an abnormal condition. Syndromes are researched, diagnosed, and treated no differently than individual diseases are.

—Wendell Anderson

See also Acquired immunodeficiency syndrome (AIDS); Acute respiratory distress syndrome (ARDS); Asperger's syndrome; Blue baby syndrome; Carpal tunnel syndrome; Chronic fatigue syndrome; Cornelia de Lange syndrome; Cushing's syndrome; Diagnosis; DiGeorge syndrome; Disease; Down syndrome; Fetal alcohol syndrome; Fragile X syndrome; Guillain-Barré syndrome; Gulf War syndrome; Hemolytic uremic syndrome; Irritable bowel syndrome (IBS); Klinefelter syndrome; Klippel-Trenaunay syndrome; Kluver-Bucy syndrome; Marfan syndrome; Metabolic syndrome; Multiple chemical sensitivity syndrome; Münchausen syndrome by proxy; Overtraining syndrome; Polycystic ovary syndrome; Prader-Willi syndrome; Premenstrual syndrome (PMS); Reiter's syndrome; Respiratory distress syndrome; Restless legs syndrome; Reye's syndrome; Rubinstein-Taybi syndrome; Severe acute respiratory syndrome (SARS); Severe combined immunodeficiency syndrome (SCID); Signs and symptoms; Sjögren's syndrome; Stevens-Johnson syndrome; Sturge-Weber syndrome; Sudden infant death syndrome (SIDS); Temporomandibular joint (TMJ) syndrome; Tourette's syndrome; Toxic shock syndrome; Turner syndrome; Wiskott-Aldrich syndrome.

For Further Information:
Kirmayer, Laurence, et al. "Explaining Medically Unexplained Symptoms." *Canadian Journal of Psychiatry* 49, no. 10 (October, 2004): 663-672.
McConnaughy, Rozalynd. "Asperger Syndrome: Living Outside the Bell Curve." *Journal of the Medical Library Association* 93, no. 1 (January, 2005): 139-140.
Pease, Roger, Jr., ed. *Merriam-Webster's Medical Desk Dictionary.* Rev. ed. Springfield, Mass.: Merriam-Webster, 2002.
Rice, Shirley. "Reye's Syndrome Isn't Just Child's Play." *Nursing* 33, no. 9 (September, 2003): 32hn1-32hn4.
Wallis, Claudia. "The Down Syndrome Dilemma." *Time* 166, no. 20 (November 14, 2005).

SYNESTHESIA

Category: Disease/Disorder
Anatomy or system affected: Brain, nervous system, psychic-emotional system
Specialties and related fields: Genetics, neurology, neuropsychology, psychiatry, psychology
Definition: A condition in which a sensory stimulus such as a letter presented visually evokes a sensation in a different modality such as a specific color.
Key terms:

functional magnetic resonance imaging(fMRI): a radiologic technique that shows regional oxygen uptake, indicating brain activity

grapheme: a written character or element-letter, word, or number

photism: in synesthesia, a vivid light or color sensation induced by a different sensory stimulus

positron emission tomography(PET): a technique that creates three-dimensional computer images from particles emitted after radioactively tagged substances are incorporated into body tissues; particle concentrations identify areas of increased energy metabolism

synesthete: a person who experiences synesthesia by virtue of having a second sensation evoked by a single stimulus

CAUSES AND SYMPTOMS

The term "synesthesia" derives from the Greek *syn-* (union/together) and *aisthesis* (sensation/perception). Regarded as an intriguing but perhaps bogus curiosity, synesthesia was once disparaged as a subjective experience unworthy of scientific interest. Since the 1980s, however, neuroimaging techniques have established the synesthetic experience as a genuine sensorineural phenomenon and a legitimate subject for scientific research. Described as rare by some and as common by others, it is estimated that approximately 4 percent of the population are synesthetes.

Various combinations of synesthetic experiences have been documented, but color is the most common concurrent perception. Of the many different types, none has been more intensively studied than grapheme-color synesthesia; specific characters written in black print induce the experience of a specific color. The induced color experiences, termed "photisms," are vivid and consistent; a specific grapheme always induces the same color in the same synesthete. A spoken word or musical note can act as the stimulus, and days of the week or months of the year also trigger colors-for some, Friday will always be chartreuse. Rarer synesthetic experiences involve touch or taste. Mirror-touch synesthesia activates a tactile sensation in the

> ## INFORMATION ON SYNESTHESIA
> **Causes:** Unknown; probably increased connectivity and cross-wiring in contiguous brain regions
> **Symptoms:** Subjective manifestations involve two or more concurrent sensory perceptions when only one has been stimulated
> **Duration:** Generally lifelong
> **Treatments:** Primarily occurs in neurologically and psychologically normal people, does not warrant medical treatment connections in synesthetic adults somehow escaped the normal pruning process of neuronal decline seen in pre-adolescents, perhaps via mutation

synesthete's body when someone within sight is touched. In tactile-emotion synesthesia, textures induce distinct emotions. Some synesthetes experience a specific taste on hearing a word or piece of music. Synesthesia has a strong genetic component, although the mode of inheritance is unclear. Familial aggregation in synesthesia was first noted by Sir Francis Galton in 1880.

One study found a greater than 40 percent prevalence of synesthesia among first-degree relatives of synesthetes. A report of monozygotic (identical) male twins discordant for grapheme-color synesthesia casts doubt on what was initially believed to be X-linked dominant inheritance; documented male-to-male transmission also argues against it. Genetic linkage studies suggest a complex pattern of inheritance, perhaps with multiple gene loci. Different types commonly coexist in the same family, and heterogeneity is characteristic. Within one type, the same word or letter evokes different colors in different individuals, and the subjective experience differs as well.

DIAGNOSIS AND DETECTION

Recognition begins with a self-report. Various psychological tests can distinguish between synesthetes and nonsynesthetes; neuroimaging is generally limited to research. Some diagnostic criteria have been generally accepted: synesthetic sensory experience is involuntary, automatic, and durable-synesthetes typically report their sensory associations as consistent over years.

Considerable evidence supports the neural basis of synesthesia. Neurologic injury can evoke synesthetic associations, and drugs such as mescaline can induce them. Brain imaging, however, identifies synesthesia as a neural phenomenon. The pattern of cerebral blood flow during a synesthetic experience, first recorded in the 1980s, was described as abnormal. Subsequent studies have used positron emission tomography (PET) and functional magnetic resonance imaging (fMRI) to show differences in brain structure and activity between synesthetes and nonsynesthetes.

Grapheme-color synesthesia has been the main focus of fMRI studies. According to posited models, increased connectivity between contiguous brain areas in the cerebral cortex facilitates cross-activation. The fusiform gyrus, involved both in color and grapheme processing, has shown increased activation in addition to increased cortical thickness, volume, and surface area. Increased white matter volume and connectivity has been observed in brains of some synesthetes compared with those of nonsynesthetic counterparts.

Can developmental mechanisms explain synesthesia? Some investigators suggest that incoming sensory information in infants is normally jumbled together, and pruning of comingled neural and synaptic connections comes with development. According to this hypothesis, sensorineural connections in synesthetic adults somehow escaped the pruning process, perhaps via mutation.

PERSPECTIVE AND PROSPECTS

Synesthesia has a long and distinguished history. Around 1710, an English ophthalmologist reported a blind patient who experienced color visions that were induced by sound. Jonathan Swift's title character in *Gulliver's Travels* (1726) encountered a group of blind apprentices taught by their blind master to mix colors by touch and smell. Swift's source was believed to be the Royal Society scientists of his day, notably Robert Boyle. Francis Galton established synesthesia as a scientific entity in 1880.

The idea that the various senses are fused could be found in literature much before it resonated in neurology. Mary Shelley described the creature in *Frankenstein* (1818) as having a difficult time separating his various sensations because he simultaneously saw, felt, heard, and smelled. Later in the nineteenth century, psychologist William James expressed his view that incoming information from different senses is fused in a child before it is later untangled. The renaissance of scientific research into synesthesia is prompted by the recognition that synesthesia can be a window into the nature of perception. Among the remaining questions is its true prevalence, which is of more than theoretical interest. Some evidence suggests that synesthetic crossmodal mechanisms are universal, even if below the level of consciousness in most adults. Human sensory experiences and their interconnections will undoubtedly continue to intrigue scientists and artists alike well into the future.

—Judith Weinblatt, MA, MS;
updated by Bryan C. Auday, PhD

See also: Hearing; Nervous system; Neurology; Neurology, pediatric; Sense organs; Smell; Taste; Touch; Vision.

For Further Information:
American Synesthesia Association. synesthesia.info. Raises awareness of synesthesia and sponsors periodic conferences that provide a forum and information source for researchers and synesthetes.
Beeli, Gian, et al. "Synaesthesia: When Coloured Sounds Taste Sweet." *Nature* 434 (March 3, 2005): 38.
Brang, David, Vilayanur S. Ramachandran. *Synesthesia*. WWW.scholarpedia.org/article/Synesthesia.
Cytowic, R. E. and David M. Eagleman. *Wednesday is indigo blue: Discovering the brain of synesthesia*. Cambridge, MA: Massachusetts Institute of Technology, 2009.
Simner, Julia and Edward M. Hubbard. Eds. *Oxford Handbook of Synesthesia*. Oxford University Press, 2014.
Ramachandran, Vilayanur, and Edward Hubbard. "Hearing Colors, Tasting Shapes." *Scientific American* 288, no. 5 (May, 2003): 42-49.
Van Campen, Cretien. *The Hidden Sense: Synesthesia in Art and Science*. Cambridge, Mass.: MIT Press, 2007.
Ward, Jamie. *The Frog Who Croaked Blue: Synesthesia and the Mixing of the Senses*. New York: Routledge, 2008.

SYPHILIS

Category: Disease/Disorder
Also known as: "Bad blood," bejel (endemic syphilis)
Anatomy or system affected: Anus, blood vessels, bones, brain, eyes, genitals, heart, joints, kidneys, mucous membranes, nervous system, reproductive system, skin
Specialties and related fields: Bacteriology, embryology, epidemiology, gynecology, internal medicine, microbiology, neonatology, neurology, obstetrics, pediatrics, public health, rheumatology
Definition: a sexually transmitted disease caused by the spirochete bacterium *Treponema pallidum* that can progress from a genital lesion to a systemic disorder involving multiple organs
Key terms:
chancre: a painless ulcer, particularly one developing on the genitals because of venereal disease
endarteritis: inflammation of the inner lining of an artery
endoflagella: whip/propeller-like structures found beneath the outer membrane of spirochetes
gumma: a small soft swelling that is characteristic of the late stages of syphilis and occurs in the connective tissue of the liver, brain, testes, and heart
spirochetes: a flexible spirally twisted bacterium, especially one that causes syphilis

CAUSES AND SYMPTOMS

Syphilis is a sexually transmitted disease (STD) resulting from infection by *Treponema pallidum*. *Treponema pallidum* is a spirochete. Spirochetes are gram-negative bacteria that are long, corkscrew-shaped cells. These bacteria are distinguished from other bacteria by endoflagella (also known as axial filaments). Endoflagella are embedded in the cell membrane and project into the periplasmic space between the cell membrane and the cell wall. In other bacteria, flagella extend through the cell wall to the exterior. As endoflagella rotate, the spirochete twists in a corkscrew fashion that helps it burrow through its medium.

The history of syphilis is unclear. Evidence exists that its origin may have been linked with a disease, yaws, found in the Western Hemisphere at the time of explorer Christopher Columbus (1451-1506). Yaws is a relatively mild disease transmitted through contaminated objects or open skin lesions, but not generally through sexual transmission; it results from infection by a subspecies of *Treponema* called *T. pallidum ssp. pertenue*. The theory suggests that this may have been the form of the disease brought back to Europe on one of Columbus's ships. Mutation and sexual transmission in the population of Europe may have produced the more serious form of the disease.

Syphilis is a disease characterized by several distinct stages. Initial exposure to the organism during sexual intercourse results in the formation of a painless skin

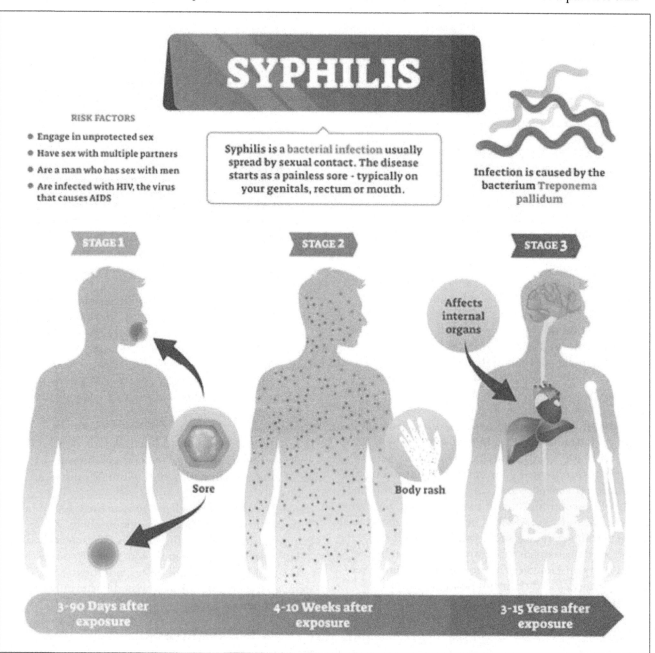

Signs and dangers of syphilis. Image via iStock/VectorMine.

lesion called a "chancre" at the site of infection (primary syphilis), developing anywhere from a week to months after infection. Spirochete bacteria usually occur within the lesion inside white blood cells (macrophages and neutrophils) that infiltrate the area. The white cells may help spread the spirochetes to other organs systems. Chancres generally heal spontaneously, leaving the impression that the disease has been eliminated.

During the weeks after the formation of the chancre, the spirochetes multiply to large numbers and become disseminated throughout the body. A second stage (secondary syphilis) often appears within two months following regression of the chancre. Symptoms are often flu-like, with malaise, headache, fever, and joint aches. A skin rash often appears, covering most of the body. Sores may develop in the mouth and throat and on many of the mucous membranes in the body. The organism is highly transmissible during this period. The rash and other symptoms generally fade over weeks.

Approximately 10 percent of untreated cases develop a third, or tertiary, stage of syphilis. The organism can infiltrate any organ or system in the body, resulting in soft tumors (gummas) in the eyes, lungs, bone, brain, or other organs. Symptoms are characteristic of the organ infected. For example, infection of the brain or other areas of the central nervous system is described as neurosyphilis or syphilitic dementia, characterized by memory loss, personality changes, and neurodegeneration. Even if tertiary syphilis is treated, the prognosis for the patient at this stage is often poor.

Cardiovascular syphilis occurs when *Treponema pallidum* affects the heart or large vessels that service it. Larger vessels have tiny arterioles that supply blood to their vessel walls called "vasa vasorum." *T. pallidum* inflames the vasa vasorum, a condition called "*endarteritis*," which deeply damages the aorta. Profound damage to the aorta wall weakens it and increases the risk of aortic aneurysms.

Treponema can cross the placenta, and the infection of a pregnant woman may result in congenital syphilis or infection of her unborn child. Infection may kill the fetus or cause it to be born with obvious deformities such as blindness or physical abnormalities. The infant may also be asymptomatic. An undiagnosed infection will likely progress, with symptoms appearing within weeks after birth. It is common for a rash to appear, with evidence of tertiary stage neurosyphilis or cardiovascular syphilis.

Syphilis diagnosis utilizes two types of tests: so-called "treponemal" tests that directly detect antibodies against specific *T. pallidum* antigens and

---

INFORMATION ON SYPHILIS

Causes: Bacterial infection transmitted through sexual contact or congenitally

Symptoms: In sexually transmitted form, painless skin lesion (chancre), malaise, headache, fever, joint aches, rash, sores in mouth and throat, and soft tumors in eyes, lungs, bone, or brain if untreated; in congenital form, stillbirth, blindness, physical abnormalities

Duration: Progressive, fatal if untreated

Treatments: Antibiotics (penicillin; also erythromycin, tetracyclines, chloramphenicol)

"non-treponemal" tests that detect antibodies the immune system makes against a cardiolipin/cholesterol/lecithin antigen. Nontreponemal tests include: 1) Rapid plasma reagin (RPR), 2) Venereal Disease Research Laboratory (VDRL), and 3) the Toluidine Red Unheated Serum Test (TRUST). Typically, nontreponemal tests are the initial tests used to determine if someone has syphilis. Healthcare providers run non-treponemal tests first because they are relatively inexpensive, easy to perform, and quantifiable, which indicates the level of infection. Unfortunately, nontreponemal tests lack specificity and sensitivity—twenty to thirty percent of individuals in the early stages of syphilis test negative with non-treponemal tests. False-positive test results result from their lack of specificity.

Traditionally, healthcare providers order treponemal tests after an initial positive non-treponemal test to corroborate it. Providers ordered treponemal tests afterward because of their complexity and expense. However, automation of newer types of treponemal tests has simplified them, and many laboratories use treponemal tests as their initial screening test for syphilis. Treponemal tests include: 1) Fluorescent treponemal antibody absorption (FTA-ABS), 2) Microhemagglutination test for antibodies to *T. pallidum* (MHA-TP), 3) *T. pallidum* particle agglutination assay (TPPA), 4) *T. pallidum* enzyme immunoassay (TP-EIA), and 5) Chemiluminescence immunoassay (CIA). Since treponemal tests detect antibodies against specific *T. pallidum* antigens, they have good specificity. However, they are not quantitative tests, only qualitative.

In cases of neurosyphilis, a positive VDRL test on cerebrospinal fluid samples confirms the diagnosis. However, VDRL has high specificity for syphilis in cerebrospinal fluid but has poor sensitivity. Therefore, after a negative VDRL test, an FTA-ABS test on the cerebrospinal sample can confirm a negative test.

Though not as specific as the VRDL, the FTA-ABS test is highly sensitive, and false negatives with this test are highly unlikely.

TREATMENT AND THERAPY
A single dose of intramuscular penicillin G benzathine is the standard treatment for most primary, secondary, and early latent syphilis cases. Treatment of tertiary syphilis eliminates the microorganism but does not reverse any potential organ damage. Treatment for related organ involvement is symptomatic.

Alternative antibiotics for people allergic to penicillin or in places where penicillin G benzathine is unavailable (e.g., Japan) include oral doxycycline, amoxicillin with probenecid, azithromycin, and intramuscular ceftriaxone. However, penicillin G benzathine is the preferred treatment for tertiary syphilis or pregnant women.

Intravenous penicillin G is the only recognized treatment for neurosyphilis.

PERSPECTIVE AND PROSPECTS
Despite the long-time existence of effective therapy, penicillin or alternative antibiotics, and the absence of any reservoir for *T. palladium* other than humans, syphilis remains the third most common sexually transmitted bacterial disease in the West. Only gonorrhea and chlamydia are more common.

As a result of effective therapy and the generally obvious symptoms of the disease, tertiary syphilis has largely disappeared. However, sexual practices continue to sustain the spread of the disease, with approximately fifty thousand cases reported each year in the United States. Three factors are primary contributors to the resurgence of the disease: prostitution, the increase in riskier sexual practices among homosexual men, and general apathy toward a relatively easy disease to treat in its early stages. An increase in congenital syphilis also reflects the presence of the disease in women of childbearing years. In the absence of condom use, both unwanted pregnancy and the spread of STDs such as syphilis may result.

No vaccine currently exists for syphilis. The inability to culture the organism in the laboratory has made research related to *Treponema* difficult. The organism does not infect animals other than humans to act as a vaccine production method. However, genetic engineering has resulted in the cloning of several bacterial gene products related to surface proteins and virulence factors, allowing the possibility for a vaccine in the future. Recent experiments demonstrated that immunizing rabbits with whole, killed spirochetes protects them against *T. pallidum* infection. Other studies with nanoparticles that deliver circular DNA molecules (plasmids) encoding *T. pallidum* outer membrane proteins to immune cells induce robust, protective immune responses in New Zealand white rabbits. Though such procedures presently are in the experimental stage, their success in the laboratory gives hope that such technologies may provide the means of developing an effective vaccine against syphilis in the future. For now, the best means of controlling syphilis remains to prevent its spread through education and safer-sex practices, and early treatment of those infected.

—*Michael A. Buratovich, PhD*

For Further Information:
Morris, Sheldon R. "Syphilis." *Merck Manual Consumer Version*, Jan. 2021, www.merckmanuals.com/home/infections/sexually-transmitted-diseases-stds/syphilis. Accessed 26 Mar. 2022.
Mroczkowski, Thomasz F. *History, Sex, and Syphilis: Famous Syphilitics and Their Private Lives.* Booklocker.com, Inc., 2016.
Syphilis. MedlinePlus, 5 Nov. 2021, medlineplus.gov/syphilis.html. Accessed 26 Mar. 2022.
Syphilis. University of Florida Health, 25 Oct. 2020, ufhealth.org/syphilis. Accessed 26 Mar. 2022.
Syphilis - CDC Fact Sheet (Detailed). Center for Disease Control and Prevention, 10 Feb. 2022. www.cdc.gov/std/syphilis/stdfact-syphilis-detailed.htm. Accessed 26 Mar. 2022.
Syphilis Tests. Testing.com, 9 Nov. 2021, www.testing.com/tests/syphilis-test/. Accessed 26 Mar. 2022.

SYSTEMIC LUPUS ERYTHEMATOSUS (SLE)

Category: Disease/Disorder
Also known as: Lupus
Anatomy or system affected: All
Specialties and related fields: Cardiology, dermatology, endocrinology, family medicine, gastroenterology, histology, immunology, internal medicine, nephrology, nutrition, orthopedics, pharmacology, physical therapy, psychiatry, psychology, pulmonary medicine, rheumatology, vascular medicine
Definition: A chronic, inflammatory autoimmune disease in which the immune system attacks the body's structures. SLE can affect any organ or body system, especially the skin, joints, blood vessels, and kidneys. It is distinguished from two other forms of lupus: drug-induced lupus, which is caused by certain prescription medications, and discoid lupus, which primarily affects the skin.

Key terms:

antibodies: proteins manufactured by the body to attack and neutralize foreign substances, such as bacteria

antinuclear antibody (ANA): an unusual antibody that is directed against structures within the nucleus of cells

autoantibodies: antibodies that attack the body's cells and tissues

autoimmune: a term describing a disease in which the body produces antibodies against its cells

connective tissue: the substance holding the body and organs together

cytotoxic: having a damaging effect on cells

discoid rash: raised red patches

erythematosus: characterized by redness of the skin

hyperlipidemia: an excess of lipids (for example, cholesterol and triglycerides) in the blood

malar rash: a redness or rash on the face covering the cheeks and the bridge of the nose; also called "butterfly rash"

photosensitivity: sensitivity to light or sunlight

Raynaud's phenomenon: discoloration and pain in the fingertips induced by cold

serositis: inflammation of the lining of the lung or heart

CAUSES AND SYMPTOMS

The cause of lupus is unknown, but scientists believe that genetic and environmental factors are involved. Although there is a genetic predisposition to lupus, and researchers have identified an associated gene in some cases, only 10 percent of lupus patients have a familial connection. Only 5 percent of children born to individuals with lupus will develop the disease. People of African, American Indian, Asian, and Hispanic origin seem to develop the disease more frequently than non-Hispanic Caucasians. Lupus affects both men and women, but the incidence is ten to fifteen times higher in women. Between 85 and 90 percent of patients are women. Most lupus diagnoses occur in young women in their late teens to thirties. Hormonal factors may play a role in this disparity because it is known that symptoms in women increase before menstrual cycles and during pregnancy. Environmental triggers include infections, exposure to ultraviolet light, extreme stress, and antibiotic usage (particularly penicillin and those in the sulfa group). Certain other drugs, particularly hydralazine, procainamide, and isoniazid, can also cause lupus. Still, this type of drug-induced lupus usually disappears after discontinuation of the offending drug.

Symptoms may begin suddenly with fever or develop gradually over months or years. The clinical course is usually marked by remissions, periods when symptoms are minimal or absent, and relapses (called "flare-ups") when the patient experiences an aggravation of symptoms and general malaise.

> **INFORMATION ON**
> **SYSTEMIC LUPUS ERYTHEMATOSUS (SLE)**
>
> **Causes:** Unclear; possibly related to paramyxoviral infection
> **Symptoms:** Red or purple facial lesions, joint pain and swelling, fatigue, low-grade fever
> **Duration:** Chronic
> **Treatments:** None; alleviation of symptoms

SLE can affect all organ systems of the body. The production of autoantibodies is the underlying physiologic problem in lupus. These autoantibodies can appear in a significant number and variety, differing from patient to patient, thus causing their varying symptoms. General symptoms include fatigue, fever, anemia, weight loss, Raynaud's phenomenon, and headaches. Joint inflammation and pain (arthritis) occur in about 90 percent of patients and are often the disease's earliest manifestation. It usually occurs intermittently and generally does not cause permanent joint damage or deformity. Skin manifestations in most patients include malar (butterfly) or discoid skin rashes; redness on the hands, fingertips, and nails; mucous membrane ulcers in the mouth and nose; and photosensitivity. Inflammation of the sac around the lungs (pleurisy) or heart (pericarditis) is frequent, resulting in pain upon deep breathing or chest pain. There may be severe complications on rare occasions, such as bleeding into the lungs, which is life-threatening, or cardiac failure. Neurologic complications may also occur, including headaches, thinking impairment, personality changes, seizures, strokes, depression, dementia, and psychosis. Kidney involvement may be either minor or progressive, leading to severe nephritis that can be fatal. Ocular changes sometimes occur, causing conjunctivitis or blurred vision. In rare cases, retinitis, inflammation of the blood vessels at the back of the eye, can occur, leading to blindness if not treated quickly.

SLE is difficult to diagnose due to its variety of symptoms and similarity to many other diseases. The constellation of symptoms appears and progresses differently for each patient and initially may seem vague and unrelated. For a positive diagnosis of SLE, a patient must have at least four of the eleven criteria established by the American College of Rheumatology: malar rash, discoid rash, photosensitivity, oral ulcers, arthritis, serositis, renal disorder, neurologic disorder, hematologic disorder, immunologic disorder, and the presence of antinuclear antibodies (ANA). Usually, patients will first see their family doctors. Upon diagnosis or discovering particular body system involvement, the family doctor may refer the patient to one or more specialists. A physician will perform several laboratory tests as part of the differential diagnostic process, including blood and urine tests and biopsies of the skin and kidney. There is no single test for lupus.

TREATMENT AND THERAPY

There is no cure for lupus. Treatment aims to minimize symptoms, reduce inflammation, and maintain normal bodily functions. The treatment approach will vary according to the individual patient's specific symptoms and organ involvement.

Preventive therapy involves lifestyle strategies aimed at reducing the risk of flare-up episodes. Patients are advised to follow a healthy diet, get adequate rest, and participate in moderate weight-bearing exercises to combat fatigue and muscle weakness. Counseling, support groups, and patient education help reduce stress and protect emotional well-being. Other recommendations include smoking cessation, limited alcohol intake, and adequate vitamin D and calcium intake. Avoidance of excessive sun exposure through protective clothing and sunscreens can reduce the occurrence of skin rashes and possibly systemic disease flares. Patients can learn to recognize the warning signs of an impending flare-up, such as increased fatigue, headaches, dizziness, stomach upset, fever, or the appearance of a rash. Regular laboratory tests can also detect an imminent flare-up. Early treatment of flare-ups can make them easier to control, prevent tissue damage, and reduce the length of time the patient is given high doses of drugs.

Medications are integral in treating lupus and fall into four main categories: nonsteroidal anti-inflammatory drugs (NSAIDs), corticosteroids, antimalarial drugs, and cytotoxic and immunosuppressive agents.

NSAIDs control symptoms and reduce muscle and joint pain and inflammation. Common NSAIDs include acetylsalicylic acid (aspirin), ibuprofen, naproxen, indomethacin, sulindac, nabumetone, tolmetin, and ketoprofen. Since these drugs can cause stomach upset, patients are usually advised to take them with meals, antacids, or prostaglandins. Some NSAIDs have prostaglandin added to the capsule. Patients taking NSAIDs must be monitored because of the potential adverse effects on the liver, kidney, and central nervous system.

Corticosteroids are synthetic hormones with excellent anti-inflammatory and immunoregulatory effects and promptly reduce symptoms. They are used to treat a spectrum of lupus manifestations, especially when organs are threatened. Prednisone is the most used, followed by hydrocortisone, methylprednisolone, and others. Topical formulations are used for skin rashes, and oral doses are given for systemic involvement. Dosages are monitored carefully and tapered after initial inflammation reduction to reduce possible side effects. Corticosteroids may also be administered by injection into the skin or joint. For severe cases, intravenous (IV) administration of large doses of methylprednisolone (called "pulse steroids") for three days is given. Unfortunately, high doses of corticosteroids over long periods can produce unpleasant side effects, such as weight gain, rounded face, acne, emotional lability, hypertension, hyperlipidemia, increased risk of infection, diabetes, and osteoporosis.

Antimalarial drugs effectively manage skin rashes, joint inflammation, and serositis. However, it may take months before their beneficial effects become apparent. They also help protect against the damaging effects of ultraviolet light. The most common agents are hydroxychloroquine (*Plaquenil*), chloroquine (*Aralen*), and quinacrine (*Atabrine*). SLE patients can take antimalarial medications combined with NSAIDs and other drugs to increase their effectiveness. They are beneficial when used with corticosteroids to decrease the dose of steroids needed. Damage to the retina is a potential side effect and is dose-related. Patients must be evaluated by an ophthalmologist twice a year.

Cytotoxic and immunosuppressive agents are potent drugs utilized in cases requiring aggressive therapy to protect major organs. They are used with, or in place of, corticosteroids to diminish the side effects of the corticosteroids. Cytotoxics are not approved by the Food and Drug Administration (FDA) for use in treating SLE; however, they are considered part of standard practice. These drugs target autoantibodies, thus suppressing the overactive immune response of lupus patients. Cyclophosphamide (*Cytoxin*) and azathioprine (*Imuran*) are used to treat lupus nephritis. They are also effective in combating blood cell deficiencies, pulmonary bleeding, vasculitis, and central nervous system disease. *Imuran* is less potent but causes fewer side effects than does *Cytoxin*. Methotrexate, mycophenolate mofetil (*CellCept*), cyclosporine, chlorambucil, and nitrogen mustard are other cytotoxic agents that have been used in the management of lupus. Intravenous immunoglobulin injections are given to some patients to increase the production of blood platelets. Side effects of cytotoxic drugs include nausea, hair loss, increased risk of certain cancers, increased risk of infection, sterility, and bone marrow suppression.

The FDA-approved belimumab (*Benlysta*) in 2011 for adults with active SLE. Belimumab is a human monoclonal antibody that blocks the binding of "soluble B-lymphocyte stimulator" (BLyS) to its receptors on B cells. BLyS is a small polypeptide that regulates B cell differentiation and stability. BLyS levels are elevated in SLE. The levels of BLyS correlate with disease activity. Inhibiting BLyS function diminishes the number of SLE flares and symptoms.

About 50 to 60 percent of patients with systemic lupus erythematosus (SLE) develop a kidney disease called "lupus nephritis." Lupus nephritis occurs during the first ten years, and up to 10 percent of these patients develop end-stage renal disease. Black and Hispanic/Latino patients have a significantly higher prevalence of lupus nephritis and generally have a more severe disease. Standard treatment for lupus nephritis includes corticosteroids plus oral or IV cyclophosphamide (*Cytoxan* and generics) or mycophenolate mofetil. Upon resolution of nephritis, maintenance treatment to prevent it from recurring consists of continuing mycophenolate mofetil (preferred) or azathioprine (Imuran and others). A new FDA-approved therapy for lupus nephritis is voclosporin (*Lupkynis*), an oral calcineurin inhibitor. Voclosporin should be used with mycophenolate mofetil (*CellCept* and generics) and a corticosteroid.

Pregnancy in a lupus patient requires special care. Even though more than 50 percent of lupus pregnancies follow an ordinary course, all lupus pregnancies are considered high risk. Doctors recommend planning pregnancy during times of remission. Recent studies contradict the traditional belief that pregnancy increases the chance of flare-ups and suggest that most flare-ups during pregnancy are mild, consisting only of rashes, fatigue, and arthritis. Frequent doctor visits are a necessity to detect and treat any problems early. The obstetrician will regularly check the baby's growth and heartbeat to detect any abnormalities that might signal problems. Some lupus medications, such as prednisone, are safe during pregnancy because they do not cross the placenta. Others, such as cyclophosphamide, need to be used with caution or discontinued during the pregnancy.

Preeclampsia is a severe condition during pregnancy. There is a sudden increase in blood pressure and protein in the urine. It requires immediate treatment of the patient and delivery of the baby. Preeclampsia affects approximately 20 percent of women with SLE during their pregnancy.

About one-third of women with lupus have antiphospholipid antibodies. These antibodies cause blood clots, which puts the patient at risk of developing them in the placenta, interfering with the baby's nourishment. Since these blood clots usually form in the placenta in the second trimester, often, the baby has developed enough to be delivered prematurely. Treating the mother with heparin reduces the chance of clots and miscarriage.

About 50 percent of lupus pregnancies result in birth before full term. Most babies born between thirty and thirty-six weeks will grow normally with no problems. Those born before thirty-six weeks are considered premature. Approximately three percent of women with lupus will have a baby with a syndrome called "neonatal lupus." This syndrome consists of a transient rash and blood count abnormalities and disappears in three to six months. Sometimes, a permanent heartbeat abnormality also occurs, but it is treatable, and the baby can grow normally.

In pregnant women with SLE, the drugs of choice are hydroxychloroquine and low-dose aspirin. During pregnancy, other safe medications with caveats include glucocorticoids (lower dose), azathioprine (do not exceed 2 mg/kg/day), and tacrolimus. For pregnancy, safe blood pressure medicines include methyldopa, labetalol, nifedipine, and hydralazine.

PERSPECTIVE AND PROSPECTS

The identification of lupus as a distinct medical entity dates to the twelfth century, when the term *lupus* (Latin for "wolf") was used to describe ulcerative facial lesions because they looked like either a wolf's bite or a wolf's facial markings. Physicians noted other descriptions of the various dermatologic manifestations of lupus over several centuries; the first medical textbook illustration occurred in 1856. The Viennese physician Moriz Kaposi, 1872, was the first physician to recognize and describe the systemic manifestations of lupus. There seemed to be two distinct forms of lupus, discoid and systemic. In 1909, Canadian physician Sir William Osler described, in detail, the major organ manifestations of SLE. In the late nineteenth century, the usefulness of quinine and salicylates in treating lupus was reported. In the mid-twentieth century, identifying antinuclear antibodies initiated the immunologic aspects of lupus. Around this same time, the first animal models were used to study lupus. Studies of animal models revealed a genetic component of lupus. A significant advance was the discovery of the effectiveness of cortisone in the treatment of systemic lupus. Corticosteroids remain the primary treatment modality, complemented by antimalarials (for skin and joint involvement) and cytotoxic agents (for severe kidney manifestations and other life-threatening complications).

The prognosis for lupus patients has improved dramatically because of earlier diagnosis and better treatment. However, the long-term prognosis for a given patient is still variable. It is often related to the severity and controllability of the initial inflammation. Also, the morbidity patterns of lupus patients have changed because of the increased usage of corticosteroids and cytotoxic drugs. Infections, accelerated atherosclerosis, and osteoporosis have become significant risk factors. However, the outlook for survival and quality of life has dramatically improved. As of 2005, more than 90 percent of lupus patients lived more than ten years postdiagnosis. Those with the organ-threatening disease had a lower rate, with only 60 percent surviving fifteen to twenty years.

A proliferation of research into the treatment of lupus that began in the 1950s continues and brings much promise for additional insight into the pathogenesis of lupus and new treatment modalities and agents. Some focus areas of current research include investigations into patterns of gene activity, the role of the protein interferon-alpha in the progression of lupus, environmental factors, immune ablation, stem cell transplantation, and the targeting of destructive white blood cells. An intensified effort by the federal government, private industry, and non-profit organizations, such as the Alliance for Lupus Research and the Lupus Foundation of America, fuels the hope that researchers will find better treatments, prevention, and ultimately a cure for lupus.

—*Michael A. Buratovich, PhD*

For Further Information:
"Belimumab (*Benlysta*) for Systemic Lupus Erythematosus." *Medical Letter on Drugs and Therapeutics*, vol. 53, no. 1366, 2011, pp. 45-46.
Herndon, Jaime. "Systemic Lupus Erythematosus." *Healthline*, 29 May 2020, www.healthline.com/health/systemic-lupus-erythematosus. Accessed 4 Apr. 2022.
Lupus. American College of Rheumatologists, Dec. 2021, www.rheumatology.org/I-Am-A/Patient-Caregiver/Diseases-Conditions/Lupus. Accessed 4 Apr. 2022.
Lupus. Mayo Clinic, 27 Jan. 2021, www.mayoclinic.org/diseases-conditions/lupus/symptoms-causes/syc-20365789. Accessed 4 Apr. 2022.
Lupus Foundation of America, www.lupus.org. www.rheumatology.org/I-Am-A/Patient-Caregiver/Diseases-Conditions/Lupus. Accessed 4 Apr. 2022.
Nevares, Alana M. "Systemic Lupus Erythematosus (SLE)." Merck Manual Consumer Version, Apr. 2020, www.merckmanuals.com/home/bone,-joint,-and-muscle-disorders/autoimmune-disorders-of-connective-tissue/systemic-lupus-erythematosus-sle?query=Systemic%20Lupus%20Erythematosus%20(SLE). Accessed 4 Apr. 2022.
Systemic Lupus Erythematosus (Lupus). National Institute of Arthritis of Musculoskeletal and Skin Diseases, Jun. 2019, www.niams.nih.gov/health-topics/lupus. Accessed 4 Apr.
Systemic Lupus Erythematosus (SLE). The Centers for Disease Control and Prevention, 17 Oct. 2018, www.cdc.gov/lupus/facts/detailed.html. Accessed 4 Apr. 2022.
"Voclosporin (*Lupkynis*) for Lupus Nephritis." *Medical Letter on Drugs and Therapeutics*, vol. 63, no. 1631, 2021, pp. 134-36.
What is Systemic Lupus Erythematosus (SLE)? Lupus Foundation of America, 18 Mar. 2021, www.lupus.org/resources/what-is-systemic-lupus-erythematosus-sle. 4 Apr. 2022.

SYSTEMIC SCLEROSIS

Category: Disease/Disorder
Also known as: Systemic scleroderma
Anatomy or system affected: All
Specialties and related fields: All
Definition: A systemic disease characterized by extensive scarring in the skin, connective tissue, and internal organs.
Key terms:
autoimmune response: an inappropriate immune response against the patient's own cells
cytokines: small proteins released by immune cells that elicit specific effects from other cells
fibroblast: an immature cell that manufactures connective tissues
fibrosis: an increase in the fibrous scar tissue deposited between cells

CAUSES AND SYMPTOMS

During the process of wound healing, specific cells known as fibroblasts deposit a protein called collagen to heal the breach in our tissues. Large areas of collagen deposition compose what we commonly call a scar. Our bodies carefully regulate collagen deposition to prevent scarring in unneeded places. People with systemic sclerosis (SSc) experience unregulated deposition of collagen.

In SSc patients, the immune system malfunctions and attacks the body's own tissues and organs. This continuous damage and inflammation leads to continuous collagen deposition and scarring, which stiffens, hardens, and thickens those tissues and organs affected by the inflammation.

Typically, the SSc-specific autoimmune response begins with damage to blood vessels, which summons immune cells to the injury site. The immune cells secrete small signaling proteins called cytokines, in particular platelet-derived growth factor (PDGF), transforming growth factor-β1 (TGF-β1), and interleukin-6 (IL-6). These cytokines signal to antibody-producing B-lymphocytes to produce antibodies against blood vessels, and also signal to fibroblasts to differentiate into myofibroblasts. In response to the tissue destruction caused by the immune response, myofibroblasts deposit collagen and other molecules in an attempt to mitigate the damage. This repeated cycle of damage and collagen deposition leads to the formation of large, stiff scars that harden the tissue or organ and compromise its function.

What causes the initial damage to blood vessels remains unknown, but several factors seem to act as triggers. Exposure to silica, organic solvents (e.g., toluene, hexane, vinyl chloride, xylene, etc.), epoxy resins, pesticides, certain drugs (e.g., bleomycin cocaine, carbidopa, and others), appetite suppressants, silicone or paraffin implants, or vibrational injuries seem to act as triggers that initiate the cascade of events that lead to SSc. Genetic factors also clearly play a vital role in the propensity someone has to develop SSc. Finally, particular viral infections (e.g., cytomegalovirus) that infect and damage blood vessels might act as triggers.

Internationally, SSc afflicts 2.3-10 people per one million, and affects women three to six times more often than men. SSc is rare in Japan and China and more common in African-American and American Indian women than in white women.

The first signs of SSc tend to be Raynaud's phenomenon or a whitening of the hands in response cold exposure, and itching (pruritus). Damage to blood vessels causes puffy, swollen hands. Afterwards, the skin begins to thicken and harden, usually beginning with the hands and face. Lack of blood flow to the hands can produce ulcers at the tips of the fingers. Also, calcium deposits form under the skin (calcinosis). Calcium deposits and thickening of the skin can restrict movement around joints, especially the smaller joints of the hand. Patients can also experience arthritis and muscle weakness.

Lung damage causes shortness of breath upon exertion and later also at rest. Elevation in blood pressures in the pulmonary arteries (pulmonary hypertension) follows. Scarring of the gastrointestinal tract usually begins with narrowing of the esophagus (peptic stricture), which causes difficulty swallowing (dysphagia), and increased scarring reduces gastrointestinal motility. Severe gastroesophageal reflux disease (GERD) follows, which predisposes the patient to esophageal cancer. Reduction in intestinal motility compromises nutrient absorption, leading to malnutrition.

In the kidney, SSc produces scleroderma renal cysts. Kidney involvement substantially raises blood pressure (malignant hypertension) and blood levels of ammonium (azotemia), and causes the leakage of blood (hematuria) and protein (proteinuria) into urine.

Heart involvement scars the heart, leading to life-threatening heart failure. Vascular damage can also induce strokes.

Those who suffer from limited cutaneous SSc usually experience symptoms restricted to the skin. However, those who have diffuse cutaneous SSc show rapid scarring (fibrosis) of the skin, and internal organs, in particular the lungs, heart, gastrointestinal tract, and kidneys.

TREATMENT AND THERAPY
Serological tests of blood from SSc patients typically reveal particular auto-antibodies or antibodies that bind to patient's own tissues; antinuclear antibodies

> ### INFORMATION ON SYSTEMIC SCLEROSIS
> **Causes:** An immune response against blood vessels leads to massive inflammation and scarring of the skin and internal organs
> **Symptoms:** Itching, Raynaud's phenomenon, difficulty swallowing, nausea, vomiting, weight loss, abdominal cramps, diarrhea, fecal incontinence, shortness of breath, chest pain, fatigue, high blood pressure, joint pain and swelling, muscle pain and weakness, blood and protein in urine
> **Duration:** Usually arises between the ages of 30 to 50 and remains for a lifetime
> **Treatments:** Skin moisturizers, avoiding cold, calcium-channel blockers, blood vessel dilating drugs, antihypertensive agents, proton pump inhibitors, immunomodulatory agents, and bone marrow transplants

are characteristic of SSc. Imaging studies can document the fibrotic changes in the lungs, heart, and gastrointestinal tract, as can histological examinations of biopsied tissues.

Treatment focuses on decreasing fibrosis and preserving organ function. To stifle fibrosis, antiscarring drugs such as D-penicillamine, interferon-α, interferon-γ, methotrexate, chlorambucil, cyclosporine, thalidomide, tacrolimus, corticosteroids, cyclophosphamide, and statins have provided some patients relief, albeit not consistently. For patients with gastrointestinal involvement, proton pump inhibitors and H2 receptor blockers can control the symptoms of GERD. To treat inflammation of muscles, high dose corticosteroids can halt the advance of fibrosis. In patients with lung involvement, calcium-channel blockers, prostaglandins such as prostacyclin, and cyclophosphamide have provided relief for some, though not all, patients. For those with kidney involvement, angiotensin-converting enzyme (ACE) inhibitors or angiotensin II receptor blockers are essential to control hypertension. For Raynaud's phenomenon, avoiding exposure to cold temperature and warm clothing can prevent the onset of symptoms.

Pulsed dye laser treatments can effectively clear fibrotic areas, but multiple treatments are required and recurrence remains a problem.

PROCEDURES AND PROSPECTS
Early paintings and written descriptions possibly recount cases of SSc, but the first codified description of SSc comes from Carlo Curzio in 1752. Curzio treated a 17-year-old woman at the Royal Hospital in Naples who suffered from a diffuse hardness of her skin. The

Milanese physician Giovambattista Fantonetti in 1836 was the first to use the term "scleroderma," which comes from a combination of the Greek words "skleros" or hard and "dermos" or skin. Fantonetti described a 30-year-old patient named Antonia Alessandri whose skin was as dark, tense, and firm as leather. Fortunately, Ms. Alessandri miraculously recovered three months later, which casts doubt on Fantonetti's diagnosis, but medical professionals continued to use the term he coined.

Perhaps the most exciting development in SSc is the use of bone marrow stem cell transplantations to treat SSc patients. Patients treated with hematopoietic stem cell transplantations (HSCTs) survive better, have significantly improved skin flexibility, and some improvements in lung function. Refining this procedure should make it more mainstream rather than experimental.

—*Michael A. Buratovich, PhD*

See also Antihypertensives; Cardiology; Dermatology; Dermopathology; Histology; Hypertension; Immunology; Immunopathology; Nephrology; Pulmonology; Raynaud's syndrome; Wounds

For Further Information:

Clearview, Darrell. *Your Scleroderma Symptoms, Treatments and Self-Help Guide.* Seattle, WA: Amazon Digital Services, 2011.
Jacob, Elliot, ed. *Medifocus Guidebook on: Scleroderma.* Silver Spring, MD: Medifocus, Inc., 2013.
Ruscitto, Louis. *Scleroderma-Understand Connective Tissue Disease.* Seattle, WA: Amazon Digital Services, 2012.

SYSTEMS AND ORGANS

Category: Anatomy
Anatomy or system affected: All
Specialties and related fields: All
Definition: Groups of tissues and organs dedicated to particular functions, all of which must work together to perform efficiently.
Key terms:
atrium: the chamber of the heart where veins terminate; the atrium receives blood returning to the heart and delivers it to the ventricle
bronchi: the airways conducting air from the mouth to the depths of the lungs
carbon dioxide: the gas produced by the body from the use of oxygen; carbon dioxide and the hydrogen ions it can create may become toxic if not excreted by the body
foodstuffs: the basic components of food that the body can use-carbohydrates (which break down to sugars, primarily to glucose), proteins (which break down to amino acids), and fat

hormone: a chemical released by a tissue to signal another tissue to modify its function
ions: small chemical substances that have a positive or negative charge; the most important ions with a positive charge are sodium, potassium, hydrogen, and calcium, while the most important negative ion is chloride
ventricles: the large chambers of the heart that pump blood into the arteries; the left ventricle pumps blood into the aorta, and the right ventricle pumps blood into the lung's arteries

STRUCTURE AND FUNCTIONS

There are essentially nine systems in the human body: the nervous, cardiovascular, respiratory, gastrointestinal, renal, endocrine, reproductive, thermoregulatory, and skeletomuscular systems. All these systems are essential to sustain life, and many work together to perform their functions efficiently. All the other systems need the nervous system to operate or to coordinate their functions. The first six of these systems will be discussed in this article.

The nervous system is composed of the central nervous system (the brain) and the peripheral nervous system (the spinal cord and nerves extending to every part of the body). The brain receives information from the body by way of the sensory nerves. It then evaluates all the information and sends out the appropriate signals to respond. For example, the ears send information to the brain that there are noises coming from behind; the brain tells the head to turn in the direction of the sounds. The eyes send the signals that the noises are coming from, for example, a gorilla. The brain must decide to run, fight, or stand and try to reason with the gorilla. Meanwhile, the brain tells the heart to beat faster and harder. It also tells the stomach and intestines to stop digestion and reduce its blood flow because blood may be needed by the muscles for running. This is called the "fight or flight" response to stress, which the nervous system controls.

Sensory information can come from any of the five senses-sight, smell, hearing, touch, or taste-but it can also come from other sensors. Sensory nerves send the brain information on pain, temperature, blood pressure, and what is going on in the stomach and intestines (hunger or a full feeling). The brain receives millions of signals each second from every part of the body and must constantly decide how to respond. Humans can choose not to respond instinctively as animals do. For example, humans often eat when they are not hungry.

Different areas of the brain are dedicated to specific functions. The upper portion of the spinal cord and lower portion of the brain (the brain stem) are dedicated to controlling involuntary functions such as breathing, the maintenance of blood pressure and heart rate, and the responses to hot and cold. The middle portion of the brain coordinates movement. The middle brain also coordinates information from upper portions of the brain and generates emotions. The uppermost and outermost portions of the brain (the cerebrum) process the information from the senses and generate responses, such as telling the body to move. The cerebrum also performs such intellectual functions as reasoning.

The cardiovascular system is composed of the heart and blood vessels. Its job is to pump blood containing oxygen and foodstuffs (sugars, proteins, and fat) to every part of the body. Blood is composed of red and white blood cells suspended in plasma, a pale yellow fluid which flows through the cardiovascular system. Red blood cells are the carriers of oxygen, the main source of energy for the body. White blood cells help fight disease and are delivered to parts of the body that are hurt or diseased. The plasma contains platelets that help blood to clot when necessary. Blood also transports wastes produced by the body from tissues to organs that can dispose of them. For example, carbon dioxide is produced by the tissues when oxygen is used for energy. Blood carries carbon dioxide back to the lungs to be removed from the body in exhaled air.

Blood is pumped by the heart in a circuit in the cardiovascular system (also called the circulatory system). The heart has four chambers, two atria and two ventricles. Blood enters the heart through the left atrium, a small pocket of muscles that help pump blood into the left ventricle. The ventricle is a larger chamber with a thick wall of muscle that can pump very hard; it pushes blood into the arteries. The left ventricle pumps blood into the main artery of the body, the aorta. The aorta branches many times into smaller arteries, which in turn branch into capillaries. Every part of the body has millions of tiny capillaries just big enough for a blood cell to pass through them; in fact, blood cells must fold to get through some capillaries. In capillaries, oxygen and foodstuffs leave the blood, and then carbon dioxide and other waste products enter the blood to be taken away. Blood flows from the capillaries into small veins, which join to make larger and larger veins. The largest veins, the venae cavae, empty into the heart, in the right atrium. The blood is pumped from the right atrium to the right ventricle. Blood is then pumped by the right ventricle through the lung and back into the left atrium to start its journey again.

The lungs are the major organ of the respiratory system. The function of the respiratory system is to bring fresh air into the lungs, getting it very close to the blood, and to expel used air. Air enters the respiratory system through the nose and mouth, which connect to the main windpipe, the trachea. The trachea branches into smaller airways called bronchi. Bronchi in turn branch into smaller airways, bronchioles. The ends of bronchioles form many rounded sacs (alveoli) that resemble a bunch of grapes. These sacs of air have very thin walls that are shared with the walls of the lung's capillaries. This close arrangement of air and blood provides a minimal distance for oxygen to travel into the blood and for carbon dioxide to leave the blood.

Air is moved into the lungs when the muscles of respiration contract and expand the lungs. The diaphragm is a large sheet of muscle which separates the chest from the abdomen. When the diaphragm contracts, it pulls the lungs down. At the same time, muscles on the chest wall contract, pulling the lungs up and out. This expansion of the lungs causes air to be sucked into and fill the air sacs. During exhalation, the respiratory muscles are relaxed, the lung collapses somewhat, and air rushes out, carrying carbon dioxide with it.

Blood, specifically red blood cells, is specialized to carry large amounts of oxygen and carbon dioxide. Red blood cells contain hemoglobin, a special substance that attaches to these gases. When the amounts of oxygen and carbon dioxide in the plasma increase, they tend to leak back into the air sacs or tissues, respectively. These gases are effectively removed from the fluid by hemoglobin, allowing more gases to enter the blood without leaking back out. Hemoglobin also coordinates the release of these gases-oxygen to the tissues and carbon dioxide to the lungs-at the correct time.

The gastrointestinal system is a multiorgan system that breaks down food to be absorbed into the blood. Initially, food is broken down by chewing and by mixing with saliva. Then it is swallowed into the esophagus, a tube which travels through the chest to empty into the stomach. The stomach adds acid and other chemicals to the food, which breaks it down even more. The food, now called chyme, passes into the upper small intestine (the duodenum). The pancreas adds enzymes; a chemical called bicarbonate, which neutralizes the acid added by the stomach; and the hormones insulin and glucagon. Insulin is the major hormone secreted by the pancreas. It is absorbed into the blood by the intestine and signals the body to get ready to receive the products of digestion, primarily sugar (glucose). Bile is also added to the contents of the upper duodenum by the liver. Bile helps to break down fat to be absorbed into the blood. As the intestinal contents move along the small intestine, from the jejunum to the ileum, water and mucus are added to help move it along, and carbohydrates are absorbed in their smallest form, glucose. Enzymes attached to the wall of the intestine break up proteins to be absorbed as their component parts, amino acids. Water in chyme is constantly being reabsorbed. Finally the colon, or large intestine, absorbs most of the remaining water. The remaining solids are excreted through the rectum.

Food is moved through the gastrointestinal system by a special type of muscle called smooth muscle. The walls of the gastrointestinal tract are composed of muscle arranged in circular fashion around the tube and along its length. Initially, a circular group of muscles contracts, narrowing a short segment of intestine. This process is called segmentation. The contraction spreads down the muscles arranged lengthwise, squeezing the contents down the length of intestine. Movement of chyme is aided by relaxation of the muscles ahead of the contraction. This motion is called peristalsis. Peristalsis is coordinated by the nervous system, but the intestines have their own set of nerves. These intestinal nerves can control the motion of the intestine without help from the central nervous system.

The kidneys are the primary organs of the renal system. It is the function of the kidneys to regulate both the amount and the composition of the fluid in the body, in spite of wide variations in the human environment and in an organism's intake of food and water. Since blood circulates everywhere in the body, the kidneys can change the composition and amount of plasma, and the other fluids of the body then equalize with it. Therefore, the kidneys can regulate all body fluids. The body has sensors for both the amount of fluid in the blood and the concentration of the important elements in the blood, such as sodium, hydrogen, and potassium.

The kidneys regulate plasma volume and composition by filtering the plasma and returning only the appropriate amounts of fluid and substances back to the blood. Arteries entering the kidneys rapidly branch into capillaries. Approximately 20 percent of all plasma flowing into the kidneys leaves the capillaries and is collected in the capsules that surround them. This fluid is funneled into specialized tubes.

Substances are taken out and put into the fluid in the tubes in order to regulate fluid volume and composition. In the beginning of the tube (the proximal tubule), most of the salt, water, glucose, and amino acids are taken back into the blood. The next sections (the loop of Henle, distal tubule, and collecting ducts) help to regulate the final amount of water excreted in urine. The collecting ducts join to form the ureter, which carries the remaining fluid, urine, to the bladder, where it is stored. From the bladder, the urine is expelled through the urethra.

The endocrine system is another multiorgan system that helps to control and modify the function of almost all other systems. Endocrine glands produce chemicals and release them into the blood to direct the functions of cells and tissues elsewhere in the body. There are

three classes of hormones: amines, peptides and proteins, and steroids. Adrenaline is an example of the amine group, insulin is a protein hormone, and estrogen is a steroid hormone. Each of these is produced by a different gland.

The adrenal glands, small glands located near the kidneys, make several hormones. The outer portion, the cortex, produces three types of steroid hormones referred to as corticosteroids: glucocorticoids, mineralocorticoids, and small amounts of androgenic hormones. The major glucocorticoid, cortisol, regulates the production and use of glucose, fats, and amino acids by many cells and tissues. It also plays a helper role for other hormonal actions, such as making them more potent during stress, and it helps prevent inflammation and swelling. The major mineralocorticoid, aldosterone, can modify the kidneys' excretion of sodium, potassium, and hydrogen. A person unable to produce mineralocorticoids will die in a few days without treatment but can be saved by aldosterone therapy. Therefore, these steroids are said to be lifesaving. The androgenic steroids can cause the development of adult male sexual characteristics, the same effect as the male sex hormone, testosterone.

The interior portion, or medulla, of the adrenal glands makes catecholamines, such as adrenaline (epinephrine). Adrenaline helps the cardiovascular system during exercise and stress. It is the hormone that stimulates much of the "fight or flight" response, making the heart beat faster and harder. Adrenaline also helps to increase blood flow to muscles, in case flight is the action of choice.

The pituitary gland, also known as the hypophysis, is located at the base of the brain and produces many hormones with a variety of actions. The pituitary is divided into two areas: the anterior lobe (also known as the adenohypophysis) and the posterior lobe (also known as the neurohypophysis). The anterior pituitary produces growth hormone, a protein that has a major influence on all metabolic activity. It causes the body to store carbohydrates, to make proteins for growth, and to use fat for energy. The other anterior pituitary hormones cause other glands to increase their production of hormones. The glands stimulated by distinct pituitary hormones are the thyroid, adrenal cortex, ovaries, testicles, and mammary glands. The posterior pituitary produces the peptide hormones antidiuretic hormone (also known as vasopressin) and oxytocin. Antidiuretic hormone (ADH) decreases the amount of water that the kidneys can excrete, which keeps the body from dehydrating. ADH can also cause the blood pressure to rise, which helps if fluid is lost as a result of bleeding. Oxytocin causes the uterus to contract during the birthing process, and it also stimulates the production of milk in new mothers. The pituitary has direct regulating control over many glands and tissues, and it regulates nearly all tissues and organs indirectly by way of its stimulating hormones. This gland is regulated in a similar fashion by the hypothalamus, a small part of the brain just above the pituitary.

The thyroid gland is located in the neck around the voice box, or larynx. The parathyroid glands are located next to the thyroid gland. Thyroid hormones (peptides) cause almost all tissues in the body to increase the use of foodstuffs for the production of proteins, aiding in growth. In addition, the thyroid gland produces calcitonin. Calcitonin and the parathyroid hormones regulate the amount of calcium in the blood. Parathyroid hormone acts by freeing calcium from bone when more calcium is needed in the blood, while calcitonin causes the opposite action. Therefore, when the level of one of these hormones goes up, the other must go down.

The sex organs are also endocrine glands. The ovaries make estrogen and progesterone, while the testes produce testosterone. These steroid hormones cause the body to develop primary and secondary sexual characteristics. When a woman is pregnant, the placenta (the part of a woman's uterus that nourishes the fetus) produces hormones that prepare her body for childbirth and breast-feeding.

DISORDERS AND DISEASES

The body has control mechanisms to ensure that its systems function properly. Many systems use what is called negative feedback to fine-tune their functioning. An example of negative feedback is the control of blood pressure. Sensors in the arteries allow the brain to monitor the body's blood pressure level. When pressure is too high, the brain tells the cardiovascular system to decrease pressure by slowing the heart and opening the blood vessels and tells the kidneys to excrete fluid. Thus, when blood pressure is high, the feedback that the brain provides is negative, because it causes a response that is opposite to the unwanted change from the normal state.

The endocrine system uses negative feedback to regulate many hormones. The simplest endocrine feedback system involves insulin and glucose. When blood glucose increases, insulin secretion increases, which in turn decreases blood glucose. A decrease in blood glucose tells the pancreas to slow down the secretion of insulin. The failure of this system results in diabetes mellitus, a disease in which the ability to regulate blood sugar is lost. When this control is lost, other systems are damaged as a result, such as the renal and cardiovascular systems.

There are also much more complex feedback control systems. The regulation of the adrenal hormone cortisol serves as an example of such a system. Cortisol

secretion is controlled by secretion of the pituitary hormone adrenocorticotropic hormone (ACTH), also called corticotropin. The secretion of ACTH is controlled by a hypothalamic hormone called corticotropin-releasing factor (CRF). Stress causes CRF to be released, which causes the release of ACTH and in turn stimulates the secretion of cortisol. In general, when the level of any of these hormones becomes too high, the release of one of the others can be shut down. High levels of cortisol turn off CRF and ACTH secretion. High levels of ACTH can turn off the secretion of the hormone that triggers its secretion, CRF. It is also thought that CRF can provide feedback to its organ of origin, the hypothalamus, and halt its own secretion. Thus, if one of the control systems fails to function, a backup system guards against total malfunction.

The systems and organs of the body are dedicated to specific functions, but each needs the others to function properly. In addition, each system requires the coordination from the central nervous system to perform efficiently. The lungs bring vital oxygen to the cardiovascular system, and all systems need the nutrients brought to them by the cardiovascular system. Some organs of the endocrine system, such as the adrenal glands, are essential to life. The kidneys keep the blood clean and maintain the body's fluid volume. The reproductive system is essential to maintaining the existence of a species. All these systems must perform their functions for the body to work well. If one system malfunctions, frequently other systems become involved and may malfunction as well.

An example of one system malfunction that causes the failure of many others is renal failure. Kidney failure can be caused by a malfunction of the cardiovascular system such as clogging of the capillaries, which prohibits the kidneys from doing their job. As a result, hydrogen and potassium ions will accumulate. The effects of high levels of hydrogen and potassium ions on the cardiovascular system are a weakened heart and lower blood pressure. The nervous system can sense the increase in hydrogen ions and will tell the respiratory system to breathe faster and deeper to rid the body of carbon dioxide and its hydrogen ions. The increase in breathing helps to lower the hydrogen ion levels in the blood but cannot completely compensate for the kidney malfunction; in fact, the increase in work by the respiratory muscles can produce more hydrogen ions. When levels of hydrogen become too high, the brain begins to malfunction. The patient may experience dizziness, have seizures, or lose consciousness. If these symptoms are not reversed, the malfunction of each system will aid in the deterioration of other systems. The brain will be irreversibly damaged, and the heart will stop.

There are several ways to treat renal failure to avoid multiple-organ sickness. Treatment of infections with antibiotics before they become severe can help to avoid early and mild kidney failure. In severe, long-term kidney failure, kidney transplantation may become necessary. The damaged kidney (or kidneys) is removed and replaced with an organ from a deceased donor or from a living donor (a person can live a normal life with only one functioning kidney). Kidneys, even from deceased donors, are rare, and many people in need of a transplant must wait for years to receive one that will not be rejected by the body's immune system. For such patients, dialysis is necessary for survival. Dialysis is the use of a machine to perform some of the functions of the kidneys. Patients with total kidney failure must be hooked up to an artificial kidney machine for several hours several times per week. Even with this treatment, they will still be very sick because the machine cannot perform all functions of the kidneys.

PERSPECTIVE AND PROSPECTS

In the Middle Ages, it was believed that "spirits" were the essence of life or "vitality"; thus, the treatment for many ailments was bloodletting, the application of leeches to remove the "evil spirit" causing the sickness. It was not until the seventeenth century that William Harvey discovered that blood circulated from arteries to veins in both the lungs and the rest of the body. Oxygen was discovered at the end of the eighteenth century by Joseph Priestley. Knowledge of chemistry, biochemistry, and physiology grew in the nineteenth century, but most of the information about systems and organs contained in this article was revealed in the twentieth century.

Many discoveries have been in the area of how the body's systems and organs interact with and influence one another. New anatomical techniques of investigation have revealed the minute structures of many organs and tissues. As a result, the presence of previously unknown nervous and other tissue parts has been recognized; their functions are under investigation. Chemical techniques have revealed many new hormone and hormonelike substances through which one tissue or organ can influence another. Research into the molecular structure of some of these biochemical signals is helping to explain how they work.

In addition, the events that occur inside a cell or group of cells have been described in greater detail. How a group of cells produces unified organ function and how this function is altered is currently under investigation. Studies into how a cell can change its function in conjunction with surrounding cells have added to the knowledge of how systems and organs can fine-tune their functions. This research involves information regarding how the genes inside cells carry messages and how these messages in turn are expressed in unified physiological functions.

—*J. Timothy O'Neill, PhD*

See also Adrenal glands; Anatomy; Brain; Circulation; Colon; Ears; Endocrine glands; Endocrine system; Eyes; Gallbladder; Gastrointestinal system; Glands; Heart; Immune system; Kidneys; Liver; Lungs; Lymphatic system; Nervous system; Pancreas; Pituitary gland; Reproductive system; Sense organs; Skin; Small intestine; Thyroid gland; Urinary system; Vascular system.

For Further Information:
Asimov, Isaac. *The Human Body: Its Structure and Operation.* Rev. ed. New York: Penguin Books, 1992. Asimov offers an easy-to-understand overview of all the body's organ functions.
Guyton, Arthur C., and John E. Hall. *Human Physiology and Mechanisms of Disease.* 6th ed. Philadelphia: W. B. Saunders, 1997. This physiology text deals with the function of the body in considerable detail. Excellent advanced reading for the physiology student.
Kittredge, Mary. *The Human Body: An Overview.* Reprint. Philadelphia: Chelsea House, 2003. This text explains the general workings of the human body. Provides background to the historical development of medical knowledge and addresses many of the pathologies that can arise in the body.
Page, Martyn, ed. *Human Body: An Illustrated Guide to Every Part of the Human Body and How It Works.* New York: DK, 2009. The first part of the book covers basic human anatomy with full color illustrations, explaining how each individual body system functions. The second part covers diseases and disorders.
Parsons, Jayne, ed. *Encyclopedia of the Human Body.* New York: DK, 2004. A beautifully illustrated and accessible guide to the human body designed for children and teens, covering anatomical concepts, disease mechanisms, and the history of medicine and its pioneers.
Thibodeau, Gary A., and Kevin T. Patton. *The Human Body in Health and Disease.* 4th ed. St. Louis, Mo.: Mosby/Elsevier, 2005. Examines the mechanisms of the human body by examining each system in detail.